HEMATOLOGY-ONCOLOGY THERAPY

MICHAEL M. BOYIADZIS, MD, MHSc
Assistant Professor of Medicine
Division of Hematology-Oncology
Department of Medicine
University of Pittsburgh School of Medicine
University of Pittsburgh Cancer Institute
Pittsburgh, Pennsylvania

PETER F. LEBOWITZ, MD, PhD
Assistant Professor of Medicine
Department of Oncology
Lombardi Comprehensive Cancer Center
Georgetown University Medical Center
Washington DC

JAMES N. FRAME, MD
Clinical Associate Professor of Medicine
Robert C. Byrd Health Sciences Center
West Virginia University School of Medicine
Medical Director, David Lee Cancer Center
Charleston Area Medical Center Health Systems
Charleston, West Virginia

TITO FOJO, MD, PhD
Senior Investigator
Medical Oncology Branch
Center for Cancer Research
National Cancer Institute
National Institutes of Health
Bethesda, Maryland

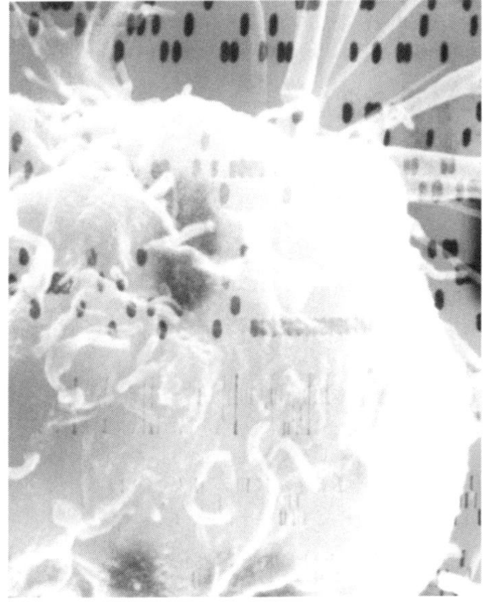

McGraw-Hill
Medical Publishing Division
New York Chicago San Francisco Lisbon London Madrid Mexico City
Milan New Delhi San Juan Seoul Singapore Sydney Toronto

Hematology-Oncology Therapy

1234567890 CCW/CCW 09876

ISBN-13:9780071434973

ISBN-10:0-07-143497-6

Notice

Medicine is an ever-changing science. As new research and clinical experience broaden our knowledge, changes in treatment and drug therapy are required. The authors and the publisher of this work have checked with sources believed to be reliable in their efforts to provide information that is complete and generally in accord with the standards accepted at the time of publication. However, in view of the possibility of human error or changes in medical sciences, neither the authors nor the publisher nor any other party who has been involved in the preparation or publication of this work warrants that the information contained herein is in every respect accurate or complete, and they disclaim all responsibility for any errors or omissions or for the results obtained from use of the information contained in this work. Readers are encourage to confirm the information contained herein with other sources. For example and in particular, readers are advised to check product information sheet included in the package of each drug they plan to administer to be certain that the information contained in this work is accurate and that changes have not been made in the recommended dose or in the contraindications for administration. This recommendation is of particular importance in connection with new or infrequently used drugs.

The editors Joe Rusko, Harriet Lebowitz, and Regina Y. Brown.
The production supervisor was Sherri Souffrance.
The book designer was Eve Siegel.
The cover designer was Elizabeth Pisacreta.

Courier Westford was printer and binder.

COVER PHOTO:

Cancer research. Colored scanning electron micrograph (SEM) of a cancer cell (white) and an autoradiogram showing the genetic code of a section of DNA (deoxyribonucleic acid). Cancer is caused by unrestrained cell growth. The pattern of bands on the autoradiogram represents the sequence of bases in the genetic code. The presence or absence of particular sections of DNA, called genes, has been linked to the development of certain forms of cancer. Finding genes, which are related to cancer development, will allow screening to take place to detect people who are at greater risk of getting cancer.

Credit: Alfred Pasieka / Photo Researchers, Inc.

Library of Congress Cataloging-in-Publication Data

Hematology-oncology therapy / Michael M. Boyiadzis . . . [et al.].
p. ; cm.
Includes index.
ISBN 0-07-143497-6
1. Blood—Diseases—Treatment. 2. Cancer—Treatment. 3. Hematology. 4. Oncology. I. Boyiadzis, Michael M.
[DNLM: 1. Neoplasms. 2. Hematologic Diseases. 3. Neoplasms—therapy. QZ 200 H487 2006]
RC633.A1H46 2006
616.99'406—dc22

2006048174

This book is printed on acid-free paper

To the patients our profession has the privilege to serve and to our colleagues whose compassionate care and research efforts continue to extend the spectrum of hope

Contents

Authors

Salah Abbasi, MD
Assistant Professor, Department of Internal Medicine, Jordan University of Science and Technology; King Abdullah University Hospital, Irbid, Jordan
Leukemia, Chronic Lymphocytic

Kenneth B. Ain, MD
Professor of Medicine, The Carmen L. Buck Professor of Oncology Research; Director, Thyroid Oncology Program, Division of Hematology & Oncology, Department of Internal Medicine, University of Kentucky Medical Center; Director, Thyroid Cancer Research Laboratory, Veterans Affairs Medical Center, Lexington, Kentucky
Thyroid Cancer

Jaffer Ajani, MD
Professor, Department of Gastrointestinal Medical Oncology, The University of Texas M.D. Anderson Cancer Center, Houston, Texas
Esophageal Cancer

Ivan Aksentijevich, MD
Fairfax Northern Virginia Hematology Oncology P.C., Alexandria, Virginia
Leukemia, Acute Lymphoblastic (Adult), Leukemia, Acute Myelogenous

Christina M. Annunziata, MD, PhD
Clinical Fellow, Medical Oncology Branch, National Cancer Institute, National Institutes of Health, Bethesda, Maryland
Lymphoma, Hodgkin

Susan Bates, MD
Head, Molecular Therapeutics Section, Senior Investigator, Medical Oncology Branch, National Cancer Institute, National Institutes of Health, Bethesda, Maryland
Renal Cell Carcinoma

Kenneth A. Bauer, MD
Professor of Medicine, Harvard Medical School; Chief, Hematology Section, VA Boston Healthcare System; Director, Thrombosis Clinical Research, Beth Israel Deaconess Medical Center, Boston, Massachusetts
The Hypercoagulable State

Ann Berger, MSN, MD
Chief, Pain and Palliatire Care Service, Warren Grant Magnuson Clinical Center Bethesda, Maryland
Cancer Pain: Assessment and Management

Michael R. Bishop, MD
Principal Investigator, Experimental Transplantation and Immunology Branch, National Cancer Institute, National Institutes of Health, Bethesda, Maryland
Complications and Follow-up After Hematopoietic Stem Cell Transplantation

Michael M. Boyiadzis, MD, MHSc
Assistant Professor of Medicine
Division of Hematology-Oncology
Department of Medicine
University of Pittsburgh School of Medicine
University of Pittsburgh Cancer Institute
Pittsburgh, Pennsylvania
Gestational Trophoblastic Neoplasia, Leukemia, Acute Lymphoblastic (Adult), Leukemia, Acute Myelogenous, Melanoma, Pancreatic Cancer, Pheochromocytoma, Renal Cell Carcinoma, Testicular Cancer, Oncologic Emergencies, Complications and Follow-up After Hematopoietic Stem Cell Transplantation, von Willebrand Disease, Aplastic Anemia, Myelodysplastic Syndromes

Jordi Bruix, MD
BCLC Group, Liver Unit, Hospital Clinic, University of Barcelona; IDIBAPS, Barcelona, Spain
Hepatocellular Carcinoma

Kathleen A. Calzone, RN, MSN, APNG
Senior Nurse Specialist (Research)
National Cancer Institute, Center for Cancer Research, Genetics Branch, National Institutes of Health, Bethesda, Maryland
Cancer Screening, Genetics of Common Inherited Cancer Syndromes

Thomas Chen, MD
New York University School of Medicine, Division of Medical Oncology; New York University Medical Center, Division of Medical Oncology, New York, New York
Vaginal Cancer

Bruce D. Cheson, MD
Professor of Medicine, Head of Hematology, Georgetown University Hospital, Washington DC
Leukemia, Chronic Lymphocytic

Barbara Conley, MD
Professor and Chief, Division of Hematology/Oncology, Department of Medicine, Michigan State University College of Human Medicine; East Lansing, Michigan
Head and Neck Cancers

William L. Dahut, MD
Principal Investigator, Medical Oncology Branch, National Cancer Institute, National Institutes of Health, Bethesda, Maryland
Bladder Cancer, Prostate Cancer

Robert Dean, MD
Associate Staff, Hematology and Medical Oncology, The Cleveland Clinic Foundation, Taussig Cancer Center, Cleveland, Ohio
Multiple Myeloma

Michael W.N. Deininger, MD, PhD
Assistant Professor, Oregon Health & Science University Cancer Institute, Portland Oregon
Leukemia, Chronic Myelogenous

Erin Donovan, MD
Clinical Fellow, Oncology/Hematology, National Cancer Institute, Medical Oncology Branch, National Institutes of Health, Bethesda, Maryland
Head and Neck Cancers

Brian J. Druker, MD
Investigator, Howard Hughes Medical Institute,
JELD-WEN Chair of Leukemia Research,
Oregon Health & Science University Cancer Institute,
Portland, Oregon
Leukemia, Chronic Myelogenous

Cynthia E. Dunbar, MD
Head, Molecular Hematopoiesis Section, Hematology Branch, National Heart, Lung and Blood Institute, National Institutes of Health, Bethesda, Maryland
Multiple Myeloma

Kieron Dunleavy, MD
Clinical Fellow, Medical Oncology Branch,
Center for Cancer Research, National Cancer Institute,
National Institutes of Health, Bethesda, Maryland
Lymphoma, Non-Hodgkin

Jennifer Eng-Wong, MD, MPH
Medical Oncology Branch, Staff Clinician, Center for Cancer Research, National Cancer Institute, National Institutes of Health, Bethesda, Maryland
Cancer Screening, Genetics of Common Inherited Cancer Syndromes

Howard Fine, MD
Branch Chief,
Neuro-Oncology Branch, Center for Cancer Research,
National Institutes of Health,
National Cancer Institute/NINDS
Bethesda, Maryland
Brain Cancer

Tito Fojo, MD, PhD
Senior Investigator
Medical Oncology Branch
Center for Cancer Research,
National Cancer Institute,
National Institutes of Health,
Bethesda, Maryland
Adrenocortical Cancer, Pheochromocytoma, Sarcomas, Oncologic Emergencies

Enriqueta Felip, MD, PhD
Medical Oncology Department;
Vall d'Hebron University Hospital, Barcelona, Spain
Lung Cancer

James N. Frame, MD
Clinical Associate Professor
Robert C. Byrd Health Sciences Center
West Virginia University School of Medicine
Medical Director
David Lee Outpatient Cancer Center
Charleston Area Medical Center Health Systems
Charleston, West Virginia
Indications for Growth Factors in the Hematology-Oncology Setting, Indications for Bisphosphonates in the Hematology-Oncology Setting, Autoimmune Hemolytic Anemia, Sickle Cell Disease: Acute Complications

Steven M. Fruchtman, MD
Associate Professor of Medicine, Department of Medicine, Mount Sinai School of Medicine; Director, Myeloproliferative Disorders Program, Department of Medicine, Mount Sinai Hospital, New York, New York
Polycythemia Vera, Essential Thrombocythemia

Barry Gause, MD
Senior Investigator, Medical Oncology Branch
Center for Cancer Research, National Cancer Institute
National Institutes of Health, Bethesda, Maryland
Melanoma

Juan C. Gea-Banacloche, MD
Chief, Infectious Diseases Consultation Service, Experimental Transplantation and Immunology Branch, National Cancer Institute, National Institute of Health, Bethesda, Maryland
Fever and Neutropenia, Complications and Follow-up After Hematopoietic Stem Cell Transplantation

James N. George, MD
George Lynn Cross Research Professor of Medicine, Hematology-Oncology Section, University of Oklahoma Health Sciences Center, Oklahoma City, Oklahoma
Thrombotic Thrombocytopenic Purpura/Hemolytic Uremic Syndrome (TTP/HUS) Idiopathic Thrombocytopenic Purpura

Giuseppe Giaccone, MD
Professor, VU University Medical Center, Department of Medical Oncology, Amsterdam, The Netherlands
Thymic Carcinoma

Eli Glatstein, MD
Professor of Radiation Oncology,
Vice Chairman and Clinical Director,
Department of Radiation of Oncology
University of Pennsylvania
Hospital of the University of Pennsylvania
Philadelphia, Pennsylvania
Radiation Complications

F. Anthony Greco
Clinical Researcher and Director
Sarah Cannon Research Institute, Nashville, Tennessee
Carcinoma of Unknown Primary

Jean Grem, MD, FACP
Professor of Medicine, Department of Internal Medicine, Section of Oncology/Hematology, University of Nebraska Medical Center, Omaha, Nebraska
Colorectal Cancer

Celia L. Grosskreutz, MD
Assistant Professor of Medicine, Hematology/Oncology Division, Department of Medicine, Mount Sinai Medical Center, New York, New York.
Polycythemia Vera, Essential Thrombocythemia

Lee Helman, MD
Acting Clinical Director and Head,
Molecular Oncology Section,
Pediatric Oncology Branch,
Center for Cancer Research,
National Cancer Institute, Bethesda, Maryland
Sarcomas

McDonald K. Horne, III
Senior Clinical Investigator, Department of Laboratory Medicine, W.G. Magnuson Clinical Center, National Institutes of Health, Bethesda, Maryland
Venous Catheter-Related Thrombosis, Heparin-Induced Thrombocytopenia (HIT) and HIT With Thromboembolic Syndrome (HITTS)

Thomas E. Hughes, PharmD, BCOP
Oncology Clinical Pharmacy Specialist, Pharmacy Department, National Institutes of Health Clinical Center, Bethesda, Maryland
Chemotherapy-Induced Nausea and Vomiting: Prophylaxis and Treatment

Eva Tiensuu Janson, MD
Associate Professor, Department of Medical Sciences, Uppsala University Hospital; Senior Consultant, Department of Endocrine Oncology, Uppsala University Hospital, Uppsala, Sweden
Carcinoid Tumors

Steven J. Jubelirer, MD
Clinical Professor of Medicine, West Virginia University, Charleston Division; Senior Scientist, Charleston Area Medical Center, Health Education and Research Institute; Medical Director, Hemophilia Treatment Center, Charleston Area Medical Center, Charleston, West Virginia
Hemophilia, Sickle Cell Disease: Acute Complications

Judith Karp, MD
Professor of Oncology and Medicine, Johns Hopkins University School of Medicine, Baltimore, Maryland
Leukemia, Acute Lymphoblastic (Adult), Leukemia, Acute Myelogenous

Lyndon Kim, MD
Staff Clinician
Neuro-Oncology Branch, NCI/NINDS, National Institutes of Health, Bethesda, Maryland
Brain Cancer

David R. Kohler, PharmD
Oncology Clinical Pharmacy Specialist, Pharmacy Department, National Institutes of Health Clinical Center, Bethesda, Maryland
Lymphoma, Non-Hodgkin, Drug Preparation and Administration, Antineoplastic Drugs: Preventing and Managing Extravasation, Indications for Bisphosphonates in the Hematology-Oncology Setting

Kiarash Kojouri, MD, MPH
Assistant Professor of Medicine, Hematology-Oncology Section, University of Oklahoma Health Sciences Center, Oklahoma City, Oklahoma
Thrombotic Thrombocytopenic Purpura/Hemolytic Uremic Syndrome (TTP/HUS), Idiopathic Thrombocytopenic Purpura

Pallavi Kumar, MD
Lapidus Cancer Institute, Baltimore, Maryland
HIV-Related Malignancies

Peter F. Lebowitz, MD, PhD
Assistant Professor of Medicine,
Lombardi Comprehensive Cancer Center,
Georgetown University Medical Center,
Washington DC
Adrenocortical Cancer, Breast Cancer, Prostate Cancer

Susan Leitman, MD
Deputy Chief, Department of Transfusion Medicine, National Institutes of Health Clinical Center, National Institutes of Health, Bethesda, Maryland
Transfusion Therapy

Gregory Leonard, MD
Consultant Medical Ongologist, Old School of Nursing, Dunmore Rono, Watorford Regional Hospital, Watorford, Ireland
Colorectal Cancer

Richard F. Little, MD
Principal Investigator, HIV and AIDS Malignancy Branch, Center for Cancer Research, National Cancer Institute, National Institutes of Health, Bethesda, Maryland
HIV-Related Malignancies

Dan L. Longo, MD
Scientific Director, National Institute on Aging, National Institutes of Health, Baltimore, Maryland
Lymphoma, Hodgkin

John Lurain, MD
John & Ruth Brewer Professor of Gynecology and Cancer Research, Department of Obstetrics and Gynecology, Northwestern University, Feinberg School of Medicine, Chicago, Illinois
Gestational Trophoblastic Neoplasia

Joan Maurel, MD
BCLC group. Hospital Clinic Barcelona, Medical Oncology Department; University of Barcelona, Barcelona, Spain
Hepatocellular Carcinoma

Robert Mayer, MD
Professor,
Department of Medicine, Harvard Medical School
Vice Chair of Academic Affairs,
Department of Adult Oncology,
Dana-Farber Cancer Institute,
Senior Physician, Department of Medicine,
Brigham and Women's Hospital
Boston, Massachusetts
Anal Cancer

Pamela W. McDevitt, PharmD
Oncology Clinical Pharmacy Specialist, David Lee Cancer Center, Charleston Area Medical Center, Charleston, West Virginia
Indications for Growth Factors in the Hematology-Oncology Setting Chemotherapy Dose Modifications

Michael Menefee, MD
Medical Fellow, National Cancer Institute, National Institutes of Health, Bethesda, Maryland
Chemotherapy Dose Modifications

Franco Muggia, MD
Professor, NYU Cancer Institute, NYU School of Medicine, New York, New York
Endometrial Cancer, Vaginal Cancer

Ashok Nambiar, MD
Assistant Professor, Department of Laboratory Medicine, University of California, San Francisco; Assistant Medical Director, Blood Bank and Donor Center, UCSF Medical Center, San Francisco, California
Transfusion Therapy

Kjell Öberg, MD
Professor, Endocrine Oncology, Dean of the Medical Faculty, Uppsala University; Professor, Department of Endocrine Oncology, Uppsala University Hospital, Uppsala, Sweden
Carcinoid Tumors

Naomi P. O'Grady, MD
Medical Director, Procedures, Vascular Access, and Conscious Sedation Services, Critical Care Medicine Department, National Institutes of Health, Bethesda, Maryland
Managing and Preventing Catheter-Related Bloodstream Infections

Deirdre O'Mahony, MD
Senior Oncology Fellow, Metabolism Branch, National Cancer Institute, National Institutes of Health, Bethesda, Maryland
Cervical Cancer, Endometrial Cancer

Karel Pacak, MD, PhD Sc
Chief, Unit of Clinical Neuroendocrinology, Reproductive Biology and Medicine Branch, National Institutes of Health, Bethesda, Maryland; Adjunct Professor of Medicine, Department of Medicine, Georgetown University, Washington DC
Pheochromocytoma

Edwin M. Posadas, MD
Instructor of Medicine and Surgery, Department of Medicine, Sections of Hematology/Oncology and Urology, University of Chicago, Pritzker School of Medicine; University of Chicago Hospitals, Department of Medicine, Chicago, Illinois
Bladder Cancer

Sheila Prindiville, MD, MPH
Staff Clinician, Head, Clinical Cancer Genetics Program, Medical Oncology Branch, Center for Cancer Research, National Cancer Institute, National Institutes of Health, Bethesda, Maryland
Cancer Screening, Genetics of Common Inherited Cancer Syndromes

Dana Rathkopf, MD
Assistant Attending Physician, Division of Solid Tumor Oncology, Memorial Sloan-Kettering Cancer Center, New York, New York
Gastric Cancer

Eddie Reed, MD
Director, Division of Cancer Prevention and Control, Centers for Disease Control and Prevention, Atlanta, Georgia
Ovarian Cancer

Margaret E. Rick, MD
Clinical Professor of Medicine, Uniformed University of the Health Sciences; Principal Investigator Assistant Chief, Department of Laboratory Medicine Department, Clinical Center, National Institutes of Health Clinical Center, National Institutes of Health, Bethesda, Maryland
von Willebrand Disease

Griffin P. Rodgers, MD, MACP
Deputy Director, Chief, Molecular and Clinical Hematology, National Institute of Diabetes, Digestive and Kidney Diseases, National Institutes of Health, Bethesda, Maryland
Sickle Cell Disease: Acute Complications

Peter Rose, MD
Professor, Case Western Reserve University School of Medicine; Section Head, Gynecology Oncology, Department of OB/Gyn, Cleveland Clinic, Cleveland, Ohio
Cervical Cancer

Rafael Rosell, MD
Associate Professor, School of Medicine, Autonomous University of Barcelona; Catalan Institute of Oncology, Hospital Germans Trias, Pujol, Badalona, Barcelona, Spain
Lung Cancer

David Ryan, MD
Assistant Professor of Medicine, Harvard Medical School; Clinical Director, Tucker Gosnell Gastrointestinal Cancer Center, Massachusetts General Hospital, Boston, Massachusetts
Anal Cancer

Verena Sagaster, MD
Department of Internal Medicine I, Division of Oncology, Vienna University Medical School; Vienna University Hospital, Vienna, Austria
Gallbladder Cancer and Cholangiocarcinoma

Scott Saxman, MD, FACP
Senior Investigator, Cancer Therapy Evaluation Program, National Cancer Institute, Bethesda, Maryland
Testicular Cancer

Werner Scheithauer, MD
Professor, Department of Internal Medicine I, Division of Oncology, Vienna University Medical School; Vienna University Hospital, Vienna, Austria
Gallbladder Cancer and Cholangiocarcinoma

Gary K. Schwartz, MD
Associate Professor of Medicine, Weill Medical College, Cornell University; Attending Physician, Department of Medicine, Memorial Sloan-Kettering Cancer Center, New York, New York
Gastric Cancer

Manish A. Shah, MD
Assistant Member, Assistant Professor of Medicine, Memorial Sloan Kettering Cancer Center; Assistant Attending Physician, Memorial Hospital for Cancer & Allied Diseases, Department of Medicine, New York, New York
Gastric Cancer

Reem A. Shalabi, PharmD, BCOP
Clinical Pharmacy Specialist, Bone Marrow Transplant, The Johns Hopkins Hospital, Baltimore, Maryland
Clinical Indications for Bisphosphonates in the Hematology-Oncology Setting

David Spigel, MD
Associate Director of Clinical Research, Sarah Cannon Research Institute, Nashville, Tennessee
Carcinoma of Unknown Primary

Diana C. Stripp, MD
Adjunct Assistant Professor, Department of Radiation Oncology, University of Pennsylvania; Adjunct Assistant Professor, Department of Radiation Oncology, Hospital of University of Pennsylvania, Philadelphia, Pennsylvania
Radiation Complications

Martin S. Tallman, MD
Professor of Medicine, Northwestern University,
Feinberg School of Medicine, Division of Hematology/Oncology;
Attending Physician, Northwestern Memorial Hospital, Chicago,
Illinois
Leukemia, Hairy Cell

Verna Vanderpuye, MD
Fellow, University of Chicago, Department of Hematology-Oncology; University Hospitals, Department of Hematology-Oncology, Chicago, Illinois
Mesothelioma

Gauri Varadhachary, MD
Assistant Professor, Department of Gastrointestinal Medical Oncology, The University of Texas M.D. Anderson Cancer Center, Houston, Texas
Esophageal Cancer

Nicholas J. Vogelzang, MD
Professor of Medicine, University of Nevada School of Medicine;
Director, Nevada Cancer Institute, Las Vegas, Nevada
Mesothelioma

Charles F. von Gunten, MD, PhD
Director, Palliative Care, Moores Cancer Center, University of California, San Diego; Medical Faculty, Department of Internal Medicine, University of California, San Diego; Director, Center for Palliative Studies, San Diego Hospice & Palliative Care, San Diego, California
Hospice Care and End-of-Life Issues

Daniel D. Von Hoff, MD, FACP
Senior Investigator, Translational Genomics Research Institute;
Clinical Professor of Medicine, University of Arizona,
Arizona Cancer Center, Phoenix, Arizona
Pancreatic Cancer

Thomas J. Walsh, MD
Chief, Immunocompromised Host Section, Pediatric Oncology Branch, National Cancer Institute, National Institutes of Health, Bethesda, Maryland
Fever and Neutropenia

Janice Walshe, MD
Consultant Medical Oncologist
Adelaide and Meath Hospital
Tallaght, Dublin
Sarcomas

David E. Weissman, MD
Professor of Internal Medicine,
Director of Palliative Care
Division of Neoplastic Diseases, Froedtert Hospital;
Medical College of Wisconsin, Milwaukee, Wisconsin
Hospice Care and End-of-Life Issues

Hanneke Wilmink, MD
Academic Medical Center Amsterdam,
Department of Medical Oncology, Amsterdam,
The Netherlands
Thymic Carcinoma

Wyndham H. Wilson, MD, PhD
Senior Investigator, Chief, Lymphoma Therapeutics Section,
Center for Cancer Research, National Cancer Institute,
National Institutes of Health, Bethesda, Maryland
Lymphoma, Non-Hodgkin

Neal S. Young, MD
Chief, Hematology Branch, National Heart, Lung, and Blood Institute, National Institutes of Health, Bethesda, Maryland
Aplastic Anemia, Myelodysplastic Syndromes

Jo Anne Zujewski, MD
Head, Breast Cancer Therapeutics,
Clinical Investigations Branch,
Cancer Treatment Evaluation Program,
National Cancer Institute,
National Institutes of Health, Bethesda, Maryland
Breast Cancer

Jeffrey Zwicker, MD
Instructor of Medicine, Division of Hematology-Oncology,
Beth Israel Deaconess Medical Center, Harvard Medical School,
Boston, Massachusetts
The Hypercoagulable State

Preface

The practical need for a readily accessible, up-to-date, comprehensive therapy resource, supported by referenced literature and the opinion of experts, was the original inspiration for *Hematology-Oncology Therapy.* Nearly 500 treatment regimens are presented in a concise and uniform format that includes oncologic disorders, non-neoplastic hematologic disorders and supportive care.

The three sections of *Hematology-Oncology Therapy* are

I. Oncology
II. Supportive Care, Drug Preparation, Complications, and Screening
III. Selected Hematologic Diseases.

Section I provides detailed information about the administration, emetogenic potential, toxicity, dose modification, monitoring, and efficacy of commonly used and recently approved chemotherapeutic regimens, drugs, and biological agents. In addition, each chapter, focused on a specific cancer, contains information about epidemiology, pathology, work-up, and staging, as well as survival data. Section II consists of topics commonly encountered in clinical hematology-oncology practice. Section III provides an authoritative guide to therapy for the principal diseases in consultative hematology.

Hematology-Oncology Therapy integrates extensive information that is critical to both office- and hospital-based clinical practice of hematology and oncology. This comprehensive approach makes the book invaluable to all practitioners involved in the care of patients with cancer or hematologic diseases. As progress in the development of new therapies continues, we look forward to updating the book regularly for the benefit of our patients and readers.

We wish to express our appreciation to the many contributors to this book, whose expert knowledge in their fields will make *Hematology-Oncology Therapy* a unique addition to the medical literature. They helped us compile the extensive and detailed information contained in this book, which are a testament to the efforts of so many to improve the treatment of patients with oncologic and hematologic diseases. We are profoundly grateful to our outstanding colleague David Kohler, Oncology Clinical Pharmacy Specialist for his dedication and untiring efforts in reviewing each treatment regimen to ensure accuracy. David's contribution in confirming the accuracy of dosage information and his innumerable suggestions regarding everything can neither be overstated nor overappreciated. We also wish to thank our editors at McGraw-Hill for having faith in our vision and concept for this book. Their professional support has earned our praise and debt of gratitude. Finally, we would like to thank those we work with and those we love for putting up with our efforts and lending their support during the writing and editing of this book.

Michael M. Boyiadzis, MD, MHSc
Peter F. Lebowitz, MD, PhD
James N. Frame, MD
Tito Fojo, MD, PhD

SECTION I. Oncology

(Continued on following page)

1. Adrenocortical Cancer

Peter F. Lebowitz, MD, PhD, and Tito Fojo, MD, PhD

Epidemiology

Incidence: 24–46 cases per year in the United States (1990–2000)
Mortality: 0.2% of cancer deaths
Median age: Bimodal median, at age 4 years and ages 40–50 years

Stage at Presentation	
Stage I:	3%
Stage II:	29%
Stage III:	19%
Stage IV:	49%

Cohn K et al. Surgery 1986;100:1170–1177
Wooten MD, King DK. Cancer 1993;72:3145–3155
http://seer.cancer.gov

Pathology

1. Unlike renal cell carcinoma, adrenocortical cancer stains positive for vimentin
2. >20 mitoses per HPF—median survival 14 months
   ≤20 mitoses per HPF—median survival 58 months
3. Tumor necrosis—poor prognosis
4. Vascular invasion—poor prognosis
5. Capsular invasion—poor prognosis

Weiss LM et al. Am J Surg Pathol 1989;13:202–206

Survival After Complete Resection

5-Year Actuarial Survival	
Stage I–II	54%
Stage III	24%
1-year survival	
Stage IV	9%

Icard P et al. Surgery 1992;112:972–980; discussion 979–980
Icard P et al. World J Surg 1992;16:753–758

Work-Up

1. CT scan of chest, abdomen, and pelvis to determine extent of disease
2. MRI of abdomen may help to identify and follow liver metastases
3. If IVC is compressed, consider IVC contrast study, ultrasound, or MRI to assess disease involvement before surgical exploration, although apparent extent of involvement should not deter exploration
4. Serum and 24-hour urinary cortisol; 24-hour urinary 17-ketosteroid
5. Additional studies can be performed to determine the functional status of the tumor including: serum estradiol, estrone, testosterone, dehydroepiandrosterone sulfate (S-DHAS), 17-OH-progesterone, and androstenedione

Staging

Stage I	<5-cm tumor confined to adrenal
Stage II	>5-cm tumor confined to adrenal
Stage III	Positive lymph nodes or local invasion with tumor outside adrenal in fat or adjacent organs
Stage IV	Distant metastasis

Macfarlane DA. Ann R Coll Surg Engl 1958;23:155–186
Sullivan M et al. J Urol 1978;120:660–665

Caveats

1. Primary therapy is complete surgical resection; when possible, local recurrences should be addressed surgically
2. Surgical resection of metastatic disease is advocated by some, and it may improve survival, although firm evidence is lacking
3. Excess hormone production should not be ignored. Do not rely on chemotherapy to relieve excess hormone production. Ketoconazole, metyrapone, and mitotane can be used to treat excess hormone production
4. Use of mitotane as adjuvant therapy is controversial, and as yet no data show clinical benefit
5. Chemotherapy is recommended for patients with metastatic disease, although evidence of survival benefit is not and will never be available

Ng L, Libertino JM. J Urol 2003;169:5–11
Vassilopoulou-Sellin R, Shultz PN. Cancer 2001;92:1113–1121
Wajchenberg BL et al. Cancer 2000;88:711–736

REGIMEN

MITOTANE (*O,'*-DDD)

Luton J-P et al. NEJM 1990;322:1195–201

Mitotane 2000–20,000 mg/day orally as a single dose or in 2–4 divided doses
Glucocorticoid replacement is necessary in all patients:
Hydrocortisone 15–20 mg orally every morning, *plus:*
Hydrocortisone 7.5–10 mg orally every evening
Mineralocorticoid replacement is also recommended:
Fludrocortisone acetate 100–200 mcg/day orally every morning, *or:*
Fludrocortisone acetate 100 mcg/day orally every morning and every evening

Emetogenic potential: Nonemetogenic to low (Emetogenicity score ≤2). See Chapter 39

Mitotane is available in the United States in tablets for oral administration containing 500 mg mitotane. Lysodren® (mitotane tablets). Bristol-Myers Squibb Company, Princeton, NJ
Hydrocortisone is available in the United States in many solid and liquid formulations, including tablets for oral administration containing 2.5, 5, 10, and 20 mg hydrocortisone
Fludrocortisone acetate is available in the United States in tablets for oral administration containing 100 mcg of fludrocortisone acetate. Florinef® Acetate (fludrocortisone acetate tablets). Monarch Pharmaceuticals, Inc, Bristol, TN

Patient Population Studied

A study of 59 patients with adrenocortical carcinoma treated with mitotane at different times in relation to surgery

Efficacy (N = 37)

Overall response rate	22%
Stable disease >12 months	5%
Clinical benefit rate	27%

Complete responses have been reported in other studies but are rare

Toxicity

Adverse Event	% Patients	No. of Patients
Anorexia/nausea	93	28
Vomiting	82	
Diarrhea	68	
Skin rash	32	
Confusion/ sleepiness	100	18
Ataxia	39	
Depression	33	
Dysarthria	28	
Tremor	22	
Visual disturbance	17	
Leukopenia	17	

Van Slooten H et al. Eur J Cancer Clin Oncol 1984; 20:47–53

Treatment Modifications

Adverse Event	Dose Modification
General Guidelines: First step with most side effects, especially if they occur as mitotane dose is advanced: (1) stop mitotane; (2) wait up to 7 days for symptoms to resolve; (3) restart mitotane at lower dose (500–1000 mg/day less than previous dose) or at previously tolerated dose; (4) increase dose in 500-mg/day increments at 1-week intervals	
Anorexia Nausea/vomiting	Administer mitotane in divided doses, and/or most of dose before bedtime. Crush tablets and dissolve in vehicle. Use antiemetics as needed. Reassess adrenal replacement
Diarrhea	Administer as divided doses. Use loperamide or diphenoxylate/ atropine
Altered mental status	Stop therapy. Follow general guidelines. Obtain imaging study only if symptoms persist after 1 week off therapy
Skin rash	If not severe, continue mitotane and treat rash with local measures and antipruritics

Therapy Monitoring

1. Check mitotane level at least every 4 weeks initially. Patients receiving long-term mitotane therapy can have monitoring reduced to every 2–3 months
2. Adrenal function can be monitored by measuring ACTH, but this alone is not reliable and should be interpreted together with clinical assessment
3. *Response assessment:* Initially every 6–8 weeks. Patients receiving long-term mitotane therapy can have monitoring reduced to every 3–6 months

Notes

1. Begin mitotane administration at a low dosage, usually no more than 2000 mg per day
2. Increase dose in increments of 500 mg to a maximum of 1000 mg per day, usually at intervals of not less than 1 week
3. Do not increase mitotane if a patient is experiencing side effects; follow General Guidelines in the Treatment Modifications section. Although mitotane is considered to have low to no emetogenic potential, it often produces low-grade nausea that is difficult to tolerate because it occurs every day. In some patients, chronic administration of antiemetics is required. See Chapter 39
4. The optimal dosage is not known; however, mitotane levels should be monitored with a goal of attaining a level of 14–20 mcg/mL. Levels greater than 20 mcg/mL are usually associated with intolerable side effects
5. A dosage of 4000–6000 mg per day usually results in a therapeutic level of mitotane in most patients after 6–10 weeks; however, some patients tolerate or require doses as high as 10,000–12,000 mg per day
6. Therapeutic levels can be achieved more quickly by administering higher doses and by increasing doses more aggressively, but this strategy usually fails because of side effects that result
7. With long-term administration of mitotane, the dosage required to maintain a therapeutic level may be substantially less, even as low as 500–1000 mg per day
8. Chronic administration results in adrenal insufficiency requiring replacement therapy, as recommended in Regimen. Some physicians prefer to begin replacement therapy at the time mitotane therapy is started; others wait until there is evidence of incipient adrenal insufficiency—usually 6–8 weeks after the start of therapy. Replacement therapy is recommended with twice-daily hydrocortisone and with once- or twice-daily fludrocortisone replacement. Measuring ACTH levels to monitor the adequacy of replacement therapy is of limited value, because normal ACTH levels are difficult if not impossible to achieve. Patients should be instructed to obtain and wear identification that warns health care providers about possible adrenal insufficiency
9. Even without effecting a reduction in tumor size, mitotane may reduce circulating hormone levels, so that mitotane therapy can be continued solely to control the signs and symptoms of hormonal excess. Furthermore, if, after a period of mitotane administration, there is evidence of disease progression, discontinuing mitotane will result in a recurrence of the signs and symptoms of hormonal excess. The latter may appear gradually as mitotane is slowly cleared, but may eventually be worse than before mitotane therapy because of interval growth of the tumor. In these patients, consider continuing mitotane or begin an alternate drug to control hormonal excess

Haak HR et al. Br J Cancer 1994;69:947–951

Hoffman DL, Mattox VR. Med Clin North Am 1972; 56:999–1012

Van Slooten H et al. Eur J Cancer Clin Oncol 1984;20: 47–53

REGIMEN

CISPLATIN + MITOTANE

Bukowski RM et al. JCO 1993;11:161–165

Hydration: ≥2000 mL 0.9% NaCl injection (0.9% NS), at ≥100 mL/hour before and after cisplatin administration. Also encourage increased oral fluid intake. Monitor and replace magnesium/electrolytes as needed.
Cisplatin 75–100 mg/m^2 by intravenous infusion in 50–250 mL of 0.9% NS over 30 minutes
Mitotane* 4000 mg/day orally, continuously

Glucocorticoid replacement is necessary in all patients:
Hydrocortisone 15–20 mg orally every morning, *plus*
Hydrocortisone 7.5–10 mg orally every evening
Mineralocorticoid replacement is also recommended
Fludrocortisone acetate 100–200 mcg/day orally every morning, *or*
Fludrocortisone acetate 100 mcg/day orally every morning and every evening

Emetogenic potential:
Day 1: High (Emetogenicity score ≥5)
Days with mitotane alone: Nonemetogenic to low (Emetogenicity score ≤2)
Potential for delayed symptoms after day 1. See Chapter 39

*Mitotane therapy may be better tolerated if started at a dose of 2000 mg/day, increasing by 500–1000 mg/day at 1-week intervals. The total daily mitotane dosage can be taken in 2–4 divided doses or as a single daily dose, which often is best tolerated at bedtime
Mitotane is available in the United States in tablets for oral administration containing 500 mg mitotane Lysodren® (mitotane tablets). Bristol-Myers Squibb Company, Princeton, NJ
Hydrocortisone is available in the United States in many solid and liquid formulations, including tablets for oral administration containing 2.5, 5, 10, or 20 mg hydrocortisone
Fludrocortisone acetate is available in the United States in tablets for oral administration containing 100 mcg of fludrocortisone acetate. Florinef® Acetate (fludrocortisone acetate tablets). Monarch Pharmaceuticals, Inc, Bristol, TN

Patient Population Studied

A trial of 42 patients with metastatic or residual adrenocortical carcinoma because complete resection was not possible. Prior therapy with mitotane was allowed

Efficacy (N = 37)

Complete response	2.7%
Partial response	27%
Median response duration	7.9 months
Median time to response	76 days

Toxicity (N = 36)

Adverse Event	% G1/2	% G3/4
Hematologic		
Anemia	8	8
Leukopenia	36	6
Thrombocytopenia	—	3
Nonhematologic		
Nausea/vomiting	75	22
Diarrhea	11	—
Mucositis	6	—
Increased bilirubin	6	—
Renal	17	8
Peripheral neuropathy	3	6
Myalgias	17	6

N = 36, but reported as percent of 37 eligible patients

Treatment Modifications

Adverse Event	Dose Modification
CrCl 30–50 mL/min	Hold cisplatin until CrCl ≥50 mL/min, then reduce dose to 75 mg/m^2 if previous dose was 100 mg/m^2 or 60 mg/m^2 if previous dose was 75 mg/m^2
CrCl <30 mL/min	Discontinue cisplatin
Unacceptable GI or neuromuscular side effects from mitotane	Reduce mitotane to 2000 mg/day
Unacceptable side effects from mitotane at 2000 mg/day	Reduce mitotane to 1000 mg/day
Unacceptable side effects from mitotane at 1000 mg/day	Discontinue mitotane

CrCl, creatinine clearance

Therapy Monitoring

1. CBC with leukocyte differential count, serum creatinine and electrolytes, serum magnesium, and LFTs on day 1
2. *Response assessment:* Repeat imaging studies every 2 cycles; 24-hour urine cortisol and 17-ketosteroids with each cycle, if abnormal at baseline
3. Mitotane level at least every 4 weeks initially. A level of 14–20 mcg/mL is desirable
4. Adrenal function can be monitored by measuring ACTH, but this alone is not reliable and should be interpreted together with clinical assessment

REGIMEN

ETOPOSIDE + DOXORUBICIN + CISPLATIN (EDP) + MITOTANE

Berruti A et al. Cancer 1998;83:2194–2200

Doxorubicin 20 mg/m^2 per dose by intravenous push injection over 3–5 minutes for 2 doses on days 1 and 8 every 4 weeks (total dosage per cycle = 40 mg/m^2)

Hydration: ≥2000 mL 0.9% NaCl injection (0.9% NS), by intravenous infusion at ≥100 mL/hour before and after cisplatin administration. Also encourage high oral intake. Monitor and replace magnesium/electrolytes as needed.
Cisplatin 40 mg/m^2 per dose intravenously in 50–250 mL of 0.9% NS over 30 minutes for 2 doses on days 2 and 9 every 4 weeks (total dosage per cycle = 80 mg/m^2)

Etoposide 100 mg/m^2 per dose intravenously in 5% dextrose injection or 0.9% NS to a concentration between 0.2 and 0.4 mg/mL over at least 60 minutes for 3 doses on days 5, 6, and 7 every 4 weeks (total dosage per cycle = 300 mg/m^2)

Mitotane 1000–4000 mg/day orally, continuously. Begin mitotane therapy at 1000–2000 mg/day, increasing by 500–1000 mg/day at 1-week intervals. The total daily mitotane dose can be taken in 2–4 divided doses or as a single daily dose, which often is best tolerated at bedtime
Glucocorticoid replacement is necessary in all patients:
Hydrocortisone 15–20 mg orally every morning, *plus*
Hydrocortisone 7.5–10 mg orally every evening
Mineralocorticoid replacement is also recommended:
Fludrocortisone acetate 100–200 mcg orally every morning, *or*
Fludrocortisone acetate 100 mcg orally every morning and every evening

Filgrastim or pegfilgrastim can be used starting on day 11 if needed
Filgrastim 5 mcg/kg per day subcutaneously until ANC has recovered to a value >2000–5000/mm^3

Emetogenic potential:
Days 1 and 8: Moderate (Emetogenicity score = 3)
Days 2 and 9: Moderately high (Emetogenicity score = 4)
Days 5–7: Low (Emetogenicity score = 2)
Days with mitotane alone: Nonemetogenic to low (Emetogenicity score ≤2)
Potential for delayed symptoms after days 2 and 9. See Chapter 39

Mitotane is available in the United States in tablets for oral administration containing 500 mg mitotane. Lysodren® (mitotane tablets). Bristol-Myers Squibb Company, Princeton, NJ
Hydrocortisone is available in the United States in many solid and liquid formulations, including tablets for oral administration containing 2.5, 5, 10, or 20 mg hydrocortisone
Fludrocortisone acetate is available in the United States as tablets for oral administration containing 100 mcg of fludrocortisone acetate. Florinef® Acetate (fludrocortisone acetate tablets). Monarch Pharmaceuticals, Inc., Bristol, TN

Patient Population Studied

A study of 28 patients with disease not amenable to resection without prior chemotherapy except mitotane

Efficacy (N = 28)

Complete response	7%
Partial response	46%
Overall response	54%
Median time to progression	24.4 months

Therapy Monitoring

1. CBC with leukocyte differential count, serum creatinine and electrolytes, serum magnesium, and LFTs on day 1
2. *Response assessment:* Repeat imaging studies every 2 cycles. 24-hour urine 17-ketosteroids and cortisol with each cycle if abnormal at baseline
3. Mitotane level at least every 4 weeks initially. A level of 14–20 mcg/mL is desirable
4. Adrenal function can be monitored by measuring ACTH, but this alone is not reliable and should be interpreted together with clinical assessment

Treatment Modifications

Adverse Event	Dose Modification
Day 1 WBC <1000/mm^3 *or* platelet count <100,000/mm^3 *or* G >2 nonhematologic toxicity	Delay chemotherapy until WBC >1000/mm^3 and platelet count >100,000/mm^3, or nonhematologic toxicity G ≤1 for a maximum delay of 2 weeks
>2-week delay in reaching WBC >1000/mm^3 *or* platelet count >100,000/mm^3 or in resolution of nonhematologic toxicity to G ≤1	Discontinue therapy
G4 ANC or G ≥3 platelet counts	Reduce dosage of all drugs by 25% except mitotane

Toxicity (N = 28)

	WHO Toxicity (% Patients)			
	G1	G2	G3	G4
Hematologic				
Neutropenia	3	21	21	3
Thrombocytopenia	—	11	—	—
Anemia	25	39	3	7
Nonhematologic				
Nausea/vomiting	28	43	11	—
Diarrhea	14	21	—	—
Mucositis	14	11	—	—
Asthenia	28	46	—	—
Myalgia	28	3	—	—
Neurologic	25	14	7	—
Renal	11	3	—	—
Hepatic	7	7	—	—

Notes

1. Response rate of 53% may not be achieved
2. Different drug administration schedules often are used, but the benefit of different schedules is not proved

REGIMEN

DOXORUBICIN

Decker RA et al. Surgery 1991;110:1006–1013

Doxorubicin 60 mg/m^2 by intravenous push injection over 3–5 minutes on day 1, every 3 weeks to a maximum cumulative lifetime dosage of 500 mg/m^2 (total dosage per cycle = 60 mg/m^2)

Emetogenic potential: Moderately high (Emetogenicity score = 4). See Chapter 39

Patient Population Studied

A study of 31 patients with unresectable adrenocortical carcinoma with ECOG PS 0–3. Fifteen of the 31 patients had been treated with mitotane immediately before doxorubicin

Efficacy (N = 31)

	Response Rate	No. of Patients
Initial treatment with chemotherapy (doxorubicin); no prior mitotane	19%	16
Tumor did not respond, or progressed when treated with mitotane	0%	15

Toxicity (N = 31)

	% Mild/ Moderate	% Severe
Bear HD et al. JCO 2003;21:4165–4174		
Hematologic		
Any hematologic	48	19
Nonhematologic		
Nausea/vomiting	45	3
Diarrhea	19	3
Skin/mucosa	16	0
Neurologic	13	0
Hepatic	6	0

Therapy Monitoring

1. CBC with leukocyte differential count, serum creatinine, electrolytes, and LFTs on day 1
2. Response assessment: Repeat imaging studies every two cycles; 24-hour urine cortisol and 17-hydroxycorticosteroids with each cycle if abnormal at baseline

Treatment Modifications

Adverse Event	Dose Modification
Day 1 ANC <1500/mm^3, platelet count <75,000/mm^3	Delay chemotherapy until ANC >1500/mm^3 and platelet counts >75,000/mm^3 for a maximum delay of 2 weeks. Use filgrastim or pegfilgrastim in subsequent cycles if delay for low ANC
Febrile neutropenia	Filgrastim or pegfilgrastim in subsequent cycles
Febrile neutropenia on filgrastim or pegfilgrastim	Reduce dosage by 25%
G ≥3 Nonhematologic toxicity	Hold therapy until resolution to G1. Reduce dosage by 25% if recovery occurs in <2 weeks

Bear HD et al. JCO 2003;21:4165–4174

Notes

The recommended limit for total cumulative lifetime doxorubicin dosage of 450–500 mg/m^2 may be exceeded, provided that adequate cardiac monitoring is conducted before every or every other chemotherapy cycle

REGIMEN

STREPTOZOCIN + MITOTANE (SO)

Khan TS et al. Ann Oncol 2000;11:1281–1287

Initial cycle:
Streptozocin 1000 mg by intravenous infusion in 100–1000 mL 0.9% NaCl injection (0.9% NS) or 5% dextrose injection (D5W), over 30–120 minutes on days 1–5 (total dosage during the first cycle = 5000 mg), followed 3 weeks later by:
Second and subsequent cycles:
Streptozocin 2000 mg by intravenous infusion in 200–1000 mL 0.9% NS or D5W, over 30–120 minutes, on day 1, every 3 weeks (total dosage per cycle = 2000 mg)

Mitotane 1000–4000 mg/day orally, continuously
Begin mitotane therapy at a dose of 1000–2000 mg/day, increasing by 500–1000 mg/day at 1-week intervals. The total daily mitotane dose can be taken in 2 to 4 divided doses or as a single daily dose, often best tolerated at bedtime
Glucocorticoid replacement is necessary in all patients:
Hydrocortisone 15–20 mg orally every morning, *plus*
Hydrocortisone 7.5–10 mg orally every evening
Mineralocorticoid replacement is also recommended:
Fludrocortisone acetate 100–200 mcg orally every morning, *or*
Fludrocortisone acetate 100 mcg orally every morning and every evening

Emetogenic potential:
Days of streptozocin administration: High (Emetogenicity score ≥5)
Days with mitotane alone: Nonemetogenic to low (Emetogenicity score ≤2). See Chapter 39

Mitotane is available in the United States in tablets for oral administration containing 500 mg mitotane. Lysodren® (mitotane tablets) product label, April 1999. Bristol-Myers Squibb Company, Princeton, NJ
Hydrocortisone is available in the United States in many solid and liquid formulations, including tablets for oral administration containing 2.5, 5, 10, and 20 mg hydrocortisone
Fludrocortisone acetate is available in the United States in tablets for oral administration containing 100 mcg of fludrocortisone acetate. Florinef® Acetate (fludrocortisone acetate tablets). Monarch Pharmaceuticals, Inc, Bristol, TN

Patient Population Studied

Forty patients with resected, recurrent, or metastatic adrenocortical carcinoma

Efficacy (N = 22)

Overall response rate	36.4%

Nonrandom comparison of patients treated after surgery with the SO regimen adjuvantly compared with those who received SO chemotherapy only after local recurrences or metastases developed showed a superior disease-free interval favoring the former group (66 months versus 22 months, respectively)

Therapy Monitoring

1. CBC with leukocyte differential count, serum creatinine, electrolytes, and LFTs on day 1; obtain creatinine clearance on day 1 if an elevation in serum creatinine is observed
2. Twenty-four-hour urine for protein on day 1
3. Response assessment: Repeat imaging studies every 2 cycles. 24-hour urine 17-ketosteroids and cortisol with each cycle if abnormal at baseline

Treatment Modifications

Adverse Event	Dose Modification
Abnormal LFTs (>2 × baseline or > twice upper limits of normal)	Hold streptozocin until LFTs return to baseline or normal; then resume treatment with same dose
Evidence of nephrotoxicity (proteinuria or decreasing creatinine clearance)	Divide streptozocin dosage into 2 days
Creatinine clearance <50 to 60 mL/min	Hold streptozocin until creatinine clearance >50 to 60 mL/min.

Toxicity (N = 40)

	% Patients
Clinical Toxicities	
Nausea with mitotane	50
Nausea with streptozocin	60
Fatigue	30
Vertigo	18
Lethargy	15
Diarrhea	13
Vomiting with mitotane	10
Vomiting with streptozocin	28
Anorexia	10
Gynecomastia	10
Polyneuropathy	5
Rash	5
Hemorrhagic cystitis	3
Laboratory Abnormalities	
Abnormal LFTs	63
Albuminuria	55
Increased creatinine	15
Autoimmune hepatitis	8

Notes

Efficacy is difficult to quantify because assessment includes patients who had undergone surgical resection and had no evidence of disease. Although a recurrence was anticipated, surgical success cannot be excluded

2. Anal Cancer

David Ryan, MD, and Robert Mayer, MD

Epidemiology

Incidence: 4660 estimated new cases in the United States in 2006
Male: 1910
Female 2750
Deaths: 620 (estimated deaths in the United States in 2005)

Stage at Presentation

Stage I–II:	>50%
Stage III:	30–40%
Stage IV:	<10%

Jemal A et al. CA Cancer J Clin 2006;56:106–30
http://seer.cancer.gov
Maggard MA et al. Dis Colon Rectum 2003;46:1517
Ryan DP et al. NEJM 2000;342:792–800

Pathology

By convention, anal cancer should now refer only to *squamous cell cancers* arising in the anus. Earlier surgical series often did not make this distinction. *Adenocarcinomas* occurring in the anal canal should be treated according to the same principles applied to rectal adenocarcinoma. Similarly, melanomas and sarcomas should be treated according to the same principles applied to those tumor types at other sites

The distal anal canal is lined by squamous epithelium, and tumors arising in this portion are often keratinizing. Around the dentate line, the mucosa transitions from squamous mucosa to the nonsquamous rectal mucosa. Tumors arising in this transitional zone are often nonkeratinizing and previously were referred to as basaloid or cloacogenic

Clark MA et al. Lancet Oncology 2004;5:149–157
Ryan DP et al. NEJM 2000;342:792–800

Work-Up

All stages
1. Sigmoidoscopy with biopsy
2. CT scan of abdomen and pelvis
3. Chest x-ray or chest CT
4. Consider HIV testing

Positive inguinal lymph node on imaging
1. Fine-needle aspiration or biopsy of node

NCCN Clinical Practice Guidelines in Oncology – V. 2. 2006
http://www.nccn.org/

Staging

Primary Tumor (T)

TX	Primary tumor cannot be assessed
T0	No evidence of primary tumor
Tis	Carcinoma in situ
T1	Tumor 2 cm or less
T2	Tumor more than 2 cm but not more than 5 cm in greatest dimension
T3	Tumor more than 5 cm in greatest dimension
T4	Tumor of any size invades adjacent organ(s), e.g. vagina, urethra, bladder

Regional Lymph Nodes (N): Clinical

NX	Regional lymph nodes cannot be assessed
N0	No regional lymph node metastases
N1	Metastasis in perirectal lymph nodes
N2	Metastasis in unilateral internal iliac and/or inguinal lymph node(s)
N3	Metastasis in perirectal and inguinal lymph nodes and/or bilateral internal iliac and/or inguinal lymph nodes

Distant Metastasis (M)

MX	Distant metastasis cannot be assessed
M0	No distant metastasis
M1	Distant Metastasis

Staging Groups

Stage 0	Tis	N0	M0
Stage I	T1	N0	M0
Stage II	T2-3	N0	M0
Stage IIIA	T1-3 T4	N1 N0	M0 M0
Stage IIIB	T4 Any T	N1 N2-3	M0 M0
Stage IV M1	Any T	Any N	

Five-Year Survival (After Chemoradiation)

All patients with stages I–III: 57–67%

Poor prognostic factors:
1. Nodal involvement
2. Skin ulceration
3. Male gender

Bartelink F et al. JCO 1997;15:2040–2049*
Flam M et al. JCO 1996;14:2527–2539; updated results in: Flam M et al Classic Papers and Current Comments: Highlights of Gastrointestinal Cancer Research 1999;3:539–552
UKCCR. Lancet 1996;348:1049–1054

Caveats

Any T, any N, M0 (stage IIIB) invasive squamous cell carcinoma of the anus

1. *Primary treatment:* Chemoradiation

   Standard chemoradiation regimen consists of fluorouracil, mitomycin, and 45–50.5 Gy of external-beam radiation therapy

2. *Treatment of persistent disease after chemoradiation or for locally recurrent disease:* Surgery

Any T, any N, M1 (stage IV) squamous cell carcinoma of the anus

1. *Local palliation:* Chemoradiation
2. *Metastatic disease:* Palliative chemotherapy with fluorouracil and cisplatin can be used

REGIMEN

MITOMYCIN + FLUOROURACIL + EXTERNAL-BEAM RADIATION THERAPY (RTOG 8704/ECOG 1289)

Flam M et al. JCO 1996;14:2527-2539

Mitomycin 10 mg/m^2 single dose (maximum dose = 20 mg) by intravenous push on day 1 every 4 weeks for 2 cycles (days 1 and 29 of radiation) (total dosage/cycle = 10 mg/m^2, but *not* greater than 20 mg)

Fluorouracil 1000 mg/m^2 per day (maximum daily dose = 2000 mg) by continuous intravenous infusion on days 1–4 every 4 weeks for 2 cycles (days 1 and 29 of radiation) (total dosage/cycle = 4000 mg/m^2, but *not* greater than 8000 mg)

External-beam radiation therapy 1.8 Gy/fraction daily 5 days/week for 5 weeks (total dose to pelvis/complete course = 45 Gy in 5 weeks)
For patients with T3, T4, or N+ lesions or T2 lesions with residual disease after 45 Gy, current RTOG protocol recommends an additional 10–14 Gy to a reduced field

Emetogenic potential: High. See Chapter 39

Treatment Modifications

Adverse Event	Dose Modification
G3/4 Diarrhea or stomatitis	Reduce fluorouracil dosage 50% during second cycle
G3 Radiation dermatitis	
G4 Radiation dermatitis	Do not give second cycle of chemotherapy
ANC <500/mm^3 or platelet <50,000/mm^3	Reduce fluorouracil and mitomycin dosages 50%
G3/4 Hematologic or nonhematologic events	Suspend chemoradiation until recovers to G ≤2

Based on RTOG protocol 98-11

Patient Population Studied

A study of 146 patients with localized (nonmetastatic) squamous cell cancer of the anal canal

Efficacy (N = 129–146)

Positive biopsy after induction	8%
5-year locoregional failure	36%
5-year colostomy rate	22%
5-year colostomy-free survival	64%
5-year disease-free survival	67%
5-year overall survival	67%

Flam M et al Classic Papers and Current Comments: Highlights of Gastrointestinal Cancer Research 1999;3:539–552

Toxicity (N = 146)

	% G4/5
Acute (≤90 days after starting treatment)	25
Hematologic	18
Nonhematologic (diarrhea, skin, mucositis)	7
Late (>90 days after starting treatment)	5
Any grade 4 adverse event	23
Toxic death rate*	2.8

*All treatment-related deaths occurred in a setting of neutropenia and sepsis
NCI CTC

Therapy Monitoring

1. *Every week*: CBC with differential
2. *Response assessment:* PE 6 weeks after completion of chemoradiotherapy. If there is regression of tumor on exam, then 12 weeks after completion of therapy repeat PE, perform sigmoidoscopy and obtain CT scan. If there is a residual mass or thickening, a biopsy should be performed. If there is residual disease at 12 weeks or if there is progression of disease on exam, consider salvage abdominoperineal resection

Notes

Severely immunocompromised patients or HIV-positive patients with low CD4 counts should be treated with caution. Consider omitting and/or reducing the dose of chemotherapy

REGIMEN

FLUOROURACIL + CISPLATIN + EXTERNAL-BEAM RADIATION THERAPY

Doci R et al. JCO 1996;14:3121–3125

Fluorouracil 750 mg/m^2 per day by continuous intravenous infusion in 500–1000 mL 0.9% NaCl injection (0.9% NS) or 5% dextrose injection (D5W) over 24 hours on days 1–4 every 21 days for 2 cycles (total dosage/cycle = 3000 mg/m^2)
(Days 1–4 and 21–24 of radiation therapy)

Hydration before cisplatin ≥1000 mL 0.9% NS over a minimum of 2–4 hours
Cisplatin 100 mg/m^2 single dose intravenously in 50–250 mL 0.9% NS over 60 minutes, day 1 every 21 days for 2 cycles (total dosage/cycle = 100 mg/m^2)
(Days 1 and 21 of radiation therapy)
Hydration after cisplatin ≥1000 mL 0.9% NS over a minimum of 2–4 hours. Also encourage high oral intake

External-beam radiation therapy 1.8 Gy/fraction daily 5 days/week up to 54–58 Gy

Emetogenic potential : High. See Chapter 39

Note: The RTOG has amended the above regimen as follows:
Two cycles of chemotherapy are given before external-beam radiation therapy commences; that is, radiation therapy begins coincident with the start of chemotherapy cycle 3
The chemotherapy regimen used has been modified as follows:
Fluorouracil 1000 mg/m^2 per day by continuous intravenous infusion in 500–1000 mL 0.9% NS or D5W over 24 hours on days 1–4 every 28 days for 4 cycles (total dosage/cycle = 4000 mg/m^2)
Cisplatin 75 mg/m^2 single dose intravenously in 250 mL 0.9% NS over 60 minutes on day 1 every 28 days for 4 cycles on days 1, 29, 57, and 85 (total dosage/cycle = 75 mg/m^2)

Patient Population Studied

A study of 35 patients with previously untreated basaloid (n = 5) or squamous cell carcinoma (n = 30) of the anus. In all patients, the cancer was located in the anal canal; in 28, the tumor extended to adjacent sites. Nine patients had nodal metastases; no patient had distant metastases

Efficacy (N = 35)

Complete response	94%
Partial response*	6%
Local recurrence	6%

At median follow-up of 37 months	
No evidence of disease	94%
Colostomy free	86%

Normal anal function preserved in 30 of 35 patients
*Two partial responses in 2 of 5 (40%) patients with T3 tumors

Toxicity[a] (N = 35)

	% G1	% G2	% G3
Hematologic (leukopenia)	40	31	—
Vomiting	40	33	10
Dermatitis, proctitis, diarrhea	8.5	88.5	3
Cardiac	—	3[b]	—

[a]Acute toxicities. Chronic toxicities not reported. No grade 4 toxicities reported
[b]Transient at end of first cycle; resolved
WHO criteria

Treatment Modifications

Adverse Event	Dose Modification
ANC <500/mm^3 or platelets <50,000/mm^3	Decrease fluorouracil and cisplatin dosages by 50%
G3/4 Diarrhea or stomatitis	Decrease fluorouracil dosage by 50%
G3 Radiation dermatitis	
G4 Radiation dermatitis	Hold radiation until resolves to G ≤ 2, and do not administer additional fluorouracil
Creatinine 1.5–2.0 mg/dL (133–177 μmol/L)	Decrease cisplatin dosage by 50%
Creatinine >2.0 mg/dL (177 μmol/L)	Hold cisplatin

Recommended by RTOG 98-11

Therapy Monitoring

1. *Before each cycle:* CBC with differential, BUN, creatinine, magnesium and electrolytes
2. *Response assessment:* PE 4–6 weeks after completion of chemoradiotherapy. Perform a biopsy only in the absence of a response to therapy. If there has been a response to therapy, reevaluate at 12 weeks with PE, sigmoidoscopy, and CT scan. If residual tumor is suspected, biopsy the affected area. If residual disease is documented at 12 weeks or if there is progression of disease on exam, consider salvage abdominoperineal resection

3. Biliary: Gallbladder Cancer and Cholangiocarcinoma

Verena Sagaster, MD, and Werner Scheithauer, MD

Epidemiology

	Gallbladder Cancer	Cholangiocarcinoma
Incidence*/100,000 (United States)	Females: 1.7	Females: 1.0
	Males: 0.9	Males: 1.5
Deaths	3340 (United States)	
Age	>70 years	50–70 years
Stage at presentation	No data reported, although cases are diagnosed in advanced stages	

*Incidence rates are much higher in certain geographic regions (Chile, northeastern Europe, and Israel)

Work-up

1. Early diagnosis of gallbladder or cholangiocellular carcinoma is nearly impossible or can only be realized in exceptional cases
2. In a patient with specific clinical symptoms or ultrasound suspicion of biliary tract cancer, a spiral CT and chest x-ray should be performed
3. Medically fit, nonjaundiced patients whose disease appears *potentially resectable* may proceed directly to surgical exploration without needle biopsy to avoid tumor spread. Consider a laparoscopic evaluation before open surgery owing to the common occurrence of otherwise nonvisible metastatic spread to the peritoneum
4. If the potential to perform a resection remains *uncertain* and for those with jaundice, a more precise assessment of tumor extent and lymph node involvement should be obtained with MRCP ± MRA which may help to rule out vascular invasion and anomalous anatomic findings for surgical planning
5. If it is obvious that a resection will *not* be possible or if distant metastases are present, fine-needle biopsy for tissue confirmation should be obtained
6. In *nonresectable jaundiced* patients, depending on the location of the biliary obstruction, a percutaneous transhepatic cholangiography (PTC) or an endoscopic retrograde cholangiography (ERC) should be considered to guide placement of a stent

Fong Y et al. Cancer of the liver and biliary tree. In: Principles and Practice of Oncology, 6th ed. Lippincott Williams & Wilkins 2001:1162–1203

Pathology

1. Gallbladder cancer
2. Cholangiocarcinoma
   - Intrahepatic 10%
   - Perihilar (Klatskin tumor) 40–60%
   - Distal 20–30%
   - Multifocal <10%

Histopathology

1. Adenocarcinoma 80–90%
   Papillary, nodular, tubular, medullary
2. Pleomorphic giant cell carcinoma >10%
3. Squamous cell carcinoma 5%
4. Mucoid carcinoma <1%
5. Anaplastic carcinoma <1%
6. Cystadenocarcinoma <1%
7. Clear cell carcinoma <1%
8. Other rare forms <1%

Lazcano-Ponce EC et al. CA Cancer J Clin 2001; 51:349–364
Nakeeb A et al. Ann Surg 1996;224:463–475

Staging

Cholangiocarcinoma

Primary Tumor (T)

TX	Primary tumor cannot be assessed
T0	No evidence of primary tumor
Tis	Carcinoma in situ
T1	Tumor is confined to the bile duct
T1a	Tumor invades lamina propria
T1b	Tumor invades the muscle layer
T2	Tumor has spread outside the bile duct but not to adjacent structures
T3	Tumor invades adjacent structures such as the liver, gallbladder, or branches of the portal vein or the hepatic artery
T4	Tumor invades into the main portal vein, or the hepatic artery, or duodenum, gallbladder, colon or stomach

Regional Lymph Nodes (N)

NX	Regional lymph nodes cannot be assessed
N0	No spread to regional lymph nodes
N1	Metastasis to lymph nodes within the hepatoduodenal ligament
N2	Metastasis to peripancreatic, periduodenal, celiac, superior mesenteric, and/or posterior pancreaticoduodenal lymph nodes

Distant Metastasis (M)

MX	Distant metastasis cannot be assessed
M0	No distant metastasis
M1	Distant metastasis

Gallbladder Cancer

Primary Tumor (T)

TX	Primary tumor cannot be assessed
T0	No evidence of primary tumor
Tis	Carcinoma in situ
T1	Tumor invades into the lamina propria or the muscle layer
T1a	Tumor invades lamina propria
T1b	Tumor invades the muscle layer
T2	Tumor invades perimuscular connective tissue
T3	Tumor perforates the serosa and/or directly invades the liver and/or one other adjacent organ
T4	Tumor invades beyond 2 cm of liver and/or several organs outside the liver

Regional Lymph Nodes (N)

NX	Regional lymph nodes cannot be assessed
NO	No spread to regional lymph nodes
N1	Metastasis to perihilar lymph nodes
N2	Metastasis to peripancreatic, periduodenal, periportal, cecal, and/or mesenteric lymph nodes

Distant Metastasis (M)

MX	Distant metastasis cannot be assessed
MO	No distant metastasis
M1	Distant metastasis

Staging Groups

Cholangiocarcinoma and Gallbladder Cancer

Stage 0	Tis	N0	M0
Stage IA	T1	N0	M0
Stage IB	T2	N0	M0
Stage IIA	T3	N0	M0
Stage IIB	T1-3	N1	M0
Stage III	T4 T4	N0 N1	M0 M0
Stage IV	Any T	Any N	M1

AJCC/System in American Cancer Society Cancer Facts & Figures 2004

Five-year Survival (Cholangiocarcinoma and Gallbladder Cancer)*

Stage IA	85–100%
Stage IB	30–40% to 70–90%
Stage II	10–60%
Stage III	10–40%
Stage IV	0%

*Statistics for gallbladder cancer not certain because few cases reported in the literature

Caveats

Gallbladder cancer

As is true for all hepatobiliary cancers, surgery remains the only curative modality for gallbladder cancer (cholecystectomy, en bloc hepatic resection, and lymphadenectomy with or without bile duct excision). Postoperative therapy for resectable patients—except those with T1, N0 disease, with negative margins who might be considered for adjuvant 5-fluorouracil (5-FU), or capecitabine-based, or gemcitabine based chemotherapy. Patients with unresectable tumor without obvious metastatic disease and without jaundice may benefit from a regimen of 5-FU- or capecitabine-based chemotherapy ± radiation. However, overall survival of such patients remains poor

Intrahepatic cholangiocarcinoma

Patients who have undergone a tumor resection with or without ablation with negative margins may be followed up with observation, because there is no definitive adjuvant regimen to improve their overall survival. For individuals whose disease is resectable but who are left with positive margins after resection: (1) consider additional resection, (2) ablative therapy, or (3) combined radiation with or without chemotherapy using either 5-FU- or capecitabine-based regimen or gemcitabine. For patients with unresectable disease, the options include depending on tumor location, spread and performance status- (1) ablative therapy with cryotherapy, radiofrequency, or microwave; (2) chemotherapy with either 5-FU or capecitabine-based regimen or gemcitabine; (3) combined radiochemotherapy; (4) or best supportive care.

Extrahepatic cholangiocarcinoma

Patients with positive margins after resection should be considered for 5-FU- or capecitabine-based chemotherapy with radiation (external-beam therapy or brachytherapy). Individuals with negative margins after resection or with negative regional nodes either can be observed or can receive 5-FU- or capecitabine-based or gemcitabine-based chemotherapy with radiation. Patients whose disease is deemed unresectable at the time of surgery should undergo biliary drainage if required, ideally non-surgically i.e. by using a stent. Given their overall poor prognosis, further options for unresectable patients include (1) a clinical trial; (2) chemoradiation (5-FU- or capecitabine-based chemotherapy/RT); (3) chemotherapy alone using either a 5-FU or capecitabine-based regimen or gemcitabine; or (4) best supportive care

National Comprehensive Cancer Network, vol. 1,2005

REGIMEN

MITOMYCIN + CAPECITABINE

Kornek GV et al. Ann Oncol 2004;15:478–483

Mitomycin 8 mg/m² by intravenous push over 2–3 minutes on day 1 every 4 weeks (total dosage/cycle = 8 mg/m²)

Capecitabine 1000 mg/m² per dose orally twice daily (approximately every 12 hours) for 14 consecutive days on days 1–14 every 4 weeks (total dosage/cycle = 28,000 mg/m²)
(Capecitabine is taken with water within 30 minutes after food ingestion)
Capecitabine is manufactured in the United States as film-coated tablets for oral administration containing either 150 mg or 500 mg capecitabine. XELODA® (capecitabine) TABLETS, Roche Laboratories Inc, Nutley, NJ

Emetogenic potential: Low (Emetogenicity score = 2). See Chapter 39

Patient Population Studied

A study of 26 chemotherapy-naive patients with advanced biliary tract cancer

Efficacy (N = 26)

Partial responses	30.8%
Stable disease	34.6%
Progressive disease	34.6%
Median progression-free survival	5.35 months
Median overall survival	9.25 months

WHO Criteria

Toxicity (N = 24)

	% G1/2	% G3
Hematologic		
Neutropenia	N/A	17
Thrombocytopenia	48	17
Nonhematologic		
Nausea/vomiting	42	—
Fatigue	42	—
Diarrhea	28	—
Hand-foot syndrome	17	—
Alopecia	12	—
Increased liver function results*	54	—
Fever without documented infection: 8%		

*Possibly due to progressive disease because >80% of patients had liver involvement
WHO criteria

Treatment Modifications

Adverse Event	Dose Modification
Nadir WBC <1000/mm³, ANC <500/mm³, or platelets <50,000/mm³	Delay chemotherapy for up to 2 weeks until adverse events G ≤ 1, then decrease subsequent mitomycin and capecitabine dosages by 25%
Any G ≥ 3 nonhematologic adverse events during the previous treatment cycle	
Duration of treatment delay >2 weeks for recovery from adverse events	Discontinue treatment

Therapy Monitoring

1. *Weekly:* CBC with differential
2. *Before each cycle:* Biochemical profile
3. *Response assessment:* Every 2 cycles

REGIMEN

GEMCITABINE

Penz M et al. Ann Oncol 2001;12:183–186

Gemcitabine 2200 mg/m² by intravenous infusion in 250 mL 0.9% NaCl injection (0.9% NS), over 30 minutes on day 1 every 2 weeks for 6 months (total dosage per 2-week cycle = 2200 mg/m²)

Emetogenic potential: Low (Emetogenicity score = 2). See Chapter 39

Patient Population Studied

A study of 32 chemotherapy-naive patients with locally advanced or metastatic biliary tract cancer

Efficacy (N = 32)

Overall response rate	21.9%
Stable disease	43.7%
Progressive disease	34.4%
Median progression-free survival	5.6 months
Median overall survival	11.5 months

WHO criteria

Toxicity (N = 32)

	% G1	% G2	% G3
Hematologic			
Neutropenia	19	22	6
Thrombocytopenia	12	3	6
Anemia	31	25	3
Nonhematologic			
Nausea/vomiting	22	22	—
Diarrhea	3	9	—
Constipation	6	3	—
Stomatitis	6	3	—
Fatigue	22	9	—
Alopecia	6	12	—
Fever	9	12	—
Cutaneous	6	3	—
Serum transaminases	12	9	—

No grade 4 toxicites
WHO criteria

Treatment Modifications

Adverse Event	Dose Modification
Nadir WBC <1000/mm³, ANC <500/mm³, or platelets <50,000/mm³	Reduce gemcitabine dosages by 25% in subsequent cycles
G ≥ 3 nonhematologic adverse event during the previous treatment cycle	
WBC <3000/mm³ or platelets <75,000/mm³ on day of treatment	Delay chemotherapy for up to 2 weeks
Treatment delay >2 weeks for recovery from hematologic adverse event	Discontinue treatment

Therapy Monitoring

1. *Every week:* CBCs with differential LFTs
2. *Before each cycle:* Complete biochemical profile
3. *Response assessment:* Every 2 months

REGIMEN

GEMCITABINE + OXALIPLATIN (GEMOX)

Maindrault-Goebel F et al. Proc Am Soc Clin Oncol 2003;22:293 [Abstract #1178]

Gemcitabine 1000 mg/m^2 by intravenous infusion in 250 mL 0.9% NaCl injection (0.9% NS) at an infusion rate of 10 mg/m^2/minute (2.5 mL/minute) on day 1 every 2 weeks (total dosage every 2 weeks = 1000 mg/m^2)

Oxaliplatin 100 mg/m^2 by intravenous infusion in 250–500 mL of 5% dextrose injection (D5W), over 2 hours on day 2 every 2 weeks (total dosage every 2 weeks = 100 mg/m^2)

Emetogenic potential: Moderately high. (Emetogenicity score = 4). See Chapter 39

Patient Population Studied

A study of 33 patients with advanced biliary tract carcinoma

Efficacy (N = 31)

Overall response rate	35.5%
Stable disease	26%
Progressive disease	38.5%
Median progression-free survival	5.7 months
Overall survival	14.3 months

Toxicity (N = 56)

G3 Neutropenia	12.5%
G3 Thrombocytopenia	9%
Peripheral sensory neuropathy	7.1%
G2 Alopecia	5.3%
G3 Nausea/vomiting	3.5%
G3 Diarrhea	—

NCI CTC

Treatment Modifications

Adverse Event	Dose Modification
Nadir WBC <1000/mm^3, ANC <500/mm^3, or platelets <50,000/mm^3	Decrease gemcitabine and oxaliplatin dosages by 25% in subsequent cycles
G ≥ 3 nonhematologic adverse event during the previous treatment cycle	
WBC <3000/mm^3 or platelets <75,000/mm^3 on day of treatment	Delay chemotherapy for up to 2 weeks
Treatment delay >2 weeks for recovery from hematologic adverse events	Discontinue treatment

Therapy Monitoring

1. *Every week:* CBCs with differential
2. *Before each cycle:* Complete biochemical profile
3. *Response assessment:* Every 2 months

4. Bladder Cancer

Edwin M. Posadas, MD, and William L. Dahut, MD

Epidemiology

Incidence: 61,420 (44,690 males; 16,730 females in 2006)
Mortality rate: 13,060 (8990 males; 4070 females in 2006)
Median age: Seventh decade
Male/female ratio: 3:1

Stage at Presentation	
Stage I:	75%
Stage II/III:	20%
Stage IV:	5%

Jemal A et al. CA Cancer J Clin 2006;56:106–30
American Cancer Society: http://www.cancer.org

Work-Up

Stage I:	H&P, cystoscopy. Upper tract imaging (IVP, retrograde pyelogram or CT). CT of abdomen and pelvis before transurethral resection of the bladder tumor (TURBT) if sessile or high-grade cytology
Stage II/III	H&P, cystoscopy. CBC, chemistry profile including alkaline phosphatase, chest x-ray, upper tract imaging with CT or MRI (including abdominopelvic CT or MRI), TURBT, bone scan if alkaline phosphatase elevated or symptoms
Stage IV:	H&P, cystoscopy, CBC, chemistry profile, chest CT, MRI or CT of abdomen & pelvis, upper tract imaging with CT or MRI, TURBT, bone scan

NCCN Clinical Practice Guidelines in Oncology – V. 1. 2006

Pathology

Transitional cell carcinoma	90–95%
Squamous cell carcinoma	3%
Adenocarcinoma	2%
Small cell carcinoma	1%

Histopathologic evaluation should include a description of cell type, grade (G1–G3), and depth of invasion. Other studies including p53 are still considered experimental. Pathologic grade is important in the management of noninvasive tumors.

Young RH. In: Vogelzang NJ, Scardino PT, Shipley WU, Coffey DS, eds. Comprehensive Textbook of Genitourinary Oncology, 2nd ed. Philadelphia: Lippincott Williams & Wilkins, 2000:310–321

Staging

Primary Tumor (T)

TX	Primary tumor cannot be assessed
T0	No evidence of primary tumor
Ta	Noninvasive papillary cancer
Tis	Carcinoma in situ (flat tumor)
T1	Tumor invades subepithelial connective tissue
T2	Tumor invades muscle
pT2a	invades superficial muscle (inner half)
pT2b	invades deep muscle (outer half)
T3	Tumor invades perivesical tissue
pT3a	microscopically
pT3b	macroscopically (extravesical mass)
T4	Tumor invades any other structures
T4a	invades prostate, uterus, vagina
T4b	invades pelvic wall or abdominal wall

AJCC Cancer Staging Manual, 6th ed. 2002:335–340

Regional Lymph nodes (N) Clinical

NX	Regional lymph nodes cannot be assessed
N0	No regional lymph node metastases
N1	Single node 2 cm or less in greatest dimension
N2	Single node more than 2 cm but not more than 5 cm; or multiple lymph nodes, none more than 5 cm
N3	Lymph nodes greater than 5 cm

Distant Metastasis (M)

MX	Distant metastasis cannot be assessed
M0	No distant metastasis
M1	Distant metastasis

AJCC Cancer Staging Manual, 6th ed. 2002:335–340

Staging Groups

Stage 0a	Ta N0 M0
Stage 0is	Tis N0 M0
Stage I	T1 N0 M0
Stage II	T2a N0 M0; T2b N0 M0
Stage III	T3a N0 M0; T3b N0 M0; T4a N0 M0
Stage IV	T4b N0 M0; any T N1 M0; any T N2 M0; any T N3 M0; any T any N M1

Reproduced, with permission, of the American Joint Committee on Cancer (AJCC), Chicago, Illinois. The original source for this material is the AJCC Cancer Staging Manual, 6th edition (2002) published by Springer-Verlag, New York, www.springeronline.com.

Five-Year Relative Survival

Stage 0	>95%
Stage I	85%
Stage II	65–75%
Stage III	30–65%
Stage IV	10–15%

American Cancer Society: http://www.cancer.org

Caveats

1. MVAC is historic standard systemic therapy for bladder cancer. However, recent phase III data suggest that gemcitabine/cisplatin may be equally efficacious with a more desirable side-effect profile
2. Because MVAC includes doxorubicin, avoid it in patients with preexisting cardiac disease unless a cardiologist is consulted who is familiar with the effects of doxorubicin
3. Consider gemcitabine/carboplatin in patients with preexisting renal disease considered candidates for chemotherapy
4. Encourage patient participation in clinical trials if systemic therapy (either adjuvant or neoadjuvant) is a consideration
5. Patients with muscle-invasive disease and good PS should be considered for adjuvant or neoadjuvant chemotherapy with a full discussion of risks and benefits of treatment

REGIMEN

METHOTREXATE + VINBLASTINE + DOXORUBICIN + CISPLATIN (MVAC)

von der Maase H et al. JCO 2000;17:3068–3077

Methotrexate 30 mg/m^2 per dose by intravenous push over 15–60 seconds on days 1, 15, and 22 every 28 days for 6 cycles (total dosage/cycle = 90 mg/m^2)

Vinblastine 3 mg/m^2 per dose by intravenous push over 1–2 minutes on days 2, 15, and 22 every 28 days for 6 cycles (total dosage/cycle = 9 mg/m^2)

Doxorubicin 30 mg/m^2 single dose by intravenous push over 3–5 minutes on day 2, every 28 days for 6 cycles (total dosage/cycle = 30 mg/m^2)

Hydration before and after cisplatin: ≥1000 mL 0.9% NaCl injection (0.9% NS) intravenously at ≥100 mL/hour before and after cisplatin administration. Also encourage high oral fluid intake. Monitor and replace magnesium/electrolytes as needed.
Cisplatin 70 mg/m^2 single dose by intravenous infusion in 100–1000 mL 0.9% NS over 1–8 hours on day 2 every 28 days for 6 cycles (total dosage/cycle = 70 mg/m^2)

Take home: Consider prophylactic filgrastim

Emetogenic potential:
Days 1, 15, and 22: Nonemetogenic (Emetogenicity score = 1)
Day 2: High (Emetogenicity score = 6). High potential for delayed symptoms after day 2. See Chapter 39

Treatment Modifications

Adverse Event	Dose Modification
Day 1 if WBC <3000/mm^3, or platelet count <100,000/mm^3	Delay chemotherapy for 1 week
Day 15 or 22 if WBC ≤2900/mm^3 or platelet count ≤74000/mm^3	Hold dose of methotrexate and vinblastine
G3/4 Mucositis*	Reduce methotrexate dosage by 33% (all remaining doses and into next cycle)
Severe neurotoxicity	Reduce vinblastine dosage by 33%
Clinical evidence of CHF	Discontinue doxorubicin

*Leucovorin may be started 24 hours after methotrexate infusion

Patient Population Studied

A study of 202 patients with locally advanced or metastatic transitional cell urothelial cancer without prior systemic chemotherapy or immunotherapy. Prior local intravesical therapy, immunotherapy, or RT were allowed. Karnofsky performance status ≥70; and measured creatinine clearance ≥60 mL/minute

Efficacy (N = 196)

Complete response	11.9%
Partial response	33.8%
Median overall survival	14.8 months
Median time to treatment failure	4.6 months
Median time to disease progression	7.4 months
Median duration of response	9.6 months

Toxicity (N = 202)

Adverse Event	% G3	% G4
Hematologic		
Anemia	15.5	2.1
Thrombocytopenia	7.7	12.9
Neutropenia	17.1	65.
Nonhematologic		
Mucositis	17.7	4.2
Nausea	19.2	1.6
Alopecia	54.2	1.0
Infection	9.9	5.2
Diarrhea	7.8	0.5
Pulmonary	2.6	3.1
Hematuria	2.3	0
Constipation	2.6	0.5
Hemorrhage	2.1	0
State of consciousness	3.1	0.5
Fever	3.1	0

WHO criteria

Therapy Monitoring

1. *Before each cycle:* CBC with differential and serum electrolytes, magnesium, BUN, creatinine, and LFTs
2. *Days 15 and 22:* CBC with differential
3. *Response evaluation:* Every 2–3 cycles—CT scan

Notes

1. Give 6 cycles unless disease progression is documented
2. Avoid it in patients with preexisting cardiac disease unless a cardiologist familiar with effects of doxorubicin is consulted

REGIMEN

CISPLATIN + GEMCITABINE

von der Maase H et al. JCO 2000;17:3068–3077

Gemcitabine 1000 mg/m^2 per dose by intravenous infusion in 50–250 mL 0.9% NaCl injection (0.9% NS) over 30–60 minutes on days 1, 8, and 15 every 28 days for a maximum of 6 cycles (total dosage/cycle = 3000 mg/m^2)

Hydration before and after cisplatin: At least 500 mL 0.9% NS intravenously over 1–4 hours before and after therapy. Also encourage high oral intake. Monitor and replace magnesium/electrolytes as needed.

Cisplatin 70 mg/m^2 single dose by intravenous infusion in 100–250 mL 0.9% NS over 60 minutes on day 2 every 28 days for a maximum of 6 cycles (total dosage/cycle = 70 mg/m^2)

Emetogenic potential:
Days 1, 8, and 15: Low (Emetogenicity score = 2)
Day 2: High (Emetogenicity score = 5)
High potential for delayed symptoms after day 2. See Chapter 39

Treatment Modifications

Adverse Event	Dose Modification
Day 1 WBC <3000/mm^3, or platelet count <100,000/mm^3	Hold chemotherapy until WBC >3000/mm^3 and platelet count >100,000/mm^3
Days 8 or 15 WBC ≤1990/mm^3, or platelet count ≤49,000/mm^3	Omit gemcitabine on that day*
Treatment delay >4 weeks	Discontinue treatment

*Missed chemotherapy doses are not given. If gemcitabine is omitted on day 15, the cycle duration may be shortened to 21 days

Patient Population Studied

A study of 203 patients with locally advanced or metastatic transitional cell urothelial cancer without prior systemic chemotherapy or immunotherapy. Prior local intravesical therapy, immunotherapy, or radiation therapy were allowed. Karnofsky performance status ≥70; measured creatinine clearance ≥60 mL/minute

Efficacy (N = 200)

Complete response	12.2%
Partial response	37.2%
Median overall survival	13.8 months
Median time to disease progression	5.4 months
Median time to treatment failure	7.8 months
Median duration of response	9.6 months

Toxicity (N = 203)

Adverse Event	% G3	% G4
Hematologic		
Anemia	23.5	3.5
Thrombocytopenia	28.5	28.5
Neutropenia	41.2	29.9
Nonhematologic		
Mucositis	1.0	0
Nausea	22	0
Alopecia	10.5	0
Infection	2.0	0.5
Diarrhea	3.0	0
Pulmonary	2.5	0.5
Hematuria	4.5	0
Constipation	1.5	0
Hemorrhage	2.0	0
State of consciousness	0.5	0
Fever	0	0

WHO criteria

Therapy Monitoring

1. *Before each cycle for 6 cycles, then every other cycle:* CBC with differential and serum electrolytes, magnesium, BUN and creatinine
2. *On all treatment days:* CBC with differential
3. *Response evaluation:* Every 2 cycles—CT scans

Notes

1. Give 6 cycles unless disease progression can be documented

REGIMEN

CARBOPLATIN + GEMCITABINE

Carles J et al. Oncology 2000;59:24–27

Carboplatin [calculated dose] AUC = 5*, single dose intravenously in 50–150 mL 5% dextrose injection (D5W) over 15–30 minutes on day 1 every 21 days for 6 cycles (total dosage/cycle calculated to produce an AUC = 5 mg/mL/min)

Gemcitabine 1000 mg/m² per dose intravenously in 50–250 mL 0.9% NaCl injection (0.9% NS) over 30 minutes on days 1 and 8, every 21 days for 6 cycles (total dosage/cycle = 2000 mg/m²)

Emetogenic potential:
Day 1: High (Emetogenicity score = 5)
Day 8: Low (Emetogenicity score = 2). See Chapter 39

*Carboplatin dose is based on a formula described by Calvert et al. to achieve a target area under the plasma concentration versus time curve (AUC)

$$\text{Total carboplatin dose (mg)} = (\text{Target AUC}) \times (\text{GFR} + 25)$$

In practice, creatinine clearance (Clcr) is used in place of glomerular filtration rate (GFR). Clcr can be calculated from the equation of Cockcroft and Gault:

$$\text{Males, Clcr} = \frac{(140 - \text{age [y]}) \times \text{body weight [kg]}}{72 \times (\text{Serum creatinine [mg/dL]})}$$

$$\text{Females, Clcr} = \frac{(140 - \text{age [y]}) \times \text{body weight [kg]}}{72 \times (\text{Serum creatinine [mg/dL]})} \times 0.85$$

Calvert AH et al. JCO 1989;7:1748–1756
Cockcroft DW, Gault MH. Nephron 1976;16:31–41
Jodrell DI et al. JCO 1992;10:520–528
Sorensen BT et al. Cancer Chemother Pharmacol 1991;28:397–401

Patient Population Studied

A study of 16 patients with one or more of the following: (1) large tumors invading the abdominal wall without involved lymph nodes or distant metastases; (2) disease involving lymph nodes; or (3) distant metastases. Also age <80 years; Karnofsky performance status >50%; normal cardiovascular and hepatic function; and creatinine clearance = 20–55 mL/min

Efficacy (N = 16)

Complete response	13%
Partial response	44%
Median overall survival	10 months
Median duration of response	7 months

Toxicity (N = 16)

Adverse Event	% G1/2	% G3/4
Hematologic		
Anemia	12	18
Granulocytopenia	12	24
Thrombocytopenia	0	18
Nonhematologic		
Vomiting	18	6
Hepatic	0	6
Alopecia	18	0
Renal impairment	6	0

Data are from a limited phase II study with only 17 patients who were evaluable for adverse events. There was one fatality due to sepsis in a setting of granulocytopenia

Treatment Modifications

Adverse Event	Dose Modification
Day 1 ANC <1500/mm³, platelets <100,000/mm³, *or* mucositis present	Hold treatment until ANC >1500/mm³, platelets >100,000/mm³, and mucositis resolves
Day 8 ANC 1000–1500/mm³, *or* platelets 75,000–99,000/mm³	Reduce gemcitabine dosage by 25%

Therapy Monitoring

1. *Day 1:* CBC with differential and serum electrolytes, BUN, and creatinine
2. *Day 8:* CBC with differential
3. *Treatment evaluation after C3 and C6:* CT scan

Notes

1. Give platelet transfusions if platelet <20,000/mm³
2. Treat for 6 cycles unless progression documented

REGIMEN

NEOADJUVANT METHOTREXATE + VINBLASTINE + DOXORUBICIN + CISPLATIN (M-VAC) BEFORE RADICAL CYSTECTOMY

Grossman HB et al. NEJM 2003;349:859–866

Methotrexate 30 mg/m² per dose by intravenous push over 15–60 seconds on days 1, 15, and 22 every 28 days for 3 cycles (total dosage/cycle = 90 mg/m²)

Vinblastine 3 mg/m² per dose by intravenous push over 1–2 minutes on days 2, 15, and 22 every 28 days for 3 cycles (total dosage/cycle = 9 mg/m²)

Doxorubicin 30 mg/m² single dose by intravenous push over 3–5 minutes on day 2, every 28 days for 3 cycles (total dosage/cycle = 30 mg/m²)

Hydration before and after cisplatin: ≥1000 mL 0.9% NaCl injection (0.9% NS) intravenously at ≥100 mL/hour before and after cisplatin administration. Also encourage high oral fluid intake. Monitor and replace magnesium/electrolytes as needed
Cisplatin 70 mg/m² single dose by intravenous infusion in 100–250 mL 0.9% NS over 70 minutes on day 2 every 28 days for 3 cycles, (total dosage/cycle = 70 mg/m²)

Emetogenic potential:
Days 1, 15, and 22: Nonemetogenic (Emetogenicity score = 1)
Day 2: High (emetogenicity score = 6). High potential for delayed symptoms after day 2. See Chapter 39

Treatment Modifications

Adverse Event	Dose Modification
On day 1 if WBC <3000/mm³, or platelet count <100,000/mm³	Delay chemotherapy for 1 week
On day 15 or 22: WBC ≤2900/mm³ or platelet count ≤74,000/mm³	Hold dose of methotrexate and vinblastine
Severe mucositis (G 3 or G 4*	Reduce methotrexate dosage by 33% (for all doses and into next cycle)
Severe neurotoxicity	Reduce vinblastine dosage by 33%
Clinical evidence of congestive heart failure	Discontinue doxorubicin

*Leucovorin may be started 24 hours after methotrexate infusion

Patient Population Studied

A study of 153 patients with muscle-invasive bladder tumors without nodal or metastatic disease eligible for radical cystectomy; no previous pelvic radiation; adequate renal, hepatic, hematologic function; SWOG performance status ≤1

Efficacy (N = 153)

(Intention-to-Treat Analysis)

Median survival	77 months
5-year survival	57%

Toxicity (N = 150)

Adverse Event	% G3[a]	% G4[b]
Hematologic		
Granulocytopenia	23	33
Thrombocytopenia	5	0
Anemia	6	1
Nonhematologic		
Nausea or vomiting	6	0
Stomatitis	10	0
Diarrhea or constipation	4	0
Renal effects	1	0
Neuropathy	2	0
Fatigue, lethargy, and malaise	3	0
All Toxicities		
Maximal grade of any adverse effect	35	37

Toxicity measured in patients who received any methotrexate, vinblastine, doxorubicin, and cisplatin
[a]Adverse events of moderate severity
[b]Severe adverse events

Therapy Monitoring

1. *Before each cycle:* CBC, with differential serum electrolytes, magnesium, BUN, creatinine, and LFTs
2. *Weekly:* CBC with differential
3. *Response evaluation:* None needed during neoadjuvant therapy

5. Brain Cancer

Lyndon Kim, MD, and Howard Fine, MD

Epidemiology

Incidence:	18,820 in 2006
Deaths:	13,100 (second leading cause of cancer deaths in 20–39 year old males, and fifth leading cause of death in 20–39 year old females in 2002)
Male: female ratio:	10,200:8100
Average age of onset: All primary brain cancer Glioblastoma and meningioma	 53 years 62 years

American Cancer Society: Cancer Statistics 2003
Central Brain Tumor Registry of US Statistical Report 2002

Pathology

I. **Neuroepithethelial Tumors**

A. Glial tumors

1. Astrocytic tumors (45–50%)
   - Glioblastoma multiforme (GBM grade IV): 50%
   - Anaplastic astrocytoma (AA grade III): 30%
   - Diffuse astrocytoma (grade II): 20%
   - Gliosarcoma (grade IV): <5% of GBM
   - Pilocytic astrocytoma (grade I): <1%
2. Oligodendrogliomas/oligoastrocytomas (5–10%)
   - Oligodendroglioma (O grade II)
   - Anaplastic oligodendroglioma (AO grade III)
   - Oligoastrocytoma (OA grade II)
   - Anaplastic oligoastrocytoma (AOA grade III)
3. Ependymal tumors (5%)
   - Myxopapillary ependymoma (grade I)
   - Ependymoma (grade II)
   - Anaplastic ependymoma (grade III)
   - Subependymoma

B. Neuronal and mixed glial-neuronal tumors (<1%)
   - Central neurocytoma
   - Dysembryoplastic neuroepithelial tumor
   - Desmoplastic infantile astrocytoma/ganglioma
   - Ganglioma
   - Paraganglioma

C. Nonglial tumors

1. Embryonal tumors (<5%)
   - Primitive neuroectodermal tumors [PNET]
   - Medulloblastoma
   - Ependymoblastoma
2. Choroid plexus tumors (<1%)
   - Choroid plexus papilloma
3. Pineal tumors (<1%)
   - Pineoblastoma
   - Pineocytoma

II. **Meningeal Tumors (15–28%)**
   - Benign meningioma (grade I): >90%
   - Atypical meningioma (grade II): 6%
   - Anaplastic meningioma (grade III): 2%
   - Hemangiopericytoma

III. **Germ Cell Tumors (<1%)**

IV. **Nerve Sheet Tumors (4–8%)**
   - Schwannoma

V. **Primary CNS Lymphoma (PCNSL) (1–5%)**

VI. **Metastatic Tumors**

Adesina A et al. Brain Cancer. BC Decker, 2001:16–47
Greenberg H et al. Brain Tumors. Oxford University Press, 1999:1–26
WHO Classification of Tumors. JARC Press, 2000:6–7

Work-Up

1. Neuroimaging study (MRI of the brain preferred over CT)

No other staging work-up is required except:

2. Primary CNS lymphoma: MRI of spine, lumbar puncture, and ophthalmologic examination
3. PNET/medulloblastoma: MRI of spine and lumbar puncture when safe to do so

Staging

[TNM staging does not apply to most brain tumors because they rarely metastasize. Ependymal tumors such as medulloblastoma are exceptions to this rule]

WHO Designation[a]	WHO Grade[a]					St. Anne—Mayo Grade[b]
	Grade	Nuclear Atypia	Mitosis	Endothelial Proliferation	Necrosis	
Pilocytic astrocytoma	I	—	—	—	—	Astrocytoma grade 1 (no criteria present)
Diffuse astrocytoma	II	+	Usually −	—	—	Astrocytoma grade 2 (1 criterion present)
Anaplastic astrocytoma	III	+	+	±	—	Astrocytoma grade 3 (2 criteria present)
Glioblastoma	IV	+	+, Active	Usually +	Usually +	Astrocytoma grade 4 (3 or 4 criteria present)

[a]The current 2000 WHO grading system stratifies previous low-grade astrocytomas (WHO grades I and II) into different subtypes. WHO grade I pilocytic astrocytoma is characteristically well circumscribed, cystic, and localized. WHO grade II diffuse astrocytoma like WHO grades III and IV that is characteristically infiltrative and progressive

[b]In the St. Anne—Mayo grading system, the grades are based on the total number of criteria present. The criteria are similar to those in the WHO system: nuclear atypia, mitosis, endothelial proliferation and necrosis

Dumas-Duport et al. Cancer 1988;62:2152–2165
Kleihues P et al. Histological Typing Tumours of the Central Nervous System, ed 2, WHO, Berlin: Springer-Verlag, 1993
WHO Classification of Tumors. JARC Press, 2000:6–7

Prognosis

Median Survival*	
Grade I	>10 years
Grade II	5–8 years
Grade III	3–5 years
Grade IV	0.9–1 year

*Because oligodendrogliomas and oligoastrocytomas are uniquely sensitive to both chemotherapy and radiation therapy with better overall survival and prognosis, every effort should be made to look for oligodendroglial cell components and provide proper treatment options based on the pathology

Burger PC et al. Cancer 1985;56:1106–1111
Piepmeier J et al. Neurosurgery 1987;67:177–181

REGIMEN

TEMOZOLOMIDE

Bower M et al. Cancer Chemother Pharmacol 1997;40:484–488

Cycle 1:
Temozolomide 150 mg/m^2 per day orally on days 1–5 of a 4-week cycle (total dosage/cycle = 750 mg/m^2)

Cycle 2 and subsequent cycles:
Temozolomide 200 mg/m^2 per day orally on days 1–5 every 4 weeks (total dosage/cycle = 1000 mg/m^2)

Temozolomide is manufactured in the United States as capsules for oral administration in the following product strengths: 5 mg, 20 mg, 100 mg, and 250 mg. TEMODAR® (temozolomide) CAPSULES Schering Corporation, Kenilworth, NJ

Emetogenic potential: Low (Emetogenicity score = 2). See Chapter 39

Treatment Modifications

Adverse Event	Dose Modification
G ≤1 myelosuppression in cycle 1	Escalate temozolomide dosage to 200 mg/m^2 per day, days 1–5
WBC <3000/mm^3 or platelets <100,000/mm^3 on day 1 of any cycle	Delay retreatment for 1 week
After a 1-week delay if WBC <2000/mm^3 or platelets <75,000/mm^3	Reduce temozolomide dosage by 25%
After a 1-week delay if WBC <1000/mm^3 or platelets <25,000/mm^3	Reduce temozolomide dosage by 50%

Patient Population Studied

A multicenter phase II trial of 103 patients with progressive or recurrent supratentorial high-grade gliomas

Efficacy (N = 103)

Objective response	11%
Stable disease	47%
Median survival	5.8 months
Progression-free survival at 6 months	22%

The study includes 18 patients not evaluable for response

Toxicity (N = 101)

	% CTC Grade				
	None	G1	G2	G3	G4
Hematologic					
Neutropenia	82	6	8	1	4
Thrombocytopenia	53	29	6	6	7
Anemia	64	32	4	0	1
Lymphopenia	12	10	20	43	16
Nonhematologic					
Nausea	40	18	21	22	0
Vomiting	41	8	27	24	1
Constipation	59	13	17	12	0
Mucositis	76	14	8	3	0
Increased ALT	53	36	9	3	0
Increased ALP	75	26	0	0	0
Increased bilirubin	95	0	5	0	1

	None	Mild	Moderate	Severe
Lethargy*	49	5	14	33
Anorexia*	64	17	10	10

*No CTC grading available

Therapy Monitoring

1. *Weekly:* CBC with differential
2. *Every 4 weeks:* Serum electrolytes, mineral panel, and LFTs

REGIMEN

TEMOZOLAMIDE WITH RADIATION THERAPY

Stupp R et al. JCO 2002;20:1375–1382
Stupp R et al. New Eng J Med 2005;352:987–96

Temozolamide with radiation therapy:
Temozolomide 75 mg/m^2 per day orally, continuously 7 days/week for 6–7 weeks in a fasting state 1 hour before radiation therapy (RT), and in the morning in a fasting state on days without RT (total dosage/6- to 7-week cycle = 3150–3675 mg/m^2)

Radiation therapy once daily at 2 Gy/fraction for 5 days/week for a total of 60 Gy

Adjuvant temozolamide after RT:
Temozolomide 200 mg/m^2 per day orally on days 1–5 every 28 days for a total of 6 cycles (total dosage/cycle = 1000 mg/m^2)

Temozolomide is manufactured in the United States as capsules for oral administration in the following product strengths: 5 mg, 20 mg, 100 mg, and 250 mg. TEMODAR® (temozolomide) CAPSULES, Schering Corporation, Kenilworth, NJ

Emetogenic potential: = Low (Emetogenicity score = 2). See Chapter 39

Treatment Modifications

Adverse Event	Dose Modification
WBC <3000/mm^3 or platelets <100,000/mm^3 on day 1 of any cycle	Delay retreatment for 1 week
After a 1-week delay if WBC <2000/mm^3 or platelets <75,000/mm^3	Reduce temozolomide dosage by 25
After a 1-week delay if WBC <1000/mm^3 or platelets <25,000/mm^3	Reduce temozolomide dosage by 50%

Adapted from Stupp R et al. JCO 2002;20; 1375–1382, with dose modification not specified

Toxicity (N = 287)

Temozolamide with Radiation Therapy (N = 287)

Toxicity	% CTC Grade	
	G2	G3/G4
Hematologic toxicity		
Leucopenia	N/A	2
Neutropenia	N/A	4
Thrombocytopenia	N/A	3
Anemia	N/A	<1
Any	N/A	7
Non-hematologic toxicity		
Fatigue	26	7
Other Constitutional symptoms	7	2
Rash/other dermatologic	9	1
Infection	1	3
Vision	14	1
Nausea/vomiting	13	<1

Adjuvant Temozolamide After RT (N = 287)

Toxicity	% CTC Grade	
	G2	G3/G4
Hematologic toxicity		
Leukopenia	N/A	5
Neutropenia	N/A	4
Thrombocytopenia	N/A	11
Anemia	N/A	1
Any	N/A	14
Non-hematologic toxicity		
Fatigue	25	6
Other constitutional symptoms	4	2
Rash/other dermatologic	5	2
Infection	2	5
Vision	10	<1
Nausea/vomiting	18	1

Patient Population Studied

A multicenter phase III trial of 573 patients with newly diagnosed GBM. 287 received temozolamide with RT

Efficacy

(N = 287)

Median Survival	14.6 months
1-year survival	61.1%
2-year survival	26.5%

Therapy Monitoring

1. *Weekly:* CBC with differential
2. *Every 4 weeks:* Serum electrolytes, chemistry panel, and LFTs

REGIMEN

CARMUSTINE [BCNU]

Levin VA et al. Cancer Treat Rep 1976;60:719–724
Walker MD et al. J Neurosurg 1978;49:333–343

Carmustine 80 mg/m^2 per dose intravenously in 100–250 mL 5% dextrose injection (D5W) over at least 60 minutes, given on days 1–3 every 6–8 weeks (total dosage/cycle = 240 mg/m^2)

or

Carmustine 200 mg/m^2 single dose intravenously in 100–500 mL D5W over at least 60 minutes, given on day 1 every 6–8 weeks (total dosage/cycle = 200 mg/m^2)
Note: Both schedules are comparable. However, there is no good rationale for the 3-day treatment schedule

Emetogenic potential: = Moderately high (Emetogenicity score = 4) See Chapter 39

Patient Population Studied

A phase III randomized study of supportive care alone in 303 patients with newly diagnosed malignant gliomas versus BCNU and/or radiation therapy

Walker MD et al. J Neurosurg 1978;49:333–343

Efficacy (N = 222)

Therapy	Median Survival
Best conventional care only	14 weeks
Carmustine only	18.5 weeks
Radiation therapy only	36 weeks
Radiation therapy + carmustine	34.5 weeks

Note: The addition of carmustine to radiation therapy failed to alter median survival significantly. However, there was a significantly greater surviving percentage of patients at the end of 18 months among those who received combination therapy

Walker MD et al. J Neurosurg 1978;49:333–343

Toxicity (N = 51 for BCNU Group)

	% Patients
Thrombocytopenia: Platelets <100,000/mm^3	54
Platelets <50,000/mm^3	30
Leukopenia: WBC <4000/mm^3	61
WBC <2000/mm^3	18
Anemia	Occasional; no profound anemia encountered
Nausea	Occasional
Vomiting	Occasional
Elevated LFTs	Occasional

Therapy Monitoring

1. *Weekly:* CBC with differential
2. *A minimum of every 6 weeks:* LFTs, BUN, creatinine
3. *Every 2–3 cycles:* Pulmonary function test

Treatment Modifications

Adverse Event	Dose Modification
Nadir prior cycle: WBC 2000–3000/mm^3 or platelets 25,000–75,000/mm^3	Delay treatment until WBC ≥3000/mm^3 and platelets ≥100,000/mm^3, then resume treatment with carmustine dosage reduced by 10–25%
Nadir prior cycle: WBC <2000/mm^3 or platelets <25,000/mm^3	Delay treatment until WBC ≥3000/mm^3 and platelets ≥100,000/mm^3, then resume treatment with carmustine dosage reduced by 25–50%
Cumulative carmustine dosage >1400 mg/m^2 or worsening forced vital capacity (FVC) or carbon monoxide diffusing capacity (DL_{co})	Discontinue carmustine

Note: Usually no more than 5–6 cycles (1000–1200 mg/m^2) of carmustine is recommended. Patients receiving >1400 mg/m^2 cumulative carmustine dosage have a higher risk of developing pulmonary toxicity. Patients with a baseline FVC or DL_{co} <70% are particularly at risk (Physicians' Desk Reference. 1999;53:768–769)

Notes

Two meta-analyses showed a survival benefit for patients treated with nitrosoureas after radiation

Fine HA et al. Cancer 1993;71:2585–2597
Stewart LA et al. Lancet 2002;359:1011–1018

REGIMEN

CARBOPLATIN (CBDCA)

Yung WK et al. JCO 1991;9:860–864

Carboplatin 400 mg/m^2, single dose intravenously over 30 minutes to 2 hours in 250 mL 5% dextrose injection (D5W) or 0.9% NaCl injection (0.9% NS) on day 1 every 4 weeks (total dosage/cycle = 400 mg/m^2)

or

Carboplatin [calculated dose] AUC = 5–7 single dose intravenously over 30 minutes to 2 hours in 250 mL D5W or 0.9% NS on day 1 every 4 weeks (total dosage/cycle calculated to produce an AUC = 5–7 mg/mL·min)

Emetogenic potential: Moderately high (Emetogenicity score = 4). See Chapter 39

Carboplatin dose is based on a formula described by Calvert et al. to achieve a target area under the plasma concentration versus time curve (AUC)

$$\text{Total carboplatin dose (mg)} = (\text{Target AUC}) \times (\text{GFR} + 25)$$

In practice, creatinine clearance (Clcr) is used in place of glomerular filtration rate (GFR). Clcr can be calculated from the equation of Cockcroft and Gault, thus:

$$\text{Males, Clcr} = \frac{(140 - \text{age [y]}) \times \text{body weight [kg]}}{72 \times (\text{Serum creatinine [mg/dL]})}$$

$$\text{Females, Clcr} = \frac{(140 - \text{age [y]}) \times \text{body weight [kg]}}{72 \times (\text{Serum creatinine [mg/dL]})} \times 0.85$$

Calvert AH et al. JCO 1989;7:1748–1756
Cockcroft DW, Gault MH. Nephron 1976;16:31–41
Jodrell DI et al. JCO 1992;10:520–528
Sorensen BT et al. Cancer Chemother Pharmacol 1991 28:397–401

Treatment Modifications

Adverse Event	Dose Modification
Day 1 WBC <3000/mm^3 or platelets <50,000/mm^3	Delay treatment until WBC ≥3000/mm^3 and platelets ≥100,000/mm^3
ANC nadir <500/mm^3 or platelets <50,000/mm^3	Reduce carboplatin dosage by 25%
Cycle 1 ANC nadir ≥1500/mm^3 and platelet nadir ≥100,000/mm^3	Increase carboplatin dosage by 12.5%

Patient Population Studied

A study of 30 patients with recurrent malignant gliomas

Efficacy (N = 29)

Partial response (PR)	7%
Minor response (MR)	7%
Stable disease (S)	34%
Median time to progression (PR/MR/S)	26 weeks
Median survival time (PR/MR/S)	50 weeks

Toxicity (N = 29)

Non-hematologic toxicity

Toxicity	Percent Cycles with Toxicity		
	Mild	Moderate	Severe
Nausea/Vomiting	8	24	2.4
Malaise	18		—

Hematologic toxicity at 400 mg/m^2

Toxicity	Percent of Patients
Neutropenia (ANC <500)	7
Thrombocytopenia* <50,000	7

*Although the incidence of thrombocytopenia in this study was low, significant thrombocytopenia often follows carboplatin treatment

Therapy Monitoring

1. *Weekly:* CBC with differential
2. *Every 28 days:* LFTs. BUN, serum creatinine, serum calcium, magnesium, and uric acid
3. *Every other cycle:* Urine for creatinine clearance
4. *When clinically indicated:* Audiogram

Notes

Adjust the dose based on hematologic toxicity and/or urine creatinine clearance

REGIMEN

PROCARBAZINE, LOMUSTINE [CCNU], VINCRISTINE (PCV)

Levin VA et al. Cancer Treat Rep 1980;64:237–241

Special instructions:
Because procarbazine is a weak monoamine oxidase inhibitor, one should restrict tyramine-containing foods in patients receiving procarbazine

DaPrada M et al. J Neural Transm 1988;26:31–56
McCabe BJ. J Am Diet Assoc 1986 86:1059–1064
Anon, Med Lett Drug Ther 1989;31:11–12

Lomustine (CCNU) 110 mg/m^2 orally, as a single dose on day 1 every 6–8 weeks (total dosage/cycle = 110 mg/m^2)
Lomustine (CCNU) is available in the United States as capsules for oral administration containing 10 mg, 40 mg, and 100 mg lomustine. CeeNU® (lomustine) Bristol Laboratories®, Princeton, NJ

Procarbazine 60 mg/m^2 per day orally for 14 consecutive days on days 8–21 every 6–8 weeks (total dosage/cycle = 840 mg/m^2)
Procarbazine is available in the United States as capsules for oral administration containing 50 mg procarbazine HCl. Matulane® brand of procarbazine hydrochloride Sigma-Tau Pharmaceuticals, Inc., Gaithersburg, MD

Vincristine 1.4 mg/m^2 per dose (maximum single dose = 2 mg) by intravenous push on days 8 and 29 every 6–8 weeks (total dosage/cycle = 2.8 mg/m^2, but *not* >4 mg/cycle)

Emetogenic potential:
Day 1: High (Emetogenicity score = 5)
Days 8–21: Moderate (Emetogenicity score = 3)
Day 29: Nonemetogenic (Emetogenicity score = 1). See Chapter 39

Treatment Modifications

Adverse Event	Dose Modification
Nadir prior cycle: WBC 2000–3000/mm^3 or platelets 25,000–75,000/mm^3	Reduce lomustine and procarbazine dosages by 10–25%
Nadir prior cycle: WBC <2000/mm^3 or platelets <25,000/mm^3	Reduce lomustine and procarbazine dosages by 25–50%
Severe neurotoxicity, eg, painful paresthesia or peripheral weakness	Discontinue vincristine
Cumulative lomustine dosage >1100 mg/m^2 or worsening forced vital capacity (FVC) or carbon monoxide diffusing capacity (DL_{co})*	Discontinue lomustine

**Note:* Usually no more than a total of 6–7 cycles (660–770 mg/m^2) of lomustine is recommended. Patients receiving >1100 mg/m^2 cumulative lomustine dosage have a higher risk of developing pulmonary toxicity. Patients with a baseline FVC or DL_{co} <70% are particularly at risk

Physicians' Desk Reference 1999;53:771–772

Patient Population Studied

A phase II study of 46 patients with recurrent malignant brain tumor

Efficacy (N = 46)

Objective response (OR)	26%
Stable disease (SD)	35%
Median time to progression (OR + SD)	26 weeks
Progression free survival at 12 months	30%

Toxicity (N = 72)

	%G1	%G2	%G3	%G4
Hematologic				
Leukopenia	14	43	15	8
Thrombocytopenia	13	17	15	11
Nonhematologic				
Nausea/vomiting	21	15	11	0
Neuropathy	15	15	8	0
Occasionally a rash is observed				

Northern California Oncology Group Criteria

Levin VA et al. J Neurosurg 1985 63:218–223. Toxicity data obtained from a similar study

Therapy Monitoring

1. *Weekly:* CBC with differential
2. *Before each treatment:* LFTs
3. *Every 3–4 cycles:* Pulmonary function test

Notes

This regimen has been particularly effective for the treatment of anaplastic oligodendrogliomas and oligoastrocytomas

Cairncross JG et al. Ann Neurol 1988;23:360–364
Kim L et al. J Neurosurg 1996;85:602–607

REGIMEN

CARMUSTINE [BCNU] + THALIDOMIDE

Fine HA et al. JCO 2003;21:2299–2304

Carmustine (BCNU) 200 mg/m^2 intravenously in 100–500 mL 5% dextrose injection (D5W) over at least 60 minutes, given on day 1 every 6 weeks (total dosage/cycle = 200 mg/m^2)

Thalidomide 200 mg per day orally as a single daily dose, and escalate by 100 mg/week as tolerated to a maximum dose of 1200 mg/day.
Note: An optimal thalidomide dose has not been identified

or

Thalidomide increase dose as tolerated 200 mg/day every 2 weeks to a maximum daily dose of 1200 mg
Initially:
Thalidomide 800 mg/day orally as a single daily dose for 2 weeks
First escalation:
Thalidomide 1000 mg/day orally as a single daily dose for 2 weeks
Second (last) escalation:
Thalidomide 1200 mg/day orally as a single daily dose continuously

Thalidomide is available in the United States as capsules for oral administration in the following product strengths: 50 mg, 100 mg, and 200 mg. THALOMID® (thalidomide capsules) 50 mg, 100 mg, and 200 mg. Celgene Corporation, Warren, NJ

Note: A prophylactic bowel regimen is recommended because thalidomide can cause severe constipation:
Docusate sodium 100 mg 1–2 tablets orally twice a day together with a high-fiber diet

Emetogenic potential:
Day 1: Moderately high (Emetogenicity score = 4). See Chapter 39

Patient Population Studied

A phase II study of 40 patients with recurrent high-grade gliomas

Efficacy (N = 38 Assessable Patients)

Complete response (CR)	3%
Partial response (PR)	21%
Stable disease	24%
Median time to progression:	
Patients with CR and PR	239 days
Patients with stable disease	172 days
Patients with disease progression	57 days
Median survival:	
Patients with CR and PR	298 days
Patients with stable disease	230 days
Patients with disease progression	133 days

Toxicity (N = 39)

	NCI CTC Grade	
	% G3	% G4
Hematologic		
Thrombocytopenia	—	3
Neutropenia (with fever)	—	8 (3)
Nonhematologic		
Maculopapular rash	5	—
Confusion[a]	8	—
Somnolence[a]	3	—
Constipation	3	—
Nausea/vomiting	3	—
Deep venous thromboses[b]	21	—
Pulmonary embolus[b]	—	18

[a]Most patients experience sedation at start of therapy but severity diminishes after first 2 weeks of therapy
[b]Uncertain if related to therapy

Note: Although clinically silent, minor–moderately decreased pulmonary diffusion capacity (DL_{co}) was measured by pulmonary function testing in some patients after 2 or more cycles of carmustine

Treatment Modifications

Adverse Event	Dose Modification
Thalidomide Modifications	
G ≥3 hematologic and nonhematologic toxicities (ie, somonolence and constipation)	Hold thalidomide until symptoms resolve to G ≤1, then resume thalidomide at dose previously tolerated. Attempt to advance dose again after 2 weeks
Peripheral neuropathy	Discontinue thalidomide as it may be irreversible. If symptom returns to baseline, resume thalidomide at dose previously tolerated*

*Physicians' Desk Reference 1999;53:3457–3462

Adverse Event	Dose Modification
Carmustine [BCNU] Modifications	
Nadir prior cycle: WBC 2000–3000/mm^3 or platelets 25,000–75,000/mm^3	Delay treatment until WBC ≥3000/mm^3 and platelets ≥100,000/mm^3, then resume treatment with carmustine dosage by reduced 10–25%
Nadir prior cycle: WBC <2000/mm^3 or platelets <25,000/mm^3	Delay treatment until WBC ≥3000/mm^3 and platelets ≥100,000/mm^3, then resume treatment with carmustine dosage reduced by 25–50%
Cumulative carmustine dosage >1400 mg/m^2 or worsening forced vital capacity (FVC) or carbon monoxide diffusing capacity (DL_{co})	Discontinue carmustine

Note: Usually no more than 5–6 cycles (1000–1200 mg/m^2) of carmustine are recommended. Patients receiving >1400 mg/m^2 cumulative dosage have a significantly high risk of developing pulmonary toxicity. Patients with a baseline FVC or DL_{co} <70% are particularly at risk

Physicians' Desk Reference 1999;53:768–769

Therapy Monitoring

1. *Weekly:* CBC with differential
2. *Every 6 weeks:* Serum electrolytes, LFTs, and renal function tests.
3. *Every 2–3 cycles:* Pulmonary function tests

REGIMEN

HIGH-DOSE TAMOXIFEN

Couldwell WT et al. Clin Cancer Res 1996;2:619–622

Initial dose and schedule:
Tamoxifen 20 mg/dose orally, twice daily for 4 days (total dose/4 days = 160 mg)
If tolerated advance dose as follows:
Increase the tamoxifen dose every week in increments of 20 mg/dose (40 mg/day) to achieve after 1 month the target doses indicated below
Target dose for females:
Tamoxifen 80 mg/dose orally, twice daily, continuously (total dose/30 days = 4800 mg)
Target dose for males:
Tamoxifen 100 mg/dose orally, twice daily, continuously (total dose/30 days = 6000 mg)
Tamoxifen is manufactured in the United States in tablets for oral administration containing either 10 mg or 20 mg tamoxifen citrate. NOLVADEX® (tamoxifen citrate), AstraZeneca Pharmaceuticals LP, Wilmington, DE

Emetogenic potential: Low (Emetogenicity score = ≤2). See Chapter 39

Patient Population Studied

A phase II study of 32 patients with recurrent malignant gliomas

Efficacy (N = 32)

Clinical and radiographic responses	25%
Stable disease	19%
Median survival	10.1 months

Toxicity (N = 32)

	% Patients
Deep vein thrombosis	6
Nausea	3
Hot flashes	3
Fatigue	6

Treatment Modifications

Adverse Event	Dose Modification
Deep venous thrombosis	Discontinue tamoxifen
Nausea/vomiting	Hold tamoxifen. Restart previously tolerated dose when symptoms G ≤1
G3 Fatigue	Hold tamoxifen. Restart previously tolerated dose when symptoms G ≤1

Therapy Monitoring

1. *Weekly:* CBC with differential
2. *Weekly while escalating dose:* LFTs, BUN, and serum creatinine
3. *Every 2 months when not escalating dose:* LFTs, BUN, and serum creatinine

REGIMEN

HIGH-DOSE METHOTREXATE FOR PRIMARY CNS LYMPHOMA

Batchelor T et al. JCO 2003;21:1044–1049

Induction phase:
Methotrexate every 14 days until complete response (CR) or a maximum of 8 cycles are delivered
Consolidation phase:
For patients achieving a CR during induction, give 2 cycles of methotrexate every 14 days, then give:
Maintenance phase:
Eleven cycles of methotrexate every 28 days

Hydration before, during and after methotrexate:
Before methotrexate administration:
5% Dextrose injection (D5W) or 5% dextrose/0.45% NaCl injection (D5W/0.45% NS) with 50–100 mEq sodium bicarbonate injection/L intravenously at 100–150 mL/hour

- Adjust infusion rate for urine output ≥100 mL/hour for ≥4 hours before starting methotrexate
- Adjust sodium bicarbonate to produce a urine pH = 7.0 for ≥4 hours before starting methotrexate

During methotrexate administration:
No additional hydration (see below)
After methotrexate administration:
D5W or D5W/0.45% NS with 50–100 mEq sodium bicarbonate injection/L intravenously at 100–150 mL/hour until serum methotrexate concentration <0.1 μmol/L

- Adjust infusion rate for urine output ≥100 mL/hour
- Adjust sodium bicarbonate for urine pH = 7.0

Methotrexate 8000 mg/m^2 intravenously over 4 hours in 500–1000 mL D5W with 50–100 mEq sodium bicarbonate every 14–28 days (total dosage/14–28 day cycle = 8000 mg/m^2) [Add sodium bicarbonate to produce a bicarbonate concentration equivalent to fluid used for hydration]

Leucovorin calcium 25 mg per dose intravenously every 6 hours for 4 doses, starting 24 hours after methotrexate administration began.
Continue intravenous leucovorin calcium every 6 hours if patient is nauseated or vomiting otherwise:
Leucovorin calcium 25 mg per dose orally every 6 hours until serum methotrexate concentration <0.1 μmol/L
Leucovorin calcium is manufactured in the United States by various pharmaceutical companies in tablets for oral administration containing 5 mg, 10 mg, 15 mg, and 25 mg leucovorin calcium

Emetogenic potential: Moderately high (Emetogenicity score = 4). See Chapter 39

Patient Population Studied

A multicenter phase II trial of 25 patients with newly diagnosed non–AIDS-related primary CNS lymphoma (PCNSL). Previous radiation therapy was not allowed

Efficacy (N = 24)

Complete response*	50%
Partial response	21%
Stable disease	4.2%
Median progression-free survival	12.8 months
Median overall survival	>22.8 months

*Median number of cycles to CR = 6

Treatment Modifications

Methotrexate dosage is based on a measured creatinine clearance before treatment commences. For any creatinine clearance <100 mL/min, methotrexate dosage is calculated by multiplying the planned dosage (8000 mg/m^2) by the ratio between the measured creatinine clearance (Clcr) and 100.

Example:
For a measured Clcr = 75 mL/min:

$$\frac{75}{100} = 0.75 \ (\textit{ie}, 75\%)$$

Thus, the adjusted methotrexate dosage is:

$$8000 \text{ mg/m}^2 \times 0.75 = 6000 \text{ mg/m}^2$$

Toxicity

(N = 25 patients; N = 287 cycles)

Toxicity	% Patients
≥One G3/4 toxicity	48
No G3/4 toxicity	52
Leukoencephalopathy	—

Batchelor T et al. JCO 2003;21:1044–1049

(N = 31 Patients; N = 375 cycles)[a]

Toxicity	% Cycles
Leukopenia (<2000 WBC/mm^3)	1
Nonoliguric acute renal failure	1
G3 mucositis	2
Leukoencephalopathy	—
Acute cerebral dysfunction	—
Delayed methotrexate clearance[b]	13

Guha-Thakurta et al. J Neurooncol 1999;43:259–268

[a]Treatment:
1. Methotrexate 8000 mg/m^2 for ≥3 induction cycles
2. Methotrexate 3500–8000 mg/m^2/cycle until CR
3. Methotrexate 3500 mg/m^2/month for 3 months
4. Methotrexate 3500 mg/m^2/3 months indefinitely

Median: 10 cycles/patient (range: 3–30 cycles)

[b]Risk factors for delayed methotrexate clearance:
1. Cycle intervals <10 days
2. Concurrent SIADH or diabetes insipidus
3. Acute renal failure
4. "Third-space" fluid compartments (eg, effusions)

Therapy Monitoring

Before each treatment cycle:
1. CBC with differential
2. Serum electrolytes
3. LFTs
4. 24-hour urine collection for creatinine clearance

During hospitalization:
1. Check urine output and pH frequently
2. Daily CBC with differential and serum electrolytes
3. Daily methotrexate levels starting the day after methotrexate administration begins and continuing until serum methotrexate concentrations are $<0.1\ \mu mol/L$. In patients with renal impairment or pleural effusion, continue checking serum methotrexate concentrations daily until methotrexate is undetectable

Notes

1. The regimen is for the treatment of primary central nervous system lymphoma for which radiation therapy has been deferred
2. In patients with renal impairment or an effusion, consider empirically continuing leucovorin calcium administration until serum methotrexate concentrations become undetectable

6. Breast Cancer

Peter F. Lebowitz, MD, PhD, and Jo Anne Zujewski, MD

Epidemiology

Incidence:	In situ: 58,490; invasive: 214,640 (estimated 2006 in United States)
Prevalence:	1,979,813 (estimated 2003 in the United States)
Deaths:	41,430 (estimated in 2006)
Median age:	50–59 years
Female/male:	Approximately 160:1

American Cancer Society, Breast Cancer Facts & Figures 2001–2002
http://seer.cancer.gov
Jemal A et al. CA Cancer J Clin 2006;56:106–30

Stage at Presentation (1999–2000)

Stage I:	49%
Stage II:	39%
Stage III:	7%
Stage IV:	5%

Pathology

Invasive Carcinoma

Ductal:	53–75%
Lobular:	5–16%
Medullary*:	3–9%
Mucinous*:	1–2%
Tubular*:	1–3%

Ductal Carcinoma in Situ (89%)

Comedo
Cribriform
Micropapillary
Papillary
Solid

Lobular Carcinoma in Situ (11%)

*Better prognosis
Better prognosis: ER+, PR+
Worse prognosis: HER2+, higher grade

Harris JR et al. Disease of the Breast, 2nd ed. Philadelphia: Lippincott Williams & Wilkins, 2000.
American Cancer Society

Work-Up

In situ:	H&P, bilateral mammogram, and pathology review
Stages I and II:	H&P, CBC, LFTs, chest x-ray, bilateral mammogram ultrasound as necessary, pathology review with ER/PR/HER2 status, bone scan and/or abdominal CT if localized symptoms, elevated alkaline phosphatase, *or* T3, N1, M0. Optional: breast MRI (for cases equivocal for breast-conserving therapy)
Stage III:	All of the above with bone scan and abdominal CT, ultrasound, or MRI
Stage IV:	All of the above with CT of chest and abdomen, biopsy at first recurrence with pathology review

Note: HER-2 testing should be done using IHC and/or FISH. An IHC resudot of 2+ should be confirmed by FISH.
NCCN Clinical Practice Guidelines, in Oncology, V. 1. 2006

Staging

Primary Tumor (T)

TX:	Primary tumor cannot be assessed
T0:	No evidence of primary tumor
Tis:	Carcinoma in situ
T1mic:	Microinvasion ≤0.1 cm in greatest dimension
T1:	(a) Tumor >0.1 cm and ≤0.5 cm (b) Tumor >0.5 cm and ≤1 cm (c) Tumor >1 cm and ≤2 cm
T2:	Tumor >2 cm but not >5 cm in greatest dimension
T3:	Tumor >5 cm in greatest dimension
T4:	Tumor of any size with direct extension to (a) chest wall, (b) skin, (c) both, or (d) inflammatory

Distant Metastasis (M)

MX:	Distant metastasis cannot be assessed
M0:	No distant metastasis
M1:	Distant metastasis

Reproduced, with permission, of the American Joint Committee on Cancer (AJCC), Chicago, Illinois. The original source for this material is the AJCC Cancer Staging Manual, 6th edition (2002) published by Springer-Verlag, New York, www.springeronline.com.

Regional Lymph Nodes (N) Clinical Classification

NX:	Regional lymph nodes cannot be assessed (eg, previously removed)
N0:	No regional lymph node metastases
N1:	Metastasis to movable ipsilateral axillary lymph node(s)
N2:	Metastasis to ipsilateral axillary lymph node(s) fixed or matted, or in clinically apparent ipsilateral internal mammary nodes in the absence of evident axillary node metastases
N3:	Metastasis to internal mammary lymph node(s) *with* axillary lymph node metastasis; or metastasis in ipsilateral infraclavicular or supraclavicular lymph node(s) with or without axillary or internal mammary nodal involvement

Reproduced, with permission, of the American Joint Committee on Cancer (AJCC), Chicago, Illinois. The original source for this material is the AJCC Cancer Staging Manual, 6th edition (2002) published by Springer-Verlag, New York, www.springeronline.com.

Staging Groups

Stage 0:	Tis N0 M0
Stage I:	T1 N0 M0*
Stage IIA:	T0 N1 M0; T1 N1 M0*;T2 N0 M0
Stage IIB:	T2 N1 M0; T3 N0 M0
Stage IIIA:	T0 N2 M0; T1 N2 M0*; T2 N2 M0; T3 N1 M0; T3 N2 M0
Stage IIIB:	T4 Any N M0
Stage IIIC:	Any T N3 M0
Stage IV:	Any T Any N M1

*Including T1mic

Adjusted Survival

	5-year	8-year
In situ	98%	97%
Stage I	96%	92%
Stage II	82%	72%
Stage III	53%	41%
Stage IV	17%	9%

SEER data (1977–1983). From Seidman H et al. CA J Clin 1987;37:5:258–290

Caveats

Criteria for Adjuvant Chemotherapy for Node-Negative Disease

1. NIH consensus	Consider for T > 1 cm		
2. St. Gallen's	*Low-risk*: ER+ (estrogen receptor-positive) and all of the following: T ≤ 2 cm, grade 1, age ≥35		
	High-risk: ER− or ER+ and one of the following: T > 2 cm, grade > 1, age < 35		
3. NCCN	T = 0–5 mm ER+: Not recommended ER−: Not recommended	T = 6–10 mm ER+: Consider* ER−: Consider*	T = 11–20 mm ER+: Consider* ER−: Recommended

*Based on other tumor characteristics such as angiolymphatic invasion, high mitotic rate, and grade

Ductal Carcinoma in Situ

- Local treatment of ductal carcinoma in situ (DCIS) consists of lumpectomy plus radiation versus mastectomy
- Tamoxifen is used to prevent recurrence and contralateral DCIS and invasive breast cancer

Early-Stage Breast Cancer

- Local treatment is lumpectomy plus radiation versus mastectomy
- Decision regarding adjuvant therapy must be individualized, but general guidelines are outlined above
- Newer computer algorithms and genetic tests have found some use in the clinic
- In general, chemotherapy should include an anthracycline-containing regimen
- In node-positive disease, a taxane should be added
- In patients with ER and/or PR (progesterone receptor)-positive disease, adjuvant hormonal therapy should be used
  - –In premenopausal women, tamoxifen is used for 5 years with or without ovarian suppression
  - –In postmenopausal women, an aromatase inhibitor should be used for at least 5 years
- In patients with HER2+ disease, recent data indicate that trastuzumab (used concomitantly with taxane treatment followed by continued use for a total of 52 weeks) should be incorporated into adjuvant regimens

Locally Advanced Breast Cancer

- Neoadjuvant chemotherapy incorporating an anthracycline and a taxane allows for higher rates of breast conservation than adjuvant chemotherapy

Metastatic Disease

Chemotherapy: In general, single-agent chemotherapy agents can be used sequentially. If a rapid clinical response is needed, combination chemotherapy regimens can be used
Hormonal therapy: For patients with ER- and/or PR-positive disease without visceral involvement or with low-volume disease, hormonal therapy is preferred
Trastuzumab: For HER2-positive disease (IHC 3+ or FISH+), a trastuzumab-containing regimen should be used

Prevention

For screening and treatment recommendations see Chapter 54, Cancer Screening

Web tools

Breast cancer risk assessment tool
http://bcra.nci.nih.gov/brc/
Adjuvant-breast cancer prognosis and benefit from adjuvant therapy
http://www.adjuvantonline.com

Carlson RW et al. Oncology 2000;14:33–49
Goldhirsch A et al. JCO 2001;19:3817–3827
NIH Consensus Statement Online 2000. Adjuvant therapy for breast cancer

ADJUVANT, NEOADJUVANT, METASTATIC REGIMEN

DOXORUBICIN + CYCLOPHOSPHAMIDE (AC)

Fisher B et al. JCO 1997;15:1858–1869

Doxorubicin HCl 60 mg/m^2 intravenously per push over 3–5 minutes, given on day 1 every 21 days for 4 cycles (total dosage/cycle = 60 mg/m^2)
Hydration before and after cyclophosphamide:
0.9% NaCl injection (0.9% NS), 500 mL before and 500 mL after cyclophosphamide
Cyclophosphamide 600 mg/m^2 intravenously in 100–500 mL 0.9% NS or 5% dextrose injection over 15–60 minutes, given on day 1 every 21 days for 4 cycles (total dosage/cycle = 600 mg/m^2)

Emetogenic potential: Moderately high (Emetogenicity score = 4). See Chapter 39 for antiemetic regimens

Efficacy (<5-Year)

Absolute Risk Reductions with Adjuvant Chemotherapy (Primarily CMF)

	% Recurrence	% Mortality
Node+, age < 50 years	15.4	12.4
Node+, age > 50 years	5.4	2.3
Node−, age < 50 years	10.4	5.7
Node−, age > 50 years	5.7	6.4

Note: Anthracycline-containing regimens may be superior to CMF (cyclophosphamide, methotrexate, and fluorouracil) with additional absolute risk reductions of 3.2% for recurrence and 2.7% for mortality

Early Breast Cancer Trialists' Collaborative Group. Lancet 1998;352:930–942

Toxicity

	% G3	% G4
Neutropenia	4.8	1.6
Infection	2.4	0.3
Sepsis	NR	3.3
Nausea	8.5	NR
Vomiting	12.4	1.2
Stomatitis	1.3	0

Other Toxicities	%
Alopecia (pronounced)	91
CHF responsive to therapy	0.1
Acute myelogenous leukemia	0.1
Myelodysplastic syndrome	0.1

NCI CTC
Fisher B et al. JCO 1997;15:1858–1869

Treatment Modifications

Adverse Event	Dose Modification
Absolute neutrophil count* (ANC) <1500/mm^3 or platelets <100,000/mm^3 at start of cycle	Delay treatment until ANC ≥ 1500/mm^3 and platelets ≥100,000/mm^3. Give filgrastim after chemotherapy during subsequent cycles
First episode of febrile neutropenia	Give filgrastim after chemotherapy during subsequent cycles
Second episode of febrile neutropenia	During subsequent cycles, consider prophylaxis with ciprofloxacin (500 mg twice daily, orally) for 7 days starting on day 5
Third episode of febrile neutropenia	Decrease both doxorubicin and cyclophosphamide dosages by 25%

*Although an ANC of 1500/mm^3 is often identified as a minimum acceptable ANC to safely proceed with treatment, recent data show that an ANC ≥ 1000/mm^3 is acceptable if filgrastim is given after chemotherapy

Bear HD et al. JCO 2003;21:4165–4174
Citron ML et al. JCO 2003;21:1431–1439

Patient Population Studied

A study of 764 patients with node-positive primary breast cancer treated with AC for adjuvant therapy. This regimen has also been studied in the neoadjuvant and metastatic settings

Fisher B et al. JCO 1997;15:1858–1869

Therapy Monitoring

1. *Before each cycle:* CBC with differential, LFTs, serum electrolytes, BUN, and creatinine.
2. A baseline left ventricular ejection fraction is recommended especially in patients at increased risk of cardiac toxicity (preexisting heart disease, cardiac risk factors, mediastinal irradiation). Subsequent evaluations should be obtained at a cumulative dose of doxorubicin of 400 to 450 mg/m^2 and periodically thereafter. A 10% decline in LVEF to below the lower limit of normal or an absolute LVEF of 40 to 45%, or a 20% decline in LVEF at any level is indicative of deterioration in cardiac function.

ADJUVANT REGIMEN

DOSE-DENSE DOXORUBICIN + CYCLOPHOSPHAMIDE, THEN PACLITAXEL (AC → P)

DOSE-DENSE DOXORUBICIN, THEN PACLITAXEL, THEN CYCLOPHOSPHAMIDE (A → P → C)

Citron ML et al. JCO 2003;21:1431–1439

Dose-Dense Doxorubicin + Cyclophosphamide, then Paclitaxel (AC → P)
Note: In the AC → P regimen, doxorubicin and cyclophosphamide are given in combination, followed sequentially by paclitaxel. Both regimens are given for 4 complete cycles

Doxorubicin HCl 60 mg/m^2 intravenously per push over 3–5 minutes, given on day 1 every 14 days for 4 cycles (total dosage/cycle = 60 mg/m^2)
Hydration before and after cyclophosphamide:
0.9% NaCl injection (0.9% NS), 500 mL before and 500 mL after cyclophosphamide
Cyclophosphamide 500 mg/m^2 intravenously in 100–500 mL 0.9% NS or 5% dextrose injection (D5W), over 15–60 minutes, given on day 1 every 14 days for 4 cycles (total dosage/cycle = 500 mg/m^2), *After 4 cycles are completed, doxorubicin + cyclophosphamide are followed by:*

Premedication for paclitaxel:
Dexamethasone 10 mg/dose orally for 2 doses 12 hours and 6 hours before paclitaxel (total dose/cycle = 20 mg), *or*
Dexamethasone 20 mg intravenously per push 30–60 minutes before paclitaxel (total dose/cycle = 20 mg)
Note: Dexamethasone doses may be gradually decreased in 2- to 4-mg increments in the absence of hypersensitivity reactions during repeated paclitaxel treatments
Diphenhydramine 50 mg intravenously per push 30–60 minutes before paclitaxel
Cimetidine 300 mg in 20–50 mL 0.9% NS or D5W over 5–20 minutes 30–60 minutes before paclitaxel
Paclitaxel 175 mg/m^2 by intravenous infusion in a volume of 0.9% NS or D5W sufficient to produce a concentration of 0.3–1.2 mg/mL over 3 hours on day 1 every 14 days for 4 cycles (total dosage/cycle = 175 mg/m^2)
Dexamethasone is marketed in the United States in numerous generic formulations for oral administration, including immediate-release tablets containing 0.25, 0.5, 0.75, 1, 2, 4, and 6 mg, and in elixirs (which contain alcohol) and solutions for oral administration

Supportive care:
Filgrastim 5 mcg/kg per day subcutaneously for 7 consecutive days on days 3–9 every 14 days for 8 cycles. Filgrastim is given in all cycles rounded to a total daily dose of either 300 or 480 mcg/dose

Dose-Dense Doxorubicin, then Paclitaxel, then Cyclophosphamide (A → P → C)
Note: In the A → P → C regimen, the individual drugs are given sequentially as single agents (doxorubicin followed by paclitaxel and subsequently cyclophosphamide); that is, each drug is given for 4 complete cycles before advancing to the next drug in sequence

Doxorubicin HCl 60 mg/m^2 intravenously per push over 3–5 minutes, given on day 1 every 14 days for 4 cycles (total dosage/cycle = 60 mg/m^2). *After 4 cycles are completed, doxorubicin is followed by:*

Premedication for paclitaxel:
Dexamethasone 10 mg/dose orally for 2 doses at 12 hours and 6 hours before paclitaxel (total dose/cycle = 20 mg), *or*
Dexamethasone 20 mg intravenously per push 30–60 minutes before paclitaxel (total dose/cycle = 20 mg)
Note: Dexamethasone doses may be gradually decreased in the absence of hypersensitivity reactions during repeated paclitaxel treatments
Diphenhydramine 50 mg intravenously per push 30–60 minutes before paclitaxel
Cimetidine 300 mg in 20–50 mL 0.9% NS or D5W over 5–20 minutes, 30–60 minutes before paclitaxel

(*continued*)

Treatment Modifications

Adverse Event	Dose Modification
ANC <1000/mm^3 or platelets <100,000/mm^3 at start of cycle	Delay treatment until ANC ≥ 1000/mm^3 and platelets ≥100,000/mm^3. If a treatment delay is >3 weeks, consider decreasing implicated drug dosage by 25%
G3 or G4 neuropathy	Discontinue treatment

Patient Population Studied

Among women with node-positive operable breast cancer, 495 patients received AC → P and 493 received A → P → C. Chemotherapy was given adjuvantly after recovery from surgery

Efficacy

	Disease-Free Survival	Overall Survival
Dose-dense regimens (N = 988)	82%	92%
Standard 3-week interval regimens (N = 985)	75%	90%

Median follow-up of 36 months

Therapy Monitoring

1. *Before each cycle:* CBC with differential, LFTs, and serum electrolytes
2. A baseline left ventricular ejection fraction is recommended especially in patients at increased risk of cardiac toxicity (pre-existing heart disease, cardiac risk factors, mediastinal irradiation). Subsequent evaluations should be obtained at a cumulative dose of doxorubicin of 400 to 450 mg/m^2 and periodically thereafter. A 10% decline in LVEF to below the lower limit of normal or an absolute LVEF of 40 to 45%, or a 20% decline in LVEF at any level is indicative of deterioration in cardiac function.

(continued)

Paclitaxel 175 mg/m^2 by intravenous infusion in a volume of 0.9% NS or D5W sufficient to produce a concentration of 0.3–1.2 mg/mL over 3 hours, on day 1 every 14 days for 4 cycles (total dosage/cycle = 175 mg/m^2). *After 4 cycles are completed, paclitaxel is followed by:*

Hydration before and after cyclophosphamide:
0.9% NS 500 mL before and 500 mL after cyclophosphamide
Cyclophosphamide 500 mg/m^2 intravenously in 100–500 mL 0.9% NS or D5W over 15–60 minutes, given on day 1 every 14 days for 4 cycles (total dosage/cycle = 500 mg/m^2)
Dexamethasone is marketed in the United States in numerous generic formulations for oral administration, including immediate-release tablets containing 0.25, 0.5, 0.75, 1, 2, 4, and 6 mg, and in elixirs (which contain alcohol) and solutions for oral administration

Supportive care:
Filgrastim 5 mcg/kg per day subcutaneously for 7 consecutive days on days 3–9 every 14 days for 8 cycles. Filgrastim is given in all cycles rounded to a total daily dose of either 300 or 480 mcg/dose

Emetogenic potential (A → P → C):
Doxorubicin cycles: Moderate (Emetogenicity score = 3)
Cyclophosphamide cycles: Moderate (Emetogenicity score = 3)
Paclitaxel cycles: Low (Emetogenicity score = 2). See Chapter 39 for antiemetic regimens
Emetogenic potential (AC → P):
Doxorubicin + cyclophosphamide cycles: Moderately high (Emetogenicity score = 4)
Paclitaxel cycles: Low (Emetogenicity score = 2). See Chapter 39 for antiemetic regimens

Toxicity

	AC → P (N = 495)	A → P → C (N = 493)
	% G3/4	% G3/4
Hematologic		
Leukopenia	6	<1
Neutropenia	9	3
Thrombocytopenia	<1	0
Anemia	<1	<1
RBC transfusions	13% of cycles	1% of cycles
Nonhematologic		
Nausea	8	7
Vomiting	6	4
Diarrhea	1	3
Stomatitis	3	1
Cardiac function	<1	1
Phlebitis/thrombosis	1	1
Sensory	4	4
Myalgias/arthralgias	5	5
Infection	3	4

ADJUVANT, NEOADJUVANT REGIMEN

DOXORUBICIN + CYCLOPHOSPHAMIDE, THEN DOCETAXEL (AC → T)

Bear HD et al. JCO 2003;21:4165–4174

Hydration before and after cyclophosphamide: 0.9% NaCl injection 500 mL before and 500 mL after cyclophosphamide
Doxorubicin HCl 60 mg/m² intravenously per push over 3–5 minutes, given on day 1 every 21 days for 4 cycles (total dosage/cycle = 60 mg/m²)
Cyclophosphamide 600 mg/m² intravenously in 100–500 mL 0.9% NS or 5% dextrose injection (D5W) over 15–60 minutes, given on day 1 every 21 days for 4 cycles (total dosage/cycle = 600 mg/m²), *After 4 cycles are completed, doxorubicin + cyclophosphamide are followed by:*

Premedication for docetaxel:
Dexamethasone 8 mg/dose orally every 12 hours for 3 days, starting 24 hours before docetaxel administration (total dose/cycle = 48 mg)

Docetaxel 100 mg/m² by intravenous infusion in a volume of 0.9% NS or D5W sufficient to produce a final docetaxel concentration of 0.3–0.74 mg/mL over 60 minutes, given on day 1 every 3 weeks for 4 cycles (total dosage/cycle = 100 mg/m²)

Dexamethasone is marketed in the United States in numerous generic formulations for oral administration, including immediate-release tablets containing 0.25, 0.5, 0.75, 1, 2, 4, and 6 mg, and in elixirs (which contain alcohol) and solutions for oral administration

Emetogenic potential (AC → T):
Doxorubicin + cyclophosphamide cycles: Moderately high (Emetogenicity score = 4)
Docetaxel cycles: Low (Emetogenicity score = 2). See Chapter 39 for antiemetic regimens

Treatment Modifications

Doxorubicin and Cyclophosphamide	
Adverse Event	**Dose Modification**
ANC <1500/mm³[a] or platelets <100,000/mm³ at start of cycle	Delay treatment until ANC ≥1500/mm³ and platelets ≥100,000/mm³. Administer filgrastim[b] during subsequent cycles
First episode of febrile neutropenia	Give filgrastim during subsequent cycles
Second episode of febrile neutropenia	Consider ciprofloxacin[c] prophylaxis in subsequent cycles
Third episode of febrile neutropenia	Decrease both doxorubicin and cyclophosphamide dosages by 25% and administer ciprofloxacin[c]
First episode of G4 documented infection	Add filgrastim[b] and ciprofloxacin[c] prophylaxis during subsequent cycles
Second episode of G4 documented infection	Decrease both doxorubicin and cyclophosphamide dosages by 25%. Administer filgrastim[b] and ciprofloxacin[c] during subsequent cycles
Third episode of G4 documented infection	Discontinued chemotherapy
Docetaxel	
ANC <1500/mm³ on day of planned treatment[a]	Delay treatment until ANC ≥1500/mm³; administer filgrastim[b] during subsequent cycles
First episode of febrile neutropenia	Reduce docetaxel dosage to 75 mg/m² during subsequent cycles (or add filgrastim[b])
Second episode of febrile neutropenia	Continue docetaxel 75 mg/m² and give filgrastim[b] during subsequent cycles
Third episode of febrile neutropenia	Add ciprofloxacin[c]
First episode of G4 documented infection	Reduce docetaxel dosage to 75 mg/m² during subsequent cycles
Second episode of G4 documented infection	Continue docetaxel at 75 mg/m² per dose and give filgrastim[b] and ciprofloxacin[c] during subsequent cycles
Third episode of G4 documented infection	Discontinue docetaxel
G3 or G4 neuropathy	Discontinue treatment

[a]Although an ANC of 1500/mm³ is often identified as a minimum acceptable ANC to safely proceed with treatment, recent data show that an ANC ≥ 1000/mm³ is acceptable if filgrastim is given after chemotherapy
[b]Filgrastim 5 mcg/kg per day subcutaneously for 8 consecutive days, days 3–10
[c]500 mg orally twice/day for 7 days, starting on day 5

Toxicity (Docetaxel) (N = 1584)

	% G3	% G4
Neutropenia	2	<0.5
Febrile neutropenia	NA	21
Infection	0.7	6
Nausea/vomiting	0.5	0.4
Stomatitis	2.2	0.4
Diarrhea	NR	0.6
Thrombosis	NR	0.7
Allergy	NR	0.3
Neuropathy	2.3	0.1

NCI CTC

Patient Population Studied

A study of 1584 women with primary breast cancer with tumor size >1 cm *or* lymph nodes with clinical evidence of malignant disease. Regimen was given as neoadjuvant therapy in this study, but it is also often given as adjuvant therapy in node-positive disease. The regimen is one of three arms in NSABP B-30

Efficacy (N = 752/1534)

Neoadjuvant Therapy	AC → T (N = 752)	AC (N = 1534)
Overall response	91%	85%
CR (pathologic)	26%	13%

Therapy Monitoring

1. *Before each cycle:* CBC with differential, LFTs, and serum electrolytes
2. A baseline left ventricular ejection fraction is recommended especially in patients at increased risk of cardiac toxicity (pre-existing heart disease, cardiac risk factors, mediastinal irradiation). Subsequent evaluations should be obtained at a cumulative dose of doxorubicin of 400 to 450 mg/m^2 and periodically thereafter. A 10% decline in LVEF to below the lower limit of normal or an absolute LVEF of 40 to 45%, or a 20% decline in LVEF at any level is indicative of deterioration in cardiac function.
3. *During dexamethasone:* monitor glucose if indicated

ADJUVANT, METASTATIC BREAST CANCER REGIMEN

DOCETAXEL + DOXORUBICIN + CYCLOPHOSPHAMIDE (TAC)

Nabholtz J-M et al. Proc Am Soc Clin Oncol 2002;21:36a [Abstract 141; adjuvant treatment]
Nabholtz JM et al. JCO 2001;19:314–321 [Treatment for metastatic disease]

Premedication for docetaxel:
Dexamethasone 8 mg/dose orally every 12 hours for 3 days, starting 24 hours before docetaxel administration (total dose/cycle = 48 mg)
Doxorubicin HCl 50 mg/m^2 intravenously per push over 3–5 minutes, given on day 1 every 3 weeks for 6 cycles (total dosage/cycle = 50 mg/m^2), *followed by:*
Hydration before and after cyclophosphamide: 0.9% NaCl injection (0.9% NS) intravenously 500 mL before and 500 mL after cyclophosphamide
Cyclophosphamide 500 mg/m^2 intravenously in 100–500 mL 0.9% NS or 5% dextrose injection (D5W), over 15–60 minutes, given on day 1 every 3 weeks for 6 cycles (total dosage/cycle = 500 mg/m^2), *followed by:*
Docetaxel 75 mg/m^2 by intravenous infusion in a volume of 0.9% NS or D5W sufficient to produce a final docetaxel concentration of 0.3–0.74 mg/mL over 60 minutes, given on day 1 every 3 weeks for 6 cycles (total dosage/cycle = 75 mg/m^2)

Note: Owing to high rates of febrile neutropenia, some clinicians administer prophylactic growth factor support with regimen:
- **Filgrastim** 5 mcg/kg per day subcutaneously for 8 consecutive days on days 3–10, *or*
- **Pegfilgrastim** 6 mg subcutaneously at least 24 hours after chemotherapy

Dexamethasone is marketed in the United States in numerous generic formulations for oral administration, including immediate-release tablets containing 0.25, 0.5, 0.75, 1, 2, 4, and 6 mg, and in elixirs (which contain alcohol) and solutions for oral administration

Emetogenic potential: High (Emetogenicity score = 5). See Chapter 39 for antiemetic regimens

Patient Population Studied

A study of 745 patients with node-positive primary breast cancer treated with adjuvant TAC and 54 patients with metastatic breast cancer and no prior chemotherapy for metastatic disease. All patients were anthracycline-naive

Nabholtz J-M et al. Proc Am Soc Clin Oncol 2002;21:36a [Abstract 141]
Nabholtz JM et al. JCO 2001;19:314–321 [Treatment for metastatic disease]

Toxicity (N = 745)

Febrile neutropenia	24%
G3/4 infection	2.8%
G3/4 asthenia	11%
G3/4 stomatitis	7%
CHF	1.2%

Efficacy

At 33 months median follow-up, patients who received TAC (N = 745) achieved superior disease-free and overall survival compared with those who received fluorouracil + doxorubicin + cyclophosphamide (FAC) (N = 746)

	TAC	FAC
Disease-free survival	82%	74%
Overall survival	TAC demonstrated a reduction in risk of 25% compared with FAC	

Treatment Modifications

Adverse Event	Dose Modification
First episode of febrile neutropenia or documented infection after treatment	Filgrastim prophylaxis administered during subsequent cycles
Second episode of febrile neutropenia or documented infection after treatment	Reduce docetaxel dosage to 60 mg/m^2 during subsequent cycles
G3 or G4 nausea, vomiting, or diarrhea despite appropriate prophylaxis	Reduce doxorubicin dosage to 40 mg/m^2 during subsequent cycles
First episode of G3 or G4 Stomatitis	Reduce doxorubicin dosage to 40 mg/m^2 during subsequent cycles
Second episode of G3 or G4 stomatitis	Reduce docetaxel dosage to 60 mg/m^2 during subsequent cycles
G3 or G4 neuropathy	Discontinue treatment
Other severe adverse events	Hold treatment until toxicity resolves to G ≤ 1, then resume at decreased dosages appropriate for the toxicity

Note: Dosages reduced for adverse events are not re-escalated

Therapy Monitoring

1. *Before each cycle:* CBC with differential, LFTs, and serum electrolytes
2. A baseline left ventricular ejection fraction is recommended especially in patients at increased risk of cardiac toxicity (pre-existing heart disease, cardiac risk factors, mediastinal irradiation). Subsequent evaluations should be obtained at a cumulative dose of doxorubicin of 400 to 450 mg/m^2 and periodically thereafter. A 10% decline in LVEF to below the lower limit of normal or an absolute LVEF of 40 to 45%, or a 20% decline in LVEF at any level is indicative of deterioration in cardiac function.
3. *During dexamethasone:* monitor glucose if indicated

ADJUVANT REGIMEN

CYCLOPHOSPHAMIDE + METHOTREXATE + FLUOROURACIL (CMF; ORAL)

Amadori D et al. JCO 2000;18:3125–34

Cyclophosphamide 100 mg/m^2 per day orally on days 1–14 every 4 weeks for 6 cycles (total dosage/cycle = 1400 mg/m^2)

Note: Encourage patients to supplement their usual oral hydration with (extra) fluid, 1000–2000 mL/day, and to void frequently while taking cyclophosphamide

Methotrexate 40 mg/m^2 per dose intravenously per push over ≤1 minute on days 1 and 8 every 4 weeks for 6 cycles (total dosage/cycle = 80 mg/m^2)

Fluorouracil 600 mg/m^2 per dose intravenously per push over 1–3 minutes, given on days 1 and 8 every 4 weeks for 6 cycles (total dosage/cycle = 1200 mg/m^2)

Cyclophosphamide is generically marketed in the United States as tablets for oral administration containing either 25 mg and 50 mg anhydrous cyclophosphamide

Emetogenic potential:
Days 1 and 8: Moderately high (Emetogenicity score = 4)
Days 2–7 and 9–14: Low (Emetogenicity score = 2). See Chapter 39 for antiemetic regimens

Patient Population Studied

A study of 281 women with node-negative resectable breast cancer. CMF was given as adjuvant therapy within 6 weeks of surgery. All patients had rapidly proliferating tumors as determined by thymidine labeling index

Amadori D et al. JCO 2000;18:3125–3134

Efficacy

Absolute risk reduction with adjuvant chemotherapy (primarily CMF)

	% 5-Year Recurrence	% 5-Year Mortality
Node+, age <50 years	15.4	12.4
Node+, age >50 years	5.4	2.3
Node–, age <50 years	10.4	5.7
Node– age >50 years	5.7	6.4

Note: Anthracycline-containing regimens may be superior to CMF with additional absolute risk reductions of 3.2% for recurrence and 2.7% for mortality

Early Breast Cancer Trialists' Collaborative Group. Lancet 1998;352:930–942

Toxicity (N = 207)

Toxicity	% of Patients
Leukocytes = 2500–3900/mm^3	67
Leukocytes <2500/mm^3	4
Platelets = 75,000–129,000/mm^3	57
Platelets <75,000/mm^3	14
Oral mucositis	18
Conjunctivitis	25
Hair loss	55
Cystitis	28
Amenorrhea	54
Febrile neutropenia	3

Boccardo F et al. JCO 2000;18:2718–2727
Bonnadonna G et al. NEJM 1976;294:405–410

Treatment Modifications

Adverse Event	Dose Modification
WBC <3500/mm^3 or platelets <100,000/mm^3 on first day of a cycle	Delay treatment for a maximum of 2 weeks until WBC >3500/mm^3 and platelets >100,000/mm^3. Continue at full dosages if counts recover within 2 weeks

If after 2 weeks WBC <3500/mm^3 or platelets <100,000/mm^3, reduce all drugs' dosages as follows:

WBC 3000–3499/mm^3 or platelets 75,000–99,999/mm^3	Reduce dosages by 25%
WBC 2500–2999/mm^3 and platelets ≥75,000/mm^3	Reduce dosages by 50%
WBC <2500/mm^3 or platelets <75,000/mm^3	Hold treatment

Therapy Monitoring

Before each cycle: CBC with differential, LFTs, and serum electrolytes

ADJUVANT, METASTATIC REGIMEN

CYCLOPHOSPHAMIDE + DOXORUBICIN + FLUOROURACIL (CAF)

Stewart DJ et al. JCO 1997;15:1897–1905

Doxorubicin HCl 50 mg/m^2 intravenously per push over 3–5 minutes, given on day 1 every 21 days for 4 cycles (total dosage/cycle = 50 mg/m^2)
Hydration before and after cyclophosphamide: 0.9% NaCl injection (0.9% NS) intravenously 500 mL before and 500 mL after cyclophosphamide
Cyclophosphamide 500 mg/m^2 intravenously in 100–500 mL 0.9% NS or 5% dextrose injection (D5W) over 15–60 minutes, given on day 1 every 21 days for 4 cycles (total dosage/cycle = 500 mg/m^2)
Fluorouracil 500 mg/m^2 intravenously per push over 1–3 minutes, given on day 1, every 21 days for 4 cycles (total dosage/cycle = 500 mg/m^2)

Emetogenic potential: High (Emetogenicity score = 5). See Chapter 39 for antiemetic regimen

or

CYCLOPHOSPHAMIDE + EPIRUBICIN + FLUOROURACIL (6 FEC 100)

French Adjuvant Study Group. JCO 2001;19:602–611

Fluorouracil 500 mg/m^2 intravenously per push over 1–3 minutes, given on day 1 every 21 days for 6 cycles (total dosage/cycle = 500 mg/m^2)
Epirubicin HCl 100 mg/m^2 intravenously per push over 3–5 minutes, given on day 1 every 21 days for 6 cycles (total dosage/cycle = 100 mg/m^2)
Hydration before and after cyclophosphamide: 0.9% NS intravenously 500 mL before and 500 mL after cyclophosphamide
Cyclophosphamide 500 mg/m^2 intravenously in 100–500 mL 0.9% NS or D5W over 15–60 minutes, given on day 1 every 21 days for 6 cycles (total dosage/cycle = 500 mg/m^2)

Emetogenic potential: Very high (Emetogenicity score = 6). See Chapter 39 for antiemetic regimen

Efficacy

Absolute risk reduction with adjuvant chemotherapy (primarily CMF)

	5-year	
	% Recurrence	% Mortality
Node+, age <50 years	15.4	12.4
Node+, age >50 years	5.4	2.3
Node−, age <50 years	10.4	5.7
Node−, age >50 years	5.7	6.4

Note: Anthracycline-containing regimens may be superior to CMF with additional absolute risk reductions of 3.2% for recurrence and 2.7% for mortality

Early Breast Cancer Trialists' Collaborative Group. Lancet 1998;352:930–942

Toxicity (N = 128)

Hematologic

	% G3	% G4
Leukopenia	56	25
Anemia	7	2
Thrombocytopenia	6	2

Nonhematologic

Toxicity	% G3/4
Gastrointestinal	20
Stomatitis	2
Cardiac*	1
Any excluding alopecia	32

*Seven percent of patients had a ≥15% decrease in ejection fraction to ≤45%

Alopecia: 55%

Cancer and Leukemia Group B Criteria

Treatment Modifications

Doxorubicin and Cyclophosphamide

Adverse Event	Dose Modification
ANC <1500/mm^3 or platelets <100,000/mm^3 at start of cycle	Delay treatment until ANC ≥1500/mm^3 and platelets ≥100,000/mm^3. Give filgrastim[a] in subsequent cycles
First episode of febrile neutropenia	Give filgrastim[a] during subsequent cycles
Second episode of febrile neutropenia	During subsequent cycles, consider prophylaxis with ciprofloxacin[b]
Third episode of febrile neutropenia	Decrease doxorubicin by 10 mg/m^2, or epirubicin by 20 mg/m^2, fluorouracil and cyclophosphamide by 100 mg/m^2, and administer filgrastim[a] + ciprofloxacin[b]
First episode of G4 documented infection	Add filgrastim[a] and ciprofloxacin[b] prophylaxis during subsequent cycles
Second episode of G4 documented infection	Decrease doxorubicin by 10 mg/m^2, or epirubicin by 20 mg/m^2, fluorouracil and cyclophosphamide by 100 mg/m^2, and administer filgrastim[a] + ciprofloxacin[b]
Third episode of G4 documented infection	Discontinue chemotherapy

[a]Filgrastim 5 mcg/kg per day subcutaneously for 8 consecutive days on days 3–10
[b]500 mg orally twice/day for 7 days starting on day 5

Patient Population Studied

A study of 128 women with metastatic breast cancer without prior chemotherapy in the metastatic setting. Patients could have had prior adjuvant chemotherapy. This regimen has also been studied in the adjuvant setting

Therapy Monitoring

1. *Weekly:* CBC with differential
2. *Before each cycle:* CBC with differential, LFTs, and serum electrolytes
3.

ADJUVANT, METASTATIC BREAST CANCER REGIMEN

DOXORUBICIN + DOCETAXEL (AT)

Nabholtz J-M et al. JCO 2003;21968–975

Note: The AT regimen is one of three arms of NSABP B-30

Premedication:

Dexamethasone 8 mg/dose orally every 12 hours for 3 days, starting 24 hours before docetaxel administration (total dose/cycle = 48 mg)

Doxorubicin HCl 50 mg/m^2 intravenously per push over 3–5 minutes, given on day 1 every 3 weeks for 8 cycles (total dosage/cycle = 50 mg/m^2), *followed after 1 hour by:*

Docetaxel 75 mg/m^2 by intravenous infusion in a volume of 0.9% NaCl injection (0.9% NS) or 5% dextrose injection (D5W) sufficient to produce a final docetaxel concentration of 0.3–0.74 mg/mL over 60 minutes, given on day 1 every 3 weeks for 8 cycles (total dosage/cycle = 75 mg/m^2)

Dexamethasone is marketed in the United States in numerous generic formulations for oral administration, including immediate-release tablets containing 0.25, 0.5, 0.75, 1, 2, 4, and 6 mg, and in elixirs (which contain alcohol) and solutions for oral administration

Emetogenic potential: Moderately high (Emetogenicity score = 4). See Chapter 39 for antiemetic regimens

Patient Population Studied

A study of 214 patients with metastatic breast cancer without prior chemotherapy for metastatic disease. This regimen is also being studied as adjuvant chemotherapy in NSABP B-30

Efficacy

AT demonstrated superior outcomes in patients with metastatic disease compared with outcomes for AC (doxorubicin + cyclophosphamide) with respect to overall response rate and time to progression.

	AT (N = 214)	AC (N = 215)
Complete response	10%	7%
Partial response	49%	39%
Time to progression	35.9 weeks	31.9 weeks

Toxicity (N = 214)

	% All Grades	% G3/4
Hematologic		
Neutropenia	97	95
Febrile neutropenia	NR	33
Thrombocytopenia	28	5
Infection	NR	8
Septic deaths	0	0
Nonhematologic		
Alopecia	95	0
Nausea	64	6
Vomiting	46	6
Stomatitis	58	8
Diarrhea	47	8
Neurosensory	28	0
Asthenia	51	8
Edema	31	0.5
Allergy	6	1.4

NCI CTC

Treatment Modifications

(In patients with metastatic disease)

Adverse Event	Dose Modification
ANC <1500/mm^3 or platelets <100,000/mm^3 at start of cycle	Delay treatment until ANC ≥1500/mm^3 or platelets ≥100,000/mm^3 Give filgrastim with remaining cycles
First episode of febrile neutropenia	Give filgrastim* during remaining cycles
Second episode of febrile neutropenia, *or* severe toxicity other than anemia	Decrease docetaxel dosage to 60 mg/m^2 and doxorubicin to 40 mg/m^2
G3/4 neuropathy	Discontinue treatment

*Filgrastim 5 mcg/kg per day subcutaneously for 8 consecutive days on days 3–10

Therapy Monitoring

1. *Before each cycle:* CBC with differential, LFTs, and serum electrolytes
2. A baseline left ventricular ejection fraction is recommended especially in patients at increased risk of cardiac toxicity (pre-existing heart disease, cardiac risk factors, mediastinal irradiation). Subsequent evaluations should be obtained at a cumulative dose of doxorubicin of 400 to 450 mg/m^2 and periodically thereafter. A 10% decline in LVEF to below the lower limit of normal or an absolute LVEF of 40 to 45%, or a 20% decline in LVEF at any level is indicative of deterioration in cardiac function.

ADJUVANT REGIMEN

DOXORUBICIN + CYCLOPHOSPHAMIDE (AC), THEN PACLITAXEL + TRASTUZUMAB (TH), THEN TRASTUZUMAB (H) (AC × 4 EVERY 3 WEEKS → TH × 12 WEEKLY → H × 40 WEEKLY)

Romond EH et al. JCO 2005;16:1673–1684
Seidman AD et al. JCO 2001;19:2587–2595

DOXORUBICIN + CYCLOPHOSPHAMIDE

Hydration:
0.9% NaCl injection (0.9% NS) 500 mL before and 500 mL after cyclophosphamide
Doxorubicin HCl 60 mg/m^2 intravenously per push over 3–5 minutes on day 1 every 21 days for 4 cycles (total dosage/cycle = 60 mg/m^2)
Cyclophosphamide 600 mg/m^2 intravenously in 100–500 mL 0.9% NS or 5% dextrose injection (D5W) over 15–60 minutes on day 1 every 21 days for 4 cycles (total dosage/cycle = 600 mg/m^2)

Emetogenic potential: Moderately high (Emetogenicity score = 4). See Chapter 39 for antiemetic regimens, *followed by:*

PACLITAXEL + TRASTUZUMAB

Shedule for week 1 of Paclitaxel + Trastuzumab
Trastuzumab 4 mg/kg (loading dose) intravenously in 250 mL 0.9% NS over at least 90 minutes 1 day before the first dose of paclitaxel is administered (total dosage during the first treatment week = 4 mg/kg)
Premedication for paclitaxel:
Dexamethasone 10 mg intravenously per push 30–60 minutes before paclitaxel (total dose/cycle = 20 mg)
Note: Dexamethasone doses may be gradually reduced in 2- to 4-mg increments if the patient has no hypersensitivity reactions during repeated paclitaxel treatments
Diphenhydramine 50 mg intravenously per push 30–60 minutes before paclitaxel
Cimetidine 300 mg in 20–50 mL 0.9% NS or 5% dextrose injection (D5W) over 5–20 minutes, 30–60 minutes before paclitaxel

Paclitaxel 80 mg/m^2 by intravenous infusion in a volume of 0.9% NS or D5W sufficient to produce a concentration of 0.3–1.2 mg/mL over 60 minutes

Schedule for weeks 2–12 of Paclitaxel + Trastuzumab
Premedication for paclitaxel:
Dexamethasone 10 mg intravenously per push 30–60 minutes before paclitaxel (total dose/cycle = 20 mg)
Note: Dexamethasone doses may be gradually reduced in 2- to 4-mg increments if the patient has no hypersensitivity reactions during repeated paclitaxel treatments
Diphenhydramine 50 mg intravenously per push 30–60 minutes before paclitaxel
Cimetidine 300 mg in 20–50 mL 0.9% NS or D5W over 5–20 minutes, 30–60 minutes before paclitaxel

Paclitaxel 80 mg/m^2 by intravenous infusion in a volume of 0.9% NS or D5W sufficient to produce a concentration of 0.3–1.2 mg/mL over 60 minutes every week continually, *followed immediately by:*
Trastuzumab 2 mg/kg per dose intravenously in 250 mL 0.9% NS over 30 to 90 minutes every week continually (total dosage/week during the second and subsequent weeks = 2 mg/kg)

Note: Administration duration may be decreased from 90 to 30 minutes if slower durations are well tolerated

Emetogenic potential: Low (Emetogenicity score = 2). See Chapter 39 for antiemetic regimens

Treatment Modifications

Doxorubicin and Cyclophosphamide

Adverse Event	Dose Modification
ANC <1500/mm^3 [a] or platelets <100,000/mm^3 at start of cycle	Delay treatment until ANC ≥1500/mm^3 and platelets ≥100,000/mm^3. Administer filgrastim[b] during subsequent cycles
First episode of febrile neutropenia	Give filgrastim during subsequent cycles
Second episode of febrile neutropenia	Consider ciprofloxacin[c] prophylaxis in subsequent cycles
Third episode of febrile neutropenia	Decrease both doxorubicin and cyclophosphamide dosages by 25% and administer ciprofloxacin[c]
First episode of G4 documented infection	Add filgrastim[b] and ciprofloxacin[c] prophylaxis during subsequent cycles
Second episode of G4 documented infection	Decrease both doxorubicin and cyclophosphamide dosages by 25%. Administer filgrastim[b] and ciprofloxacin[c] during subsequent cycles
Third episode of G4 documented infection	Discontinued chemotherapy

Weekly Paclitaxel + Trastuzumab

Adverse Event	Dose Modification
ANC ≤800/mm^3 or platelets ≤50,000/mm^3	Hold treatment until ANC >800/mm^3 and platelets >50,000/mm^3, then resume with weekly paclitaxel dosage reduced by 10 mg/m^2
G2 Motor or sensory neuropathies	Reduce weekly paclitaxel dosage by 10 mg/m^2 without interrupting planned treatment
Other nonhematologic adverse events G2 or G3	Hold treatment until adverse events resolve to G ≤ 1, then resume with weekly paclitaxel dosage reduced by 10 mg/m^2
Patients who cannot tolerate paclitaxel at 60 mg/m^2 per week	Discontinue treatment

(*continued*)

TRASTUZUMAB

Schedule for weeks 1–40 of Trastuzumab

Trastuzumab 2 mg/kg per dose intravenously in 250 mL 0.9% NS over 30 to 90 minutes every week continually (total dosage/week = 2 mg/kg) for 40 weeks

Note: Administration duration may be decreased from 90 to 30 minutes if slower durations are well tolerated

Dexamethasone is marketed in the United States in numerous generic formulations for oral administration, including immediate-release tablets containing 0.25, 0.5, 0.75, 1, 2, 4, and 6 mg, and in elixirs (which contain alcohol) and solutions for oral administration

Efficacy

(Adjuvant AC → paclitaxel + trastuzumab, combined analysis of NSABP B-31 and NCCTG N98310

	AC → Paclitaxel (N = 1679)	AC → TH → H (N = 1672)	Hazard Ratio (First Event)
Disease-free survival (4 year)	67.1%	85.3%	0.48
Overall survival (4 year)	91.4%	86.6%	0.67

Romond EH et al JCO 2005;16:1673–1684

Therapy Monitoring

For AC

Each cycle: CBC with differential, serum electrolytes, LFTs

For weekly paclitaxel

1. *Every week:* CBC with differential
2. *Periodically:* LFTs, serum electrolytes, calcium, and magnesium

For trastuzumab

Every 3–4 months: Evaluate cardiac ejection fraction

- In NSABP B31 and NCCTG N9831, cardiac ejection fraction was assessed before entry after completion of AC, and 6, 9, and 18 months after initiation of trastuzumab
- Initiation of trastuzumab required cardiac ejection fraction to be in the normal range with no more than a 16% point decrease from baseline
- At 6 and 9 months, if the cardiac ejection fraction had declined 10–15% to below normal, or by ≥16% below baseline, even if still in the normal range, trastuzumab was held for 4 weeks and reassessed. Trastuzumab could be restarted if cardiac ejection fraction recovered. See table below

Relationship of LVEF to LLN		Absolute Decrease	
	<10%	10%–15%	≥16%
Within normal limits	Continue	Continue	Hold[a]
1%-5% below LLN	Continue	Hold[a]	Hold[a]
≥6% brlow LLN	Continue[1]	Hold[a]	Hold[a]

LLN = lower limit of normal; LVEF = left ventricular ejection fraction

[a]Repeat LVEF assessment after 4 weeks. If criteria for continuation were met, trastuzumab was resumed. If two consecutive holds or a total of three holds occurred, trastuzumab was discontinued

Treatment Modifications (*continued*)

Treatment delay >2 weeks	Decrease weekly paclitaxel dosage by 10 mg/m^2 or consider discontinuing treatment
G3/4 Neurotoxicity	Discontinue treatment

Patient Population Studied

A study of 1672 patients with HER2 3+ or FISH+, node-positive, or high-risk node-negative (>2 cm tumor of ER/PR+, or >1 cm tumor for ER/PR−) primary breast cancer

Toxicity

	Incidence of NYHA Class III or IV CHF	
	No Trastuzumab	Trastuzumab
NSABP B31	0.8%	4.1%
NCCTG N9831	0%	2.9%

Rare cases of interstitial pneumonitis were reported in both trials, which may be related to trastuzumab therapy

METASTATIC REGIMEN

WEEKLY DOCETAXEL

Burstein HJ et al. JCO 2000;18:1212–1219

Premedication:
Dexamethasone 8 mg/dose orally for 3 doses at approximately 12 hours and 1 hour before docetaxel, and 12 hours after docetaxel administration (total dose/cycle = 24 mg)
Docetaxel 40 mg/m^2 by intravenous infusion in a volume of 0.9% NaCl injection (0.9% NS) or 5% dextrose injection (D5W) sufficient to produce a final docetaxel concentration of 0.3–0.74 mg/mL over 60 minutes every week for 6 consecutive weeks every 8 weeks (total dosage/cycle = 240 mg/m^2)

Dexamethasone is marketed in the United States in numerous generic formulations for oral administration, including immediate-release tablets containing 0.25, 0.5, 0.75, 1, 2, 4, and 6 mg, and in elixirs (which contain alcohol) and solutions for oral administration

Emetogenic potential: Low (Emetogenicity score ≤2). See Chapter 39 for antiemetic regimens

Patient Population Studied

A study of 29 women with metastatic breast cancer with prior treatment of metastatic disease limited to one prior chemotherapy regimen. No limitation on prior hormonal therapy

Efficacy (N = 29)

Partial response	41%
Stable disease ≥6 months	17%

Toxicity (N = 29)

	% G1/2	% G3/4
Hematologic		
Neutropenia	28	14
Anemia	86	0
Nonhematologic		
Nausea/Vomiting	34	3
Gastritis	24	3
Diarrhea	24	3
Stomatitis	17	0
Constipation	3	3
Alopecia	66	0
Fatigue	59	14
Excessive lacrimation	52	0
Fluid retention	45	0
Pleural effusion	31	0
Dysgeusia	24	0
Sensory neuropathy	17	3
Arthralgia	14	0
Dry mouth	14	0
Phlebitis	14	0
Hypersensitivity	3	0

NCI CTC

Treatment Modifications

Adverse Event	Dose Modification
G2 Neurotoxicity	Decrease docetaxel dosage by 25%*
Febrile neutropenia	
G4 Thrombocytopenia	
Any G3 nonhematologic adverse event	
G4 Nonhematologic toxicity	Consider discontinuing treatment
ANC <1000/mm^3	Hold treatment until ANC >1000/mm^3, platelets >100,000/mm^3, bilirubin normalizes, and AST <1.5 ULN. If delay > 3 weeks, consider discontinuing therapy
Platelets <100,000/mm^3	
Bilirubin > upper limit of normal range (ULN)	
AST > 1.5 ULN	
ANC <1000/mm^3 for >2 weeks	Consider adding filgrastim during subsequent cycles
Patients who miss 1–2 weekly treatments in a cycle, but remain eligible for retreatment	Consider retreatment during week 7 of the affected cycle

*Do not re-escalate dose after a dosage decrease

Therapy Monitoring

1. *Weekly, before each docetaxel dose:* CBC with differential
2. *Every other week:* LFTs

METASTATIC REGIMEN

EVERY 3 WEEKS DOCETAXEL

Chan S et al. JCO 1999;17:2341–2354
Taxotere® (docetaxel) Injection Concentrate product label, April 2003. Aventis Pharmaceuticals, Inc. Bridgewater, NJ

Premedication:
Dexamethasone 8 mg/dose orally every 12 hours for 3 days, starting 24 hours before docetaxel administration (total dose/cycle = 48 mg)
Docetaxel 100 mg/m² by intravenous infusion in a volume of 0.9% NaCl injection (0.9% NS) or 5% dextrose injection (D5W) sufficient to produce a final docetaxel concentration of 0.3–0.74 mg/mL over 60 minutes, given on day 1 every 3 weeks (total dosage/cycle = 100 mg/m²)

Dexamethasone is marketed in the United States in numerous generic formulations for oral administration, including immediate-release tablets containing 0.25, 0.5, 0.75, 1, 2, 4, and 6 mg, and in elixirs (which contain alcohol) and solutions for oral administration

Emetogenic potential: Low (Emetogenicity score = 2). See Chapter 39 for antiemetic regimens

Patient Population Studied

A study of 159 women with metastatic breast cancer limited to one prior chemotherapy regimen for metastatic disease. No prior taxoid treatment

Efficacy (N = 148)

Overall response	52%
Complete response	7.4%

Toxicity

	% G3/4	Overall %
Hematologic		
Neutropenia	93.5	97.4
Anemia	4.4	88.6
Thrombocytopenia	1.3	4.4
Febrile neutropenia	—	5.7
Infection	2.5	—
Nonhematologic		
Nausea	3.1	39.6
Vomiting	3.1	22.6
Stomatitis	5	59.7
Diarrhea	10.7	50.3
Skin toxicity	1.9	37.7
Allergy	2.5	17.6
Alopecia	—	91.2
Asthenia	14.5	59.7
Nail disorder	2.5	44
Neurosensory	5	42.8
Neuromotor	5	18.2
Fluid retention	5	59.7

NCI CTC

Treatment Modifications

Adverse Event	Dose Modification
First episode of hematologic or nonhematologic adverse events G ≥ 3 other than alopecia and anemia	Reduce docetaxel dosage from 100 mg/m² to 75 mg/m²
Second episode of hematologic or nonhematologic adverse events G3 other than alopecia and anemia	Reduce docetaxel dosage from 75 mg/m² to 55 mg/m²

Therapy Monitoring

1. *Weekly:* CBC with differential
2. *Before each docetaxel dose:* CBC with differential, LFTs, and serum electrolytes
3. *During dexamethasone:* monitor glucose if indicated

METASTATIC REGIMEN

WEEKLY PACLITAXEL

Perez EA et al. JCO 2001;19:4216–4223
Seidman AD et al. JCO 1998;16:3353–3361

Premedication:
Dexamethasone 10 mg/dose orally for 2 doses at 12 hours and 6 hours before paclitaxel (total dose/cycle = 20 mg) or
Dexamethasone 20 mg intravenously per push 30–60 minutes before paclitaxel (total dose/cycle = 20 mg)

Note: Dexamethasone doses may be gradually decreased in 2- to 4- mg increments in the absence of hypersensitivity reactions during repeated paclitaxel treatments
Diphenhydramine 50 mg intravenously per push 30–60 minutes before paclitaxel
Cimetidine 300 mg in 20–50 mL 0.9% NaCl injection (0.9% NS) or 5% dextrose injection (D5W) over 5–20 minutes, 30–60 minutes before paclitaxel
Paclitaxel 80 mg/m^2 per dose by intravenous infusion in a volume of 0.9% NS or D5W sufficient to produce a concentration of 0.3–1.2 mg/mL over 1 hour weekly for 4 consecutive weeks every 4 weeks (total dosage/cycle = 320 mg/m^2)

Dexamethasone is marketed in the United States in numerous generic formulations for oral administration, including immediate-release tablets containing 0.25, 0.5, 0.75, 1, 2, 4, and 6 mg, and in elixirs (which contain alcohol) and solutions for oral administration

Emetogenic potential: Low (Emetogenicity score ≤2). See Chapter 39 for antiemetic regimens

Treatment Modifications

Adverse Event	Dose Modification
ANC ≤ 800/mm^3 or platelets ≤ 50,000/mm^3	Hold treatment until ANC >800/mm^3 and platelets >50,000/mm^3, then resume with weekly paclitaxel dosage reduced by 10 mg/m^2
G2 Motor or sensory neuropathies	Reduce weekly paclitaxel dosage by 10 mg/m^2 without interrupting planned treatment
Other nonhematologic adverse events G2 or G3	Hold treatment until adverse events resolve to G ≤ 1, then resume with weekly paclitaxel dosage reduced by 10 mg/m^2
Patients who cannot tolerate paclitaxel at 60 mg/m^2 per week	Discontinue treatment
Treatment delay >2 weeks	Decrease weekly paclitaxel dosage by 10 mg/m^2 or consider discontinuing treatment

Patient Population Studied

A study of 212 women with metastatic breast cancer who had previously received 1–2 chemotherapy regimens for metastatic disease. Prior taxane treatment was allowed

Perez EA et al. JCO 2001;19:4216–4223

A study of 23 women with metastatic breast cancer who had not previously received treatment with a taxane

Seidman AD et al. JCO 1998;16:3353–3361

Efficacy (N = 212)

Partial response	19.2%
Complete response	2.3%
Overall response	21.5%
Stable disease	41.8%

Perez EA et al. JCO 2001;19:4216–4223

Toxicity

Toxicity	% G1/2	% G3	% G4
Hematologic			
Neutropenia	40	10	5
Thrombocytopenia	25	0.5	0.5
Anemia	83	9	0
Febrile neutropenia	0	1	0
Infection	3	0	0
Nonhematologic			
Anaphylaxis	1	0.5	0.5
Neuropathy	59	9	0
Arthralgia/myalgia	23	2	0
Asthenia	44	4	0
Edema	16	0.5	0
Nausea	25	1	0
Vomiting	9	1	0
Diarrhea	22	0.5	0
Stomatitis	19	0.5	0
Alopecia	43	0	0
Nail changes	20	0	0
Rash	18	0.5	0

Perez EA et al. JCO 2001;19:4216–4223
NCI CTC

Therapy Monitoring

1. *Weekly:* CBC with differential
2. *Periodically during therapy:* LFTs and serum electrolytes

METASTATIC REGIMEN

EVERY 3 WEEKS PACLITAXEL

Nabholtz J-M et al. JCO 1996;14:1858–1867

Premedication for paclitaxel:
Dexamethasone 10 mg/dose orally for 2 doses at 12 hours and 6 hours before paclitaxel (total dose/cycle = 20 mg) **or**
Dexamethasone 20 mg intravenously per push 30–60 minutes before paclitaxel (total dose/cycle = 20 mg)

Note: Dexamethasone doses may be gradually decreased in 2- to 4- mg increments in the absence of hypersensitivity reactions during repeated paclitaxel treatments
Diphenhydramine 50 mg intravenously per push 30–60 minutes before paclitaxel
Cimetidine 300 mg in 20–50 mL 0.9% NaCl injection (0.9% NS) or 5% dextrose injection (D5W) over 5–20 minutes, 30–60 minutes before paclitaxel
Paclitaxel 175 mg/m² by intravenous infusion in a volume of 0.9% NS or D5W sufficient to produce a concentration of 0.3–1.2 mg/mL over 3 hours, given on day 1 every 3 weeks (total dosage/cycle = 175 mg/m²), *or*
Paclitaxel 135 mg/m² by intravenous infusion in a volume of 0.9% NS or D5W sufficient to produce a concentration of 0.3–1.2 mg/mL over 3 hours, given on day 1 every 3 weeks (total dosage/cycle = 135 mg/m²)

Dexamethasone is marketed in the United States in numerous generic formulations for oral administration, including immediate-release tablets containing 0.25, 0.5, 0.75, 1, 2, 4, and 6 mg, and in elixirs (which contain alcohol) and solutions for oral administration

Emetogenic potential: Low (Emetogenicity score = 2). See Chapter 39 for antiemetic regimens

Treatment Modifications

Adverse Event	Dose Modification
WHO G3/4 neutropenia for ≥7 days	Decrease paclitaxel dosage by 25%
Any thrombocytopenia for ≥7 days	
Febrile neutropenia, documented infection, or hemorrhage	
WHO G3 mucositis	
WHO G >2 paresthesias	Discontinue therapy
Symptomatic arrhythmia or heart block >first-degree	
Other major organ toxicities WHO G >2	
Severe hypersensitivity reaction	

Patient Population Studied

A study of 471 women with measurable metastatic breast cancer who had received one prior chemotherapy regimen (as adjuvant therapy or for metastatic disease) or two prior chemotherapy regimens (one adjuvant and one metastatic)

Efficacy (N = 471)

	175 mg/m²	135 mg/m²
Complete response	5%	2%
Partial response	24%	20%
Stable disease (>4 weeks)	43%	42%
Progressive disease	27%	36%

Toxicity (N = 471)

	175 mg/m²	135 mg/m²
Hematologic		
Leukopenia G3 or G4	34%	24%
Neutropenia G3 or G4	67%	50%
Neutropenia G3/4 for ≥7 days	11%	5%
Thrombocytopenia G3 or G4	3%	2%
Anemia G3 or G4	4%	2%
Febrile neutropenia	4%	2%
Infection any grade	23%	15%
Nonhematologic		
Severe hypersensitivity*	—	<1%
Bradycardia <50 bpm	3%	4%
Peripheral neuropathy G3 or G4	7%	3%
Arthralgia/myalgia G3	16%	9%
Edema, any grade	13%	16%
Nausea/vomiting G3 or G4	5%	5%
Mucositis G3	3%	<1%

*Includes any of the following: hypotension requiring vasopressors, angioedema, respiratory distress requiring bronchodilators, or generalized urticaria
WHO Criteria

Therapy Monitoring

Before each cycle: CBC with differential, LFTs and serum electrolytes

METASTATIC REGIMEN

CAPECITABINE

Blum JL et al. Cancer 2001;92:1759–1768
Reichardt P et al. Ann Oncol 2003;14:1227–1233

Capecitabine 1250 mg/m^2 per dose orally twice daily with approximately 200 mL of water within 30 minutes after a meal for 28 doses on days 1–14 every 3 weeks (total dosage/cycle = 35,000 mg/m^2)

Notes:

- Capecitabine is given for 2 consecutive weeks followed by 1 week without treatment
- Doses are given as combinations of 500-mg and 150-mg tablets
- If a dose is missed, do not double the next dose, continue with original schedule
- In practice, treatment often is begun with capecitabine 1000 mg/m^2 per dose twice daily for 28 doses on days 1–14 every 3 weeks owing to a high rate of dose reduction with higher doses

Ancillary medications:

Antidiarrheal regimen: **Loperamide** 4 mg orally as needed for diarrhea followed by **loperamide** 2 mg with each loose stool to maximum of 24 mg/24 hours

Capecitabine is manufactured in the United States as film-coated tablets for oral administration containing either 150 mg or 500 mg capecitabine. XELODA® (capecitabine) TABLETS

Emetogenic potential: Low (Emetogenicity score = 2). See Chapter 39 for antiemetic regimens

Patient Population Studied

A trial of 75 patients with metastatic breast cancer who developed disease progression during or after taxane-containing chemotherapy

Efficacy (N = 75)

Intention-to-treat overall response	26%
Intention-to-treat stable disease >6 weeks	31%
Median duration of response	8.3 mos

Blum JL et al. Cancer 2001;92:1759–1768

Treatment Modifications

Episode	Action	Dose Modification as % of Initial Dosage
First G2	Hold capecitabine and resume after adverse events resolve to G ≤ 1	No change
Second G2		Reduce by 25%
Third G2		Reduce by 50%
Fourth G2	Discontinue capecitabine	
First G3	Hold capecitabine and resume after adverse events resolve to G ≤ 1	Reduce by 25%
Second G3		Reduce by 50%
Third G3	Discontinue capecitabine	
First G4	Hold capecitabine and resume after adverse events resolve to G ≤ 1	Reduce by 50%
Second G4	Discontinue capecitabine	

Toxicity

Adverse Event	% All Grades	% G3/4
Hematologic		
Neutropenia	26	4
Anemia	72	4
Thrombocytopenia	24	4
Nonhematologic		
Diarrhea	57	15
Hand-foot syndrome	57	11
Nausea	53	4
Fatigue	41	8
Vomiting	37	4
Stomatitis	24	7
Anorexia	23	3
Hyperbilirubinemia	22	11
Constipation	15	1

XELODA® (capecitabine) tablets product label, April 2003. Roche Laboratories, Inc; Nutley, NJ

Therapy Monitoring

Before starting each cycle: CBC with differential, serum electrolytes, and LFTs

Notes

Advise patient to stop taking capecitabine and contact doctor if develops:

1. Diarrhea: An additional 4 bowel movements in a day above what is normal or any diarrhea at night
2. Vomiting: More than once in a 24 hour period
3. Nausea or anorexia
4. Stomatitis
5. Hand-and-Foot syndrome
6. Fever or infection

METASTATIC REGIMEN

DOCETAXEL + CAPECITABINE

O'Shaughnessy JO et al. JCO 2002;12:2812–2823

Premedication:
Dexamethasone 8 mg/dose orally twice daily for 3 days, starting 24 hours before docetaxel administration (total dose/cycle = 48 mg)
Docetaxel 75 mg/m^2 by intravenous infusion in a volume of 0.9% NaCl injection (0.9% NS) or 5% dextrose injection (D5W) sufficient to produce a final docetaxel concentration of 0.3–0.74 mg/mL over 60 minutes, given on day 1 every 3 weeks for 4 cycles (total dosage/cycle = 75 mg/m^2)
Capecitabine 1250 mg/m^2 per dose orally twice daily with approximately 200 mL water within 30 minutes after a meal for 28 doses on days 1–14, every 3 weeks (total dosage/cycle = 35,000 mg/m^2)

Notes:
- Capecitabine is given for 2 consecutive weeks followed by 1 week without treatment
- Doses are given as combinations of 500-mg and 150-mg tablets
- If a dose is missed, do not double the next dose, continue with original schedule
- In practice, treatment often is begun with capecitabine 1000 mg/m^2 per dose twice daily for 28 doses on days 1–14 every 3 weeks because of a high rate of dose reduction with higher doses

Ancillary medications:
Antidiarrheal regimen: Loperamide 4 mg orally as needed for diarrhea followed by **loperamide** 2 mg with each loose stool to maximum of 24 mg/24 hours

Capecitabine is manufactured in the United States as film-coated tablets for oral administration containing either 150 mg or 500 mg capecitabine. XELODA® (capecitabine) TABLETS
Dexamethasone is marketed in the United States in numerous generic formulations for oral administration, including immediate-release tablets containing 0.25, 0.5, 0.75, 1, 2, 4, and 6 mg, and in elixirs (which contain alcohol) and solutions for oral administration

Emetogenic potential: Low (Emetogenicity score = 2). See Chapter 39 for antiemetic regimens

Treatment Modifications

Modifications for Both Capecitabine and Docetaxel

Dosage[b]			
Capecitabine	**Docetaxel**	**Episode[a]**	**Action**
No change		First G2	Hold and resume chemotherapy > adverse events resolve to G ≤ 1
Reduce by 25%		Second G2	Hold and resume chemotherapy > adverse events resolve to G ≤ 1
Reduce by 50%	Discontinue	Third G2	Hold and resume **only** capecitabine after adverse events resolve to G ≤ 1
		Fourth G2	Discontinue therapy
Reduce by 25%		First G3	Hold and resume chemotherapy > adverse events resolve to G ≤ 1
Reduce by 50%	Discontinue	Second G3	Hold and resume **only** capecitabine after adverseevents resolve to G ≤ 1
		Third G3	Discontinue therapy
Reduce by 50%	Discontinue	First G4	Hold and resume **only** capecitabine after adverse events resolve to G ≤ 1
		Second G4	Consider discontinuing therapy

[a]Except isolated neutropenia
[b]Dosage modification as percent of initial dosage

Modifications for Docetaxel Only

Adverse Event	Dose Modification
ANC <1500/mm^3 on day 1 of cycle	Hold docetaxel until ANC recovers to ≥ 1500/mm^3
ANC <500/mm^3 for >1 week OR febrile neutropenia (≥38°C)	Hold docetaxel until ANC ≥ 1500/mm^3, then reduce dosage to 55 mg/m^2
Adverse events attributable to docetaxel that do not recover to G ≤ 1 within 2 weeks after planned re-treatment	Discontinue docetaxel
G3/4 Neurotoxicity	Discontinue docetaxel

Patient Population Studied

A trial of 255 patients with metastatic breast cancer with prior anthracycline, no prior docetaxel, and less than three prior chemotherapy regimens

Efficacy (N = 255)

Overall response	42%
Complete response	5%
Stable disease >6 wks	38%

Superior Efficacy Compared with 100 mg/m^2 Docetaxel

	Docetaxel + Capecitabine	Docetaxel 100 mg/m^2
Objective response	30%	42%
Time to progression	4.2 months	6.1 months
Overall survival	11.5 months	14.5 months

Toxicity

Toxicity	% G3	% G4
Neutropenia	17	69
Anemia	70	10
Thrombocytopenia	38	3
Febrile neutropenia	NA	16
Diarrhea	53	14
Stomatitis	50	17
Hand-foot syndrome	39	24
Nausea	35	7
Alopecia	35	6
Edema	31	2
Vomiting	31	4
Asthenia	22	4
Fatigue	18	4
Constipation	18	2
Arthralgia/myalgia	13	2
Anorexia	12	1
Lacrimation	12	0
Hyperbilirubinemia	11	9
Peripheral neuropathy	6	0

XELODA® (capecitabine) tablets product label, April 2003. Roche Laboratories, Inc
Taxotere® (docetaxel) Injection Concentrate product label, April 2003. Aventis Pharmaceuticals, Inc
NCI of Canada CTC

Therapy Monitoring

Start of each cycle: CBC with differential, LFTs, and serum electrolytes

Notes

Advise patient to stop taking capecitabine and contact doctor if develops:

1. Diarrhea: An additional 4 bowel movements in a day above what is normal or any diarrhea at night
2. Vomiting: More than once in a 24 hour period
3. Nausea or anorexia
4. Stomatitis
5. Hand-and-Foot syndrome
6. Fever or infection

METASTATIC REGIMEN

WEEKLY VINORELBINE

Fumoleau P et al. JCO 1993;11:1245–1252
Nisticò C et al. Breast Cancer Res Treat 2000;59:223–229
Romero A et al. JCO 1994;12:336–341

Vinorelbine 20–30 mg/m² per dose by intravenous infusion in 100 mL 0.9% NaCl injection (0.9% NS) over 20 minutes every week, continually (total dosage/week = 20–30 mg/m²)

Emetogenic potential: Nonemetogenic (Emetogenicity score = 1). See Chapter 39 for antiemetic regimens

Patient Population Studied

A study of 40 women with metastatic breast cancer with prior treatment with at least one anthracycline-containing regimen

Efficacy (N = 36)

Overall response	53%
Complete response	13%
Partial response	40%
Median duration of response	10 months

Toxicity

	% G1/2	% G3/4
Hematologic		
Neutropenia	58	25
Anemia	63	10
Thrombocytopenia	8	0
Nonhematologic		
Nausea/vomiting	30	0
Mucositis	10	0
Neuropathy	23	0
Phlebitis	45	15
Constipation	40	0
Mild asthenia	13	
Moderate asthenia	48	
Severe asthenia	18	

Nisticò C et al. Breast Cancer Res Treat 2000;59: 223–229
WHO criteria

Therapy Monitoring

1. *Before each dose:* CBC with differential count
2. *Every other week:* LFTs

Treatment Modifications

Adverse Event	Dose Modification
ANC >1250/mm³ and platelets >100,000/mm³ on treatment day	Give starting dose
ANC 750–1250/mm³ or platelets 50,000–99,000/mm³ on treatment day	Reduce vinorelbine dosage to 75% of starting dose
ANC <750/mm³ or platelets <50,000/mm³	Hold vinorelbine dose until ANC >750/mm³ and platelets >50,000/mm³, then resume at dose as determined by ANC and platelets
Treatment delays for neutropenia ≥2 weeks	Add filgrastim
For treatment delays >3 weeks	Consider discontinuing treatment
Total bilirubin 2–3 mg/dL (34.2–51.3 μmol/L)	Give vinorelbine at 12.5 mg/m²
Total bilirubin >3 mg/dL (51.3 μmol/L)	Hold vinorelbine
G2 Neurologic adverse events	Hold vinorelbine until adverse events resolve to G ≤ 1, then resume treatment with 25% dose reduction
G3 Nonhematologic adverse events	Hold vinorelbine dose until adverse events resolve to G ≤ 1, then resume treatment with 25% dose reduction
G4 Nonhematologic adverse events	Consider discontinuing treatment

Burstein HJ et al. JCO 2001;19:2722–2730
Nisticò C et al. Breast Cancer Res Treat 2000;59:223–229

METASTATIC REGIMEN

DOXORUBICIN HCL LIPOSOME INJECTION (LIPOSOMAL DOXORUBICIN)

Perez AT et al. Cancer Invest 2002;20(suppl 2):22–29
Ranson MR et al. Crit Rev Oncol Hematol 2001;37:115–120
Ranson MR et al. JCO 1997;15:3185–3191

Doxorubicin HCl liposome injection 40–50 mg/m^2 by intravenous infusion in 250 mL (doses ≤90 mg) or 500 mL (doses >90 mg) 5% dextrose injection (D5W) over 60 minutes, given on day 1 every 3 weeks (total dosage/cycle = 40–50 mg/m^2)

Emetogenic potential: Low (Emetogenicity score = 2). See Chapter 39 for antiemetic regimens

Patient Population Studied

A study of 40 women with metastatic breast cancer. Half of the patients had been treated previously with doxorubicin; more than half had received ≥ two prior chemotherapy regimens

Perez AT et al. Cancer Invest 2002;20(suppl 2):22–29

Efficacy (N = 37)

Partial response	25%
Stable disease >6 months	18%

Toxicity (N = 40)

	% G1/2	% G3/4
Neutropenia	22	25
Thrombocytopenia	6	3
Anemia	71	0
Mucositis	38	31
Palmar-plantar erythrodysesthesia	13	3

NCI CTC
DOXIL® (doxorubicin HCl liposome injection) product label, February 2003. Ortho Biotech Products LP, Raritan, NJ

Therapy Monitoring

1. *Before each dose:* CBC with differential.
2. *Periodically during therapy:* LFTs, serum electrolytes, cardiac function by ECHO

Treatment Modifications

Adverse Event	Dose Modification
Palmar-Plantar Erythrodysesthesia (PPE)	
G2	Delay treatment until PPE resolves to G ≤ 1
G3/4	Delay treatment until PPE resolves to G ≤ 1, then resume treatment with liposomal doxorubicin dosage reduced by 25%
Delay >2 weeks due to PPE	Discontinue treatment
Hematologic Adverse Events	
ANC 500–1500/mm^3 or platelets 25,000–75,000/mm^3	Delay treatment until ANC >1500/mm^3 and platelets >75,000/mm^3, then resume treatment at the same dosage and schedule
ANC <500/mm^3 or platelets <25,000/mm^3	Delay treatment until ANC >1500/mm^3 and platelets >75,000/mm^3, then resume treatment with dosage reduced by 25% from the last dose administered, *or* add hematopoietic growth factor
Stomatitis	
G2	Delay treatment until stomatitis resolves to G ≤ 1
G3/4	Delay treatment until stomatitis resolves to G ≤ 1, then resume treatment with liposomal doxorubicin dosage decreased by 25%
For delays >2 weeks due to stomatitis	Discontinue treatment
Other G3 adverse events (except nausea, vomiting, or alopecia)	Delay treatment until stomatitis resolves to G1, then resume treatment with liposomal doxorubicin dosage decreased by 25%

DOXIL® (doxorubicin HCl liposome injection) product label, February 2003. Ortho Biotech Products LP

METASTATIC REGIMEN

WEEKLY DOXORUBICIN OR EPIRUBICIN

Gasparini G et al. Am J Clin Onvol 1991;14:38–44
Torti FM et al. Ann Intern Med 1983;99:745–749

Doxorubicin HCl 20 mg/m^2 per dose intravenously per push over 3–5 minutes every week continually (total dosage/week = 20 mg/m^2)

Note: Evaluate left ventricular end-diastolic function (LVEF) after patients receive a cumulative doxorubicin dosage approximately equal to, but not more than 550 mg/m^2. Additional treatment is given on a case-by-case basis

or

Gasparini G et al. Am J Clin Oncol 1991;14:38–44

Epirubicin HCl 20 mg/m^2 per dose intravenously per push over 3–5 minutes every week continually (total dosage/week = 20 mg/m^2)

Note: Evaluate left ventricular end-diastolic function after patients receive a cumulative epirubicin dosage approximately equal to, but not more than 650 mg/m^2. Additional treatment is given on a case-by-case basis

Emetogenic potential: Moderate (Emetogenicity score = 3). See Chapter 39 for antiemetic regimens

Treatment Modifications

Adverse Event	Dose Modification
WBC <3000/mm^3, platelets <100,000/mm^3	Hold treatment for at least 1 week
LVEF (cardiac ejection fraction) <40%, or symptomatic congestive heart failure	Discontinue therapy

Gasparini G et al. Am J Clin Oncol 1991;14:38–44

Patient Population Studied

A study of 21 women with metastatic breast cancer with prior treatment with CMF

Efficacy (N = 21)

Overall response	38%
Complete response	5%
Partial response	33%
Median duration of response	7 months

Toxicity

	% G1/2	% G3/4
Hematologic		
Leukopenia	57	33
Anemia	10	0
Thrombocytopenia	2	0
Nonhematologic		
Nausea/vomiting	48	5
Stomatitis	43	0
Alopecia	38	5
Phlebitis	45	15
Acute arrhythmias	14	0
Cardiac function	0	5

The incidence of cardiac toxicity was reduced with weekly doxorubicin in comparison with an every-3-week schedule

Gasparini G et al. Am J Clin Oncol 1991;14:38–44
Torti FM et al. Ann Intern Med 1983;99:745–749

Therapy Monitoring

1. *Before each doxorubicin dose:* CBC with differential
2. *Periodically:* Liver function tests
3. *LVEF:* After patients receive a total cumulative lifetime doxorubicin dosage ≥450 mg/m^2 or a total cumulative lifetime epirubicin dosage ≥650 mg/m^2 and after each additional 100 mg/m^2

METASTATIC REGIMEN

GEMCITABINE

Blackstein M et al. Oncology 2002;62:2–8
Carmichael J et al. JCO 1995;13:2731–2736

Gemcitabine 800–1200 mg/m^2 per dose by intravenous infusion in 50–250 mL 0.9% NaCl injection (0.9% NS) over 30 minutes, given on days 1, 8, and 15 every 28 days for up to 8 cycles (total dosage/cycle = 2400–3600 mg/m^2)

Emetogenic potential: Low (Emetogenicity score = 2). See Chapter 39 for antiemetic regimens

Patient Population Studied

A trial of 39 patients with metastatic breast cancer who had not previously received chemotherapy for metastatic disease

Efficacy (N = 35)

Overall response rate	37.1%
Complete response rate	5.7%
Partial response rate	31.4%

Blackstein M et al. Oncology 2002;62:2–8

Toxicity (N = 39)

	% G1/2	% G3/4
Hematologic		
Anemia	61	9
Neutropenia	36	30
Thrombocytopenia	25	6
Nonhematologic		
Alkaline phosphatase	35	0
Alanine aminotransferase	59	6
Allergic	13	0
Cutaneous	31	3
Diarrhea	23	0
Fever	15	0
Infection	10	3
Nausea/vomiting	41	10
Pulmonary	13	5
Alopecia	46	0

Blackstein M et al. Oncology 2002;62:2–8
WHO criteria

Treatment Modifications

Adverse Event	Dose Modification
ANC = 1000–1499/mm^3, WBC = 1000–1999/mm^3, or platelets 50,000–99,999/mm^3 on day of treatment	Reduce dosage by 25%
ANC and WBC <1000/mm^3, or platelets <50,000/mm^3 on day of treatment	Hold treatment until ANC and WBC >1000/mm^3, and platelets >50,000/mm^3. Resume treatment with gemcitabine dosage reduced by 50%
ANC and WBC <500/mm^3, or platelets <25,000/mm^3 on day of treatment	Consider discontinuing therapy
WHO G3 nonhematologic adverse events (excluding nausea/vomiting and alopecia)	Decrease dosage by 50% or withhold treatment until recover to G ≤ 1
WHO G4 nonhematologic adverse events	Hold treatment until resolution to G ≤ 1 then resume with 50% dose reduction

Therapy Monitoring

Before starting each treatment: CBC with differential, LFTs, and serum electrolytes

METASTATIC REGIMEN

CARBOPLATIN + DOCETAXEL

Mavroudis D et al. Oncology 2003;64:207–212

Premedication:
Dexamethasone 8 mg/dose orally twice daily for 3 days, starting the day before docetaxel administration (total dose/cycle = 48 mg)
Docetaxel 75 mg/m^2 by intravenous infusion in a volume of 0.9% NaCl injection (0.9% NS) or 5% dextrose injection (D5W) sufficient to produce a final docetaxel concentration of 0.3–0.74 mg/mL over 60 minutes, given on day 1 every 21 days (total dosage/cycle = 75 mg/m^2)
Carboplatin [calculated dose] AUC = 6* intravenously in at least 250 mL 0.9% NS or D5W over 30 minutes, immediately after docetaxel on day 1 every 21 days (total dosage/cycle calculated to produce an AUC = 6 mg/mL·min)

Dexamethasone is marketed in the United States in numerous generic formulations for oral administration, including immediate-release tablets containing 0.25, 0.5, 0.75, 1, 2, 4, and 6 mg, and in elixirs (which contain alcohol) and solutions for oral administration

Emetogenic potential: High (Emetogenicity score = 5). See Chapter 39 for antiemetic regimens

Carboplatin dose is based on a formula described by Calvert et al. to achieve a target area under the plasma concentration versus time curve (AUC)

$$\text{Total carboplatin dose (mg)} = (\text{Target AUC}) \times (\text{GFR} + 25)$$

In application, creatinine clearance (Clcr) is used in place of glomerular filtration rate (GFR). Clcr can be calculated from the equation of Cockcroft and Gault, thus:

$$\text{Males, Clcr} = \frac{(140 - \text{age [y]}) \times (\text{body weight [kg]})}{72 \times (\text{Serum creatinine [mg/dL]})}$$

$$\text{Females, Clcr} = \frac{(140 - \text{age [y]}) \times (\text{body weight [kg]})}{72 \times (\text{Serum creatinine [mg/dL]})} \times 0.85$$

Calvert AH et al. JCO 1989;7:1748–1756
Cockcroft DW, Gault MH. Nephron 1976;16:31–41
Jodrell DI et al. JCO 1992;10:520–528
Sorensen BT et al. Cancer Chemother Pharmacol 1991;28:397–401

Patient Population Studied

A study of 36 patients with metastatic breast cancer with prior anthracycline or taxane therapy in the metastatic setting

Efficacy (N = 36)

(Intention-to-treat analysis)

Complete response	8%
Partial response	53%
Overall response rate	61%
Median duration of response	8 months

Treatment Modifications

Adverse Event	Dose Modification
ANC <1500/mm^3, platelets <100,000/mm^3 at start of cycle	Delay treatment until ANC ≥1500/mm^3 (consider adding filgrastim with next cycle) and platelet count ≥100,000/mm^3
First episode of febrile neutropenia or G3/4 neutropenia	Give filgrastim prophylaxis with remaining cycles
Second episode of febrile neutropenia or G3/4 neutropenia	Decrease both drug dosages by 25%
G3/4 thrombocytopenia	Decrease carboplatin dosage by 25%
G3/4 neuropathy	Discontinue therapy

TOXICITY (N = 36)

	% G1/2	% G3/4
Hematologic		
Neutropenia	19	44
Anemia	83	8
Thrombocytopenia	47	11
Febrile neutropenia	0	19
Nonhematologic		
Nausea/vomiting	22	6
Mucositis	14	3
Diarrhea	19	0
Asthenia	50	0
Neurotoxicity	11	3
Allergic reaction	8	0
Fluid retention	6	0

NCI CTC

Therapy Monitoring

Before each cycle: CBC with differential, LFTs, and serum electrolytes

METASTATIC REGIMEN

TRASTUZUMAB

Esteva FJ et al. JCO 2002;20:1800–1808
Leyland-Jones B et al. JCO 2003;21:3965–3971
Vogel CL et al. JCO 2002;20:719–726

Trastuzumab 4 mg/kg initial (loading) dose intravenously in 250 mL 0.9% NaCl injection (0.9% NS), over at least 90 minutes (total initial dosage = 4 mg/kg), *followed at weekly intervals by:*
Trastuzumab 2 mg/kg per dose intravenously in 250 mL 0.9% NS over 30–90 minutes every week, continually (total dosage/week = 2 mg/kg)
Note: Administration duration may be decreased from 90 to 30 minutes if slower durations are well tolerated

or

Trastuzumab 8 mg/kg initial (loading) dose intravenously in 250 mL 0.9% NS over at least 90 minutes (total initial dosage = 8 mg/kg), *followed 3 weeks later by:*
Trastuzumab 6 mg/kg per dose intravenously in 250 mL 0.9% NS over 30–90 minutes every 3 weeks, continually (total dosage/3-week cycle = 6 mg/kg)
Note: Administration duration may be decreased from 90 to 30 minutes if slower durations are well tolerated

Emetogenic potential: Nonemetogenic (Emetogenicity score = 1). See Chapter 39

Therapy Monitoring

Every 3–4 months: Evaluate cardiac ejection fraction
Adapting guidelines from NSABP B31 and NCCTG N9831, initiation of trastuzumab requires cardiac ejection fraction to be in the normal range. At any evaluation if the cardiac ejection fraction has declined 10% to 15% to below normal or ≥16% below baseline, even if still in the normal range, hold trastuzumab for 4 weeks and reasses

Relationship of LVEF to LLN	Absolute Decrease		
	<10%	10%–15%	≥16%
Within normal limits	Continue	Continue	Hold[a]
1%–5% below LLN	Continue	Hold[a]	Hold[a]
≥6% below LLN	Continue[1]	Hold[a]	Hold[a]

LLN = lower limit of normal; LVEF = left ventricular ejection fraction
[a]Repeat LVEF assessment after 4 weeks. If criteria for continuation were met, trastuzumab was resumed. If two consecutive holds or a total of three holds occurred, trastuzumab was discontinued

Efficacy (N = 84[1])

Overall response[b]	35%[a]
Complete response[b]	8%[a]
Clinical benefit[c]	48%[a]

[a]Patients with 3+ HER2 overexpression by IHC
[b]>50% of objective responses lasted >12 months
[c]CR, PR, MR, or stable disease for >6 months

Vogel CL et al. JCO 2002;20:719–726

Treatment Modifications

Adverse Event	Dose Modification
Left ventricle ejection fraction <45%, or symptomatic congestive heart failure	Discontinue trastuzumab

Patient Population Studied

A study of 84 women with HER2-overexpressing (IHC 3+) metastatic breast cancer with no prior cytotoxic chemotherapy for metastatic disease. Twenty-seven women with HER2 (IHC 2+) metastatic breast cancer were also enrolled

Vogel CL et al. JCO 2002;20:719–726

Toxicity

	Severity	
Cardiac Toxicity		
	Any	NYHA Classes III/IV
Cardiac dysfunction	3–7%	2–4%
Noncardiac Toxicity		
	Any	Severe
Pain	59%	8%
Asthenia	53%	7%
Nausea	37%	3%
Fever	36%	2%
Chest pain	25%	3%
Chills	22%	0
Rash	20%	0
Dyspnea	15%	0

Seidman A et al. JCO 2002;20:1215–1221
Vogel CL et al. JCO 2002;20:719–726

METASTATIC REGIMEN

WEEKLY DOCETAXEL + TRASTUZUMAB

Esteva FJ et al. JCO 2002;20:1800–1808

Initial treatment (first cycle)
Trastuzumab 4 mg/kg (loading dose) intravenously in 250 mL 0.9% NaCl injection (0.9% NS), over at least 90 minutes 1 day before the first dose of docetaxel is administered (total initial dosage = 4 mg/kg)
Premedication for docetaxel:
Dexamethasone 8 mg/dose orally for 3 doses at approximately 12 hours and 1 hour before docetaxel, and 12 hours after docetaxel administration (total dose/cycle = 24 mg)
Docetaxel 35 mg/m^2 per dose by intravenous infusion in a volume of 0.9% NS or 5% dextrose injection (D5W), sufficient to produce a final docetaxel concentration of 0.3–0.74 mg/mL over 30 minutes every week for 3 consecutive weeks (days 1, 8, and 15) every 4 weeks (total dosage/cycle = 105 mg/m^2)

Second and subsequent treatments
Premedication for docetaxel:
Dexamethasone 8 mg /dose orally
Dexamethasone schedule
- Initially, every 12 hours for 3 doses, starting the evening before docetaxel administration
- If no significant fluid retention or hypersensitivity reactions occur during the first 2 cycles, give dexamethasone 8 mg/dose for 2 doses on the day of docetaxel administration
- If there is no evidence of fluid retention after a fourth cycle, give single-dose dexamethasone 8 mg just before docetaxel administration

Docetaxel 35 mg/m^2 per dose by intravenous infusion in a volume of 0.9% NS or D5W sufficient to produce a final docetaxel concentration of 0.3–0.74 mg/mL over 30 minutes every week for 3 consecutive weeks (days 1, 8, and 15) every 4 weeks (total dosage/cycle = 105 mg/m^2), *followed immediately by:*
Trastuzumab 2 mg/kg per dose intravenously in 250 mL 0.9% NS over 30–90 minutes every week, continually (total dosage/week = 2 mg/kg)
Note: Administration duration may be decreased from 90 to 30 minutes if slower durations are well tolerated

Dexamethasone is marketed in the United States in numerous generic formulations for oral administration, including immediate-release tablets containing 0.25, 0.5, 0.75, 1, 2, 4, and 6 mg, and in elixirs (which contain alcohol) and solutions for oral administration

Emetogenic potential: Low (Emetogenicity score = 2). See Chapter 39

Patient Population Studied

A study of 30 women with HER2-overexpressing (FISH+ or IHC 3+) metastatic breast cancer who had not received > three prior chemotherapy regimens. No limitation on prior hormonal therapy

Efficacy (N = 30)

Overall response	63%
Complete response	None
Partial response	63%
Minor response	7%
Stable disease >4 months	20%

Therapy Monitoring

1. *Before each docetaxel dose:* CBC with differential and LFTs
2. *Periodically:* Serum electrolytes, calcium, magnesium
3. *Every 3–4 months:* Cardiac ejection fraction

Treatment Modifications

Adverse Event	Dose Modification*
ANC < 500/mm^3	Reduce docetaxel dosage by 5 mg/m^2
Febrile neutropenia	
Platelets <50,000/mm^3	
G2 Nonhematologic adverse events	
G3 Nonhematologic adverse events (except fatigue)	Reduce docetaxel dosage by 10 mg/m^2
G3 Fatigue	Reduce docetaxel dosage by 5 mg/m^2
Left ventricle ejection fraction <45% or congestive heart failure	Discontinue trastuzumab
G3/4 neurotoxicity	Discontinue docetaxel

*Minimum dosage to continue treatment = 20 mg/m^2

Toxicity (N = 30)

	% G1/2	% G3	% G4
Hematologic			
Neutropenia	49	16	10
Anemia	56	0	0
Thrombocytopenia	3	0	0
Febrile neutropenia	0	3	0
Nonhematologic			
Left ventricle dysfunction	26	3	0
Diarrhea	60	6	0
Alopecia	80	NR*	NR*
Fatigue	62	20	0
Excessive lacrimation	93	0	0
Edema	46	0	0
Pleural effusion	26	3	0
Myalgia	60	NR*	NR*
Neuropathy	36	3	0
Onycholysis	50	0	0
Hypersensitivity	0	6	0

*NR, not reported
NCI of Canada CTC

METASTATIC REGIMEN

TRASTUZUMAB + PACLITAXEL (EVERY 3 WEEKS)

Leyland-Jones B et al. JCO 2003;21:3965–3971
Slamon DJ et al. NEJM 2001;344:783–792

Premedication for paclitaxel:
Dexamethasone 20 mg/dose orally for 2 doses at 12 hours and 6 hours before paclitaxel (total dose/cycle = 40 mg)
Diphenhydramine 50 mg intravenously per push 30–60 minutes before paclitaxel
Cimetidine 300 mg in 20–50 mL 0.9% NaCl injection (0.9% NS) or 5% dextrose injection (D5W) over 5–20 minutes, 30–60 minutes before paclitaxel

Paclitaxel 175 mg/m^2 by intravenous infusion in a volume of 0.9% NS or D5W sufficient to produce a concentration of 0.3–1.2 mg/mL over 3 hours every 3 weeks for 6 cycles (total dosage/cycle = 175 mg/m^2)
Trastuzumab 4 mg/kg (loading dose) intravenously in 250 mL 0.9% NS over at least 90 minutes (total initial dosage = 4 mg/kg), *followed by:*
Trastuzumab 2 mg/kg per dose intravenously in 250 mL 0.9% NS over 30–90 minutes every week, starting 1 week after the initial dose (total dosage/cycle during the first 3-week cycle = 8 mg/kg; total dosage/cycle during subsequent cycles = 6 mg/kg)

Dexamethasone is marketed in the United States in numerous generic formulations for oral administration, including immediate-release tablets containing 0.25, 0.5, 0.75, 1, 2, 4, and 6 mg, and in elixirs (which contain alcohol) and solutions for oral administration

Emetogenic potential: Low (Emetogenicity score = 2). See Chapter 39 for antiemetic regimens

Treatment Modifications

Adverse Event	Dose Modification
G3/4 ANC for ≥7 days	Reduce paclitaxel dosage by 25%
Any thrombocytopenia for >7 days	Reduce paclitaxel dosage by 25%
Febrile neutropenia, documented infection, or hemorrhage	Reduce paclitaxel dosage by 25%
G3 Mucositis	Reduce paclitaxel dosage by 25%
G3/4 Neuropathy	Discontinue paclitaxel
Symptomatic arrhythmia or heart block other than first degree	Discontinue trastuzumab
Left ventricle ejection fraction <45% or NYHA class III/IV cardiac dysfunction	Discontinue trastuzumab
Severe hypersensitivity reaction	Discontinue trastuzumab

Nabholtz JM et al. JCO 1996;14:1858–1867

Patient Population Studied

A study of 92 women with HER2 (IHC 2+, IHC 3+, or FISH+) progressive metastatic breast cancer that had not previously received chemotherapy for metastatic disease

Leyland-Jones B et al. JCO 2003;21:3965–3971

Efficacy (N = 92)

Overall response	60%
Complete response	13%
Partial response	47%
Median duration of response	10.5 months

Leyland-Jones B et al. JCO 2003;21:3965–3971

Toxicity

	% All	% Severe
Hematologic		
Leukopenia	24	6
Anemia	14	1
Infection	46	1
Nonhematologic		
Cardiac dysfunction	13	2*
Anorexia	24	1
Asthenia	62	8
Fever	47	2
Chills	47	1
Back pain	36	8
Chest pain	30	3
Constipation	25	0
Diarrhea	45	1
Nausea	50	3
Vomiting	37	9
Stomatitis	10	0
Alopecia	56	26
Arthralgia	37	9
Myalgia	38	7
Paresthesia	47	2
Rash	38	1

*NYHA classes III/IV
Slamon DJ et al. NEJM 2001;344:783–792

Therapy Monitoring

1. *Every 3 weeks:* CBC with differential, LFTs, and serum electrolytes
2. *Every 3–4 months:* Cardiac ejection fraction

METASTATIC REGIMEN

WEEKLY PACLITAXEL + TRASTUZUMAB

Seidman AD et al. JCO 2001;19:2587–2595

Initial treatment (first week)
Trastuzumab 4 mg/kg (loading dose) intravenously in 250 mL 0.9% NaCl injection (0.9% NS) over at least 90 minutes 1 day before the first dose of paclitaxel is administered (total dosage during the first treatment week = 4 mg/kg)
Premedication for paclitaxel:
Dexamethasone 10 mg intravenously per push 30–60 minutes before paclitaxel (total dose/cycle = 20 mg)

Note: Dexamethasone doses may be gradually reduced in 2–4 mg increments if the patient has no hypersensitivity reactions during repeated paclitaxel treatments
Diphenhydramine 50 mg intravenously per push 30–60 minutes before paclitaxel
Cimetidine 300 mg in 20–50 mL 0.9% NS or 5% dextrose injection (D5W) over 5–20 minutes, 30–60 minutes before paclitaxel

Paclitaxel 90 mg/m^2 by intravenous infusion in a volume of 0.9% NS or D5W sufficient to produce a concentration of 0.3–1.2 mg/mL over 60 minutes (total dosage during the first treatment week = 90 mg/m^2)

Schedule for second and subsequent weeks
Premedication for paclitaxel:
Dexamethasone 10 mg intravenously per push 30–60 minutes before paclitaxel (total dose/cycle = 20 mg)

Note: Dexamethasone doses may be gradually reduced in 2- to 4-mg increments if the patient has no hypersensitivity reactions during repeated paclitaxel treatments
Diphenhydramine 50 mg intravenously per push 30–60 minutes before paclitaxel
Cimetidine 300 mg in 20–50 mL 0.9% NS or D5W over 5–20 minutes 30–60 minutes before paclitaxel

Paclitaxel 90 mg/m^2 by intravenous infusion in a volume of 0.9% NS or D5W sufficient to produce a concentration of 0.3–1.2 mg/mL over 60 minutes every week, continually (total dosage/week = 90 mg/m^2), *followed immediately by:*
Trastuzumab 2 mg/kg per dose intravenously in 250 mL 0.9% NS over 30 minutes every week, continually (total dosage/week during the second and subsequent weeks = 2 mg/kg)

Note: Administration duration may be decreased from 90 to 30 minutes if slower durations are well tolerated

Dexamethasone is marketed in the United States in numerous generic formulations for oral administration, including immediate-release tablets containing 0.25, 0.5, 0.75, 1, 2, 4, and 6 mg, and in elixirs (which contain alcohol) and solutions for oral administration

Emetogenic potential: Low (Emetogenicity score = 2). See Chapter 39

Patient Population Studied

A study of 95 women with metastatic breast cancer who had not previously received treatment with more than three chemotherapy regimens. At least 1 year elapsed since prior taxane treatment. Only 50% of these patients had HER2 overexpression (ie, 3+ by immunohistochemistry)

Efficacy (N = 40–95)

Overall response	75%[a]
Intention-to-treat complete response	4%[b]
Intention-to-treat partial response	53%[b]

[a]In FISH-positive patients, N = 40
[b]In all patients, N = 95

Treatment Modifications

Adverse Event	Dose Modification
ANC <1000/mm^3 or platelets <100,000/mm^3 on day of planned treatment	Hold paclitaxel until ANC ≥1000/mm^3 and platelets ≥100,000/mm^3
If >2 weeks are required for recovery to ANC ≥1000/mm^3 and platelets ≥100,000/mm^3	Reduce paclitaxel dosage by 20 mg/m^2
Platelet nadir count ≤50,000/mm^3	
Documented infection	
G2 Nonhematologic adverse events	Reduce paclitaxel dosage by 10 mg/m^2
G3 Nonhematologic adverse events	Hold paclitaxel until toxicity resolves to G ≤ 2, and reduce paclitaxel dosage by 20 mg/m^2 during subsequent treatments
Left ventricle ejection fraction <45% or NYHA classes III or IV cardiac dysfunction	Discontinue trastuzumab
G3/4 Neurotoxicity	Discontinue paclitaxel

Toxicity (N = 95)

	% G1/2	% G3/4
Hematologic		
Neutropenia	29	6
Anemia	41	2
Thrombocytopenia	4	0
Infection	19	1
Febrile neutropenia	0	2
Nonhematologic		
Neuropathy	63	29
Myalgia	44	3
Arthralgia	13	0
Infusion reaction	9	1
Edema	38	5
Diarrhea	61	4
Nausea	43	3
Asthenia	52	7
Skin	9	1
Onycholysis	34	0
Cardiac Dysfunction		
Asymptomatic >20% decrease in ejection fraction	7	
Serious Cardiac Events		
Myocardial infarction	1	
Congestive heart failure	1	
Arrythmia	1	

NCI of Canada CTC

Therapy Monitoring

1. *Every week:* CBC with differential
2. *Periodically:* LFTs, serum electrolytes, calcium and magenesium
3. *Every 3–4 months:* Cardiac ejection fraction

METASTATIC REGIMEN

WEEKLY VINORELBINE + TRASTUZUMAB

Jahanzeb M et al. Oncologist 2002;7:410–417

First cycle:
Trastuzumab 4 mg/kg (loading dose) intravenously in 250 mL 0.9% NaCl injection (0.9% NS) over at least 90 minutes, given on day −1 (1 day before the first dose of vinorelbine is administered)
Trastuzumab 2 mg/kg per dose intravenously in 250 mL 0.9% NS over 30 minutes for 3 doses on days 8, 15, and 22 before vinorelbine administration (total dosage during the first cycle = 10 mg/kg)
Note: Administration duration may be decreased from 90 to 30 minutes if slower durations are well tolerated
Vinorelbine 30 mg/m² per dose intravenously diluted in 0.9% NS or 5% dextrose injection (D5W) to a concentration of 1.5–3 mg/mL by peripheral or central venous access over 6–10 minutes for 4 doses on days 1, 8, 15, and 22 every 28 days (total dosage/cycle = 120 mg/m²)

Second and subsequent cycles:
Trastuzumab 2 mg/kg per dose intravenously in 250 mL 0.9% NS over 30 minutes for 4 doses on days 1, 8, 15, and 22 before vinorelbine administration every 28 days (total dosage/cycle = 8 mg/kg)
Note: Administration duration may be decreased from 90 to 30 minutes if slower durations are well tolerated
Vinorelbine 30 mg/m² per dose intravenously diluted in 0.9% NS or D5W to a concentration of 1.5–3 mg/mL by peripheral or central venous access over 6–10 minutes for 4 doses on days 1, 8, 15, and 22 every 28 days (total dosage/cycle = 120 mg/m²)

Alternate Regimen

Burstein HJ et al. JCO 2001;19:2722–2730

First week:
Trastuzumab 4 mg/kg (loading dose intravenously in 250 mL 0.9% NS before vinorelbine over at least 90 minutes (total dosage during the first week = 4 mg/kg)
Vinorelbine 25 mg/m² per dose intravenously diluted in 0.9% NS or D5W to a concentration between 1.5 and 3 mg/mL by peripheral or central venous access over 6–10 minutes into the side-arm of a freely-flowing parenteral solution, weekly after trastuzumab administration, continually (total dosage/week = 25 mg/m²)

Second and subsequent weeks:
Trastuzumab 2 mg/kg per dose intravenously in 250 mL 0.9% NS over 30 minutes, weekly before vinorelbine administration, continually (total dosage during the second and subsequent weeks = 2 mg/kg)
Note: Administration duration may be decreased from 90 to 30 minutes if slower durations are well tolerated
Vinorelbine 25 mg/m² per dose intravenously diluted in 0.9% NS or D5W to a concentration between 1.5 and 3 mg/mL by peripheral or central venous access over 6–10 minutes into the side-arm of a freely-flowing parenteral solution, weekly after trastuzumab administration, continually (total dosage/week = 25 mg/m²)

Emetogenic potential: Nonemetogenic (Emetogenicity score = 1). See Chapter 39 for antiemetic regimens

Treatment Modifications

Adverse Event	Dose Modification
ANC >1250/mm³ or platelets >100,000/mm³ on day of treatment	No modification, give 100% doses
ANC 750–1250/mm³ or platelets 50,000–99,000/mm³ on day of treatment	Reduce vinorelbine dosage to 15 mg/m²
ANC <750/mm³ or platelets <50,000/mm³ on day of treatment	Delay vinorelbine dose until ANC >750/mm³ or platelets >50,000/mm³
Treatment delay of ≥2 weeks due to ANC <750/mm³	Consider adding filgrastim prophylaxis after subsequent treatments
Treatment delay >3 weeks due to ANC <750/mm³	Consider discontinuing treatment
Total bilirubin 2–3 mg/dL (34.2–51.3 μmol/L)	Reduce vinorelbine dosage to 12.5 mg/m²
Total bilirubin >3 mg/dL (51.3 μmol/L)	Hold vinorelbine
G2 Neurologic adverse events	Consider treatment delay until resolved to G ≤ 1. If no prior dose reductions, can reduce vinorelbine dosage to 15 mg/m² until toxicity resolves to G ≤ 1
G3 Nonhematologic adverse events	Hold vinorelbine until toxicity resolves to G ≤ 1
G4 Nonhematologic adverse events	Consider discontinuing treatment
Left ventricle ejection fraction <45% or congestive heart failure	Discontinue trastuzumab

Burstein HJ et al. JCO 2001;19:2722–2230
Jahanzeb M et al. Oncologist 2002;7:410–417

Patient Population Studied

A study of 40 women with HER2-overexpressing metastatic breast cancer who had not previously received more than 2 chemotherapy regimens for metastatic disease

Efficacy (N = 40)

Overall response	75%
Complete response	8%
Partial response	68%
Stable disease >6 months	5%

Burstein HJ et al. JCO 2001;19:2722–2730

Toxicity

	% G1/2	% G3/4
Hematologic		
Leukopenia	51	38
Neutropenia	28	43
Anemia	86	3
Thrombocytopenia	15	0
Febrile neutropenia	NA	3
Nonhematologic		
Cardiac dysfunction	26	0
Nausea/vomiting	63	0
Constipation	18	0
Stomatitis	20	0
Diarrhea	28	0
Rash	18	0
Thrombosis	0	3
Pancreatitis	0	3
Fatigue	66	5
Infusion reaction	38	0
Neuropathy	48	0

Burstein HJ et al. JCO 2001;19:2722–2730
NCI CTC

Therapy Monitoring

1. *Weekly:* CBC with differential and LFTs
2. *Every 3–4 months:* Cardiac ejection fraction

ADJUVANT/METASTATIC REGIMENS

HORMONAL THERAPY AGENTS

Selective estrogen-receptor modulators
Tamoxifen 20 mg daily orally

Selective estrogen-receptor down-regulator
Fulvestrant 250 mg monthly intramuscularly

Aromatase inhibitors
Anastrozole 1 mg daily orally
Letrozole 2.5 mg daily orally
Exemestane 25 mg daily orally

Progestins
Megestrol Acetate 40 mg 4 times daily orally

LHRH agonists
Goserelin 3.6 mg implant every 28 days subcutaneously
Goserelin 10.8 mg implant every 3 months subcutaneously

Anastrozole is available in the United States for oral administration as immediate-release tablets containing 1 mg anastrozole [Arimidex®]

Exemestane is available for oral administration as immediate-release tablets containing 25 mg exemestane [AROMASIN®]

Fulvestrant is marketed in the United States in two product configurations for intramuscular injection, as (1) a clear-glass syringe barrel containing 250 mg fulvestrant/5 mL (50 mg/mL); and (2) two half-full clear-glass syringe barrels each containing 125 mg fulvestrant/2.5 mL (50 mg/mL). [FASLODEX®]
Notes for the 2-barrel product: Both syringes must be administered to deliver the recommended monthly 250-mg dose. The syringes are presented in a tray with polystyrene plunger rod and safety needles for connection to the barrel

Goserelin acetate is available in the United States in two sustained-release formulations for subcutaneous administration, which deliver either 3.6 mg (1-month supply) or 10.8 mg (3-month supply) of goserelin. The delivery systems contain goserelin acetate dispersed in a sterile, white- to cream-colored 1-mm (3.6 mg) or 1.5-mm (10.8 mg) diameter biodegradable polymer cylinder preloaded in a single-use syringe with a siliconized needle and sealed in a light- and moisture-proof aluminum foil laminate pouch

Letrozole is available in the United States for oral administration as film-coated tablets containing 2.5 mg letrozole. [Femara®]

Megestrol acetate is available in the United States for oral administration as tablets containing either 20 mg or 40 mg of megestrol acetate, and as a lemon-lime flavored oral suspension containing micronized megestrol acetate 40 mg/mL [Megace®]

Tamoxifen citrate is available in the United States for oral administration as immediate-release tablets containing either 10 mg or 20 mg of tamoxifen base [Nolvadex®]

Efficacy

Tamoxifen	
Prevention:	50% reduction in breast cancer (invasive and noninvasive) in women at increased risk (5-year risk of 1.66%)
Adjuvant:	50% reduction in recurrence, 28% reduction in mortality
Metastatic:	Response rate 30–70% depending on ER/PR status: ER-positive/PR-positive >ER-positive/PR-negative >ER-negative/PR-positive
Fulvestrant	
Metastatic:	At least equivalent to anastrozole
Anastrozole	
Adjuvant:	Superior disease-free survival vs. tamoxifen when used as initial therapy or after 2–3 years of tamoxifen
Metastatic:	Likely superior to tamoxifen
Letrozole	
Neoadjuvant:	Superior to tamoxifen
Adjuvant:	Improved disease-free survival when started after 5 years of tamoxifen
Metastatic:	Superior to tamoxifen
Exemestane	
Adjuvant:	Superior to tamoxifen when used after 2–3 years of tamoxifen therapy
Metastatic:	Superior to megestrol acetate
Progestins	
Metastatic:	Equivalent to tamoxifen
LHRH agonists	
Adjuvant/ Metastatic	Evidence of efficacy in combination with tamoxifen for premenopausal women

The ATAC Trialists' Group. Lancet 2002;359:2131–2139
Ellis MJ et al. JCO 2001;19:3808–3816
Fisher B et al. J Natl Cancer Inst 1998;90:1371–1388
Goss PE et al. NEJM2003;349:1793–1802
Kaufmann M et al. JCO 2000;18:1399–1411
Klijn JGM et al. JCO 2001;19:343–353
Mouridsen H et al. JCO 2001;19:2596–2606
Nabholtz JM et al. JCO 2000;18:3758–3767
Osborne CK et al. JCO 2002;20:3386–3395

Toxicity

Note: Pregnancy is contraindicated with all hormonal therapies

Tamoxifen

	Increase Over Placebo Group	
Endometrial cancer	1.39 per 1000 women/yr	
Pulmonary embolism	0.46 per 1000 women/yr	
Deep venous thrombosis	0.5 per 1000 women/yr	
Cerebrovascular accident	0.53 per 1000 women/yr	
Cataracts	3.1 per 1000 women/yr	
	Tamoxifen	Placebo
Hot flashes	45.7%	28.7%
Vaginal discharge	29.0%	13.0%

Tamoxifen (ATAC Data)

Hot flashes	39.7%
Vaginal bleeding	8.2%
Endometrial cancer	0.7%
Venous thromboembolism (VTE)	3.5%
Fractures	3.7%
Musculoskeletal	21.3%

Fulvestrant

Toxicities similar to anastrozole without musculoskeletal side effects. Injection site reaction

Anastrozole (ATAC Data)

Hot flashes	34.3%
Vaginal bleeding	4.5%
Endometrial cancer	0.1%
VTE	2.1%
Fractures	5.9%
Musculoskeletal	27.8%

Letrozole

Toxicities similar to anastrozole

Exemestane

Toxicities similar to anastrozole with weight gain

Megestrol

Weight gain/edema
Hyperglycemia
Sedation
Thromboemboli

Goserelin

Hot flashes	70%
Tumor flare	23%
Nausea	11%
Edema	5%

The ATAC Trialists' Group. Lancet 2002; 359:2131–2139
Fisher B et al. J Natl Cancer Inst 1998;90:1371–1388
Stuart NSA et al. Eur J Cancer 1996;32A:1888–1892
Robertson JFR et al. Cancer 2003;98:229–238
AROMASIN® exemestane tablets product label, September 2004. Distributed by Pharmacia & Upjohn Company, Division of Pfizer, Inc, New York, NY
FASLODEX® fulvestrant Injection product label, August 2004. Manufactured by Vetter Pharma-Fertigung GmbH & Co. KG, Ravensburg, Germany. Manufactured for AstraZeneca UK Ltd, Macclesfield, England. Distributed by AstraZeneca Pharmaceuticals LP, Wilmington, DE
Femara® (letrozole tablets) 2.5-mg Tablets product label, November 2004. Novartis Pharmaceuticals Corporation, East Hanover, NJ
Megace® (megestrol acetate tablets) and Megace® Oral Suspension (megestrol acetate) product labels, July 2002. Bristol-Myers Squibb Company, Princeton, NJ
Zoladex® 3.6 mg goserelin acetate implant Equivalent to 3.6 mg goserelin and Zoladex® 10.8 mg goserelin acetate implant 3-month product labels, March 2004. Manufactured by AstraZeneca UK Ltd., Macclesfield, England. Manufactured for AstraZeneca Pharmaceuticals LP, Wilmington, DE

Therapy Monitoring

Tamoxifen

1. LFTs >1 month, then every 3–6 months
2. Serum chemistries every 6 months

Fulvestrant

1. Clinic visit at 1 month
2. Serum chemistries and LFTs every 6 months

Anastrozole

1. Clinic visit at 1 month
2. Bone density scan at baseline and every 6–12 months when used as adjuvant therapy
3. Serum chemistries and LFTs every 6 months

Letrozole

1. Clinic visit at 1 month
2. Bone density scan at baseline and every 6–12 months when used as adjuvant therapy
3. Serum chemistries and LFTs every 6 months

Exemestane

1. Clinic visit at 1 month
2. Bone density scan at baseline and every 6–12 months when used as adjuvant therapy
3. Serum chemistries and LFTs every 6 months

Megestrol

1. Clinic visit, serum chemistries, and LFTs at 1 month, then every 3–6 months
2. Monitor adrenal function every 3 months

Note: Consider replacement (or stress dose) steroids with withdrawal or physiologic stress

LHRH Agonists (Goserelin)

1. Clinic visit at 1 month
2. Serum chemistries and LFTs every 6 months

7. Carcinoid Tumors

Eva Tiensuu Janson, MD, and Kjell Öberg, MD

Epidemiology

Incidence: *Foregut*
Bronchial: 0.6–0.8/100,000
Thymic: 0.01/100,000
Stomach: 0.1–0.2/100,000
Midgut
Small intestine: 1–2/100,000
Appendix: 0.05–0.1/100,000
Hindgut
Colon: 0.15/100,000
Rectum: 0.35/100,000 (1.2/100,000 African Americans)

Male/female ratio: 1:1

Modlin IM et al. Cancer 2003;97:934–959

Pathology

Bronchial (lung) carcinoid tumors

1. *Typical bronchial carcinoid:* Constitute about 85 % of bronchial carcinoid tumors; display a highly organized architecture. Mitoses are rare <2 per 10 high-power field [HPF]). Usually benign
2. *Atypical bronchial carcinoid:* Constitute about 15 % of bronchial carcinoid tumors. Less well organized cell architecture. High mitotic frequency (2–10 mitosis per 10 HPF). Presence of necrosis. Usually malignant

Thymic carcinoid tumor

The histopathologic pattern may vary from highly differentiated tumors to poorly differentiated neuroendocrine carcinomas. Usually malignant

Stomach carcinoid tumors

1. *Type 1 gastric carcinoid:* Associated with hypergastrinemia and chronic atrophic gastritis. Single or multiple polyps, usually <1 cm. Usually benign, the tumors consist of ECL-cells
2. *Type 2 gastric carcinoid:* Associated with MEN 1 and Zollinger-Ellison syndrome. Single or multiple polyps. Can be malignant
3. *Type 3 gastric carcinoid:* Sporadic tumor of >2 cm, not associated with hypergastrinemia. Often malignant, the tumors consist of ECL, EC, and gastrin-producing cells
4. *Type 4 gastric neuroendocrine carcinoma:* Highly malignant, poorly differentiated with high proliferation index. All tumors are malignant

Intestinal carcinoid tumors

1. *Duodenal carcinoid:* Usually single tumors. Most are malignant and may be part of the MEN 1 syndrome (gastrinoma) or Recklinghausen´s syndrome (somatostatinoma)
2. *Small intestinal (classical midgut) carcinoid:* Presentation with four different histopathologic patterns: insular, acinar, trabecular, or mixed growth pattern. Low proliferation rate. Usually malignant and presentation may be with metastases several years after the primary diagnosis
3. *Appendiceal carcinoid:* Small tumor with a low proliferation rate. Usually benign. If >2 cm or located at the base of the appendix, there is a risk of malignancy
4. *Colon carcinoid:* Usually highly malignant tumors with a poorly differentiated neuroendocrine carcinoma (small cell tumors)
5. *Rectal carcinoid:* Small well-differentiated tumors, usually showing a trabecular growth pattern. Low proliferation index. Usually benign. If >2 cm, increased risk of malignancy

Rindi G et al. J Mol Med 1998;76:413–420
Travis WD. Clin Chest Med 2002;23:65–81

Work-Up

Radiology/nuclear medicine

1. Thoracic and abdominal CT or MRI
2. Somatostatin receptor scintigraphy (Octreoscan®)
3. In selected cases, PET with 5-hydroxy tryptophane or 18-fluorodeoxyglucose as tracer to localize small primary tumors or recurrences

Tumor markers

1. *All patients with a suspicion of carcinoid tumor.* Measure plasma chromogranin A levels
2. *Bronchial (lung) carcinoid patients:* Measure p-ACTH, u-kortisol, GH and IGF-1 levels
3. *Foregut carcinoid patients:* Measure histamine metabolites in urine as well as gastrin and somatostatin in selected cases
4. *Midgut carcinoid patients.* Two 24-hour collections of urine to measure the serotonin metabolite, 5-hydroxyindoleacetic acid (5-HIAA), and plasma for neuropeptide K and substance P (peptides belonging to the tachykinin family)
5. *Patients with colon or rectum carcinoids:* Pancreatic polypeptide (PP) can be measured

Diagnostic biopsies

Biopsies should be obtained if tumor lesions are found with radiology or nuclear medicine imaging techniques:

1. *All patients:* When possible, an ultrasound-guided needle biopsy (1.2 mm) should be performed to obtain material of histopathologic examination
2. *For gastric carcinoid tumors:* Gastroscopy with biopsies is preferred
3. *For rectal carcinoid tumors:* Rectoscopy (sigmoidoscopy) should be performed to obtain biopsies

Schnirer II et al. Acta Oncol 2003;42:672–692

Staging and 5-year Survival

	Localized Disease	Regional Metastases	Distant Metastases
Bronchial	81	77	26
Thymus	60–100	40	29
Stomach	69	38	21
Classical midgut	64	72	50
Appendix	81	88	31
Colon	80	50	5
Rectum	91	49	32

Caveats

Debulking Therapy

1. *Surgical resection* of the primary tumor should be considered for every patient with a carcinoid tumor, regardless of the site of the primary tumor. Debulking surgery with resection of liver and lymph node metastases should also be discussed whenever possible. Resection of the primary tumor seems to be favorable for survival (midgut carcinoid 7.4 versus 4.0 years)

Ferguson MK et al. E J Cardiothorac Surg 2000;18:156–161; Hellman P et al. W J Surg 2002;8:991–997; Modlin IM et al. Surg Oncol 2003;2:153–172

2. *Radiofrequency ablation* of liver metastases up to 3–5 cm in diameter can be considered both intraoperatively and percutaneously by ultrasound guidance

Hellman P et al. W J Surg 2002;8:1052–1056

3. *Liver transplantation* can be considered for patients with midgut carcinoid tumors with only liver metastases. A thorough pretransplantation examination should be performed, including somatostatin receptor scintigraphy and, if possible, 5-HTP-PET to rule out extrahepatic metastases. In a small series (15 patients with midgut carcinoid tumor), liver transplantation had up to 69% 5-year survival

Le Treut YP et al. Ann Surg 1997;225:355–364

4. *Liver embolization* can be considered in patients with massive liver involvement. Patients with excessive hormone production should receive infusion of a somatostatin analogue after the procedure to reduce the risk of hormone crises; 40–50% of the patients have a biochemical response with >50% reduction in hormone levels, whereas about 40% show a reduction in tumor size

Eriksson BK et al. Cancer 1998;83:2293–2301

Symptomatic Treatment of Diarrhea

1. **Loperamide** 2 mg/dose orally up to 16 mg/day
2. **Tincture of opium** orally; dose is individually titrated. Begin with 2–4 drops dissolved in water administered orally 2–3 times per day, and titrate dropwise as needed
3. **Cholestyramine** 4 g/dose orally, 2–6 doses/day (up to 24 g/day) [Especially in patients who have undergone an ileocecal resection]

REGIMEN

SOMATOSTATIN ANALOGUES

Kvols LK et al. NEJM 1986;315:663–666 Öberg K, ERiksson B. Ann Oncol 2004;15:966–973

Octreotide acetate injection 100–500 mcg per dose subcutaneously 2 or 3 times daily, doubling the dose at 3- to 4-day intervals until maximum control of symptoms is achieved

or

Octreotide acetate for injectable suspension 10–30 mg per dose intragluteally every 4 weeks [Avoid intramuscular injection into the deltoids]

or

Lanreotide acetate (powder for suspension for injection) 30 mg per dose intramuscularly every 10–14 days (not available in the United States)

Emetogenic potential: **Nonemetogenic** (Emetogenicity score = 1). See Chapter 39

Supplemental therapy for all somatostatin analogues: Pancreatic enzymes to avoid steatorrhea. Individualize dosage by giving the number of tablets or capsules that optimally minimize steatorrhea (see Notes)

Treatment Modifications

(Patients receiving octreotide acetate for injectable suspension or lanreotide acetate)

Escape from antisecretory response	Administer octreotide acetate injection 100–500 mcg per dose subcutaneously 2 or 3 times daily. Increase dose or reduce interval between doses of the long-acting preparation as needed
Steatorrhea	Increase dose of pancreatic enzyme supplement to 3 capsules with every meal

Patient Population Studied

Primary symptomatic treatment in 25 patients with hormonally active tumors

Efficacy (N = 25)

(Octreotide 150 mcg/dose 3 times daily; 18 months follow-up)

Biochemical response[a]	72%
Biochemical stable disease	28%
Tumor size stable (n = 13)	100%
Symptomatic relief[b]	76%

[a]>50% decrease in 24-hour urinary 5-HIAA
[b]>50% decrease in flushing and diarrhea

Kvols LK et al. NEJM 1986;315:663–666

Toxicity (N = 25)

Steatorrhea[ab]	Frequent (~ 66%)
Loose stools[b]	Common
Nausea[b]	Common
Abdominal cramps[b]	Common
Flatulence[b]	Common
Hyperglycemia[c]/hypoglycemia	<10%
Gallbladder stone/sludge	50%
Bradycardia	<2%
Pain/erythema at injection site	Occasional
Gastric atony	Very rare

[a]Occurs frequently unless pancreatic enzyme supplements are administered. Etiology is presumed to be transient inhibition of pancreatic exocrine function and malabsorption of fat
[b]Start within hours of the first sc injection and usually subside spontaneously within the first few weeks of treatment
[c]From transient inhibition of insulin secretion

Kvols LK et al. NEJM 1986;315:663–666
Öberg K et al. Ann Oncol 2004;15:966–973

Therapy Monitoring

1. *Every 3 months:* Complete history and physical examination
2. *Every 3–6 months:* Conventional imaging (CT, MRI, or ultrasound), serum electrolytes, and serum glucose
3. *Every year:* Somatostatin receptor scintigraphy (Octreoscan®) is controversial
4. *New symptoms:* Somatostatin receptor scintigraphy (Octreoscan®)

Notes

1. Performing an Octreoscan® provides information about the somatostatin receptor status of the patient's tumor and should be performed before treatment with a somatostatin analogue is initiated. Patients with receptor-positive tumors more frequently respond to such treatment than those with receptor-negative tumors
2. Because of adverse events, administration of the immediate-release formulation is recommended before administration of the intramuscular depot formulation
3. Patients should begin therapy with octreotide acetate injection subcutaneously for 3–7 days to test for tolerability before receiving a long-acting formulation (octreotide acetate for injectable suspension or lanreotide acetate) intramuscularly
4. Increase the dosage of the short-acting octreotide acetate injection until control of symptoms is achieved by doubling the dosage at 3- to 4-day intervals
5. Patients who are considered to be "responders" to the drug and who tolerate the short-acting formulation can then receive octreotide acetate for injectable suspension or lanreotide acetate
6. The subcutaneous injections should be continued for 10–14 days after the start of the long-acting formulation to allow time for therapeutic levels to be achieved
7. Conversion to the long-acting formulation provides greater patient convenience. If the dose of the short-acting formulation was 200–600 mcg per day, begin with a 20-mg dose of the long-acting formulation. If the dose of the short-acting formulation was 750–1500 mcg per day, begin with a 30-mg dose of the long-acting formulation
8. Supplementary ("rescue") administration of the short-acting octreotide acetate injection should be given to patients escaping the antisecretory effects of the long-acting octreotide acetate for injectable suspension. If the rescue therapy is required during the week before the next dose of the long-acting formulation, a reduction in the dosing interval by 1 week is recommended. If the rescue medication is administered sporadically throughout the month, then increasing the dose of octreotide acetate for injectable suspension stepwise by 10 mg per month up to 60 mg per month should be tried

Supplemental therapy for all somatostatin analogues:
Pancreatic enzymes to avoid steatorrhea

Individualize dosage by giving the number of tablets or capsules that optimally minimize steatorrhea.
Select Pancrelipase products with a high lipase content to avoid steatorrhea. In some patients, enteric-coated enzyme tablets may not dissociate as intended and may pass through the bowel intact
Administer Pancrelipase with meals or snacks. Individualize dosage by giving the number of tablets or capsules that optimally minimize steatorrhea. Adjust doses slowly; monitor symptoms and response

- Do not crush or chew enteric-coated products or the enteric-coated contents of opened capsules
- Capsules may be opened and shaken onto a small quantity of soft food that is not hot and does not require chewing
- Pancrelipase should be immediately swallowed without chewing to prevent mucosal irritation
- Ingested doses should be followed with a glass of juice or water to ensure complete ingestion
- Avoid mixing Pancrelipase with foods that have a pH >5.5, which can dissolve enteric coatings

REGIMEN

INTERFERON ALFA

Öberg K. Acta Oncol 1991;30:519–522

Recombinant interferon alfa-2b 3–6 million units/dose subcutaneously 3 times per week indefinitely (total dose/week = 9–18 million units)
Note: Median dose is 3–6 million units/dose. Median duration of therapy is 30 months

Ancillary medications:
Primary antipyretic prophylaxis:
Acetaminophen 650–1000 mg orally

or

Ibuprofen 400–600 mg orally starting 1 hour before the administration of interferon, then every 4 hours as needed
Secondary antiemetic prophylaxis:
If required as secondary prophylaxis, then use as primary prophylaxis with subsequent doses

Emetogenic potential: Nonemetogenic (Emetogenicity score = 1). See Chapter 39

Note: If effectiveness of recombinant interferon alfa-2b diminishes and the WBC returns to normal, development of antibodies against the interferon should be suspected. A change to Alferon N Injection® (interferon alfa-n3; human leukocyte derived) should be considered

Treatment Modifications

Adverse Event	Dose Modification
WBC >3000/mm³	Increase interferon alfa
WBC <2000/mm³	Decrease interferon alfa

First occurrence of a DLT	Hold dose until resolution, then decrease interferon alfa by 33%
Second occurrence of a DLT	Hold dose until resolution, then decrease interferon alfa by 66%
Third occurrence of a DLT	Discontinue interferon alfa therapy

Definitions of Dose-Limiting Toxicities (DLTs)

Hematologic DLT	ANC <500/mm³
Hepatic DLT	SGPT (ALT) or SGOT (AST) >5 times upper limit of normal (ULN)

Patient Population Studied

A study including 111 patients with midgut carcinoid tumors with liver metastases. Sixty-eight received chemotherapy as first-line therapy and then alfa-interferon. Forty-three received alfa-interferon as first-line therapy

Efficacy (N = 111)

Biochemical Response	
Objective response[a]	42%
Stable disease	39%
Progressive disease	19%
Tumor Size Response	
Objective response[b]	14%
Stable disease	67%
Progressive disease	19%
Subjective Response	
Symptomatic relief[c]	68%

[a]>50% reduction in hormone levels
[b]>50% reduction in tumor size
[c]Improvement of diarrhea, flush

Toxicity (N = 111)

Nonhematologic	
Flu-like symptoms	89%
Fatigue	70%
Weight loss	59%
Increased blood lipids	32%
Increased liver enzymes	31%
Liver steatosis	19%
Thyroid autoantibodies[a]	15%
Antinuclear factor[a]	15%
Worsening psoriasis[a]	3%
Hematologic	
Anemia (<11 g/dL)	31%
Leukopenia (<2000/mm³)	3%
Thrombocytopenia (<150,000/mm³)	14%

[a]Manifestations of autoimmune phenomena

WHO Criteria

Note: Adverse reactions are very common, especially at the initiation of treatment, but most are transient and can be managed with dose reductions

Therapy Monitoring

Every third month: CBC with differential

Notes

Interferon alfa is suggested as primary antitumoral treatment in midgut carcinoid tumors

REGIMEN

STREPTOZOCIN + FLUOROURACIL

Adapted from Moertel CG. Cancer Clin Trials 1979;2:327–334
Kalsas GA et al. Endocr Rev 2004;25:458–511

Induction course:
Streptozocin 1000 mg per day by rapid intravenous injection over 1–2 minutes days 1–5 (total dosage/cycle = 5000 mg)

Fluorouracil 400 mg/m^2 per day by rapid intravenous injection over 1–2 minutes days 1–3 (total dosage/cycle = 1200 mg/m^2)

Subsequent courses:
Streptozocin 2000 mg by rapid intravenous injection over 1–2 minutes, given on day 1 every 3 weeks (total dosage/cycle = 2000 mg)

Fluorouracil 400 mg/m^2 by rapid intravenous injection over 1–2 minutes, given on day 1 every 3 weeks (total dosage/cycle = 400 mg/m^2)

Emetogenic potential:
Induction, days 1–3: Very high (Emetogenicity score = 6)
Induction, days 4 and 5: High (Emetogenicity score = 5).
Subsequent courses, day 1: Very high (Emetogenicity score = 6). See Chapter 39

Patient Population Studied

A study of 44 patients with unresectable metastatic carcinoid with significant symptoms associated with their malignant disease

Efficacy

Biochemical response	30%
Tumor size response	<10%

Kalsas GA et al. Endocr Rev 2004;25:458–511

Toxicity (N = 22–49)

	% of Patients
Nausea and Vomiting (n = 49)	
Mild	43
Moderate	27
Severe	14
WBC Nadir (n = 25)	
≥2000 < 3000/mm^3	8
≥1000 < 2000/mm^3	4
<1000/mm^3	8
Platelet Nadir (n = 22)	
<50,000/mm^3	5
Serum Creatinine (n = 38)	
>1.2 ≤ 1.5 mg/dL	16
>1.5 ≤ 2.0 mg/dL	3
>2.0 mg/dL	3
Liver Enzymes	
Increase in bilirubin	<10

Treatment Modifications

Adverse Event	Dose Modification
Pretreatment urinary 5-HIAA >150 mg/24 hours *or* Carcinoid syndrome with florid symptoms	Consider reducing streptozocin and fluorouracil dosages in first cycle by 50%. If well tolerated, dosages may be escalated to 100% during subsequent cycles as tolerated
Hematologic toxicities	Streptozocin and fluorouracil dosages are titrated to produce mild-to-moderate hematologic toxicities
Evidence of nephrotoxicity (proteinuria or decreasing glomerular filtration rate)	Streptozocin dose should be divided in 2 days
Persistent or severe nephrotoxicity	Discontinue streptozocin

Therapy Monitoring

1. *Before each cycle:* WBC with differential and platelet count, renal and liver function tests, and fasting blood glucose
2. *Every 6 weeks:* Response evaluation: Measure indicator lesions and obtain 24-hour urine for 5HIAA determination

Notes

Use in a patient with a carcinoid tumor if the proliferation index is less than 10%; should not be used as first-line therapy for midgut carcinoid tumors, but can be considered for foregut carcinoid tumors

REGIMEN

CARBOPLATIN + ETOPOSIDE

Adapted from Fjällskog M-LH et al. Cancer 2001;92:1101–1107

Carboplatin [calculated dose] AUC = 4–5 by intravenous infusion in 50–150 mL 5% dextrose injection (D5W) over 15–30 minutes on day 1 every 3–4 weeks (total dosage/cycle calculated to produce an AUC = 4–5 mg/mL/min)

Etoposide 100 mg/m^2 by intravenous infusion diluted in 0.9% NS to a concentration of 0.2–0.4 mg/mL over 60 minutes on days 1, 2, and 3 every 3–4 weeks (total dosage/cycle = 300 mg/m^2)

Emetogenic potential: Moderately high (Emetogenicity score = 4). See Chapter 39

Note: Carboplatin dose is based on Calvert's formula to achieve a target area under the plasma concentration versus time curve (AUC) [AUC units = mg/m/min]

$$\text{Total carboplatin dose (mg)} = (\text{Target AUC}) \times (\text{GFR} + 25)$$

In practice, creatinine clearance (Clcr) is used in place of glomerular filtration rate (GFR). Clcr can be calculated from the equation of Cockcroft and Gault:

$$\text{Males, Clcr} = \frac{(140 - \text{age}[y]) \times \text{body weight}[kg]}{72 \times (\text{Serum creatinine}[mg/dL])}$$

$$\text{Females, Clcr} = \frac{(140 - \text{age}[y]) \times \text{body weight}[kg]}{72 \times (\text{Serum creatinine}[mg/dL])} \times 0.85$$

Calvert AH et al. JCO 1989;7:1748–1756
Cockcroft DW, Gault MH. Nephron 1976;16:31–41
Jodrell DI et al. JCO 1992;10:520–528
Sorensen BT et al. Cancer Chemother Pharmacol 1991;28:397–401

Patient Population Studied

Patients with bronchial carcinoid tumors

Efficacy (N = 18)

Biochemical response	22%
Biochemical stable disease	66%
Tumor size response	39%
Tumor size stable	50%

Toxicity (N = 36)

Nephrotoxicity	53%
G3/4 neutropenia	64%
G1/2 peripheral neuropathy	17%
Ototoxicity (mild)	8%
Alopecia	100%

WHO criteria

Treatment Modifications

Adverse Event	Dose Modification
Day 1 ANC <1500/mm^3 or platelets <100,000/mm^3	Delay treatment 1 week or until ANC >1500/mm^3 and platelets >100,000/mm^3. Then, retreat at 100% doses
ANC nadir <500/mm^3	Administer filgrastim during subsequent cycles on days 4–11 (8 days)
Nadir platelet count <50,000/mm^3	Reduce carboplatin dosage by 25%
Cycle 1 ANC nadir ≥1500/mm^3 and platelet nadir ≥100,000/mm^3	Increase carboplatin dosage by 12.5%

Therapy Monitoring

1. *At least weekly:* CBC with differential
2. *Every cycle:* LFTs, BUN, serum creatinine, serum calcium, magnesium, and uric acid
3. *Every other cycle:* Urine for creatinine clearance
4. *When clinically indicated*: Audiogram

Notes

Use in a patient with a carcinoid tumor if the proliferation index is greater than 15%, especially in a patient with a bronchial carcinoid tumor

REGIMEN

[^{177} Lutetium-DOTA^0,TYR^3] octreotate (^{177}Lu-octreotate)

Kwekkeboom DJ et al. Eur J Nucl Med Mol Imaging 2003;30:417–422

Amino acid mixture (containing lysine 2.5%, arginine 2.5%) in 1000 mL 0.9 NaCl injection (0.9% NS) by continuous intravenous infusion at 250 mL/hour, starting 30 minutes before administering ^{177}Lu-octreotate and continuing for up to 3.5 hours after ^{177}Lu-octreotate administration

^{177}Lu-octreotate 100 mCi/dose by intravenous infusion over 20 minutes every 6–9 weeks for 7–8 doses (total cumulative dose after 8 doses = 800 mCi [29.6 Gbq])

Emetogenic potential: Unknown but probably nonemetogenic (Emetogenicity score = 1). See Chapter 39

Efficacy (N = 12)

Tumor size decrease	33%
Tumor size stabilization	50%

Toxicity

Nonhematologic	
Nausea	30%
Vomiting	14%
Abdominal pain	11%

Hematologic (WHO)	% Grade I	% Grade II
Anemia	8	0
Leukopenia	5	1
Thrombocytopenia	3	1

Patient Population Studied

A study of 12 patients with carcinoid tumors with metastases

Therapy Monitoring

Every 2–4 weeks: CBC with differential, and serum creatinine

Notes

Tumor-targeting therapy with radiolabeled somatostatin analogues is still under development. However, it may be used in selected patients with a tracer uptake at the time of somatostatin receptor scintigraphy (Octreoscan®)

8. Carcinoma of Unknown Primary

David Spigel, MD and F. Anthony Greco, MD

Epidemiology

Incidence: Unknown* (estimated at 80,000–90,000 patients/year)

Mortality rate: Varies by histology and clinical subsets

1-year survival:	35–40%
2-year survival:	15–20%
3-year survival:	10–15%
5-year survival:	10%
8-year survival:	<10%

Median age: Varies by histology (usually sixth decade)

Male/female ratio: M ≅ F

Stage at Presentation

Local/regional:	<10%
≥2 sites:	>90%

*Due to patient heterogeneity and tumor registry misclassification

Greco FA, Hainsworth JD. In: DeVita VT, Jr, Hellman S, Rosenberg SA, eds. Cancer: Principles & Practice of Oncology, 6th ed. Lippincott; 2001:2537–2560
Hainsworth JD, Greco FA. NEJM 1993;329:257–263
Hainsworth JD et al. JCO 1991;9:1931–1938

Pathology

Histology	%
Adenocarcinoma (well differentiated or moderately differentiated)	60%
Poorly differentiated carcinoma/ (± features of adenocarcinoma)	30%
Poorly differentiated malignant neoplasm	5%
Squamous carcinoma	5%

Hainsworth JD, Greco FA. NEJM 1993;329:257–263

Work-Up

Clinical evaluation

- H&P, including pelvic, breast, and rectal exams
- CBC
- Comprehensive metabolic profile
- Urinalysis
- Occult blood in feces
- Lactate dehydrogenase (LDH)
- Serum human chorionic gonadotropin (β-HCG)
- Alpha fetoprotein (AFP)
- Carcinoembryonic antigen (CEA)
- CA 19-9, CA 27–29 (or CA 15-3), CA 125
- Chest/abdominal/pelvic CT

Where appropriate:

- Positron emission tomography (PET)
- Prostate specific antigen (PSA)
- Mammography, bronchoscopy, and panendoscopy (particularly for squamous carcinomas)

Pathologic studies

- Immunohistochemistry analyses for:
  - –PSA in men
  - –Estrogen receptor (ER) in women
  - –Progesterone receptor (PR) in women
  - –HER2/neu overexpression in women
  - –CD 117

Where appropriate:

- Electron microscopy
- Cytogenetic analysis

Focused Work-Up

Presentation	Men	Women
Head and neck or supraclavicular adenopathy	• ENT exam • Chest/abdominal CT • PSA, testicular ultrasound	• ENT exam • Chest/abdominal CT • Mammography, ER/PR • Pathologic evaluation
Axillary adenopathy	• Chest/abdominal CT • PSA	• Chest/abdominal CT • Mammography, ER/PR • (Consider ultrasound or MRI)
Mediastinal involvement	• Chest/abdominal CT • βHCG/AFP • PSA	• Chest/abdominal CT • βHCG/AFP • Mammography, ER/PR

(continued)

(continued)

Presentation	Men	Women
Chest (effusion and/or nodules) involvement	• Chest/abdominal CT • PSA	• Chest/abdominal/pelvic CT • Mammography, ER/PR • CA 125
Peritoneal involvement	• Chest/abdominal/pelvic CT • PSA	• Chest/abdominal/pelvic CT • Mammography, ER/PR • CA 125
Retroperitoneal mass	• Chest/abdominal/pelvic CT • PSA • βHCG/AFP • Testicular ultrasound	• Chest/abdominal/pelvic CT • Mammography, ER/PR • CA 125
Inguinal adenopathy	• Abdominal/pelvic CT • PSA	• Abdominal/pelvic CT • Mammography, ER/PR • CA 125
Hepatic involvement	• Chest/abdominal/pelvic CT • Colonoscopy • AFP • PSA	• Chest/abdominal/pelvic CT • Colonoscopy • AFP • Mammography, ER/PR
Skeletal involvement	• Bone scan • PSA	• Bone scan • Mammography, ER/PR
Brain involvement	• Chest/abdominal CT	• Chest/abdominal CT • Mammography, ER/PR

Greco FA, Hainsworth JD. In: DeVita VT Jr, Hellman S, Rosenberg SA, eds. Cancer: Principles & Practice of Oncology, 6th ed. Lippincott. 2001:2537–2560
Occult Primary Cancer. In: NCCN Clinical Practice Guidelines in Oncology, May 2003. © National Comprehensive Cancer Network, Inc., 2001, 2002, 2003

Caveats

Axillary nodal metastases in a woman	Treatment appropriate for stage II breast cancer to include surgery ± radiation, chemotherapy, and hormonal therapy where applicable. If additional sites, manage patient as you would a patient with metastatic breast cancer
Peritoneal carcinomatosis in a woman	Metastases outside the peritoneal cavity are unusual. Appropriate initial treatment as for advanced ovarian cancer including adequate surgical cytoreduction
Suspected prostate cancer	Treatment appropriate for advanced prostate cancer to include androgen deprivation and, potentially, chemotherapy
Solitary sites of metastases	Definitive local treatment (surgery, radiation, or both), followed by empiric adjuvant systemic chemotherapy regimens, as listed in this chapter
Tumor with features of extragonadal germ cell tumors in a young man	Treatment appropriate for poor-prognosis germ cell tumors Platinum-based regimen (eg, BEP regimen: bleomycin, etoposide, and cisplatin) preferred
Cervical adenopathy involved by squamous carcinoma	Definitive local therapy: Radiation ± surgery ± chemotherapy
Inguinal adenopathy involved by squamous carcinoma	Definitive local therapy: Radiation ± surgery ± chemotherapy
Poorly differentiated neuroendocrine carcinoma	Empiric combination chemotherapy regimens appropriate for small cell lung cancer
Well-differentiated neuroendocrine carcinoma	Treatment appropriate for metastatic carcinoid tumors
Poorly differentiated carcinoma	Empiric combination chemotherapy regimens as listed in this chapter

REGIMEN

PACLITAXEL + CARBOPLATIN + ETOPOSIDE

Hainsworth JD et al. JCO 1997;15:2385–2393

Premedication:
Dexamethasone 20 mg per dose orally 12 hours and 4 hours before starting paclitaxel
Diphenhydramine 50 mg intravenously per push, over 30–60 minutes before starting paclitaxel
Cimetidine 300 mg intravenously in 25–100 mL of 0.9% NaCl injection (0.9% NS) or 5% dextrose injection (D5W) over 30–60 minutes before starting paclitaxel
Dexamethasone 20 mg intravenously per push 30 minutes before starting paclitaxel

Paclitaxel 200 mg/m^2 intravenously diluted in 0.9% NS or D5W to a concentration between 0.3 and 1.2 mg/mL, over 1 hour, before starting carboplatin on day 1 every 21 days (total dosage/cycle = 200 mg/m^2)

Carboplatin [calculated dose] AUC = 6 intravenously diluted in 0.9% NS or D5W to a concentration >0.5 mg/mL over 20–30 minutes, on day 1 every 21 days (total dosage/cycle calculated to produce an AUC = 6 mg/mL/min)

Etoposide 50 mg per dose orally on days 1, 3, 5, 7, and 9, alternating with:
Etoposide 100 mg per dose orally on days 2, 4, 6, 8, and 10 (total dose/cycle = 750 mg)

Emetogenic potential:
Day 1: High (Emetogenicity score ≥5).
Days 2–10: Low (Emetogenicity score ~2).
Potential for delayed symptoms after day 1. See Chapter 39

Carboplatin dose is based on a formula described by Calvert et al. to achieve a target area under the plasma concentration versus time curve (AUC)

$$\text{Total carboplatin dose (mg)} = (\text{Target AUC}) \times (\text{GFR} + 25)$$

In practice, creatinine clearance (Clcr) is used in place of glomerular filtration rate (GFR). Clcr can be calculated from the equation of Cockcroft and Gault:

$$\text{Males, Clcr} = \frac{(140 - \text{age [y]}) \times \text{body weight [kg]}}{72 \times (\text{Serum creatinine [mg/dL]})}$$

$$\text{Females, Clcr} = \frac{(140 - \text{age [y]}) \times \text{body weight [kg]}}{72 \times (\text{Serum creatinine [mg/dL]})} \times 0.85$$

Calvert AH et al. JCO 1989;7:1748–1756
Cockcroft DW, Gault MH. Nephron 1976;16:31–41
Jodrell DI et al. JCO 1992;10:520–528
Sorensen BT et al. Cancer Chemother Pharmacol 1991;28:397–401

Etoposide is available in the United States in capsules containing 50 mg etoposide. VePesid® (etoposide) for injection and capsules. Manufactured by R.P. Scherer GmbH Oncology Products, Eberback/Baden, Germany for Bristol Laboratories® Oncology products, A Bristol-Myers Squibb Co., Princeton, NJ

Treatment Modifications

Adverse Event	Dose Modification
Day 21: ANC >1500/mm^3 and platelets ≥100,000/mm^3	Administer 100% doses
Day 21: ANC <1500/mm^3 or platelets <100,000/mm^3	Delay treatment 1 week or until ANC >1500/mm^3 and platelets >100,000/mm^3 Then, retreat at 100% doses
Day 8: ANC ≥1000/mm^3 and platelets ≥ 75,000/mm^3	Complete 10 days of etoposide
Day 8: ANC < 1000/mm^3 *or* platelets < 75,000/mm^3	Hold day 8, 9, and 10 etoposide doses
Hospitalization for febrile neutropenia	Administer 75% of paclitaxel and carboplatin and first 8 days of etoposide in all subsequent cycles
Reversible G3 or G4 nonhematologic toxicity (except for alopecia, nausea, and vomiting)	Decrease the dose of the suspected offending drug(s) by 25% during subsequent cycles

Hematopoietic growth factors are used as secondary prophylaxis at the discretion of a treating physician, but should not substitute for recommended dose modifications

Patient Population Studied

A study of 55 patients with carcinoma of unknown primary site were treated and available for assessment. Responding patients received 4 courses of treatment. The following histologies were included: adenocarcinoma (n = 30); poorly differentiated carcinoma or poorly differentiated adenocarcinoma (n = 21); poorly differentiated neuroendocrine carcinoma (n = 3); and squamous carcinoma (n = 1)

Efficacy

Complete response	6%
Partial response	30%
Median actuarial survival	9.1 months
1-year survival	38%
2-year survival	19%
3-year survival	12%
5-year survival	8%
8-year survival	6%

Greco FA, Hainsworth JD. In: DeVita VT Jr, Hellman S, Rosenberg SA, eds. Cancer: Principles & Practice of Oncology, 6th ed. Lippincott; 2001:2537–2560

Toxicity (N = 55)

	% G3	% G4
Hematologic		
Leukopenia	56	20
Thrombocytopenia	15	11
Febrile neutropenia	—	13
Nonhematologic		
Nausea/vomiting	7	2
Peripheral neuropathy	7	—
Fatigue	7	—
Arthralgia/myalgia	2	—
Hypersensitivity reaction	—	2

Hainsworth JD et al. JCO 1997;15:2385–2393

Therapy Monitoring

1. *Weekly:* CBC with differential platelet count
2. *Response evaluation:* after 2 treatment cycles. If objective response or stable disease with symptomatic improvement recorded, administer 2 more cycles for a total of 4 cycles

Notes

1. Responses are similar in adenocarcinoma and poorly differentiated carcinoma
2. This regimen is easier to administer and less toxic than cisplatin-based regimens
3. Toxicity is primarily myelosuppression

REGIMEN

GEMCITABINE + IRINOTECAN

Doss HH et al. Proc Am Soc Clin Oncol 2004;23:354 [Abstract 4167]
Greco FA et al. Proc Am Soc Clin Oncol 2002;21:161a [Abstract 642]
Hainsworth JD et al. Cancer Invest 2001;19:335–339
Ryo H et al. Gan To Kagaku Ryoho 2003;30:237–242

Premedication (suggested antiemetic regimen):
Granisetron 1 mg orally or intravenously per push (or comparable dose of another 5-HT_3-receptor antagonist) 30 minutes before chemotherapy
Dexamethasone 20 mg orally or intravenously per push 15–30 minutes before chemotherapy

Gemcitabine 1000 mg/m^2 intravenously diluted with 0.9% NaCl (0.9% NS) injection to a concentration ≥0.1 mg/mL over 30 minutes, given on days 1 and 8 every 21 days (total dosage per cycle: 2000 mg/m^2)

Irinotecan 100 mg/m^2 intravenously diluted with 5% dextrose injection (D5W) to a concentration within the range of 0.12–2.8 mg/mL over 90 minutes, given on days 1 and 8 every 21 days (total dosage per cycle = 200 mg/m^2)
Management of irinotecan diarrhea:
Loperamide 4 mg orally at first onset of diarrhea. Followed with loperamide 2 mg orally every 2 hours, continuously until diarrhea resolves for at least 12 hours. During sleep, change schedule to loperamide 4 mg orally every 4 hours

Emetogenic potential: Moderately high (Emetogenicity score = 4). See Chapter 39

Treatment Modifications[a]

Adverse Event	Dose Modification[b]
ANC >1500/mm^3 *and* platelet count >100,000/mm^3	Administer 100% dosage
ANC 1000–1500/mm^3 *or* platelet count 75,000–100,000/mm^3	Reduce gemcitabine and irinotecan dosages by 25%
ANC <1000/mm^3 *or* platelet count <75,000/mm^3	Delay treatment one week, or until ANC >1000/mm^3 *and* platelets >100,000/mm^3, then administer 75% dosage
G3/4 Diarrhea[c]	Hold irinotecan until diarrhea G ≤ 1; reduce irinotecan dosage to 75% for all subsequent doses
Other reversible G3/4 nonhematologic toxicity	Administer 75% dosage of the offending drug in subsequent courses

[a] Hematopoietic growth factors are used as secondary prophylaxis at the discretion of a treating physician, but should not substitute for recommended dose modifications
[b] Parameters for both day 1 and day 8
[c] G1/2 diarrhea administer 100% irinotecan dosage

Patient Population Studied

A multicenter community-based trial of 31 patients with previously treated (one prior regimen) CUP (adenocarcinoma, poorly differentiated carcinoma, poorly differentiated adenocarcinoma, or poorly differentiated neuroendocrine carcinoma) who received gemcitabine + irinotecan every 21 days for 6 cycles

Doss HH et al. Proc Am Soc Clin Oncol 2004;23:354 [Abstract 4167]

Efficacy (N = 31)

Complete response	4%
Partial response	11%
Stable disease	41%
Median time to progression	3.5 months
Median survival*	4 months
1-year survival	15%

*After a median follow-up of 7 months

Doss HH et al. Proc Am Soc Clin Oncol 2004;23:354 [Abstract 4167]

Toxicity (N = 31)

	% G3/4
Hematologic	
Neutropenia	30
Thrombocytopenia	8
Anemia	9
Febrile neutropenia	3
Nonhematologic	
Diarrhea	8
Nausea/vomiting	8
Fatigue	8

Therapy Monitoring

1. *Before each cycle:* CBC, serum electrolytes, BUN, creatinine, and LFTs
2. *Response evaluation:* Every 2 cycles

9. Cervical Cancer

Deirdre O'Mahony, MD, and Peter Rose, MD

Epidemiology

Incidence: 9,710 (estimated new cases in United States 2006)

Deaths: 3,700 (estimated deaths in United States in 2006)

Stage at Presentation	
Localized:	55%
Regional:	32%
Distant:	8%
Unstaged:	6%

National Cancer Institute, Surveillance, Epidemiology and End Results (SEER) program 1995–2001
Jemal A et al. CA Cancer J Clin 2006; 56:106–30

Work-Up

Stage IA/Stage IB1:	• H&P • CBC with platelet count, LFTs, BUN, creatinine • Cervical biopsy (pathologic review) • Cone biopsy as indicated • Chest x-ray, intravenous pyelogram, or CT/MRI optional
Stage IB2 or greater:	• Chest x-ray, intravenous pyelogram, or CT/MRI ± PET ± lymphangiogram • Consider examination under anesthesia
Stage III/IV:	• Consider cystoscopy/proctoscopy

Reproduced, with permission, of the American Joint Committee on Cancer (AJCC), Chicago, Illinois. The original source for this material is the AJCC Cancer Staging Manual, 6th edition (2002) published by Springer-Verlag, New York, www.springeronline.com.

Pathology

Squamous cell carcinomas • Large cell, keratinizing • Large cell, nonkeratinizing • Small cell (not neuroendocrine) • Verrucous carcinoma	75–80%
Adenocarcinomas • Adenoma malignum • Mucinous • Papillary • Endometrioid • Clear cell • Adenoid cystic	15–20%
Adenosquamous	Rare
Glassy cell carcinoma	Rare
Neuroendocrine small cell carcinoma	Rare

Hunter RD. In: Souhami RL, Tannock I, Hohenberger P, Horiot J-C, editors. Oxford Textbook of Oncology, 2nd ed. New York: Oxford University Press; 2002: 1835–1837

Histologic Grade

Gx	Cannot be assessed
G1	Well differentiated
G2	Moderately differentiated
G3	Poorly differentiated
G4	Undifferentiated

Staging

Primary Tumor

Stage		Description
TNM	FIGO	
Tx		Tumor cannot be assessed
T0	0	No evidence of primary tumor
Tis		Carcinoma in situ
T1	I	Tumor confined to corpus uteri
T1a	IA	Invasive tumor diagnosed only by microscopy. Stromal invasion with a maximum depth of 5 mm measured from the base of the epithelium and a horizontal spread of ≤7 mm
T1a1	IA1	Stromal invasion of ≤3 mm and ≤7 mm in horizontal spread
T1a2	IA2	Stromal invasion of >3 mm but <5 mm, and ≤7 mm in horizontal spread
T1b	IB	Clinically visible tumor confined to the cervix or microscopic lesion greater than T1a
T1b1	IB1	Clinically visible lesion ≤4 cm in greatest dimension
T1b2	IB2	Clinically visible lesion >4 cm in greatest dimension
T2	II	Tumor invades beyond uterus but not to pelvic wall or lower third of vagina
T2a	IIA	Tumor without parametrial invasion
T2b	IIB	Tumor with parametrial invasion
T3	III	Tumor extends to pelvic wall ± involves lower third of vagina ± causes hydronephrosis or nonfunctioning kidney
T3a	IIIA	Tumor involves lower third of vagina, no extension to pelvic wall
T3b	IIIB	Tumor extends to pelvic wall ± causes hydronephrosis or non-functioning kidney
T4	IVA	Tumor invades bladder mucosa or rectum ± extends beyond true pelvis

Regional Lymph Nodes

Nx	Regional nodes cannot be assessed
N0	No regional nodes involved
N1	Regional lymph node metastasis

Distant Metastasis

Mx	Distant metastasis cannot be assessed
M0	No distant metastasis
M1	Distant Metastasis

AJCC Stage Grouping

Stage	T	N	M
0	Tis	N0	M0
IA	T1	N0	M0
IA1	T1a1	N0	M0
IA2	T1a2	N0	M0
IB	T1b	N0	M0
IB1	T1b1	N0	M0
IB2	T1b2	N0	M0
II	T2	N0	M0
IIA	T2a	N0	M0
IIB	T2b	N0	M0
III	T3	N0	M0
IIIA	T3a	N0	M0
IIIB	T1	N1	M0
	T2	N1	M0
	T3a	N1	M0
	T3b	N1	M0
IVA	T4	Any N	M0
IVB	Any T	Any N	M1

AJCC Cancer Staging Manual, 6th ed. New York: Springer-Verlag, 2002:259–265

Overall 5-year Survival Relative to Figo Disease Stage

Stage	% Survival
IA1	94.6
IA2	92.6
IB	80.7
IB1	90.4
IB2	79.8
IIA	76
IIB	73.3
IIIA	50.5
IIIB	46.4
IVA	29.6
IVB	22

Caveats

1. The use of concurrent chemotherapy and radiation has reduced the overall mortality rate by nearly 50%
2. Concurrent chemoradiation should be given to women with high-risk local disease or regionally advanced disease
3. In cervical cancer, survival rates and rates of local control appear to correlate with radiation dose and the time of administration. Better results are achieved with higher radiation doses and shorter periods of administration
4. Chemotherapy agents with single-agent activity include:
   - **Cisplatin:** Considered the most active drug with response rates of 20–30%. At a dosage of 50 mg/m^2, cisplatin remains the platinum compound of choice despite less toxicity with carboplatin
   - **Ifosfamide:** Active in patients who have not received prior chemotherapy with response rates of 16–40% (Coleman RE et al. Cancer Chemother Pharmacol 1986;18:280–283; Meanwell CA et al. Cancer Treat Rep 1986;70:727–730; Sutton GP et al. Am J Obstet Gynecol 1993;168:805–807)
   - **Paclitaxel:** 17% response rate in GOG trial (McGuire WP et al. JCO 1996;14:792–795)
   - **Vinorelbine:** 18% response rate in patients with recurrent/metastatic carcinoma of the cervix (Morris M et al. JCO 1998;16:1094–1098; Lacava JA et al. JCO 1997;15:604–609); and 45% response rate in patients with previously untreated, locally advanced cervical cancer (Lhommé et al. Eur J Cancer 2000;36:194–199)
   - **Toptecan:** 18.6% response rate in advanced, recurrent, or persistent squamous cell carcinoma of the uterine cervix (Muderspach LI et al. Gynecol Oncol 2001;81:213–215)
   - **Gemcitabine:** 11–18% response rate in patients with advanced disease with symptomatic relief in 69–90% of patients (Goedhals L et al. [abstract 819] Proc Am Soc Clin Oncol 1996;15:296; Hansen HH. [abstract 058] Ann Oncol 1996;7[suppl 1]:29)
   - **Irinotecan;** 13.3% response rate in patients with recurrent squamous carcinoma of the cervix (Look KY et al. Gynecol Oncol 1998;70:334–338)
5. Despite activity, single agents have not had much impact on survival
6. Combination chemotherapy is essential if systemic treatment is to have an impact on survival
7. Platinum combinations yield high response rates, particularly in patients with no prior radiation therapy
8. Two randomized trials have shown improvement in progression-free survival (Long HJ III et al. JCO 2005;26:4626–4633, Moore DH et al. JCO 2004;22:3113–3119), with one trial demonstrating an improvement in survival (Long HJ III et al. JCO 2005;26:4626–4633) for combinations
9. The GOG is currently conducting a randomized trial comparing four cisplatin-based combinations with paclitaxel, topotecan, vinorelbine and gemcitabine

REGIMEN FOR INITIAL THERAPY

CONCURRENT RADIATION THERAPY + CHEMOTHERAPY/WEEKLY CISPLATIN

Keys HM et al. NEJM 1999;340:1154–1161
Rose PG et al. NEJM 1999;340:1144–1153

Note: Chemotherapy is given concomitantly with radiation therapy

Cisplatin 40 mg/m^2 per dose intravenously in 50–250 mL of 0.9% NaCl injection (0.9% NS) over 60 minutes weekly for 6 doses during weeks 1–6 (days 1, 8, 15, 22, 29, and 36) starting 4 hours before radiation therapy (total dosage/week = 40 mg/m^2)
Optional hydration with cisplatin: ≥500 mL 0.9% NS at ≥100 mL/hour before and after cisplatin administration. Also, encourage high oral intake and provide potassium and magnesium supplementation

Emetogenic potential: Moderately high (Emetogenicity score = 4). See Chapter 39 for antiemetic regimens

Patient Population Studied

Women with untreated invasive squamous cell carcinoma, adenosquamous carcinoma, or adenocarcinoma of the cervix of International Federation of Gynecology and Obstetrics stage IIB (localized disease with parametrial involvement) stage II (extension of tumor to the pelvic wall) or stage IVB (involvement of the bladder and rectal mucosa). Patients with disease outside the pelvis and those with metastases to para-aortic lymph nodes or intraperitoneal disease were not eligible

Efficacy (N = 176)

	%	*P* value[a]
Probability of progression-free survival at 48 months	62	0.001
Probability of survival at 48 months	66.5	0.004
Progression-free survival at 24 months	67[2]	—
Local progression	19[b]	—
Lung metastases	20[b]	—

[a]Compared with control group (RT + hydroxyurea)
[b]In control group (RT + hydroxyurea), progression-free survival at 24 mo = 47%, local progression = 30% and lung metastases = 10%

Rose PG et al. NEJM 1999;340:1144–1153

Toxicity (N = 176)

	% G1	% G2	% G3	% G4
Hematologic				
Leukopenia	17	26	21	2
Thrombocytopenia	15	4	2	0
Other hematologic	13	27	10	5
Nonhematologic				
Gastrointestinal	32	28	8	4
Genitourinary	11	6	3	2
Cutaneous	7	6	1	1
Neurologic	6	8	1	0
Pulmonary	0	1	0	0
Cardiovascular	0	0	0	0
Fever	2	4	0	0
Fatigue	5	3	0	0
Pain	2	2	0	0
Weight loss	2	2	1	0
Hypomagnesemia	3	2	2	1
Other*	5	2	1	2

NCI CTC

*Includes G3 renal abnormalities (serum creatinine 3.1–6 times institutional upper limit of normal), G3 electrolyte imbalance, G3 dehydration, G3 hepatic infection, G4 lymphopenia, G4 vaginal necrosis, G4 edema, and G4 renal abnormalities (serum creatinine >6 times institutional upper limit of normal)

G1, minimal; G2, mild; G3, moderate; G4, severe

Rose PG et al. NEJM 1999;340:1144–1153

Treatment Modifications

Adverse Event	Dose Modification
WBC <2000/mm^3	Delay radiation therapy for up to 1 week until WBC >2000/mm^3
Radiation-related gastrointestinal or genitourinary toxicity	Delay radiation therapy for up to 1 week until symptoms resolve
WBC <2500/mm^3 or platelet count <50,000/mm^3	Hold cisplatin until WBC >2500/mm^3 and platelet >50,000/mm^3
G2 Neurotoxicity	Reduce cisplatin dosage to 30 mg/m^2 per dose
≥ G3 Neurotoxicity	Discontinue cisplatin
Serum creatinine ≥2 mg/dL (177 micromol/L)	Reduce cisplatin dosage to 30 mg/m^2 per dose
Serum creatinine ≥2 mg/dL (177 micromol/L) despite reduction of cisplatin dosage to 30 mg/m^2	Discontinue cisplatin

Therapy Monitoring

Every week: CBC with differential, serum magnesium, BUN, and creatinine

Notes

1. Number of cycles of chemotherapy:

No. of Cycles	% of Patients
0	0.6
1	1.1
2	1.1
3	4
4	10.2
5	33.5
≥6	49.4

2. Radiation therapy (RT) administered:

Percentage of patients who received ≥85% of prescribed RT to both points A and B	90%
Median delay in patients receiving ≥85% of prescribed RT	8 days
Median duration of treatment	9 weeks

3. The rate of local recurrences was significantly lower than the comparison arm with hydroxyurea, whereas the rate of distant recurrences, especially in the lungs, was only slightly less. These results suggest that the principal effect of cisplatin is radiosensitization

REGIMEN FOR INITIAL THERAPY

CONCURRENT RADIATION THERAPY + CHEMOTHERAPY/CISPLATIN + FLUOROURACIL

Morris M et al. NEJM 1999;340:1137–1143
Peters WA III et al. JCO 2000;18:1606–1613
Whitney CW et al. JCO 1999;17:1339–1348

Notes:

- Chemotherapy is given concomitantly with radiation therapy (begin within 16 hours after the first radiation fraction is administered)
- One cycle is administered at the time of the second intracavitary insertion

Cisplatin 50–75 mg/m² per dose intravenously in 100–500 mL of 0.9% NaCl injection (0.9% NS) over 4 hours every 3 weeks for 3 cycles. Administration commences within 16 hours after starting radiation therapy (total dosage/3-week cycle = 50 – 75 mg/m²)
Optional hydration with cisplatin: ≥500 mL 0.9% NS at ≥100 mL/hour before and after cisplatin administration. Also, encourage high oral intake and provide potassium and magnesium supplementation

Fluorouracil 1000 mg/m² per day by continuous intravenous infusion in 100–1000 mL 0.9% NS or 5% dextrose injection (D5W) over 24 hours daily for 4 consecutive days (96-hour infusion) every 3 weeks (starting on days 1, 22, and 43). Administration commences immediately after completing cisplatin infusion (total dosage/cycle = 4000 mg/m²)

For delayed diarrhea:*
Loperamide 2 mg orally every 2 hours during waking hours (4 mg orally every 4 hours during hours of sleep). Continue for at least 12 hours after diarrhea resolves
If diarrhea persists >48 hours despite loperamide:
Stop loperamide and hospitalize patient for IV hydration
For persistent diarrhea:
Octreotide 100–150 mcg subcutaneously 3 times daily. Maximum total daily dose = 1500 mcg
Antibiotic therapy:
Ciprofloxacin 500 mg orally twice daily if absolute neutrophil count <500/mm³ (even with no fever or diarrhea), or if patient is febrile in association with diarrhea. Antibiotics should also be administered if patient is hospitalized with prolonged diarrhea and should be continued until diarrhea resolves

Emetogenic potential:
Day 1: Very high (Emetogenicity score = 6). Potential for delayed symptoms
Days 2 and 3: Low–moderate (Emetogenicity score = 2 – 3). See Chapter 39 for antiemetic regimens

*Rothenberg ML et al. JCO 2001;19:3801–3807
Wadler S et al. JCO 1998;16:3169–3178

Patient Population Studied

Women of all ages with squamous cell carcinoma, adenocarcinoma, or adenosquamous carcinoma of the cervix who had stages IIB through IVA according to the staging system of the International Federation of Gynecology and Obstetrics or stage IB or IIA with a tumor diameter of at least 5 cm or biopsy-proven metastases to the pelvic lymph nodes. Women were excluded who had disease outside the pelvic area or disease that had spread to para-aortic lymph nodes

Efficacy (N = 195)

5-year survival[a]	73%	$P = .004$[b]
5-year disease-free survival[a]	67%	$P = .001$[b]
Rate of distant relapse	14%	$P < .001$[b]
Rate of locoregional recurrence	19%	$P < .001$[b]

[a]Estimated from Kaplan-Meier curves
[b]*P* value compared with radiation therapy alone with estimated 5-year survival = 58%; estimated 5-year disease-free survival = 40%; rate of distant relapse = 33%; and rate of locoregional recurrence = 35%

Morris M et al. NEJM 1999;340:1137–1143

Treatment Modifications

Adverse Event	Dose Modification
WBC <2000/mm³	Delay radiation therapy for up to 1 week until WBC >2000/³
Radiation-related gastrointestinal or genitourinary toxicity	Delay radiation therapy for up to 1 week until symptoms resolve
WBC <2500/mm³ or platelet count <50,000/mm³	Hold cisplatin until WBC >2500/mm³ and platelet >50,000/mm³
WBC <3000/mm³ or platelet count <100,000/mm³	Hold fluorouracil until WBC >3000/³ and platelet >100,000/³
G3 WBC	Reduce fluorouracil dosage to 750 mg/m²
G4 WBC	Reduce fluorouracil dosage to 500 mg/m²
G3 Platelet count	Reduce fluorouracil dosage to 750 mg/m²
G4 Platelet count	Reduce fluorouracil dosage to 500 mg/m²
G3 Stomatitis or diarrhea	Reduce fluorouracil dosage to 750 mg/m²
G4 Stomatitis or diarrhea	Reduce fluorouracil dosage to 500 mg/m²
G2 Neurotoxicity	Reduce cisplatin dosage to 30 mg/m²
G ≥3 Neurotoxicity	Discontinue cisplatin
Serum creatinine ≥2 mg/dL (177 micromol/L)	Reduce cisplatin dosage to 30 mg/m²
Serum creatinine ≥2 mg/dL (177 micromol/L) despite reduction of cisplatin dosage to 30 mg/m²	Discontinue cisplatin

Toxicity (N = 193, 195)

Worst side effects reported during treatment or within 60 days after completion of treatment (N = 195)

	% G3	% G4	% G5
Skin abnormalities	2	1	0
Nausea and vomiting	7.2	1.5	0
Bowel/rectal abnormalities	6.2	2.6	0
Bladder abnormalities	1	0	0
Hematologic effects	29.2	8.2	0
Other	4.1	1.5	1
Maximal grade of toxicity	33	11	1
Maximal grade of nonhematologic toxicity	8	2	1

G3, moderate toxicity; .G4 severe toxicity; G5, fatal

Worst side effects of treatment occurring or persisting more than 60 days after completion of treatment (N = 193)

	% G3	% G4
Skin or subcutaneous tissue	0.5	0
Small bowel	0.5	2.1
Large bowel or rectum	2.1	6.7
Bladder	2.1	0.5
Uterus	0.5	1
Other	1	0.5
Maximal grade of toxicity	4	8

G3, moderate toxicity; G4, severe toxicity; G5, fatal

Morris M et al. NEJM 1999;340:1137–1143
Cooperative Group Common Toxicity Criteria
Acute Radiation Morbidity Scoring Criteria
Late Radiation Morbidity Scoring Scheme of the Radiation Therapy Oncology Group (RTOG) and the European Organization for Research and Treatment of Cancer (EORTC)

Therapy Monitoring

1. *Weekly during treatment:* Clinical assessment, CBC with differential and platelet count, and pelvic examination
2. *Before each cycle of chemotherapy:* CBC with differential and platelet count, serum magnesium, creatinine, urea nitrogen, alanine aminotransferase, alkaline phosphatase, and bilirubin
3. *At time of each intracavitary treatment:* Pelvic examination under anesthesia

Notes

Chemotherapy with cisplatin and fluorouracil is more effective than pelvic and para-aortic radiation alone

REGIMEN FOR INITIAL THERAPY

CONCURRENT RADIATION THERAPY + CHEMOTHERAPY/WEEKLY CARBOPLATIN

Duenas-Gonzalez A et al. Int J Radiat Oncol Biol Phys 2003;56:1361–1365
Higgins RV et al. Gynecol Oncol 2003;89:499–503

Carboplatin (calculated dose) AUC = 2* by intravenous infusion in 50–150 mL 5% dextrose injection (D5W) over 30 minutes on day 1 every 3 weeks (total dosage/cycle calculated to produce an AUC = 2 mg/mL/min)

Not routinely used but can be used if clinically indicated:
Filgrastim 5 mcg/kg per day subcutaneously daily until ANC has recovered to a value >2000–5000/mm^3

Emetogenic potential: Moderately high (Emetogenicity score = 4). See Chapter 39 for antiemetic regimens

*Carboplatin dose is based on Calvert's formula to achieve a target area under the plasma concentration versus time curve (AUC) [AUC units = mg/mL·min]

$$\text{Total carboplatin dose (mg)} = (\text{target AUC}) \times (\text{GFR} + 25)$$

In practice, creatinine clearance (Clcr) is used in place of glomerular filtration rate (GFR). Clcr can be calculated from the equation of Cockcroft and Gault:

$$\text{Females, Clcr} = \frac{(140 - \text{age[y]}) \times \text{body weight [kg]}}{72 \times (\text{Serum creatinine [mg/dl]})} \times 0.85$$

Calvert AH et al. JCO 1989;7:1748–1756
Cockcroft DW, Gault MH. Nephron 1976;16:31–41
Jodrell DI et al. JCO 1992;10:520–528
Sorensen BT et al. Cancer Chemother Pharmacol 1991;28:397–401

Efficacy (N = 31)

Complete response	90%
Disease-free at median follow-up 12 months	74%

Higgins RV et al. Gynecol Oncol 2003;89:499–503

Toxicity (N = 29)

	% G1	% G2	% G3	% G4
Hematologic				
Leukopenia	27.6	34.5	10.3	0
Neutropenia	41.4	20.7	3.4	0
Thrombocytopenia	17.2	3.4	6.9	0
Anemia	37.9	27.6	0	0
Nonhematologic				
Gastrointestinal	48.3	6.9	0	0
Genitourinary	34.5	13.8	0	0
Cutaneous	3.4	3.4	0	0

Higgins RV et al. Gynecol Oncol 2003;89:499–503

Treatment Modifications

Adverse Event	Dose Modification
ANC <500/mm^3 or platelet count <50,000/mm^3	Delay therapy for 1 week until ANC >500/^{3} and platelet count >50,000/mm^3
ANC 500–999/mm^3 or platelet count 50,000 >100,000/mm^3	Administer radiation therapy without carboplatin

Note: Do not reduce or escalate the dose of carboplatin

Patient Population Studied

Patients with stages IB-1, IB-2, IIA, IIB, IIIA, IIIB, IVA primary, invasive squamous cell carcinoma or adenocarcinoma, or adenosquamous carcinoma of the uterine cervix, not previously treated, without evidence of para-aortic nodal involvement by radiography or surgical evaluation

Therapy Monitoring

1. *Weekly during treatment:* Clinical assessment, CBC with differential and platelet count, and pelvic examination
2. *Weekly or every other week during treatment:* Serum creatinine, urea nitrogen, alanine aminotransferase, alkaline phosphatase, and bilirubin

Notes

Success rate in administering planned carboplatin treatments was 94%

REGIMEN FOR ADVANCED/ RECURRENT CERVICAL CANCER

CISPLATIN + VINORELBINE

Gebbia V et al. Oncology 2002;63:31–37

Hydration before cisplatin: ≥500 mL 0.9% NaCl injection (0.9% NS) at ≥100 mL/hour before and after cisplatin administration. Also, encourage high oral intake and provide potassium and magnesium supplementation
Mannitol diuresis: May be given to patients who have received adequate hydration. Administer 250 mL of a 15–25% mannitol solution intravenously over 1 hour before starting cisplatin or simultaneously with cisplatin. Continued hydration is essential with adequate fluid input during and for a minimum of 4 hours after the administration of mannitol

Note: Original study recommended 18% mannitol. Although this can be compounded, commercially available (ready-to-use) parenteral products in the United States include 5%, 10%, 15%, and 25% solutions

Cisplatin 80 mg/m^2 intravenously in 500 mL of 0.9% NS over 60 minutes on day 1 every 21 days (total dosage per cycle = 80 mg/m^2)

Vinorelbine 25 mg/m^2 per dose by intravenous infusion in a volume of 0.9% NS or 5% dextrose injection sufficient to produce a solution with a concentration of 1.5–3 mg/mL over 6–10 minutes for 2 doses on days 1 and 8 every 21 days (total dosage/cycle = 50 mg/m^2)

Emetogenic potential:
Day 1: High (Emetogenicity score = 5)
Day 8: Nonemetogenic (Emetogenicity score = 1). See Chapter 39 for antiemetic regimens

Patient Population Studied

A study of women with stage IV de novo or metastatic/recurrent cervical cancer no longer amenable to surgery and/or radiation therapy, with adequate hematopoietic, hepatic, and renal parameters, and a GOG performance status of 0–2

Efficacy (N = 42)

Complete response	12%
Partial response	36%
Median time to progression	5.6 months
Median overall survival	9.1 months

WHO Criteria

Toxicity (N = 42)

	% G1/2	% G3	% G4
Hematologic			
Neutropenia	26	21	12
Thrombocytopenia	19	—	—
Anemia	12	12	5
Nonhematologic			
Vomiting	52	21	—
Mucositis	14	—	—
Diarrhea	5	—	—
Constipation	38	—	—
Peripheral neuropathy	19	—	—
Alopecia	12	—	—

WHO Toxicity Criteria

Treatment Modifications

Adverse Event	Dose Modification
WBC <4000/mm^3 or platelet count <100,000/mm^3	Delay therapy for 1 week until WBC >4000/mm^3 and platelet count >100,000/mm^3
>G2 Neutropenia on day 8	Omit day 8 vinorelbine, and reduce all subsequent doses by 5 mg/m^2
Day 8 platelet count <50,000/mm^3	Omit vinorelbine dose
G2 Neurotoxicity	Reduce cisplatin dosage by 20 mg/m^2 and vinorelbine dosage by 5 mg/m^2
>G2 Neurotoxicity	Hold vinorelbine until neurotoxicity ≤G1; then reduce cisplatin dosage by 20 mg/m^2 and vinorelbine dosage by 5 mg/m^2
G1 Renal toxicity	Reduce all subsequent cisplatin dosages by 20 mg/m^2
≥G2 Renal toxicity	Hold cisplatin dose until renal toxicity ≤G1; then reduce all subsequent cisplatin dosages by 20 mg/m^2
G4 Nonhematologic toxicity	Discontinue therapy

Therapy Monitoring

1. *Before each cycle:* PE, CBC with differential, serum electrolytes, magnesium, BUN, and creatinine
2. *Every week:* CBC with differential, serum electrolytes, magnesium, BUN, and creatinine
3. *Response evaluation:* Every 3 cycles

REGIMEN FOR ADVANCED/ RECURRENT CERVICAL CANCER

CISPLATIN + TOPOTECAN

Long HJ III et al. JCO 2005;23:4626–4633 (GOG 204)

Topotecan HCl 0.75 mg/m² per day by intravenous infusion in 50–250 mL 0.9% NaCl injection (0.9% NS) or 5% dextrose injection (D5W) over 30 minutes for 3 consecutive days on days 1–3 every 21 days (total dosage/cycle = 2.25 mg/m²)

Hydration before and after cisplatin: ≥1000 mL 0.45% NaCl injection (0.45% NS) by intravenous infusion over a minimum of 2–4 hours
Cisplatin 50 mg/m² intravenously in 50–250 mL 0.9% NS at 1 mg/minute on day 1 every 21 days (total dosage/cycle = 50 mg/m²)
Note: Administer cisplatin within 4 hours after completing topotecan administration

Filgrastim (use only if indicated according to **Treatment Modifications**):
Filgrastim 5 mcg/kg per day subcutaneously starting 24–48 hours after completion of chemotherapy (days 4 or 5), until ANC count recovers to ≥10,000/mm³
Supportive care: Monitor and replace calcium, magnesium, and potassium as needed

Emetogenic potential:
Day 1: Very high (Emetogenicity score = 6). Potential for delayed symptoms
Days 2 and 3: Low (Emetogenicity score = 2). See Chapter 39 for antiemetic regimens

Patient Population Studied

A study of women with advanced (stage IVB), recurrent or persistent carcinoma of the uterine cervix, who were unsuitable candidates for curative treatment with surgery and/or radiation therapy. Histologic types included squamous, adenosquamous, and adenocarcinoma. Prior cisplatin therapy was allowed

Treatment Modifications

Cisplatin Dose Levels	
Initial dosage	50 mg/²
Dose level −1	37.5 mg/m²
Dose level −2	25 mg/m²

Toptecan Dose Levels	
Initial dosage	50 mg/m²
Dose level −1	37.5 mg/m²
Dose level −2	25 mg/m²

Topotecan Dosage Modifications

Total Bilirubin (mg/dL)	% Starting Topotecan Dosage
≤2.0	100
2.1–3.0	50
>3.0	25

Adverse Event	Dose Modification
Day 1 ANC <1500/mm³ or platelet count <100,000/mm³	Hold chemotherapy until ANC ≥1500/mm³ and platelet count ≥100,000/mm³
G4 Thrombocytopenia	Reduce topotecan dosage 1 level; continue with same cisplatin dosage
G3/4 ANC with fever	
G3/4 ANC with fever despite 1 dose level reduction	Administer filgrastim with all subsequent courses
G2/3/4 Nephrotoxicity	Hold cisplatin until serum creatinine ≤1.5 mg/dL (133 μmol/L); then resume treatment. If creatinine >1.5 mg/dL (133 μmol/L) >2 weeks beyond scheduled start of next cycle, discontinue cisplatin
G2 Peripheral neuropathy or ototoxicity*	Reduce cisplatin dosage by 2 levels
G3/4 Peripheral neuropathy or ototoxicity	Hold cisplatin until neuropathy ≤G1; then reduce cisplatin dosage by 2 levels. If G3/4 toxicity persists >2 weeks beyond scheduled start of next cycle, discontinue cisplatin
G4 Gastrointestinal toxicity	Continue cisplatin at same dosage
Second event of G4 gastrointestinal toxicity	Reduce cisplatin dosage by 1 level
G2/3 Mucositis or diarrhea	Reduce topotecan dosage by 1 level
G4 Mucositis or diarrhea	Reduce topotecan dosage by 1–2 levels
Recurrent mucositis or diarrhea despite dosage reduction or persistence of mucositis/ diarrhea >2 weeks beyond scheduled start of next cycle	Discontinue topotecan

*G2 ototoxicity consists of tinnitus and symptomatic hearing loss

Toxicity (N = 147)

	% G3	% G4
Hematologic		
Leukopenia	39.4	23.8
Granulocytopenia	24.5	45.6
Thrombocytopenia	24.5	6.8
Anemia	40	6.1
Other hematologic	11.6	2.7
Nonhematologic		
Infection	14.2	3.4
Renal	6.1	6.1
Nausea	12.2	1.4
Emesis	13.6	1.4
Other gastrointestinal	10.9	2.7
Metabolic	8.8	4.8
Neuropathy	0.7	—
Other neurologic	2	0.7
Cardiovascular	4.8	4.1
Pulmonary	2.7	—
Pain	19	2
Constitutional	7.5	—
Hemorrhage	5.4	0.7
Hepatic	3.4	1.4

NCI CTC

Efficacy (N = 147)

Complete response	10%
Partial response	16%
Stable disease	45%
Median progression-free survival	4.6 months
Median survival	9.4 months

GOG Criteria

Therapy Monitoring

1. *Once per week:* CBC with differential
2. *Before the start of a cycle:* CBC with differential, serum calcium, magnesium, potassium, bilirubin, and creatinine

REGIMEN FOR ADVANCED/ RECURRENT CERVICAL CANCER

CISPLATIN + PACLITAXEL

Moore DH et al. JCO 2004;22:3113–3119 (GOG 204)

Premedication for paclitaxel:
Dexamethasone 20 mg/dose orally or intravenously for 2 doses at 12 hours and 6 hours before paclitaxel
Note: If patient has no acute toxicities to paclitaxel, the dexamethasone doses at 12 hours and 6 hours before paclitaxel may eventually be omitted, *plus*
Dexamethasone 20 mg intravenously per push or in 10–50 mL 0.9% NaCl injection (0.9% NS) or 5% dextrose injection (D5W) over 10–15 minutes, 30 minutes before paclitaxel
Diphenhydramine 50 mg intravenously per push 30 minutes before paclitaxel
Cimetidine 300 mg or **ranitidine** 50 mg, *or*
Famotidine 20 mg intravenously in 20–50 mL 0.9% NS or D5W over 5–20 minutes, 30 minutes before paclitaxel

Paclitaxel 135 mg/m² by continuous intravenous infusion in a volume of 0.9% NS or D5W sufficient to produce a concentration of 0.3–1.2 mg/mL over 24 hours on day 1 every 3 weeks for 6 cycles (total dosage/cycle = 135 mg/m²)

Hydration before and after cisplatin:
≥1000 mL 0.45% NaCl injection by intravenous infusion over a minimum of 2–4 hours
Cisplatin 50 mg/m² intravenously in 50–250 mL 0.9% NS at a rate of 1 mg/minute on day 1 every 3 weeks for 6 cycles (total dosage/cycle = 50 mg/m²)
Note: Begin cisplatin within 4 hours after completing paclitaxel administration

Filgrastim (use only if indicated according to **Treatment Modifications***):*
Filgrastim 5 mcg/kg per day subcutaneously, starting 24–48 hours after chemotherapy is completed. Continue daily administration until ANC count recovers to ≥10,000/mm³
Supportive care: Monitor and replace calcium, magnesium, and potassium as needed

Emetogenic potential:
Day 1: Very high (Emetogenicity score = 6). Potential for delayed symptoms. See Chapter 39 for antiemetic regimens

Treatment Modifications

Cisplatin Dose Levels	
Initial dosage	50 mg/m²
Dose level −1	37.5 mg/²
Dose level −2	25 mg/m²

Paclitaxel Dose Levels	
Initial dosage	135 mg/m²
Dose level −1	110 mg/m²
Dose level −2	90 mg/m²

Adverse Event	Dose Modification
Day 1 ANC <1500/mm³ or platelet count <100,000/mm³	Hold chemotherapy until ANC ≥1500/mm³ and platelet count ≥100,000/mm³
ANC <1500/mm³ or platelet count <100,000/mm³ persist ≥2 weeks beyond the scheduled start of cycle	Discontinue therapy
G4 Thrombocytopenia	Reduce paclitaxel dosage by 1 level; continue with same cisplatin dosage
G3/4 ANC with fever[a]	
G3/4 ANC with fever despite 1 dose level reduction	Administer filgrastim with all subsequent courses
G3/4 ANC with fever despite paclitaxel dose reduction and filgrastim	Reduce paclitaxel dosage by 1 level or 20%; continue with same cisplatin dosage
G2 Peripheral neuropathy	Reduce paclitaxel dosage by 2 levels
G3/4 Peripheral neuropathy	Hold paclitaxel until neuropathy ≤G1; then reduce paclitaxel dosage by 2 levels. If G3/4 toxicity persists >2 weeks beyond scheduled start of next cycle, discontinue paclitaxel
G2 Hepatic toxicity	Hold paclitaxel until toxicity ≤G1; then reduce paclitaxel dosage by 1 level
G3/4 Hepatic toxicity	Hold paclitaxel until toxicity ≤G1; then reduce paclitaxel dosage by 1–2 levels. If G3/4 toxicity persists >2 weeks beyond scheduled start of cycle, discontinue paclitaxel
G2/3/4 Nephrotoxicity	Hold cisplatin until serum creatinine ≤1.5 mg/dL (133 μmol/L); then resume treatment.

(*continued*)

Treatment Modifications (*continued*)

Adverse Event	Dose Modification
	Discontinue cisplatin if creatinine >1.5 mg/dL (133 μmol/L) >2 weeks beyond scheduled start of next cycle
G2 Peripheral neuropathy or ototoxicity[b]	Reduce cisplatin dosage by 2 levels
G3/4 Peripheral neuropathy or ototoxicity	Hold cisplatin until neuropathy ≤G1 then reduce cisplatin dosage by 2 dose levels. If G3/4 toxicity persists >2 weeks beyond scheduled start of next cycle, discontinue cisplatin
G4 Gastrointestinal toxicity	Continue cisplatin at same dosage
Second event of G4 gastrointestinal toxicity	Reduce cisplatin dosage 1 level

[a]Use filgrastim if felt beneficial
[b]G2 Ototoxicity consisits of tinnitus and symptomatic hearing loss

Note: Management of paclitaxel hypersensitivity reaction:
1. Discontinue infusion
2. Wait for symptoms to resolve
3. If symptoms were not life-threatening repeat premedications (dexamethasone, diphenhydramine, and cimetidine or ranitidine or famotidine) in preparation for restarting infusion
4. Administer 1 mL of the original paclitaxel solution diluted in 100 mL of the same base solution over 1 hour, *then*
5. Administer 5 mL of the original paclitaxel solution diluted in 100 mL of the same base solution over 1 hour, *then*
6. Administer 10 mL of the original paclitaxel solution diluted in 100 mL of the same base solution over 1 hour, *then*
7. Administer the remaining original solution at the original infusion rate

Patient Population Studied

A study of women with advanced (stage IVB), recurrent, or persistent squamous cell carcinoma of the uterine cervix. Twenty-four percent had received prior chemotherapy and radiation

Efficacy (N = 130)

Complete response	15%
Partial response	21%
Overall response rate (ORR)	36%
ORR, prior chemoradiotherapy (n = 31)	32%
ORR, no prior chemoradiotherapy (n = 99)	37%
Progression-free survival	4.8 months
Progression-free survival, no prior therapy	4.9 months
Median survival	9.7 months
Median survival, no prior therapy	9.9 months

Toxicity (N = 129)

	% G1	% G2	% G3	% G4
Hematologic				
Leukopenia	12.4	22.5	35.7	17
Granulocytopenia	7.8	7.8	20.9	45.7
Thrombocytopenia	30.2	3.1	1.6	2.3
Anemia	10.9	31	22.5	5.4
Nonhematologic				
Nausea/vomiting	29.5	20.9	9.3	0.8
Other gastrointestinal	14	9.3	6.2	0.8
Cardiac	1.6	1.6	1.6	0
Neurologic	19.4	13.2	3.1	0
Fever	1.6	13.2	0	0.8
Dermatologic	2.3	1.6	1.6	0.8
Alopecia	11.6	52.7	0	0
Genitourinary	6.2	10.9	0.8	0
Renal	4.7	7	2.3	0

Therapy Monitoring

1. *Every 15 minutes for the first hour of the paclitaxel infusion:* Vital signs including blood pressure, respiratory rate, and temperature
2. *Once per week:* CBC with differential
3. *Before the start of a cycle:* CBC with differential, serum calcium, magnesium, potassium, bilirubin, and creatinine

REGIMEN FOR ADVANCED/ RECURRENT CERVICAL CANCER

CISPLATIN + GEMCITABINE

Burnett AF et al. Gynecol Oncol 2000;76:63–66 (GOG 204)

Gemcitabine 1000 mg/m^2 per dose intravenously diluted to a concentration ≥0.1 mg/mL in 0.9% NaCl injection (0.9% NS) over 30 minutes for 2 doses on days 1 and 8 every 21 days (total dosage/cycle = 2500 mg/m^2)

Note: After gemcitabine administration, flush the patient's vascular access device with 75–125 mL of 0.9% NS

Hydration before and after cisplatin: ≥1000 mL 0.45% NaCl injection (0.45% NS) by intravenous infusion over a minimum of 2–4 hours

Cisplatin 50 mg/m^2 intravenously in 100 mL 0.9% NS over 60 minutes on day 1 every 21 days (total dosage/cycle = 50 mg/m^2)

Note: Administer cisplatin within 4 hours after completing gemcitabine.

Filgrastim (use only if indicated according to* Treatment Modifications*):

Filgrastim 5 mcg/kg per day subcutaneously, starting 24–48 hours after chemotherapy is completed. Continue daily administration until ANC recovers to ≥10,000/mm^3

Supportive care: Monitor and replace calcium, magnesium, and potassium as needed

Emetogenic potential:

Day 1: High (Emetogenicity score = 6).

Day 8: Low (Emetogenicity score = 2). See Chapter 39 for antiemetic regimens

Patient Population Studied

Phase II trial in patients with advanced, persistent, or recurrent squamous cell carcinoma of the cervix

Treatment Modifications

Cisplatin Dose Levels	
Initial dosage	50 mg/m^2
Dose level −1	37.5 mg/m^2
Dose level −2	25 mg/m^2

Gemcitabine Dose Levels	
Initial dosage	1000 mg/m^2
Dose level −1	800 mg/m^2
Dose level −2	600 mg/m^2

Gemcitabine Dosage Modification

Total Bilirubin (mg/dL)	% of Starting Gemcitabine Dosage
≤2.0	100
2.1–3.0	50
>3.0	25

Note: Gemcitabine dose reductions at any time after day 1 of cycle 1 will be continued throughout the rest of the study

Adverse Event	Dose Modification
Day 1 ANC <1500/mm^3 or platelet count <100,000/mm^3	Hold chemotherapy until ANC ≥1500/mm^3 and platelet count ≥100,000/mm^3
ANC <1500/mm^3 or platelet count <100,000/mm^3 that persist ≥3 weeks beyond the scheduled start of cycle	Discontinue therapy
>2-weeks delay until ANC ≥1500/mm^3 and platelet count ≥100,000/mm^3	Reduce gemcitabine by 1 dosage level
Day 8 ANC ≥1500/mm^3 or platelet count ≥100,000/mm^3	Administer day 1 gemcitabine dosage on day 8
Day 8 ANC 1000–1499/mm^3 or platelet count 75,000–99,000/mm^3	Reduce gemcitabine by 1 dosage level from day 1 level on day 8
Day 8 ANC <1500/mm^3 or platelet count <100,000/mm^3	Hold day 8 gemcitabine dosage; reduce gemcitabine dosage by 1 level in ensuing cycles on day 8
G4 Thrombocytopenia	Reduce gemcitabine by dosage 1 level; continue with same cisplatin dosage
G3/4 ANC with fever[a]	Reduce gemcitabine dosage by 1 level; continue with same cisplatin dosage
G3/4 ANC with fever despite 1 dose level reduction	Administer filgrastim with all subsequent courses
G3/4 ANC with fever despite gemcitabine dose reduction and filgrastim	Reduce gemcitabine dosage 1 level or 20%; continue with same cisplatin dosage
G1 Mucositis or diarrhea	Hold gemcitabine until toxicity resolves; then resume with same dosage
G2/3 Mucositis or diarrhea	Hold gemcitabine until toxicity ≤G1; reduce subsequent dosages by 1 level

(continued)

Treatment Modifications (*continued*)

Adverse Event	Dose Modification
Mucositis or diarrhea that is G4 or that persists >2 weeks, or repeated episodes of persistent toxicity ≥G2	Hold gemcitabine until toxicity ≤G1; consider discontinuing gemcitabine
G2/3/4 Nephrotoxicity	Hold cisplatin until serum creatinine ≤1.5 mg/dL (133 μmol/L) then resume treatment. If creatinine >1.5 mg/dL (133 μmol/L) >2 weeks beyond scheduled start of next cycle, discontinue cisplatin
G2 Peripheral neuropathy or ototoxicity[b]	Reduce cisplatin dosage by 2 levels
G3/4 Peripheral neuropathy or ototoxicity	Hold cisplatin and gemcitabine until neuropathy ≤G1 then reduce cisplatin dosage by 2 dose levels. If G3/4 toxicity persists >2 weeks beyond scheduled start of next cycle, discontinue cisplatin
G4 Gastrointestinal toxicity	Continue cisplatin at same dosage
Second event of G4 gastrointestinal toxicity	Reduce cisplatin dosage 1 level

[a]Use filgrastim if felt beneficial
[b]G2 Ototoxicity consists of tinnitus and symptomatic hearing loss. If neurotoxicity occurs, it will most likely be cisplatin-related

Efficacy (N = 17)

Complete response	5.9%
Partial response*	35.3%
Median survival patients with response	12 months
Median survival patients without response	7 months

*Six patients; three had received prior radiation therapy
GOG Response Criteria

Toxicity (N = 82 cycles)

	% G3	% G4
Hematologic		
Neutropenia	7.3	2.4
Anemia	1.2	1.2
Median leukocyte nadir	3145/mm³	
Median platelet nadir	174,000/mm³	
Nonhematologic		
Gastrointestinal	2.4	0

Therapy Monitoring

1. *Once per week:* CBC with differential
2. Before start of a cycle: CBC with differential, serum calcium, magnesium, potassium, bilirubin, and creatinine

REGIMEN FOR ADVANCED/ RECURRENT CERVICAL CANCER

CISPLATIN + IRINOTECAN

Chitapanarux I et al. Gynecol Oncol 2003;89:402–407

Irinotecan 60 mg/m^2 per dose intravenously diluted in a volume of 5% dextrose injection (D5W) or 0.9% NaCl injection (0.9% NS) sufficient to produce a concentration of 0.12–2.8 mg/mL over 90 minutes for 3 doses on days 1, 8, and 15 every 28 days, (total dosage/cycle = 180 mg/m^2)
Hydration before and after cisplatin:
≥1000 mL 0.45% NaCl injection by intravenous infusion over a minimum of 2–4 hours
Note: Encourage high oral intake and provide potassium and magnesium supplementation

Cisplatin 60 mg/m^2 intravenously in 500 mL of 0.9% NS over 90 minutes on day 1 after completing irinotecan administration every 28 days (total dosage per cycle = 60 mg/m^2)

Regimen for delayed diarrhea:
Loperamide 4 mg orally after first loose stool, *then*:
Loperamide 2 mg orally with each loose stool to a maximum daily dose of 24 mg until 12 hours after the last loose stool or for a maximum of 48 hours—whichever condition occurs first
If diarrhea persists >24 hours despite loperamide: Add oral prophylactic broad-spectrum antibiotic.
Ciprofloxacin 500 mg orally twice daily if absolute neutrophil count <500/mm^3 (even in the absence of fever or diarrhea) or if patient is febrile in association with diarrhea. Antibiotics should also be administered if patient is hospitalized with prolonged diarrhea and should be continued until resolution of diarrhea
If diarrhea persists >48 hours despite loperamide: Stop loperamide and hospitalize patient for IV hydration. Consider an alternative antidiarrheal treatment:
Octreotide 100–150 mcg subcutaneously 3 times daily. Maximum total daily dose = 1500 mcg
Regimen for acute cholinergic syndrome:
Atropine sulfate 0.25–1 mg subcutaneously. If symptoms are severe, add prophylaxis during subsequent cycles

Emetogenic potential:
Day 1: Very high (Emetogenicity score = 6)
Days 8 and 15: Moderate (Emetogenicity score = 3). See Chapter 39 for antiemetic regimens

Patient Population Studied

Chemotherapy-naive women with metastatic or recurrent cervical cancer, with measurable disease, adequate hematopoietic, renal, and hepatic function, and with a WHO performance status of 0–2

Efficacy (N = 30)

Complete response	6.7%
Partial response	60%
Median survival	16.9 months
Median time to progression	13.4 months

WHO Criteria

Toxicity (N = 30)

	% G1	% G2	% G3	% G4
Hematologic				
Neutropenia	26.7	26.7	30	—
Anemia	13.3	46.6	16.7	—
Thrombocytopenia	—	—	—	—
Nonhematologic				
Alopecia	50	50	—	—
Acute diarrhea	16.7	3.3	—	—
Late-onset diarrhea	33.3	10	—	—
Nausea/vomiting	30	40	23.3	—
Renal	3.3	20	20	6.7

With respect to nonhematologic toxicity, renal dysfunction was the most significant; 2 patients developed G4 creatinine elevations
NCI CTC

Treatment Modifications

Adverse Event	Dose Modification
WBC <4000/mm^3, platelet count <100,000/mm^3, or diarrhea	Delay start of cycle by 1 week until WBC >4000/mm^3, platelet count >100,000/mm^3, and no diarrhea
Day 8 or 15 WBC <3000/mm^3 or platelet count <100,000/mm^3	Hold irinotecan
>G1 Diarrhea	Hold irinotecan
If WBC <1000/mm^3, platelet count <50,000/mm^3, or diarrhea >G2 at any time in cycle	Reduce subsequent irinotecan dosage by 50%
Serum creatinine >1.5 × upper limits of normal	Reduce cisplatin to 50 mg/m^2

Therapy Monitoring

1. *Before each cycle:* PE, CBC with differential, serum magnesium, BUN, creatinine, electrolytes, and liver function tests
2. *Weekly:* CBC with differential and serum creatinine
3. *Response evaluation:* After cycles 1 and 2 and every 2 cycles thereafter

10. Colorectal Cancer

Gregory Leonard, MD, and Jean Grem, MD

Epidemiology

Incidence: Male: Female:	Age-adjusted 1997–2001 63.4/100,000 46.4/100,000
Prevalence: Colon Rectal	 106,680 estimated new cases in 2006 41,930 estimated new cases in 2006
Mortality rate:	55,170 estimated deaths from colon and rectal cancer in 2006
Median age:	65 years
Male/female ratio:	Slight increase in incidence in males
Stage at presentation:	Stage I: 15% Stage II: 20–30% Stage III: 30–40% Stage IV: 20–25%

www.seer.cancer.gov
Jemal A et al. CA Cancer J Clin 2006;56:106–30
Skibber JM et al. Cancer of the colon. In: Devita VT Jr, Hellman S, Rosenberg SA, eds. Cancer: Principles and Practice of Oncology, 6th ed. Philadelphia: Lippincott Williams & Wilkins, 2001:1216–1270

Pathology

World Health Organization Classification

1. Adenocarcinoma (>90%)
2. Mucinous adenocarcinoma
3. Adenosquamous carcinoma
4. Small cell carcinoma
5. Medullary carcinoma
6. Signet ring adenocarcinoma
7. Squamous cell carcinoma
8. Undifferentiated
9. Other

Skibber JM et al. Cancer of the colon. In: Devita VT, Jr, Hellman S, Rosenberg SA, editors. Cancer: Principles and Practice of Oncology, 6th ed. Philadelphia: Lippincott Williams & Wilkins, 2001:1216–1270

Work-Up

In situ and Stage I	H&P, carcinoembryonic antigen (CEA), full colonoscopy, and pathology review
Stage II	H&P, CBC, serum electrolytes, LFTs, serum creatinine, BUN, and CEA. Full colonoscopy, chest x-ray, CT scan of abdomen, and pelvis, pathology review *Rectal lesions:* Transrectal ultrasound. MRI may also be useful
Stage III	As above for stages I–II. If patient has potentially resectable disease, additional studies may be needed before laparotomy to confirm resectability, including spiral CT scan, contrast MRI, PET scan, angiography, and laparoscopy
Stage IV	As above plus CT scan of chest

Skibber JM et al. Cancer of the colon. In: Devita VT, Jr, Hellman S, Rosenberg SA, editors. Cancer: Principles and Practice of Oncology, 6th ed. Philadelphia: Lippincott Williams & Wilkins, 2001:1216–1270

TNM Staging

Primary Tumor (T)

TX	Primary tumor cannot be assessed
TO	No evidence of primary tumor
T1s	Carcinoma in situ
T1	Tumor invades submucosa
T2	Tumor invades muscularis propria
T3	Tumor invades through the muscularis propria into the subserosa, or into nonperitonealized, pericolic, or perirectal tissues
T4	Tumor directly invades other organs or structures, and/or perforates visceral peritoneum

Reproduced, with permission, of the American Joint Committee on Cancer (AJCC), Chicago, Illinois. The original source for this material is the AJCC Cancer Staging Manual, 6th edition (2002) published by Springer-Verlag, New York, www.springeronline.com.

Regional Lymph Nodes (N)

NX	Regional lymph nodes cannot be assessed
N0	No regional lymph node metastasis
N1	Metastasis in 1–3 regional lymph nodes
N2	Metastasis in ≥4 regional lymph nodes

Distant Metastasis (M)

MX	Distant metastasis cannot be assessed
M0	No distant metastasis
M1	Distant metastasis

TNM Stage/Dukes Stage

TNM Stage		Dukes Stage
Stage 0	Tis N0 M0	—
Stage I	T1-2 N0 M0	A
Stage IIA	T3 N0 M0	B
Stage IIB	T4 N0 M0	B
Stage IIIA	T1-2 N1 M0	C
Stage IIIB	T3-4 N1 M0	C
Stage IIIC	Any T N2 M0	C
Stage IV	Any T Any N M1	D

Five-Year Survival

	Colon	Rectal
I	>90%	>90%
II	75–85%	70–85%
IIIA	59%	55%
IIIB	42%	35%
IIIC	27%	24%
IV	<5%	<5%

AJCC Cancer Staging Manual, 6th ed. New York: Springer-Verlag, 2002:113–123
Greene FL et al. Ann Surg 2002;236:416–421
Greene FL et al. [Abstract 1007] Proc Am Soc Clin Oncol 2003;22:251

Caveats

Stage II colon cancer: An American Society of Clinical Oncology Panel, in collaboration with the Cancer Care Ontario Practice Guideline Initiative, found no evidence of a statistically significant survival benefit of adjuvant chemotherapy for stage II patients. Consequently, the routine use of adjuvant chemotherapy for medically fit patients with stage II colon cancer is not recommended. However, there are populations of patients with stage II disease that could be considered for adjuvant therapy, such as patients with inadequately sampled nodes, T4 lesions, perforation, or poorly differentiated histology

Stage III colon cancer: Systemic combined chemotherapy is the principal adjuvant therapy for stage III colon cancer. Such treatment is associated with ~30% reduction in the risk of disease recurrence, and 22–32% reduction in mortality rate. For patients with stage III, the NCCN panel recommends 5-fluorouracil/leucovorin, capecitabine, or 5-fluorouracil/leucovorin/oxaliplatin–based adjuvant therapy

Stage IV colon cancer: The choice of therapy is based on consideration of the type and timing of the prior therapy that has been administered and the differing toxicity profiles of the constituent drugs. Patients with previously untreated advanced or metastatic disease should be treated with FOLFOX or FOLFIRI or 5-fluorouracil/leucovorin plus bevacizumab or capecitabine. Patients with progressive disease who have received 5-fluorouracil-based first-line therapy should be treated with second- or third-line chemotherapy consisting of FOLFIRI, FOLFOX, or irinotecan in combination with cetuximab. Current data do not support the use of bevacizumab in second- or third-line regimens after progression on a first-line bevacizumab-containing regimen

Rectal cancer: Either preoperative chemoradiation or postoperative chemoradiotherapy is standard for patients with suspected or proven serosal invasion (pT3) and/or regional node involvement. Patients with recurrent localized disease should be considered for resection with or without radiotherapy. Chemotherapy regimens (FOLFOX, FOLFIRI, 5-fluorouracil/leucovorin, IFL, CapOX or irinotecan) with or without bevacizumab/cetuximab should be considered for patients with distant metastasis

Benson Al B et al JCO;2004;22:1–12
Meyerhardt JA et al NEJM 2005;352:476–487
National Comprehensive Cancer Network, vol. 2,2006

ADJUVANT AND ADVANCED REGIMEN

BOLUS FLUOROURACIL + LEUCOVORIN (ROSWELL PARK REGIMEN)

Petrelli N et al. JCO 1989;7:1419–1426
Wolmark N et al. JCO 1999;17:3553–3559

Adjuvant therapy:
Leucovorin calcium 500 mg/m^2 intravenously in 250 mL 0.9% NaCl injection (0.9% NS) over 2 hours once per week for 6 consecutive weeks (weeks 1–6) every 8 weeks (total dosage/cycle = 3000 mg/m^2)
Fluorouracil 500 mg/m^2 intravenously per push over 1–2 minutes, starting 1 hour after leucovorin once per week for 6 consecutive weeks (weeks 1–6) every 8 weeks (total dosage/cycle = 3000 mg/m^2)

Advanced colorectal cancer:
Leucovorin calcium 500 mg/m^2 intravenously in 250 mL 0.9% NS over 2 hours once per week for 6 consecutive weeks (weeks 1–6) every 8 weeks (total dosage/cycle = 3000 mg/m^2)
Fluorouracil 600 mg/m^2 intravenously per push over 1–2 minutes, starting 1 hour after leucovorin once per week for 6 consecutive weeks (weeks 1–6) every 8 weeks (total dosage/cycle = 3600 mg/m^2)

*Management of diarrhea**
For delayed diarrhea:
Loperamide 2 mg orally every 2 hours during waking hours (4 mg orally every 4 hours during hours of sleep). Continue for at least 12 hours after diarrhea resolves
If diarrhea persists >48 hours despite loperamide: Stop loperamide and hospitalize patient for intravenous hydration
For persistent diarrhea:
Octreotide 100–150 mcg subcutaneously 3 times daily. Maximum total daily dose = 1500 mcg
Antibiotic therapy:
Ciprofloxacin 500 mg orally twice daily if absolute neutrophil count <500/mm^3 (even with no fever or diarrhea) or if patient is febrile in association with diarrhea. Antibiotics should also be administered if patient is hospitalized with prolonged diarrhea and should be continued until diarrhea resolves

Emetogenic potential: Low (Emetogenicity score = 2). See Chapter 39 for antiemetic regimens

*Rothenberg ML et al. JCO 2001;19:3801–3807
*Wadler S et al. JCO 1998;16:3169–3178

Treatment Modifications

Adverse Event	Dose Modification*
Any G1 toxicity	Maintain dose
Any G2 toxicity	Hold treatment until toxicity resolves to G ≤1. If toxicity occurs after the fourth weekly dose, stop until the next cycle; then resume at same dosage. If diarrhea occurs, reduce fluorouracil to 400 mg/m^2 per dose
Any G3/4 toxicity	Hold treatment until toxicity resolves to G ≤ 1. If toxicity occurs after the fourth weekly dose, stop until next cycle; then resume at 400 mg/m^2 per dose. If diarrhea occurs, reduce fluorouracil to 350 mg/m^2 per dose
Further toxicity	Reduce fluorouracil to 300 mg/m^2 per dose. If diarrhea occurs, reduce fluorouracil to 250 mg/m^2 dose

*Leucovorin dosage remains constant at 500 mg/m^2 per dose

Adapted from NSABP C-07 protocol
Wolmark et al. Proc Am Soc Clin Oncol 2005;23:246S Abstract 3500

Patient Population Studied

Patients with stage II (Dukes' B) or III (Dukes' C) colorectal cancer after potentially curative resection (duration of therapy was 4 cycles)

Wolmark N et al. JCO 1999;17:3553–3559

Efficacy (N = 691)

	5-Year DFS	5-Year Overall Survival
All patients	65%	74%
Stage II	75%	84%
Stage III	57%	67%

DFS, disease-free survival

Toxicity (N ≅ 691)

Most Common Toxicities by Grade

Toxicity	% G0	% G1	% G2	% G3	% G4
Overall	4	16	45	26	9
Diarrhea	21	15	37	22	5
Stomatitis	72	18	9	1	<1
Vomiting	66	14	15	3	2
Hematologic				<2	
Neurologic				2% ataxia	
Death					4 patients

Wolmark N et al. JCO 1999;17:3553–3539

Therapy Monitoring

1. *Before each cycle:* H&P, CBC with differential, CEA, serum electrolytes, creatinine, BUN, and LFTs
2. *Every 2–3 months:* CT scans to assess cancer status in patients presenting with advanced colorectal cancer

ADJUVANT AND ADVANCED REGIMEN

BOLUS FLUOROURACIL (MAYO CLINIC)

Francini G et al. Gastroenterology 1994;106:899–906
Poon MA et al. JCO 1989;7:1407–1418
Van Cutsem E et al. JCO 2001;19:4097–4106

Leucovorin calcium 20 mg/m^2 per day by intravenous injection over 30 seconds on 5 consecutive days, given on days 1–5 every 4 weeks for 6 cycles (total dosage/cycle = 100 mg/m^2)
Fluorouracil 425 mg/m^2 per day intravenously per push over 1–2 minutes after leucovorin on 5 consecutive days, given on days 1–5 every 4 weeks for 6 cycles (total dosage/cycle = 2125 mg/m^2)

or

Leucovorin calcium 200 mg/m^2 per day by intravenous injection over 30 seconds on 5 consecutive days, given on days 1–5 every 4 weeks for 6 cycles (total dosage/cycle = 1000 mg/m^2)
Fluorouracil 400 mg/m^2 per day intravenously per push over 1–2 minutes after leucovorin on 5 consecutive days, given on days 1–5 every 4 weeks for 6 cycles (total dosage/cycle = 2000 mg/m^2)

*Management of diarrhea**
For delayed diarrhea:
Loperamide 2 mg orally every 2 hours during waking hours (4 mg orally every 4 hours during hours of sleep). Continue for at least 12 hours after diarrhea resolves
If diarrhea persists >48 hours despite loperamide: Stop loperamide and hospitalize patient for IV hydration
For persistent diarrhea:
Octreotide 100–150 mcg subcutaneously 3 times daily. Maximum total daily dose = 1500 mcg
Antibiotic therapy:
Ciprofloxacin 500 mg orally twice daily if absolute neutrophil count <500/mm^3 (even without fever or diarrhea) or if patient is febrile in association with diarrhea. Antibiotics should also be administered if patient is hospitalized with prolonged diarrhea and should be continued until diarrhea resolves

Emetogenic potential: Low (Emetogenicity score = 2). See Chapter 39 for antiemetic regimens

*Rothenberg ML et al. JCO 2001;19:3801–3807
*Wadler S et al. JCO 1998;16:3169–3178

Patient Population Studied

Patients with stage II or III colorectal cancer after potentially curative resection, or with advanced colorectal cancer

Efficacy (N = 301)

Complete response	0.7%
Partial response	14.3%
Stable disease	55.5%
Mean duration of response	9.4 months
Median time to progression	4.7 months
Median survival	12.1 months

Van Cutsem E et al. JCO 2001;19:4097–4106

Treatment Modifications

Adverse Event	Dose Modification*
No toxicity	Optional escalation of fluorouracil dosage by 10%
G1 Toxicity	Maintain dose
G2 Nonhematologic adverse events	Reduce fluorouracil dosage by 20%
G3 Hematologic adverse events	Reduce fluorouracil dosage by 20%
G3/4 Nonhematologic adverse events	Reduce fluorouracil dosage by 30%
G4 Hematologic adverse events	Reduce fluorouracil dosage by 30%

*Leucovorin dosage remains constant at 500 mg/m^2 per dose
Van Cutsem E et al. JCO 2001;19:4097–4106

Toxicity (N = 299)

	% All G	% G3	% G4
Nonhematologic			
Stomatitis	55	13	0.3
Diarrhea	48	9.4	1
Nausea	39	—	—
Vomiting	25	—	—
Fatigue	12	—	—
Hand-foot syndrome	7	0.3	—
Increased bilirubin*	—	3	3.3
Hematologic			
Anemia	—	0.7	0.3
Neutropenia	—	9.4	10.4
Thrombocytopenia	—	0	0.3

*G3 and G4 correspond to G2 and G3 in updated NCIC CTC

Van Cutsem E et al. JCO 2001;19:4097–4106

Therapy Monitoring

1. *Before each cycle:* H&P, CBC with differential, CEA, serum electrolytes, creatinine, BUN, and LFTs
2. *Every 2–3 months:* CT scans to assess cancer status

ADJUVANT AND ADVANCED REGIMEN

CAPECITABINE

Twelves C et al. NEJM 2005;352:2696–2704
Van Cutsem E et al. JCO 2001;19:4097–4106

Capecitabine 1250 mg/m^2 per dose orally with water within 30 minutes after a meal twice daily for 28 doses, on days 1–14 every 3 weeks (total dosage/cycle = 35,000 mg/m^2)

Notes:

- Capecitabine is given for 2 consecutive weeks followed by 1 week without treatment
- Doses are rounded down to approximate a calculated dose using combinations of 500-mg and 150-mg tablets
- In practice, treatment often is begun with capecitabine 1000 mg/m^2 per dose twice daily for 28 doses on days 1–14 (total dosage/cycle = 28,000 mg/m^2. Dosage may be increased during subsequent cycles if initial treatment at a lesser dosage is tolerated

Capecitabine is manufactured in the United States as film-coated tablets for oral administration containing either 150 mg or 500 mg capecitabine XELODA (capecitabine) TABLETS

For delayed diarrhea:
Loperamide 4 mg orally after first loose stool, then:
Loperamide 2 mg orally with each loose stool to a maximum daily dose of 24 mg

Emetogenic potential: Low (Emetogenicity score = 2). See Chapter 39 for antiemetic regimens

Treatment Modifications

Adverse Event	Dose Modification
First occurrence of a G2 toxicity	No dose reduction*
Second occurrence of a given G2 toxicity	Reduce dosage by 25%*
First occurrence of a G3 toxicity	
Third occurrence of a given G2 toxicity	Reduce dosage by 50%*
Second occurrence of a given G3 toxicity	
Any G4 toxicity	
Fourth occurrence of a given G2 toxicity	Discontinue capecitabine
Third occurrence of a given G3 toxicity	
Second occurrence of a given G4 toxicity	
Both G4 hematologic and G4 nonhematologic toxicity	

*Interrupt capecitabine treatment until is toxicity resolves to G ≤ 1

NCI Canada CTC

Patient Population Studied

Patients receiving first-line treatment for metastatic colorectal cancer and adjuvant therapy for early-stage colorectal cancer. Equivalent to bolus fluorouracil + leucovorin

Efficacy (N = 301)

Complete response	0.3%
Partial response	18.6%
Stable disease	56.8%
Mean duration of response	7.2 months
Median time to progression	5.2 months
Median survival	13.2 months

Van Cutsem E et al. JCO 2001;19:4097–4106

Toxicity (N = 297)

	% All G	% G3	% G4
Nonhematologic			
Diarrhea	50.2	9.4	1.3
Hand-foot syndrome	48	16.2	0
Nausea	37.7	—	—
Stomatitis	21.9	1	0.3
Vomiting	18.5	—	—
Fatigue	10	—	—
Increased bilirubin[a,b]	—	23.6	4.7
Hematologic			
Anemia	—	2.7	0
Neutropenia	—	0	2
Thrombocytopenia	—	0.7	0.3

[a]G3 and G4 correspond to G2 and G3 in updated NCIC CTC
[b]Eight (10%) of patients with G3/4 hyperbilirubinemia also had G3 abnormalities in ALT or AST

Van Cutsem E et al. JCO 2001;19:4097–4106

Therapy Monitoring

1. *Before each cycle:* H&P, CBC with differential, CEA, serum electrolytes, creatinine, BUN, and LFTs
2. *Every 2–3 months:* CT scans to assess cancer status in patients presenting with advanced colorectal cancer

METASTATIC DISEASE REGIMEN

INFUSIONAL FLUOROURACIL

Hansen RM et al. J Natl Cancer Inst 1996;88:668–674

Fluorouracil 300 mg/m^2 per day by continuous intravenous infusion in 50–1000 mL 0.9% NaCl injection (0.9% NS) or 5% dextrose injection (D5W) (total dosage/week = 2100 mg/m^2). Treatment is continued indefinitely until toxicity/disease progression

*Management of diarrhea**
For delayed diarrhea:
Loperamide 2 mg orally every 2 hours during waking hours (4 mg orally every 4 hours during hours of sleep). Continue for at least 12 hours after diarrhea resolves
If diarrhea persists >48 hours despite loperamide: Stop loperamide and hospitalize patient for intravenous hydration

For persistent diarrhea:
Octreotide 100–150 mcg subcutaneously 3 times daily. Maximum total daily dose = 1500 mcg
Antibiotic therapy:
Ciprofloxacin 500 mg orally twice daily if absolute neutrophil count <500/mm^3 (even with no fever or diarrhea) or if patient is febrile in association with diarrhea. Antibiotics should also be administered if patient is hospitalized with prolonged diarrhea and should be continued until diarrhea resolves

Emetogenic potential = Low (Emetogenicity score = 2). See Chapter 39 for antiemetic regimens

*Rothenberg ML et al. JCO 2001;19:3801–3807
*Wadler S et al. JCO 1998;16:3169–3178

Treatment Modifications

Adverse Event	Dose Modification
G2 Nonhematologic toxicity	Reduce fluorouracil dosage by 50 mg/m^2 per day
G3 Nonhematologic toxicity	Reduce fluorouracil dosage by 100 mg/m^2 per day
Hematologic toxicity	No modifications

Patient Population Studied

A study of 159 patients with previously untreated metastatic adenocarcinoma of the colon or rectum

Efficacy (N = 159)

Overall response	28%
Complete response	5%
Median survival	13 months

Toxicity (N = 159)

Requiring Treatment Interruption	
G2 Stomatitis	35%
G3 Stomatitis	5%
G2/3 Hand-foot syndrome	36%
G3 Vomiting and diarrhea	3%
G3/4 Hematologic	6%
All toxicities	
None	2%
Mild	15%
Moderate	52%
Severe	27%
Life-threatening	4%
Lethal	1%

Therapy Monitoring

1. *Before each cycle:* H&P, CBC with differential, CEA serum electrolytes, and LFTs
2. *Weekly:* CBC with differential count
3. *Every 2–3 months:* CT scans to assess response

METASTATIC DISEASE REGIMEN

SINGLE-AGENT IRINOTECAN (CPT-11)

Cunningham D et al. Lancet 1998;352:1413–1418

Irinotecan 350 mg/m^2 intravenously over 90 minutes in 250 mL 5% dextrose injection (D5W), given on day 1 every 3 weeks (total dosage/cycle = 350 mg/m^2)

Note: Reduce dosage to 300 mg/m^2 for patients ≥70 years or whose WHO performance status = 2

Alternative
Irinotecan 100–125 mg/m^2 intravenously over 90 minutes in 250 mL 0.9% NS or D5W every week for 4 consecutive weeks every 6 weeks (total dosage/cycle = 400–500 mg/m^2)

Note: Four weeks of treatment followed by 2 weeks without treatment

Pitot HC. Oncology 1998;12(8 suppl 6):48–53

For delayed diarrhea:
Loperamide 4 mg orally after first loose stool, *then:*
Loperamide 2 mg orally with each loose stool to a maximum daily dose of 24 mg until 12 hours after the last loose stool or for a maximum of 48 hours, whichever condition occurs first
If diarrhea persists >24 hours despite loperamide:
Add oral prophylactic broad-spectrum antibiotic
Ciprofloxacin 500 mg orally twice daily if absolute neutrophil count <500/mm^3 (even in the absence of fever or diarrhea) or if patient is febrile in association with diarrhea. Antibiotics should also be administered if patient is hospitalized with prolonged diarrhea and should be continued until resolution of diarrhea
If diarrhea persists >48 hours despite loperamide:
Stop loperamide and hospitalize patient for intravenous hydration. Consider an alternative antidiarrheal treatment
Octreotide 100–150 mcg subcutaneously 3 times daily. Maximum total daily dose = 1500 mcg

For acute cholinergic syndrome:
Atropine sulfate 0.25–1 mg subcutaneously. If symptoms are severe, add prophylaxis during subsequent cycles

Emetogenic potential: Moderate (Emetogenicity score = 3). See Chapter 39 for antiemetic regimens

Patient Population Studied

A study of 189 patients with metastatic colorectal cancer with documented disease progression within 6 months of fluorouracil-based treatment

Treatment Modifications

(Camptosar, irinotecan hydrochloride injection product label, July 2005. Pharmacia & Upjohn Company, Division of Pfizer, Inc., New York, NY)

Three-Week Irinotecan

Notes:
- Dose modifications are based on the NCI CTC
- Before beginning a treatment cycle, patients should have baseline bowel function without antidiarrheal therapy for 24 hours, ANC ≥1500/mm^3, and platelet ≥100,000/mm^3
- Treatment should be delayed 1–2 weeks to allow for recovery from treatment-related toxicities. If a patient has not recovered after 2 weeks, consider stopping therapy

Toxicity in Previous Cycle	Dosage at the Start of a 3-Week Cycle
Neutropenia/Thrombocytopenia	
G1 ANC (1500–1999/mm^3) or G1 thrombocytopenia	Maintain dose and schedule
G2 ANC (1000–1499/mm^3) or G2 thrombocytopenia	Maintain dose and schedule
G3 ANC (500–999/mm^3) or G3 thrombocytopenia	Reduce dosage by 50 mg/m^2
G4 ANC (<500/mm^3) or G4 thrombocytopenia	Reduce dosage by 50 mg/m^2
Febrile neutropenia	Hold until neutropenia resolves. Resume treatment with irinotecan dosage reduced by 50 mg/m^2
Diarrhea	
G1 (2–3 stools/day > baseline)	Maintain dose and schedule
G2 (4–6 stools/day > baseline)	Maintain dose and schedule
G3 (7–9 stools/day > baseline)	Reduce irinotecan dosage by 50 mg/m^2
G4 (≥10 stools/day > baseline)	Reduce irinotecan dosage by 50 mg/m^2
Other Nonhematologic Toxicities	
Any G1 toxicity	Maintain dose and schedule
Any G2 toxicity	Maintain dose and schedule
Any G3 toxicity	Reduce dosage by 50 mg/^{2}
Any G4 toxicity	Reduce dosage by 50 mg/m^2

(*continued*)

Treatment Modifications (*continued*)

Weekly Irinotecan—4 of Every 6 Weeks

Notes:
- Dose modifications are based on the NCI CTC
- Before beginning a treatment cycle, patients should have baseline bowel function without antidiarrheal therapy for 24 hours, ANC ≥1500/mm^3, and platelet ≥100,000/mm^3
- Treatment should be delayed 1–2 weeks to allow for recovery from treatment-related toxicities. If a patient has not recovered after 2 weeks, consider stopping therapy

Toxicity	Weekly Dosage Based on Intracycle Toxicity	Dose at Start of a 6-Week Cycle
	Neutropenia/Thrombocytopenia	
G1 ANC (1500–1999/mm^3) or G1 thrombocytopenia	Maintain dose and schedule	Maintain dose and schedule
G2 ANC (1000–1499/mm^3) or G2 thrombocytopenia	Decrease weekly dosage by 25 mg/m^2	Maintain dose and schedule
G3 ANC (500–999/mm^3) or G3 thrombocytopenia	Omit weekly dose until toxicity G ≤2, then reduce irinotecan dosage by 25 mg/m^2	Reduce dosage by 25 mg/m^2
G4 ANC (<500/mm^3) or G4 thrombocytopenia	Omit weekly dose until toxicity G ≤2, then reduce irinotecan dosage by 50 mg/m^2	Reduce dosage by 50 mg/m^2
Febrile neutropenia	Omit weekly dose until neutropenia G ≤2, then reduce irinotecan dosage by 50 mg/m^2	Reduce dosage by 50 mg/m^2
	Diarrhea	
G1 (2–3 stools/day > baseline)	Delay treatment until diarrhea resolves to baseline; then resume irinotecan treatment	Maintain dose and schedule
G2 (4–6 stools/day > baseline)	Delay until diarrhea resolves to baseline, then reduce irinotecan dosage by 25 mg/m^2	Maintain dose and schedule
G3 (7–9 stools/day > baseline)	Delay until diarrhea resolves to baseline, then reduce irinotecan dosage by 25 mg/m^2	Reduce dosage by 25 mg/m^2
G4 (≥ 10 stools/day > baseline)	Delay until diarrhea resolves to baseline, then reduce irinotecan dosage by 50 mg/m^2	Reduce dosage by 50 mg/m^2
	Other Nonhematologic Toxicities	
Any G1 toxicity	Maintain dose and schedule	Maintain dose and schedule
Any G2 toxicity	Delay until toxicity resolves to G ≤1, then reduce irinotecan dosage by 25 mg/m^2	Maintain dose and schedule
Any G3 toxicity	Delay until toxicity resolves to G ≤2, then reduce irinotecan dosage by 25 mg/m^2	Reduce dosage by 25 mg/m^2
Any G4 toxicity	Delay until toxicity resolves to G ≤2, then reduce irinotecan dosage by 50 mg/m^2	Reduce dosage by 50 mg/m^2

Efficacy (N = 189)

	Irinotecan	BSC
Partial response	4%	0.7%
Partial or minor response	10.5%	4.4%
Median survival	9.2 months	6.5 months

BSC, best supportive care

Toxicity (N = 183)

Toxicity	% G3/4
Any G3/4 toxicity	79
Nonhematologic	
Diarrhea	22
Nonabdominal pain	19
Asthenia	15
Abdominal pain	14
Nausea	14
Vomiting	14
Neurologic symptoms	12
Cholinergic symptoms*	12
Constipation	10
Infection without G3/4 ANC	9
Anorexia	5
Mucositis	2
Cutaneous signs	2
Hematologic	
Leukopenia/neutropenia	22
Anemia	7
Thrombocytopenia	1
Fever/infection with G3 ANC	3

*Cholinergic syndrome: flushing, diaphoresis, abdominal pain, and diarrhea

Cunningham D et al. Lancet 1998;352:1413–1418

Therapy Monitoring

1. *Before each cycle:* H&P, CBC with differential, CEA, serum electrolytes, and LFTs
2. *Weekly:* CBC with differential count
3. *Every 2–3 months:* CT scans to assess response

METASTATIC DISEASE REGIMEN

IRINOTECAN + BOLUS FLUOROURACIL + LEUCOVORIN (IFL)

Saltz LB et al. NEJM 2000;343:905–914

Irinotecan 125 mg/m^2 intravenously in 250 mL 5% dextrose injection (D5W) over 90 minutes, given weekly for 4 consecutive weeks every 6 weeks (total dosage/cycle = 500 mg/m^2)

Leucovorin calcium 20 mg/m^2 per dose by intravenous injection over 30 seconds, given weekly for 4 consecutive weeks every 6 weeks (total dosage/cycle = 80 mg/m^2)
Fluorouracil 500 mg/m^2 per dose intravenously per push over 1–2 minutes after leucovorin, given weekly for 4 consecutive weeks every 6 weeks (total dosage/cycle = 2000 mg/m^2)

*Management of diarrhea**
For delayed diarrhea:
Loperamide 2 mg orally every 2 hours during waking hours (4 mg orally every 4 hours during hours of sleep). Continue for at least 12 hours after diarrhea resolves
If diarrhea persists >48 hours despite loperamide:
Stop loperamide and hospitalize patient for IV hydration
For persistent diarrhea:
Octreotide 100–150 mcg subcutaneously 3 times daily. Maximum total daily dose = 1500 mcg
Antibiotic therapy:
Ciprofloxacin 500 mg orally twice daily if absolute neutrophil count <500/mm^3 (even with no fever or diarrhea) or if patient is febrile in association with diarrhea. Antibiotics should also be administered if patient is hospitalized with prolonged diarrhea and should be continued until diarrhea resolves

For acute cholinergic syndrome:
Atropine sulfate 0.25–1 mg subcutaneously. If symptoms are severe, add prophylaxis during subsequent cycles

Emetogenic potential: Moderately high (Emetogenicity score = 4). See Chapter 39 for antiemetic regimens

*Rothenberg ML et al. JCO 2001;19:3801–3807
*Wadler S et al. JCO 1998;16:3169–3178

Treatment Modifications

(Camptosar, irinotecan hydrochloride injection product label, July 2005. Pharmacia & Upjohn Company, Division of Pfizer, Inc, New York, NY)

	Dosage Levels		
	Initial	−1	−2
Irinotecan	125 mg/m^2	100 mg/m^2	75 mg/m^2
Leucovorin	20 mg/m^2		
Fluorouracil	500 mg/m^2	400 mg/m^2	300 mg/m^2

Notes:
- Dose modifications are based on the NCI CTC
- Before beginning a treatment cycle, patients should have baseline bowel function without antidiarrheal therapy for 24 hours, ANC ≥1500/mm^3, and platelet ≥100,000/mm^3
- Treatment should be delayed 1–2 weeks to allow for recovery from treatment-related toxicities. If a patient has not recovered after 2 weeks, consider stopping therapy
- If toxicity occurs despite 2 dose reductions (ie, on level −2) discontinue therapy

Toxicity	Weekly Dosage Based on Intracycle Toxicity	Dosage at the Start of a 6-Week Cycle
Neutropenia/Thrombocytopenia		
G1 ANC (1500–1999/mm^3) or G1 thrombocytopenia	Maintain dose and schedule	Maintain dose and schedule
G2 ANC (1000–1499/mm^3) or G2 thrombocytopenia	Reduce weekly dosage by 1 dosage level	Maintain dose and schedule
G3 ANC (500–999/mm^3) or G3 thrombocytopenia	Hold treatment until toxicity G ≤ 2, then reduce weekly dosage by 1 dosage level	Reduce weekly dosage by 1 dosage level
G4 ANC (<500/mm^3) or G4 thrombocytopenia	Hold treatment until toxicity G ≤ 2, then reduce weekly dosage by 2 dosage levels	Reduce weekly dosage by 2 dosage levels
Febrile neutropenia	Hold treatment until toxicity resolves, then reduce weekly dosage by 1 dosage level	
Diarrhea		
G1 (2–3 stools/day > baseline)	Maintain dose and schedule	Maintain dose and schedule
G2 (4–6 stools/day > baseline)	Hold until diarrhea resolves to baseline, then reduce weekly dosage by 1 level	Maintain dose and schedule
G3 (7–9 stools/day > baseline)	Delay until diarrhea resolves to baseline, then reduce weekly dosage by 1 level	Reduce weekly dosage by 1 dosage level
G4 (≥10 stools/day > baseline)	Delay until diarrhea resolves to baseline then reduce weekly dosage by 2 levels	Reduce weekly dosage by 2 dosage levels

(continued)

Treatment Modifications (*continued*)

Other Nonhematologic Toxicities		
Any G1 toxicity	Maintain dose and schedule	Maintain dose and schedule
Any G2 toxicity	Hold treatment until toxicity G ≤ 1, then reduce weekly dosage by 1 dosage level	Maintain dose and schedule
Any G3 toxicity	Hold treatment until toxicity G ≤ 1, then reduce weekly dosage by 1 dosage level	Reduce weekly dosage by 1 dosage level
Any G4 toxicity	Hold treatment until toxicity G ≤ 1, then reduce weekly dosage by 2 dosage levels	Reduce weekly dosage by 2 dosage levels
G2–4 Mucositis	Reduce fluorouracil by 1 dosage level (do not alter irinotecan)	

Goldberg RM et al. JCO 2004;22:23–30
Saltz LB et al. NEJM 2000;343:905–914

Efficacy (N = 231)

(Intention-to-treat analysis)

Confirmed objective response	39%
Median duration of response	9.2 months
Median progression-free survival	7 months
Median overall survival	14.8 months

Toxicity (N = 225)

	% G3	% G4
Diarrhea	15.1	7.6
Vomiting	5.3	4.4
Mucositis	2.2	0
Neutropenia	29.8	24
Fever/neutropenia		7.1
Fever/infection		1.8
Therapy discontinued due to toxicity		7.6
Drug-related death		0.9

Patient Population Studied

A study of 231 patients with metastatic colorectal cancer who had not previously received chemotherapy except adjuvant therapy that was completed more than 12 months before study entry. Patients had not previously received pelvic radiation

Therapy Monitoring

1. *Before each cycle:* H&P, CBC with differential, CEA, serum electrolytes, and LFTs
2. *Weekly:* CBC with differential count and safety assessment
3. *Every 6 weeks* × *4 (24 weeks), then every 12 weeks:* CT scans to assess response

METASTATIC DISEASE REGIMEN

LEUCOVORIN + INFUSIONAL FLUOROURACIL + IRINOTECAN (FOLFIRI)

Douillard JY et al. Lancet 2000;355:1041–1047
Tournigand C et al. JCO 2004;22:229–237

Irinotecan 180 mg/m^2 intravenously over 90 minutes in 500 mL 5% dextrose injection (D5W), given on day 1 every 2 weeks (total dosage/cycle = 180 mg/^{2}), *and*

Leucovorin calcium 200 mg/m^2 over 2 hours in 25–500 mL 0.9% NaCl injection (0.9% NS) or D5W , given on days 1 and 2 every 2 weeks (total dosage/cycle = 400 mg/m^2)
Fluorouracil 400 mg/m^2 intravenously per push over 1–2 minutes after leucovorin, given on days 1 and 2 every 2 weeks, *followed by:*
Fluorouracil 600 mg/m^2 by continuous intravenous infusion over 22 hours in 100–1000 mL 0.9% NS or D5W, given on day 1 every 2 weeks (total dosage/cycle = 1400 mg/m^2), *or*
Leucovorin calcium 200 mg/m^2 intravenously over 2 hours in 25–500 mL 0.9% 0.9% NS or D5W on day 1 every 2 weeks
Fluorouracil 400 mg/m^2 per push over 1–2 minutes after leucovorin, given on day 1 every 2 weeks, *followed by:*
Fluorouracil 2400 mg/m^2 by continuous intravenous infusion over 46 hours in 100–1000 mL 0.9% NS or D5W, given on day 1 every 2 weeks (total dosage/cycle = 2800 mg/m^2)

Management of diarrhea*
For delayed diarrhea:
Loperamide 2 mg orally every 2 hours during waking hours (4 mg orally every 4 hours during hours of sleep). Continue for at least 12 hours after diarrhea resolves
If diarrhea persists >48 hours despite loperamide:
Stop loperamide and hospitalize patient for intravenous hydration
For persistent diarrhea:
Octreotide 100–150 mcg subcutaneously 3 times daily. Maximum total daily dose = 1500 mcg
Antibiotic therapy:
Ciprofloxacin 500 mg orally twice daily if absolute neutrophil count <500/mm^3 (even with no fever or diarrhea) or if patient is febrile in association with diarrhea. Antibiotics should also be administered if patient is hospitalized with prolonged diarrhea and should be continued until diarrhea resolves

(continued)

Patient Population Studied

A study of 199 patients with previously untreated advanced colorectal cancer

Treatment Modifications

(Camptosar, irinotecan hydrochloride injection product label, July 2005. Pharmacia & Upjohn Company, Division of Pfizer, Inc, New York, NY)

	Dosage Levels		
	Initial	−1	−2
Irinotecan	180 mg/m^2	150 mg/m^2	120 mg/m^2
Leucovorin	200 mg/m^2		
Bolus fluorouracil	400 mg/m^2	320 mg/m^2	240 mg/m^2
Infusional fluorouracil	600 mg/m^2	480 mg/m^2	360 mg/m^2
Infusional fluorouracil	2400 mg/m^2	2000 mg/m^2	1600 mg/m^2

Notes:

- Dose modifications are based on the NCI CTC
- Before beginning a treatment cycle, patients should have baseline bowel function without antidiarrheal therapy for 24 hours, ANC ≥1500/mm^3, and platelet ≥100,000/mm^3
- Treatment should be delayed 1–2 weeks to allow for recovery from treatment-related toxicities. If a patient has not recovered after 2 weeks, consider stopping therapy

If toxicity occurs despite 2 dose reductions (ie, on level −2), discontinue therapy

Toxicity	Modifications for Irinotecan and Fluorouracil
Neutropenia/Thrombocytopenia	
G1 ANC (1500–1999/mm^3) or G1 thrombocytopenia	Maintain dose and schedule
G2 ANC (1000–1499/mm^3) or G2 thrombocytopenia	Reduce dosage by 1 dosage level
G3 ANC (500–999/mm^3) or G3 thrombocytopenia	Hold treatment until toxicity resolves to G ≤ 2, then reduce dosage by 1 dosage level
G4 ANC (<500/mm^3) or G4 thrombocytopenia	Hold treatment until toxicity resolves to G ≤ 2, then reduce dosage by 2 dosage levels
Febrile neutropenia	Hold treatment until neutropenia resolves, then reduce dosage by 2 dosage levels
Diarrhea	
G1 (2–3 stools/day > baseline)	Maintain dose and schedule
G2 (4–6 stools/day > baseline)	Delay until diarrhea resolves to baseline then reduce dosage by 1 dosage level
G3 (7–9 stools/day > baseline)	Delay until diarrhea resolves to baseline then reduce dosage by 1 dosage level
G4 (≥10 stools/day > baseline)	Delay until diarrhea resolves to baseline then reduce dosage by 2 dosage levels

(continued)

(*continued*)

For acute cholinergic syndrome:
Atropine sulfate 0.25–1 mg subcutaneously. If symptoms are severe, add prophylaxis during subsequent cycles

Emetogenic potential: Moderately high (Emetogenicity score = 4). See Chapter 39

*Rothenberg ML et al. JCO 2001;19:3801–3807

Efficacy (N[a] = 169/198)

Confirmed overall response	40.8% (34.8%)[b]
Complete response	3.6% (3.0%)
Partial response	37.3% (31.8%)
Median time to progression	6.7 months
Median survival	17.4 months

[a] Evaluable = 169 patients; intention-to-treat = 198 patients. Both totals include patients receiving weekly and 2-weekly regimens
[b] % of evaluable patients (% of intention-to-treat patients)

Douillard JY et al. Lancet 2000;355:1041–1047

Treatment Modifications (*continued*)

Other Nonhematologic Toxicities

Any G1 toxicity	Maintain dose and schedule
Any G2 toxicity	Hold treatment until toxicity resolves to G ≤ 1, then reduce dosage by 1 dosage level
Any G3 toxicity	Hold treatment until toxicity resolves to G ≤1, then reduce dosage by 1 dosage level
Any G4 toxicity	Hold treatment until toxicity resolves to G ≤1, then reduce dosage by 2 dosage levels
G2–4 Mucositis	Decrease only fluorouracil by 20%

André T et al. Eur J Cancer 1999;35:1343–1347
Douillard JY et al. Lancet 2000;355:1041–1047
Tournigand C et al. JCO 2004;22:229–237

Toxicity (N = 54)

	% All G	% G3/4
Nonhematologic		
Diarrhea	68.3	13.1
Nausea	58.6	2.1
Alopecia	56.6	—
Asthenia	44.8	6.2
Vomiting	41.4	2.8
Mucositis	38.6	4.1
Cholinergic syndrome	28.3	1.4
Anorexia	17.2	2.1
Pain other than abdominal	9.7	0.7
Non-abdominal pain	8.3	—
Hand-foot syndrome	9	0.7
Hematologic		
Anemia	97.2	2.1
Neutropenia	82.5	46.2
Fever with G3/4 neutropenia	—	3.4
Infection with G3/4 neutropenia	—	2.1

Douillard JY et al. Lancet 2000;355:1041–1047

Therapy Monitoring

1. *Before each cycle:* H&P, CBC with differential, CEA serum electrolytes, and LFTs
2. *Every 2–3 months:* CT scans to assess response

METASTATIC OR ADJUVANT REGIMEN

LEUCOVORIN + INFUSIONAL FLUOROURACIL + OXALIPLATIN (FOLFOX)

André T et al. NEJM 2004;350:2343–2351
de Gramont A et al. JCO 2000;18:2938–2947
Rothenberg et al. JCO 2003;21:2059–2069
Tournigand C et al. JCO 2004;22:229–237

FOLFOX 4 (de Gramont A et al):
Oxaliplatin 85 mg/m^2 intravenously over 2 hours in 250 mL 5% dextrose injection (D5W), given on day 1 every 2 weeks, concurrently with leucovorin administration (total dosage/cycle = 85 mg/m^2)

Note: Oxaliplatin must not be mixed with NaCl injection. Therefore, when leucovorin and oxaliplatin are given concurrently via a Y-connector, both drugs must be administered in D5W

Leucovorin calcium 200 mg/m^2 per dose intravenously over 2 hours in 25–500 mL D5W on 2 consecutive days, given on days 1 and 2 every 2 weeks (total dosage/cycle = 400 mg/m^2), *followed by:*
Fluorouracil 400 mg/m^2 per dose intravenously per push over 1–2 minutes after leucovorin given on days 1 and 2 every 2 weeks, *followed by:*
Fluorouracil 600 mg/m^2 per dose by continuous intravenous infusion over 22 hours in 100–1000 mL 0.9% NaCl injection (0.9% NS) or D5W on 2 consecutive days, given on days 1 and 2 every 2 weeks (total dosage/cycle = 2000 mg/m^2)

FOLFOX 6 (Tournigand C et al):
Oxaliplatin 100 mg/m^2 intravenously over 2 hours in 250 mL D5W , given on day 1 every 2 weeks, concurrently with leucovorin administration (total dosage/cycle = 100 mg/m^2)

Note: Oxaliplatin must not be mixed with NaCl injection. Therefore, when leucovorin and oxaliplatin are given concurrently via a Y-connector, both drugs must be administered in D5W

Leucovorin calcium 200 mg/m^2 intravenously over 2 hours in 25–500 mL 0.9% NS or D5W, given on day 1 every 2 weeks
Fluorouracil 400 mg/m^2 intravenously per push over 1–2 minutes after leucovorin on day 1 every 2 weeks, *followed by:*
Fluorouracil 2400 mg/m^2 by continuous intravenous infusion over 46 hours in 100–1000 mL 0.9% NS or D5W on day 1, every 2 weeks (total dosage/cycle = 2800 mg/m^2)

Management of diarrhea*
For delayed diarrhea:
Loperamide 2 mg orally every 2 hours during waking hours (4 mg orally every 4 hours during hours of sleep). Continue for at least 12 hours after diarrhea resolves
If diarrhea persists >48 hours despite loperamide: Stop loperamide and hospitalize patient for intravenous hydration
For persistent diarrhea:
Octreotide 100–150 mcg subcutaneously 3 times daily. Maximum total daily dose = 1500 mcg
Antibiotic therapy:
Ciprofloxacin 500 mg orally twice daily if absolute neutrophil count <500/mm^3 (even with no fever or diarrhea) or if patient is febrile in association with diarrhea. Antibiotics should also be administered if patient is hospitalized with prolonged diarrhea and should be continued until diarrhea resolves

Emetogenic potential: Moderately high (Emetogenicity score = 4). See Chapter 39 for antiemetic regimens

*Rothenberg ML et al. JCO 2001;19:3801–3807
*Wadler S et al. JCO 1998;16:3169–3178

Treatment Modifications (Folfox 4)

Adverse Event	Dose Modification
Any G2/3/4 nonhematologic toxicity	Delay start of next cycle until the severity of all toxicities are G ≤ 1
ANC ≤ 1500/mm^3 or platelet count ≤100,000/mm^3	Delay start of next cycle until ANC >1500/mm^3 and platelet count > 100,000/mm^3
G3/4 Non-neurologic	Reduce fluorouracil and oxaliplatin dosages by 20%
G3/4 ANC	Reduce oxaliplatin dosage by 20%
Persistent (≥ 14 days) paresthesias	Reduce oxaliplatin dosage by 20%
Temporary (7–14 days) painful paresthesias	
Temporary (7–14 days) functional impairment	
Persistent (≥14 days) painful paresthesias	Discontinue oxaliplatin
Persistent (≥14 days) functional impairment	

de Gramont A et al. JCO 2000;18:2938–2947

Treatment Modifications (Folfox 6)

Adverse Event	Dose Modification
ANC ≤ 1500/mm^3 or platelet count ≤100,000/mm^3 or persistent nonhematologic toxicity ≥G2	Delay start of next cycle until ANC >1500/mm^3 and platelet count >100,000/mm^3
≥G3 Toxicity	Reduce fluorouracil dosage to 2000 mg/m^2
G4 ANC, G3/4 thrombocytopenia or G4 diarrhea	Reduce oxaliplatin dosage to 75 mg/m^2
G2 Paresthesias (persistent paresthesia or dysesthesia without functional impairment)	Reduce oxaliplatin dosage to 75 mg/m^2
Persistent G2 paresthesia/dysesthesia	Reduce oxaliplatin dosage to 50 mg/m^2

(*continued*)

Treatment Modifications (Folfox 6) (*continued*)

Persistent painful paresthesia or G3 neurotoxicity (persistent paresthesia or dysesthesia with persistent functional impairment)	Discontinue oxaliplatin

Tournigand C et al. JCO 2004;22:229–237

Patient Population Studied

Patients with previously untreated advanced colorectal cancer

Efficacy (N = 210)

Intent-to-Treat Analysis	
Objective response	50%
Complete response	1.4%
Partial response	48.6%
Stable disease	31.9%
Progressive disease	10%
Median survival	16.2 months

de Gramont A et al. JCO 2000;18:2938–2947
WHO Criteria

Toxicity (N = 209) (Folfox 4)

	% G1	% G2	% G3	% G4
Nonhematologic				
Nausea	44	22.5	5.7	NA
Vomiting	24	24.4	4.3	1.5
Diarrhea	30.6	16.3	8.6	3.3
Mucositis	24.9	12.9	5.3	0.5
Cutaneous	19.6	9.1	0	0
Alopecia	15.8	1.9	NA	NA
Neurologic	20.6	29.2	18.2	NA
Hematologic				
Neutropenia	14.3	14.3	29.7	12
Thrombocytopenia	62.2	11.5	2	0.5
Anemia	59.8	23.5	3.3	0

de Gramont A et al. JCO 2000;18:2938–2947

Toxicity (N = 110) (Folfox 6)

	% G1	% G2	% G3	% G4
Nonhematologic				
Nausea	39	25	3	0
Vomiting	22	17	3	0
Diarrhea	28	13	9	2
Mucositis	35	10	1	0
Cutaneous	17	5	2	0
Alopecia	19	9	NA	NA
Neurologic[a]	26	37	34	NA
Fatigue	17	15	3	0
Hematologic				
Neutropenia	18	20	31	13
Thrombocytopenia	57	21	5	0
Anemia	39	12	3	0

[a]Neurotoxicity scale:
G1 = Short-lasting paresthesia with complete regression by next cycle
G2 = Persistent paresthesia or dysesthesia without functional impairment
G3 = Persistent functional impairment

Tournigand C et al. JCO 2004;22:229–237

Therapy Monitoring

1. *Before each cycle:* H&P, CBC with differential, CEA serum electrolytes, and LFTs
2. *Every 2–3 months:* CT scans to assess response in patients presenting with advanced colorectal cancer

METASTATIC DISEASE REGIMEN

BEVACIZUMAB + LEUCOVORIN + BOLUS FLUOROURACIL + IRINOTECAN

Hurwitz H et al. NEJM 2004;350:2335–2342

Bevacizumab 5 mg/kg intravenously in 100 mL 0.9% NaCl injection (0.9% NS) every 2 weeks (total dosage/6-week cycle = 15 mg/kg)

Note: Administration duration for the initial dose is 90 minutes. If administration is well tolerated, the administration duration may be decreased stepwise during subsequent administrations to 60 minutes and, finally, to a minimum duration of 30 minutes

Irinotecan 125 mg/m^2 intravenously in 250 mL 5% dextrose injection (D5W) over 90 minutes weekly for 4 consecutive weeks every 6 weeks (total dosage/6-week cycle = 500 mg/m^2)

Leucovorin calcium 20 mg/m^2 intravenously over 2 hours in 25–500 mL 0.9% NS or D5W, given weekly for 4 consecutive weeks every 6 weeks (total dosage/6-week cycle = 80 mg/m^2), *followed by:*
Fluorouracil 500 mg/m^2 intravenously per push over 1–2 minutes, after leucovorin, weekly for 4 consecutive weeks, given every 6 weeks (total dosage/cycle = 2000 mg/m^2)

*Management of diarrhea**
Loperamide 2 mg orally every 2 hours during waking hours (4 mg orally every 4 hours during hours of sleep). Continue for at least 12 hours after diarrhea resolves
If diarrhea persists >48 hours despite loperamide: Stop loperamide and hospitalize patient for intravenous hydration
For persistent diarrhea:
Octreotide 100–150 mcg subcutaneously 3 times daily. Maximum total daily dose = 1500 mcg
Antibiotic therapy:
Ciprofloxacin 500 mg orally twice daily if absolute neutrophil count <500/mm^3 (even without fever or diarrhea) or if patient is febrile in association with diarrhea. Antibiotics should also be administered if patient is hospitalized with prolonged diarrhea and should be continued until diarrhea resolves
For acute cholinergic syndrome:
Atropine sulfate 0.25–1 mg subcutaneously. If symptoms are severe, add prophylaxis during subsequent cycles

Emetogenic potential: Moderately high (Emetogenicity score = 4). See Chapter 39 for antiemetic regimens

*Rothenberg ML et al. JCO 2001;19:3801–3807
*Wadler S et al. JCO 1998;16:3169–3178

Treatment Modifications

Adverse Event	Dose Modification
Gastrointestinal perforation, serious bleeding	Discontinue bevacizumab permanently
Wound dehiscence requiring medical intervention	
Nephrotic syndrome	
Hypertensive crisis	
Moderate to severe proteinuria	Hold bevacizumab pending further evaluation (eg, 24-hour urine protein or workup and treatment of hypertension)
Severe hypertension not controlled with medical management	

Note: Bevacizumab should be suspended at least several weeks before elective surgery and should not be resumed until a surgical incision is fully healed

Information from Product Label:
http://www.gene.com/gene/products/information/pdf/avastin-prescribing.pdf or
http://www.fda.gov/cder/approval/index.htm

Standard intracycle and intercycle dose modifications of irinotecan and fluorouracil according to the package insert were permitted in patients with treatment-related adverse events. Suggestions include the following:

(Camptosar®, irinotecan hydrochloride injection product label, July 2005. Pharmacia & Upjohn Company, Division of Pfizer, Inc, New York, NY)

	Dosage Levels		
	Initial	**−1**	**−2**
Irinotecan	125 mg/m^2	100 mg/m^2	75 mg/m^2
Leucovorin	20 mg/m^2		
Fluorouracil	500 mg/^{2}	400 mg/m^2	300 mg/m^2

Notes:

- Dose modifications are based on the NCI CTC
- Before beginning a treatment cycle, patients should have baseline bowel function without antidiarrheal therapy for 24 hours, ANC ≥ 1500/mm^3, and platelet ≥100,000/mm^3
- Treatment should be delayed 1–2 weeks to allow for recovery from treatment-related toxicities. If a patient has not recovered after 2 weeks, consider stopping therapy
- If toxicity occurs despite 2 dose reductions (ie, on level −2) discontinue therapy

Toxicity	Weekly Dosage Based on Intracycle Toxicity	Dosage at Start of a 6-Week Cycle
Neutropenia/Thrombocytopenia		
G1 ANC (1500–1999/mm^3) or G1 thrombocytopenia	Maintain dose and schedule	Maintain dose and schedule
G2 ANC (1000–1499/mm^3) or G2 thrombocytopenia	Reduce weekly dosage by 1 dosage level	Maintain dose and schedule
G3 ANC (500–999/mm^3) or G3 thrombocytopenia	Hold treatment until toxicity G ≤ 2, then reduce weekly dosage by 1 dosage level	Reduce weekly dosage by 1 dosage level

(continued)

Patient Population Studied

First-line therapy of metastatic colorectal cancer. Exclusion criteria included prior chemotherapy or biologic therapy for metastatic disease, although adjuvant or radiosensitizing use of fluoropyrimidines with or without leucovorin or levamisole was permitted

Efficacy (N = 402)

Overall response rate	44.8%
Complete response	3.7%
Partial response	41%
Median survival	20.3 months
Progression-free survival	10.6 months

RECIST Criteria

Toxicity (N = 393)

Adverse events occurred with greater incidence (≥2%) among patients who received bevacizumab + bolus IFL than those who received bolus IFL + placebo

Toxicity	% of Patients
Any G3/4 toxicity	85
Cardiovascular	
Any thrombosis	19.4
Deep venous thrombosis	8.9
Pulmonary embolus	3.6
Any hypertension	22.4
G3 Hypertension	11
Digestive	
G3/4 Diarrhea	32.4
Hematologic	
G3/4 Leukopenia	37
Other Toxicities (G1–4)	
Proteinuria	26.5
G2/3 Proteinuria	3.1/0.8

Treatment Modifications (*continued*)

Toxicity	Weekly Dosage Based on Intracycle Toxicity	Dosage at Start of a 6-Week Cycle
Neutropenia/Thrombocytopenia		
G4 ANC (<500/mm³) or G4 thrombocytopenia	Hold treatment until toxicity G ≤2, then reduce weekly dosage by 2 dosage levels	Reduce weekly dosage by 2 dosage levels
Febrile neutropenia	Hold treatment until toxicity resolves, then reduce weekly dosage by 1 dosage level	
Diarrhea		
G1 (2–3 stools/day > baseline)	Maintain dose and schedule	Maintain dose and schedule
G2 (4–6 stools/day > baseline)	Hold until diarrhea resolves to baseline, then reduce weekly dosage by 1 level	Maintain dose and schedule
G3 (7–9 stools/day > baseline)	Delay until diarrhea resolves to baseline, then reduce weekly dosage by 1 level	Reduce weekly dosage by 1 dosage level
G4 (≥10 stools/day > baseline)	Delay until diarrhea resolves to baseline, then reduce weekly dosage by 2 levels	Reduce weekly dosage by 2 dosage levels
Other Nonhematologic Toxicities		
Any G1 toxicity	Maintain dose and schedule	Maintain dose and schedule
Any G2 toxicity	Hold treatment until toxicity G ≤ 1, then reduce weekly dosage by 1 dosage level	Maintain dose and schedule
Any G3 toxicity	Hold treatment until toxicity G ≤ 1, then reduce weekly dosage by 1 dosage level	Reduce weekly dosage by 1 dosage level
Any G4 toxicity	Hold treatment until toxicity G ≤ 1, then reduce weekly dosage by 2 dosage levels	Reduce weekly dosage by 2 dosage levels
G2–4 Mucositis	Reduce fluorouracil by 1 dosage level (do not alter irinotecan)	

Goldberg RM et al. JCO 2004;22:23–30
Saltz LB et al. NEJM 2000;343:905–914

Therapy Monitoring

1. *Before each cycle:* H&P, CBC with differential, serum electrolytes, CEA BUN, creatinine, and LFTs. Urine for protein analysis including 24-hour urine for protein if needed
2. *Twice per week initially, then at a minimum of once per week:* Blood pressure
3. *Every 6 weeks for the first 24 weeks:* CT scans to assess response

METASTATIC DISEASE REGIMEN

CETUXIMAB

Cunningham et al. NEJM 2004;351:337–345
Saltz et al. JCO 2004;22:1201–1208

Warning: Despite the use of prophylactic antihistamines, severe infusion reactions occur with the administration of cetuximab in about 3% of patients, rarely with fatal outcome (<1 in 1000). Approximately 90% of severe infusion reactions are associated with initial cetuximab administration and are characterized by the rapid onset of airway obstruction (bronchospasm, stridor, hoarseness), urticaria, and/or hypotension. Exercise caution with every cetuximab infusion

Notes:

(1) Test doses do not reliably predict hypersensitivity reactions to cetuximab administration and are not recommended

(2) Mild to moderate infusion reactions
- Interrupt or slow the cetuximab infusion rate
- Permanently decrease administration rate by 50%
- Give antihistamine prophylaxis before repeated treatments

(3) Severe reactions
- Immediately interrupt cetuximab therapy
- Administer epinephrine, glucocorticoids, intravenous antihistamines, bronchodilators, and oxygen as needed
- Permanently discontinue further treatment

Cetuximab premedication:
Diphenhydramine 50 mg intravenously per push before cetuximab administration (other H_1-receptor antagonists may be substituted)

Initial cetuximab dose:
Cetuximab 400 mg/m^2 intravenously over 120 minutes (maximum infusion rate = 5 mL/min) as a single dose (total initial dosage = 400 mg/m^2)

Maintenance cetuximab doses:
Cetuximab 250 mg/m^2 intravenously over 60 minutes (maximum infusion rate = 5 mL/min) every week (total weekly dosage = 250 mg/m^2)

Notes:
- Cetuximab is intended for direct administration and should not be diluted
- Maximum infusion rate = 5 mL (10 mg)/minute

(*continued*)

Treatment Modifications

(ERBITUX™ (Cetuximab) product label, June 2004. Manufactured by ImClone Systems Incorporated, Branchburg, NJ. Distributed and Marketed by Bristol-Myers Squibb Company, Princeton, NJ)

Infusion Reactions	
Mild/moderate (G1/2)	Permanently decrease administration rates by 50%
Severe (G3/4)	Immediately and permanently discontinue cetuximab

Severe (G3/4) Dermatologic Toxicity

Occurrence	Cetuximab	Improvement	Cetuximab Dosage
First	Delay infusion 1–2 weeks	Yes	Continue at 250 mg/m^2
		No	Discontinue
Second	Delay infusion 1–2 weeks	Yes	Decrease to 200 mg/m^2
		No	Discontinue
Third	Delay infusion 1–2 weeks	Yes	Decrease to 150 mg/m^2
		No	Discontinue
Fourth	Discontinue		

Information from the product label:
http://www.bms.com/cgi-bin/anybin.pl?sql=select%20PPI%20from%20TB_PRODUCT_PPI%20where%20PPI_SEQ=106&key=PPI
or
http://www.fda.gov/cder/approval/index.htm

Patient Population Studied

A study of patients with metastatic colorectal cancer whose tumor expresses EGFR and whose disease had progressed after receiving an irinotecan-containing regimen

Efficacy

	Cetuximab + Irinotecan	Cetuximab
Response	22.9%	10.8%
Progression-free survival	4.1 months	1.5 months

Cunningham et al. NEJM 2004;351:337–345

(continued)

- Administer cetuximab through a low protein-binding in-line filter with pore size = 0.22 micrometers
- Use 0.9% NaCl injection to flush vascular access devices after administration is completed

Emetogenic potential: Nonemetogenic

In the pivotal trial, cetuximab was given alone or in combination with irinotecan. All patients received a 20-mg test dose on day 1, then cetuximab was given at 400 mg/m^2 intravenously as an initial dose, followed by 250 mg/m^2 per week intravenously until disease progression or unacceptable toxicity. Cetuximab was added to irinotecan using the same dose and schedule for irinotecan on which the patient's tumor had previously progressed

Toxicity

Toxicity	% G3/4	
	Cetuximab + Irinotecan	Cetuximab Alone
Asthenia/malaise	14	10
Abdominal pain	3	5
Fever	2	0
Infusion reaction	0	4
Acne like rash	9	5
Nausea/vomiting	7	4

Therapy Monitoring

1. *Before each cycle:* H&P, CBC with differential, CEA serum electrolytes, BUN, creatinine, and LFTs. Urine for protein analysis including 24-hour urine for protein if needed
2. *Every 6 weeks for the first 24 weeks:* CT scans to assess response

RECTAL CANCER REGIMEN

ADJUVANT OR NEOADJUVANT CHEMOTHERAPY + RADIATION

O'Connell MJ et al. NEJM 1994;331:502–507
Tepper JE et al. JCO 1997;15:2030–2039

Chemotherapy Before or After Radiation

Fluorouracil + calcium leucovorin (Roswell Park, Mayo Clinic, *or* infusional fluorouracil) or FOLFOX

Note: Systemic chemotherapy is usually administered 4 weeks before or after surgery or chemoradiotherapy

Radiation + Chemotherapy

Fluorouracil 225 mg/m^2 per day by continuous intravenous infusion in 50–1000 mL 0.9% NaCl injection (0.9% NS) or 5% dextrose injection (D5W) over 24 hours daily throughout radiation therapy (total dosage/week = 1575 mg/m^2)
Radiation therapy 180 cGy per fraction for 25 fractions (total dose = 4500 cGy), followed by boost of 540 cGy, followed by a second boost of 360 cGy if all small bowel can be excluded from the field

Emetogenic potential:
Chemotherapy before or after radiation:
Fluorouracil ± leucovorin: Low (Emetogenicity score = 2)
FOLFOX: Moderately high (Emetogenicity score = 4)
Radiation + chemotherapy: Moderate (Emetogenicity score ≤3)
See Chapter 39 for antiemetic regimens

Treatment Modifications

Adverse Event	Dose Modification
G ≥ 3 Gastrointestinal toxicity	Interrupt radiation treatments. Resume when the toxicities decrease to G ≤ 2
G ≥ 3 Hematologic toxicity	
G ≥ 3 Gastrointestinal toxicity	Interrupt fluorouracil infusion. Resume when the toxicities decrease to G ≤ 2
G ≥ 3 Hematologic toxicity	

Patient Population Studied

A study of patients with surgically resected stages II or III rectal cancer with the inferior edge of tumor at or below the level of sacral promontory or within 12 cm of the anal verge

Efficacy (N = 328)

Bolus fluorouracil for 2 cycles ± semustine before and after RT with fluorouracil by continuous infusion during radiation

4-year relapse-free survival	63%
4-year overall survival	70%

O'Connell MJ et al. NEJM 1994;331:502–507

Therapy Monitoring

1. *Before each cycle and weekly during RT:* H&P, CBC with differential, serum electrolytes, BUN, creatinine, and LFTs
2. *Every 2–3 months:* CT scans to assess response

11. Endometrial Cancer

Deirdre O'Mahony, MD, and Franco Muggia, MD

Epidemiology

Incidence: 41,200 (estimated new cases in the United States 2006)
Deaths: 7350 (estimated deaths in United States in 2006)

Stage at Presentation

Localized:	72%	Stage I:	79%
Regional:	16%	Stage II:	12.5%
Distant:	8%	Stage III:	13.3%
Unstaged:	4%	Stage IV:	4%

Jemal A et al. CA cancer J Clin 2006;56:106–30
National Cancer Institute. Surveillance, Epidemiology and End Results (SEER) program 1995–2001
Modified from Creasman WT et al. J Epidemiol Biostat 2001;6:47–86

Pathology

Endometrioid • Ciliated adenocarcinoma • Secretory adenocarcinoma • Papillary or villoglandular • Adenocarcinoma with squamous differentiation –Adenocanthoma –Adenosquamous	75–80%
Serous	<10%
Clear cell	4%
Mucinous	1%
Squamous	<1%
Mixed	10%
Undifferentiated	

International Society of Gynecologic Pathologist: Classification of Endometrial Carcinomas

Histopathology: Degree of Differentiation

G1	≤5% of nonsquamous or nonmorular solid growth pattern
G2	6–50% of a nonsquamous or nonmorular solid growth pattern
G3	>50% nonsquamous or nonmorular solid growth pattern

Note:

1. Cases may be defined according to the degree of differentiation of the adenocarcinoma
2. Nuclear atypia, inappropriate for the architecture grade, raises the grade to 3
3. Serous, clear cell, and mixed mesodermal tumors are high risk and considered grade 3
4. Adenocarcinomas with benign squamous elements are graded according to the nuclear grade of the glandular component

AJCC Cancer Staging Manual, 6th ed. New York: Springer-Verlag, 2002:267–273

Work-Up

Stage I	H&P CBC with platelet count Chest x-ray Cervical cytology
Stage II	Consider endocervical curettage or cervical biopsy
Stage III/IV	CA-125 MRI/CT as clinically indicated

NCCN Clinical Practice Guidelines in Oncology, V. 1. 2006

Staging

Stage I	Tumor limited to the uterine fundus
Stage IA	The uterine cavity measures ≤8 cm
Stage IB	The length of the uterine cavity is >8 cm
Stage II	The tumor extends to the uterine cervix
Stage III	The tumor has spread to the adjacent pelvic structures
Stage IV	Bulky disease or distant spread is present
Stage IVA	Tumor invades the mucosa of the bladder or rectosigmoid
Stage IVB	Distant metastases are present

International Federation of Gynecology and Obstetrics, 1971

Primary Tumor

Tx	Tumor cannot be assessed
T0	No evidence of primary tumor
Tis	Carcinoma in situ
T1	Tumor confined to corpus uteri
T1a	Tumor limited to endometrium
T1b	Tumor invades <50% myometrium
T1c	Tumor invades >50% myometrium
T2	Tumor invades cervix but not beyond uterus
T2a	Endocervical glandular involvement only
T2b	Cervical stromal invasion
T3	Local and/or regional spread
T3a	Tumor invades uterine serosa ± adnexa ± malignant peritoneal washings
T3b	Vaginal involvement (direct extension or metastasis)
T4	Tumor invades bladder mucosa ± bowel mucosa

Regional Lymph Nodes

Nx	Regional nodes not assessed
N0	No regional nodes involved
N1	Metastasis to the pelvic ± para-aortic lymph nodes

Distant Metastasis

Mx	Distant metastasis not assessed
M0	No distant metastasis
M1	Distant metastasis

Reproduced, with permission, of the American Joint Committee on Cancer (AJCC), Chicago, Illinois. The original source for this material is the AJCC Cancer Staging Manual, 6th edition (2002) published by Springer-Verlag, New York, www.springeronline.com.

Surgical Figo Staging: 1988

Stage/grade	T	N	M	
Stage Ia G1/G2/G3	T1a	N0	M0	Tumor limited to endometrium
Stage Ib G1/G2/G3	T1b	N0	M0	Tumor invades <50% myometrium
Stage Ic G1/G2/G3	T1c	N0	M0	Tumor invades >50% myometrium
Stage IIa G1/G2/G3	T2a	N0	M0	Endocervical glandular involvement only
Stage IIb G1/G2/G3	T2b	N0	M0	Cervical stromal invasion
Stage IIIa G1/G2/G3	T3a	N0	M0	Tumor invades uterine serosa ± adnexa ± malignant peritoneal washings
Stage IIIb G1/G2/G3	T3b	N0	M0	
Stage IIIc G1/G2/G3	T1	N1	M0	Vaginal involvement (direct extension or metastasis)
	T2	N1	M0	Metastasis to pelvic ± para-aortic nodes
	T3	N1	M0	
Stage IVa G1/G2/G3	T4	Any N	M0	Tumor invasion of bladder ± bowel mucosa
Stage IVb G1/G2/G3	Any T	Any N	M1	Distant metastases including intra-abdominal ± inguinal lymph nodes

AJCC Cancer Staging Manual, 6th ed. New York: Springer-Verlag, 2002:267–273

Overall 5-Year Survial: Relative To Figo Disease Stage

Stage	% Survival
Ia	88.9
Ib	90
Ic	80.7
IIa	79.9
IIb	72.3
IIIa	63.4
IIIb	38.8
IIIc	51.1
IVa	19.9
IVb	17.2

Caveats

1. FIGO staging has replaced clinical staging in clinical trials since 1988
2. Consistent activity has been noted for anthracyclines (mainly doxorubicin), platinums (both cis- and carboplatin), and taxanes (mainly paclitaxel) in phase II and phase III studies
3. Vinca alkaloids and alkylating agents have shown some activity in phase II trials, but their contribution is uncertain in phase III trials
4. Several phase II studies have shown that combination regimens in general produce improved response rates with limited improvement in progression-free survival and overall survival
5. Well-differentiated tumors metastasize infrequently, but endocrine therapy has established efficacy and may be tried before chemotherapy
6. Combination chemotherapy regimens based on platinum, anthracycline, and taxanes are shown to be superior to radiation as adjuvants in stage III/IV resected disease
7. For patients with advanced disease, a combination of chemotherapy with radiation may be the best option
8. Patients with advanced or recurrent endometrial carcinoma should be considered for systemic therapy. Patients who have grade I tumor and/or known progesterone positive disease should be treated with a progestin. Those with a grade 2–3 tumor and/or known progesterone receptor–negative disease should beconsidered for initial treatment with single-agent chemotherapy or combination chemotherapy. Chemotherapy should be also considered for patients who do not respond to initial hormonal therapy

REGIMEN

PACLITAXEL, DOXORUBICIN, CISPLATIN (TAP)

Fleming GF et al. JCO 2004;22:2159–2166

Doxorubicin 45 mg/m^2 intravenously per push over 3–5 minutes on day 1 every 21 days (total dosage/cycle = 45 mg/m^2)
Followed immediately by:

Cisplatin 50 mg/m^2 intravenously in 250 mL 0.9% NaCl injection (0.9% NS) over 1 hour after doxorubicin administration on day 1 every 21 days (total dosage/cycle: 50 mg/m^2)

Paclitaxel 160 mg/m^2 by intravenous infusion in a volume of 0.9% NS or 5% dextrose injection (D5W) sufficient to produce a concentration of 0.3–1.2 mg/mL over 3 hours on day 2 every 21 days (total dosage/cycle = 160 mg/m^2)

Filgrastim 5 mcg/kg per day subcutaneously beginning on day 3 and continuing through day 12

Notes:
- No modifications to starting drug doses based on age or history of pelvic radiation therapy
- Women with a BSA >2 m^2 received treatment as if their BSA were equal to only 2 m^2

Emetogenic potential:
Day 1: Very high (Emetogenicity score = 6)
Day 2: Low (Emetogenicity score = 2). See Chapter 39 for antiemetic regimens

Treatment Modifications

Adverse Event	Dose Modification
G3/4 Thrombocytopenia or G4 ANC	Reduce cisplatin and paclitaxel dosages by 20%
G3 Peripheral neuropathy	Hold therapy until neuropathy ≤G1. Restart therapy with paclitaxel and cisplatin doses reduced by 20%
Recurrent G3 neurologic toxicity	Discontinue therapy
LVEF <45% or a fall in LVEF of 20% from baseline	Discontinue therapy
Toxicity-related delay in administration of >3 weeks	Discontinue therapy

Patient Population Studied

Chemotherapy-naive women with histologically documented measurable stage III or stage IV or recurrent endometrial carcinoma of any cell type plus a GOG performance status of 0–2

Efficacy (N = 134)

Complete response*	22%
Partial response*	35%
Median progression-free survival	8.3 months
Median overall survival	15.3 months

*Histologic subtype was not related to the probability of response
GOG Response Criteria

Toxicity (N = 131)

	% of Patients		
	G2	G3	G4
Nonhematologic			
Auditory	7	0	0
LVEF	10	2	0
Pulmonary	5	2	0
Deep venous thrombosis	1	6	0
Constitutional	31	10	2
Vomiting	23	10	2
Diarrhea	8	8	1
Mucositis or stomatitis	7	1	0
Genitourinary/renal	3	3	1
Metabolic	8	12	7
Sensory peripheral neuropathy	27	12	0
Hematologic			
Neutropenia	13	23	36
Thrombocytopenia	21	20	2

Treatment was considered to have contributed to 5 deaths
NCI CTC

Therapy Monitoring

1. *Every cycle:* Pelvic examination and serum electrolytes, calcium, magnesium, BUN, and creatinine
2. *Every other cycle:* Tumor measurements by radiologic examination
3. *Every third cycle:* Left ventricular ejection fraction

Notes

TAP produced significantly longer progression-free survival (8.5 versus 5.3 months) and survival (15.3 versus 12.3 months) than doxorubicin + cisplatin (AC). Toxicity was also greater with TAP (24% discontinued therapy)

REGIMEN

CISPLATIN + VINORELBINE

Gebbia V et al. Ann Oncol 2001;12:767–772

Hydration before cisplatin:
≥500 mL 0.9% NaCl injection (0.9% NS) at ≥100 mL/hour before and after cisplatin administration. Also, encourage high oral intake and provide potassium and magnesium supplementation
Mannitol diuresis:
May be given to patients who have received adequate hydration. Administer 250 mL of a 15–25% mannitol solution intravenously over 1 hour before starting cisplatin or simultaneously with cisplatin. Continued hydration is essential with adequate fluid input during and for a minimum of 4 hours after administration of mannitol
Note: Original study recommended 18% mannitol. Although this can be compounded, commercially available (ready-to-use) parenteral products in the United States include 5%, 10%, 15%, and 25% solutions

Cisplatin 80 mg/m^2 intravenously in 500 mL of 0.9% NS over 60 minutes on day 1 every 21 days (total dosage/cycle = 80 mg/m^2)

Vinorelbine 25 mg/m^2 per dose by intravenous infusion in a volume of 0.9% NS or 5% dextrose injection (D5W) sufficient to produce a solution with concentration within the range 1.5–3 mg/mL, over 6–10 minutes for 2 doses on days 1 and 8 every 21 days (total dosage/cycle = 50 mg/m^2)

Emetogenic potential:
Day 1: High (Emetogenicity score = 5)
Day 8: Nonemetogenic (Emetogenicity score = 1).
See Chapter 39 for antiemetic regimens

Efficacy (N = 35)

Overall response	57% (20 patients)
Complete response	11% (4 patients)
Partial response	46% (16 patients)
Stable disease	17% (6 patients)
Median overall survival	240 days (8 months)

Patient Population Studied

Patients with advanced endometrial adenocarcinoma no longer amenable to radical surgery and/or radiation therapy with measurable disease and a Karnofsky performance status >60%

Treatment Modifications

Adverse Event	Dose Modification
WBC < 4000/mm^3 or platelet count <100,000/mm^3	Delay therapy for 1 week until WBC >4000/mm^3 and platelet count >100,000/mm^3
>G2 Neutropenia on day 8	Omit day 8 vinorelbine, and reduce all subsequent doses by 5 mg/m^2
Day 8 platelet count <50,000/mm^3	Omit vinorelbine dose
G2 Neurotoxicity	Reduce cisplatin dosage by 20 mg/m^2 and vinorelbine dosage by 5 mg/m^2
>G2 Neurotoxicity	Hold vinorelbine until neurotoxicity ≤G1; then reduce cisplatin dosage by 20 mg/m^2 and vinorelbine dosage by 5 mg/m^2
G1 Renal toxicity	Reduce all subsequent cisplatin dosages by 20 mg/m^2
≥G2 Renal toxicity	Hold cisplatin dose until renal toxicity ≤G1; then reduce all subsequent cisplatin dosages by 20 mg/m^2
G4 Nonhematologic toxicity	Discontinue therapy

Toxicity (N = 35)

Toxicity	% G1	% G2	% G3	% G4
Hematologic				
Anemia	14	20	6	—
Leukopenia	20	23	12	6
Thrombocytopenia	6	6	9	—
Nonhematologic				
Vomiting	18	20	18	—
Stomatitis	6	—	—	—
Diarrhea	9	3	—	—
Neurotoxicity	14	-	—	—
Constipation	14	6	—	—
Pain	3	—	—	—
Alopecia	11	3	—	—
Phlebitis	14	—	—	—
Laboratory Abnormalities				
↑ BUN	18	—	—	—
↑ Creatinine	9	—	—	—
↑ ALT/AST	3	—	—	—

Notes

In the absence of disease progression and unacceptable toxicity, therapy was continued for a total of 8 cycles

Therapy Monitoring

1. *Day 1 every cycle:* Pelvic examination, CBC with differential, serum electrolytes, magnesium, BUN, and creatinine
2. *Day 8 every cycle:* CBC with differential
3. *Every month:* ECG, serum chemistries, and CBC
4. *Every 2–3 cycles:* Tumor measurement by radiologic examination

12. Esophageal Cancer

Gauri Varadhachary, MD, and Jaffer Ajani, MD

Epidemiology

Incidence:	14,550 (estimated for 2006 in the United States)
Mortality:	13,770 (estimated for 2006)
Median age*:	Squamous cell esophageal carcinoma: 53.4 years Adenocarcinoma of the esophagus: 62.6 years
Male/female ratio:	3:1 for squamous cell carcinoma and 7:1 for adenocarcinoma
Stage at presentation:	Accuracy improves with invasive staging (endoscopic ultrasound, laparoscopy) Locoregional disease: 50% Distant metastasis: 50%

Jemal A et al. CA Cancer J Clin 2006;56:106–30

*Kelsen DP et al. Textbook of Gastrointestinal Oncology: Principles and Practice. Lippincott Williams & Williams, 2001

Pathology

Upper to midthoracic esophagus:	Predominantly squamous cell carcinoma
Distal esophagus and GE junction:	Predominantly adenocarcinoma
Other rare pathology:	Basaloid-squamous carcinoma (1.9%)[a] or small cell carcinomas

Especially in white men, the incidence of adenocarcinoma of the GE junction has risen significantly in the United States, whereas that of squamous cell carcinoma has slightly decreased. In the 1960s, squamous cell cancer accounted for 90% or more of esophageal cancer.[b] Data from 1996 suggested that they occur with equal frequency, and in 2004 the trend has changed further so that adenocarcinoma now accounts for at least 75% of esophageal cancers. This is thought to be related to increase in body mass index and Barrett's esophagus

[a]Abe K et al. Am J Surg Pathol 1996;20:453–461
[b]Daly JM et al. National Cancer Data Base Report on Esophageal Carcinoma. Cancer 1996;78:1820–1828

Work-Up

1. H&P, esophagogastroduodenoscopy, barium swallow, CBC, serum electrolytes, BUN, creatinine, LFTs and mineral panel, CT scan of chest and abdomen
2. Endoscopic ultrasound is highly recommended if there is no evidence of distant metastases, with FNA if indicated
3. For local-regional cancer at or above the carina, a bronchoscopy must be considered
4. In selected patients with local-regional GE junction cancer, a laparoscopic staging of the peritoneal cavity may be warranted
5. In patients with local-regional cancer, PET/CT scan is strongly recommended. Suspicious metastatic cancer should be confirmed
6. In addition, for patients with local-regional cancer (stage I–III), a multidisciplinary evaluation is required, including nutritional assessment. The need for supplementation depends on the severity of dysphagia, and the overall nutritional status (>10% weight loss). Enteral nutritional support is preferred (PEG is avoided if surgery is a consideration)
7. A barium enema or a colonoscopy should be performed if colon interposition or bypass is planned. Consider arteriogram if performing colon interposition

NCCN Clinical Practice Guidelines in Oncology, –V. 1. 2006

Staging

Note that the TNM staging reflects pathologic staging and does not have information on the number of nodes involved. Clinical staging usually incorporates radiologic imaging (CT staging) as well as the endoscopic ultrasound staging, which helps direct treatment. Clinical staging, although improving, remains suboptimal

Primary Tumor (T)

TX	Primary tumor cannot be assessed
T0	No evidence of primary tumor
Tis	Carcinoma in situ
T1	Tumor invades lamina propria or submucosa
T2	Tumor invades muscularis propria
T3	Tumor invades adventitia
T4	Tumor invades adjacent structures

Cancer Staging Manual, 6th ed. Springer-Verlag, 2002

Regional Lymph Nodes (N)

NX	Regional lymph nodes cannot be assessed
N0	No regional lymph node metastasis
N1	Regional lymph node metastasis

Cancer Staging Manual, 6th ed. Springer-Verlag, 2002

Stage Grouping

Stage 0	Tis N0 M0
Stage I	T1 N0 M0
Stage IIA	T2 N0 M0 T3 N0 M0
Stage IIB	T1 N1 M0 T2 N1 M0
Stage III	T3 N1 M0 T4 Any N M0
Stage IV	Any T Any N M1
Stage IVA	Any T Any N M1a
Stage IVB	Any T Any N M1b

Reproduced, with permission, of the American Joint Committee on Cancer (AJCC), Chicago, Illinois. The original source for this material is the AJCC Cancer Staging Manual, 6th edition (2002) published by Springer-Verlag, New York, www.springeronline.com.

Distant Metastasis (M)

MX	Distant metastasis cannot be assessed
M0	No distant metastasis
M1	Distant metastasis
Tumors of the lower thoracic esophagus	
M1a	Metastasis in celiac lymph nodes
M1b	Other distant metastasis
Tumors of the midthoracic esophagus	
M1a	Not applicable
M1b	Nonregional lymph nodes and/ or other distant metastasis
Tumors of the upper thoracic esophagus	
M1a	Metastasis in the upper cervical nodes
M1b	Other distant metastasis

Reproduced, with permission, of the American Joint Committee on Cancer (AJCC), Chicago, Illinois. The original source for this material is the AJCC Cancer Staging Manual, 6th edition (2002) published by Springer-Verlag, New York, www.springeronline.com.

Five-Year Survival

Stage 0	100%
Stage I	75%
Stage IIA	40% 25%
Stage IIB	15% 15%
Stage III	10% 10%
Stage IV	<5–10%
Stage IVA	5–10%
Stage IVB	<5%

Caveats

1. Patients with high-grade dysplasia (HGD): Check p53 status and ploidy. Treatment options include surgery, photodynamic therapy, and observation. Clinical trial is preferred
2. Treatment options for patients with carcinoma in situ (TIS) and T1N0M0: Definitive chemoradiation, surgery, photodynamic therapy, and endoscopic mucosal resection. Clinical trial is preferred
3. Local-regional cancer
   a. Defined as:
      - Potentially resectable, or
      - Unresectable, which includes T4 lesion, supraclavicular adenopathy, and celiac nodal metastasis in patients with upper or mid thoracic esophageal cancer
   b. Considerations in treatment:
      - Preoperative chemoradiation followed by surgery is a common practice in the United States
      - There are no data comparing definitive chemoradiation with preoperative chemeradiation + surgery versus surgery alone. Overall 5-year-survival rates for surgery alone and definitive chemoradiation are similar (~20%)
4. Patients with distal esophageal and GE junction carcinomas with regional and/or celiac axis lymphadenopathy should not necessarily be considered to have unresectable disease due to metastases. These patients are often offered curative-intent therapy

REGIMEN

FLUOROURACIL + CISPLATIN + RADIATION

Herskovic A et al. NEJM 1992;326:1593–1598
Minsky BD et al. JCO 2002 20:1167–1174 (INT 0123; RTOG 94-05)

Hydration before cisplatin: ≥1000 mL 0.9% NaCl injection (0.9% NS) at ≥100 mL/hour before and after cisplatin administration. Also encourage high oral intake. Monitor and replace magnesium/electrolytes as needed.
Mannitol diuresis: May be given to patients who have received adequate hydration. A bolus dose of 12.5–25 g mannitol can be administered as an intravenous push before cisplatin or in the same container as cisplatin. Continued hydration is essential
In an inpatient or "day hospital" setting, additional mannitol can be administered in the form of an infusion: 100–200 mL 20% mannitol injection administered intravenously over 4–8 hours. This can be done either during or immediately after cisplatin, but requires maintenance of adequate fluid input during and for hours after mannitol administration

Cisplatin 75 mg/m^2 intravenously in 50–250 mL of 0.9% NaCl injection (0.9% NS) over 30 minutes, given on day 1 during weeks 1, 5, 9, and 13 (total dosage per 28-day cycle [1 dose] = 75 mg/m^2)

Fluorouracil 1000 mg/m^2 per day by continuous intravenous infusion in 500–1000 mL 0.9% NS or 5% dextrose injection (D5W) on days 1–4 during weeks 1, 5, 9, and 13 (total dosage per 28-day cycle [4 doses] = 4000 mg/m^2)

Radiation 1.8 Gy/day for 5 days/week
Starts concurrently with chemotherapy
Planned cumulative dose = 50.4 Gy (duration of planned treatment is 5 weeks, 3 days)

Take home: Mouthwash regimen for mucositis

Emetogenic potential:
Day 1: High (Emetogenicity score = 6)
Days 2–4: Low–moderate (Emetogenicity score = 3). High potential for delayed symptoms after day 1. See Chapter 39

Patient Population Studied

A clinical trial of 236 patients with AJCC clinical stage T1–4 N0–1 M0 primary squamous cell or adenocarcinoma of the cervical, mid, or distal esophagus selected for a nonsurgical (definitive chemoradiation) approach. Patients received combined-modality therapy consisting of chemotherapy with concurrent radiation therapy. Patients were randomized to receive either 64.8 Gy or 50.4 Gy. The higher radiation dose did not increase survival or local/regional control

Efficacy (N = 109)

Median duration of response	4.2 months
Alive/no failure	25%
Loco-regional failure at 2 years	52%
Distant failure	16%
Treatment-related death	2%

Therapy Monitoring

1. *Weekly:* H&P
2. *Before each cycle:* CBC with differential and serum electrolytes, BUN, creatinine, and magnesium
3. *Response evaluation:* 5 to 6 weeks after completion of therapy

Toxicity (N = 109/99)

Grade	% Acute Toxicities	% Late Toxicities
1	1	20
2	26	22
3	43	24
4	26	13
5	2	0

Maximum toxicity per patient based on RTOG morbidity scale. N = 109 for acute toxicity and 99 for late toxicity

Treatment Modifications

Adverse Event	Dose Modification
G3/4 toxicity	A minimum 1-week treatment delay. Resume when toxicity is grade ≤2. Continue radiation if toxicity is unrelated to radiation therapy (RT)
If during weeks 1, 5, 9, or 13, day 1: ANC ≥ 2000/mm^3 but <3000/mm^3, or platelets ≥ 75,000/mm^3 but <100,000/mm^3	Reduce cisplatin and fluorouracil dosages by 25%; continue RT
If during weeks 1, 5, 9, or 13, day 1: ANC <2000/mm^3, or platelets <75,000/mm^3	Hold chemotherapy and RT until toxicity resolves, then reduce cisplatin and fluorouracil dosages by 50%
ANC < 1000/mm^3, or platelets ≤75,000/mm^3 between cycles on days chemotherapy is not administered	Reduce cisplatin and fluorouracil dosages by 50%
Serum creatinine = 1.6–2.0 mg/dL (140–176 micromol/L)	Reduce cisplatin dosage by 50%
Creatinine >2.0 mg/dL (176 μmol/L	Cisplatin discontinued; continue RT
G3/4 stomatitis during fluorouracil treatment	Do not administer additional fluorouracil during that cycle. Reduce all subsequent fluorouracil dosages by 25%
G3/4 stomatitis on days chemotherapy not administered	Reduce all subsequent fluorouracil dosage by 25%
G ≥ 3 RT-related toxicity	Hold RT, and resume when toxicity is G ≤ 2

Notes

1. Doses for this regimen and other data based on Minsky et al
2. Patients who cannot tolerate cisplatin are treated with carboplatin (AUC = 5)

REGIMEN

IRINOTECAN + CISPLATIN

Ilson DH et al. JCO 1999;17:3270–3275

Primary antiemetic prophylaxis before starting chemotherapy:
(1) **Granisetron** 2 mg orally 60 minutes before starting chemotherapy
(2) **Dexamethasone** 20 mg intravenously per push 5–60 minutes before starting chemotherapy
Granisetron is manufactured in the United States in tablets for oral administration containing 1 mg granisetron and as an oral solution containing 2 mg granisetron/10 mL. KYTRIL® (granisetron hydrochloride) Tablets, Oral Solution. Roche Laboratories, Inc, Nutley, NJ
Hydration before cisplatin: 5% dextrose/0.9% NaCL injection (D5W/0.9% NS) or 0.9% NS ≥500 mL intravenously over a minimum of 1 hour. Also encourage high oral intake. Monitor and replace magnesium/electrolytes as needed.
Cisplatin 25–30 mg/m² per dose intravenously in 25–100 mL of 0.9% NS over 30–60 minutes weekly for 4 consecutive weeks [days 1, 8, 15, and 22] followed by 20 days [days 23–42] without cisplatin (total dosage/cycle = 100–120 mg/m²) followed by:

Irinotecan 50–65 mg/m² per dose intravenously in a volume of 5% dextrose injection (D5W) sufficient to produce a solution with concentration of 0.12–2.8 mg/mL over 30 minutes, weekly, for 4 consecutive weeks [days 1, 8, 15, and 22] followed by 20 days [days 23–42] without irinotecan (total dosage/cycle = 200–260 mg/m²)
Secondary prophylaxis for diarrhea or abdominal cramping that occurs within 1 hour after irinotecan administration:
Atropine 0.25–1 mg subcutaneously as premedication. Administer the first time in response to symptoms and as primary prophylaxis during subsequent cycles
Antidiarrheal regimen*:
Loperamide 2 mg every 2 hours orally; continue until free from diarrhea for 12 hours
If diarrhea persists more than 48 hours despite loperamide, stop loperamide and hospitalize patient for intravenous hydration
For persistent diarrhea:
Octreotide 100–150 mcg subcutaneously 3 times per day. Maximum total daily dose = 1500 mcg
*Wadler S et al. JCO 1998;16:3169–3178

Emetogenic potential:
On days of cisplatin + irinotecan administration: High (Emetogenicity score = 5). See Chapter 39

Patient Population Studied

A study of 35 patients with advanced (unresectable or metastatic) esophageal adenocarcinoma or squamous cell carcinoma with good performance status

Efficacy (N = 35)

Complete response	6%
Partial response	51%
Minor response	20%
Stable disease	20%
Disease progression	3%
Median duration of response	4.2 months

Treatment Modifications

Adverse Event	Dose Modification
G3/4 Diarrhea or mucositis	Reduce irinotecan dosage by 10 mg/m² per dose
G4 Fatigue >3 days	
On the day of re-treatment if ANC < 1000/mm³, WBC < 3000/mm³ or platelet <100,000/mm³	Hold treatment until ANC ≥ 1000/mm³, WBC ≥3000/mm³ and platelet ≥100,000/mm³ No dosage reductions for treatment delays ≤1 week. Reduce irinotecan dosage 10 mg/m² per dose if treatment delayed >2 weeks, for febrile neutropenia, or for bleeding from thrombocytopenia
If blood counts on day 22 do not permit administering the 4th week of planned chemotherapy	Shorten treatment to a 5-week cycle: 3 consecutive weeks of treatment (days 1, 8, and 15), followed by 20 consecutive days without chemotherapy (days 16–35)
Serum creatinine >1.7 mg/dL (150 μmol/L), but <2.0 mg/dL (177 μmol/L)	Reduce cisplatin dosage to 15 mg/m² per dose
G ≥ 2 diarrhea/mucositis on treatment days	Hold treatment for 1 week

Note: If toxicities warrant holding either drug, both drugs are held

One-week treatment delays are common owing to leukocyte counts <3000/mm³ and ANC <1000/mm³ on treatment days

Toxicity (N = 35)

	% G1/2	% G3/4
Hematologic		
Neutropenia	43	46
Anemia	69	31
Thrombocytopenia	57	0
Nonhematologic		
Diarrhea	74	11
Fatigue	97	3
Nausea	94	6
Vomiting	45	3
Cardiac	0	3
Renal	60	3
Pulmonary/dyspnea	52	0
Neurosensory	54	0
Neurocerebellar	0	3
Skin	43	0
Stomatitis	20	0
Increased bilirubin	3	0

NCI CTC

Reported as percent of patients experiencing toxicity at any time during therapy

Therapy Monitoring

1. *Pretreatment:* Complete H&P, 12-lead ECG, CBC, PT, PTT, serum electrolytes, BUN, creatinine, mineral panel and LFTs, urinalysis, chest x-ray, ± double-contrast barium esophagram, and chest and abdominal CT
2. *Before each cycle:* CBC and serum electrolytes, magnesium BUN, creatinine, mineral panel, and LFTs, with weekly intracycle CBC and serum creatinine
3. *Response evaluation:* After the first and second cycles and after every second cycle thereafter

Notes

Alternate infusion schedule of 2 weeks on and 1 week off may be better for some patients (days 1 and 8 every 21 days)

REGIMEN

EPIRUBICIN + CISPLATIN + FLUOROURACIL (ECF)

Findlay M et al. Ann Oncol 1994;5:609–616
Ross P et al. JCO 2002;20:1996–2004

All chemotherapy is given through a central vascular access device
Warfarin 1 mg/day orally continuously (prophylaxis against vascular access device occlusion)

Epirubicin 50 mg/m² by intravenous push just before cisplatin on day 1 every 3 weeks for up to 8 cycles (total dosage/3-week cycle = 50 mg/m²)

Hydration before cisplatin: 1000 mL 0.9% NaCl injection (0.9% NS) with 20 mEq KCl + 16 mEq $MgSO_4$ intravenously over 80 minutes (~750 mL/hour) with:
Furosemide 40 mg orally or intravenously followed by 500 mL 0.9% NS with 8 mEq $MgSO_4$ intravenously over 40 minutes (~750 mL/hour)
Cisplatin 60 mg/m² intravenously in 1000 mL 0.9% NS with 20 mEq KCl + mannitol 20,000 mg over 4 hours on day 1, every 3 weeks for up to 8 cycles (total cisplatin dosage/3-week cycle = 60 mg/m²) followed by:
Hydration after cisplatin: 1000 mL 0.9% NS with 20 mEq KCl + 16 mEq $MgSO_4$ intravenously over 6 hours (~167 mL/hour)

Fluorouracil 200 mg/m per day as a continuous intravenous infusion in 500–1000 mL of 0.9% NS or 5% dextrose injection (D5W) over 24 hours for up to 24 weeks, starting on the same day as the first of epirubicin and cisplatin (total dosage/3-week cycle = 4200 mg/m²)

General hydration: Encourage high oral intake. Monitor and replace magnesium/electrolytes as needed.

Emetogenic potential:
Day 1: High (Emetogenicity score = 6)
Days 2–21: Low (Emetogenicity score = 2)
High potential for delayed symptoms after day 1 chemotherapy. See Chapter 39

Patient Population Studied

A study of 429 (290 + 139) previously untreated patients with good performance status and locally advanced or metastatic adenocarcinoma or squamous cell carcinoma of the esophagus

Efficacy (N = 278/128)

Complete response	11%[a]	12%[b]
Partial response	32%[a]	59%[b]
Stable disease	23%[a]	
Disease progression/died	29%[a]	10%[b]
Median failure-free survival	7 months	

[a]Ross P et al. JCO 2002;20:1996–2004; N = 278
[b]Findlay M et al. Ann Oncol 1994;5:609–616; N = 128

Treatment Modifications

Adverse Event	Dose Modification
Palmar/plantar erythema (PPE)	Add oral pyridoxine 50 mg 3 times daily. If PPE does not improve, discontinue fluorouracil for 1 week, then restart at 150 mg/m² per day (25% decrease)
G1/2 Mucositis or diarrhea	Hold fluorouracil until toxicity resolves, then restart at 150 mg/m² per day (25% reduction)
G3/4 Mucositis or diarrhea	Hold fluorouracil until toxicity resolves, then restart at 100 mg/m² per day (50% reduction)
Creatinine clearance ≥60 mL/min[b]	Cisplatin 60 mg/m² (100%)
Creatinine clearance 40–60 mL/min[b]	Cisplatin X milligrams/m² where X = absolute value of creatinine clearance
Creatinine clearance <40 mL/min[b]	Hold cisplatin
EF[a] ≥ 50%	Epirubicin 50 mg/m² per dose
EF[a] < 50%	Not eligible to receive epirubicin
First episode of ANC <2000/mm³ or platelets <100,000/mm³ on the day of epirubicin + cisplatin treatment	Delay treatment for 1 week, or until ANC ≥ 2000/mm³ and platelets ≥100,000/mm³
Second episode of ANC < 2000/mm³ or platelets <100,000/mm³ on the day of epirubicin + cisplatin treatment, or febrile tropenia after previous treatment	Delay treatment until ANC ≥2000/mm³ and platelets ≥100,000/mm³ then reduce epirubicin dosage to 38.5 mg/m² per dose (25% reduction) in subsequent cycles

[a]Obtain baseline multigated cardiac scan to determine left ventricular ejection fraction (EF) for evidence of cardiovascular disease
[b]Creatinine clearance as a measure of glomerular filtration rate (GFR)

Toxicity (N = 272/139)

	% G1/2/3/4		% G3/4	
Hematologic				
Leukopenia	62[a]	—	13[a]	21[b]
Neutropenia	67[a]	—	32[a]	—
Thrombocytopenia	15[a]	—	4[a]	8[b]
Anemia	73[a]	—	9[a]	—
Nonhematologic				
Mucositis/stomatitis	55[a]	24[b]	5[a]	7[b]
Plantar-palmar erythema	30[a]	27[b]	1[a]	1[b]
Nausea	81[a]	—	10[a]	—
Vomiting	—	58[b]	—	13[b]
Diarrhea	44[a]	26[b]	6[a]	4[b]
Alopecia	87[a]	100[b]	—	—
Lethargy	89[a]	—	18[a]	—
Infection	38[a]	19[b]	6[a]	6[b]
Fever	14[a]	—	1[a]	—
Reduced GFR	—	73[b]	—	5[b]
Increased serum creatinine	—	18[b]	—	1[b]

[a]NCI Common Toxicity Criteria (Ross P et al, JCO 2002;20:1996–2004; N = 272)
[b]WHO criteria (Findlay M et al. Ann Oncol 1994;5:609–616; N = 139)

Therapy Monitoring

1. *Before each chemotherapy cycle:* CBC with differential, platelet count, serum electrolytes, magnesium BUN, creatinine, LFTs, and mineral panel
2. *Response evaluation:* After cycles 3, 6, and 8, CT scan and endoscopy
3. Obtain a baseline multigated cardiac scan to determine left ventricular ejection fraction for evidence of cardiovascular disease

REGIMEN

FLUOROURACIL + CISPLATIN

Bleiberg H et al. Eur J Cancer 1997;33:1216–1220

Hydration before cisplatin: ≥1000 mL 0.9% NaCl injection (0.9% NS) at ≥100 mL/hour before and after cisplatin administration. Also encourage high oral intake. Monitor and replace magnesium/electrolytes as needed.
Cisplatin 75–100 mg/m² intravenously in 250 mL 0.9% NS over 60 minutes, given on day 1 every 3 weeks (total dosage/cycle = 75–100 mg/m²)
Take home: Potassium and magnesium oral supplements to use as needed, guided by laboratory monitoring

Fluorouracil 750–1000 mg/m² per day by continuous intravenous infusion in 2000 mL 5% dextrose injection (D5W) over 24 hours on days 1–5 every 3 weeks (total dosage/cycle = 3750–5000 mg/m²)

Emetogenic potential:
Day 1: High (Emetogenicity score = 6)
Days 2–5: Low–moderate (Emetogenicity score = 3)
High potential for delayed symptoms after day 1. See Chapter 39

Patient Population Studied

A study of 44 patients with advanced squamous cell carcinoma of the esophagus.

Efficacy (N = 34)

Complete response	3%
Partial response	32%
Stable disease	29%
Disease progression	18%
Early death	15%
Median failure free survival	7 months

Toxicity (N = 44)

	% G3/4
Hematologic	
Leukopenia	14
Thrombocytopenia	14
Nonhematologic	
Nausea/vomiting*	27
Vascular thrombosis	9
Mucositis	5
Diarrhea	2

*The high rate of nausea and vomiting observed in the original 1997 study should be reduced considerably by using currently available serotonin receptor (5-HT$_3$ antagonist and other antiemetics
WHO criteria

Therapy Monitoring

1. *Before each cycle:* H&P, chest x-ray, CBC with differential, serum electrolytes, BUN, creatinine, and mineral panel
2. *Response evaluation:* Every 2 cycles

Treatment Modifications

Adverse Event	Dose Modification
ANC nadir <1000/mm³ or platelet nadir <50,000/mm³ after treatment	Delay treatment until ANC >1000/mm³ and platelet >50,0000/mm³, then decrease cisplatin dosage by 25% and decrease daily fluorouracil dosages by 50% during subsequent cycles*
Serum creatinine >1.5 mg/dL (133 μmol/L), but <3 mg/dL (265 μmol/L) or creatinine clearance >40 mL/min, but <60 mL/min[0]	Delay treatment until serum creati nine <1.5 mg/dL (133 μmol/L), then decrease cisplatin dosage by 50%*
Serum creatinine >3 mg/dL (265 μmol/L) or creatinine clearance <40 mL/min	Stop cisplatin
G >2 Stomatitis or diarrhea	Decrease fluorouracil dosage by 50%

*Treatment delays for unresolved adverse events of ≥3 weeks warrant discontinuation of treatment

Notes

1. This regimen should be used in selected patients with good performance status
2. Also used for metastatic adenocarcinoma of the distal esophagus and GE junction
3. Patients who cannot tolerate cisplatin can be treated with carboplatin (AUC = 5)

REGIMEN

DOCETAXEL + CISPLATIN + FLUOROURACIL (DCF)

Ajani JA et al. Proc Am Soc Clin Oncol 2003;22:249 [abstract 999]

Docetaxel 75 mg/m^2 intravenously in a volume of 0.9% NaCl injection (0.9% NS) or 5% dextrose injection (D5W) sufficient to produce a solution with concentration within the range 0.3–0.74 mg/mL over 60 minutes, given on day 1 every 3 weeks (total dosage/cycle = 75 mg/m^2)

Hydration before cisplatin: ≥1000 mL 0.9% NS at ≥100 mL/hour before and after cisplatin administration. Also encourage high oral intake. Monitor and replace magnesium/electrolytes as needed.
Cisplatin 75 mg/m^2 intravenously in 25–250 mL of 0.9% NS over 15 – 60 minutes, given on day 1 every 3 weeks (total dosage/cycle = 75 mg/m^2)

Fluorouracil 750 mg/m^2 per day by continuous intravenous infusion in 250–1000 mL of 0.9% NS or D5W over 24 hours on days 1–5 every 3 weeks (total dosage/cycle = 3750 mg/m^2)

Emetogenic potential:
Day 1: High (Emetogenicity score = 6)
Days 2–5: Low–moderate (Emetogenicity score = 2). High potential for delayed symptoms after day 1. See Chapter 39

Patient Population Studied

A study of 115 patients with metastatic or locally unresectable gastric or gastroesophageal junction adenocarcinoma and measurable or evaluable disease

Toxicity (N = 115)

	% Patients
Any G3/4 adverse events	82
Complicated neutropenia	30
Death rate from all causes within 30 days after the last treatment	11.7

Efficacy (N = 115)

Overall response rate	39%
One year survival	44%
Time to progression	5.2 months
Median overall survival	10.2 months

Therapy Monitoring

1. *Before each cycle:* H&P, chest x-ray, CBC with differential, serum electrolytes, BUN, creatinine, and mineral panel
2. *Response evaluation:* Every 2 cycles

Treatment Modifications

Adverse Event	Dose Modification
G3/4 Hematologic adverse events	Use hematopoietic growth factors or decrease doses of docetaxel, cisplatin and fluorouracil by 25% for subsequent cycles
G3/4 Nonhematologic adverse events	Reduce doses of docetaxel, cisplatin and fluorouracil by 25% for subsequent cycles

Notes

1. Reported DCF data reflects interim analysis
2. This regimen is not recommended for patients with WHO/ECOG performance status >1
3. For patients who cannot tolerate cisplatin, DCF is not recommended; however, substitutes such as oxaliplatin or carboplatin have been used
4. Primary prophylaxis with filgrastim or pegfilgrastim may also be considered for qualifying patients

REGIMEN

SINGLE-AGENT VINORELBINE

Conroy T et al. JCO 1996;14:164–170

Vinorelbine 25 mg/m^2 per week intravenously in 50 mL 0.9% NaCl injection (0.9% NS) over 20 minutes (total dosage/week = 25 mg/m^2

Emetogenic potential: Nonemetogenic (Emetogenicity score = 1). See Chapter 39

Patient Population Studied

A study of 46 patients with metastatic squamous cell carcinoma of the esophagus-30 without prior chemotherapy and 16 pretreated with cisplatin-based chemotherapy

Efficacy (N = 46)

	Overall	Naive*
Complete response	2%	0
Partial response	13%	20%
Stable disease	35%	37%
Disease progression	44%	37%
Median duration of response	21 weeks	

*Patients not previously treated with chemotherapy; N = 16 of 46 overall

Toxicity (N = 46)

	% G1	% G2	% G3	% G4
Granulocytopenia[a]	10	17	47	10
Granulocytopenia[b]	6	19	38	25
Thrombocytopenia[a]	0	0	0	0
Thrombocytopenia[b]	6	6	6	0
Anemia[a]	43	13	7	3
Anemia[b]	38	38	13	0
Mucositis	9	4	0	0
Infection	11	11	4	0
Alopecia	11	2	2	0
Diarrhea	11	2	0	0
Nausea/vomiting	20	9	5	0
Liver toxicity	5	0	2	0
Asthenia[a]	30	10	3	0
Asthenia[b]	19	12	0	0
Constipation[a]	10	10	0	0
Constipation[b]	6	6	13	0
Peripheral neurotoxicity[a]	20	0	0	0
Peripheral neurotoxicity[b]	38	0	0	0

[a]No prior chemotherapy
[b]Prior cisplatin-based therapy

WHO criteria

Treatment Modifications

Adverse Event	Dose Modification
G2 Peripheral neurotoxicity	Reduce vinorelbine dosage by 20% during subsequent treatments
G3 Peripheral neurotoxicity	Discontinue therapy
Paralytic ileus	Hold vinorelbine treatment until bowel function recovers, then decrease subsequent vinorelbine dosage by 50%
ANC <1000/mm^3 or platelet count <50,000/mm^3	Hold vinorelbine treatment until ANC >1000/mm^3 and platelet >50,000/mm^3 Adjust subsequent, vinorelbine dosages to patient's tolerance
Patients with histologically-proven cirrhosis	Initial vinorelbine dosage 20 mg/m^2 per week for 4 weeks. If tolerated well, increase dosage to 25 mg/m^2 per week
Injection pain or phlebitis after administration through peripheral venous access	Recommend subsequent treatments through a central vascular access device

Therapy Monitoring

1. *After every fourth weekly treatment:* CBC with differential, serum electrolytes, BUN, creatinine, and mineral panel
2. *Response evaluation:* Every 8 weeks of treatment

Notes

Although the recommended starting dosage is 25 mg/m^2 per week, dose reductions and delays for hematologic toxicity may result in a dose intensity of 20 mg/m^2 per week in heavily pretreated patients or those who have received radiation therapy. Treat responding patients for at least 6 months or until disease progression

13. Gastric Cancer

Manish A. Shah, MD, Dana Rathkopf, MD, and Gary K. Schwartz, MD

Epidemiology

	United States	Worldwide
Incidence	22,280	876,000
Deaths	11430	647,000
Age	65–74 years	
Male:female ratio	2.3:1.0 [mortality in men is approximately doubled]	

Stage at Presentation*	
Localized	23%
Regional	32%
Distant	32%

*Categories do not total 100% because sufficient information is not available to assign a stage to all cancer cases

Jemal A et al. CA Cancer J Clin 2006; 56:106–30

Pathology

Borrman Classification

Gross appearance is the basis for the first classification system of stomach cancers. Any of the four types may coexist:

Type I: Polypoid
Type II: Fungating
Type III: Ulcerated
Type IV: Infiltrative

Lauren Classification

Pattern of local invasion based on histologic features:

(1) Intestinal: composed of cohesive neoplastic cells that form glands and tubular structures
(2) Diffuse: scattered neoplastic cells that invade individually with minimal intercellular cohesion
(3) Mixed

World Health Organization Classification

(1) Adenocarcinoma (intestinal type, diffuse type)
(2) Papillary adenocarcinoma
(3) Tubular adenocarcinoma
(4) Mucinous adenocarcinoma
(5) Signet ring cell carcinoma
(6) Adenosquamous carcinoma
(7) Squamous cell carcinoma
(8) Undifferentiated carcinoma
(9) Unclassified carcinoma

Goseki Classification

Based on histologic architecture, differentiation, and mucin-staining properties:

Group I: Well differentiated, poor mucin content
Group II: Well differentiated, rich mucin content
Group III: Poorly differentiated, poor mucin content
Group IV: Poorly differentiated, rich mucin content

Noffsinger A et al. Gastric Cancer: Pathology. In: Kelsen DP et al, eds. Gastrointestinal Oncology: Principles and Practice. Lippincott Williams & Wilkins, 2002:360–362

Work-Up

1. Multidisciplinary evaluation
2. History and physical examination
3. CBC, platelets, serum electrolytes, BUN, creatinine, mineral panel, and LFTs
4. CT chest, abdomen, and pelvis
5. Esophagogastroduodenoscopy

Locoregional (M0):

1. Medically fit for surgery
   a. Laparoscopy for preoperative assessment to exclude metastatic disease
   b. If considering preoperative therapy, conduct endoscopic US to confirm locally advanced disease
2. Medically unfit for surgery
   a. If considering chemoradiation, conduct laparoscopy to rule out peritoneal spread

Stage IV (M1):

1. No further work-up necessary

NCCN Clinical Practice Guidelines, In Oncology – V. 1. 2006

Pathologic Staging

Primary Tumor (T)

Tx	Primary tumor cannot be assessed
T0	No evidence of primary tumor
Tis	Carcinoma in situ: intraepithelial tumor without invasion of the lamina propria
T1	Tumor invades lamina propria or submucosa
T2	Tumor invades muscularis propria or subserosa[a]
T2a	Tumor invades muscularis propria
T2b	Tumor invades subserosa
T3	Tumor penetrates the serosa (visceral peritoneum) without invasion of adjacent structures[b,c]
T4	Tumor invades adjacent structures[b,c]

Regional Lymph nodes (N)

NX	Regional lymph node(s) cannot be assessed
N0	No regional lymph node metastasis
N1	Metastasis in 1–6 regional lymph nodes
N2	Metastasis in 7–15 regional lymph nodes
N3	Metastasis in >15 regional lymph nodes

Distant Metastasis (M)

MX	Distant metastasis cannot be assessed
M0	No distant metastasis
M1	Distant metastasis

[a]A tumor may penetrate the muscularis propria with extension into the gastrocolic or gastrohepatic ligaments, or into the greater or lesser omentum, without perforation of the visceral peritoneum covering these structures. In this case, the tumor is classified as T2. If there is perforation of the visceral peritoneum covering the gastric ligaments or the omentum, the tumor should be classified as T3

[b]The adjacent structures of the stomach include the spleen, transverse colon, liver, diaphragm, pancreas, abdominal wall, adrenal gland, kidneys, small intestine, and retroperitoneum

[c]Intramural extension of disease to the duodenum or esophagus is classified by the depth of greatest invasion in any of these sites, including the stomach

Staging Groups

Stage 0 (in situ)	T1s	N0	M0
Stage IA	T1	N0	M0
Stage IB	T1	N1	M0
	T2a/b	N0	M0
Stage II	T1	N2	M0
	T2a/b	N1	M0
	T3	N0	M0
Stage IIIA	T2a/b	N2	M0
	T3	N1	M0
	T4	N0	M0
Stage IIIB	T3	N2	M0
Stage IV	T4	N1-2	M0
	Any T	N3	M0
	Any T	Any N	M1

Reproduced, with permission, of the American Joint Committee on Cancer (AJCC), Chicago, Illinois. The original source for this material is the AJCC Cancer Staging Manual, 6th edition (2002) published by Springer-Verlag, New York, www.springeronline.com.

Treatment and Survival by Stage

Stage	Treatment	5-Year Survival Rate
Stage 0 (in situ)	Surgery	>90%
Stage IA	Surgery	60–80%
Stage IB	Surgery ± chemoradiation therapy	50–60%
Stage II	Surgery + chemoradiation therapy	30–50%
Stage IIIA	Surgery + chemoradiation therapy	~20% (distal tumors)
Stage IIIB	Surgery + chemoradiation therapy	~10%
Stage IV	Palliative chemotherapy, radiation therapy	~5%

Adapted from Bonin SR et al. Gastric cancer. In: Pazdur R et al, eds. Cancer Management: A Multidisciplinary Approach, 7th ed. © The Oncology Group, 2003:259–270

Hundahl SA et al. The National Cancer Data Base Report on Poor Survival of U.S. Gastric Carcinoma Patients Treated with Gastrectomy. Cancer 2000;88(4):921–932

Surgery

Surgical options:

1. Distal (body + antrum): subtotal gastrectomy preferred
2. Proximal (cardia): total or proximal gastrectomy, as indicated (total gastrectomy avoids reflux gastritis)
3. A >5 cm proximal and distal margin from gross tumor is desired
4. Avoid splenectomy if possible
5. Consider placing a feeding tube

Extent of lymph node dissection:

A minimum of 15 lymph nodes should be evaluated

1. D0: unacceptable
2. D1: standard
3. D2: remains debated

NCCN Oncology Practice Guidelines, vol 1, 2003
Bonenkamp JJ et al. Extended lymph-node dissection for gastric cancer. Dutch Gastric Cancer Group. NEJM 1999;340:908–914
Cuschieri et al. Lancet 1996;347:995–999.

Caveats

1. Diffuse gastric histology and peritoneal spread may adversely affect the motility of the gastrointestinal tract. Consider promotility agents
2. Common sites of metastatic spread:

   Lymphatic: M1 lymph nodes include para-aortic nodes. Supradiaphragmatic and mediastinal nodes may also be involved. Rare involvement of the left supraclavicular nodes occurs via the thoracic duct

   Blood-borne: Distant metastases to the liver, lungs, bone, and skin. Either hematogenous spread or neoplastic seeding of the peritoneum, mesentery, and omentum can result in massive bilateral involvement of the ovaries (Krukenberg tumor)
3. Consider investigational agents as first-line therapy because the relative 5-year survival rate for all stages is 22%
4. Adjuvant chemoradiation is recommended following surgery

Bonin SR et al. Gastric cancer. In: Pazdur R et al, eds. Cancer Management: A Multidisciplinary Approach, 7th ed. The Oncology Group, 2003:259–270
Noffsinger A et al. Gastric cancer: Pathology. In: Kelsen DP et al, eds. Gastrointestinal Oncology: Principles and Practice. Lippincott Williams & Wilkins, 2002:365
D' Angelica et al Patterns of initial recurrence in completely resected gastric adenocarcinoma. Ann Surg 2004; 240:808–16

ADJUVANT REGIMEN

ADJUVANT CHEMORADIATION: FLUOROURACIL, LEUCOVORIN, AND RADIATION

Macdonald JS et al. NEJM 2001;345:725–730

Chemotherapy before radiation:
Fluorouracil 425 mg/m^2 per day by intravenous infusion in 25–100 mL of 0.9% NaCl injection (0.9% NS) or 5% dextrose injection (D5W) over 5–30 minutes on days 1–5 (total dosage/cycle = 2125 mg/m^2)
Leucovorin 20 mg/m^2 per day by intravenous infusion in 25–100 mL of 0.9% NS or D5W over 5–15 minutes on days 1–5 (total dosage/cycle = 100 mg/m^2)

Chemotherapy plus radiation:
[Starts 28 days after last chemotherapy (ie, day 29)]
Fluorouracil 400 mg/m^2 per day by intravenous infusion in 25–100 mL of 0.9% NS or D5W over 5–30 minutes on days 1–4 during the first week of radiation therapy (total dosage during first week of combined chemoradiation = 1600 mg/m^2)
Leucovorin 20 mg/m^2) per day by intravenous infusion in 25–100 mL of 0.9% NS or D5W over 5–15 minutes on days 1–4 during the first week of radiation therapy (total dosage during the first week of combined chemoradiation = 80 mg/m^2)
Radiation 180 cGy/day for 5 days/week for 5 consecutive weeks (total dose 4500 cGy in 25 fractions)

- Radiation fields must be evaluated carefully
- One-third of patients require field adjustments

Fluorouracil 400 mg/m^2 per day by intravenous infusion in 25–100 mL of 0.9% NS or D5W over 5–30 minutes on days 3–5 during the fifth week of radiation therapy (total dosage during the fifth week of combined chemoradiation = 1200 mg/m^2)
Leucovorin 20 mg/m^2 per day by intravenous infusion in 25–100 mL of 0.9% NS or D5W over 5–15 minutes on days 3–5 during the fifth week of radiation therapy (total dosage during the fifth week of combined chemoradiation = 60 mg/m^2)

Chemotherapy after radiation:
[Starts 1 month after completing radiation therapy]
Fluorouracil 425 mg/m^2 per day by intravenous infusion in 25–100 mL of 0.9% NS or D5W over 5–30 minutes on days 1–5 every 4 weeks, for 2 cycles (total dosage/cycle = 2125 mg/m^2)
Leucovorin 20 mg/m^2 per day by intravenous infusion in 25–100 mL of 0.9% NS or D5W over 5–15 minutes on days 1–5, every 4 weeks for 2 cycles (total dosage/cycle = 100 mg/m^2)

Emetogenic potential: Low (Emetogenicity score = 2). See Chapter 39

Treatment Modifications

Dose modification as clinically indicated based on the most significant toxicity

Dosage level −1	Fluorouracil 350 mg/m^2
Dosage level −2	Fluorouracil 300 mg/m^2

Note: These recommendations apply to all four chemotherapy phases

Toxicity (N = 273)

	No. of Patients (%) (Grade ≥ 3)
Hematologic	148 (54)
Gastrointestinal	89 (33)
Influenza-like	25 (9)
Infection	16 (6)
Neurologic	12 (4)
Cardiovascular	11 (4)
Pain	9 (3)
Metabolic	5 (2)
Hepatic	4 (1)
Lung-related	3 (1)
Death*	3 (1)

*One patient died from a cardiac event, one from pulmonary fibrosis, and one from sepsis complicating myelosuppression

Cessation of Chemoradiotherapy (N = 281)

Reason	No. of Patients (%)
Protocol treatment completed	181 (64)
Toxic effects	49 (17)
Patient declined further treatment	23 (8)
Progression of disease	13 (5)
Death	3 (1)
Other	12 (4)

Patient Population Studied

A study of 556 evaluable patients with stage IB-IV M0 gastric cancer who had undergone curative surgery were randomly assigned to receive adjuvant chemoradiation or observation alone. Patients essentially had completely recovered from resection and were no longer losing weight. Locoregional radiation therapy plus fluorinated pyrimidine-based chemotherapy as adjuvant treatment significantly improved overall and relapse-free survival among patients with gastric cancer

Efficacy (N = 281)

Intention-to-Treat Analysis

Median overall survival	36 months
3-year disease-free survival	48%
Median relapse free survival	30 months

Therapy Monitoring

1. *Prior to each cycle:* Interval history with emphasis on clinical toxicities, PE, CBC with differential, serum creatinine, and LFTs before each cycle
2. *Response evaluation:* One month after completing radiation therapy, then at chemotherapy completion. Subsequent follow-up as clinically indicated, including EGD and CT imaging

ADVANCED DISEASE REGIMEN

EPIRUBICIN, CISPLATIN, AND FLUOROURACIL (ECF)

Webb A et al. JCO 1997;15:261–267

Epirubicin 50 mg/m^2 by intravenous push over 3–20 minutes on day 1 every 3 weeks for a maximum of 8 cycles (total dosage/3-week cycle = 50 mg/m^2)

Hydration before cisplatin: ≥1000 mL 0.9% NaCl injection (0.9% NS) infused over a minimum of 3–4 hours. Monitor and replace magnesium/electrolytes as needed
Mannitol diuresis: **Mannitol** may be given to patients who have received adequate hydration. A bolus dose of 12.5 g mannitol can be administered as an intravenous push before starting cisplatin or in the same container as cisplatin. Continued hydration is essential
Cisplatin 60 mg/m^2 by intravenous infusion in 100–500 mL of 0.9% NS over 30–60 minutes on day 1 every 3 weeks for a maximum of 8 cycles (total dosage/3-week cycle = 60 mg/m^2)
Hydration after cisplatin: ≥1000 mL 0.9% NS infused over a minimum of 3–4 hours. Also, encourage high oral intake. Goal is to achieve a urine output of ≥100 mL/hour

Fluorouracil 200 mg/m^2 by continuous intravenous infusion in 50–1000 mL 0.9% NS, or 5% dextrose injection (D5W) over 24 hours, starting on cycle 1, day 1, continuously for a maximum duration of 6 months (total dosage/3-week cycle = 4200 mg/m^2)

Emetogenic potential:
Day 1: Very high (Emetogenicity score = 7)
High potential for delayed symptoms after day 1
During fluorouracil continuous infusion: Nonemetogenic (Emetogenicity score <2). See Chapter 39

Patient Population Studied

A trial of 274 patients with previously untreated advanced esophagogastric cancer randomized to receive epirubicin, cisplatin, and fluorouracil (ECF; N = 137) compared with fluorouracil, doxorubicin, and methotrexate (FAMTX; N = 137). The ECF regimen resulted in a survival and response advantage, tolerable toxicity, and better quality of life and cost-effectiveness

Efficacy (N = 111–126)

	N = 111	Intent to Treat = 126
CR	6%	5.5%
PR	39%	34%
SD	21%	18%
PD	20%	17%
Insufficient Treatment		
Early death	6%	
Toxic death	1%	
Toxicity	3.5%	
Patient request	3.5%	
Median survival		8.9 months
1-year survival		36%
2-year survival		11%
Median failure-free survival		7.4 months

WHO criteria

Treatment Modifications

(Treatment delays in 32% of patients. Dose reductions in 41% of patients)

Adverse Event	Dose Modification
Plantar/palmar erythema (PPE)	Give pyridoxine 50 mg orally three times daily. If PPE does not improve, hold fluorouracil for 1 week, then resume at 150 mg/m^2 per day by continuous infusion
G ≤ 2 Mucositis or diarrhea	Interrupt chemotherapy until mucositis and diarrhea resolve, then resume fluorouracil with daily dosage reduced by 50 mg/m^2
G3/4 Mucositis or diarrhea	Interrupt chemotherapy until mucositis and diarrhea resolve, then resume fluorouracil with daily dosage reduced by 100 mg/m^2
Creatinine clearance[a] 40–60 mL/min	Reduce cisplatin so that dose in milligrams equals the creatinine clearance[a] value in mls/min[b]
Creatinine clearance[a] <40 mL/min	Hold cisplatin
Day 1 WBC <2000/mm^3 or platelet count <100,000/mm^3	Delay cisplatin and epirubicin for 1 week or until myelosuppression resolves
Second treatment delay due to myelosuppression	Delay cisplatin and epirubicin for 1 week, or until myelosuppression resolves, then decrease epirubicin dosage by 25% during subsequent treatments
Sepsis during an episode of neutropenia	

[a]Creatinine clearance used as a measure of glomerular filtration rate
[b]This also applies to patients with creatinine clearance (GFR) of 40–60 mL/min at the outset of treatment

Findlay M et al. Ann Oncol 194;5:609–616

Toxicity (N = Unclear/63)

	% All Grades	%G3/4
Hematologic		
Leukopenia	61	12
Neutropenia	68	36[b]
Thrombocytopenia	10	4
Anemia	68	8
Nonhematologic		
Mucositis	49	6
Plantar-palmar erythema	31	3
Nausea/vomiting	88	17
Diarrhea	38	6
Infection	40	8
Renal	12	1
Peripheral neuropathy	20	—
Alopecia	93 (56[a])	—

[a]G2 alopecia, pronounced or total hair loss
[b]Treatment-related death in one patient due to sepsis during period of neutropenia

NCI CTC

Therapy Monitoring

1. *Before each cycle:* PE with attention to clinical toxicities, CBC with differential, serum sodium, potassium, magnesium, creatinine, BUN, and LFTs before each cycle
2. *Before repeated cisplatin treatments:* Monitor serum creatinine for calculated creatinine clearance (CrCl). Measure CrCl with either a 12- or a 24-hour urine collection

ADVANCED DISEASE REGIMEN

IRINOTECAN + CISPLATIN

Ajani JA et al. Cancer 2002;94:641–646

Irinotecan 65 mg/m^2 by intravenous infusion diluted in 5% dextrose injection (D5W) to a concentration of 0.12–2.8 mg/mL over 90 minutes weekly, during weeks 1–4 every 6 weeks (total dosage/cycle = 260 mg/m^2)
Early-onset diarrhea (within 24 hours after irinotecan administration):
Atropine 0.5 mg by intravenous push. The dose may be repeated after 15 minutes if diarrhea, abdominal cramping, or diaphoresis persists
Note. If atropine is given, include atropine 0.5 mg by intravenous push in primary prophylaxis during all subsequent cycles
Late-onset diarrhea ≥24 hours after irinotecan administration:
Loperamide 4 mg orally at the first onset of loose stools, followed by:
Loperamide 2 mg orally every 2 hours around-the-clock until the patient is free from diarrhea for 12 hours
Loperamide is available in the United States as capsules and tablets containing 2 mg loperamide, and in liquid formulations containing loperamide 1 mg/mL or 5 mg/mL

Hydration before cisplatin: ≥1000 mL 0.9% NaCl injection (0.9% NS) infused over a minimum of 3–4 hours
Cisplatin 30 mg/m^2 intravenously after irinotecan in 100–250 mL 0.9% NS over 60 minutes, weekly on weeks 1–4, every 6 weeks (total dosage/cycle = 120 mg/m^2)
Note: Irinotecan and cisplatin are administered weekly for 4 consecutive weeks followed by a recovery period of 2 weeks without treatment

Emetogenic potential: High (Emetogenicity score = 5). See Chapter 39

Patient Population Studied

A phase II trial of 36 evaluable patients with advanced untreated gastric or gastroesophageal junction carcinoma

Efficacy (N = 36)

Complete response	11%
Partial response	47%
Minor response	14%
Progressive disease	22%
Stable disease	6%
Median time to progression	24 weeks
Median survival	9 months

Toxicity (N = 36)

	% G1	% G2	% G3	% G4
Diarrhea	27	21	17	5
Fatigue	13	16	27	14
Myalgia	13	2	2	0
Nausea	18	32	15	1
Emesis	22	19	4	2
Neuropathy	6	2	0	0
Alopecia	36	33	0	0
Dizziness	1	2	0	0
Neutropenia	15	18	12	15
Febrile neutropenia	0	3	4	0

Treatment-related death: 1 patient neutropenia and sepsis

Therapy Monitoring

1. *Cycle 1:* CBC with differential, serum electrolytes, magnesium, calcium, BUN, and LFTs on days 1 and 22
2. *Before repeated cycles:* PE, CBC with differential, serum electrolytes, magnesium, calcium, BUN, and LFTs

Treatment Modifications

	Dosage Level	
Cisplatin	Level 0	30 mg/m^2
	Level −1	20 mg/m^2
Irinotecan	Level 0	65 mg/m^2
	Level −1	50 mg/m^2
	Level −2	40 mg/m^2

Adverse Event	Dose Modification
If on day 1 of a cycle, WBC <3000/mm^3, ANC <1000/mm^3, or platelet < 100,000/mm^3	Hold irinotecan and cisplatin for 1 week, then resume treatment if WBC ≥3000/mm^3, ANC ≥1000/mm^3 platelet ≥100,000/mm^3, serum creatinine <1.5 mg/dL (133 μmol/L) and nonhematologic toxicity including gastrointestinal toxicity or stomatitis ≤ G1
If on day 1 of a cycle, G ≥ 2 nonhematologic adverse event, or serum creatinine ≥1.8 mg/dL (158 μmol/L)	Hold cisplatin and irinotecan for 1 week, then resume at cisplatin dose level −1 if creatinine ≤1.5 mg/dL (133 μmol/L)
G4 Neutropenia (with or without fever)	Add primary prophylaxis with filgrastim during all subsequent cycles
Febrile neutropenia despite filgrastim support	Hold treatment until adverse event resolves, then resume chemotherapy with irinotecan or cisplatin dosage reduced by one dose level
G3/4 Nonhematologic adverse events (except nausea or vomiting), G3/4 diarrhea despite loperamide, G4 ANC, or thrombocytopenia during cycle 1	

Modified from Ajani JA et al. Cancer 2002;94:641–646
Saltz LB et al. JCO 1998;16:3858–3865

ADVANCED DISEASE REGIMEN

CISPLATIN + FLUOROURACIL (FUP)

Vanhoefer U et al. JCO 2000;18:2648–2657

Fluorouracil 1000 mg/m² by continuous intravenous infusion in 50–1000 mL of 0.9% NaCl injection (0.9% NS) or 5% dextrose injection (D5W) over 24 hours on days 1–5 every 28 days (total dosage/cycle = 5000 mg/m²)

Hydration before cisplatin: ≥1000 mL 0.9% NS infused over a minimum of 3–4 hours. Monitor and replace magnesium/electrolytes as needed.
Optional mannitol diuresis: **Mannitol** may be given after adequate hydration. A dose of 12.5 g mannitol can be administered as an intravenous push before starting cisplatin or in the same container as cisplatin (through an in-line filter with pore size ≤5 micrometers). Continued hydration is essential
Cisplatin 100 mg/m² intravenously in 100–500 mL of 0.9% NS over 1 hour on day 2 every 28 days (total dosage/cycle = 100 mg/m²)
Hydration after cisplatin: ≥1000 mL 0.9% NS infused over a minimum of 3–4 hours. Also, encourage high oral intake. Goal is to achieve a urine output of ≥100 mL/hour. "Hyperhydration" encouraged in anticipation of mucositis
Optional mannitol diuresis: **Mannitol** 12.5 g intravenously at 60 mL/hour for 5 hours after cisplatin (through an in-line filter with pore size = 1.2 micrometer)

Emetogenic potential:
During fluorouracil continuous infusion: Low (Emetogenicity score ~2)
Day 2: Very high (Emetogenicity score = 7)
High potential for delayed symptoms after day 2. See Chapter 39

Patient Population

A trial of 245 eligible patients with advanced adenocarcinoma of the stomach randomized to receive sequential high-dose methotrexate, fluorouracil, and doxorubicin (FAMTX) versus etoposide, leucovorin, and fluorouracil (ELF) versus infusional fluorouracil and cisplatin (FUP). The overall response rate in patients with measurable disease was 12% (FAMTX), 9% (ELF), and 20% (FUP). Final report of EORTC trial 40902

Efficacy (n = 81)

Eligible Patients with Measurable Disease	
Partial response	20%
No change	43%
Progressive disease	21%
Intention-to-treat analyses (N = 134)	
Progression-free survival	4.1 months
Median survival	7.2 months
Probability at 1 year for survival	27%

WHO Response Criteria

Toxicity (n = 127)

Adverse Event	% Patients with G3 or G4
Leukopenia	17
Neutropenia	35
Thrombocytopenia	9
Infection	5
Nausea/vomiting	26
Mucositis	12
Diarrhea	6
Renal	2
Peripheral neuropathy	<1
Alopecia	16

Treatment-related death in 2 patients

WHO criteria

Treatment Modifications

Dosage Levels		
Cisplatin	Level 0	100 mg/m²
	Level −1	75 mg/m²
	Level −2	50 mg/m²
Fluorouracil	Level 0	1000 mg/m²/day for 5 days
	Level −1	800 mg/m²/day for 5 days
	Level −2	600 mg/m²/day for 5 days

Adverse Event	Dose Modification
G3/4 Diarrhea or stomatitis	Reduce fluorouracil one dose level
Reduction in creatinine clearance[a] to ≤ 60% of on study value	Delay therapy 1 week. If creatinine clearance does not recover to pretreatment values, then reduce cisplatin one dose level
Peripheral neuropathy	Delay therapy 1 week. If symptoms do not resolve to G ≤ 1, reduce cisplatin one dose level

Other dose modifications as clinically indicated based on the most significant toxicity

[a]Creatinine clearance used as a measure of glomerular filtration rate

Therapy Monitoring

1. *Before each cycle*: PE, CBC with differential, and serum electrolytes, magnesium, calcium, BUN, and LFTs before repeated cycles
2. *Response evaluation*: Every 2 cycles

ADVANCED DISEASE REGIMEN

DOCETAXEL, CISPLATIN, AND FLUOROURACIL (DCF)

Moiseynko VM et al. Proc Am Soc Clin Oncol 2005;23:4002

Docetaxel 75 mg/m^2 by intravenous infusion diluted in 0.9% NaCl injection (0.9% NS) or 5% dextrose injection (D5W) sufficient to produce a docetaxel concentration of 0.3–0.74 mg/mL over 30–60 minutes on day 1 every 3 weeks (total dosage/cycle = 75 mg/m^2)

Hydration before cisplatin: ≥1000 mL 0.9% NS infused over a minimum of 3–4 hours. Monitor and replace magnesium/electrolytes as needed
Optional mannitol diuresis: **Mannitol** may be given to patients who have received adequate hydration. A bolus 12.5 g mannitol can be administered as an intravenous push before starting cisplatin or in the same container as cisplatin. Continued hydration is essential
Cisplatin 75 mg/m^2 by intravenous infusion in 100—250 mL 0.9% NS over 30–60 minutes on day 1 every 3 weeks (total dosage/cycle = 75 mg/m^2)
Hydration after cisplatin: ≥1000 mL 0.9% NS infused over a minimum of 3–4 hours. Also, encourage high oral intake. Goal is to achieve a urine output of ≥100 mL/hour

Fluorouracil 750 mg/m^2 per day by continuous intravenous infusion in 50–1000 mL 0.9% NS or D5W over 24 hours on days 1–5 every 3 weeks (total dosage/cycle = 3750 mg/m^2)

Emetogenic potential:
Day 1: Very high (Emetogenicity score ~ 9)
High potential for delayed symptoms after day 1
During fluorouracil continuous infusion: Low (Emetogenicity score = 2). See Chapter 39

Patient Population Studied

A trial of 445 evaluable patients with chemotherapy-naive metastatic or locally recurrent, unresectable gastric carcinoma randomly assigned to receive DCF or cisplatin and fluorouracil (FUP). The DCF regimen resulted in a significantly longer time to progression, survival and higher response rate than FUP, but G3/4 adverse events were significant in both arms

Efficacy

Time to disease progression	5.6 months (4.9–5.9)
Median overall survival	9.2 months
Response rate	36.7%

Toxicity (n ≃ 110)

Adverse Event	% Patients G ≥3
Neutropenia	82
Febrile neutropenia or infection with neutropenia	66
Neurosensory	17
Infection	36
Anorexia	29
Nausea	35
Vomiting	33
Lethargy	47
Diarrhea	45
Stomatitis	46
Death rate due to all causes within 30 days > last chemotherapy cycle	10.4%

Treatment Modifications

	Dosage Level	
Docetaxel	Level −1	55 mg/m^2
Cisplatin	Level −1	60 mg/m^2
Fluorouracil	Level −1	500 mg/m^2/day for 5 days

Adverse Event	Dose Modification
G3/4 Diarrhea or stomatitis	Reduce fluorouracil one dose level
Reduction in creatinine clearance[a] to <60% of on-study value	Delay therapy 1 week. If creatinine clearance does not recover to pretreatment values, then reduce cisplatin one dose level
Peripheral neuropathy	Delay therapy 1 week. If symptoms do not resolve to G ≤ 1, reduce cisplatin and/or docetaxel one dose level

[a]Creatinine clearance used as a measure of glomerular filtration rate.
Other dose modifications as clinically indicated based on the most significant toxicity

Therapy Monitoring

1. *Before each cycle:* PE, CBC with differential, serum electrolytes, magnesium, calcium, BUN, and LFTs.
2. *Response evaluation:* Every 2 cycles

14. Gestational Trophoblastic Neoplasia

Michael M. Boyiadzis, MD, MHSc, and John Lurain, MD

Epidemiology

Incidence:*

Hydatidiform mole: 1 in 1000–2000 pregnancies (United States and Europe)
Choriocarcinoma: 1 in 20,000–40,000 pregnancies (United States and Europe)
Gestational trophoblastic neoplasia (GTN) lesions are nearly always disorders of the reproductive years. The incidence is higher in women <20 years and >40 years

*The reported incidence of hydatidiform mole and choriocarcinoma varies widely throughout the world, being greatest in Asia, Africa, and Latin America and substantially lower in North America and Europe

Blaustein's Pathology of the Female Genital Tract, 5th ed. Chapter 24, 2002

Pathology

Hydatidiform Mole

Benign (80%)	**GTN (20%)**
Complete hydatidiform mole	Invasive mole (18%)
Partial hydatidiform mole	Choriocarcinoma (2%)*
	Placental site trophoblastic tumor (rare)
	Epitheloid trophoblastic tumors (rare)

**Note:* Half of all choriocarcinomas occur in association with nonmolar pregnancies

Gestational Trophoblastic Neoplasia

- Potential for local invasion and metastases
- Most commonly develops after a molar pregnancy, but can arise de novo after any gestational experience: spontaneous or induced abortion, ectopic pregnancy, or preterm or term pregnancy
- The most common sites of metastases are lungs (80%), brain (10%) liver (10%), and vagina (~5%)

Cheung AN-Y. Best Pract Res Clin Obstet Gynaecol 2003;17:849–868
Wong LC et al. Asia-Oceania J Obstet Gynecol 1990;16:123–126

Work-Up

Once a diagnosis of GTN has been made, it is necessary to determine the extent of disease
Once the initial work-up is completed, patients are categorized (see Staging below)

1. H&P
2. Serum β-hCG

Note: For staging purposes, the β-hCG level that is important is that obtained immediately before instituting treatment and not the β-hCG obtained at the time of the previous molar evacuation

3. CBC, LFT, serum electrolytes, BUN, creatinine, PTT, and PT
4. Chest x-ray
5. CT of chest, abdomen, and pelvis
6. MRI brain (especially in patients with lung lesions. Asymptomatic patients with a normal chest x-ray are unlikely to have brain metastasis)
7. TSH, T_4 (elevations of thyroid tests are not common in patients with GTN but can occur mostly in association with hydatidiform mole)

Soper JT. Clin Obstet Gynecol 2003;46:570–578
Soper JT et al. Gynecol Oncol 2004;93:575–585

Staging

FIGO Anatomic Staging System for GTN

Stage	Extent of GTN [GTT]
I:	Confined to the uterus
II:	Extends outside the uterus, but is limited to the genital structures (adnexa, vagina, broad ligament)
III:	Extends to the lungs, with or without known genital tract involvement
IV:	All other metastatic sites

Revised 2000 FIGO Scoring System[a] (Modified WHO Scoring System)

[*Note:* This scoring system does not apply to patients with placental site trophoblastic tumors]

Prognostic factor	0	1	2	4
Age (years)	≤39	>39	—	—
Antecedent pregnancy	Hydatidiform mole	Abortion	Term pregnancy	—
Interval from index pregnancy	<4 months	4–6 months	7–12 months	>12 months
Pretreatment β-hCG level (units/L)	<1000	1000–10,000	>10,000–100,000	>100,000
Largest tumor size including uterus	—	3–4 cm	5 cm	—
Sites of metastases	Lung[b]	Spleen, kidney	GI tract	Brain, liver
Number of metastases identified[b]	0	1–4	4–8	>8
Previous ineffective chemotherapy	—	—	Single drug	≥2 drugs

[a]FIGO staging system includes a modification of the WHO prognostic index score for risk assessment
[b]Chest x-ray is used to count the number of metastases for risk score assessment

Note: Total score for a patient is obtained by adding individual scores for each prognostic factor

Total Score	Risk
0–6	Low risk
≥7	High risk

Both the **FIGO Anatomic Staging System** and the **Modified WHO SCORING System** are often used. By convention, the FIGO system is depicted by a Roman numeral and should be followed by the Modified WHO Score depicted by an Arabic numeral. The two values are separated by a colon. Example: III:9

Clinical Assessment

Note: **Previously used clinical classification schema should not be used for staging**

Metastatic GTN
(Any extrauterine metastases)

Low-risk metastatic GTN = no risk factors:

- Short disease duration (<4 months from antecedent pregnancy)
- Pretherapy β-hCG <40,000 units/L
- No brain or liver metastases
- No antecedent term pregnancy
- No prior chemotherapy

High-risk metastatic GTN = any risk factor:

- Long disease duration (>4 months from antecedent pregnancy)
- Pretherapy β-hCG >40,000 units/L
- Brain or liver metastases
- Antecedent term pregnancy
- Prior chemotherapy

Hancock BW. Best Pract Res Clin Obstet Gynaecol 2003; 17:869-83
Soper JT. Clin Obstet Gynecol 2003; 46:570-78
Kohorn EI. Int J Gynecol Cancer 2001; 11:73-7
Kohorn EI et al, International Journal of Gynecological Cancer 2000; 10:84-88

Survival

GTN can be cured predictably even in the presence of widespread metastases. Overall survival is >95%, with survival rates approaching 100% for stage I and stage II/III or WHO score <7 and 80–90% for stage IV or WHO score ≥7 disease

Caveats

Nonmetastatic (FIGO Stage I) and low-risk metastatic (FIGO Stages II and III; WHO Score <7) GTN

1. Excellent prognosis. Remission rates with chemotherapy approach 100%. Hysterectomy can be used as part of initial therapy in patients who no longer wish to preserve fertility
2. A majority can achieve a remission with **single-agent chemotherapy**. The most active single agents include methotrexate, actinomycin-D, and etoposide
3. Begin therapy with methotrexate. Switch chemotherapy:
   - *To alternate single-agent (actinomycin-D):* If β-hCG values plateau after and initial good response *or*
   - *To multi-agent chemotherapy:* If no response or a rise in β-hCG

High-risk metastatic GTN (FIGO Stage IV; WHO Score ≥7)

1. Standard treatment is combination chemotherapy. The most commonly used regimen is EMA/CO, consisting of a combination of etoposide, methotrexate, actinomycin-D, cyclophosphamide, and vincristine
2. Salvage chemotherapy consists of a regimen combining platinum agents (cisplatin or carboplatin) and etoposide with methotrexate and actinomycin-D (EP/EMA), bleomycin (BEP), ifosfamide (VIP, ICE), or paclitaxel
3. Although effective chemotherapy of metastatic GTN is available, physicians must be vigilant for possible secondary malignancies. The risk of treatment-related leukemia has been reported to be increased 16.6-fold with 80% of cases occurring within 5 years after etoposide exposure. An increased incidence of colon, melanoma, and breast cancers has also been reported at 5, 10, and 25 years, respectively, after treatment. Because not only the intensity of therapy, but also the duration of therapy may be important, keep the duration to <6 months whenever possible
4. Fertility seems to be preserved in a majority of patients without an excess of fetal abnormalities

Placental site trophoblastic tumors

1. Placental site trophoblastic tumor is a rare form of GTN that can infiltrate locally, spread via lymphatics and metastasize to other sites, most commonly the lung. Placental site trophoblastic tumor is excluded from the FIGO scoring system and should be managed separately because biological behavior is different from typical GTN
2. When disease is limited to the uterus, the treatment of choice is hysterectomy
3. EP/EMA is currently the chemotherapy regimen of choice for patients with metastatic disease or associated poor prognostic factors
4. Important adverse determinants of outcome in patients with metastatic disease are interval from prior pregnancy >2 years and a high mitotic rate (>5 mitosis/10 HPF)

β-hCG levels

1. GTN always produces measurable β-hCG that can be detected with a sensitive assay, allowing for precise monitoring of disease and response to therapy
2. Use a radioimmunoassay that detects intact β-hCG as well as the various degradation products. Assays must be able to detect degraded forms of β-hCG because they are produced in larger amounts in patients with GTN compared with those with a normal pregnancy
3. Treatment decisions should be based on measurements of serum β-hCG because there is higher background interference in urine samples
4. Complete remission is diagnosed after obtaining 3 consecutive weekly β-hCG levels within the normal range
5. Resistance to treatment is defined as a plateau of β-hCG levels on two consecutive measurements or a β–hCG rise after a course of treatment
6. *Following remission:* β–hCG levels are obtained monthly for 12 months and every 3 months during the second year

Follow-up

Patients are advised not to become pregnant for 1 year after completion of successful treatment

Lurain JT. Expert Opin Pharmacother 2003;4:2005–2017
Newlands ES. Best Pract Res Clin Obstet Gynaecol 2003;17:905–923
Newlands ES et al. [Abstract] Proc Am Soc Clin Oncol 1995;14:269
Soper JT et al. Gynecol Oncol 2004;93:575–585

REGIMEN FOR LOW-RISK GTN

METHOTREXATE

Lurain JR, Elfstrand EP. Am J Obstet Gynecol 1995;172:574–579

Methotrexate 0.4 mg/kg (maximum daily dose = 25 mg) per day intravenously per push, daily for 5 days on days 1–5 every 2 weeks (total dosage/14-day cycle = 2 mg/m^2, maximum dose/14-day cycle = 125 mg)

Supportive care:
Mouth care primary prophylaxis for stomatitis

Recommendations:
1. Administer treatment courses as often as toxicity permits, usually every 14 days
2. Encourage increased oral fluid intake or, if NPO, give parenteral hydration
3. Avoid drugs that can alter methotrexate elimination, such as nonsteroidal anti-inflammatory drugs, omeprazole (and possibly other proton pump inhibitors), penicillins, probenecid, and salicylates
4. Administer two additional cycles after the first normal β-hCG level

Emetogenic potential:
Days 1–5: Nonemetogenic (Emetogenicity score = 1). See Chapter 39

Patient Population Studied

Retrospective review of 253 patients with nonmetastatic gestational trophoblastic tumors [invasive mole (209) or choriocarcinoma (44)] treated from 1962 to 1990. Antecedent pregnancy was hydatidiform mole (230), abortion (16), and term or preterm delivery (7). A mean of 4.7 courses (range 1–7) of single-agent methotrexate was administered

Efficacy (N = 253)

Treatment	% Complete Response
Methotrexate alone	89.3*
Methotrexate™ actinomycin D	8.7
Multiagent chemotherapy or surgery	2.0
Survival	100

*Six patients (2.4%) had a relapse 1–9 months after achieving a complete response. All were placed into a permanent remission with additional chemotherapy

Toxicity (N = 253)

Stomatitis	G3 (16 patients) Mild to moderate (many)
Conjunctivitis	3 patients
Pleuritic/peritoneal pain	3 patients
Hair loss	None
Nausea/vomiting	Not common
Toxicity requiring dose reduction	11 patients (4.3%)
Toxicity requiring change in therapy*	12 patients (4.7%)

*Reasons: G3 stomatitis (5), rash and stomatitis (4); prolonged neutropenia (2), elevated LFTs (1)

Treatment Modifications

Adverse Event	Dose Modification
G ≤ 1 toxicity	Continue therapy if easy to manage
G2 toxicity	Consider a 20% reduction in methotrexate dosage
G ≥ 3 toxicity	Discontinue methotrexate and institute other therapy

Therapy Monitoring

1. *Every other week:* PE, CBC with differential, serum electrolytes, LFTs, serum creatinine, BUN, and β-hCG
2. *Methotrexate levels:* Not routinely performed
3. *Complete remission:* 3 consecutive weekly β-hCG levels within normal range
4. *Resistance to treatment:* β-hCG plateau over 2 consecutive treatments or a β-hCG rise after any treatment
5. *Following remission:* β-hCG levels are obtained monthly for 12 months, and every 3 months during the second year

Notes

1. Pretreatment β-hCG levels >40–50,000 units/L, nonmolar antecedent pregnancy and clinicopathologic diagnosis of choriocarcinoma are associated with development of resistance
2. Determination of glomerular filtration rate before treatment does not predict for methotrexate clearance and potential toxicity, but serum creatinine that is within normal limits and a GFR (creatinine clearance) ≥60 mL/min are generally accepted as reasonable criteria for adequate renal function

REGIMEN FOR LOW-RISK GTN

METHOTREXATE WITH FOLINIC ACID (MTX-FA)

Bagshawe KD et al. Br J Obstet Gynecol 1989;96:795–802
Berkowitz RS et al. Gynecol Oncol 1986;23:111–118
Wong LC et al. Am J Obstet Gynecol 1985;152:59–62

Methotrexate 1 mg/kg (maximum daily dose = 50 mg) per day intramuscularly or intravenously per push on days 1, 3, 5, and 7 every 2 weeks (total dosage/14-day cycle = 4 mg/m^2, or 200 mg)
Leucovorin calcium 0.1 mg/kg orally or intramuscularly on days 2, 4, 6, and 8, beginning 24 hours after the methotrexate administration every 2 weeks (total dose/cycle = 60 mg).

Supportive care:
Mouth care primary prophylaxis for stomatitis

Notes:
1. Administer treatment courses as often as toxicity permits after a minimum rest period of 7 days (usually every 14 days)
2. Encourage increased oral fluid intake or, if NPO, give parenteral hydration
3. Avoid drugs that can alter methotrexate elimination, such as nonsteroidal anti-inflammatory drugs, omeprazole (and possibly other proton pump inhibitors), penicillins, probenecid, and salicylates
4. Administer two additional cycles after the first normal β-hCG level

Emetogenic potential:
Days 1, 3, 5, and 7: Nonemetogenic (Emetogenicity score = 1). See Chapter 39

Patient Population Studied

Patients with low-risk GTN

Efficacy (N = 348)

Treatment	Complete Response
Changed treatment for drug resistance	20%
Relapsed	4%
Survival	99.7%[1]

One death due to concurrent non-Hodgkin lymphoma
Bagshawe KD et al. Br J Obstet Gynecol 1989;96:795–802

Toxicity (N = 185)

	% Patients
Hepatotoxicity; normalized in 1 week	14.1%
Granulocytopenia without infection or need for antibiotics	5.9%; no secondary infections
Thrombocytopenia without need for platelets	1.6%; without infections
Pleuritic chest pain	3.1%
Nausea/vomiting	1%; requiring intravenous therapy
Alopecia	0%
Toxicity requiring change in therapy*	6%

Berkowitz RS et al. Gynecol Oncol 1986;23:111–118
Bagshawe KD et al. Br J Obstet Gynecol 1989;96:795–802

Treatment Modifications

Adverse Event	Dose Modification
G ≤ 1 toxicity	Continue therapy if easy to manage
G2 toxicity including LFTs	Consider a 20% reduction in methotrexate dosage
G ≥ 3 toxicity including LFTs	Discontinue methotrexate and institute other therapy

Therapy Monitoring

1. *Every morning before methotrexate:* CBC and LFTs
2. *Every other week:* PE, CBC with differential, serum electrolytes, LFTs, serum creatinine, BUN, and β-hCG
3. *Methotrexate levels:* Not routinely performed
4. *Complete remission:* 3 consecutive weekly β-hCG levels within normal range
5. *Resistance to treatment:* β-hCG plateau over 2 consecutive treatments or a β-hCG rise after any treatment
6. *Following remission:* β-hCG levels are obtained monthly for 12 months and every 3 months during the second year

REGIMEN FOR LOW-RISK GTN

ACTINOMYCIN-D

Osathanondh R et al. Cancer 1975;36:863–866

Actinomycin-D 12 mcg/kg per day intravenously per push over 1–2 minutes for 5 consecutive days on days 1–5 (total dosage/cycle = 60 mcg/kg)

Notes:

1. Treatment delivered over 5 days and repeated as needed every 2 weeks
2. Patients who did not respond after 2 consecutive courses were classified as having resistant disease

Emetogenic potential:
Days 1–5: Moderate (Emetogenicity score = 3). See Chapter 39

Alternate regimen:
Actinomycin-D 1.25 mg/m² intravenously per push over 1–2 minutes, given on day 1 every 2 weeks (total dosage/cycle = 1.25 mg/m²)

Petrilli ES et al. Cancer 1987;60:2173–2176

Note: This is an acceptable regimen for the treatment of nonmetastatic postmolar GTN, but should not be used for metastatic disease, known choriocarcinoma or as secondary therapy to treat methotrexate-resistant disease

Emetogenic potential:
Day 1: Moderate (Emetogenicity score = 3). See Chapter 39

Efficacy (N = 70[a])

Nonmetastatic gestational trophoblastic neoplasia (GTN) = 31
Metastatic gestational trophoblastic neoplasia (GTN) = 39

	Nonmetastatic GTN			Metastatic GTN		
	Non-CCA	CCA	Total	Non CCA	CCA	Total
CR*	93%	100%	94%	76%	56%	67%

[a]CCA, choriocarcinoma
[b]CR (complete response) = β-hCG in normal range for 3 consecutive weeks off therapy

Patient Population Studied

A study of 70 patients (previously untreated) with nonmetastatic (31) and metastatic gestational trophoblastic disease (39) accrued from 1965 to 1973

Toxicity (N = 32)

Toxicity	% of Patients
Hematologic	
WBC <2500/mm³	25
ANC <1500/mm³	38
Platelets <100,000/mm³	16
Nonhematologic	
SGOT level >50 units	22
Nausea and vomiting	66
Stomatitis	38
Skin rash	34
Alopecia	44

Goldstein DP et al. Obstet Gynecol 1972;39:341–345

Treatment Modifications

Adverse Event	Dose Modification
WBC <3000/mm³	Hold actinomycin-D until WBC >2500/mm³
ANC <1500/mm³	Hold actinomycin-D until ANC >1500/mm³
Platelet count <100,000/mm³	Hold actinomycin-D until platelet >100,000/mm³
Hepatotoxicity before or during treatment (LFTs ≥ 3 × ULN)	Hold actinomycin-D until LFTs ≤ 1.5 × ULN
Increasing β-hCG level	Discontinue actinomycin-D
Plateau in β-hCG levels after 2 cycles of actinomycin-D	Discontinue actinomycin-D

Therapy Monitoring

1. *Every other week:* PE, CBC with differential, serum electrolytes, LFTs, serum creatinine, BUN and β-hCG
2. *Complete remission:* 3 consecutive weekly β-hCG levels within normal range
3. *Resistance to treatment:* β-hCG plateau over 2 consecutive treatments or a β-hCG rise after any treatment
4. *Following remission:* β-hCG levels are obtained monthly for 12 months and every 3 months during the second year

Notes

1. In current practice, actinomycin-D is most frequently used as secondary therapy after the development of methotrexate resistance rather than as primary therapy, because it causes more nausea and alopecia than methotrexate and produces local tissue injury if extravasation occurs while administered
2. Appropriate as primary therapy for patients with liver or renal disease or with large effusions that are relative contraindications to methotrexate

REGIMEN FOR HIGH-RISK GTN

ETOPOSIDE + METHOTREXATE + ACTINOMYCIN-D + CYCLOPHOSPHAMIDE + VINCRISTINE (EMA/CO)

Bower M et al. JCO 1997;15:2636–2643
Escobar PF et al. Gynecol Oncol 2003;91:552–557
Newlands ES et al. Br J Obstet Gynecol 1986;93:63–69

EMA component (days 1–3):
Actinomycin-D 0.5 mg (fixed dose) per day intravenously per push over 1–2 minutes for 2 consecutive days on days 1 and 2 every 2 weeks (total dose/cycle = 1 mg)
Etoposide 100 mg/m^2 per day intravenously in 250–500 mL 0.9% NaCl injection (0.9% NS) over 30 minutes for 2 consecutive days on days 1 and 2 every 2 weeks (total dosage/cycle = 200 mg/m^2)
Methotrexate 100 mg/m^2 intravenously per push or in 25 mL 0.9% NS or 5% dextrose injection (D5W) over 5 minutes, given on day 1, *followed immediately afterward by:*
Methotrexate 200 mg/m^2 intravenously in ≥1000 mL 0.9% NS over 12 hours on day 1 every 2 weeks (total dosage/cycle = 300 mg/m^2). *Note:* See dose adjustment for CNS metastases below
Leucovorin calcium 15 mg orally or intramuscularly every 12 hours for 4 doses on days 2 and 3, beginning 24 hours after the start of methotrexate infusion every 2 weeks (total dose/cycle = 60 mg). *Note:* See dose adjustment for CNS metastases below

CO component (day 8):
Vincristine 0.8 mg/m^2 (maximum dose, 2 mg) intravenously per push over 1–2 minutes, given on day 8 every 2 weeks (total dosage/cycle = 0.8 mg/m^2; maximum dose/cycle = 2 mg)
Cyclophosphamide 600 mg/m^2 intravenously in 250 mL 0.9% NS over 30 minutes, given on day 8 every 2 weeks (total dosage/cycle = 600 mg/m^2)

CNS treatment for patients with documented cranial metastases:
3000 cGy whole-brain radiation in fifteen 200-cGy fractions given 5 times per week for 3 weeks
Dexamethasone as needed, 4 mg orally every 6 hours while radiation is administered, tapering over 2–4 weeks after the completion of radiation
Alternative approach: Surgical excision followed by stereotactic radiation
Methotrexate 1000 mg/m^2 by continuous intravenous infusion over 24 hours in 1000 mL 0.9% NS on day 1 every 2 weeks (total dosage/cycle = 1000 mg/m^2)
Leucovorin calcium 30 mg orally, intramuscularly, or intravenously every 12 hours for 6 doses on days 2–5, beginning 32 hours after the start of methotrexate infusion every 2 weeks (total dose/cycle = 180 mg)

Note: During CNS therapy, the methotrexate dose is increased to 1000 mg/m^2 *for 2 to 3 cycles*, and the leucovorin calcium is increased to 30 mg

Duration of therapy:
Repeat EMA alternating weekly with CO to serologic remission (serum β-hCG <5 units/L), then administer for an additional 4–8 weeks (2–4 cycles) of therapy. In the report by Escobar of 45 high-risk GTT patients, 4–7 cycles were administered with a mean of 5.5 cycles

Note: Encourage increased oral fluid intake or, if NPO, give parenteral hydration

Emetogenic potential:
Days 1 and 2: High (Emetogenicity score = 5)
Day 8: Moderate (Emetogenicity score = 3). See Chapter 39

Treatment Modifications

Adverse Event	Dose Modification
WBC <3000/mm^3, platelets <100,000/mm^3, liver transaminases >1.5 × ULN	Hold therapy until WBC ≥3000/mm^3, platelets ≥100,000/mm^3, liver transaminases ≤1.5 × ULN
More than one treatment delay for WBC <3000/mm^3	Administer filgrastim 300 mcg/day subcutaneously on days 9–14 of all subsequent cycles
Hgb <10 g/dL	Transfuse as needed and administer erythropoietin
Peripheral neuropathy >G2	Discontinue vincristine

Patient Population Studied

Women with high-risk GTN. Almost one-half had received prior chemotherapy

Efficacy (N = 272)

	All Patients	Prior Therapy No	Prior Therapy Yes
Complete response	78.3%[a]	78%	79%
Progressive disease	17.2%[b]	14%	21%
Early deaths	4.5%	8%	—
Cumulative overall 5-year survival rate		86%	
Disease-specific 5-year survival survival rate		88%	

[a]16/213 patients suffered relapse after attaining a complete response
[b]Forty-seven patients developed resistance to EMA/CO. 16/21 (76%) patients without prior therapy and 17/26 (65%) patients with prior therapy underwent successful salvage treatment and were alive and in remission at the time of publication

Bower M et al. JCO 1997;15:2636–2643

(N = 45)

	All Patients	Prior Therapy No	Prior Therapy Yes
Initial complete response	71%	76%	65%
Successful salvage therapy	20%[a]	—	—
Died of disease	9%	—	—
Survival[b]	91%	92%	90%

[a]All achieved remission with cisplatin-based therapy
[b]Median follow-up 36 months

Escobar PF et al. Gynecol Oncol 2003;91:552–557 (N = 45)

Toxicity (N = 257 cycles)

	% Cycles G1	% Cycles G2	% Cycles G3
Anemia	0.8	8.5	5.8
Neutropenia	6.6	5.4	1.6
Thrombocytopenia	1.6	—	—
Alopecia	All patients		

Gastrointestinal toxicity [nausea, vomiting, diarrhea and stomatitis] occurred in some patients, but was G3 requiring hospitalization in only one

Escobar PF et al. Gynecol Oncol 2003;91:552–557

Bower M et al, 1997 (N = 272):
Two cases of AML FAB subtypes M1 and M5

Therapy Monitoring

1. *Every other week*: PE, CBC with differential, serum electrolytes, LFTs, serum creatinine, BUN, and β-hCG
2. *Methotrexate levels:* Not routinely performed
3. *Complete remission*: 3 consecutive weekly β-hCG levels within normal range
4. *Resistance to treatment:* β-hCG plateau over 2 consecutive treatments or a β-hCG rise after any treatment
5. *Following remission:* β-hCG levels are obtained monthly for 12 months, and every 3 months during the second year

REGIMEN FOR REFRACTORY GTN

ETOPOSIDE + METHOTREXATE + ACTINOMYCIN-D + CISPLATIN (EP/EMA)

Bower M et al. JCO 1997;15:2636–2643
Newlands ES et al. JCO 2000;18:854–859

EP component (day 1:)
Etoposide 150 mg/m² intravenously in 250–500 mL 0.9% NaCl injection (0.9% NS) over 30 minutes, given on day 1 every 2 weeks
Cisplatin 75 mg/m² + 20 mEq potassium chloride per dose in 1000 mL 0.9% NS by intravenous infusion over 4 hours followed by 2000 mL 0.9% NS with 20 mEq/L potassium chloride by intravenous infusion over 8 hours (total duration of infusion is 12 hours) on day 1, every 2 weeks (total dosage/2-week cycle = 75 mg/m²)
Hydration after cisplatin: Encourage high oral intake if possible. Monitor and replace magnesium/electrolytes as needed.

EMA component (days 8–10)
Actinomycin-D 0.5 mg (total dose) intravenously per push over 1–2 minutes, given on day 8 every 2 weeks (total dose/2-week cycle = 0.5 mg)
Etoposide 100 mg/m² intravenously in 250–500 mL 0.9% NS over 30 minutes, given on day 8 every 2 weeks (total dosage/2-week cycle = 250 mg/m² [sum of EP + EMA regimens])
Methotrexate 100 mg/m² intravenously per push or in 25 mL 0.9% NS or D5W over 5 minutes, given on day 8, *followed immediately afterward by:*
Methotrexate 200 mg/m² intravenously in ≥ 1000 mL 0.9% NS over 12 hours on day 8 every 2 weeks (total dosage/cycle = 300 mg/m²).

Leucovorin calcium 15 mg orally or intramuscularly every 12 hours for 4 doses on days 9 and 10, beginning 24 hours after the start of methotrexate infusion every 2 weeks (total dose/cycle = 60 mg).

Recommendations:
1. EP and EMA components of treatment are alternated at weekly intervals
2. Encourage increased oral fluid intake or, if NPO, give parenteral hydration
3. Avoid concomitant use of drugs that can alter methotrexate elimination, such as nonsteroidal anti-inflammatory drugs, omeprazole (and perhaps other proton pump inhibitors), penicillins, probenecid, and salicylates
4. Most patients need filgrastim (G-CSF)

Emetogenic potential:
Day 1: High (Emetogenicity score = 6)
Day 8: High (Emetogenicity score = 5). See Chapter 39

Treatment Modifications

Adverse Event	Dose Modification
WBC <2000/mm³, platelets <75,000/mm³	Hold therapy until WBC ≥ 2000/mm³ and platelets ≥ 75,000/mm³
Serum creatinine >1.5 × ULN	Obtain creatinine clearance (CrCl) and reduce cisplatin dose by the same percentage as the reduction in CrCl clearance from baseline
G ≥ 2 Mucositis	Double the dose of folinic acid and double the duration of administration before considering methotrexate dose reduction
More than one treatment delay for WBC <2000/mm³	Administer filgrastim 300 mcg/day, subcutaneously on days 9–14 of all subsequent cycles

Patient Population Studied

A study of 42 women with high-risk GTN refractory to or relapsing after EMA/CO chemotherapy. Patients either (1) had improvement while receiving EMA-CO but a persistently low β-hCG level or (2) developed a re-elevation of β-hCG after having a complete response to prior treatment with EMA-CO. The mean age was 30.8 years (range 18–47 years)

Efficacy

Response	Alive in Remission
β-hCG plateau on EMA/CO[a] (n = 22)	
—	21 (95%)
Resistant to or relapsed after EMA/CO[b] (n = 12)	
12 (100%)	9 (75%)
Placental site trophoblastic tumor (n = 8)	
—	4 (50%)
All patients (N = 42)	
—	34 (81%)

[a] β-hCG sufficiently close to normal range, but not possible to evaluate response
[b] >1 log decline in β-hCG

Surgical Procedures in Patients Receiving EP/EMA

	Effect on β-hCG Response		
Operation	Decreased	None	Not assessed
Hysterectomy	2	4	4
Thoracotomy	1	3	5
Craniotomy	2	0	1
Total	5 (23%)	7 (32%)	10 (45%)

Toxicity*

	% G3	% G4
Hematologic (n = 25)		
Anemia	20	—
Leukopenia	48	20
Thrombocytopenia	24	16
Ten patients (40%) had multiple G3/4 toxicities		
Nonhematologic (n = 22)		
Elevated BUN	32%	9%

*Complete results on patients treated before 1988 were no longer available. In the 42 patients:
- Treatment delays due to myelosuppression were observed in 37/42 patients (88%)
- Dose reductions were required in 16/42 patients (38%)
- Filgrastim was administered to 13/42 patients (31%)

NCI CTC

Therapy Monitoring

1. *Every other week:* PE, CBC with differential, serum electrolytes, LFTs, serum creatinine, BUN, and β-hCG
2. *Methotrexate levels:* Not routinely performed
3. *Complete remission:* 3 consecutive weekly β-hCG levels within normal range
4. *Resistance to treatment:* β-hCG plateau over 2 consecutive treatments or a β-hCG rise after any treatment
5. *Following remission:* β-hCG levels are obtained monthly for 12 months and every 3 months during the second year

15. Head and Neck Cancers

Erin Donovan, MD, and Barbara Conley, MD

Epidemiology

- **Yearly incidence:** 40,000–50,000 cases; head and neck cancers account for 3–5% of all cancers diagnosed in the United States each year
- **Age:** Most patients are older than 50 years. Incidence increases with age
- **Male:female ratio:** 2.5:1
- These cancers present most commonly in the oral cavity, oropharynx, and larynx
- Over 50% of head and neck cancers have spread to regional nodes at the time of diagnosis
- Metastatic disease outside the head/neck area is present in only 10% at presentation, but 20% of those treated for cure with surgery and/or radiation or with chemoradiation develop metastatic disease outside the locoregional area, commonly concurrent with a locoregional recurrence
- Patients cured of the initial tumor have a 2–6% per year incidence of second primary tumors, commonly diagnosed in the upper aerodigestive tract
- Smoking and alcohol abuse are risk factors, but tumors do occur in patients with no history of these risk factors

AJCC Cancer Staging Manual, 6th ed. New York: Springer-Verlag, 2002:17–75
Jemal A et al. CA Cancer J Clin 2006;56:106–30

Pathology

1. Squamous carcinomas (90%)
2. Lymphomas
3. Salivary gland tumors (adenocarcinoma, adenoid cystic carcinoma, mucoepidermoid carcinoma)
4. Sarcomas
5. Melanomas

Work-Up

1. History and physical examination
2. ENT examination
3. Laryngoscopy with biopsy of suspicious lesions
4. CT and/or MRI of the head and neck
5. X-ray or CT of chest (to rule out metastatic disease or second primary tumor)
6. Needle biopsy of lymph node not associated with obvious primary tumor

Organ Site Specific Workup

a. Ethmoid sinus: H&P, CT and/or MRI, CXR, pathology review if diagnosis with incomplete excision

b. Maxillary sinus: H&P, Head and neck CT with contrast ± MRI, CXR, dental/prosthetic consultation as indicated

c. Salivary glands: H&P, CT/MRI, CXR, pathology review

d. Lip, oral cavity: H&P, CT/MRI, parorex, biopsy, preanesthesia studies, dental evaluation

e. Hypopharynx: H&P, biopsy, CXR or chest CT, CT with contrast or MRI of primary and neck, examination under anesthesia with laryngoscopy/esophagoscopy, preanesthesia studies, dental evaluation, multidisciplinary consultation as indicated

f. Glottic larynx: Same work up as for hypopharynx + CT scan with contrast and thin cuts of the larynx or MRI of primary, speech and swallowing studies

NCCN Clinical Practice Guidelines in Oncology V. 1. 2006

Staging

Primary Tumor (T)

- Differs for each site (refer to AJCC staging manual)
- Lesions in the oral cavity, hypopharynx, and oropharynx >4 cm are T3
- For larynx and hypopharynx cancers, vocal cord paralysis indicates at least T3
- Local invasion of adjacent structures indicates T4

Regional Lymph Nodes (N)

Nx	Cannot be assessed
N0	No clinically evident node
N1	Single ipsilateral node ≤3 cm diameter
N2a	Single ipsilateral node >3 cm but <6 cm in diameter
N2b	Multiple ipsilateral nodes, none >6 cm in diameter
N2c	Bilateral or contralateral lymph nodes, none >6 cm in diameter
N3	Lymph node >6 cm in diameter

Distant Metastases (M)

MX	Distant metastases cannot be assessed
M0	No distant metastases
M1	Distant metastases

Staging Groups

(Cancers of Oral Cavity, Oropharynx, Hypopharynx, and Larynx*)

Stage	T (Primary)	N	M
I	T1	N0	M0
II	T2	N0	M0
III	T3	N0	M0
	T1–3	N1	M0
IVA	T4a (resectable)	N0-1	M0
	T1–4a	N2	M0
IVB	T4b (unresectable)	Any N	M0
	Any T	N3	M0
IVC	Any T	Any N	M1

Note: Tumor grade is not considered when staging head and neck cancers because it is not associated with outcome

*The same for all primary sites, except nasopharynx

Reproduced, with permission, of the American Joint Committee on Cancer (AJCC), Chicago, Illinois. The original source for this material is the AJCC Cancer Staging Manual, 6th edition (2002) published by Springer-Verlag, New York, www.springeronline.com.

Survival (5-year)

Stage I	>80%
Stage II	30–70%
Stage III*	20–50%
Stage IV*	20–50%

*A palpable lymph node in the neck generally decreases survival by 50% compared with that expected without node involvement

Caveats

Squamous cell cancers of the head and neck:

- Stages I and II may be treated with either surgery or radiation with equally good results
- Locoregionally advanced cancers are best treated with a multidisciplinary approach, involving surgery, radiation, chemotherapy, nutrition, and dentistry
- Stages III and IVA (resectable) locally advanced cancers in patients with good performance status may be treated with surgery followed by radiation therapy with or without concurrent chemotherapy, *or* by initial concomitant chemoradiation therapy followed by surgery, if necessary for salvage. *Note:* Sequential chemotherapy followed by radiation is not currently recommended for organ preservation in a patient fit enough to undergo concomitant chemoradiation
- Stage IVB (unresectable) is treated with concomitant chemoradiation in patients able to tolerate such treatment, or with radiation alone or palliative chemotherapy in patients with poor performance status
- Stage IVC is usually treated with systemic chemotherapy alone unless there is a need for local palliation that could be effected by radiation or by surgery
- Locally recurrent squamous cell cancers are resected if possible. If the time to recurrence is longer than 6 months after initial chemoradiation, re-irradiation may be possible and is being studied in several centers
- Treatment of either locally recurrent or metastatic disease with systemic chemotherapy has been somewhat disappointing. Initially robust response is seen, especially in a patient who has not received chemotherapy previously, but the time to progression is often short—about 2–4 months—with a median survival of 6–9 months. Although response rates are improved with combination chemotherapy, it has not been shown to improve survival compared with single-agent chemotherapy. Some recent phase II studies of multiagent chemotherapy, however, have reported encouraging median survivals of 9–10 months for patients with a good performance status. The choice of systemic therapy for metastatic disease should be guided by a patient's performance status, the goals of treatment (as assessed by the patient and caregiver), and the expected toxicity and beneficial effect of the proposed regimen
- It is recommended that all patients who are to receive concomitant chemoradiation be evaluated for dental problems and extractions should be performed before starting treatment
- Concomitant chemoradiation regimens are associated with increased efficacy but also with increased toxicity compared with sequential chemoradiation
- Patients should be followed up closely for dehydration, electrolyte abnormalities, and adequacy of nutritional intake
- Most centers place enteral feeding tubes prophylactically before the start of treatment for patients undergoing concomitant chemoradiation, because the incidence of grade 3 or greater mucositis is 70–80%
- The incidence of hypothyroidism in patients receiving radiation for head and neck squamous cancers is about 50%. Thyroid function studies should be assessed at baseline and followed up 3–4 times yearly for the lifetime of a patient after completion of radiation therapy. Thyroid replacement therapy should be instituted as indicated before development of symptomatic hypothyroidism

Adelstein DJ et al. JCO 2003;21:92–98
Cooper JS et al. Int J Radiat Oncol Biol Phys 1989;17:449–456
Forastiere AA et al. NEJM 2003;349:2091–2098
Garden AS et al. JCO 2004;22:2856–2864
Kao J et al. Cancer Treat Rev 2003;29:21–30
Pignon JP et al. Lancet 2000;355:949–955

CONCOMITANT CHEMORADIATION REGIMENS

CISPLATIN WITH RADIATION THERAPY

Adelstein DJ et al. JCO 2003;21:92–98
Forastiere AA et al. NEJM 2003;349:2091–2098

Pretreatment:
Dental evaluation; percutaneous feeding tube; nutrition evaluation
Hydration:
Pre- and post-cisplatin hydration with 1000 mL 0.9% NaCl injection (0.9% NS). Add potassium and magnesium as needed based on pretreatment electrolytes
Cisplatin 100 mg/m^2 intravenously in 100–1000 mL 0.9% NS over 30–120 minutes on days 1, 22, and 43 of radiation therapy (total dosage during radiation therapy: 300 mg/m^2)
Radiation at least 70 Gy to primary site and clinically positive nodes given in daily (Mon–Fri) fractions of 2 Gy/day over 7 weeks; at least 50 Gy to entire neck

Emetogenic potential:
Days 1, 22, and 43: High (Emetogenicity score ≥ 5). See Chapter 39 for antiemetic regimens

Efficacy (N = 259)

Organ Preservation (n = 172); Unresectable (n = 87)

	% Organ Preservation	% Unresectable
Complete response	90	40
Laryngeal preservation*	84	—
Estimated overall survival (OS) 2 years	74	
Estimated OS 5 years	54	
Estimated disease-free survival (DFS) 2 years	61	
Estimated DFS 5 years	36	
OS 3 years		37
Disease-specific survival		51
Median survival		19 months
Compliance		85

*At 3.8 years
Adelstein DJ et al. JCO 2003;21:92–98
Forastiere AA et al. NEJM 2003;349:2091–2998

Treatment Modifications

Adverse Event	Dose Modification[a]
Creatinine clearance <50 mL/min	Ineligible for therapy
Day 1, 22, or 43 ANC <1500/mm^3 or platelets <100,000/mm^3	Delay cisplatin until ANC >1500/mm^3 and platelets >100,000/mm^3, for up to 3 weeks. Discontinue cisplatin if recovery has not occurred after a 3-week delay
ANC nadir <500/mm^3	Reduce cisplatin dosage to 75 mg/m^2
Platelet nadir <25,000/mm^3	
G1 Neurotoxicity or ototoxicity	
Serum creatinine 1.5–2.0 mg/dL (133–177 μmol/L)	Hold cisplatin[b], then reduce dosage to 75 mg/m^2
ANC nadir <500/mm^3 with a cisplatin dosage of 75 mg/m^2	Reduce cisplatin dosage to 50 mg/m^2
Platelet nadir <25,000/mm^3 with a cisplatin dosage of 75 mg/m^2	
G2 Neurotoxicity or ototoxicity	
Serum creatinine 2.1–3.0 mg/dL (186–265 μmol/L)	Hold cisplatin[b], then reduce dosage to 50 mg/m^2
ANC nadir <500/mm^3 with a cisplatin dosage of 50 mg/m^2	Discontinue cisplatin
Platelet nadir <25,000/mm^3 with a cisplatin dosage of 50 mg/m^2	
Serum creatinine >3.0 mg/dL (> 265 μmol/L)	
G3/4 Neurotoxicity or ototoxicity	

[a]The use of colony-stimulating factors is discouraged
[b]Hold cisplatin dosage until serum creatinine <1.5 mg/dL or within 0.2 mg/dL (17.7 μmol/L) of baseline

Patient Population Studied

Organ preservation: Patients with previously untreated stage III or stage IV squamous cell carcinoma of the glottic or supraglottic larynx, the surgical treatment of which would require total laryngectomy. The disease had to be considered curable with surgery and postoperative radiation therapy. Karnofsky PS at least 60%; adequate organ function; creatinine clearance at least 50 mL/minute
Unresectable: Patients with stage III/IV unresectable squamous cancer excluding nasopharyngeal cancer, or cancers of the paranasal sinuses or parotid glands. ECOG PS 0–1, adequate organ function

Toxicity (N = 266)

Organ Preservation (n = 171);
Unresectable (n = 95)

	% G3/4/5 Toxicity	
Toxicity	**Organ Preservation**	**Unresectable**
Hematologic	47	
Leukopenia		42
Anemia		18
Thrombocytopenia		3
Mucosal	43	45
Pharyngeal/esophageal	35	—
Nausea or vomiting	20	16
Laryngeal	18	—
Dermatologic*	7	7
Infection	4	—
Renal/genitourinary	4	8
Neurologic	5	—
Other (not specified)	40	—
G5 Toxicity	5	4

*Within radiation field

Therapy Monitoring

1. *Before cisplatin and weekly after treatment:* CBC with differential, serum electrolytes, calcium, and magnesium
2. *Weekly follow-up recommended during therapy:* Attention to signs and symptoms of dehydration as supplemental hydration and nutritional support often are required
3. *Every 4–6 months:* Thyroid function studies

CONCOMITANT CHEMORADIATION REGIMENS

CISPLATIN + PACLITAXEL WITH RADIATION THERAPY

Garden AS et al. Preliminary results of RTOG 97-03. JCO 2004;22:2856–2864

Pretreatment:
Dental evaluation; percutaneous feeding tube; nutrition evaluation
Premedication:
Dexamethasone 8–20 mg intravenously per push 30 minutes before paclitaxel
Diphenhydramine 50 mg intravenously per push 30–60 minutes before paclitaxel
Ranitidine 150 mg in 20–50 mL 0.9% NaCl injection (0.9% NS), or 5% dextrose injection (D5W) over 5–20 minutes, given 30–60 minutes before paclitaxel
Paclitaxel 30 mg/m^2 per dose intravenously in a volume of 0.9% NS or D5W sufficient to produce a concentration of 0.3–1.2 mg/mL over 3–24 hours weekly, on day 1 for 7 consecutive weeks (total dosage/7-week cycle = 210 mg/m^2)
Optional: **Dexamethasone** 4 mg orally every 6 hours for 4 doses following paclitaxel with glucose monitoring if indicated
Cisplatin 20 mg/m^2 per dose intravenously in 100–1000 mL 0.9% NS over 15–60 minutes weekly on day 2 for 7 consecutive weeks (total dosage/7 week cycle = 140 mg/m^2)
Radiation at least 70 Gy to primary site and clinically positive nodes given in daily (Mon–Fri) fractions of 2 Gy/day over 7 weeks

Dexamethasone is marketed in the United States in numerous formulations for oral administration, such as 0.25-, 0.5-, 0.75-, 1-, 2-, 4-, and 6-mg tablets, and in elixirs (which contain alcohol) and solutions for oral administration

Emetogenic potential:
Day 1 (with paclitaxel): Low (Emetogenicity score = 2)
Day 2 (with cisplatin): Moderately high (Emetogenicity score = 4). See Chapter 39 for antiemetic regimens

Treatment Modifications

Adverse Event	Dose Modification
Creatinine clearance <50 mL/min (<0.83 mL/s)	Ineligible for therapy
ANC <1000/mm^3 or platelets <75,000/mm^3 at the time of chemotherapy administration	Delay chemotherapy until ANC >1000/mm^3 and platelets >75,000/mm^3. Discontinue chemotherapy if recovery has not occurred after a 3-week delay
Serum creatinine >1.5 mg/dL (>133 μmol/L) or 20% higher than baseline value if baseline >1.5 mg/dL	Hold cisplatin dosage until serum creatinine <1.5 mg/dL (<133 μmol/L) or within 0.2 mg/dL (17.7 μmol/L) of baseline
G2 Neurotoxicity or ototoxicity	Hold cisplatin and paclitaxel until neurotoxicity resolves to G ≤ 1
G3/4 Neurotoxicity or ototoxicity	Discontinue chemotherapy

Patient Population Studied

A study of 77 patients with stage III or stage IV, M0 squamous cancer of oral cavity, oropharynx, or hypopharynx, previously untreated, assigned to one of three arms in a randomized phase II RTOG trial. ECOG PS at least 70% and adequate organ function are required

Efficacy (N = 77)

Complete response	82%
Estimated 2-year disease-free survival	51.3%
Estimated 2-year overall survival	66.6%

Toxicity (N = 77)

	% G3/4
Nonhematologic	84
Hematologic	39
Mucositis	10 (G4)
Skin	3 (G4)
% Late Grade 4 Toxicities* (N = 72)	
Bone	4.2
Mucous membrane	1.4
Pharynx and esophagus	1.4
Larynx	1.4
Spinal cord	1.4
Skin	0
Subcutaneous tissue	0

*No grade 5 toxicities

Therapy Monitoring

1. *Weekly:* CBC with differential, serum electrolytes, calcium, and magnesium. Weekly follow-up recommended during therapy with attention to signs and symptoms of dehydration because supplemental hydration and nutritional support are often required
2. *Every 4–6 months:* Thyroid function studies

CONCOMITANT CHEMORADIATION REGIMENS

CARBOPLATIN + FLUOROURACIL WITH RADIATION THERAPY

Calais G et al. J Natl Cancer Inst 1999;91:2081–2086

Pretreatment:
Dental evaluation; percutaneous feeding tube; nutrition evaluation

Carboplatin 70 mg/m^2 intravenously in 50–100 mL 5% dextrose injection (D5W) or 0.9% NaCl injection (0.9% NS) over 15–30 minutes for 4 consecutive days, given on days 1–4 every 3 weeks (total dosage/cycle = 280 mg/m^2)
Fluorouracil 600 mg/m^2 by continuous intravenous infusion in 50–1000 mL 0.9% NS or D5W over 24 hours for 4 consecutive days, given on days 1–4 every 3 weeks (total dosage/cycle = 2400 mg/m^2)
Radiation 2 Gy/day, 5 fractions per week to tumor and clinically positive nodes to a total dose of 70 Gy

For delayed diarrhea:
Loperamide 2 mg orally every 2 hours during waking hours (4 mg orally every 4 hours during hours of sleep). Continue for at least 12 hours after diarrhea resolves
If diarrhea persists > 48 hours despite loperamide: Stop loperamide and hospitalize patient for intravenous hydration
For persistent diarrhea:
Octreotide 100–150 mcg subcutaneously 3-times-daily. Maximum total daily dose = 1500 mcg
Antibiotic therapy:
Ciprofloxacin 500 mg orally twice daily if absolute neutrophil count < 500/mm^3 (even in the absence of fever or diarrhea) or if patient is febrile in association with diarrhea. Antibiotics should also be administered if patient is hospitalized with prolonged diarrhea and should be continued until diarrhea resolves

Rothenberg ML et al. JCO 2001;19:3801–3807
Wadler S et al. JCO 1998;16:3169–3178

Emetogenic potential: High (Emetogenicity score = 5). See Chapter 39 for antiemetic regimens

Patient Population Studied

A study of 109 patients with previously untreated stage III or stage IV squamous cell carcinoma of the oropharynx without evidence of distant metastases. Patients were assigned to the chemoradiation arm of a randomized phase III trial with Karnofsky PS at least 60% and adequate organ function

Efficacy (N = 109)

Locoregional control	66%
3-year overall survival	51%
3-year disease-free survival	42%
Median survival	29.2 months

Therapy Monitoring

1. *Weekly:* CBC with differential, serum electrolytes, calcium, and magnesium. Weekly follow-up recommended during therapy with attention to signs and symptoms of dehydration because supplemental hydration and nutritional support are often required
2. *Every 4–6 months:* Thyroid function studies

Treatment Modifications

Adverse Event	Dose Modification
Creatinine clearance <50 mL/min	Ineligible for therapy
ANC <1000/mm^3 or platelets <75,000/mm^3 at time of chemotherapy administration	Delay chemotherapy until ANC >1000/mm^3 and platelets >75,000/mm^3
G ≥ 2 Neurotoxicity	Hold carboplatin until neurotoxicity resolves to G ≤ 1
G3/4 Neurotoxicity	Discontinue carboplatin
G ≥ 2 Diarrhea (4–6 stools/day > baseline)	Delay until diarrhea resolves to baseline
G ≥ 2 Mucositis	Delay chemotherapy until toxicity resolves to G ≤ 1
G ≥ 2 Nonhematologic toxicity	

Toxicity (N = 109)

	% of Patients
Acute Nonhematologic Toxicity	
G3/4 Mucositis	71
Erythema/pruritis/dry desquamation	44
Moist desquamation	23
Weight loss > 10% body mass	14
Need for feeding tube	36
G5 Toxicities	0.9
Acute Hematologic Toxicity	
G3/4 Neutropenia	4
G3/4 Thrombocytopenia	6
G3/4 Anemia	3
Late Toxicities	
G3/4 Xerostomia	10
Severe cervical fibrosis	12

CONCOMITANT CHEMORADIATION REGIMEN

CISPLATIN WITH RADIATION THERAPY FOLLOWED BY CISPLATIN + FLUOROURACIL

Al-Sarraf M et al. JCO 1998;16:1310–1317

Pretreatment:
Dental evaluation; percutaneous feeding tube; nutrition evaluation

Hydration + mannitol before, during, and after cisplatin administration:

- Pre-cisplatin hydration with 2000 mL 5% dextrose and 0.45% NaCl injection (D5W/0.45% NS) with potassium chloride 40 mEq intravenously over 24 hours. Monitor and replace magnesium/electrolytes as needed
- *Mannitol diuresis:* May be given to patients who have received adequate hydration. A bolus dose of mannitol 12.5–25 g can be administered as an intravenous push before starting cisplatin or prepared as an admixture with cisplatin. Continued hydration is essential
- *Continued mannitol diuresis:* In an inpatient or day-hospital setting, one can administer additional mannitol in the form of an infusion: mannitol 25 g in 1000 mL D5W/0.45% NS + potassium chloride 30 mEq intravenously over 4 hours. This can be done either during or immediately after cisplatin, but requires maintenance of adequate fluid input during and for hours after the administration of mannitol
- Post-cisplatin hydration with 2000 mL D5W/0.45% NS with potassium chloride 40 mEq intravenously over 24 hours starting after second mannitol dose is completed

During radiation therapy:
Cisplatin 100 mg/m^2 per dose intravenously in 25–250 mL of 0.9% NaCl injection (0.9% NS) over 15–20 minutes every 21 days for 3 cycles, given on days 1, 22, and 43 of radiation therapy (total dosage during radiation therapy = 300 mg/m^2)
Radiation 1.8–2 Gy/day, 5 fractions per week to tumor and clinically positive nodes to a total dose of 70 Gy. A total of 50 Gy to entire neck is recommended

After radiation therapy:
Note: Start 4 weeks after radiation therapy or the last dose of cisplatin, regardless of response to cisplatin + radiation
Cisplatin 80 mg/m^2 per dose intravenously in 25–250 mL of 0.9% NS over 15–30 minutes every 28 days for 3 cycles, given on days 71, 99, and 127 (total dosage/cycle = 80 mg/m^2)
Fluorouracil 1000 mg/m^2 per day by continuous intravenous infusion in 100–1000 mL 0.9% NS or 5% dextrose injection (D5W) over 24 hours for 4 consecutive days every 4 weeks for 3 cycles (96-hour infusion; on days 71–74, 99–102, and 127–130) (total dosage/cycle = 4000 mg/m^2)

For delayed diarrhea:
Loperamide 2 mg orally every 2 hours during waking hours (4 mg orally every 4 hours during hours of sleep). Continue for at least 12 hours after diarrhea resolves
If diarrhea persists > 48 hours despite loperamide: Stop loperamide and hospitalize patient for intravenous hydration
For persistent diarrhea:
Octreotide 100–150 mcg subcutaneously 3 times daily. Maximum total daily dose = 1500 mcg
Antibiotic therapy:
Ciprofloxacin 500 mg orally twice daily if absolute neutrophil count < 500/mm^3 (even with no fever or diarrhea) or if patient is febrile in association with diarrhea. Antibiotics should also be administered if patient is hospitalized with prolonged diarrhea and should be continued until diarrhea resolves

Rothenberg ML et al. JCO 2001;19:3801–3807
Wadler S et al. JCO 1998;16:3169–3178

Emetogenic potential:
During radiation therapy: High (Emetogenicity score ≥5)
After radiation therapy: High (Emetogenicity score 6). See Chapter 39 for antiemetic regimens

Treatment Modifications

Adverse Event	Dose Modification
ANC <2000/mm^3 or platelet count <100,000/mm^3	Hold chemotherapy until ANC ≥2000/mm^3 and platelet count ≥100,000/mm^3
ANC nadir ≥1500/mm^3 or platelet count nadir ≥75,000/mm^3	No dose modification
ANC nadir 1000–1499/mm^3 and/or platelet nadir 50,000–74,999/mm^3	Reduce cisplatin dosage to 80 mg/m^2
ANC nadir <1000/mm^3 and/or platelet nadir <50,000/mm^3	Hold chemotherapy until ANC >2000/mm^3 and platelet >100,000/mm^3 and then reduce cisplatin dosage to 60 mg/m^2
Serum creatinine ≤2.0 mg/dL (≤177 μmol/L) or creatinine clearance ≥ 60 mL/min (≥1.00 mL/s)	No dose modification
Serum creatinine 2.1–4 mg/dL (186–354 μmol/L) or creatinine clearance 40–59 mL/min (0.67–0.98 mL/s)	Hold cisplatin dosage until serum creatinine <1.5 mg/dL (<133 μmol/L), then reduce cisplatin dosage to 80 mg/m^2
Serum creatinine >4 mg/dL (>354 μmol/L) or creatinine clearance <40 mL/min	Discontinue cisplatin
G ≥ 2 Diarrhea (4–6 stools/day > baseline)	Hold fluorouracil until diarrhea resolves to baseline
G ≥ 2 Mucositis	Hold fluorouracil until toxicity resolves to G ≤ 1
G ≥ 2 Neurotoxicity	Hold cisplatin until neurotoxicity resolves to G ≤ 1
G3/4 Neurotoxicity	Discontinue cisplatin

Patient Population Studied

A study of 78 patients with stages III or stage IV nasopharyngeal cancer without evidence of systemic metastasis and no history of previous radiation therapy or chemotherapy. Patients were randomized to the combined modality arm of a 2-arm randomized phase III trial

Efficacy (N = 78)

Complete remission	49%
3-year overall survival	78%
Median overall survival	>2.7 years
Estimated 3-year progression-free survival	69%

Therapy Monitoring

1. *Weekly:* CBC with differential, serum electrolytes, calcium, and magnesium. Weekly follow-up recommended during therapy with attention to signs and symptoms of dehydration, as supplemental hydration and nutritional support are often required
2. *For 2 days, starting the day after cisplatin administration, and as needed:* Serum electrolytes and magnesium
3. *Every 4–6 months:* Thyroid function studies

Toxicity (N = 78/53)

	% G3/4 Toxicities	
	Chemotherapy + Radiation (N = 78)	Adjuvant Chemotherapy (N = 53)
Hematologic		
Anemia	0	5.7
Leukopenia	29.5	22.6
Granulocytopenia	6.4	3.8
Thrombocytopenia	1.3	0
Nonhematologic		
Stomatitis	37.2	20.8
Nausea	17.9	9.4
Vomiting	14.1	1.9
Impaired hearing	11.5	11.3
Weight loss	6.4	0
Infection	2.6	1.9
Renal	0	0
Desquamation, RT field	2.6	N/A

No grade 5 toxicities with either part of regimen

INITIAL OR METASTATIC DISEASE REGIMEN

CETUXIMAB ± RADIATION

Bonner JA, et al. NEJM 2006; 354:567–78
ERBITUX® (Cetuximab) product label, March 2006. Manufactured by ImClone Systems Incorporated, Branchburg, NJ; Distributed and Marketed by Bristol-Myers Squibb Company, Princeton, NJ

Premedication:
Diphenhydramine 50 mg (or an equivalent [H_1] antihistamine) administer IV per push or as a short infusion 30 minutes prior to cetuximab administration.
Note: Severe infusion reaction can occur with the administration of cetuximab. Approximately 90% of severe reactions were associated with the first infusion despite the use of prophylactic antihistamines

Initial Dose:
Cetuximab 20 mg **test dose,** administer intravenously over 20 minutes, followed by a 30 minute observation period, then
Cetuximab 400 mg/m^2, administer intravenously over 120 minutes 1 week prior to radiation therapy

Maintenance Doses:
Cetuximab 250 mg/m^2, administer intravenously over 60 minutes, weekly ± **radiation**
Note: If administering radiation, administer cetuximab weekly for the duration of radiation

Radiation regimens used in the randomized trial

Regimen	Total Radiation Dose	Once-Daily Fractions	Twice-Daily Fractions
Once daily	70.0 Gy 35 fractions	2.0 Gy/fraction 5 fractions/week 7 weeks	Not applicable
Twice daily	72.0–76.8 Gy 60–64 fractions	Not applicable	1.2 Gy/fraction; 10 fractions/week for 6.0–6.5 week
Concomitant boost	72.0 Gy 42 fractions	32.4 Gy 1.8 Gy/fraction 5 fractions/week 3.6 weeks	Morning dose: 21.6 Gy; 1.8 Gy/fraction; 5 fractions/week; 2.4 weeks Afternoon dose: 18.0 Gy; 1.5 Gy/fraction; 5 fractions/week; 2.4 weeks

Emetogenic potential:
Cetuximab alone: Low (Emetogenicity score = 2)
Cetuximab + RT: Low – Moderate (Emetogenicity score = ≤ 3). See Chapter 39 for antiemetic regimens

Dose Modification

Infusion Reaction Severity	
G1/2	Reduce dosage by 50%
G3/4	Discontinue Cetuximab

Severe Acneiform Rash*	Cetuximab	Subsequent Treatment Modifications by Outcome	
		Improvement	No improvement
1st occurrence	Delay repeated treatment for 1 to 2 weeks	Resume with cetuximab 250 mg/m^2, weekly	Discontinue cetuximab
2nd occurrence		Resume with cetuximab 200 mg/m^2, weekly	
3rd occurrence		Resume with cetuximab 150 mg/m^2, weekly	
4th occurrence		Discontinue Cetuximab	

*In patients with mild and moderate skin toxicity treatment should continue without dose modification

Patient Population Studied

424 patients with stage III or IV non-metastatic measurable squamous cell carcinoma of the oropharynx, hypopharynx, or larynx were randomly assigned to receive high dose radiotherapy alone (n = 213) or high-dose radiotherapy plus cetuximab (n = 211)

Efficacy (N = 211)

	Radiotherapy alone (N = 213)	Radiotherapy plus Cetuximab (N = 211)
Loco-regional control		
Median duration (months)	14.9	24.4
Median duration of loco-regional control according to site (months)		
Oropharynx	23	49
Larynx	11.9	12.9
Hypopharynx	10.3	12.5
Median duration of loco-regional control according to stage		
Stage III	16.2	38.9
Stage IV	13.5	20.9
Progression free survival		
Median duration (months)	12.4	17.1
Rate at 2 y (%)	37	46
Overall survival (OS)		
Median duration (months)	29.3	49
Median duration of OS according to site		
Oropharynx	30.3	>66
Larynx	31.6	32.8
Hypopharynx	13.5	13.7
Median duration of OS according to stage		
Stage III	42.9	55.2
Stage IV	24.2	47.4
Median duration of OS according to radiotherapy regimen (months)		
Once daily	15.3	18.9
Twice daily	53.3	58.9
Concomitant boost	31	>66

Therapy Monitoring

Weekly: CBC with differential, serum electrolytes, calcium, and magnesium weekly during radiation

Toxicity (N = 208)

	Radiotherapy alone (N = 212)		Radiotherapy plus Cetuximab (N = 208)	
Adverse Event	**% All grades**	**% G3–5**	**% All grades**	**% G3–5**
Mucositis	94	52	93	56
Acneiform rash*	10	1	87	17
Radiation dermatitis	90	18	86	23
Weight loss	72	7	84	11
Xerostomia	71	3	72	5
Dysphagia	63	30	65	26
Asthenia	49	5	56	4
Nausea	37	2	49	2
Constipation	30	5	35	5
Taste perversion	28	0	29	0
Vomiting	23	4	29	2
Pain	28	7	28	6
Anorexia	23	2	27	2
Fever	13	1	26	1
Pharyngitis	19	4	26	3
Dehydration	19	8	25	6
Oral Candidiasis	22	0	20	0
Coughing	19	0	20	<1
Voice alteration	22	0	19	2
Diarrhea	13	1	19	2
Headache	8	<1	19	<1
Pruritus	4	0	16	0
Infusion reaction*	2	0	15	3
Insomnia	14	0	15	0
Dyspepsia	9	1	14	0
Increased sputum	15	1	13	<1
Infection	9	1	13	1
Anxiety	9	1	11	<1
Chills	5	0	11	0
Anemia	13	6	3	1

*With the exception of acneiform rash and infusion-related events, the incidence rates of G3–5 reactions were similar in the two treatment groups

Note: Four patients discontinued cetuximab because of hypersensitivity reactions after the test dose or first dose

Notes

1. *Indications:*

Cetuximab, in combination with radiation therapy, is indicated for the treatment of locally or regional advanced squamous cell carcinoma of the head and neck.

Bonner JA et al. NEJM 2006; 354:567–78

Cetuximab as a single agent is indicated for the treatment of patients with recurrent or metastatic squamous cell carcinoma of the head and neck after prior platinum based therapy has failed

Trigo J, et al. [Abstract 5502] Proc Am Soc Clin Oncol 2004; 23:487:

Evaluated the efficacy of cetuximab monotherapy in 103 patients with platinum-refractory, recurrent or metastatic squamous cell carcinoma of the head and neck in a multicenter phase II study. An initial dose of cetuximab 400 mg/m^2 was followed by cetuximab 250 mg/m^2 weekly, until disease progression, with an option to switch to cetuximab plus the same platinum agent on which patients' disease had previously progressed after disease progression occurred with cetuximab monotherapy. Drug-related adverse events in >10% of pts included: skin rash/acne 80% (1% G3), fatigue 24% (4% G3), fever/chills 19% (2% G3), nail changes 15% (all G1/2) and nausea 13% (1% G3). There was one treatment-related death due to a hypersensitivity reaction in a patient for whom mechanical ventilation was not suitable. Preliminary efficacy data were as follows: 5 CR, 12 PR, 38 SD, 47 PD and 1 not assessable, for an overall objective response rate of 16.5% (95% CI: 9.9%–25.1%). The disease control rate was 53.4% (95% CI: 43.3%–63.3%). Median TTP and median survival were 85 days and 175 days, respectively

METASTATIC DISEASE REGIMEN

METHOTREXATE

Forastiere AA et al. JCO 1992;10:1245–1251

Methotrexate 40 mg/m^2 intravenously per push over 15–30 seconds, or as a short infusion in 10–100 mL 0.9% NaCl injection (0.9% NS) or 5% dextrose injection (D5W) over 5–15 minutes every week, continually (total dosage/week = 40 mg/m^2)

Note: Increase methotrexate dosage to 50 mg/m^2 weekly if patients experience only grade 0 (zero) mucositis or myelosuppression after 40 mg/m^2

Emetogenic potential: Low (Emetogenicity score = 2). See Chapter 39 for antiemetic regimens

Treatment Modifications

Adverse Event	Dose Modification
G ≥ 2 Hematologic or nonhematologic toxicity	Reduce methotrexate dosage by 10 mg/m^2

Patient Population Studied

A study of 88 patients with squamous cancer of the head and neck, which was recurrent after attempted cure with surgery and radiation therapy, or with newly diagnosed disease with distant metastasis. Those with recurrence had received no prior chemotherapy for their recurrent disease; they had a history of induction chemotherapy 6 months or more before study entry was allowed. Patients were randomly assigned to the methotrexate arm of a 3-arm phase III randomized trial. Performance status SWOG ≤ 2 and adequate organ function were required, including creatinine clearance ≥50 mL/min (≥0.83 mL/s)

Efficacy (N = 88)

Complete response	2%
Partial response	8%
Stable disease	50%
Median duration of response	4.1 months

Toxicity (N = 87)

	% G1/2	% G3/4
Hematologic		
Anemia	25.3	3.4
Granulocytopenia	8	6.9
Neutropenia	28.7	16.1
Thrombocytopenia	9.2	5.7
Nonhematologic		
Diarrhea	3	0
Stomatitis	34	10
Nausea/vomiting	38	8
Ototoxicity	2	0
Renal	3	3

G5 toxicity = 1.1%

Therapy Monitoring

Weekly: CBC with differential. Serum creatinine and LFTs as needed

Notes

Median duration of therapy is 8 weeks

METASTATIC DISEASE REGIMEN

CISPLATIN

Jacobs C et al. JCO 1992;10:257–263

Hydration + mannitol before, during, and after cisplatin administration:

- Pre-cisplatin hydration with 2000 mL 5% dextrose and 0.45% NaCl injection (D5W/0.45% NS) with potassium chloride 40 mEq intravenously over 24 hours. Monitor and replace magnesium/electrolytes as needed
- *Mannitol diuresis:* May be given to patients who have received adequate hydration. A bolus dose of mannitol 12.5–25 g can be administered as an intravenous push before starting cisplatin, or it can be prepared as an admixture with cisplatin. Continued hydration is essential
- *Continued mannitol diuresis:* In an inpatient or day-hospital setting, one can administer additional mannitol in the form of an infusion: mannitol 25 g in 1000 mL D5W/0.45% NS + potassium chloride 30 mEq intravenously over 4 hours. This can be done either during or immediately after cisplatin, but requires maintenance of adequate fluid input during and for hours after the administration of mannitol
- *Optional:* Post-cisplatin hydration with 1000–2000 mL D5W/0.45% NS with potassium chloride 40 mEq intravenously over 12–24 hours after second mannitol dose is completed

Cisplatin 100 mg/m^2 intravenously in 25–250 mL of 0.9% NS over 15–20 minutes every 21 days (total dosage/cycle = 100 mg/m^2)

Emetogenic potential: High (Emetogenicity score = 5). See Chapter 39 for antiemetic regimens

Patient Population Studied

A study of 84 patients with unresectable recurrent disease or newly diagnosed distant metastatic disease who had received no prior chemotherapy, who were randomized to the cisplatin alone arm of a 3-arm phase III randomized trial. WHO Performance status <4 and good organ function were required. Thirty-six percent had performance status of 2 or 3

Efficacy (N = 83)

Complete response	3.6%
Partial response	13.3%
Median duration of response	2 months
Median survival	5.7 months

Toxicity (N = 83)

	% G1/2	% G3/4
Hematologic		
Neutropenia	35	1
Thrombocytopenia	11	1
Anemia (Hgb < 8 g/dL)	NR	11
Nonhematologic		
Vomiting	54	18
Diarrhea	17	0
Mucositis	3	2
Ototoxicity	3	1
Magnesium < 1.5 mg/dL	= 22%	
Creatinine > 2 mg/dL (>177 µmol/L)	= 14%	
G > 1 Cardiovascular toxicity	= 5%	
Alopecia	= 4%	

Therapy Monitoring

1. *Weekly:* CBC with differential
2. *Before each cycle:* serum electrolytes, creatinine, calcium, magnesium, and liver function tests

Treatment Modifications

Adverse Event	Dose Modification
Creatinine clearance <50 mL/min (<0.83 mL/s)	Ineligible for therapy
Day 1 ANC <1500/mm^3 or platelets <100,000/mm^3	Delay cisplatin until ANC >1500/mm^3 and platelets >100,000/mm^3 for up to 3 weeks. Discontinue cisplatin if recovery has not occurred after a 3-week delay
ANC nadir <500/mm^3	Reduce dosage to 75 mg/m^2
Platelet nadir <25,000/mm^3	
G1 Neurotoxicity or ototoxicity	
Serum creatinine 1.5–2.0 mg/dL (133–177 µmol/L)	Hold cisplatin*, then reduce dosage to 75 mg/m^2
ANC nadir <500/mm^3 with a cisplatin dosage of 75 mg/m^2	Reduce dosage to 50 mg/m^2
Platelet nadir <25,000/mm^3 with a cisplatin dosage of 75 mg/m^2	
G2 Neurotoxicity or ototoxicity	
Serum creatinine 2.1–3.0 mg/dL (186–265 µmol/L)	Hold cisplatin*, then reduce cisplatin dosage to 50 mg/m^2
ANC nadir <500/mm^3 with a cisplatin dosage of 50 mg/m^2	Discontinue cisplatin
Platelet nadir <25,000/mm^3 with a cisplatin dosage of 50 mg/m^2	
Serum creatinine >3.0 mg/dL (>265 µmol/L)	
G3/4 Neurotoxicity or ototoxicity	

*Hold cisplatin until serum creatinine <1.5 mg/dL (<133 µmol/L) or within 0.2 mg/dL (17.7 µmol/L) of baseline

METASTATIC DISEASE REGIMEN

DOCETAXEL (TAXOTERE®)

Catimel G et al. Ann Oncol 1994;5:533–537

Premedication:
Dexamethasone 5–10 mg orally every 12 hours for 3 days, starting the day before docetaxel administration
Diphenhydramine 25–50 mg intravenously per push, given 30–60 minutes before docetaxel
Docetaxel 100 mg/m² intravenously after dilution in a volume of 0.9% NaCl injection or 5% dextrose injection sufficient to produce a final docetaxel concentration of 0.3–0.74 mg/mL, given over 60 minutes every 21 days (total dosage/cycle = 100 mg/m²)

Dexamethasone is marketed in the United States in numerous formulations for oral administration, such as 0.25-, 0.5-, 0.75-, 1-, 2-, 4-, and 6-mg tablets, and in elixirs (which contain alcohol) and solutions for oral administration

Emetogenic potential: Low (Emetogenicity score = 2). See Chapter 39 for antiemetic regimens

Treatment Modifications

Adverse Event	Dose Modification
G ≥ 2 Cutaneous toxicity without recovery to G ≤ 1 at time of retreatment	Reduce docetaxel dosage 25%
G ≥ 2 Peripheral neuropathy without recovery to G ≤ 1 at time of retreatment	
G4 Granulocytopenia lasting more than 7 days or associated with fever >38.5°C	
G3/4 Nonhematologic toxicity	

Patient Population Studied

A trial of 40 patients with unresectable recurrent disease following attempted cure with surgery and/or radiation therapy (may have received neoadjuvant chemotherapy) or newly diagnosed with distant metastases treated in a phase II trial. Performance status WHO ≤2, age <75 years, and adequate organ function were required

Efficacy (N = 37)

Complete response	5.4%
Partial response	27%
Stable disease	35%
Median duration of response	6.5 months

Toxicity (N = 39 pts/166 cycles)

	G1/2 (% Cycles)	G3/4 (% Cycles)
Hematologic		
Leukopenia	23 (43)	74 (48)
Neutropenia	5 (20)	87 (61)
Anemia	74 (61)	5 (1)
Thrombocytopenia	13 (5)	0 (0)
% Nonhematologic		
Skin toxicity	46	7.5
Asthenia	46	23
Peripheral neuropathy	41	—
Nausea	33	2.5
Edema	30.7	—
Vomiting	28.5	2.5
Stomatitis	25.6	13
Diarrhea	25.6	2.5
Phlebitis	23	—
Hypersensitivity	20.5	2.5
Myalgia	13	—

Therapy Monitoring

1. *Weekly:* CBC with differential
2. *During dexamethasone:* monitor glucose if indicated

METASTATIC DISEASE REGIMEN

GEFITINIB (IRESSA) OR ERLOTINIB (TARCEVA) (ORAL EPIDERMAL GROWTH FACTOR INHIBITOR)

Cohen EEW et al. JCO 2003;21:1980–1987
Soulieres D et al. JCO 2004;22:77–85

Gefitinib 500 mg orally once daily, continually
or
Erlotinib 150 mg orally once daily, continually

Note: Patients unable to swallow tablets or those with silicone-based feeding tubes may dissolve gefitinib or erlotinib tablets in distilled water

Erlotinib is manufactured in the United States in film-coated tablets for oral administration containing 25 mg, 100 mg, and 150 mg erlotinib. Tarceva erlotinib tablets product label, November 2004. Manufactured by Schwarz Pharma Manufacturing, Seymour, IN. Manufactured for OSI Pharmaceuticals Inc, Melville, NY. Distributed by Genentech Inc, South San Francisco, CA
Gefitinib is manufactured in the United States in film-coated tablets for oral administration containing 250 mg gefitinib. IRESSA (gefitinib tablets) 250 mg product label, June 2005. Manufactured by AstraZeneca UK Limited, Macclesfield, Cheshire, England. Manufactured for AstraZeneca Pharmaceuticals LP, Wilmington, DE

Emetogenic potential:
Erlotinib: Low (Emetogenicity score = 2)
Gefitinib: Low (Emetogenicity score = 2). See Chapter 39 for antiemetic regimens

Patient Population Studied

Gefitinib: 52 patients with recurrent or metastatic disease considered ineligible for curative surgery or radiation therapy who had received ≤1 prior systemic therapy. Performance status ECOG ≤2 and adequate organ function were required
Erlotinib: 115 patients with locally recurrent and/or metastatic head and neck squamous cell carcinoma regardless of their HER1/EGFR status. ECOG performance status 0–2

Efficacy (N = 47/115)

	Gefitinib (N = 47)	Erlotinib (N = 115)
Complete response	2.1%	0
Partial response	8.5%	4.3%
Stable disease	42.6%	38.3%
Median duration of response	1.6 months	
Median time to progression	3.4 months	9.6 weeks
Median survival	8.1 months	6 months
1-year survival	29.2%	50%

Treatment Modifications

Adverse Event	Dose Modification
Gefitinib	
G2 Skin rash, nausea, or diarrhea:	Hold gefitinib until toxicity G ≤1
Repeat G2 skin rash, nausea, or diarrhea	Reduce gefitinib dose to 250 mg per day
Other nonhematologic G2 toxicities	Hold gefitinib until toxicity G ≤1, then reduce dose to 250 mg per day
Any G3/4 toxicity	Hold gefitinib until toxicity resolves to G ≤ 1, then resume with dose reduced to 250 mg daily
Toxicity not resolved to G ≤ 1 after interrupting treatment for 2 weeks, or a second dose reduction indicated	Discontinue treatment
Erlotinib	
G2 Skin rash	Hold erlotinib until toxicity G ≤ 1
Repeat G2 skin rash	Reduce erlotinib dose to 100 mg per day
Other nonhematologic G2/3 toxicities	Hold erlotinib until toxicity G ≤ 1, then reduce erlotinib dose to 100 mg per day
G4 Toxicity	Discontinue erlotinib

Toxicity (N = 50/115)

	Gefitinib (N = 50)		Erlotinib (N = 115)	
	% G1/2	% G3/4	% G1/2	% G3/4
Skin rash	48	0	34	6
Diarrhea	44	6	17	2
Anorexia	20	6		
Nausea	14	4	9	0
Vomiting	12	0	N/A	
Dyspnea	6	0	N/A	
Keratitis	4	0	N/A	
↑AST	12	0		
↑ALT	4	0	24	2
↑Alkaline phosphatase	4	0		
↑Creatinine	2	0	10	
Hypercalcemia	14	6		

Therapy Monitoring

1. *Every 8 weeks:* Tumor response evaluation
2. *Shortness of breath:* Stop gefitinib and evaluate for pneumonitis

Notes

Protocol for managing rash:

- Mild soap and lukewarm water to wash affected area
- Moisturize area with mild lotion
- Limit direct sun exposure. Use a sunscreen appropriate for sensitive skin (SPF15 or higher)
- Avoid over the counter acne treatments
- Remove makeup

METASTATIC DISEASE REGIMEN

CISPLATIN + FLUOROURACIL

Forastiere AA et al. JCO 1992;10:1245–1251

Hydration + mannitol before, during, and after cisplatin administration:

- Pre-cisplatin hydration with 1000 mL 0.9% NaCl injection (0.9% NS) with potassium and magnesium added as needed based on pretreatment values
- *Mannitol diuresis:* May be given to patients who have received adequate hydration. A bolus dose of mannitol 12.5–25 g can be administered as an intravenous push before starting cisplatin or prepared as an admixture with cisplatin. Continued hydration is essential
- *Continued mannitol diuresis:* In an inpatient or day-hospital setting, one can administer additional mannitol in the form of an infusion: mannitol 12.5–25 g in 1000 mL 5% dextrose and 0.45% NaCl injection (D5W/0.45% NS) + potassium chloride 30 mEq intravenously over 4 hours. This can be done either during or immediately after cisplatin, but it requires maintenance of adequate fluid input during and for hours after the administration of mannitol
- Post-cisplatin hydration with 1000 mL 0.9% NS with potassium and magnesium added as needed based on measured values

Cisplatin 100 mg/m^2 intravenously in 25–250 mL of 0.9% NS over 15–30 minutes, given on day 1 every 21 days (total dosage/cycle = 100 mg/m^2)
Fluorouracil 1000 mg/m^2 by continuous intravenous infusion in 100–1000 mL 0.9% NS or 5% dextrose injection (D5W) over 24 hours for 4 consecutive days (96-hour infusion), given on days 1–4 every 21 days (total dosage/cycle = 4000 mg/m^2)

For delayed diarrhea:
Loperamide 2 mg orally every 2 hours during waking hours (4 mg orally every 4 hours during hours of sleep). Continue for at least 12 hours after diarrhea resolves
If diarrhea persists > 48 hours despite loperamide: Stop loperamide and hospitalize patient for intravenous hydration
For persistent diarrhea:
Octreotide 100–150 mcg subcutaneously 3 times daily. Maximum total daily dose = 1500 mcg
Antibiotic therapy:
Ciprofloxacin 500 mg orally twice daily if absolute neutrophil count < 500/mm^3 (even with no fever or diarrhea) or if patient is febrile in association with diarrhea. Antibiotics should also be administered if patient is hospitalized with prolonged diarrhea and should be continued until diarrhea resolves

Emetogenic potential:
Day 1: Very high (Emetogenicity score = 6)
Days 2–5: Low (Emetogenicity score = 2). See Chapter 39 for antiemetic regimens

Patient Population Studied

A study of 87 patients with squamous head and neck cancer either with unresectable recurrence after attempted cure with surgery and radiation therapy or with newly diagnosed disease with distant metastases. Those with recurrence had received no prior chemotherapy for recurrent disease. A history of induction chemotherapy 6 months or more before study entry was allowed. Patients were entered randomly onto the cisplatin + fluorouracil arm of a 3-arm, randomized, phase III trial. Performance status SWOG ≤ 2 and adequate organ function were required

Efficacy (N = 87)

Complete response	6%
Partial response	26%
Stable disease	37%
Median duration of response	4.2 months

Treatment Modifications

Adverse Event	Dose Modification
G ≥2 Mucosal or skin toxicity	Reduce fluorouracil dosage 20%
G ≥2 Diarrhea (4–6 stools/day > baseline)	Hold fluorouracil until diarrhea resolves to baseline
G3 Myelosuppression	Reduce cisplatin dosage 25%. Do not change fluorouracil dosage
G4 Myelosuppression	Reduce cisplatin dosage 40%. Do not change fluorouracil dosage
Creatinine clearance <50 mL/min (<0.83 mL/s)	Do not administer therapy
Serum creatinine >1.5 mg/dL (>133 μmol/L) or 20% higher than baseline if >1.5 mg/dL (>133 μmol/L)	Hold cisplatin dosage until serum creatinine <1.5 mg/dL (<133 μmol/L) or within 0.2 mg/dL (17.7 μmol/L) of baseline
Serum creatinine 1.5–2.0 mg/dL (133–177 μmol/L) immediately before a cycle	Hold cisplatin*, then reduce cisplatin dosage by 25% during subsequent cycles
Serum creatinine 2.1–3.0 mg/dL (186–265 μmol/L) immediately before a cycle	Hold cisplatin*, then reduce cisplatin dosage by 50% during subsequent cycles
Serum creatinine >3.0 mg/dL (>265 μmol/L) immediately before a cycle	Hold cisplatin
G2 Neurotoxicity or ototoxicity	Hold cisplatin until neurotoxicity resolves to G ≤ 1
G3/4 Neurotoxicity or ototoxicity	Discontinue chemotherapy

*Hold cisplatin until serum creatinine <1.5 mg/dL (< 133 μmol/L), or within 0.2 mg/dL (17.7 μmol/L) of baseline

Toxicity (N = 85)

	% G1/2	% G3/4
Hematologic		
Anemia	55.3	4.7
Leukopenia	42.4	30.6
Granulocytopenia	31.8	8.2
Thrombocytopenia	12.9	5.9
Nonhematologic		
Nausea/vomiting*	68	8
Stomatitis	19	14
Diarrhea	12	2
Renal toxicity	18	9
Ototoxicity	8	4
Peripheral neuropathy	5	1
G5 Toxicities	1.1%	

*Current antiemetics not available at the time of trial
SWOG Criteria

Therapy Monitoring

1. *Before each cycle:* PE, CBC, LFTs, serum electrolytes, calcium, and magnesium
2. *One week after treatment:* Serum electrolytes, calcium, and magnesium
3. *Weekly follow-up recommended during at least the first cycle:* Attention to signs and symptoms of dehydration as supplemental hydration is often required

METASTATIC DISEASE REGIMEN

CARBOPLATIN + FLUOROURACIL

Forastiere AA et al. JCO 1992;10:1245–1251

Carboplatin 300 mg/m² intravenously in 50–500 mL 5% dextrose injection (D5W) or 0.9% NaCl injection (0.9% NS) over at least 15 minutes, given on day 1 every 28 days (total dosage/cycle = 300 mg/m²)
Fluorouracil 1000 mg/m² by continuous intravenous infusion in 100–1000 mL 0.9% NS or D5W over 24 hours for 4 consecutive days (96-hour infusion), given on days 1–4 every 28 days (total dosage/cycle = 4000 mg/m²)

For delayed diarrhea:
Loperamide 2 mg orally every 2 hours during waking hours (4 mg orally every 4 hours during hours of sleep). Continue for at least 12 hours after diarrhea resolves
If diarrhea persists > 48 hours despite loperamide: Stop loperamide and hospitalize patient for intravenous hydration
For persistent diarrhea:
Octreotide 100–150 mcg subcutaneously 3 times daily. Maximum total daily dose = 1500 mcg
Antibiotic therapy:
Ciprofloxacin 500 mg orally twice daily if absolute neutrophil count < 500/mm³ (even with no fever or diarrhea) or if patient is febrile in association with diarrhea. Antibiotics should also be administered if patient is hospitalized with prolonged diarrhea and should be continued until diarrhea resolves

Emetogenic potential: High (Emetogenicity score = 5). See Chapter 39 for antiemetic regimens

Patient Population Studied

A study of 86 patients with squamous head and neck cancer and recurrence after attempted cure with surgery and radiation therapy or with newly diagnosed disease with distant metastases. Those with recurrence had not previously received chemotherapy for their recurrent disease. A history of induction chemotherapy was allowed 6 months or more before study entry. Patients were randomly assigned to the carboplatin + fluorouracil arm of a 3-arm, randomized, phase III trial. Performance status of SWOG ≤ 2 and adequate organ function were required, including creatinine clearance ≥ 50 mL/min (≥ 0.83 mL/s)

Efficacy (N = 86)

Complete response	2%
Partial response	19%
Stable disease	42%
Median duration of response	5.1 months

Toxicity (N = 86)

	% G1/2	% G3/4
Hematologic		
Leukopenia	50	12
Anemia	42	14
Granulocytopenia	21	2
Thrombocytopenia	19	13
Nonhematologic		
Nausea/vomiting*	48	6
Stomatitis	28	15
Diarrhea	6	2
Ototoxicity	2	0
Peripheral neuropathy	2	0
Renal toxicity	1	1
G5 Toxicity	1.2%	

*Current antiemetics not available at the time of trial
SWOG Criteria

Treatment Modifications

Adverse Event	Dose Modification
G ≥ 2 Mucosal or skin toxicity	Reduce fluorouracil dosage by 20%
G ≥ 2 Diarrhea (4–6 stools/day > baseline)	Hold fluorouracil until diarrhea resolves
G3/4 Toxicity myelosuppression	Reduce carboplatin dosage by 20%. Do not change fluorouracil dosage
G0/1 Myelosuppression	Increase carboplatin dosage by 20% to 360 mg/m² on the same administration schedule

Therapy Monitoring

1. *Weekly:* PE, CBC, serum electrolytes, LFTs calcium, and magnesium
2. *Weekly follow-up recommended during at least the first cycle:* Attention to signs and symptoms of dehydration as supplemental hydration is often required

METASTATIC DISEASE REGIMEN

DOCETAXEL + CISPLATIN

Glisson BS et al. JCO 2002;20:1593–1599

Premedication:
Dexamethasone 8 mg orally or intravenously every 12 hours for 3 days starting the day before docetaxel infusion

Hydration + mannitol before, during, and after cisplatin administration:
- Pre-cisplatin hydration with 1000 mL 0.9% NaCl injection (0.9% NS) with potassium and magnesium added as needed based on pretreatment values
- *Mannitol diuresis:* May be given to patients who have received adequate hydration. A bolus dose of mannitol 12.5–25 g can be administered as an intravenous push before starting cisplatin or prepared as an admixture with cisplatin. Continued hydration is essential
- *Continued mannitol diuresis:* In an inpatient or day-hospital setting, one can administer additional mannitol in the form of an infusion: mannitol 12.5–25 g in 1000 mL 5% dextrose and 0.45% NaCl injection (D5W/0.45% NS) + potassium chloride 30 mEq intravenously over 4 hours. This can be done either during or immediately after cisplatin, but it requires maintenance of adequate fluid input during and for hours after the administration of mannitol
- Post-cisplatin hydration with 1000 mL 0.9% NS with potassium and magnesium added as needed based on measured values

Docetaxel 75 mg/m^2 intravenously after dilution in a volume of 0.9% NS or 5% dextrose injection sufficient to produce a final docetaxel concentration of 0.3–0.74 mg/mL over 60 minutes, given on day 1 every 21 days (total dosage/cycle = 75 mg/m^2), *followed by*
Cisplatin 75 mg/m^2 intravenously in 25–250 mL 0.9% NS over 30 minutes on day 1 every 21 days (total dosage/cycle = 75 mg/m^2)

Dexamethasone is marketed in the United States in numerous formulations for oral administration, such as 0.25-, 0.5-, 0.75-, 1-, 2-, 4-, and 6-mg tablets, and in elixirs (which contain alcohol) and solutions for oral administration

Emetogenic potential: Very high (Emetogenicity score = 6). See Chapter 39 for antiemetic regimens

Patient Population Studied

A study of 36 patients with recurrent disease or disease deemed incurable, who had not previously received chemotherapy for recurrent disease and had never received a taxane, were entered in a multicenter phase II trial. Performance status ECOG 0–1 and adequate organ function were required, including creatinine clearance ≥ 50 mL/min (≥0.83 mL/s)

Efficacy (N = 86)

Complete response	6%
Partial response	34%
Stable disease	34%
Median duration of response	4.9 months
Median time to response	5 weeks
Median time to treatment failure	3 months
Median survival	9.6 months
1-year survival	28%
2-year survival	19%

Treatment Modifications

Adverse Event	Dose Modification
ANC < 1500/mm^3 or platelets <100,000/mm^3 at the time of chemotherapy administration	Delay chemotherapy until ANC >1500/mm^3 and platelets >100,000/mm^3. Discontinue if recovery has not occurred after a 3-week delay
Creatinine clearance <50 mL/min (<0.83 mL/s)	Do not administer therapy
Serum creatinine >1.5 mg/dL (>133 μmol/L) or 20% higher than baseline value if baseline >1.5 mg/dL (>133 μmol/L)	Hold cisplatin until serum creatinine <1.5 mg/dL (<133 μmol/L) or within 0.2 mg/dL (17.7 μmol/L) of baseline
Serum creatinine 1.5–2.0 mg/dL (133–177 μmol/L) immediately before a cycle	Hold cisplatin*, then reduce cisplatin dosage by 25% during subsequent cycles
Serum creatinine 2.1–3.0 mg/dL (186–265 μmol/L) immediately before a cycle	Hold cisplatin*, then reduce cisplatin dosage by 50% during subsequent cycles
Serum creatinine >3.0 mg/dL (>265 μmol/L) immediately before a cycle	Hold cisplatin
G2 Neurotoxicity or ototoxicity	Hold cisplatin until neurotoxicity resolves to G ≤ 1
G3/4 Neurotoxicity or ototoxicity	Discontinue chemotherapy

*Hold cisplatin until serum creatinine < 1.5 mg/dL (<133 μmol/L) or within 0.2 mg/dL (17.7 μmol/L) of baseline

Toxicity (N = 35/36)

	% G1/2	% G3/4
Hematologic (N = 35)		
Neutropenia	NR	80
Thrombocytopenia	NR	3
Anemia	NR	14
Nonhematologic (N = 36)		
Nausea	56	11
Asthenia	53	25
Stomatitis	44	3
Vomiting	41	8
Neurosensory	39	3
Diarrhea	38	6
Infection	27	17
Skin	19	0
Neurosensory, hearing	17	0
Pulmonary	14	8
Allergy	14	8
Neuromotor	14	3
Hypotension	14	0
G5 Toxicity	2.8%	

NR = Not reported

NCI CTC

Therapy Monitoring

1. *Weekly:* CBC with differential
2. *Before each cycle:* Serum electrolytes, creatinine, calcium, magnesium, LFTs, and urinalysis
3. *During dexamethasone:* monitor glucose if indicated

METASTATIC DISEASE REGIMEN

PACLITAXEL + CARBOPLATIN

Pivot X et al. Oncology 2001;60:66–71

Premedication:

Prednisone 60 mg orally twice daily for a total of 4 doses, starting the day before chemotherapy
Cimetidine 300 mg by intravenous infusion in 25–100 mL 0.9% NaCl injection (0.9% NS) or 5% dextrose injection (D5W) over 5–30 minutes, given 30 minutes before paclitaxel
Diphenhydramine 50 mg intravenously per push given 30–60 minutes before paclitaxel
Paclitaxel 175 mg/m^2 by intravenous infusion in a volume of 0.9% NS or D5W sufficient to produce a concentration of 0.3–1.2 mg/mL over 3 hours on day 1 every 21 days (total dosage/cycle = 175 mg/m^2) *followed by*
Carboplatin [calculated dose] AUC = 6 by intravenous infusion in 500 mL of 0.9% NS over 2 hours on day 1 every 21 days (total dosage/cycle calculated to produce an AUC of 6 mg/mL·min)

Prednisone is marketed in the United States in numerous solid formulations for oral administration, such as in tablets containing 1, 2.5, 5, 10, 20, and 50 mg prednisone, and in solutions and syrups for oral administration

Emetogenic potential: High (Emetogenicity score = 5). See Chapter 39 for antiemetic regimens

Carboplatin doses were determined according to the Chatelut formula (Chatelut E et al. J Natl Cancer Inst 1995;87:573–580):

$$\text{Carboplatin clearance (females)} = (0.134 \times \text{wt}) + [(218 \times \text{wt}) \times (1 - 0.00457 \times \text{age}) \times 0.686]/\text{Serum creatinine}$$

$$\text{Carboplatin clearance (males)} = (0.134 \times \text{wt}) + [(218 \times \text{wt}) \times (1 - 0.00457 \times \text{age})]/\text{Serum creatinine}$$

Weight (wt) is in kilogram units; age is in years; and serum creatinine is in micromoles/liter

Treatment Modifications

Adverse Event	Dose Modification
G3/4 Mucositis	Reduce paclitaxel dosage by 20%
G3 Thrombocytopenia	Reduce paclitaxel dosage by 20%
G4 Thrombocytopenia	Reduce paclitaxel dosage by 50%
G4 Neutropenia >5 days	Reduce paclitaxel dosage by 20%
ANC < 1500/mm^3 or platelets <100,000/mm^3 at the time of chemotherapy administration	Delay chemotherapy until ANC >1500/mm^3 and platelets >100,000/mm^3. Discontinue chemotherapy if recovery has not occurred after a 2-week delay
Creatinine clearance (Clcr) <45 mL/min (<not> 0.75 mL/s)	Delay treatment until Clcr >45 mL/min. Discontinue therapy if has not recovered by 6 weeks
G2 neurotoxicity	Hold paclitaxel until neurotoxicity resolves to G ≤ 1
G 3/4 neurotoxicity	Discontinue chemotherapy

Patient Population Studied

A study of 27 patients with unresectable recurrent disease or distant metastatic disease. Previous radiation treatment and concomitant or induction chemoradiation were allowed. ECOG performance status 0–2 and adequate organ function were required, including creatinine clearance ≥45 mL/min (≥0.75 mL/s)

Efficacy (N = 27)

Complete response	7.4%
Partial response	22.2%
Stable disease	11.1%
Median duration of response	4.4 months
Median survival	7.2 months

SWOG Criteria

Therapy Monitoring

1. *Before each cycle:* CBC with differential, serum electrolytes, calcium, magnesium, and LFTs
2. *Weekly:* CBC with differential

Toxicity (N = 27)

	% G2	% G3/4
Hematologic		
Anemia	40.7	11.1
Neutropenia	14.8	62.9
Febrile neutropenia	—	18.5
Thrombocytopenia	11.1	14.8
Nonhematologic		
Alopecia	29.6	44.4
Neurotoxicity (neuropathy)	11.1	7.4
Mucositis	11.1	7.4
Nausea/vomiting	7.4	7.4
Cardiotoxicity		3.7
G5 Toxicity	3.7%*	

*One patient with neutropenia and sepsis
NCI CTC

METASTATIC DISEASE REGIMEN

PACLITAXEL, IFOSFAMIDE, AND CARBOPLATIN

Shin DM et al. Cancer 2001;91:1316–1323

Premedication:
Dexamethasone 20 mg intravenously per push 30–60 minutes before paclitaxel
Cimetidine 300 mg by intravenous infusion in 25–100 mL 0.9% NaCl injection (0.9% NS) or 5% dextrose injection (D5W) over 5–30 minutes, given 30–60 minutes before paclitaxel
Diphenhydramine 50 mg intravenously per push 30–60 minutes before paclitaxel

Paclitaxel 175 mg/m^2 by intravenous infusion in a volume of 0.9% NS or D5W sufficient to produce a concentration of 0.3–1.2 mg/mL over 3 hours, given on day 1 every 3 to 4 weeks (total dosage/cycle = 175 mg/m^2), *followed by*
Mesna 200 mg/m^2 per day as a slow intravenous push before ifosfamide on 3 consecutive days, given on days 1–3 every 3–4 weeks (total dosage/cycle = 600 mg/m^2)
Ifosfamide 1000 mg/m^2 per day intravenously in a volume of 0.9% NS or D5W sufficient to produce a concentration between 0.6 and 20 mg/mL over 2 hours on 3 consecutive days, given on days 1–3 every 3–4 weeks (total dosage/cycle = 3000 mg/m^2)
Mesna 400 mg/m^2 per day by continuous intravenous infusion in 250–1000 mL 0.9% NS or D5W over 24 hours, during and after ifosfamide administration on 3 consecutive days, given on days 1–3 every 3 to 4 weeks (total dosage/cycle = 1200 mg/m^2)
Carboplatin [calculated dose] AUC = 6* by intravenous infusion in 500 mL 0.9% NS over 30 minutes on day 1 every 3–4 weeks (total dosage/cycle calculated to produce an AUC = 6 mg/mL·min)
Dexamethasone 4 mg orally every 6 hours for 4 doses on day 1, following paclitaxel (total dose administered/cycle, including premedication = 36 mg)

Note: Consider hematopoietic growth factor support

Dexamethasone is marketed in the United States in numerous formulations for oral administration, such as 0.25-, 0.5-, 0.75-, 1-, 2-, 4-, and 6-mg tablets, and in elixirs (which contain alcohol) and solutions for oral administration

Emetogenic potential: Very high (Emetogenicity score = 6). See Chapter 39 for antiemetic regimens

*Carboplatin dose is based on Calvert's formula to achieve a target area under the plasma concentration versus time curve (AUC) [AUC units = mg/mL·min]

$$\text{Total carboplatin dose (mg)} = (\text{Target AUC}) \times (\text{GFR} + 25)$$

In practice, creatinine clearance (Clcr) is used in place of glomerular filtration rate (GFR). Clcr can be calculated from the equation of Cockcroft and Gault:

$$\text{Males, Clcr} = \frac{(140 - \text{age[y]}) \times \text{body weight [kg]}}{72 \times (\text{Serum creatinine [mg/dL]})}$$

$$\text{Females, Clcr} = \frac{(140 - \text{age [y]}) \times \text{body weight [kg]}}{72 \times (\text{Serum creatinine [mg/dL]})} \times 0.85$$

Calvert AH et al. JCO 1989;7:1748–1656
Cockcroft DW, Gault MH. Nephron 1976;16:31–41
Jodrell DI et al. JCO 1992;10:520–528
Sorensen BT et al. Cancer Chemother Pharmacol 1991;28:397–401

Treatment Modifications

Agent		Dose Level			
	Day	−2	−1	0	1
Paclitaxel (mg/m^2)	1	135	175	175	175
Ifosfamide (mg/m^2)	1–3	1000			
Mesna (mg/m^2)	1–3	200/400			
Carboplatin (AUC)	1	4	5	6	7

Adverse Event	Dose Modification
ANC < 1500/mm^3 or platelets <100,000/mm^3 at time of next cycle of chemotherapy	Delay chemotherapy until ANC > 1500/mm^3 and platelets > 100,000/mm^3
G ≥ 3 Nonhematologic toxicity	Reduce paclitaxel and carboplatin dosages one dose level
G4 Hematologic toxicity lasting >7 days	
Neutropenic fever with or without documented infection	
10–15 RBCs/high-power field (HPF) on urinalysis	Administer an additional dose of mesna at 400 mg/m^2
>50 RBCs/HPF on urinalysis	Administer mesna at 1000 mg/m^2 and hold ifosfamide until red blood cells are <10/HPF

Patient Population Studied

A study of 55 patients with unresectable recurrent disease after surgery and/or radiation or with distant metastatic disease. Patients with recurrent disease had not previously received chemotherapy for the recurrence. ECOG performance status 0–2 and adequate organ function were required

Efficacy (N = 54)

Complete response	17%
Partial response	43%
Median duration of response	3.7 months
Median survival	9.1 months
Estimated 1-year survival	36%
Estimated 2-year survival	13%

WHO criteria

Toxicity (N = 54)

	% G1	% G2	% G3	% G4
Nonhematologic				
Fatigue	30	22	6	
Nausea/vomiting	28	9	4	
Peripheral neuropathy	28	7	2	
Weight loss	13	11	0	
Anorexia	13	9	4	
Stomatitis/mucositis	6	2	0	
Myalgia/arthralgia	9	7	2	
Renal toxicity	2	0	2	
Hematologic				
Neutropenia	NR	NR	G3/4 = 92%	
Neutropenia and fever	30%			
Anemia	13% required RBC transfusion			
Thrombocytopenia	7% required platelet transfusion			

NCI CTC

Therapy Monitoring

1. *Weekly:* CBC with differential, serum electrolytes, creatinine calcium, and LFTs
2. *Days 2 and 3 of each cycle:* Monitor for red blood cells in urine for toxic effects of ifosfamide
3. *Before each cycle:* H&P, tumor measurements, and toxicity assessment

16. Hepatocellular Carcinoma

Joan Maurel, MD, and Jordi Bruix, MD

Epidemiology

Incidence*: 5000 per year

Male:female ratio: Men are far more likely to develop hepatocellular carcinoma (HCC) than women

Age: In the United States, liver cancer occurs more often in people over age 60 than in younger people

Stage at Presentation	
Stage A:	35%
Stage B:	20%
Stage C:	20%
Stage D	25%

*The incidence of HCC varies widely according to geographic location. The distribution also differs among ethnic groups and regions within the same country

The annual international incidence of the disease is 1 million cases

Parkin DM et al. Int J Cancer 2001;94:153–6

Bruix J and Sherman M. Hepatology 2005;42:1208–36

Pathology

Hepatocellular carcinoma:	99%
Fibrolamelar hepatocellular carcinoma:	<1%

Nakashima T, Kojiro M. Hepatocellular Carcinoma. Tokyo: Springer Verlag, 1987

Work-Up

1. Alfa fetoprotein (AFP)
2. Chest x-ray
3. Abdominal spiral CT and/or dynamic liver MRI and/or ultrasound

Note: Specific clinical scenarios such as selection for liver transplantation may also require chest CT to accurately exclude lung metastases, but there are no robust data supporting the cost-efficiency of this policy

Diagnostic criteria for HCC

1. Cytohistologic criteria
2. Noninvasive diagnostic criteria (restricted to patients with cirrhosis and tumors > 1 cm):
   - 1–2 cm: Two coincidental dynamic imaging techniques (contrast us, CT or MRI) showing arterial uptake with contrast washout in the delayed venous phase
   - >2 cm: One dynamic imaging technique showing the specific HCC pattern (arterial uptake with washout in delayed venous phase)

Note: AFP determination has almost no role. A non-specific dynamic pattern should prompt a tumor biopsy since AFP may also be increased in cholangiocarcinoma and metastatic disease

Bruix J and Sherman M. Hepatology 2005;42:1208–36

Staging

Primary Tumor (T)

TX	Primary tumor cannot be assessed
T0	No evidence of primary tumor
T1	Solitary tumor without vascular invasion
T2	Solitary tumor 5 cm or less in greatest dimension with vascular invasion, or multiple tumors none more than 5 cm in greatest dimension.
T3	Multiple tumors more than 5 cm or with vascular invasion (portal or hepatic vein)
T4	Direct tumor invasion or visceral peritoneum perforation

Reproduced, with permission, of the American Joint Committee on Cancer (AJCC), Chicago, Illinois. The original source for this material is the AJCC Cancer Staging Manual, 6th edition (2002) published by Springer-Verlag, New York, www.springeronline.com.

Regional Lymph Nodes (N): Clinical

NX	Regional lymph nodes cannot be assessed
N0	No regional lymph node metastases
N1	Metastasis to regional lymph nodes

Distant Metastasis (M)

MX	Distant metastasis cannot be assessed
M0	No distant metastasis
M1	Distant metastases

Reproduced, with permission, of the American Joint Committee on Cancer (AJCC), Chicago, Illinois. The original source for this material is the AJCC Cancer Staging Manual, 6th edition (2002) published by Springer-Verlag, New York, www.springeronline.com.

Staging Groups

Stage A	Single nodule <5 cm or 3 nodules <3 cm without symptoms (PS 0); Okuda <3; Child-Pugh A-B
Stage B	Large/multinodular without symptoms (PS 0) and/or vascular invasion or extrahepatic spread without symptoms (PS 0); Okuda <3; Child-Pugh A-B
Stage C	Any size with symptoms (PS 1-2) or vascular invasion/extrahepatic spread with symptoms (PS 1-2); Okuda <3; Child-Pugh A-B
Stage D	Any size Okuda 3 or Child-Pugh C or PS >2

Bruix J and Sherman M. Hepatology 2005;42:1208–36

Three-Year Survival (BCLC)

Stage A	60–75%
Stage B	50%
Stage C	10%
Stage D	0%

Bruix J and Sherman M. Hepatology 2005;42:1208–36
Llovet JM et al. Lancet 2003;362:1907–1917

Caveats

Patients diagnosed at an early stage (BCLC A: One small HCC or up to 3 nodules <3 cm and preserved liver function) should be considered for one of the following options:

1 Tumor resection
2 Liver transplantation from cadaveric or live donor
3 Percutaneous ablation by ethanol injection or radiofrequency ablation

Llovet JM et al. Lancet 2003;362:1907–1917
Bruix J and Sherman M. Hepatology 2005;42:1208–36

REGIMEN

CHEMOEMBOLIZATION WITH DOXORUBICIN

Llovet JM et al. Lancet 2002;359:1734–1739

Doxorubicin dose adjusted to serum bilirubin concentration (see table below) prepared as an emulsion with 10 mL ethiodized oil injection administered intra-arterially followed by mechanical obstruction achieved by intra-arterial injection of gelatin sponge fragments suspended in radiologic contrast media until flow stagnation occurred. Chemoembolization was performed at baseline, repeated 2 months and 6 months later, and then every 6 months until disease progression

Note: Doxorubicin dosage was based on serum total bilirubin concentration as per the table below:

Total Bilirubin		Doxorubicin Dosage
(μmol/L)	(mg/dL)	
<25.6	<1.5	75 mg/m^2
25.6–51.3	1.5–3	50 mg/m^2
51.3–85.5	3–5	25 mg/m^2

Emetogenic potential: Low (Emetogenicity score = 2). See Chapter 39

Treatment Modifications

Doxorubicin dosage modifications were based on serum total bilirubin concentrations before treatment

Patient Population Studied

A study of 112 patients with intermediate BCLC stage (stage B or C) randomized to conservative treatment (n = 35), embolization (n = 37), or chemo-embolization (n = 40)

Efficacy

1. Chemoembolization induced objective responses sustained for at least 6 months in 35% (14) of cases, and was associated with a significantly lower rate of portal vein invasion than conservative treatment
2. Probability of portal vein invasion reduced from 58% in control to 17% in patients with chemoembolization
3. Survival probabilities at 1 year and 2 years were 75% and 50% for embolization; 82% and 63% for chemoembolization and 63% and 27% for control

Toxicity (N = 40)

Adverse Event	No. of Patients
Cholecystitis	2
Leukopenia	2
Ischemic biliary stricture	1
Hepatic infarction	1
Spontaneous bacterial peritonitis	1
Bacteremia	1
Septic shock	1
Allergic dermatitis	1
Severe alopecia	1

Therapy Monitoring

1. *Every 3 months:* CBC with differential, LFTs, serum creatinine, and BUN
2. *Every 6 months:* CT and ultrasound to evaluate efficacy

REGIMEN

CHEMOEMBOLIZATION WITH CISPLATIN

Lo C-M et al. Hepatology 2002;35:1164–1171

Premedication:
Hydrate before and after cisplatin by administering 0.9 NaCl injection (0.9% NS) as continuous intravenous infusion at 100 mL/hour. Begin 12 hours before cisplatin and continue for 6 hours after the cisplatin dose is administered
Amoxicillin with clavulanic acid 1200 mg intravenously before chemoembolization
Mannitol 20 g intravenously before chemoembolization
Tropisetron 5 mg intravenously before chemoembolization

Chemoembolization:
Cisplatin (1 mg/mL) emulsified with ethiodized oil injection in equivalent volumes (1:1)
- Administer cisplatin intra-arterially via the left or right hepatic artery as appropriate for tumor vascularization. If selective catheterization is not possible, the cisplatin emulsion is injected into the hepatic artery, distal to the gastroduodenal artery
- The emulsion is injected slowly under fluoroscopic monitoring to a maximum volume of 60 mL (≤30 mg cisplatin) at a controlled rate to prevent retrograde flow, followed by mechanical obstruction achieved by intra-arterial injection of gelatin sponge pellets 1 mm in diameter mixed with gentamicin 40 mg

Chemoembolization is repeated every 2–3 months until comorbid pathologies, adverse events, or disease progression are observed

Medications after the procedure:
Amoxicillin-clavulonic acid (250 mg/125 mg) orally 3 times daily for 3 days and sucralfate 500 mg orally 4 times daily for 3 days

Emetogenic potential: Low–moderate (Emetogenicity score = 3). See Chapter 39

Treatment Modifications

Withhold or discontinue chemoembolization for:
- Hepatic artery thrombosis
- Main portal vein thrombosis
- Arteriovenous shunting
- Hepatic encephalopathy
- Ascites not controlled by diuretics
- Variceal bleeding within the last 3 months
- Serum total bilirubin >50 μmol/L (>2.9 mg/dL)
- Serum albumin <28 g/L (<2.8 /dL)
- Prothrombin time 4 seconds >control

Patient Population Studied

A study of 80 patients with Okuda Stage I–II HCC and no contraindications for chemoembolization; 40 assigned to chemoembolization and 39 assigned to control. Chemoembolization resulted in a marked tumor response and the actuarial survival was significantly better in the chemoembolization group than in the control group. Although death from liver failure was more frequent in patients who received chemoembolization, the liver functions of the survivors were not significantly different

Efficacy

Patients with measurable disease	
Partial response	39%
Patients with measurable AFP	
Objective response in AFP	72%
All patients	
1-year survival	57%
2-year survival	31%
3-year survival	26%

Toxicity (N = 40 Patients/192 Courses)

	% Cycles
Fevers ≥38°C	32.8
Abdominal pain	26
Vomiting	16.7
Ascites	5.2
Gastrointestinal bleeding	4.2
Bleeding at femoral puncture	1.6
Encephalopathy	1.6
Ruptured tumor	1
Pleural effusion	1
Liver abscess	0.5
Hematuria	0.5
Hypotension	0.5
Bradycardia	0.5

Therapy Monitoring

Every 3 months: CBC with differential, LFTs, serum creatinine, and BUN; CT scan to evaluate efficacy

17. HIV-Related Malignancies

Pallavi Kumar, MD, and Richard F. Little, MD

Kaposi's Sarcoma (KS)

Epidemiology of KS

Incidence/100,000

United States	
Males:	2.1
Females:	0.11
Africa	
Males:	39.3
Females:	21.8

Stage at Presentation in HAART Era (Based on ACTG* Modified TIS Staging)

Poor risk:	25%
Good risk:	75%

*ACTG: AIDS Clinical Trials Group

Deaths due to AIDS since advent of HAART have decreased by over 50%

Nasti G et al. JCO 2003;21:2876–2882

Pathology

1. All KS is caused by human herpesvirus 8 (HHV-8), also called the Kaposi's sarcoma–associated herpesvirus (KSHV), a gamma herpesvirus first identified in 1994
2. Pathology shows a highly vascular tumor with spindle-shaped cells staining positive for KSHV

Moore PS, Chang Y. NEJM 1995;332:1181–1185

Work-Up

1 Biopsy to confirm diagnosis

2 HIV serology

3 CD4 and HIV-1 viral load

4 Assessment of tumor extent:

- Physical examination of the skin and lymph nodes
- Chest x-ray
- Chest CT scan not routinely indicated unless x-ray is abnormal
- For GI symptoms, work-up as indicated, procedures to consider include endoscopy, colonoscopy and CT of abdomen

Staging (Validated ACTG TIS Staging for AIDS-KS)*

Good Risk: Stage 0 [Stage 0—All criteria below]	Poor Risk: Stage 1 [Stage 1—Any criterion below]
Tumor (T)	
Confined to skin and/or lymph nodes	Tumor-associated edema or ulceration Extensive oral KS Gastrointestinal KS KS in other non-nodal viscera
Immune System (I)*	
CD4 cells >150/mm^3	CD4 cells <150/mm^3
Systemic Illness (S)	
• No history of opportunistic infection or thrush	• History of opportunistic infections, thrush, or both
• No B symptoms persisting >2 weeks: 1 Unexplained fever 2 Night sweats 3 >10% involuntary weight loss 4 Diarrhea	• B symptoms present
• Performance status >70 (Karnofsky)	• Performance status <70 (Karnofsky) • Other HIV-related illness (eg, neurologic disease, lymphoma)

Staging example:
A patient with KS restricted to the skin, CD4 count of 10 cells/μL, and a history of *Pneumocystis carinii* pneumonia would be T0 I1 S1

*According to the AIDS Clinical Trials Group (ACTG). Staging takes into account tumor extent (T), immune status (I), and systemic illness (S)

Notes:
1. In the HAART era, immune status may not be prognostically predictive. However, in patients with resistant HIV, immune status may be relevant
2. In the HAART era, poor prognosis is T1 S1. All other stages are considered good prognosis. See survival table

Krown SE et al. JCO 1997;15:3085–3092
Nasti G et al. JCO 2003;21:2876–2882

Survival

Stage	3-Year Survival (%)
T0 S0	88
T1 S0	80
T0 S1	81
T1 S1	53

Nasti G, et al. J Clin Oncol 2003; 21: 2876–82

REGIMEN [HIV REGIMENS]

HIGHLY ACTIVE ANTIRETROVIRAL THERAPY (HAART)

HAART should be considered as fundamental oncologic care in patients with AIDS-KS. Unless there is some overwhelming reason not to administer it, HAART should be given in essentially all AIDS-KS patients

Antiretroviral drugs are classified according to the type of compound and the part of the viral life cycle that the drug inhibits. The HAART regimen generally comprises a combination of three or more drugs from at least two different classes as defined by these criteria. The treatment goal is potent inhibition of HIV replication to levels <50 copies HIV mRNA/μL. HAART should be considered part of the fundamental oncologic therapy for AIDS-KS

Examples:
Zidovudine 300 mg orally twice daily
Lamivudine 150 mg orally twice daily
Lopinavir/ritonavir 400 mg/100 mg orally twice daily

or

Stavudine 40 mg orally twice daily
Lamivudine 150 mg orally twice daily
Efavirenz 600 mg orally once daily at bedtime

or

Other regimens available at http://www.aidsinfo. nih.gov/

Toxicity

Zidovudine	
Common[a]	Nausea, anorexia, vomiting, headache, malaise
Infrequent[b]	Constipation, asthenia
Rare[c]	G3/4 anemia, granulocytopenia, increased liver transaminases
Lamivudine	
Common	Headache
Infrequent	Depression, dizziness, hyperamylasemia, nasal stuffiness, malaise/fatigue
Rare	Hyperbilirubinemia, neuropathy, anemia, granulocytopenia, pancreatitis, increased liver transaminases, lactic acidosis, rash
Lopinavir/Ritonavir	
Common	Mild–moderate diarrhea, nausea, lipodystrophy (with chronic use)
Infrequent	Abdominal pain, nausea, asthenia, rash, increased liver transaminases, total cholesterol and triglycerides
Rare	Hyperbilirubinemia, neuropathy, pancreatitis, hyperglycemia, exacerbation or new-onset diabetes, lactic acidosis
Stavudine	
Common	Headache, peripheral sensory neuropathy, diarrhea, nausea, vomiting, rash, lipodystrophy (with chronic use)
Infrequent	Increased liver transaminases, sleep disorders
Rare	Anemia, pancreatitis, lactic acidosis
Efavirenz	
Common	Dizziness, insomnia, diarrhea, nausea, vomiting, rash, lipodystrophy (with chronic use)
Infrequent	Impaired concentration, somnolence, abnormal dreams, hyperlipidemia, increased liver transaminases, immune reconstitution syndrome, hyperamylasemia
Rare	Hallucinations, depression, suicidal ideation, increased total cholesterol, pancreatitis

HAART is generally well tolerated. Less than 5% have toxicity >G1. Toxicity is regimen specific
[a]Common: >10%
[b]Infrequent: 3–10%
[c]Rare: <3%

Treatment Modifications

Antiretroviral drugs should be managed by physicians with expertise in the care of patients with HIV disease. Certain drug combinations can be antagonistic and should not be used. Dose modifications must be done with caution because inadequate plasma drug levels increase the potential to develop resistant mutant HIV. At least 3 medications are required for HAART: If toxicity requiring dosing cessation is ascribed to one medication, patients should be instructed to stop all medications to avoid resistance

Patient Population Studied

Patients without previous HIV or KS therapy

Efficacy

1. For initial therapy of KS, a trial of HAART is reasonable in many cases. Up to 74% of treatment-naive cases (eg, never previously treated for either HIV or KS) can have a substantial tumor response to HAART
2. Responses may be seen within 3–6 months
3. Those most likely to respond are those with:
   - Minimal tumor burden
   - HIV viral load suppression to very low levels
   - CD4 cell increases ≥150 cells/mm^3 above pretreatment levels
4. Response durations can be long-lasting, although progressive diseases may occur early

Therapy Monitoring

1. *Monthly for first 3 months:* Clinical evaluation, assessment of tumor burden, viral titers, immunologic assessment (CD4 cells) CBC with differential, liver function tests, BUN, creatinine, amylase, and lipase
2. *Every 3 months after first 3 months (if clinically improving):* Clinical evaluation, assessment of tumor burden, viral titers, immunologic assessment (CD4 cells), CBC with differential, liver function tests, BUN, creatinine, amylase, and lipase

REGIMEN

LOCAL THERAPY: ELECTRON-BEAM RADIATION, INTRALESIONAL THERAPY, CRYOTHERAPY (LIQUID NITROGEN, ALITRETINOIN GEL (TOPICAL all-*TRANS*RETINOIC ACID), PHOTODYNAMIC THERAPY

Ramirez-Amador et al. Oral Oncol 2002;38:460–467
Von Roenn JH. Hematol Oncol Clin North Am 2003;17:747–762

Important: Administer HAART to all patients

Electron-beam radiation:
Dosing varies; radiation therapy may be more toxic in HIV patients

Intralesional therapy:
Vinblastine 0.1 mL of 0.1 mg/mL [or 0.2 mg/mL per 1 cm^2 of lesion surface area] intralesionally every 1–2 weeks, *or*
3% Sodium tetradecyl sulfate (Sotradecol®) injection 0.1–0.3 mL intralesionally every 1–2 weeks

Cryotherapy (liquid nitrogen):
Liquid nitrogen is effective for treatment of small cosmetically disturbing lesions, particularly in the face. Liquid nitrogen is applied to the lesion to achieve a thaw time of approximately 40 seconds. High response rates have been reported lasting from 6 weeks to 6 months. Treatment-related hypopigmentation may be cosmetically unacceptable, particularly in dark-skinned patients

Alitretinoin gel:
Alitretinoin 0.1% gel topically to affected areas 3–5 times per day

Photodynamic therapy:
Doses vary

Note: Surgical resection is not generally useful. Clear margins are not meaningful

Patient Population Studied

Most studies were conducted before the widespread use of HAART in patients with minimal disease

Efficacy

1 Local therapy is rarely useful except with limited disease
2 Local recurrence is common
3 Patients who benefit favorably from HAART may have better long-term outcome in terms of tumor recurrence
4 Patients who derive no benefit from HAART are likely to have new tumors or recurrent tumors relatively quickly in the treatment fields

Electron-beam radiation:
Recurrence within the radiation field is common
Intralesional injections:
Useful for small lesions of cosmetic import. Not feasible for multiple lesions
Cryotherapy:
Not feasible for multiple lesions
Alitretinoin gel:
Reported response rate up to 40%
May be most useful for patients with minimal disease
Photodynamic therapy:
For limited disease can be very effective

Treatment Modifications

1. HIV infection may render certain tissues more vulnerable to toxic effects of radiation
2. Radiation therapy of oral disease should be reserved for symptomatic oral KS because of the high incidence of radiation-induced mucositis

Toxicity

Electron-beam radiation:
Poor cosmetic outcome: Hyperpigmentation and telangiectasia
Chronic lymphedema
Intralesional injections: Very painful
Cryotherapy:
Avoid in dark skinned patients; permanently destroys melanocytes, leaving a white spot
Alitretinoin gel:
Can cause local irritation
Photodynamic therapy:
Burning sensation during treatment

Therapy Monitoring

Monitor for efficacy; no specific monitoring required

REGIMEN

INTERFERON ALFA-2B

Krown SE. Curr Opin Oncol 2001;13:374–381
Von Roenn JH. Hematol Oncol Clin North Am 2003;17:747–762

Important: Administer HAART to all patients

Interferon alfa-2b 5–10 million UNITS subcutaneously or intramuscularly daily (total dose/week = 35–70 million UNITS)

or

Interferon alfa-2b 5–10 million UNITS subcutaneously or intramuscularly 3 times per week (total dose/week = 15–30 million UNITS)

or

Interferon alfa-2b 1 million UNITS subcutaneously daily or twice weekly (total dose/week = 2–7 million UNITS)

Ancillary medications:

1. Primary antipyretic prophylaxis:
   Acetaminophen 650–1000 mg orally

   or

   Ibuprofen 400–600 mg orally starting 1 hour before interferon, then every 4 hours as needed
2. Secondary antiemetic prophylaxis:
   If required as secondary prophylaxis, use as primary prophylaxis with subsequent doses. See Chapter 39

Emetogenic potential: Nonemetogenic (Emetogenicity score = 1). See Chapter 39

Patient Population Studied

Patients with HIV-related KS

Treatment Modifications

Adverse Event	Dose Modification
First occurrence of WHO G ≥3 toxicity	Hold dose until toxicity G ≤1, then reduce interferon alfa dosage by 33%
Second occurrence of WHO G ≥3 toxicity	Hold dose until toxicity G ≤1, then decrease interferon alfa dosage by 66%
Third occurrence of WHO G ≥3 toxicity	Hold dose until toxicity G ≤1, then reduce interferon alfa dosage to 1 million UNITS
WHO G ≥3 toxicity at 1 million UNITS	Discontinue interferon alfa therapy
Life-threatening or persistent, severe toxic reactions	
Hypotension resistant to intravenous vasopressors	Stop treatment. Resume cautiously if blood pressure recovers

(1) Most treatment withdrawals occur in the first 4 months of treatment, after which discontinuation of therapy due to toxicity is unusual

(2) A response to other adverse events is determined largely by the patient and the treating physician. Side effects are rarely life-threatening and should not lead to discontinuation if appropriate and proactive supportive care is provided

Definitions of dose-limiting toxicities (DLTs):
Hematologic DLT: Granulocyte count <500/mm^3
Hepatic DLT: SGPT (ALT) or SGOT (AST) >5 times ULN (upper limit of normal)

Efficacy

- Response rates to interferon as a single agent vary from 20% to 60%
- Multiple studies combining interferon and zidovudine reported response rates of ≥40%

Notes:

1. Combine interferon with HAART for best outcome
2. Patients with CD4 counts ≥200/mm^3 have better response
3. Higher doses may be associated with better efficacy, but because of the complexity of interactions regarding status of underlying HIV disease and response potential, not all patients require high doses

Toxicity

Low-dose group: 35 patients treated with interferon-alfa-2b 1 million UNITS once daily with didanosine* 125–200 mg orally every 12 hours
Intermediate-dose group: 33 patients treated with interferon alfa-2b 10 million UNITS once daily with didanosine* 125–200 mg orally every 12 hours

*125 mg if weight <60 kg; 200 mg if weight ≥60 kg. By amendment, other antiretroviral therapies were subsequently substituted for or added to didanosine

	Low-Dose Group	Intermediate-Dose Group
	% G3/4	% G3/4
Neutropenia	3	21
Hyperamylasemia	9	18
Anemia	<10	<10
Thrombocytopenia	<10	<10
Elevated LFT	<10	<10
Hypertriglyceridemia	<10	<10

Notes:

- Grade 2/3 chills, fatigue, and fever occurred significantly more often in the intermediate-dose than in the low-dose group
- Additional adverse events included cough, dyspnea, headache, anorexia, myalgias, and rash

Krown SE et al. J Interferon Cytokine Res 2002;22:295–303

Therapy Monitoring

1. *Every 2 weeks initially, then once per month:* CBC with differential and serum electrolytes, BUN, creatinine, LFTs, and mineral panel
2. *Response evaluation:* Patients are evaluated for response every 4–8 weeks

REGIMEN

DAUNORUBICIN CITRATE LIPOSOME INJECTION (LIPOSOMAL DAUNORUBICIN)

Gill PS et al. JCO 1996;14:2353–2364

Important: Administer HAART to all patients

Daunorubicin citrate liposome injection 40 mg/m^2 intravenously in a volume of 5% dextrose injection (D5W) equivalent to the volume of liposomal daunorubicin over 60 minutes as a single dose every 2 weeks (total dosage/cycle = 40 mg/m^2)

Ancillary medications: Secondary prophylaxis for neutropenia at discretion of health care provider
Filgrastim 5 mcg/kg per day subcutaneously, starting 24 hours after chemotherapy is completed. Continue until ANC post-nadir is ≥10,000/mm^3. Resume filgrastim if ANC decreases to <1500/mm^3 before subsequent cycle. Many patients do not require daily filgrastim, and often only a few injections during the cycle are needed

Emetogenic potential: Low (Emetogenicity score = 2). [Antiemetics generally are not required unless patient has a history of nausea or vomiting to DaunoXome®. See Chapter 39]

Patient Population Studied

Advanced AIDS-KS pre-HAART. A prospective randomized phase III trial of 232 patients randomly assigned to receive liposomal daunorubicin 40 mg/m^2 or a combination chemotherapy regimen of doxorubicin 10 mg/m^2, bleomycin 15 units, and vincristine 1 mg (ABV). Both regimens were administered every 2 weeks

Efficacy (N = 116)

Complete response	2.6%
Partial response	22.4%
Median response duration	175 days
Median survival	369 days

Toxicity (N = 116)

	% G1/2	% G3/4
Hematologic[a]		
Neutropenia	12/55	36/15
Leukopenia	12/79	33/5
Thrombocytopenia	93/12	0/1
Anemia	62/55	9/2
Nonhematologic		
Fatigue	43	6
Fever	42	5
Diarrhea	34	4
Nausea	51	3
Vomiting	20	3
Abdominal pain	20	3
Dyspnea	23	3
Headache	22	3
Anorexia	21	2
Cough	26	2
Neuropathy	12	1
Alopecia	8	
Back pain/flushing/chest tightness	14%	
Reduced ejection fraction[b]	0	

[a]Some patients experienced toxicity on ≥1 cycle
[b]Occurred within 5 minutes of infusion; subsided if discontinued; did not recur if resumed at slower rate

Treatment Modifications

Treatment proceeds as planned if pretreatment ANC is ≥750/mm^3 and platelet count ≥75,000/mm3

Adverse Event	Dose Modification
ANC ≤750/mm^3	Delay liposomal daunorubicin until ANC > 750/mm^3. Consider adding filgrastim or neulasta during subsequent cycles
Cardiac toxicity (≥20% reduction in ejection fraction)	Discontinue therapy
Pulmonary toxicity	Discontinue therapy
Liver dysfunction*	Dosage modifications indicated, but not specified

*DaunoXome® (daunorubicin citrate liposome injection) labeling indicates dose modifications for increased bilirubin, but some protease inhibitors (eg, indinavir, atazanavir) cause mild hyperbilirubinemia); dose adjustment may not be required in this setting

Therapy Monitoring

1. *Before therapy:* CBC with differential, LFTs, BUN, serum creatinine, and ejection fraction
2. *Before each cycle:* CBC with differential LFTs. BUN and serum creatinine
3. *Cumulative daunorubicin or doxorubicin dosage ≥500 mg/m^2:* Ejection fraction

Notes

1. Trial conducted in the pre-HAART era. 95% received antiretroviral drugs as monotherapy or 2 drugs concurrent with liposomal daunorubicin
2. Chronic therapy may be required; patients responding to HAART may have long-term progression-free survival and require fewer (eg, 4–6) cycles of chemotherapy

REGIMEN

DOXORUBICIN HCL LIPOSOME INJECTION (LIPOSOMAL DOXORUBICIN)

Northfelt DW et al. JCO 1998;16:2445–2451

Important: Administer HAART to all patients

Doxorubicin HCl liposome injection 20 mg/m^2 intravenously by peripheral venous access into a freely running infusion of 5% dextrose injection (D5W) over 30 minutes as a single dose every 2–3 weeks (total dosage/cycle = 20 mg/m^2)

Premedication: Generally not required
Ancillary medications: Secondary prophylaxis for neutropenia at discretion of health care provider: **Filgrastim** 5 mcg/kg per day subcutaneously starting 24 hours after chemotherapy is completed. Continue until ANC post-nadir is ≥10,000/mm^3. Resume filgrastim use if ANC decreases to ≤1500/mm^3 before the subsequent cycle. Many patients do not require daily filgrastim, and often only a few injections during the cycle are needed

Emetogenic potential: Low (Emetogenicity score = 2). Antiemetics generally are not required. See Chapter 39

Patient Population Studied

A trial of 258 patients pre-HAART with advanced AIDS-KS randomly assigned to either pegylated-liposomal doxorubicin 20 mg/m^2 or a doxorubicin, bleomycin, and vincristine (ABV) regimen. Both regimens were administered every 14 days for 6 cycles

Efficacy (N = 133)

Complete response	0.8%
Partial response	45.1%
• Flattening of lesions	37%
• Decreased sum of products of largest perpendicular diameters	6%
• Reduced number and flattening of lesions	1%
• Reduced size and flattening of lesions	1%
Median response duration	90 days
Median survival	160 days

Modified AIDS Clinical Trials Group

Toxicity (N = 133)[a]

	% G3/4
At least one G3/4 toxicity	92
Hematologic	
Leukopenia[b]	36%
ANC ≤ 500/mm^3	6%
Febrile with ANC ≤ 500/mm^3	0%
Anemia	9.8%
Thrombocytopenia	3%
Septic episodes	6%
Nonhematologic	
Nausea or vomiting	15%
Mucositis/stomatitis	5%
Peripheral neuropathy	6%
Alopecia	1%
Palmar-plantar erythrodysesthesia	4%
Infusion-related reactions[c]	4.5
Cardiac ejection fraction decreased ≥ 20% from baseline (n = 47)[d]	2 patients

[a]Percent of patients experiencing G3/4 toxicity
[b]44% received G-CSF or GM-CSF
[c]Flushing, chest pain, dyspnea, difficulty swallowing, hypotension, back pain
[d]One death due to cardiomyopathy

WHO Criteria

Treatment Modifications

Adverse Event	Dose Modification
G3 Toxicity other than granulocytopenia	Delay treatment for up to 14 days
ANC ≤750/mm^3 on cycle day 1	Delay treatment until ANC recovers. Consider adding filgrastim
Palmar-plantar erythrodysesthesia	Delay treatment. May require dosage reductions

Although Doxil® (doxorubicin HCl liposome injection; Alza Corporation) product labeling indicates dose modifications for increased bilirubin, some protease inhibitors (eg, indinavir, atazanavir) cause a mild hyperbilirubinemia, in which cases dose adjustment may not be necessary

Therapy Monitoring

1. *Before therapy:* CBC with differential, LFTs, BUN and serum creatinine, and ejection fraction
2. *Before each cycle:* CBC with differential, LFTs, BUN, serum creatinine, and response assessment
3. *Cumulative daunorubicin or doxorubicin dosage dose ≥500 mg/m^2:* Ejection fraction

Notes

1. Trial conducted in the pre-HAART era
2. Chronic therapy may be required

REGIMEN

PACLITAXEL (TAXOL®)

Saville MW et al. Lancet 1995;346:26–28
Gill PS et al. JCO 1999;17:1876–1883

Important: Administer HAART to all patients

Premedication: Primary prophylaxis against hypersensitivity reactions from paclitaxel:
Dexamethasone 10 mg/dose for 2 doses orally 14 and 7 hours before paclitaxel, plus:
Diphenhydramine 50 mg for 1 dose by intravenous push 30 minutes before paclitaxel, *and:*
Ranitidine 50 mg or **cimetidine** 300 mg for 1 dose by intravenous infusion in 25–100 mL 0.9% NACl injection (0.9% NS) or 5% dextrose injection (D5W) over 5–30 minutes, 30 minutes before paclitaxel

Paclitaxel 135 mg/m^2 intravenously in an amount of 0.9% NS or D5W sufficient to produce a concentration of 0.3–1.2 mg/mL over 3 hours every 21 days (total dosage/cycle = 135 mg/m^2)

or

Premedication: Primary prophylaxis against hypersensitivity reactions from paclitaxel:
Dexamethasone 20 mg for 1 dose intravenously prior to paclitaxel (reduce to 8 mg if no hypersensitivity reactions occur during cycle 1), *plus:*
Diphenhydramine 50 mg for 1 dose by intravenous push 30 minutes before paclitaxel, *and:*
Ranitidine 50 mg for 1 dose or **cimetidine** 300 mg for 1 dose by intravenous infusion in 25–100 mL 0.9% NS or D5W over 5–30 minutes, 30 minutes before paclitaxel

Paclitaxel 100 mg/m^2 intravenously in an amount of 0.9% NS or D5W sufficient to produce a concentration of 0.3–1.2 mg/mL over 3 hours every 14 days (total dosage/cycle = 100 mg/m^2)

Ancillary medications: Secondary prophylaxis for neutropenia at discretion of health care provider:
Filgrastim 5 mcg/kg per day subcutaneously starting 24 hours after chemotherapy is completed. Continue until ANC post-nadir is ≥10,000/mm^3. Resume filgrastim if ANC decreases to <1500/mm^3 before start of subsequent cycle. Many patients do not require daily filgrastim, and often only a few injections during the cycle are needed

Emetogenic potential: Low (Emetogenicity score = 2). See Chapter 39

Treatment Modifications

Adverse Event	Dose Modification
Intracycle ANC consistently >1000/mm^3	Increase paclitaxel dosage by 20 mg/m^2 to a maximum of 175 mg/m^2 per cycle
G4 Hematologic toxicity	Decrease paclitaxel dosage by 25%

Saville MW et al. Lancet 1995;346:26–28

Adverse Event	Dose Modification
Cycle, day 1 ANC <1000/mm^3, or platelet count <50,000/mm^3	Delay treatment until ANC >1000/mm^3, or platelet count >50,000/mm^3
ANC < 500/mm^3 for 7 days	Reduce paclitaxel dosage by 20%
G1/2 Peripheral neuropathy*	Reduce paclitaxel dosage by 20%
G3/4 Peripheral neuropathy*	Discontinue therapy
Total bilirubin >3.0 mg/dL (51.3 μmol/L)	Delay treatment until bilirubin <3.0 mg/dL (51.3 μmol/L), then reduce dosage by 20%
Liver transaminases >5 × the upper limit of normal range	Delay treatment until liver transaminases <3 × upper limit of normal, then reduce dosage by 20%

*Increased neuropathy reported when using stavudine

Gill PS et al. JCO 1999;17:1876–1883

Patient Population Studied

Data from phase II trials with advanced KS in highly immunosuppressed patients treated pre-HAART

Efficacy

Objective responses (Saville et al)	71%
Objective responses (Gill et al)	59%
Median response duration (Saville et al)	2.5 months
Median duration of response (Gill et al)	10.4 months

Toxicity

	G1/2	G3/4
Neutropenia[a]	—	61%
Diarrhea	—	12%
Fever	—	11%
Nausea	—	6%
Peripheral neuropathy	45%	4%
Rash	—	2%

Alopecia: Common; complete in 10%

[a]Growth factors not used routinely
Saville MW et al. Lancet 1995;346:26–28 (N = 20) (NCI CTC)

	% G1/2[a]	% G3	%G4
Hematologic			
Neutropenia[b]	33	25	36
Anemia	45	22	5
Thrombocytopenia	25	4	2
Nonhematologic			
Alopecia	78	9	—
Fatigue	50	23	2
Rash ± pruritus	9	0	—
Myalgia	21	16	—
Nausea/vomiting	57	13	0
Diarrhea	57	14	2
Neuropathy	45	2	0
Mucositis	18	2	0
Elevated AST	35	5	0

[a]Includes patients with unknown grades
[b]Although 50% of patients on G-CSF on entry
Welles L et al. JCO 1998;16:1112–1121
Gill PS et al. JCO 1999;17:1876–1883 (N = 56) (Southwest Oncology Group Toxicity Criteria)

Therapy Monitoring

Before each cycle: CBC with differential, LFTs, BUN, serum creatinine, and physical examination with careful attention to peripheral nerves

Notes

1. Chronic therapy may be required
2. Active in patients who did not benefit from other therapies

HIV-Related Lymphoma (ARL)

Epidemiology

Incidence

- 43 cases/10,000 person-years in HIV-positive individuals
- Approximately 3% of HIV-infected patients develop ARL as the AIDS-defining diagnosis
- 10–15% of patients with AIDS develop ARL
- Since the advent of HAART, ARL has decreased by 50% owing to CD4 cell preservation; however, incidence within CD4 strata has not been changed by HAART

Stage at presentation

- Over 60% have advanced stage III–IV disease with B-cell symptoms
- Extranodal involvement common
- Among HIV-infected patients with non-Hodgkin lymphoma (NHL), 80% of NHL are aggressive; by comparison, 30% of non–HIV-associated lymphomas are aggressive

Besson C et al. Blood 2001;98:2339–2344

Pathology

Distribution of histologic subtypes tracks with CD4 cells and has been influenced by HAART-induced immune preservation. Specifically, since HAART, fewer immunoblastic subtypes are seen

1 Diffuse large B-cell lymphoma (DLBCL): 70%
   - Centroblastic: 20–30% associated with Epstein-Barr virus (EBV)
   - Immunoblastic: 80% associated with EBV
   - Primary central nervous system lymphoma: 100% associated with EBV

2 Burkitt's lymphoma: 20%
   - 0–50% associated with EBV

3 Other (eg, primary effusion lymphoma [PEL], plasmablastic lymphoma of the oral cavity [PBOC]): 10%
   - 70% associated with EBV

Jaffe ES, Harris NL, Stein H, Vardiman JW. World Health Organization Classification of Tumors: Pathology & Genetics: Tumors of Haematopoietic and Lymphoid Tissues. Lyon: IARC Press, 2001:351

Work-Up

1 Assessment of hematologic and biochemical parameters
2 CT scans of chest, abdomen, and pelvis
3 Bone marrow biopsy
4 CNS assessment with head MRI and lumbar puncture
5 CD4 cell count
6 FDG-PET scans optional but useful

If primary brain lymphoma suspected:

1. Must rule out peripheral disease
2. Slit-lamp exam of optic nerve
3. Minimally invasive diagnosis combining FDG-PET (or SPECT) with assessment of EBV presence in the CSF by polymerase chain reaction can be used in some cases rather than biopsy
   - If both tests are positive: 100% positive predictive value for primary brain lymphoma
   - If both tests are negative: 100% negative predictive value for brain lymphoma
   - If these tests are discordant: Biopsy is required to establish diagnosis

Antinori A et al. JCO 1999;17:554–560
Levine AM. Semin Oncol 1990;17:104–112

Staging

Ann Arbor Staging System for Lymphomas

Stage	Description
I	Single lymph node region
IE	Single extralymphatic organ or site
II	Two or more lymph node regions on the same side of the diaphragm
IIE	Single extranodal site + adjacent nodes
III	Nodal regions on both sides of the diaphragm (III)
IIIE	Nodal regions on both sides of the diaphragm + single extranodal site
IIIS	Nodal regions on both sides of the diaphragm + involvement of spleen
IIISE	Nodal regions on both sides of the diaphragm + single extranodal site + involvement of spleen
IV	Diffuse or disseminated involvement of one or more extralymphatic organs Bone marrow involvement Liver involvement Brain involvement

Absence of associated symptoms is designated A
Presence of symptoms is designated B. B symptoms include unexplained fevers, unexplained >10% weight loss, sweats

Survival

Overall survival is generally poor in most reports, but has improved since the advent of HAART:

1 *Diffuse large B-cell lymphoma (DLCBL):*
   - Pre-HAART 4–18 months
   - Since HAART–21 months
   - Recent phase II trial of DA-EPOCH demonstrated survival equivalent to non-AIDS, bcl-2 negative DLBCL

2 *PEL:* Median survival around 4–6 months with therapy

3 *PBOC:* Initial reports suggested poor survival due to low CR, but clinical heterogeneity of these cases is becoming more evident, and some may have favorable outcome

4 CD4 cell count is the primary prognostic determinant

Besson C et al. Blood 2001;98:2339–2344

REGIMEN

ETOPOSIDE + PREDNISONE + VINCRISTINE + CYCLOPHOSPHAMIDE + DOXORUBICIN (DOSE-ADJUSTED EPOCH: DA-EPOCH)

Little RF et al. Blood 2003;101:4653–4659

Important Note: HAART is suspended until all cycles are completed, then optimized on/after day 6 of final cycle. Some recommend continuing HAART for patients already on a stable regimen

Etoposide 50 mg/m^2 per day for 4 days by continuous intravenous infusion over 24 hours* on days 1–4 every 21 days for a maximum of 6 cycles (total dosage/cycle = 200 mg/m^2)

Doxorubicin 10 mg/m^2 per day for 4 days by continuous intravenous infusion over 24 hours* on days 1–4 every 21 days for a maximum of 6 cycles (total dosage/cycle = 40 mg/m^2)

Vincristine 0.4 mg/m^2 per day for 4 days by continuous intravenous infusion over 24 hours* on days 1–4 every 21 days for a maximum of 6 cycles (total dosage/cycle = 1.6 mg/m^2)
**Note:* See Special Instructions below for preparing a 3-in-1 admixture with etoposide, doxorubicin, and vincristine

Prednisone 60 mg/m^2 per day orally on days 1–5 every 21 days for a maximum of 6 cycles (total dosage/cycle = 300 mg/m^2)
Prednisone is marketed in the United States in numerous generic formulations for oral administration, including immediate-release tablets containing 1, 2.5, 5, 10, 20, or 50 mg and solutions and syrups for oral administration

Cyclophosphamide single dose on day 5 intravenously in 100 mL of 0.9% NaCl injection (0.9% NS) or 5% dextrose injection (D5W) over 30 minutes every 21 days for a maximum of 6 cycles (total dosage/cycle = 187–375 mg/m^2)
Note: Baseline CD4+ lymphocyte count determines cycle 1 cyclophosphamide dose

Baseline CD4+ Count	Cyclophosphamide Dosage
<100/mm^3	187 mg/m^2
≥100/mm^3	375 mg/m^2

Note: After cycle 1, cyclophosphamide dosage is increased or decreased in increments of 187 mg/m^2 (to a maximum 750 mg/m^2) to achieve an ANC nadir of ≅ 500/mm^3

Ancillary medications:
Filgrastim 5 mcg/kg per day continuously from cycle day 6 until ANC is >5000/mm^3 or until cycle day 20—whichever occurs first

Antimicrobial prophylaxis
Anti–*Pneumocystis carinii* prophylaxis: **Cotrimoxazole** (trimethoprim 160 mg + sulfamethoxazole 800 mg) orally twice daily for 3 days per week continuously throughout treatment (eg, Monday, Wednesday, and Friday)
Mycobacterium avium-intracellulare complex prophylaxis for patients with CD4+ counts <100/mm^3: **Azithromycin** 1200 mg orally once weekly

Emetogenic potential:
Days 1–4: Low (Emetogenicity score ≤2)
Day 5: Moderate (Emetogenicity score ≤3). See Chapter 39

CNS prophylaxis:
Methotrexate 12 mg per dose intrathecally in a volume of **preservative-free** 0.9% NaCl injection (PF 0.9% NS) equivalent to the amount of CSF removed (eg, 5–12 mL) via intraventricular catheter or reservoir (eg, Ommaya) on days 1 and 5 every 21 days during cycles 3, 4, 5, and 6 (total dose/cycle = 24 mg)

(*continued*)

Treatment Modifications

Adverse Event	Dose Modification
ANC nadir during previous cycle ≥500/mm^3	Increase cyclophosphamide dosage by 187 mg/m^2 to a maximum of 750 mg/m^2 per cycle
ANC nadir during previous cycle <500/mm^3	Reduce cyclophosphamide dosage by 187 mg/m^2
Platelet count nadir during previous cycle <25,000/mm^3	Reduce cyclophosphamide dosage by 187 mg/m^2

Patient Population Studied

Phase II trial of 39 patients with previously untreated ARL. Median CD4 cells/mm^3: 198 (range 3–1182). Median potential follow-up of 53 months

Efficacy

Complete response	74%
Partial response	13%
Complete response [CD4+ cells >100/mm^3]	87%
Complete response [CD4+ cells ≤100/mm^3]	56%
At 53 Months' Potential Follow-up	
Disease-free survival of patients achieving a CR	92%
Overall survival	60%
Overall survival [CD4+ cells >100/mm^3]	87%
Overall survival [CD4+ cells ≤100/mm^3]	16%

(*continued*)

CNS treatment (confirmed CNS disease):*
Methotrexate 6 mg per dose, *plus*
Cytarabine 30 mg per dose, *plus*
Hydrocortisone 15 mg per dose

Induction: All three drugs are given together twice weekly for at least 4 consecutive weeks, or for 2 weeks after CSF specimens show no evidence of lymphoma. Administer intrathecally in a volume of PF 0.9% NS equivalent to the amount of CSF removed (eg, 5–12 mL) via intraventricular catheter or reservoir (eg, Ommaya). Total doses/week: **Methotrexate** = 12 mg; **Cytarabine** = 60 mg; **Hydrocortisone** = 30 mg

Consolidation: All three drugs are given together once weekly for 6 weeks. Administer intrathecally in a volume of PF 0.9% NS equivalent to the amount of CSF removed (eg, 5–12 mL) via intraventricular catheter or reservoir (eg, Ommaya). Total doses/week: **Methotrexate** = 6 mg; **Cytarabine** = 30 mg; **Hydrocortisone** = 15 mg

Maintenance: All three drugs are given together, once monthly for 6 months. Administer intrathecally in a volume of PF 0.9% NS equivalent to the amount of CSF removed (eg, 5–12 mL). Total doses/month: **Methotrexate** = 6 mg; **Cytarabine** = 30 mg; **Hydrocortisone** = 15 mg

**Note:* Monotherapy with methotrexate or cytarabine may be feasible in patients with sensitive disease

Toxicity (N = 209 Cycles/39 Patients)

	% of Cycles
Hematologic	
G4 neutropenia (ANC <500/mm^3)	30*
Febrile neutropenia	13
G3/4 anemia	17
G3/4 thrombocytopenia	21
Nonhematologic	
G3/4 constipation	3
G3/4 stomatitis	3
G3 neuropathy	2 patients

*Despite filgrastim 5 mcg/kg per day
ECOG Criteria

Therapy Monitoring

1. *Day 1 each cycle:* CBC with differential count, LFTs, BUN, and serum creatinine
2. *Twice-weekly during chemotherapy*: CBC with differential
3. *Cycle 4 and at end of cycle 6:* CD4+ cell count (modify opportunistic infection prophylaxis therapy in response to findings)
4. *After cycles 4 and 6:* Tumor restaging
5. *End of cycle 6:* Viral load
6. *Every 3 months thereafter:* CD4+ cell count and viral load as baseline to starting/resuming HAART

Special Instructions

General instructions:
To prepare a 3-in-1 admixture with etoposide + doxorubicin + vincristine, dilute all three drug products in 0.9% NaCl injection (0.9% NS) as follows:

Total Dose of Etoposide	Volume of 0.9% NS
≤62 mg	250 mL
62.1–125 mg	500 mL
>125mg	1000 mL

Etoposide (base) + doxorubicin + vincristine 3-in-1 admixtures:
Etoposide 50 mg/m^2, doxorubicin hydrochloride 10 mg/m^2, and vincristine sulfate 0.4 mg/m^2 admixtures diluted in 0.9% NS to produce a final etoposide concentration <250 mcg/mL, in polyolefin-lined infusion bags are stable and compatible for 72 hours at 23°–25°C, and at 31°–33° C when protected from exposure to light

Wolfe JL et al. Am J Health Syst Pharm 1999;56:985–989

Etoposide (PHOSphate) + doxorubicin + vincristine 3-in-1 admixtures:
Etoposide PHOSphate, doxorubicin hydrochloride, and vincristine sulfate admixtures diluted in 0.9% NS, to produce a final etoposide concentration <250 mcg/mL in polyolefin-lined infusion bags are stable and compatible for up to 124 hours at 2°–6°C and 35°–40°C in the dark and in regular fluorescent light. In admixtures stored at 35°–40°C and exposed to light, the initial drug concentrations decreased slightly, but remain within acceptable concentrations

Yuan P et al. Am J Health Syst Pharm 2001;58:594–598

A 3-in-1 admixture does not prevent microbial growth after exposure to bacterial and fungal contamination. With respect to product sterility, expiration dating should be determined by the aseptic techniques used in preparation and local and national guidelines

REGIMEN

CYCLOPHOSPHAMIDE + DOXORUBICIN (HYDROXYLDAUNORUBICIN) + VINCRISTINE (ONCOVIN®) + PREDNISONE (CHOP)

Kaplan L. Proceedings of the 7th International Conference on Malignancies in AIDS and Other Immunodeficiencies [online]; 2003 Apr 28-29 [cited 2004 Feb 25]; Bethesda, Maryland, Abstract S17. Available from: URL: http://cancer.gov/dctd/aids/2003icmaoi_abs.pdf

Important: Recommendations below are for CHOP chemotherapy without rituximab. CHOP-rituximab cannot be recommended as standard of care in ARL. See NOTES below
Important: Administer HAART to all patients

Cyclophosphamide 750 mg/m² single dose intravenously in 100 mL of 0.9% NaCl injection (0.9% NS) or 5% dextrose injection (D5W) over 30 minutes, given on day 1 every 21 days (total dosage/cycle = 750 mg/m²)
Doxorubicin 50 mg/m² single dose intravenously per push over 3–5 minutes, given on day 1 every 21 days (total dosage/cycle = 50 mg/m²)
Vincristine 1.2 mg/m² single dose intravenously per push over 1 minute on day 1 every 21 days (total dosage/cycle = 1.2 mg/m²)
Prednisone 100 mg/day for 5 days orally on days 1–5 every 21 days (total dose/cycle = 500 mg)
Prednisone is marketed in the United States in numerous generic formulations for oral administration, including immediate-release tablets containing 1, 2.5, 5, 10, 20, and 50 mg, and in solutions and syrups for oral administration

Ancillary medications: Primary prophylaxis for neutropenia beginning with cycle 1:
Filgrastim 5 mcg/kg per day subcutaneously starting 24 hours after chemotherapy is completed. Continue until absolute neutrophil count post-nadir is ≥10,000/mm³. Resume filgrastim if ANC decreases to <1500/mm³ before the start of the subsequent cycle. Alternatively, some oncologists recommend **pegfilgrastim**

Prophylaxis with antifungal, antibacterial, and antiviral agents as appropriate:
Fluconazole 100 mg orally once daily
Cotrimoxazole (trimethoprim 160 mg + sulfamethoxazole 800 mg) orally once daily
Rifabutin 300 mg orally once daily

Fluconazole is available in the United States in various formulations for oral administration, including immediate-release tablets containing 50 mg, 100 mg, 150 mg, and 200 mg, and in powdered fluconazole for preparing liquid suspensions
Cotrimoxazole (trimethoprim + sulfamethoxazole in 1-mg:5-mg ratio) is generically available in the United States in a variety of formulations and product strengths, including immediate-release tablets containing 80 mg trimethoprim + 400 mg sulfamethoxazole or 160 mg trimethoprim + 800 mg sulfamethoxazole, and as a powder for preparing an oral suspension containing 40 mg trimethoprim/5 mL + 200 mg sulfamethoxazole/5 mL
Rifabutin is available in the United States as 150-mg capsules for oral administration

Emetogenic potential: High (Emetogenicity score = 5). See Chapter 39

Patient Population Studied

A study of 95 patients on the CHOP-rituximab arm and 47 patients on the CHOP arm in a 2:1 randomization. Median CD4+ lymphocyte count was 133 cells/mm³; 79% of patients had stages III/IV disease

Efficacy (N = 47)

47 Patients Treated with CHOP

Complete response	50%
Median time to response	9 weeks

Treatment Modifications

Adverse Event	Dose Modification
ANC < 1000/mm³	Administer filgrastim in subsequent cycles
Platelet count < 75,000/mm³	Reduce vincristine dose 25%
Other nonhematologic G3/4 toxicity	Reduce dose of all agents by 25%

Toxicity (N = 47)

	% Patients
G3/4 neutropenia	17
Fever and ANC <100/mm³	8.5
Death due to infection	2

NCI CTC

Therapy Monitoring

1. *Day 1 of each cycle:* CBC with differential count
2. *Twice-weekly during chemotherapy:* CBC with differential
3. *Every 2 cycles:* Tumor restaging

Notes

	CHOP-R	CHOP	P Value
Complete response	58%	50%	0.371
G3/4 neutropenia	39%	17%	
Infection + neutropenia	10.5%	0	
Death due to infection	15%	2%	

At the present time, CHOP-Rituximab cannot be recommended as standard of care in ARL

REGIMEN

INFUSIONAL CYCLOPHOSPHAMIDE + DOXORUBICIN + ETOPOSIDE WITH RITUXIMAB (R-ICDE)

Sparano JA et al. JCO 1996;14:3026–3035
Tirelli U et al. Recent results. Cancer Res 2002;159:149–153

Important notes:
(1) Although the regimen reported is for iCDE + rituximab, at present rituximab cannot be recommended as standard of care in ARL
(2) HAART is administered to all patients
(3) Treat for 2 cycles > CR, or a maximum of 6 cycles

Rituximab premedication (See "Important notes" above):
(1) **Acetaminophen** 650 mg orally 30 minutes before rituximab
(2) **Diphenhydramine** 50 mg by intravenous push 30 minutes before rituximab
Rituximab 375 mg/m^2 intravenously in 0.9% NaCl injection (0.9% NS) or 5% dextrose injection (D5W) diluted to a concentration of 1–4 mg/mL on day 1 every 28 days for 5–6 cycles (total dosage/cycle = 375 mg/m^2)
Infusion rates:
- Initially, 50 mg/hour. If hypersensitivity or infusion reactions do not occur during the first 30 minutes, increase the rate by 50 mg/hour every 30 minutes to a maximum rate of 400 mg/hour
- Subsequently, if previous administration was well tolerated, start at 100 mg/hour and increase by 100 mg/hour every 30 minutes to a maximum rate of 400 mg/hour

Cyclophosphamide 200 mg/m^2 per day for 4 consecutive days by continuous intravenous infusion over 24 hours (see Admixture Note below) on days 2–5 every 28 days for 5–6 cycles (total dosage/cycle = 800 mg/m^2)

Doxorubicin 12.5 mg/m^2 per day for 4 consecutive days by continuous intravenous infusion over 24 hours (see Admixture Note below) days 2–5 every 28 days for 5–6 cycles (total dosage/cycle = 50 mg/m^2)
Admixture note: A 24-hour supply of cyclophosphamide + doxorubicin may be combined as a single admixture in 1000 mL 0.9% NS or D5W for 4 consecutive days. Administered via a central vascular access device (VAD)

Etoposide 60 mg/m^2 per day for 4 consecutive days by continuous intravenous infusion in 1000 mL 0.9% NS or D5W over 24 hours on days 2–5 every 28 days for 5–6 cycles (total dosage/cycle = 240 mg/m^2)
Note: Etoposide is administered via a VAD lumen different from the one used to administer doxorubicin + cyclophosphamide, or via peripheral venous access

Filgrastim 5 mcg/kg per day subcutaneously starting 24 hours after infusional chemotherapy is completed (day 7). Continue until ANC post-nadir is ≥10,000/mm^3. Resume filgrastim if ANC decreases to <1500/mm^3 before start of subsequent cycle

CNS prophylaxis [in patients with small non–cleaved-cell lymphoma or lymphomatous bone marrow involvement]:
Cytarabine 45 mg/m^2 single dose intrathecally in a volume of **preservative-free** 0.9% NaCl injection (PF 0.9% NS), equivalent to the amount of CSF removed (eg, 5–12 mL), on day 1 during cycles 1 and 2 (total dose/cycle = 45 mg/m^2)
Methotrexate 12 mg per dose intrathecally in a volume of PF 0.9% NS equivalent to the amount of CSF removed (eg, 5–12 mL) on days 3 and 5 during cycles 1 and 2 (total dose/cycle = 24 mg/m^2)
Leucovorin 15 mg every 6 hours for 6 doses orally or intravenously in 10–50 mL of 0.9% NS or D5W over 10–30 minutes, starting 12 hours after each methotrexate injection
Leucovorin calcium is available generically in the United States in various formulations for oral administration, including immediate-release tablets containing 5 mg, 10 mg, 15 mg, and 25 mg leucovorin calcium

(continued)

Treatment Modifications

R-iCDE is repeated every 28 days if ANC is ≥1500/mm^3 and platelet count ≥50,000/mm^3

Adverse Event	Dose Modification
First episode of febrile neutropenia, or platelet nadir <25,000/mm^3	Reduce doxorubicin, cyclophosphamide, and etoposide dosages by 25%
Second and subsequent episodes of febrile neutropenia, or platelet nadir <25,000/mm^3	Reduce doxorubicin, cyclophosphamide, and etoposide dosages by 10%
Total serum bilirubin 1.6–2.9 mg/dL (27.4–49.6 μmol/L)	Reduce doxorubicin dosage by 50%
Total serum bilirubin 3.0–4.9 mg/dL (51.3–83.4 μmol/L)	Reduce doxorubicin dosage by 75%
Total serum bilirubin ≥5 mg/dL (85.5 μmol/L)	Hold doxorubicin
Creatinine clearance* <60 mL/min	Decrease etoposide dosage in proportion to the percentage decrement in creatinine clearance from 60 mL/min

*Creatinine clearance is used as a measure of the glomerular filtration rate

Patient Population Studied

Phase II trial with 29 patients. Median CD4+ lymphocyte count 132/mm^3; median follow-up of 9 months

Efficacy (N = 28)

Complete response	86%
Partial response	4%
Actuarial survival at 2 years	80%

Tirelli U et al. Recent results. Cancer Res 2002;159: 149–153
Modified Eastern Cooperative Group (ECOG) Response Criteria

(continued)

Treatment of lymphomatous meningitis:
Cytarabine 45 mg/m^2 single dose intrathecally in a volume of PF 0.9% NS equivalent to the amount of CSF removed (eg, 5–12 mL), *alternating three times weekly with:*
Methotrexate 12 mg per dose intrathecally in a volume of PF 0.9% NS equivalent to the amount of CSF removed (eg, 5–12 mL)
***Leucovorin** 15 mg every 6 hours for 6 doses orally or intravenously in 10–50 mL of 0.9% NS or D5W over 10–30 minutes, starting 12 hours after each methotrexate injection
Leucovorin calcium is available generically in the United States in various formulations for oral administration, including immediate-release tablets containing 5 mg, 10 mg, 15 mg, and 25 mg leucovorin calcium
Note: After two consecutive CSF specimens are obtained without evidence of lymphoma, chemotherapy administration is decreased to twice weekly for 2 weeks, then once weekly for 4 weeks, then once monthly for 6 months
Whole-brain irradiation 2 Gy/fraction, 5 fractions per week for 12 total fractions (total dose = 24 Gy)
Prophylaxis with antifungal, antibacterial, and antiviral agents:
Fluconazole 100 mg orally once daily
Clotrimazole (trimethoprim 160 mg + sulfamethoxazole 800 mg) orally once daily
Rifabutin 300 mg orally once daily

Fluconazole is available in the United States in various formulations for oral administration, including immediate-release tablets containing 50 mg, 100 mg, 150 mg, and 200 mg and as powdered fluconazole for preparing liquid suspensions
Clotrimazole (trimethoprim + sulfamethoxazole in 1-mg:5-mg ratio) is generically available in the United States in a variety of formulations and product strengths, including immediate-release tablets containing 80 mg trimethoprim + 400 mg sulfamethoxazole or 160 mg trimethoprim + 800 mg sulfamethoxazole, and as a powder for preparing an oral suspension containing 40 mg trimethoprim/5 mL + 200 mg sulfamethoxazole/5 mL
Rifabutin is available in the United States as capsules for oral administration containing 150 mg rifabutin
Emetogenic potential:
Day 1: Nonemetogenic (Emetogenicity score 1)
Days 2–5: Moderate (Emetogenicity score ≤4). See Chapter 39 for antiemetic regimens

Toxicity (N = 29)

	% G3/4
Hematologic	
Neutropenia	79
Anemia	45
Thrombocytopenia	34
Nonhematologic	
Bacterial infection	34
Opportunistic infection	7
Mucositis	17

Treatment dose reductions were required in 22% of patients

3 deaths from lymphoma at 9 months' median follow-up

Tirelli U et al. Recent results. Cancer Res 2002;159: 149–153

Therapy Monitoring

1. *Day 1 each cycle:* CBC with differential count, LFTs, BUN, and serum creatinine
2. *Twice-weekly during chemotherapy:* CBC with differential
3. *Every 2 cycles:* Tumor restaging

18. Leukemia, Acute Lymphoblastic (ADULT)

Ivan Aksentijevich, MD, Michael M. Boyiadzis, MD, MHSc, and Judith Karp, MD

Epidemiology

Incidence: 3930; adults 1300 in the United States in 2006
Deaths: 1490; death rate in adults 60–80 % in 2006
Median age: Most new cases—age 2–5 years. A bimodal age-specific incidence pattern then ensues with a continuously decreasing rate through young adulthood until the age 50 when the incidence rate again rise
Male/female ratio: Slight male predominance: 1.3:1

Cao TM, Coutre SE: Wintrobe's Clinical Hematology, 11th ed, Chapter 78. Lippincott Williams & Wilkins, 2003:2077–2096
Jemal A et al. CA Cancer J Clin 2006;56:106–30

Pathology

French-American-British (FAB) Classification

	FAB L1	FAB L2	FAB L3
Morphology			
Size	Small and homogenous	Larger and pleomorphic	Medium and homogenous
N/C ratio	Higher in >75% of cells	Lower in >25% of cells	Variable
Nucleoli	Inconspicuous, 0–1	Prominent, ≥1	Multiple and prominent
Vacuolization	Not prominent	Not prominent	Sharply defined
Basophilia	Moderate	Moderate	Deep
Cytochemistry			
MPO	–	–	–
NSE	±	±	–
PAS	+	+	–
AP	+	+	–
Frequency (%)			
Adults	30%	60%	10%

N/C, nuclear-to-cytoplasmic; MPO, myeloperoxidase; NSE, nonspecific esterase; PAS, periodic acid-Schiff; AP, acid phosphatase

Immunophenotype of Adult ALL

B-Lineage-ALL

Lineage	% Frequency	TdT	HLA-DR	CD34	CD19	CD22	CD79a	CD10	cyμ	cyκ/λ	sIgH/sIgL
Precursor B-cell ALL	5–10										
Pro-B ALL	40–50	+	+	+	+	+	+	–	–	–	–
cALL	10	+	+	–	+	+	–	+	–	–	–
Pre-B ALL	1	+	+	–	+	+	–	±	+	–	–
Transitional precursor B-cell ALL	1	±	+	–	+	+	–	–	–	–	+*
Mature B-cell ALL	5	–	+	–	+	±	–	–	–	+	+

T-Lineage-ALL

Lineage	Frequency %	cyCD3	CD7	CD1a	CD2	CD5	sCD3
Pro-T ALL	5	+	+	–	–	–	–
Pre-T ALL		+	+	–	+	+	–
Cortical-T ALL	10—15	+	+	+	+	+	–
Mature-T ALL	5—10	+	+	–	+	+	+

*Usually no surface light chain (L) expression
TdT, terminal deoxynucleotidyl transferase; cy, cytoplasmic; s, surface; IgH, immunoglobulin heavy chain; IgL, immunoglobulin light chain; ALL, acute lymphoblastic leukemia; cALL, common acute lymphoblastic leukemia

Note: ALL blasts co-express myeloid markers in 15–50% of adults. Most frequently co-expressed myeloid markers are CD13 and CD33. The co-expression of myeloid markers does not have any worse prognostic significance

Frequency of Cytogenetics in Adult ALL	
t(9;22)	20–25%
t(v;11)	7%
t(1;19)	3%
t(12;21)	2–3%
Hyperdiploidy	5–10%
Random	25–30%
Normal	15–34%

v: variant

Adverse Prognostic Factors in Adult ALL

- Age >60 years
- WBC count >50,000/mm^3
- Prolonged time to complete remission (CR) (>4–6 weeks)
- Adverse cytogenetics:
  t(9;22)
  t(4;11)
  Trisomy 8
  Hypodiploidy

Work-Up

1. History and physical examination
2. CBC with differential, platelets, electrolytes, mineral panel, LDH, uric acid, PT, PTT, fibrinogen
3. Lumbar puncture at diagnosis should be performed if no mass/lesion is detected on imaging studies
4. Bone marrow biopsy/aspiration with cytogenetics, immunophenotyping, and/or cytochemistry
5. Chest x-ray and/or chest CT scan
6. HLA Typing (in patients considered potential bone marrow transplantation [BMT] candidates)
7. MUGA scan or echocardiogram

Bassan R et al Crit Rev Oncol/Hematol 2004;50:223–261

Staging

WHO Classification of ALL

Precursor B-cell ALL/lymphoma
Cytogenetic subgroups:
- t(9;22)(34q;11)
- 11q23 MLL
- t(1;19)(q23;p23) E2A/PBX1
- t(12;21)(p12;q12) ETV/CBF-alpha

Precursor T-cell ALL/lymphoma
Burkitt-cell leukemia/lymphoma

The WHO classification suggests that the distinction of L1, L2, L3 morphologies be abandoned because L1 and L2 morphologies do not predict immunophenotype, genetic aberrations, or clinical behavior

Response Criteria for ALL

Complete remission
- ANC >1500/mm^3
- Hemoglobin >10 g/dL
- Platelet >100,000/mm^3
- No circulating blast cells
- Bone marrow with >25% cellularity and <5% blast
- Extramedullary disease resolved
- Cytogenetics normal in those with previously abnormal cytogenetics
- Negative molecular studies in patients with Ph+ leukemia

Patients who do not achieve a complete response are considered to have resistant disease. Relapse after a complete response is defined as reappearance of leukemic blasts in the peripheral blood or the finding of >5% blasts in the bone marrow, not attributable to another cause

Survival

	% Overall	% Standard Risk (25% of Adults)	% Poor Risk (75% of Adults)
Complete remission rate	65–85	65–85	65–85
Long-term disease-free survival	20–30	50–60	<20
Adult cure rate	20–30	50	<20

Faderi S et al. Cancer 2003;98:1337–1354
Harris NL et al. Histopathology 2000;36:69–86
Hoelzer D et al. Crit Rev Oncol/Hematol 2000;36:49–58
Pui CH, Evans WE. NEJM 1998;339:605–615

Caveats

There is no standard of care for ALL that is as yet satisfactory. All patients with ALL should be considered for enrollment in a clinical trial
Treatment regimens for ALL have evolved empirically into complex schemes that use numerous agents in various doses, combinations, and schedules, and few of the individual components have been tested rigorously in randomized trials. The backbone of chemotherapy for ALL remains the sequence of induction, consolidation/intensification, and prolonged maintenance

Remission induction: Vincristine, a glucocorticoid, and an anthracycline are the principal agents used in current remission induction regimens. The combination of these three agents results in a CR rate of 70–90%. Most modern induction regimens have also incorporated cyclophosphamide and or L-asparaginase, although neither has been proved by controlled trials to be beneficial in adult patients when added to initial induction regimen. There is no proof that high-dose regimens that differ from vincristine + steroid + anthracycline ± cyclophosphamide ± L-asparaginase are in any way superior

There are variants of ALL that may benefit from more specific treatments:
Mature B-cell ALL: Patients with mature B-cell ALL (Burkitt cell leukemia, L3) experience improvement in survival rate when high doses of cyclophosphamide, methotrexate, and cytarabine are incorporated early in the treatment. The probability of leukemia-free survival improved from 35% with standard ALL induction to 60–70% with high doses of cyclophosphamide, methotrexate, and cytarabine
Philadelphia chromosome-positive ALL: Philadelphia chromosome-positive ALL is consider a high-risk adult ALL and carries a poor prognosis. Imatinib mesylate should be considered in the treatment of this ALL subtype

Consolidation/intensification: Eradication of minimal residual disease during hematologic remission is the primary aim of the consolidation/intensification phase. It is difficult to assess the value of individual components of the treatment because the number, schedule, and combination of cytostatic drugs vary considerably among studies. A general feature of the regimens used during this phase is the alternate use of active drugs at variable dosage for some months

Maintenance: The maintenance regimen consists of a combination of 6-mercaptorunine, methotrexate, vincristine, and corticosteroid given for 2–3 years. Extension of maintenance beyond 3 years has not shown additional benefits. No maintenance therapy is given to patients with mature B-cell ALL. These patients respond well to short-term dose-intensive regimens, and disease recurrence beyond the first year of remission is rare

Allogeneic BMT: Although the role of allogeneic BMT for treatment of patients with adult ALL in first remission is controversial, it is often recommended for those in high-risk groups. Outcome data from most uncontrolled individual trials indicate disease-free survival between 40% and 60% with matched-sibling allogeneic BMT

Patients who suffer a relapse with ALL have a poor prognosis with standard salvage therapy. Response rates to salvage chemotherapy range from 30% to 70%, but responses are generally short-lived with a median survival of 6 months. Patients in second CR should be considered for allogeneic BMT

Evaluation and treatment of CNS leukemia:

- For patients who do not have CNS involvement at the time of diagnosis, prophylactic treatment should be administered. The cumulative risk of CNS leukemia in patients who do not receive prophylactic treatment can be as high as 30% (7% during induction, 14% while in remission, and 5% simultaneously with marrow relapse). Effective prophylaxis can be achieved with the use of intrathecal chemotherapy with or without cranial radiation therapy (per specific regimen see below)
- Up to 10% of adults with ALL present with CNS involvement at the time of diagnosis. The risk is higher in patients with T-lineage ALL, mature ALL, high WBC count, elevated LDH serum, a high proportion of bone marrow cells in a proliferative state (>14% of cells in S+G2M phase of the cell cycle)
- Adult ALL patients with CNS involvement at diagnosis require CNS-directed therapy, starting with induction therapy. Administer therapy either with 15 mg methotrexate + 50 mg hydrocortisone or 100 mg cytarabine + 50 mg hydrocortisone intrathecally or via an Ommaya reservoir weekly until CNS clearance. If clearance is slow, one may treat with all three drugs combined (same doses). Once CNS involvement is negative, patients should continue treatment as specified in the regimen

Hyperleukocytosis in ALL:

- The frequency of hyperleukocytosis (conventionally and arbitrarily defined as a WBC count or blast count >100,000/mm^3) ranges from 10% to 30% in adult patients with ALL
- Symptoms may arise from the involvement of any organ, but intracranial hemorrhages and respiratory failure account for most deaths (cautiously interpret ABGs: spuriously low PaO_2 can result from rapid consumption of plasma oxygen by the markedly increased number of WBCs)
- Factors associated with hyperleukocytosis in ALL include T-cell phenotype, 11q23 rearrangements and t(9;22)(q34;q11)
- Symptoms of leukostasis are rarely seen in ALL (2–6%). In many patients, leukostasis becomes evident a few days after diagnosis, and sometimes after the first leukocytoreduction. Clinical deterioration and death may occur after the blast count has been significantly reduced, suggesting that, although leukocytoreduction is an important step in the management of leukostasis, additional measures are needed to prevent leukostasis-related deaths

(continued)

Caveats *(continued)*

- *Treatment*
  - –Prompt leukocytoreduction, initiation of chemotherapy, and supportive care. Leukocytoreduction can be achieved by the use of hydroxyurea, which should be started immediately in all patients with hyperleukocytotic ALL. Hydroxyurea 12.5–25 mg/kg per dose 4 times daily, *or* 17–33 mg/kg per dose 3 times daily reduces the WBC count by 50–80% within 24–48 hours. Hydroxyurea is discontinued as the other agents begin to have an effect
  - –Leukopheresis is rarely performed in ALL unless symptoms of leukostasis or blast counts >300,000/mm^3 are seen. The disadvantages of leukopheresis are that it requires the placement of a large-caliber central venous catheter that is not always available, and it may worsen the thrombocytopenia. In addition, because leukopheresis is not cytostatic, rebound leukocytosis may occur in association with this procedure. There are no guidelines that identify the absolute WBC concentration to be achieved by leukopheresis, which correlate with reversal of the signs and symptoms of leukostasis. The most consistent success has been achieved using a continuous-flow procedure in which large volumes (8–10 L) of patient blood are processed

Grima KM. J Clin Apher 2000;15:28–52
Porcu P et al. Ther Apher 2002;6:15–23

REGIMEN FOR PROPHYLAXIS AGAINST AND TREATMENT OF TUMOR LYSIS SYNDROME

HYDRATION, HYPERURICEMIA AND HYPERPHOSPHATEMIA

1. Hydration

2500–3000 mL/day as tolerated, 5% dextrose/0.45% NaCl injection (D5W/0.45% NS) with sodium bicarbonate injection 100 mEq/1000 mL intravenously at 100–150 mL/hour (2500–3000 mL/day)

Notes about hydration:

- **Potassium** is *not* added to parenteral hydration solutions during the first few days of induction therapy unless serum potassium decreases to <3.0 mEq/dL
- **Furosemide** 20–40 mg intravenously every 12–24 hours to maintain fluid balance. Diuresis is maintained for at least the first 72 hours after starting chemotherapy in the absence of metabolic aberrations or after metabolic complications normalize

2. Hyperuricemia

Hyperuricemia develops within 24–48 hours after initiating chemotherapy when the excretory capacity of the renal tubules is exceeded. In the presence of an acid pH, uric acid crystals form in the renal tubule, leading to intraluminal renal tubular obstruction, an acute renal obstructive uropathy, and renal dysfunction

Administer **allopurinol** orally or intravenously, starting 12 hours to 3 days (preferably 2–3 days) before initiating cytoreductive chemotherapy

Urinary alkalization: Increases the solubility and excretion of uric acid and helps avoid **uric acid crystallization** in renal tubules; however, alkalinization is not uniformly recommended because:

- It favors precipitation of calcium/phosphate complexes in renal tubules, a concern in patients with concomitant hyperphosphatemia
- The metabolic alkalemia that may result from the administration of bicarbonate can worsen the neurologic manifestations of hypocalcemia
- At urine pH > 6.5, the solubility of **xanthine** and **hypoxanthine** significantly decreases, leading to the development of urinary xanthine crystals during and after allopurinol therapy

Initial dosage

100 mg/m^2 per dose orally every 8 hours (maximum daily dose = 800 mg), *or*
3.3 mg/kg per dose orally every 8 hours (maximum daily dose = 800 mg), *or*
200–400 mg/m^2 per day intravenously (maximum daily dose = 600 mg)

Maintenance doses: Should be based on serum uric acid determinations performed approximately 48 hours after initiation of allopurinol therapy and periodically thereafter. Continue administering allopurinol until leukemic blasts have been cleared from the peripheral blood

Allopurinol dose adjustments for impaired renal function:

Creatinine Clearance	Oral Allopurinol Dose
10–20 mL/min	200 mg/day
3–10 mL/min	100 mg/day
<3 mL/min	100 mg every 36–48 hours

Notes:

- The incidence of allergic reactions is increased in patients receiving amoxicillin, ampicillin, or thiazide diuretics
- Allopurinol inhibits the metabolism of **azathioprine and mercaptopurine**: decrease azathioprine and mercaptopurine doses by 65–75% when they are used concomitantly with allopurinol
- Side effects include rash (1.5%), nausea (1.3%), vomiting (1.2%), and renal insufficiency (1.2%)

3. Hyperphosphatemia

Correction of hyperphosphatemia (and hypocalcemia):

Hyperphosphatemia develops within 24–48 hours after initiation of chemotherapy. It may result in tissue precipitation of calcium phosphate resulting in hypocalcemia, intrarenal calcifications, nephocalcinosis and acute obstructive uropathy. Treatment of hyperphosphatemia usually corrects any related hypocalcemia; thus, calcium administration should be given only to patients with symptoms related to hypocalcemia

Oral phosphate binders: **Aluminium hydroxide** 15–30 mL orally every 6 hours

Hemodialysis is the most effective therapeutic strategy. Consider hemodialysis if hyperphosphatemia is severe, especially in the setting of renal failure and symptomatic hypocalcemia. The clearance of phosphorus is better after hemodialysis compared with continuous venovenous hemofiltration and compared with continuous peritoneal dialysis

See also Chapter 46, Oncologic Emergencies

LARSON REGIMEN (CALGB STUDY 9111)

CALGB STUDY 9111 (LARSON REGIMEN)

Larson RA et al Blood 1998;92:1556–1564

See Regimen for Prophylaxis Against and Treatment of Tumor Lysis Syndrome earlier in chapter. Also see Chapter 46, Oncologic Emergencies

Induction (1 course, 4 weeks in duration)

Treatment Strata by Patient's Age	
<60 Years	≥60 Years
Cyclophosphamide 1200 mg/m² intravenously in 100—250 mL 0.9% NaCl injection (0.9% NS) or 5% dextrose injection (D5W) over 15–30 minutes on day 1 (total dosage/course = 1200 mg/m²) **Daunorubicin** 45 mg/m² per day intravenously per push over 3–5 minutes for 3 consecutive days on days 1–3 (total dosage/course = 135 mg/m²) **Prednisone** 60 mg/m² per day orally for 21 consecutive days on days 1–21 (total dosage/course = 1260 mg/m²)	**Cyclophosphamide** 800 mg/m² intravenously in 100–250 mL 0.9% NaCl injection (0.9% NS) or 5% dextrose injection (D5W) over 15–30 minutes on day 1 (total dosage/course=800 mg/m²) **Daunorubicin** 30 mg/m² per day intravenously per push over 3–5 minutes for 3 consecutive days on days 1–3 (total dosage/course = 90 mg/m²) **Prednisone** 60 mg/m² per day orally for 7 consecutive days on days 1–7 (total dosage/course = 420 mg/m²)

All Patients

Vincristine 2 mg per dose intravenously per push over 1–2 minutes for 4 doses on days 1, 8, 15, and 22 (total dose/course = 8 mg)
Asparaginase 6000 units/m² per dose intramuscularly, or intravenously in 10–50 mL 0.9% NS or D5W over at least 30 minutes for 6 doses on days 5, 8, 11, 15, 18, and 22 (total dosage/course = 36,000 units/m²)

Filgrastim 5 mcg/kg per day subcutaneously for at least 7 consecutive days. Start on day 4 at least 12 hours after the last dose of daunorubicin, and continue until the ANC is ≥ 1000/mm³ after the ANC nadir for 2 consecutive days (24 hours apart)

Emetogenic potential during induction:
Day 1: High (Emetogenicity score = 5). Potential for delayed symptoms
Days 2 and 3: Moderate (Emetogenicity score = 3)
Days 5, 8, 11, 15, 18, and 22: Low (Emetogenicity score = 2). See Chapter 39 for antiemetic regimens

Early intensification (2 courses, 4 weeks each in duration)
Methotrexate 15 mg intrathecally via lumbar puncture in 6–15 mL *preservative-free* 0.9% NS on day 1 every 4 weeks for 2 courses (total dose/course = 15 mg)
Cyclophosphamide 1000 mg/m² intravenously in 100–250 mL 0.9% NS or D5W over 15–30 minutes on day 1 every 4 weeks for 2 courses (total dosage/course = 1000 mg/m²)
Mercaptopurine 60 mg/m² per day orally for 14 consecutive days on days 1–14 every 4 weeks for 2 courses (total dosage/course = 840 mg/m²)
Cytarabine 75 mg/m² per dose subcutaneously for 8 doses on days 1–4 and days 8–11 every 4 weeks for 2 courses (total dosage/course = 600 mg/m²)
Vincristine 2 mg per dose intravenously per push over 1–2 minutes for 2 doses on days 15 and 22 every 4 weeks for 2 courses (total dose/course = 4 mg)
Asparaginase 6000 units/m² per dose intramuscularly or intravenously in 10–50 mL 0.9% NS or D5W over at least 30 minutes for 4 doses on days 15, 18, 22, and 25 every 4 weeks for 2 courses (total dosage/course = 24,000 units/m²)
Filgrastim 5 micrograms/kg per day subcutaneously for at least 14 consecutive days. Start on day 2, and continue until the ANC is ≥5000/mm³ after the ANC nadir for 2 consecutive days (24 hours apart)

(continued)

Treatment Modifications

Adverse Event	Dose Modification
Serum creatinine >3 mg/dL (264 µmol/L) Bilirubin 3–5.0 mg/dL (51.3–81.5 µmol/L)	Reduce daunorubicin dosage by 50%
Bilirubin >5 mg/dL (81.5 µmol/L)	Hold daunorubicin
Bilirubin >3 mg/dL	Reduce vincristine dosage by 50%
Elevated amylase or pancreatitis	Stop asparaginase
Serum creatinine levels 1.5–2.0 mg/dL (132–176 µmol)	Reduce methotrexate dosage by 25%
Serum creatinine levels >2.0 mg/dL (176 µmol/L)	Reduce methotrexate dosage by 50%
Bilirubin 3–5 mg/dL (51.3–81.5 µmol/L)	Reduce methotrexate dosage by 25%
Bilirubin >5 mg/dL (81.5 µmol/L)	Hold methotrexate

Patient Population Studied

A study of 102 patients (median age 35 years) with newly diagnosed ALL

Efficacy (N = 102)

Induction Course	
Complete remission	87%
≥ 60 years (n = 21)	81%
< 60 years	83%
Refractory disease	8%
Died during induction	5%
Median disease-free survival (DFS)	2.3 years
Median DFS Ph + patients	0.8 years
Median overall survival	2.4 years

(continued)
Note: In all cases, filgrastim should be discontinued at least 2 days before cyclophosphamide administration resumes on the first day of course 2

Emetogenic potential during early intensification:
Day 1: Moderately high (Emetogenicity score = 4)
Days 15, 18, 22, and 25: Low (Emetogenicity score = 2). See Chapter 39 for antiemetic regimens

CNS prophylaxis and interim maintenance (1 course, 12 weeks in duration)
Cranial irradiation 2400 cGy (total dose) delivered during 12 consecutive days on days 1–12
Methotrexate 15 mg per dose intrathecally via lumbar puncture or Ommaya reservoir in 6–15 mL *preservative-free* 0.9% NaCl injection (0.9% NS) for 5 doses on days 1, 8, 15, 22, and 29 (total dose/course = 75 mg)
Mercaptopurine 60 mg/m^2 per day orally for 70 consecutive days on days 1–70 (total dosage/course = 4200 mg/m^2)
Methotrexate 20 mg/m^2 per dose orally for 5 doses on days 36, 43, 50, 57, and 64 (total dosage/course = 100 mg/m^2)

Emetogenic potential during CNS prophylaxis and interim maintenance:
Days 1–12: Moderate (Emetogenicity score = 3)
Days 15, 22, and 29: Low (Emetogenicity score = 2). See Chapter 39 for antiemetic regimens

Late intensification (1 course, 8 weeks in duration)
Doxorubicin 30 mg/m^2 per dose intravenously per push over 3–5 minutes for 3 doses on days 1, 8, and 15 (total dosage/course = 90 mg/m^2)
Vincristine 2 mg per dose intravenously per push over 1–2 minutes for 3 doses on days 1, 8, and 15 (total dose/course = 6 mg)
Dexamethasone 10 mg/m^2 per day orally for 14 consecutive days on days 1–14 (total dosage/course = 140 mg/m^2)
Cyclophosphamide 1000 mg/m^2 intravenously in 100–250 mL 0.9% NS or D5W over 15–30 minutes on day 29 (total dosage/course = 1000 mg/m^2)
Thioguanine 60 mg/m^2 per day orally for 14 consecutive days on days 29–42 (total dosage/course = 840 mg/m^2)
Cytarabine 75 mg/m^2 per dose subcutaneously for 8 doses on days 29–32 and days 36–39 (total dosage/course = 600 mg/m^2)

Emetogenic potential during late intensification: Nonemetogenic (Emetogenicity score = 1). See Chapter 39 for antiemetic regimens

Prolonged maintenance (courses are 4 weeks in duration, and are repeated until 24 months after diagnosis)
Vincristine 2 mg per dose intravenously per push over 1–2 minutes on day 1 every 4 weeks (total dose/course = 4 mg)
Prednisone 60 mg/m^2 per day orally for 5 consecutive days on days 1–5 every 4 weeks (total dosage/course = 300 mg/m^2)
Mercaptopurine 60 mg/m^2 per day orally for 28 consecutive days on days 1–28 (total dosage/course = 1680 mg/m^2)
Methotrexate 20 mg/m^2 per dose orally for 4 doses on days 1, 8, 15, and 22 (total dosage/course = 80 mg/m^2)

Emetogenic potential during prolonged maintenance: Low (Emetogenicity score = 2). See Chapter 39 for antiemetic regimens

Dexamethasone is marketed in the United States in numerous generic formulations for oral administration, including prompt-release tablets containing 0.25, 0.5, 0.75, 1, 2, 4, and 6 mg, and in elixirs (which contain alcohol) and solutions for oral administration
Mercaptopurine is available in the United States generically formulated as prompt-release tablets for oral administration, containing 50 mg
Methotrexate is available in the United States generically in a variety of formulations and product strengths for oral administration, including prompt-release tablets containing 2.5 mg, 5 mg, 7.5 mg, 10 mg, and 15 mg
Prednisone is marketed in the United States in numerous generic formulations for oral administration, including prompt-release tablets containing 1, 2.5, 5, 10, 20, and 50 mg, and in solutions and syrups for oral administration
Thioguanine is formulated in the United States as prompt-release tablets for oral administration, containing 40 mg. TABLOID® brand Thioguanine 40-mg Scored Tablets product label, December 2004. Manufactured by DSM Pharmaceuticals, Inc., Greenville, NC. Manufactured for GlaxoSmithKline, Research Triangle Park, NC

Toxicity of Remission Induction (N = 100)

	% G3/4/5
Leukopenia	98
Thrombocytopenia	97
Anemia	93
Infection	78
Nausea	23
↑ Bilirubin	44
↑ Transaminases	35
Malaise/fatique	16
Motor neuropathy	18
Pain	21
Hyperglycemia	33
Hypofibrinogenemia	26

CALGB

Toxicity of Intensification and Maintenance (N = 197)

Data are from 197 newly diagnosed ALL patients who were treated with the same chemotherapy regimen but did not receive filgrastim

G3/4	% Intensification	% Maintenance
Leukopenia	97	75
Thrombocytopenia	84	32
Anemia	84	26
Hemorrhage	4	0
Infection	49	25
Nausea/vomiting	17	8
Stomatitis	9	7
Diarrhea	3	1
Hepatic	28	30
Pulmonary	5	4
Cardiac	1	6
Genitourinary	2	1
CNS	13	6
Peripheral nervous system	12	7
Skin	1	2
Allergy	1	1

CALGB

Larson RA et al. Blood 1995:85:2025–2037

Therapy Monitoring

1. CBC with differential daily during chemotherapy and every other day after recovery of WBC $>500/\text{mm}^3$ until either normal differential or persistent leukemia is documented. Platelets every day while in hospital until patients no longer require platelet transfusions
2. Electrolytes, mineral panel, uric acid at least daily during active treatment until the risk of tumor lysis is past
3. Amylase and fibrinogen levels before asparaginase administration. If fibrinogen level is <100 mg/dL, administer fresh frozen plasma or cryoprecipitate. See Chapter 45, Transfusion Therapy
4. Bone marrow aspirate/biopsy at day 29 of the initial induction course. If no CR is achieved, consider clinical trial or reinduction with another regimen
5. When in CR, bone marrow biopsy/aspirate should be performed at the end of each consolidation cycle (or, at the very least, every other cycle) and every 3 months during maintenance

Notes

1. An additional group of 96 patients in the Larson study (Blood 1998) did not receive filgrastim after randomization. The median time to recover neutrophils ≥ 1000 mm^3 during the remission induction course was 16 days for the patients assigned to receive filgrastim and 22 days for the patients who were assigned to placebo. Patients in the filgrastim group had a significantly shorter duration of neutropenia and thrombocytopenia and fewer days on the hospital compared with patients receiving placebo. The patients assigned to receive filgrastim had a higher CR rate and fewer deaths during remission induction than those receiving placebo. Overall toxicity was not lessened by the use of filgrastim. After a median follow-up of 4.7 years, no significant difference in the overall survival between the two groups was found
2. In Larson's study, lumbar puncture was performed at diagnosis only in symptomatic patients. Symptomatic patients with CNS leukemia should receive therapy either with 15 mg methotrexate + 50 mg hydrocortisone or 100 mg cytarabine + 50 mg hydrocortisone intrathecally or via an Ommaya reservoir weekly until the CSF clears. If clearance is slow, one may treat with all three drugs combined (same doses). After there is no evidence of disease in the CSF, patients should continue treatment as specified in the regimen
3. Asparaginase has been associated with severe reactions, including anaphylaxis and sudden death. This reaction may occur with the first dose or after successive doses of the drug. Retreatment with asparaginase in patients who have received a course of the drug may result in an increased risk of hypersensitivity reactions. Because of allergic reactions to asparaginase, an intradermal skin test should be performed before the initial injection of the drug or when the drug is given after an interval of a week or more between doses. However, note that test doses of asparaginase before repeated asparaginase treatment are not reliable for predicting hypersensitivity because too many false-negative test results occur (Ohnuma T et al. Cancer Res 1970; 30:2297–2305). The product label notes: Acute reactions have occurred in the absence of a positive skin test and during continued maintenance of therapeutic serum levels. See Chapter 40, Drug Preparation and Administration, for information on additional testing and on what constitutes a positive result
4. Leukocyte-depleted blood products should be used for transfusion. Irradiation of all blood products is advised to reduce the risk of graft-versus-host disease in all immunosuppressed patients
5. Routine gut decontamination and/or prophylactic antimicrobials should be administered according to institutional guidelines. The choice for antimicrobial prophylaxis varies among care providers

LINKER REGIMEN

LINKER REGIMEN

Linker C et al. JCO 2002;20:2464–2471

See Regimen for Prophylaxis Against and Treatment of Tumor Lysis Syndrome earlier in chapter. Also see Chapter 46, Oncologic Emergencies

Treatment Sequence

1A → 1B → 1C → 2A → 2B → 2C → 3C → Maintenance Therapy

Induction (course 1A, DVP/Asp)
Daunorubicin 60 mg/m^2 per day intravenously per push over 3–5 minutes for 3 consecutive days on days 1–3 (total dosage/course after 3 doses = 180 mg/m^2)

Note: If day 14 bone marrow evaluation reveals residual leukemia, give a fourth dose of **daunorubicin** 60 mg/m^2 intravenously per push over 3–5 minutes on day 15 (total dosage/course after 4 doses = 240 mg/m^2)

Vincristine
Patients ≤40 years: 1.4 mg/m^2 per dose intravenously per push over 1–2 minutes for 4 doses on days 1, 8, 15, and 22 (total dosage/course = 5.6 mg/m^2)
Patients >40 years: 1.4 mg/m^2 per dose (maximum single dose = 2 mg) intravenously per push over 1–2 minutes for 4 doses on days 1, 8, 15, and 22 (total dosage/course = 5.6 mg/m^2; maximum dose/course = 8 mg)
Prednisone 60 mg/m^2 per day orally for 28 consecutive days on days 1–28 (total dosage/course = 1680 mg/m^2)
Asparaginase 6000 units/m^2 per day intramuscularly, or intravenously in 10–50 mL 0.9% NaCl injection (0.9% NS) or 5% dextrose injection (D5W) over at least 30 minutes for 12 consecutive days on days 17–28 (total dosage/course = 72,000 units/m^2)

Methotrexate 12 mg intrathecally via lumbar puncture in 5–12 mL *preservative-free* 0.9% NaCl injection (see Caveats in the general information section before the individual regimens)

Filgrastim 5 micrograms/kg subcutaneously daily starting on day 14 of chemotherapy and continuing until the ANC is >1500/mm^3 for 2 days (24 hours apart) after the ANC nadir

Emetogenic potential during induction:
Days 1–3: Moderate (Emetogenicity score = 3)
Days 17–28: Low (Emetogenicity score = 2). See Chapter 39 for antiemetic regimens

Consolidation (courses 1B and 2B, HD-cytarabine + etoposide)
Cytarabine 2000 mg/m^2 per day intravenously in 100–1000 mL 0.9% NaCl injection (0.9% NS) or 5% dextrose injection (D5W) over 2 hours for 4 consecutive days on days 1–4 (total dosage/course = 8000 mg/m^2)
Etoposide 500 mg/m^2 per day intravenously diluted in 0.9% NS or D5W to a concentration of 0.2–0.4 mg/mL over 3 hours for 4 consecutive days on days 1–4 (total dosage/course = 2000 mg/m^2)

Emetogenic potential during consolidation (cytarabine + etoposide):
Days 1–4: High (Emetogenicity score = 5). Potential for delayed symptoms. See Chapter 39 for antiemetic regimens

Consolidation (course 2A, DVP/Asp)
Daunorubicin 60 mg/m^2 per day intravenously per push over 3–5 minutes for 3 consecutive days on days 1–3 (total dosage/course = 180 mg/m^2)
Vincristine
Patients ≤40 years: 1.4 mg/m^2 per dose intravenously per push over 1–2 minutes for 3 doses on days 1, 8, and 15 (total dosage/course = 4.2 mg/m^2)
Patients >40 years: 1.4 mg/m^2 per dose (maximum single dose = 2 mg) intravenously per push over 1–2 minutes for 3 doses on days 1, 8, and 15 (total dosage/course = 4.2 mg/m^2; maximum dose/course = 6 mg)
Prednisone 60 mg/m^2 per day orally for 21 consecutive days on days 1–21 (total dosage/course = 1260 mg/m^2)

(continued)

Treatment Modifications

Adverse Event	Dose Modification
Serum creatinine >3 mg/dL (264 µmol/L) Bilirubin 3–5.0 mg/dL (51.3–85.5 µmol/L)	Reduce daunorubicin dosage by 50%
Bilirubin >5 mg/dL (85.5 µmol/L)	Hold daunorubicin
Bilirubin >3 mg/dL (51.3 µmol/L)	Reduce vincristine dosage by 50%
Elevated amylase or pancreatitis	Stop asparaginase
Serum creatinine levels 1.5–2.0 mg/dL (132–176 µmol)	Reduce methotrexate dosage by 25%
Serum creatinine levels >2.0 mg/dL (176 µmol/L)	Reduce methotrexate dosage by 50%
Bilirubin 3–5 mg/dL (51.3–85.5 µmol/L)	Reduce methotrexate dosage by 25%

Patient Population Studied

A study of 84 newly diagnosed adult patients with ALL (median age 27 years)

Efficacy (N = 84)

Induction	%
Complete remission*	93%
5-Year event free survival	48% ± 13%
5-Year overall survival	47% ± 13%
5-Year event free survival for patients achieving remission	52% ± 13%
5-Year disease-free survival (DFS) for patients achieving remission	54% ± 13%
Nine patients with high risk who did not undergo transplantation	Relapsed with median time to relapse 2.5 months
Standard-risk B-precursor disease 5-year DFS	66% ± 16%
All precursor B-cell 5-year event-free survival	55%

*One treatment-related death and 5 patients with resistant disease

(continued)

Asparaginase 12,000 units/m^2 per dose intramuscularly, or intravenously in 10–50 mL 0.9% NS or D5W over at least 30 minutes for 3 doses/week (eg, Monday, Wednesday, and Friday) for 2 consecutive weeks (total dosage/course = 72,000 units/m^2)
Emetogenic potential during consolidation (DVP/Asp):
Days 1–3: Moderate (Emetogenicity score = 3). See Chapter 39 for antiemetic regimens
Emetogenic potential with asparaginase: Low (Emetogenicity score = 2). See Chapter 39 for antiemetic regimens

Consolidation (courses 1C, 2C, and 3C, HD-methotrexate + mercaptopurine)
Hydration with methotrexate: 1500–3000 mL/m^2 per day. Use a solution containing a total amount of sodium not greater than 0.9% NaCl injection (ie, 154 mEq/1000 mL) by intravenous infusion during methotrexate administration and for at least 24 hours afterward
Fluid administration may commence 2–12 hours before starting methotrexate, depending on a patient's fluid status

Notes:

- Urine output should be at least 100 mL/hour before starting methotrexate infusion
- Maintain hydration at a rate that maintains urine output of at least 100 mL/hour until the serum methotrexate concentration is <0.05 micromol/L

Sodium bicarbonate 50–150 mEq/1000 mL is added to the parenteral solution to maintain urine pH ≥7.0

Base Solution	Base Solution Sodium Content	Sodium Bicarbonate Additive	Total Sodium Content
0.45% NaCl injection (0.45% NS)	77 mEq/L	50–75 mEq	127–152 mEq/L
0.2% NaCl injection (0.2% NS)	34 mEq/L	100–125 mEq	134–159 mEq/L
5% Dextrose injection (D5W)	0 mEq/L	125–150 mEq	125–150 mEq/L
D5W/0.45% NS	77 mEq/L	50–75 mEq	125–152 mEq/L
D5W/0.2% NS	34 mEq/L	100–125 mEq	134–159 mEq/L

Methotrexate 220 mg/m^2 per dose intravenously in 25–100 mL 0.9% NaCl injection (0.9% NS) over 1 hour every 2 weeks on days 1 and 15, *followed by:*
Methotrexate 60 mg/m^2 per hour by continuous intravenous infusion for 36 hours every 2 weeks on days 1 and 15 (total dosage/administration event, bolus + infusion = 2380 mg/m^2; total dosage/course [not including intrathecal methotrexate] = 4760 mg/m^2)

Note: For logistical practicality and efficiency, parenteral admixtures containing methotrexate may include a portion or all the fluid and sodium bicarbonate needed to meet hydration and urinary alkalinization requirements during methotrexate administration

Leucovorin calcium 50 mg/m^2 per dose intravenously in 25–250 mL 0.9% NS or D5W over 15–30 minutes, starting immediately after methotrexate is completed (37 hours after methotrexate administration began) every 6 hours for 3 doses every 2 weeks on days 2 and 16, *then:*
Leucovorin calcium 50 mg/m^2 per dose orally starting 6 hours after the last intravenously-administered dose of leucovorin every 6 hours until serum methotrexate concentrations are <0.05 micromol/L ($<5 \times 10^{-8}$ mol/L, or < 50 nmol /L) every 2 weeks
Mercaptopurine 75 mg/m^2 per day orally for 28 consecutive days on days 1–28 (total dosage/course = 2100 mg/m^2)

Emetogenic potential during consolidation (high-dose methotrexate):
Days 1, 2, 15, and 16: Moderately high (Emetogenicity score = 4). See Chapter 39 for antiemetic regimens

(continued)

(continued)

Maintenance chemotherapy:
Mercaptopurine 75 mg/m^2 per day orally continually until complete remission is sustained for 30 months (total dosage/week = 525 mg/m^2)
Methotrexate 20 mg/m^2 per dose orally once weekly until complete remission is sustained for 30 months (total dosage/week = 20 mg/m^2)

Emetogenic potential during maintenance: Nonemetogenic (Emetogenicity score = 1). See Chapter 39 for antiemetic regimens

Leucovorin calcium is manufactured in the United States in tablets for oral administration containing 5 mg, 10 mg, 15 mg, and 25 mg leucovorin calcium by various pharmaceutical manufacturers
Mercaptopurine is available in the United States generically formulated as prompt-release tablets for oral administration, containing 50 mg
Methotrexate is available in the United States generically in a variety of formulations and product strengths for oral administration, including: prompt-release tablets containing 2.5 mg, 5 mg, 7.5 mg, 10 mg, and 15 mg
Prednisone is marketed in the United States in numerous generic formulations for oral administration, including prompt-release tablets containing 1, 2.5, 5, 10, 20, and 50 mg, and in solutions and syrups for oral administration

Supportive care:
PCP prophylaxis: **Cotrimoxazole** (trimethoprim 160 mg + sulfamethoxazole 800 mg) orally twice daily on two days per week

Toxicity (N = 53–84)

	1A DVP/Asp (n = 84)	1B HDAC/ Etoposide (n = 79)	2A DVP/Asp (n = 59)	2B HDAC/ Etoposide (n = 53)
No. of Days to Hematologic Recovery				
ANC				
>500/mm^3	18	19	16	20
>1000/mm^3	23	20	17	20
No. of days ANC <500	14	12	5	12
Platelets				
>20,000/mm^3	15	19	1	22
>50,000/mm^3	18	21	20	27
>100,000/mm^3	22	24	29	29
No. of platelet transfusions	4	3	0	4
No. of RBC transfusions	6	7	2	6

Therapy Monitoring

1. CBC with differential daily during chemotherapy and every other day after recovery of WBC >500/mm^3 until either normal differential or persistent leukemia is documented. Platelets every day while in hospital until patient no longer requires platelet transfusions
2. Electrolytes, mineral panel, and uric acid at least daily during active treatment until the risk of tumor lysis is past
3. Amylase and fibrinogen levels before asparaginase administration. If fibrinogen level <100 mg/dL, administer fresh frozen plasma or cryoprecipitate
4. Bone marrow aspirate/biopsy at day 14 of the initial induction course and before first consolidation
5. If no CR is achieved, consider clinical trial or reinduction with another regimen
6. When in CR, bone marrow biopsy/aspirates should be performed at the end of each consolidation cycle (or, at the very least, every other cycle) and every 3 months during maintenance

Notes

1. In the study by Linker et al, patients received CNS prophylaxis with intrathecal methotrexate during the initial diagnostic lumbar puncture. Five subsequent doses began with the first course of post-remission chemotherapy and were delivered weekly as tolerated. Patients with CNS disease at diagnosis received intensified CNS therapy: 10 intrathecal treatments, and cranial irradiation 18 Gy was given after bone marrow remission was achieved

CNS prophylaxis/treatment:
Methotrexate 12 mg per dose intrathecally via lumbar puncture in 5–12 mL *preservative-free* 0.9% NaCl injection

Methotrexate	Prophylaxis	Treatment
Total number of doses Total dose/course	6* 72 mg	10* 120 mg
Cranial irradiation	None	1800 cGy after bone marrow CR

*First dose given at the start of induction course 1A. Second and subsequent doses start concurrently with post-CR chemotherapy, and continue on a weekly schedule

2. Asparaginase has been associated with severe reactions, including anaphylaxis and sudden death. This reaction may occur with the first dose or after successive doses of the drug. Retreatment with asparaginase in patients who have received a course of the drug may result in an increased risk of hypersensitivity reactions. Because of the occurrence of allergic reactions to **asparaginase**, an intradermal skin test should be performed before the initial injection of the drug or when the drug is given after an interval of a week or more between doses. However, note that test doses of asparaginase before repeated asparaginase treatment are not reliable for predicting hypersensitivity because too many false-negative test results occur (Ohnuma T et al. Cancer Res 1970; 30:2297–2305). The product label notes: Acute reactions have occurred in the absence of a positive skin test and during continued maintenance of therapeutic serum levels. See Chapter 40, Drug Preparation and Administration, for information on additional testing and on what constitutes a positive result
3. Leukocyte-depleted blood products should be used for transfusion. Irradiation of all blood products is advised to reduce the risk of graft-versus-host disease in all immunosuppressed patients
4. Routine gut decontamination and/or prophylactic antimicrobials should be administered according to institutional guidelines. The choice for antimicrobial prophylaxis varies among care providers
5. *Keratitis prophylaxis*: Steroid eye drops (prednisolone 1% or dexamethasone 0.1%) daily until 24 hours after high-dose cytarabine is completed

DOSE-INTENSIVE REGIMEN

HYPER-CVAD

Kantarjian HM et al. JCO 2000;18:547–561

See Regimen for Prophylaxis Against and Treatment of Tumor Lysis Syndrome earlier in chapter. Also see Chapter 46, Oncologic Emergencies

Dose-intensive chemotherapy
The dose-intensive phase consists of 8 cycles of hyper-CVAD alternating with high-dose methotrexate and cytarabine every 3–4 weeks (when WBC count is >3000/mm^3 and platelet count is >60,000/mm^3)

Hyper-CVAD (cycles 1, 3, 5, and 7)
Cyclophosphamide 300 mg/m^2 per dose intravenously over 3 hours in 500 mL 0.9% NaCl injection (0.9% NS) or 5% dextrose injection (D5W) every 12 hours for 6 doses on days 1–3 for 4 cycles, cycles 1, 3, 5, and 7 (total dosage/cycle = 1800 mg/m^2)
Mesna 600 mg/m^2 per day by continuous intravenous infusion in 1000 mL 0.9% NS over 24 hours for approximately 69 hours for 4 cycles, cycles 1, 3, 5, and 7. Mesna administration starts concurrently with cyclophosphamide on day 1 and continues until 6 hours after the last dose of cyclophosphamide is completed (total dosage/cycle ~1725 mg/m^2)
Vincristine 2 mg/dose by intravenous push over 1–3 minutes for 2 doses on days 4 and 11 for 4 cycles, cycles 1, 3, 5, and 7 (total dose/cycle = 4 mg)
Doxorubicin 50 mg/m^2 intravenously via central venous access in 25–250 mL 0.9% NS or D5W over 2 hours on day 4 for 4 cycles, cycles 1, 3, 5, and 7 (total dosage/cycle = 50 mg/m^2)
Dexamethasone 40 mg per dose orally, or by intravenous infusion in 25–150 mL 0.9% NS or D5W over 15–30 minutes for 8 doses on days 1–4 and days 11–14, for 4 cycles, cycles 1, 3, 5, and 7 (total dose/cycle = 320 mg)

Filgrastim 5 micrograms/kg subcutaneously every 12 hours, starting on day 5 (24 hours after the last dose of chemotherapy). Continue until post-nadir WBC count >3000/mm^3 and platelet count is >60,000/mm^3. If platelet recovery is delayed, filgrastim is continued unless the WBC count exceeds 30,000/mm^3

Supportive care: Antimicrobial prophylaxis
Ciprofloxacin 500 mg orally twice daily, *or* **levofloxacin** 500 mg orally once daily
Fluconazole 200 mg orally once daily but *withhold* fluconazole on days when vincristine is administered
Acyclovir 200 mg orally twice daily, *or* **valacyclovir** 500 mg orally once daily

Emetogenic potential with hyper-CVAD (cycles 1, 3, 5, and 7):
Days 1–4: Moderately high (Emetogenicity score = 4). Potential for delayed symptoms. See Chapter 39 for antiemetic regimens

High-dose methotrexate + cytarabine (cycles 2, 4, 6, and 8)
Hydration: with 5% dextrose injection/0.45% NS (D5W/0.45% NS) with sodium bicarbonate injection 100 mEq/1000 mL intravenously at 100–150 mL/hour (2400–3600 mL/day)
Methotrexate 200 mg/m^2 per dose intravenously in 25–100 mL 0.9% NS over 2 hours, *followed by:*
Methotrexate 800 mg/m^2 by continuous intravenous infusion over 24 hours on day 1 for 4 cycles, cycles 2, 4, 6, and 8 (total dosage/cycle, bolus + infusion = 1000 mg/m^2)

Note: For logistical practicality and efficiency, parenteral admixtures containing methotrexate may include a portion or all of the fluid and sodium bicarbonate needed to meet hydration and urinary alkalinization requirements during methotrexate administration

Leucovorin calcium 15 mg/m^2 per dose intravenously in 25–250 mL 0.9% NS or D5W over 15–30 minutes, starting 48 hours after methotrexate administration began (24 hours after methotrexate administration ends) every 6 hours for 8 doses (total dosage/cycle = 120 mg/m^2)

(continued)

Treatment Modifications During the Induction Phase

Adverse Effect	Dose Modification
Bilirubin >2 mg/dL (>34.2 μmol/L)	Reduce vincristine to 1 mg
Bilirubin level 2–3 mg/dL (34.2–51.3 μmol/L)	Reduce doxorubicin dosage by 25%
Bilirubin level 3–4 mg/dL (51.3–68.4 μmol/L)	Reduce doxorubicin dosage by 50%
Bilirubin level >4mg/dL (>68.4 μmol/L)	Reduce doxorubicin dosage by 75%
Serum creatinine 1.5–2.0 mg/dL (132–176 μmol)	Reduce methotrexate dosage by 25%
Serum creatinine >2.0 mg/dL (176 μmol)	Reduce methotrexate dosage by 50%
Bilirubin level 3–5 mg/dL (51.3–85.5 μmol/L)	Reduce methotrexate dosage by 25%
Bilirubin >5 mg/dL (>85.5 μmol/L)	Hold methotrexate
Serum creatinine level >2.0 mg/dL (>176 μmol/L)	Reduce cytarabine dosage to 1000 mg/m^2

Patient Population Studied

A study of 204 newly diagnosed ALL adult patients (median age: 39.5 years). No exclusions were made because of performance status, cardiac, hepatic, renal function, or concomitant active infection.

Efficacy (N = 204)

Complete response (CR)	91%
CR <30 years	98%
CR >60 years	79%
Resistant disease	3%
Died during induction	6%
Median survival time	35 months
5-Year estimated survival rate	39%
5-Year estimated survival for patients <30 years	54%
3-Year estimated survival for patients >60 years	25%
CR for Ph-positive disease	91%

(continued)

Note: If serum methotrexate concentrations are:

>20 micromol/L at hour 24 (end of methotrexate administration)

>1 micromol/L at hour 48 (24 hours after methotrexate administration ends), *or*

>0.1 micromol/L at hour 72 (48 hours after methotrexate administration ends), *then*:

leucovorin doses are escalated to 50 mg/dose intravenously every 6 hours until serum concentrations are < 0.1 micromol/L

Cytarabine

Patients < 60 years: 3000 mg/m² per dose intravenously in 50–500 mL 0.9% NS or D5W over 2 hours every 12 hours for 4 doses on days 2 and 3, for 4 cycles, cycles 2, 4, 6, and 8 (total dosage/cycle [not including intrathecal cytarabine] = 12,000 mg/m²)

Patients ≥ 60 years: 1000 mg/m² per dose intravenously in 50–500 mL 0.9% NS or D5W over 2 hours every 12 hours for 4 doses on days 2 and 3 for 4 cycles, cycles 2, 4, 6, and 8 (total dosage/cycle [not including intrathecal cytarabine] = 4000 mg/m²)

Methylprednisolone 50 mg intravenously twice daily for 6 doses on days 1–3 (total dose/cycle = 300 mg)

Filgrastim 5 mcg/kg per dose subcutaneously, every 12 hours, starting on day 4 (24 hours after the last dose of chemotherapy) and continue until post-nadir WBC count > 3000/mm³ and platelet count is > 60,000/mm³. If platelet recovery is delayed, filgrastim is continued unless the WBC count exceeds 30,000/mm³

Supportive care: Antimicrobial prophylaxis

Ciprofloxacin 500 mg orally twice daily, *or* **levofloxacin** 500 mg orally once daily

Fluconazole 200 mg orally once daily

Acyclovir 200 mg orally twice daily, *or* **valacyclovir** 500 mg orally once daily

Emetogenic potential with high-dose methotrexate and cytarabine (cycles 2, 4, 6, and 8):

Days 1–3: Moderately high (Emetogenicity score = 4). Potential for delayed symptoms. See Chapter 39 for antiemetic regimens

Maintenance phase

Mercaptopurine 50 mg orally on an empty stomach 3 times daily for 2 years (total dose/4 weeks = 4200 mg)

Methotrexate 20 mg/m² orally once weekly for 2 years (total dosage/4 weeks = 80 mg/m²)

Vincristine 2 mg intravenously per push over 1–2 minutes once monthly for 2 years (total dose/month = 2 mg)

Prednisone 200 mg per day orally for 5 consecutive days every month, starting on the day vincristine is given (total dose/month = 1000 mg)

Supportive care: Antimicrobial prophylaxis:

Cotrimoxazole (trimethoprim 160 mg + sulfamethoxazole 800 mg) orally twice daily on weekends

Acyclovir 200 mg orally daily or 3 times weekly for the first 6 months of maintenance therapy, *or*

Valacyclovir 500 mg orally once daily or 3 times weekly for the first 6 months of maintenance therapy

Emetogenic potential during maintenance chemotherapy: Nonemetogenic (Emetogenicity score = 1). See Chapter 39 for antiemetic regimens

Mercaptopurine is available in the United States generically formulated as prompt-release tablets for oral administration, containing 50 mg

Methotrexate is available in the United States generically in a variety of formulations and product strengths for oral administration, including: prompt-release tablets containing 2.5 mg, 5 mg, 7.5 mg, 10 mg, and 15 mg

Prednisone is marketed in the United States in numerous generic formulations for oral administration, including prompt-release tablets containing 1, 2.5, 5, 10, 20, and 50 mg, and in solutions and syrups for oral administration

Toxicity (N = 204)

Induction Chemotherapy (First Course of Hyper-CVAD)	
Myelosuppression	
Median time to granulocytes >1000/mm³	18 days
Median time to platelets >100,000 mm³	21 days
Hospitalization	63%
Sepsis	15%
Pneumonia	22%
Fungal infection	4%
Fever of unknown origin	45%.
Neurotoxicity	6%
Moderate–severe mucositis	6%
Moderate–severe diarrhea	3%
Ileus	2%
Disseminated intravascular coagulopathy	2%
Consolidation Courses (Second Course of Hyper-CVAD)	
Median time to recovery of counts	20 days
Pneumonia	2%
Hospitalization	18%
Neurotoxicity	8%
Mucositis	2%
Diarrhea	2%
Sepsis	3%
Fever of unknown origin	8%.
High-Dose Methotrexate + Cytarabine Therapy	
Sepsis	11%
Pneumonia	5%
Fever of unknown origin	23%
Neurotoxicity	5%
Minor infections	7%
Hospitalization	42%
Mucositis	5%
Rash and desquamation of palms and feet	3%
Diarrhea	1%
Maintenance Therapy	
Sepsis	5%
Pneumonia	7%
Fever of unknown origin	7%
Moderate hepatotoxicity	10%
Herpes zoster or varicella	8%
Cytomegalovirus infection	10%
Mucositis	5%
Diarrhea	5%

Therapy Monitoring

1. CBC with differential daily during chemotherapy and every other day after recovery of WBC >500/mm^3 until either normal differential or persistent leukemia is documented. Platelets every day
2. Electrolytes, mineral panel, uric acid at least daily during active treatment until the risk of tumor lysis is past
3. Bone marrow aspirate/biopsy after induction course
4. If no CR is achieved, consider clinical trial or re-induction with another regimen
5. When in CR, bone marrow biopsy/aspirate should be performed every 3 months for the first 2 years

Notes

1. In the study by Kantarjian et al, patients had a diagnostic lumbar puncture on day 2 of the first course of treatment
   a. Patients with CNS disease at the time of diagnosis receive intrathecal therapy with:
      - Intrathecal **methotrexate** 12 mg/dose via lumbar puncture or 6 mg/dose via intraventricular route twice weekly until CSF cell count normalizes and cytology becomes negative for malignant disease, then administer intrathecally during subsequent cycles on day 2 *and*
      - Intrathecal **cytarabine** 100 mg via lumbar puncture or intraventricular route twice weekly until CSF cell count normalizes and cytology becomes negative for malignant disease then administer intrathecally during subsequent cycles on day 2

   b. Patients with cranial nerve root involvement receive radiation 24–30 Gy in 10–12 fractions to the base of the skull or whole brain

   c. Patients with no evidence of CNS disease should receive CNS prophylaxis based on the prognostic factors for CNS leukemia

CNS prophylaxis

	Risk Categories		
Risk Factors	**High**	**Low**	**Unknown**
LDH	>600 units/L	Within normal limits	Unknown
Proliferative index (% S + G2M)	≥14%		
Histology	Mature B-cell ALL	Not applicable	

	Treatment by Risk Category		
Intrathecal Prophylaxis	**High**	**Unknown**	**Low**
Methotrexate 12 mg intrathecally via lumbar puncture or intraventricular route on day 2	For 8 cycles, cycles 1–8	For 4 cycles, cycles 1–4	For 2 cycles, cycles 1 and 2
Cytarabine 100 mg intrathecally via lumbar puncture or intraventricular route on day 8			

2. Patients with mature B-cell ALL received no maintenance therapy
3. Patients who receive high-dose cytarabine need to be closely monitored for changes in renal function. Renal dysfunction is highly correlated with an increased risk of cellebellar toxicity. Patients need to be monitored for nystagmus, dysmetria, and ataxia before each dose of cytarabine
4. *Keratitis prophylaxis*: Steroid eye drops (prednisolone 1% or dexamethasone 0.1%) daily until 24 hours after high-dose cytarabine is completed
5. Leukocyte-depleted blood products should be used for transfusion. Irradiation of all blood products is advised to reduce the risk of graft-versus-host disease in all immunosuppressed patients
6. Routine gut decontamination and/or prophylactic antimicrobials should be administered according to institutional guidelines. The choice for antimicrobial prophylaxis varies among care providers

REGIMEN

HOELZER REGIMEN (B-NHL86 STUDY)

Hoelzer D et al. Blood 1996;87:495–508

See Regimen for Prophylaxis Against and Treatment of Tumor Lysis Syndrome earlier in chapter. Also see Chapter 46, Oncologic Emergencies

Cytoreductive (Preinduction) Phase
Cyclophosphamide 200 mg/m² per day intravenously in 50–250 mL 0.9% NaCl injection or 5% dextrose injection over 15–60 minutes daily for 5 consecutive days on days 1–5 (total dosage/course = 1000 mg/m²)
Prednisone 60 mg/m² per day orally for 5 consecutive days on days 1–5 (total dosage/course = 300 mg/m²)

Emetogenic potential during preinduction phase:
Days 1–5: Moderate (Emetogenicity score = 3). See Chapter 39 for antiemetic regimens

Induction (Six Alternating 5-Day Cycles: Block A → Block B)

Block A (cycles 1, 3, and 5)
Vincristine 2 mg by intravenous push over 1–2 minutes on day 1 (total dose/cycle = 2 mg)
Hydration with methotrexate:

- Administer 1500–2000 mL/m² per day. Use a solution containing a total amount of sodium not greater than 0.9% NaCl injection (ie, 154 mEq/1000 mL) by intravenous infusion during methotrexate administration and for at least 24 hours afterward
- Fluid administration may commence 2–12 hours before starting methotrexate, depending upon a patient's fluid status
- Urine output should be at least 100 mL/h before starting methotrexate infusion
- Maintain hydration at a rate that maintains urine output of at least 100 mL/h until leucovorin use is completed

Methotrexate
Patients <50 years: 150 mg/m² loading dose intravenously in 25–100 mL 0.9% NS or D5W over 30 minutes on day 1, *followed by:*
1350 mg/m² by continuous intravenous infusion in 250–1000 mL 0.9% NS or D5W over 23.5 hours on day 1 (total dosage/cycle, not including intrathecally administered doses = 1500 mg/m²)
Patients 50–65 years: 50 mg/m² loading dose intravenously in 25–50 mL 0.9% NS or D5W over 30 minutes on day 1, *followed by:*
450 mg/m² by continuous intravenous infusion in 100–1000 mL 0.9% NS or D5W over 23.5 hours on day 1 (total dosage/cycle, not including intrathecally administered doses = 500 mg/m²)
Notes:

- Measure serum methotrexate concentrations at *hours* 42 and 68 after methotrexate administration began
- The intensity and administration route for leucovorin are directed by serum methotrexate concentrations (see below)

Leucovorin calcium 30 mg/m² intravenously in 25–250 mL 0.9% NS or D5W over 15–30 minutes at 36 hours after methotrexate administration began (12 hours after methotrexate administration ends), *then:*
Leucovorin calcium 30 mg/m² orally at 42 hours after methotrexate administration began, *then:*
Leucovorin calcium 15 mg/m² orally at 48 hours after methotrexate administration began, *then:*
Leucovorin calcium 5 mg/m² per dose orally for 3 doses at 54, 68, and 78 hours after methotrexate administration began

(continued)

Treatment Modifications

Adverse Event	Dose Modification
Bilirubin >2 mg/dL (34.2 μmol/L)	Reduce vincristine to 1 mg
Bilirubin 2–3 mg/dL (34.2–51.3 μmol/L)	Reduce doxorubicin dosage by 25%
Bilirubin 3–4 mg/dL (51.3–68.4 μmol/L)	Reduce doxorubicin dosage by 50%
Bilirubin level >4 mg/dL (>68.4 μmol/L)	Reduce doxorubicin dosage by 75%
Creatinine levels 1.5 to 2.0 mg/dL (133–176 μmol/L)	Reduce methotrexate dosage by 25%
Creatinine levels >2.0 mg/100 mL (>176 micromol/L)	Reduce methotrexate dosage by 50%
Bilirubin 3–5 mg/dL (51.3–85.5 μmol/L)	Reduce methotrexate dosage by 25%
Bilirubin >5 mg/dL (>85.5 μmol/L)	Hold methotrexate

Patient Population Studied

A study of 35 patients (median age 36 years) with newly diagnosed L3 ALL

Efficacy (N = 35)

Complete response	74%
No response	17%
Relapse	23%
Leukemia-free survival at 4 years	71%
Overall survival at 4 years	51%

(continued)

Note: Leucovorin rescue is intensified for delayed methotrexate clearance:

Time After Methotrexate Began	Serum Concentrations	Leucovorin Regimen
Hour 42	>0.5–5 micromol/L	Leucovorin calcium 50 mg/m^2 per dose intravenously every 6 hours for up to 60 hours
Hour 68	>0.01 micromol/L	Leucovorin calcium 30 mg/m^2 per dose intravenously every 6 hours for 4 doses

An admixture containing **ifosfamide** 800 mg/m^2 + **mesna** 160 mg/m^2 per day intravenously in a volume of 0.9% NS or D5W sufficient to produce ifosfamide concentrations between 0.6 and 20 mg/mL over 60 minutes for 5 consecutive days on days 1–5 (total ifosfamide dosage/cycle = 4000 mg/m^2) *then:*
Mesna 160 mg/m^2 per dose intravenously diluted with 0.9% NS or D5W to a concentration of 1–20 mg/mL over 15 minutes for 2 doses per day at 4 hours and 8 hours after ifosfamide administration is completed for 5 consecutive days on days 1–5 (total mesna dosage/cycle = 2400 mg/m^2)
Teniposide 100 mg/m^2 per day intravenously diluted with either D5W or 0.9% NS to produce a final teniposide concentration of 0.1 mg/mL, 0.2 mg/mL, 0.4 mg/mL, or 1 mg/mL over 60 minutes for 2 consecutive days on days 4 and 5 (total dosage/cycle = 200 mg/m^2)
Cytarabine 150 mg/m^2 per dose intravenously in 25–250 mL 0.9% NS or D5W over 15–30 minutes every 12 hours for 4 doses on days 4 and 5 (total dosage/cycle = 600 mg/m^2)
Dexamethasone 10 mg/m^2 per day orally for 5 consecutive days on days 1–5 (total dosage/cycle = 50 mg/m^2)

CNS prophylaxis during block A:
Methotrexate 15 mg intrathecally via lumbar puncture in 6–15 mL *preservative-free* 0.9% NaCl injection (0.9% NS) on day 1 (total dose after 6 cycles, not including intravenously administered doses = 90 mg)
Cytarabine 40 mg intrathecally via lumbar puncture in 3–10 mL *preservative-free* 0.9% NS on day 1 (total dose after 6 cycles, not including intravenously administered doses = 240 mg)
Preservative-free dexamethasone 4 mg intrathecally via lumbar puncture in 4–10 mL *preservative-free* 0.9% NS on day 1 (total dose after 6 cycles = 24 mg)

Emetogenic potential during induction, block A:
Day 1 with methotrexate 1500 mg/m^2: High (Emetogenicity score = 5)
Day 1 with methotrexate 500 mg/m^2: Moderately high (Emetogenicity score = 4)
Days 2 and 3: Moderate (Emetogenicity score = 3)
Days 4 and 5: Moderately high (Emetogenicity score = 4). Potential for delayed symptoms. See Chapter 39 for antiemetic regimens

Block B (cycles 2, 4, and 6)
Vincristine 2 mg by intravenous push over 1–2 minutes on day 1 (total dose/cycle = 2 mg)
Hydration with methotrexate:

- Administer 1500–2000 mL/m^2 per day. Use a solution containing a total amount of sodium not greater than 0.9% NaCl injection (ie, 154 mEq/1000 mL) by intravenous infusion during methotrexate administration and for at least 24 hours afterward
- Fluid administration may commence 2–12 hours before starting methotrexate, depending on a patient's fluid status
- Urine output should be at least 100 mL/hour before starting methotrexate infusion
- Maintain hydration at a rate that maintains urine output of at least 100 mL/hour until leucovorin use is completed

(continued)

Toxicity (N = 35)

	% All G	% G3/4
Neutropenia		81
Thrombocytopenia		35
Anemia		42
Mucositis	53	20
Infections		9
Pain		9
Elevated transaminases	13	

Therapy Monitoring

1. CBC with differential daily during chemotherapy and every other day after recovery of WBC > 500/mm^3 until either normal differential or persistent leukemia is documented. Platelet count every day while in hospital until patient no longer requires platelet transfusions
2. Electrolytes, mineral panel, serum creatinine, BUN, and uric acid at least daily during active treatment until the risk of tumor lysis has passed
3. Bone marrow aspirate/biopsy after each of the first 2 cycles
4. When in CR, bone marrow biopsy/aspirate should be perform every 3 months for the first 2 years

(continued)

Methotrexate
Patients <50 years: 150 mg/m² loading dose intravenously in 25–100 mL 0.9% NS or D5W over 30 minutes on day 1, *followed by:*
1350 mg/m² by continuous intravenous infusion in 250–1000 mL 0.9% NS or D5W over 23.5 hours on day 1 (total dosage/cycle, not including intrathecally administered doses = 1500 mg/m²)
Patients 50–65 years: 50 mg/m² loading dose intravenously in 25–50 mL 0.9% NS or D5W over 30 minutes on day 1, *followed by:*
450 mg/m² by continuous intravenous infusion in 100–1000 mL 0.9% NS or D5W over 23.5 hours on day 1 (total dosage/cycle, not including intrathecally administered doses = 500 mg/m²)

Notes:
- Measure serum methotrexate concentrations at *hours* 42 and 68 after methotrexate administration began
- The intensity and administration route for leucovorin are directed by serum methotrexate concentrations (see below)

Leucovorin calcium 30 mg/m² intravenously in 25–250 mL 0.9% NS or D5W over 15–30 minutes at 36 hours after methotrexate administration began (12 hours after methotrexate administration ends), *then:*
Leucovorin calcium 30 mg/m² orally at 42 hours after methotrexate administration began, *then:*
Leucovorin calcium 15 mg/m² orally at 48 hours after methotrexate administration began, *then:*
Leucovorin calcium 5 mg/m² per dose orally for 3 doses at 54, 68, and 78 hours after methotrexate administration began

Note: Leucovorin rescue is intensified for delayed methotrexate clearance

Time After Methotrexate Began	Serum Concentrations	Leucovorin Regimen
Hour 42	>0.5–5 micromol/L	Leucovorin calcium 50 mg/m² per dose intravenously every 6 hours for up to 60 hours
Hour 68	>0.01 mocromol/L	Leucovorin calcium 30 mg/m² per dose intravenously every 6 hours for 4 doses

Cyclophosphamide 200 mg/m² per day intravenously in 50–250 mL 0.9% NS or D5W over 15–60 minutes for 5 consecutive days on days 1–5 (total dosage/course = 1000 mg/m²)
Teniposide 100 mg/m² per day intravenously diluted with either D5W or 0.9% NS to produce a final teniposide concentration = 0.1 mg/mL, 0.2 mg/mL, 0.4 mg/mL, or 1 mg/mL over 60 minutes for 2 consecutive days on days 4 and 5 (total dosage/cycle = 200 mg/m²)
Doxorubicin 25 mg/m² per day intravenously via central venous access in 25–100 mL 0.9% NS or D5W over 15 minutes daily for 2 consecutive days on days 4 and 5 (total dosage/cycle = 50 mg/m²)
Dexamethasone 10 mg/m² per day orally for 5 consecutive days on days 1–5 (total dosage/cycle = 50 mg/m²)

CNS prophylaxis during block B:
Methotrexate 15 mg intrathecally via lumbar puncture in 6–15 mL *preservative-free* 0.9% NaCl injection (0.9% NS) on day 1 (total dose after 6 cycles, not including intravenously administered doses = 90 mg)
Cytarabine 40 mg intrathecally via lumbar puncture in 3–10 mL *preservative-free* 0.9% NS on day 1 (total dose after 6 cycles, not including intravenously administered doses = 240 mg)
Preservative-free dexamethasone 4 mg intrathecally via lumbar puncture in 4–10 mL *preservative-free* 0.9% NS on day 1 (total dose after 6 cycles = 24 mg)

(continued)

(continued)

Emetogenic potential during induction, block B:
Day 1 with methotrexate 1500 mg/m^2: High (Emetogenicity score = 5)
Day 1 with methotrexate 500 mg/m^2: Moderately high (Emetogenicity score = 4)
Days 2 and 3: Moderate (Emetogenicity score = 3)
Days 4 and 5: Moderately high (Emetogenicity score = 4). Potential for delayed symptoms. See Chapter 39 for antiemetic regimens

Supportive care: Antimicrobial prophylaxis
Routine gut decontamination and/or prophylactic antimicrobials should be administered according to institutional guidelines. The choice for antimicrobial prophylaxis varies among care providers (from day 1 until ANC > 500/mm^3):
Norfloxacin 400 mg orally twice daily, *or*
Valacyclovir 500 mg orally every 8 hours, *or*
Vancomycin 1 g intravenously daily

Dexamethasone is marketed in the United States in numerous generic formulations for oral administration, including prompt-release tablets containing 0.25, 0.5, 0.75, 1, 2, 4, and 6 mg, and in elixirs (which contain alcohol) and solutions for oral administration
Leucovorin calcium is manufactured in the United States in tablets for oral administration containing 5 mg, 10 mg, 15 mg, and 25 mg leucovorin calcium by various pharmaceutical manufacturers
Prednisone is marketed in the United States in numerous generic formulations for oral administration, including prompt-release tablets containing 1, 2.5, 5, 10, 20, and 50 mg, and in solutions and syrups for oral administration

Notes

1. If no CR is achieved, consider clinical trial or re-induction with another regimen
2. In the B-NHL86 study, patients in CR received additional CNS prophylaxis with 24 Gy cranial irradiation administered after the completion of the first 2 cycles (one A and one B)
3. Leukocyte-depleted blood products should be used for transfusion. Irradiation of all blood products is advised to reduce the risk of graft-versus-host disease in all immunosuppressed patients
4. Teniposide must be prepared and administered with containers and administrations sets that are not made of phthalate-plasticized polyvinyl chloride. Polyolefin and polyolefin lined containers and administrations generally are appropriate

REGIMEN FOR RELAPSED OR REFRACTORY T-LINEAGE (ALL) OR LYMPHOBLASTIC LYMPHOMA (LBL)

NELARABINE (ARRANON; 506U78)

De Angelo DJ et al. Blood 2002;100:198a, abstract 743 [CALGB Study 19801]
Gandhi V et al. JCO 2001;19:2142–2152
Prescribing information for Nelarabine Injection
www.fda.gov

Nelarabine 1500 mg/m^2 intravenously in 0.45% NaCl injection (0.45% NS) diluted to a concentration of 8 mg/mL over 2 hours on days 1, 3, and 5 every 21 days (total dosage/cycle = 4500 mg/m^2)

Emetogenic potential: Low–moderate (Emetogenicity score = 2–3). See Chapter 39 for antiemetic regimens

Treatment Modifications

None specified. Physician should be guided by toxicity profile

Toxicity (N = 39)

	% G3/4
Thrombocytopenia	47
Neutropenia	43
Anemia	26
Peripheral motor neuropathy	3
Depressed level of consciousness	3

Patient Population Studied

A study of 40 patients (22 with ALL and 18 with lymphoblastic lymphoma). Patients with > 25% lymphoblasts within the bone marrow were considered to have ALL. The lymphoblasts had to express at least two T-cell antigens. All patients were refractory to at least one induction regimen or in first or greater relapse after achieving a CR. Patients could not have evidence of CNS disease and had to have a calculated creatinine clearance of >50 mL/minute

Efficacy (N = 28)

Adult Patients with ≥2 Prior Chemotherapy Regimens	
Complete response (CR)	18%
CR*	4%
CR + CR*	22%
Duration of CR plus CR*	4 to 195+ weeks
Median overall survival	20.6 weeks
Survival at 1 year	29%

CR* complete response without hematologic recovery

Therapy Monitoring

1. *Weekly and before a treatment cycle:* CBC with differential, serum electrolytes, mineral panel
2. Response evaluation: Every 2 cycles

Notes

1. Preclinical studies have demonstrated that immature T lymphocytes and T lymphoblasts are extremely sensitive to the cytotoxic effects of deoxyguanosine and its derivative, ara-G (9-β-D-arabinofuranosylguanine). However ara-G is difficult to synthesize and poorly water-soluble. Nelarabine (2-amino-9-β-D-arabinofuranosyl-6-methoxy-9H-purine) is a water-soluble prodrug of ara-G. Nelarabine is rapidly demethylated in the serum by adenosine deaminase to ara-G and is converted to ara-GTP in T lymphoblasts
2. Nelarabine is indicated for the treatment of patients with T-cell ALL and T-cell lymphoblastic lymphoma whose disease has not responded to or has relapsed after treatment with at least two chemotherapy regimens. This use is based on the induction of complete responses
3. The alternate-day schedule is based on the prolonged intracellular retention ($t_{1/2}$, >24 hours) of ara-GTP, indicating that cytotoxic levels of ara-GTP may be retained for as long as 48 hours, thereby preventing the need for daily nelarabine infusions [Gandhi V et al. JCO 1998;16:3607–3615]. The alternate-day schedule of administering nelarabine as a single agent has demonstrated clinical efficacy in the setting of indolent leukemias [O'Brien S et al. Blood 1998;92:490a–491a]
4. Severe neurologic events have been reported with nelarabine. These events have included altered mental status including severe somnolence, central nervous system effects including convulsions, and peripheral neuropathy ranging from numbness to paresthesias to motor weakness and paralysis. There have also been reports of events associated with demyelination, and ascending peripheral neuropathies similar in appearance to Guillain-Barré syndrome

19. Leukemia, Acute Myelogenous

Ivan Aksentijevich, MD, Michael M. Boyiadzis, MD, MHSc, and Judith Karp, MD

Epidemiology

Incidence: 11,930 (2006)
Deaths: 9040 (2006)
Overall incidence: 2.5 cases per 100,000
Median age: 64 years (40 years for acute promyelocytic leukemia)
Male/female ratio: Male predilection slightly higher only in the elderly

Jemal A et al. CA Cancer J Clin 2006;56:106–30
Rohatiner A, Lister TA. Acute myelogenous leukemia. In: Henderson ES, Lister TA, Greaves MF, eds. Leukemia, 7th ed. Philadelphia: Saunders, 2002:485–517

Pathology

Type (Prevalence)	Characteristic	MPO	SB	NSE	Cytogenetics
M0 (3%)	No myelogenous differentiation (must demonstrate CD13 or CD33)	−	−	−	inv3q26,t(3;3)
M1 (15–20%)	Minimal evidence of granulocytic differentiation. MPO, azurophilic granules, and Auer rods	+	+	−	
M2 (25–30%)	Maturation beyond the promyelocytes. Promonocytes and monocytes <20%. Cells contain azurophilic granules and Auer rods	+	+	−	t(8;21),t(6;9)
M3, M3v (5–10%)	Abnormal promyelocytes with heavy granulation (variant has granulation that are not visible by light microscopy). The nuclei varies in size and shape and are often bi-lobed	+	+	−	t(15;17),t(5;17), t(11;17)
M4 (20%)	Granulocytic and monocytic differentiation. Promonocytes and monocytes > 20%	+	+	+	11q23,inv3q26, t(3;3)
M4eo (5–10%)	Same as M4 with variable number of abnormal eosinophils	+	+	+	inv16,t(16;16)
M5 (2–9%)	Large blasts with delicate lacy chromatin and occasional prominent vesicular nucleoli. The cytoplasm is basophilic	−	−	+	11q23, t(8;16)
M6 (3–5%)	Erythropoietic component exceeds 50% of all nucleated cells	+	+	−	t(1;22)
M7v (3–12%)	Blasts look like immature megakaryocytes; stain positive for factor VIII. Often marrow myelofibrosis	−	−	+	

MPO, myeloperoxydase; NSE, nonspecific esterase; SB, Sudan black
Löwenberg B et al. NEJM 1999;341:1051–1062

Work-Up

- H&P
- CBC, platelets, electrolytes, mineral panel, PT, PTT, fibrinogen, LDH
- Bone marrow biopsy with cytogenetics
- Immunophenotyping or cytochemistry
- HLA Typing (in patients considered potential bone marrow transplantation candidates)
- Cardiac scan if prior cardiac history or prior anthracycline use
- Lumbar puncture if symptomatic (should be performed if no mass/lesion is detected on imaging studies)
- FLT3 mutation evaluation is recommended

NCCN Clinical Practice Guidelines in Oncology, V. 1. 2006

Pathology (*continued*)

WHO Proposed Classification of Myelogenous Neoplasia

1. **AMLs with recurrent genetic abnormalities**
   - AML with t(8;21)(q22;q22), AML1 (AML1/ETO)
   - AML with abnormal bone marrow eosinophils and inv(16)(p13q22) or t(16;16)(p13;q11),CBFβ/MYH11X
   - Acute promyelocytic leukemia (AML with t(15;17)(q22;q11-12) and variants
   - AML with 11q23 (MLL) abnormalities
2. **AML with multilineage dysplasia**
   - Following prior myelodysplastic syndrome or myeloproliferative disorder
   - Without prior myelodysplastic syndrome or myeloproliferative disorder, but with dysplasia in at least 50% of cells in 2 or more lineages
3. **AML and myelodysplastic syndromes, therapy-related**
   - Alkylating agent-/radiation–related type
   - Topoisomerase II inhibitor–related type
   - Other types
4. **AML not otherwise categorized**
   - AML minimally differentiated
   - AML without maturation
   - AML with maturation
   - Acute myelomonocytic leukemia
   - Acute monocytic leukemia
   - Acute erythroid leukemia
   - Acute megakaryocytic leukemia
   - Acute basophilic leukemia
   - Acute panmyelosis with myelofibrosis
   - Myelogenous sarcoma
5. **Acute biphenotypic leukemias**

Vardiman JW et al. Blood 2002;100:2292–2302

Response Criteria for Acute Myelogenous Leukemia

Morphologic leukemia-free state
Bone marrow <5% blasts in an aspirate with spicules
No blasts or Auer rods or persistence of extramedullary disease

Complete remission (CR)
Morphologic leukemia-free state *and*

- Absolute neutrophil count $>1000/mm^3$
- Platelets $\geq 100{,}000/mm^3$
- No residual evidence of extramedullary disease

Notes:
Morphologic CR—patient independent of transfusions
Cytogenetic CR—cytogenetics normal (in those with previously abnormal cytogenetics)
Molecular CR—negative molecular studies in patients with acute promyelocytic leukemia or Ph+ leukemia

Patients who fail to achieve a CR are considered treatment failures. Relapse after a CR is defined as reappearance of leukemic blasts in the peripheral blood or the finding of more than 5% blasts in the bone marrow, not attributable to another cause
Cheson BD et al. JCO 2003;21:4642–4649

Cytogenetic Risk Groups

Favorable	Inv(16); t(15;17) with any abnormality; t(8;21) lacking del(9q) or complex karyotype
Standard	Normal or +8 or +21 or others
Unfavorable	−5del(5q); −7del(7q); inv(3q), abnormality of 11q, 20q, 21q, 17p, del(9q), t(6;9), t(9;22); complex karyotype with ≥3 abnormalities

Predictor of Poor Response to Induction	Predictor of Relapse
1. Unfavorable cytogenetics	1. Unfavorable cytogenetics
2. Age > 60 years	2. Age >60 years
3. MDR expression	3. MDR expression
4. CNS involvement	4. CNS involvement
5. AML in patient with history of MDS	5. Delayed response to induction therapy
6. AML secondary to chemotherapy	6. WBC $>20{,}000/mm^3$
7. Unfavorable immunophenotype	7. Female sex
8. CD34+	8. Increased LDH
9. Poor performance status	

	% Complete Response to Induction Chemotherapy	% 5-Year Overall Survival
Overall	50–75	10–30
Patient ≤60 years with standard and favorable cytogenetics	85	60–70
Patient ≤60 years with unfavorable cytogenetics	75	<20
Patient >60 years with standard and favorable cytogenetics	50	<20 at 2 years
Patient >60 years with unfavorable cytogenetics or poor performance status or >80 years	30	<10

Grimwade D et al. Blood 1998;92:2322–2333
Löwenberg B et al. NEJM 1999;341:1051–1062

Caveats

All patients with AML should be considered for enrollment in a clinical trial. In contrast to those with APL for whom the standard of care may achieve a higher cure rate, no satisfactory standard of care is yet available for those with AML

AML Other Than Acute Promyelocytic Leukemia (APL)

Patients ≤60 years, initial presentation
Induction therapy: **Cytarabine**, and either **daunorubicin, idarubicin, or mitoxantrone**
Note: The addition of etoposide to daunorubicin or mitoxantrone and cytarabine has improved complete response (CR) rates but not disease-free survival and overall survival. In addition, secondary leukemias may be induced
Postremission therapy: Required in all patients to prevent relapse
- ***Intermediate or poor risk cytogenetics:*** If an HLA-compatible sibling is available, allogeneic hematopoietic stem cell transplantation (HSCT) can be considered either immediately after induction or after a single intensive postremission therapy; this may include cytarabine 3000 mg/m^2 every 12 hours for 6 days *or* 3000 mg/m^2 every 12 hours on days 1, 3, and 5. If no HLA-compatible sibling is available after remission is achieved, consider a clinical trial or 2–4 additional cycles of cytarabine as described above
- ***Favorable risk cytogenetics:*** Multiple cycles of cytarabine are recommended over allogeneic HSCT. The role of autologous HSCT in such patients is not yet established

Patients >60 years, initial presentation
Induction therapy: Standard doses of **cytarabine**, and either **daunorubicin, idarubicin, or mitoxantrone**
Consolidation therapy: Either standard-dose cytarabine or cytarabine 1000–1500 mg/m^2 twice daily on days 1, 3, and 5, or for 6 days for 1–2 cycles. Lower doses may as effective. For patients > 70 years, 1000–1500 mg/m^2 for 5–6 days is reasonable, but lower doses may be equally effective. Autologous HSCT and low-intensity matched HSCT may be considered

Patients ≤60 years in first relapse
- *CR duration >6—12 months:* Re-treat with either the induction regimen they last received or a high-dose cytarabine-containing regimen. After a second CR, patients should be considered for an allogeneic HSCT or for autologous transplantation using autologous marrow that had been stored during the first remission
- *CR duration <6 months:* Enroll in a clinical trial or treat with matched-sibling allogeneic transplantation. The latter may provide the best outcome.

Patients >60 years in first relapse
Salvage therapy with gemtuzumab ozogamicin, enrollment in a clinical trial, or re-treatment with the previous induction regimen if the patient has achieved a long duration of remission

Acute Promyelocytic Leukemia

Initial presentation
Although treatment for other subtypes of AML need not necessarily start emergently, treatment for APL with all-*trans* retinoic acid should start as soon as the diagnosis is suspected because of the significant risks of bleeding, particularly intracranial bleeding. If t(15;17) is not confirmed, discontinue all-*trans* retinoic acid and treat as for other forms of AML
Note: Leukopheresis should not be performed in APL patients

(continued)

Caveats (*continued*)

Induction therapy: **All *trans*-**retinoic acid 45 mg/m^2 per day and an anthracycline-based chemotherapy (**idarubicin** 12 mg/m^2 per dose every other day for 4 doses, or **daunorubicin** 50–60 mg/m^2 per day for 3 days). If induction fails, consider a clinical trial, for example, with arsenic trioxide, matched-sibling HSCT, or alternative-donor HSCT.
Consolidation therapy: Patients who achieve a CR during induction should receive consolidation therapy with at least 2 cycles of an anthracycline-based chemotherapy—either **idarubicin** or **daunorubicin.** This should be followed by maintenance therapy with all-*trans* retinoic acid (45 mg/m^2 per day) either 1 week on followed by 1 week off, or treatment given during 15 consecutive days every 3 months. The **all-*trans*** retinoic acid is combined with **mercaptopurine** (60 mg/m^2 daily) + **methotrexate** (20 mg/m^2 for 1 dose per week). The duration of maintenance therapy is 1–2 years
Monitoring for residual disease: Polymerase chain reaction (PCR) should be routinely performed to monitor residual disease: every 3 months for 2 years, then every 6 months for 2–3 years. If the PCR converts from negative to positive, a confirmatory test should be done within 4–6 weeks

Tretinoin (all-*trans* retinoic acid; ATRA) is manufactured in the United States in capsules for oral administration, which contain 10 mg tretinoin. VESANOID® (tretinoin) CAPSULES. Distributed by Roche Laboratories, Inc, Nutley, NJ
Mercaptopurine is manufactured in the United States in capsules for oral administration, which contain 50 mg mercaptopurine (Generic formulations and Purinethol®, GlaxoSmithKline, Research Triangle Park, NC)

APL in first relapse

Treat with arsenic trioxide to a second CR followed by autologous HSCT with reinfusion of molecularly negative PBSCs or allogeneic HSCT in younger patients if a suitable donor is available

Evaluation and Treatment of CNS Leukemia

Asymptomatic patients: Routine lumbar puncture should not be performed in asymptomatic newly diagnosed patients with AML
Symptomatic patients: Symptomatic patients should have imaging studies first to exclude CNS bleeding or infiltrative or mass lesions (chloromas). A lumbar puncture should be performed in symptomatic patients after coagulopathy has been corrected and imaging studies have not detected any mass or other lesion. In patients with cytologically positive CSF, an Ommaya reservoir should be placed, if possible, to administer intrathecal therapy with cytarabine (30 mg), methotrexate (15 mg), and hydrocortisone (15 mg) twice weekly until the CSF is clear, then weekly for 6 weeks. Induction chemotherapy should be started concurrently. Radiation therapy should be considered in patients with a chloroma that causes focal neurologic deficits
Patients in remission: Routine lumbar puncture should not be performed in patients in remission except for those with FAB M4 or M5 morphology or with WBC counts >100,000/mm^3 at diagnosis. Patients with positive cytology should be treated with intrathecal therapy with cytarabine (30 mg), methotrexate (15 mg), and hydrocortisone (15 mg) twice weekly until clear, then weekly for 6 weeks, *or* reevaluated for CNS disease or clearance after the first cycle of high-dose cytarabine therapy

Kimby E et al. Acta Oncologica 2001;40:231–252
Löwenberg B, Griffin JD, Tallman MS. Acute myeloid leukemia and acute promyelocytic leukemia. Hematology 2003:82–101
Tallman MS et al. Blood 2005;106:1154–1163
NCCN Clinical Practice Guidelines in Oncology, vol. 1, 2006

Hyperleukocytosis in AML

Incidence: The frequency of hyperleukocytosis (conventionally and arbitrarily defined as a WBC count or blast count >100,000/mm^3) ranges from 5% to 13% in adult patients with AML
Risk factors: Factors associated with hyperleukocytosis in AML include FAB M4, M5, APL microgranular variant, 11q23 rearrangements, inv(16),(p13q22), and chromosome 6 abnormalities
Symptoms: Symptoms may arise from the involvement of any organ, but intracranial hemorrhages and respiratory failure account for most deaths (cautiously interpret ABGs: spuriously low PaO_2 can result from rapid consumption of plasma oxygen by the markedly increased number of WBCs). In many patients, leukostasis becomes evident a few days after diagnosis and sometimes after the first leukocytoreduction. Clinical deterioration and death may occur after the blast count has been significantly reduced.
Note: This suggests that although leukocytoreduction is an important step in the management of leukostasis, additional measures are needed to prevent leukostasis-related deaths
Treatment: Prompt leukocytoreduction, initiation of chemotherapy, and supportive care. *Leukocytoreduction* can be achieved with hydroxyurea or leukopheresis.

1. **Hydroxyurea** should be started immediately in all patients with hyperleukocytic AML. Hydroxyurea 12.5–25 mg/kg per dose orally 4 times daily, *or* 17–33 mg/kg per dose orally 3 times daily, reduces the WBC count 50–80% within 24–48 hours

Hydroxyurea is marketed in the United States as capsules for oral administration containing hydroxyurea 200, 300, or 400 mg, Droxia™ (hydroxyurea capsules); and as capsules for oral administration containing hydroxyurea 500 mg, Hydrea™ (hydroxyurea capsules

(*continued*)

Caveats (*continued*)

2. **Leukopheresis** is recommended for patients with WBCs >100,000/mm^3 and symptoms of leukostasis. Disadvantages of leukopheresis are:
    - It requires a large-caliber central venous catheter that is not always available
    - It may worsen the thrombocytopenia
    - Because it is not cytostatic, rebound leukocytosis may occur
    - No guidelines area available for the absolute WBC to be achieved

Note: The most consistent success has been achieved using a continuous-flow procedure in which large volumes (8–10 L) of patient blood are processed

Grima KM. J Clin Apher 2000;15:28–52
Porcu P et al. Ther Apher 2002;6:15–23

REGIMEN FOR PROPHYLAXIS AGAINST AND TREATMENT OF TUMOR LYSIS SYNDROME

HYDRATION, HYPERURICEMIA AND HYPERPHOSPHATEMIA

Prophylaxis Against Tumor Lysis Syndrome

See also Chapter 46, Oncologic Emergencies

1. Hydration

2500–3000 mL/day as tolerated, 5% dextrose/0.45% NaCl injection (D5W/0.45% NS) with sodium bicarbonate injection 100 mEq/1000 mL intravenously at 100–150 mL/hour (2400–3600 mL/day)

Notes:

- **Potassium** is not added to parenteral hydration solutions during the first few days of induction therapy unless serum potassium decreases to <3.0 mEq/dL
- **Furosemide** 20–40 mg intravenously every 12–24 hours to maintain fluid balance. Diuresis is maintained for at least the first 72 hours after starting chemotherapy in the absence of metabolic aberrations or after metabolic complications normalize

2. Hyperuricemia

Hyperuricemia develops within 24–48 hours after initiating chemotherapy when the excretory capacity of the renal tubules is exceeded. In the presence of an acid pH, uric acid crystals form in the renal tubule, leading to intraluminal renal tubular obstruction, an acute renal obstructive uropathy, and renal dysfunction

Urinary alkalization

Increases the solubility and excretion of uric acid and helps avoid **uric acid** crystallization in renal tubules; however, alkalinization is not uniformly recommended because:

- It favors precipitation of calcium/phosphate complexes in renal tubules, a concern in patients with concomitant hyperphosphatemia
- The metabolic alkalemia that may result from the administration of bicarbonate can worsen the neurologic manifestations of hypocalcemia
- At urine pH >6.5, the solubility of **xanthine** and **hypoxanthine** significantly decreases, leading to urinary xanthine crystals during and after allopurinol therapy

Administer allopurinol Orally or intravenously starting 12 hours to 3 days (preferably 2–3 days) before starting cytoreductive chemotherapy

Initial dosage:

- 100 mg/m^2 per dose orally every 8 hours (maximum daily dose = 800 mg), *or*
- 3.3 mg/kg per dose orally every 8 hours (maximum daily dose = 800 mg), *or*
- 200–400 mg/m^2 per day intravenously (maximum daily dose = 600 mg)

Maintenance dosage: Should be based on serum uric acid determinations performed approximately 48 hours after initiation of allopurinol therapy and periodically thereafter. Continue administering allopurinol until leukemic blasts have been cleared from the peripheral blood

Allopurinol dose adjustments for impaired renal function:

Creatinine Clearance	Oral Allopurinol Dose
10–20 mL/min	200 mg/day
3–10 mL/min	100 mg/day
<3 mL/min	100 mg every 36–48 hours

Notes:

- The incidence of allergic reactions is increased in patients receiving amoxicillin, ampicillin, or thiazide diuretics
- Side effects include rash (1.5%), nausea (1.3%), vomiting (1.2%), and renal insufficiency (1.2%)

Allopurinol is available in the United States generically as immediate-release tablets for oral administration containing 100 mg or 300 mg allopurinol

3. Hyperphosphatemia

Correction of hyperphosphatemia (and hypocalcemia):

Hyperphosphatemia develops within 24–48 hours after of initiation of chemotherapy and may lead to tissue precipitation of calcium phosphate, resulting in hypocalcemia, intrarenal calcifications, nephrocalcinosis, and acute obstructive uropathy. Treatment of hyperphosphatemia usually corrects any related hypocalcemia. Therefore, calcium administration should be given only to patients with symptoms related to hypocalcemia

Oral phosphate binders: **Aluminum hydroxide** 15–30 mL orally every 6 hours

Hemodialysis is the most effective therapeutic strategy. Consider hemodialysis if hyperphosphatemia is severe, especially in the setting of renal failure and symptomatic hypocalcemia. The clearance of phosphorus is better with hemodialysis than with continuous venovenous hemofiltration or continuous peritoneal dialysis

REGIMEN

STANDARD-DOSE CYTARABINE + DAUNORUBICIN

Wiernik PH et al. Blood 1992;79:313–319

See Regimen for Prophylaxis Against and Treatment of Tumor Lysis Syndrome earlier in chapter. Also see Chapter 46, Oncologic Emergencies

Cytarabine 100 mg/m^2 per day by continuous intravenous infusion in 100–1000 mL 0.9% NaCl Injection (0.9% NS) or 5% dextrose injection (D5W) over 24 hours for 7 consecutive days on days 1–7 (total dosage/cycle = 700 mg/m^2)
Daunorubicin 45 mg/m^2 per day intravenously per push over 3–5 minutes for 3 consecutive days on days 1–3 (total dosage/cycle = 135 mg/m^2).
Note: The optimal induction dose of daunorubicin is unknown. Daunorubicin 45–60 mg/m^2 is typically used

Supportive care: Antimicrobial prophylaxis
Routine gut decontamination and/or prophylactic antimicrobials should be administered according to institutional guidelines. The choice for antimicrobial prophylaxis varies among care providers (from day 1 until ANC >500/mm^3):

Norfloxacin 400 mg orally twice daily, *or*
Valacyclovir 500 mg orally every 8 hours, *or*
Vancomycin 1 g intravenously daily

Note:
Multiple studies have established the safety of hematopoietic growth factors when administered after induction therapy to reduce the period of neutropenia. Growth factors should be initiated in patients only after BM biopsy demonstrates a hypoplastic bone marrow following induction therapy. However, G-CSF (or other forms of G-CSF) should be discontinued for at least 7 days before obtaining bone marrow to document a response

Emetogenic potential:
Days 1–3: Moderately high (Emetogenicity score = 4)
Days 4–7: Low (Emetogenicity score = 2). See Chapter 39 for antiemetic regimens

Patient Population Studied

A study of 113 patients (median age 55 years) with newly diagnosed AML

Efficacy (N = 111)

Complete Response (CR)	%
<50 years	70
51–59 years	65
>60 years	44
Induction CR	58
With 1 course	38

Treatment Modifications

Adverse Event	Dose Modification
Serum creatinine >3 mg/dL (>264 µmol)	Reduce daunorubicin dosage by 50%
Bilirubin 2.5–5.0 mg/dL (43–85.5 µmol/L)	
Bilirubin >5 mg/dL (>85.5 µmol/L)	Hold daunorubicin

Toxicity (N = 111)

Adverse Event	% Patients
Fever	100
Infection	92
Nausea	82
Diarrhea	78
Anorexia	71
Vomiting	66
Stomatitis	63
Hemorrhage	56
Hyperbilirubinemia (>1.25 × ULN)	45
Alopecia (G3/4)	37
Dysphagia	18
Esophagitis	13
Phlebitis	7
WBC< 1000/mm^3	Median 22.5 days (range: 0–240 days)
Platelets < 50,000/mm^3	Median 29 days (range: 0–239 days)

Note: Most toxicities reported were grades 1–2: 21 deaths (23%) occurred during induction therapy; 2 patients died from intracranial bleeding; 7 patients died from hypoplastic marrow; 2 patients died from progressive disease; 12 patients died of unknown causes

Therapy Monitoring

1. CBC with differential daily during chemotherapy and every other day after recovery of WBC >500/mm^3 until either normal differential or persistent leukemia is documented. Platelet count every day while in hospital until patient no longer requires platelet transfusions
2. Electrolytes, mineral panel, uric acid at least daily during active treatment until risk of tumor lysis has passed
3. Bone marrow aspirate/biopsy 7–10 days after chemotherapy is completed to document hypoplasia. If hypoplasia is not documented or indeterminate, repeat biopsy in 7–14 days to identify whether leukemia persists. If bone marrow is hypoplastic, repeat the biopsy at the time of hematologic recovery to document a remission

Notes

1. A standard regimen that is effective in all cytogenetic subtypes
2. Leukocyte-depleted blood products should be used for transfusion. Irradiation of all blood products is advised to reduce the risk of graft-versus-host disease in all immunosuppressed patients
3. Cumulative lifetime daunorubicin dosages >550 mg/m^2 are associated with an increased risk of drug-induced congestive heart failure in adults. In patients who received radiation therapy that encompassed the heart, daunorubicin-induced heart failure has occurred at cumulative lifetime dosages of 400 mg/m^2. The total daunorubicin dosage should take into account previous and current therapies with other potentially cardiotoxic agents, particularly related compounds such as doxorubicin
4. Screening lumbar puncture should be considered at first remission for patients with FAB M4 or M5 morphology or WBC counts >100,000/mm^3 at diagnosis
5. If the bone marrow has residual blasts (≥ 5%), give additional therapy with either standard-dose cytarabine and an anthracycline or high-dose cytarabine. Reinduction should be initiated without delay

REGIMEN

STANDARD-DOSE CYTARABINE + IDARUBICIN

Vogler WR et al. Blood 1992;10:1103–1011

See Regimen for Prophylaxis Against and Treatment of Tumor Lysis Syndrome earlier in chapter. Also see Chapter 46, Oncologic Emergencies

Cytarabine 100 mg/m^2 per day by continuous intravenous infusion in 100–1000 mL 0.9% NaCl injection (0.9% NS) or 5% dextrose injection (D5W) over 24 hours for 7 consecutive days on days 1–7 (total dosage/cycle = 700 mg/m^2)
Idarubicin 12 mg/m^2 per day intravenously diluted to a concentration of 1–10 mg/100 mL in 0.9% NS or D5W over 15–30 minutes for 3 consecutive days on days 1–3 (total dosage/cycle = 36 mg/m^2)

Supportive care: Antimicrobial prophylaxis
Routine gut decontamination and/or prophylactic antimicrobials should be administered according to institutional guidelines. The choice for antimicrobial prophylaxis varies among care providers (from day 1 until ANC >500/mm^3):

Norfloxacin 400 mg orally twice daily, *or*
Valacyclovir 500 mg orally every 8 hours, *or*
Vancomycin 1 g intravenously daily)

Notes:
Multiple studies have established the safety of hematopoietic growth factors when administered after induction therapy to reduce the period of neutropenia. Growth factors should be initiated in patients only after BM biopsy demonstrates a hypoplastic bone marrow following induction therapy. However, G-CSF (or other forms of G-CSF) should be discontinued for at least 7 days before obtaining bone marrow to document a response

Emetogenic potential:
Days 1–3: Moderately high (Emetogenicity score = 4)
Days 4–7: Low (Emetogenicity score = 2). See Chapter 39 for antiemetic regimens

Patient Population Studied

A study of 111 patients (median age 60 years) with newly diagnosed AML

Efficacy (N = 105)

Complete Response (CR)	%
15–50 years (n = 29)	86
51–60 years (n = 24)	71
>60 years (n = 52)	63
Induction CR	69
With 1 course	77
Median time to CR	42 days

Toxicity (N = 105)

Adverse Event	%G1/2	%G3/4
Nausea and vomiting	76	6
Diarrhea	57	16
Mucositis	43	7
Skin rash	41	5
Hair loss	37	40
Cardiac	5	11
↑ SGOT	47	5
↑ Alkaline phosphatase	52	5
↑ Serum creatinine	29	2

	Mean Duration of Aplasia (days)
WBC < 1000/mm^3	31.2
Platelets < 50,000/mm^3	35.1

Treatment Modifications

Adverse Event	Dose Modification
Serum creatinine >3 mg/dL (>364 µmol/L	Reduce idarubicin dosage by 50%
Bilirubin 2.5–5.0 mg/dL (43–85.5 µmol/L)	Reduce idarubicin dosage by 50%
Bilirubin > 5 mg/dL (>85.5 µmol/L)	Hold idarubicin

Therapy Monitoring

1. CBC with differential daily during chemotherapy and every other day after recovery of WBC > 500/mm^3 until either normal differential or persistent leukemia is documented. Platelet count every day while in hospital until the patient no longer requires platelet transfusions
2. Electrolytes, mineral panel, uric acid at least daily during active treatment until risk of tumor lysis has passed
3. Bone marrow aspirate/biopsy 7–10 days after chemotherapy is completed to document hypoplasia. If hypoplasia is not documented or indeterminate, repeat biopsy in 7–14 days to identify whether leukemia persists. If bone marrow is hypoplastic, repeat the biopsy at the time of hematologic recovery to document a remission

Notes

1. Leukocyte-depleted blood products should be used for transfusion. Irradiation of all blood products is advised to reduce the risk of graft-versus-host disease in all immunosuppressed patients
2. Screening lumbar puncture should be considered at first remission for patients with FAB M4 or M5 morphology or WBC counts >100,000/mm^3 at diagnosis
3. If the bone marrow has residual blasts (≥5%), give additional therapy with either standard-dose cytarabine and anthracycline or high-dose cytarabine. Reinduction should be initiated without delay

REGIMEN

STANDARD-DOSE CYTARABINE + MITOXANTRONE

Arlin Z et al. Leukemia 1990;4:177–183

See Regimen for Prophylaxis Against and Treatment of Tumor Lysis Syndrome earlier in chapter. Also see Chapter 46, Oncologic Emergencies

Cytarabine 100 mg/m^2 per day by continuous intravenous infusion in 100–1000 mL 0.9% NaCl injection (0.9% NS) or 5% dextrose injection (D5W) over 24 hours for 7 consecutive days on days 1–7 (total dosage/cycle = 700 mg/m^2)
Mitoxantrone 12 mg/m^2 per day intravenously in 50–100 mL 0.9% NS or D5W over 15–30 minutes for 3 consecutive days on days 1–3 (total dosage/cycle = 36 mg/m^2)

Supportive care: Antimicrobial prophylaxis
Routine gut decontamination and/or prophylactic antimicrobials should be administered according to institutional guidelines. The choice for antimicrobial prophylaxis varies among care providers (from day 1 until ANC >500/mm^3):

- **Norfloxacin** 400 mg orally twice daily, *or*
- **Valacyclovir** 500 mg orally every 8 hours, *or*
- **Vancomycin** 1 g intravenously daily

Notes:
Multiple studies have established the safety of hematopoietic growth factors when administered after induction therapy to reduce the period of neutropenia. Growth factors should be initiated in patients only after BM biopsy demonstrates a hypoplastic bone marrow following induction therapy. However, G-CSF (or other forms of G-CSF) should be discontinued for at least 7 days before obtaining bone marrow to document a response

Emetogenic potential:
Days 1–3: Moderately high (Emetogenicity score = 4)
Days 4–7: Low (Emetogenicity score = 2). See Chapter 39 for antiemetic regimens

Treatment Modifications

Adverse Event	Dose Modification
Bilirubin 2.5–5.0 mg/dL	Reduce mitoxantrone dosage by 50%
Bilirubin >5 mg/dL	Hold mitoxantrone

Therapy Monitoring

1. CBC with differential daily during chemotherapy and every other day after recovery of WBC >500/mm^3 until either normal differential or persistent leukemia is documented. Platelets every day while in hospital until patient no longer requires platelet transfusions
2. Electrolytes, mineral panel, uric acid at least daily during active treatment until the risk of tumor lysis has passed
3. Bone marrow aspirate/biopsy 7–10 days after chemotherapy is completed to document hypoplasia. If hypoplasia is not documented or indeterminate, repeat biopsy in 7–14 days to identify whether leukemia persists. If bone marrow is hypoplastic, repeat the biopsy at the time of hematologic recovery to document a remission

Patient Population Studied

A study of 108 patients (median age 60 years) with newly diagnosed AML

Efficacy (N = 98)

Overall complete response (CR)	63%
CR <60 years	80%
CR ≥60 years	46%
Median time to CR	35 days

Toxicity (N = 97)

	% of Patients
Fever	82
Infections	80
Nausea/vomiting	78
Alopecia	50
Sepsis	49
Bleeding	44
Stomatitis/mucositis	38
Hepatic	17

Notes

1. Leukocyte-depleted blood products should be used for transfusion. Irradiation of all blood products is advised to reduce the risk of graft-versus-host disease in all immunosuppressed patients
2. Screening lumbar puncture should be considered at first remission for patients with M4 or M5 morphology or WBC counts >100,000/mm^3 at diagnosis
3. If the bone marrow has residual blasts (≥5%), give additional therapy with either standard-dose cytarabine and anthracycline or high-dose cytarabine. Reinduction should be initiated without delay

REGIMEN

HIGH-DOSE CYTARABINE + DAUNORUBICIN

Weick JK et al. Blood 1996;88:2841–2851

See Regimen for Prophylaxis Against and Treatment of Tumor Lysis Syndrome earlier in chapter. Also see Chapter 46, Oncologic Emergencies

Cytarabine 2000 mg/m² per dose by intravenous infusion as undiluted drug or diluted in 50–250 mL 0.9% NaCl injection (0.9% NS) or 5% dextrose injection (D5W) over 60 minutes every 12 hours for 12 doses, days 1–6 (total dosage/cycle = 24,000 mg/m²)
Daunorubicin 45 mg/m² per day intravenously per push over 3–5 minutes for 3 consecutive days on days 7–9 (total dosage/cycle = 135 mg/m²)

Supportive care:
- Keratitis prophylaxis: steroid eye drops (prednisolone 1% or dexamethasone 0.1%) daily until 24 hours after completing high-dose cytarabine therapy
- Routine gut decontamination and/or prophylactic antimicrobials should be administered according to institutional guidelines. The choice for antimicrobial prophylaxis varies among care providers (from day 1 until ANC >500/mm³):
  Norfloxacin 400 mg orally twice daily, *or*
  Valacyclovir 500 mg orally every 8 hours, *or*
  Vancomycin 1 g intravenously daily

Notes:
Multiple studies have established the safety of hematopoietic growth factors when administered after induction therapy to reduce the period of neutropenia. Growth factors should be initiated in patients only after BM biopsy demonstrates a hypoplastic bone marrow following induction therapy. However, G-CSF (or other forms of G-CSF) should be discontinued for at least 7 days before obtaining bone marrow to document a response

Emetogenic potential:
Days 1–6: Moderately high (Emetogenicity score = 4)
Days 7–9: Moderate (Emetogenicity score = 3). See Chapter 39 for antiemetic regimens

Toxicity

Adverse Event	n = 84, <50 years			n = 86, 50–64 years		
	G3	G4	G5	G3	G4	G5
Hepatic/abnormal LFTs	5	4	0	6	2	0
Neurologic	6	0	1	4	0	0
Mucositis	3	0	0	1	0	0
Nausea, vomiting, anorexia	3	0	0	4	0	0
Infection	1	1	9	2	2	14
Fatal hemorrhage	0	0	2	0	0	1

G3, severe; G4, life-threatening; G5, death

Note:
- Onset of cerebellar toxicity generally occurs 5–10 days after the start of therapy; findings include nystagmus, ataxia, and dysarthria. Symptoms usually resolve over 2–3 weeks after completing treatment; however, recovery can be delayed for months
- Ophthalmologic toxicity with high-dose cytarabine is common. Patients develop conjunctivitis and corneal toxicity consisting of photophobia, redness, tearing, and blurred vision. Visual acuity may decrease. Prophylactic topical ophthalmic corticosteroid products decrease the severity of ocular complications

Bolwell BJ et al. Leukemia 1988;2:253–260

Treatment Modifications

Dose Adjustments Based on Renal Function*

Serum Creatinine	Cytarabine Dosage
<1.5 mg/dL (<133 μmol/L) doses	2000 mg/m² every 12 hours for 12 doses
1.5–1.9 mg/dL (133–168 μmol/L), or an increase from baseline by 0.5–1.2 mg/dL (44–106 μmol/L)	1000 mg/m² every 12 hours for 12 doses
≥2.0 mg/dL (177 μmol/L), or an increase >1.2 mg/dL (106 μmol/L)	100 mg/m² per day by continuous infusion over 24 hours for up to 6 days

*The risk of neurotoxicity with high-dose cytarabine is directly related to renal function throughout therapy

Adverse Event	Dose Modification
Bilirubin 1.5–2.9 mg/dL	Reduce daunorubicin dosage by 50%
Bilirubin >3 mg/dL (>51.3 μmol/L)	Hold daunorubicin
Neurologic toxicity	Hold cytarabine. Patients who develop CNS symptoms should not subsequently receive high-dose cytarabine
Patients with rapidly rising serum creatinine due to tumor lysis	Hold cytarabine

Patient Population Studied

A study of 172 patients (median age 50 years) with newly diagnosed AML

Efficacy (N = 172)

Complete response <50 years	55%
Complete response 50–64 years	45%

Therapy Monitoring

1. CBC with differential daily during chemotherapy and every other day after recovery of WBC >500/mm^3 until either normal differential or persistent leukemia is documented. Platelet count every day while in hospital until patient no longer requires platelet transfusions
2. Electrolytes, serum creatinine and BUN, mineral panel, uric acid at least daily during active treatment until the risk of tumor lysis has passed
3. Bone marrow aspirate/biopsy 7–10 days after chemotherapy is completed to document hypoplasia. If hypoplasia is not documented or indeterminate, repeat biopsy in 7–14 days to determine whether leukemia persists. If bone marrow is hypoplastic, repeat the biopsy at the time of hematologic recovery to document a remission

Notes

1. Patients who receive high-dose cytarabine need to be closely monitored for changes in renal function. Renal dysfunction is highly correlated with an increased risk of cerebellar toxicity. Patients must be monitored for nystagmus, dysmetria, and ataxia before each dose of high-dose cytarabine
2. Leukocyte-depleted blood products should be used for transfusion. Irradiation of all blood products is advised to reduce the risk of graft-versus-host disease in all immunosuppressed patients
3. Screening lumbar puncture should be considered at first remission for patients with FAB M4 or M5 morphology or WBC counts >100,000/mm^3 at diagnosis
4. If the bone marrow has residual blasts (5%), give additional therapy. Additional high-dose cytarabine is unlikely to achieve remission. If a sibling donor has been identified, an allogeneic HSCT may salvage 25–30% of patients with induction failure. If a donor is not immediately available, patients should be considered for a clinical trial

REGIMEN

HIGH-DOSE CYTARABINE

Bloomfield CD et al. Cancer Res 1998;56:4173–4179
Mayer RJ et al. NEJM 1994;331:896–903

See Regimen for Prophylaxis Against and Treatment of Tumor Lysis Syndrome earlier in chapter. Also see Chapter 46, Oncologic Emergencies

Cytarabine 3000 mg/m^2 per dose by intravenous infusion in 100–1000 mL 0.9% NaCl injection (0.9% NS) or 5% dextrose injection (D5W) over 3 hours every 12 hours (12-hour interval between the start of each dose; 2 doses per day) for 6 doses on days 1, 3, and 5 every 28 days for 4 cycles (total dosage/cycle = 18,000 mg/m^2)

Supportive care:

- Keratitis prophylaxis: steroid eye drops (prednisolone 1% or dexamethasone 0.1%) daily until 24 hours after high-dose cytarabine is completed
- Routine gut decontamination and/or prophylactic antimicrobials should be administered according to institutional guidelines. The choice for antimicrobial prophylaxis varies among care providers (from day 1 until ANC >500/mm^3):

  Norfloxacin 400 mg orally twice daily, *or*

  Valacyclovir 500 mg orally every 8 hours, *or*

  Vancomycin 1 g intravenously daily

Emetogenic potential:
Days 1, 3, and 5: High (Emetogenicity score ~5). Potential for delayed symptoms. See Chapter 39 for antiemetic regimens

Patient Population Studied

A study of 596 patients in complete remission after induction chemotherapy (daunorubicin + cytarabine) randomly assigned to receive 4 cycles of cytarabine at one of three 5-day dosage schedules: low-dose cytarabine by continuous infusion, moderate-dose cytarabine by continuous infusion, or high-dose cytarabine administered intermittently

Treatment Modifications

Dose Adjustments Based on Renal Function*

Serum Creatinine	Cytarabine Dosage
<1.5 mg/dL (<133 μmol/L)	2000 mg/m^2 every 12 hours for 12 doses
1.5–1.9 mg/dL (133–168 μmol/L), or an increase from baseline by 0.5–1.2 mg/dL (44–106 μmol/L)	1000 mg/m^2 every 12 hours for 12 doses
≥2.0 mg/dL (177 μmol/L), or an increase >1.2 mg/dL (106 μmol/L)	100 mg/m^2 per day by continuous infusion over 24 hours for up to 6 days

*The risk of neurotoxicity with high does cytarabine is directly related to renal function throughout therapy

Adverse Event	Dose Modification
Neurologic toxicity	Hold cytarabine. Patients who develop CNS symptoms should not receive subsequent high dose cytarabine
Patients with rapidly rising serum creatinine due to tumor lysis	Hold cytarabine

Efficacy

4 Years After Randomization	Cytarabine		
	% LD	% MD	% HD
Alive	31	35	46
Continuous CR (<60 years)	24	29	44
Disease-free (≥60 years)	<16	<16	<16

Cytogenetics	Disease-Free 4 Years After High-Dose Cytarabine
Good-risk	60%
Intermediate risk	30%
Poor risk	12%

LD, low-dose cytarabine: 100 mg/m^2 by continuous intravenous infusion over 24 hours for 5 days
MD, moderate-dose cytarabine: 400 mg/m^2 by continuous infusion over 24 hours
HD, high-dose cytarabine: 3000 mg/m^2 over 3 hours twice daily on days 1, 3, and 5 for 6 doses
Bloomfield CD et al. Cancer Res 1998;56:4173–4179
Mayer RJ et al. NEJM 1994;331:896–903

Toxicity

	% Patients Who Received 4 Planned Cycles		
	LD CIVI	MD CIVI	HD Int
All patients	76	74	56
Patients ≤60 years	78	76	62

Cytarabine Regimens	% Cycles in Which Patients Were Hospitalized	% Serious CNS Toxicity	% Deaths During Remission
LD CIVI	16	0	1
MD CIVI	59	0	6
HD Int	71	12%	5

LD CIVI, low dose continuous intravenous infusion; cytarabine 100 mg/m^2 per day by continuous intravenous infusion over 24 hours for 5 days on days 1–5
MD CIVI, moderate dose by continuous intravenous infusion; cytarabine 400 mg/m^2 per day by continuous intravenous infusion over 24 hours for 5 days on days 1–5
HD Int, high dose by intermittent administration schedule; 3000 mg/m^2 per dose by intravenous infusion over 3 hours twice daily on days 1, 3, and 5 for 6 doses

Therapy Monitoring

1. CBC with differential and platelet count daily during chemotherapy
2. Electrolytes, serum creatinine, BUN, LFTs, mineral panel daily during chemotherapy
3. Outpatient monitoring after chemotherapy: CBC with differential, platelet count, and electrolytes 2–3 times weekly until recovery
4. Bone marrow biopsy/aspirate only if peripheral blood counts are abnormal or failure to recover counts within 5 weeks

Notes

1. This trial of postremission therapy for AML demonstrated a significant dose-response effect for cytarabine. Patients ≤60 years who received high-dose cytarabine were more likely to remain in remission and to survive longer than similar patients who received lower doses
2. Patients who receive high-dose cytarabine need to be closely monitored for changes in renal function. Renal dysfunction is highly correlated with increased risk of cerebellar toxicity. Patients need to be monitored for nystagmus, dysmetria, and ataxia before each dose of cytarabine

REGIMEN

GEMTUZUMAB OZOGAMICIN

Larson RA et al. Leukemia 2002;16:1627–1636

See Regimen for Prophylaxis Against and Treatment of Tumor Lysis Syndrome earlier in chapter. Also see Chapter 46, Oncologic Emergencies

Premedication and Supportive care:
Diphenhydramine 50 mg orally 60 minutes before starting gemtuzumab ozogamicin
Acetaminophen 650–1000 mg orally 60 minutes before starting gemtuzumab ozogamicin, *plus*
Acetaminophen 650–1000 mg orally every 4 hours for 2 doses as needed for febrile reactions to gemtuzumab ozogamicin

Gemtuzumab ozogamicin 9 mg/m^2 by intravenous infusion in 100–1000 mL 0.9% NaCl injection (0.9% NS) over 2 hours every 14 days (total of 2 doses = 18 mg/m^2)

Emetogenic potential: Low (Emetogenicity score = 2). See Chapter 39 for antiemetic regimens

Treatment Modifications

Renal Impairment

There are no controlled trials demonstrating the efficacy and safety of gemtuzumab ozogamicin in patients with renal function impairment. In one case report, gemtuzumab ozogamicin was administered in a patient receiving hemodialysis. After receiving two infusions, no excessive toxicities were seen, and a bone marrow biopsy revealed a normocellular marrow

Hepatic Impairment

Patients with a serum total bilirubin >2 mg/dL (34.2 μmol/L) were not studied. Extra caution should be used when administering gemtuzumab ozogamicin to patients with any hepatic impairment. Full hematologic recovery is not required to give a second dose

Patient Population Studied

A study of 101 patients >60 years (median age 69 years) with CD33-positive AML in first relapse

Efficacy (N = 101)

	Median Time to Remission	Remission Rates	Median Relapse-Free Survival
Overall		28%	3.3 months
Complete response (CR)	65 days	13%	6.8 months
CRp (complete response with incomplete platelet recovery)	75 days	15%	2.2 months

Toxicity (N = 101)

Infusion-Related Adverse Events

Chills	10%
Hypotension	6%
Fever	4%

Adverse Events After Treatment

	% G3/4
Neutropenia	99
Thrombocytopenia	99
Hyperbilirubinemia	24
AST/ALT elevation	15
Death[a]	14
Fever	14
Severe bleeding[b]	11
Anemia	13
Chills	13
Dyspnea	12
Hypertension	12
Nausea/vomiting	12
Hypotension	6

[a]The causes of death included disease progression (n = 9), cerebral hemorrhage (n = 2), sepsis (n = 2), and infection (n = 1)

[b]Most frequently cerebral hemorrhage (3%) and epistaxis (3%)

Notes:

1. Hepatic veno-occlusive disease (VOD) has been reported in association with gemtuzumab ozogamicin taken as a single agent, as part of a combination chemotherapy regimen, and in patients without a history of liver disease or HSCT
2. Patients who receive gemtuzumab ozogamicin either before or after HSCT, patients with underlying hepatic disease or abnormal liver function, and patients receiving gemtuzumab ozogamicin in combinations with other chemotherapy may have an increased risk of developing severe VOD
3. Gemtuzumab ozogamicin administration can result in severe hypersensitivity reactions (including anaphylaxis) and other infusion-related reactions, which may include severe pulmonary events. Infrequently, hypersensitivity reactions and pulmonary events have been fatal. In most cases, infusion-related symptoms occurred during the infusion or within 24 hours of administration of gemtuzumab ozogamicin

Therapy Monitoring

1. CBC, electrolytes, BUN, serum creatinine, and LFT daily for 2 weeks or until neutrophil/platelet recovery
2. Bone marrow aspiration/biopsy if clinically indicated to evaluate disease status either between doses or after completion of the 2 doses. If patients are stable based on blood counts, bone marrow biopsy may not need to be performed

Notes

1. Because tumor lysis syndrome may occur as a result of treatment, leukocyte reduction with hydroxyurea or leukophoresis should be considered to reduce the peripheral WBC to $<30,000/mm^3$ before administering gemtuzumab ozogamicin
2. Patients should be monitored closely for signs and symptoms of VOD: rapid weight gain, ascites, hepatomegaly, and right upper quadrant pain

REGIMEN

TRETINOIN (ALL-*TRANS* RETINOIC ACID; ATRA) + IDARUBICIN

Sanz MA et al. Blood 1999;94:3015–3021

See Regimen for Prophylaxis Against and Treatment of Tumor Lysis Syndrome earlier in chapter. Also see Chapter 46, Oncologic Emergencies

Tretinoin 22.5 mg/m^2 per dose orally every 12 hours until hematologic CR, but *not* for >90 days (total dosage/week = 315 mg/m^2)
Idarubicin 12 mg/m^2 per dose intravenously, diluted to a concentration of 1–10 mg/100 mL in 0.9% NaCl injection (0.9% NS) or 5% dextrose injection (D5W) over 15–30 minutes for 4 doses on days 2, 4, 6, and 8 (total dosage/induction course = 48 mg/m^2)

Tretinoin (all-*trans* retinoic acid; ATRA) is manufactured in the United States in capsules for oral administration, which contain 10 mg tretinoin. VESANOID® (tretinoin) CAPSULES. Distributed by Roche Laboratories, Inc, Nutley, NJ

Emetogenic potential:
Tretinoin alone: Moderate (Emetogenicity score = 3)
Days 2, 4, 6, and 8: Moderately high (Emetogenicity score = 4). See Chapter 39 for antiemetic regimens

Treatment Modifications

Adverse Event	Dose Modification
Serum creatinine >3 mg/dL (>264 micromol/L).	Reduce idarubicin dosage by 50%
Bilirubin 2.6–5.0 mg/dL (44.5–85.5 μmol/L)	Reduce idarubicin dosage by 50%
Bilirubin >5 mg/dL (>85.5 μmol/L)	Hold idarubicin
ATRA or APL syndrome (see Notes that follow)	Hold ATRA and treat with dexamethasone 10 mg IV every 12 hours for ≥3–5 days, with subsequent taper over 1 week. Restart ATRA when symptoms and signs improve

Patient Population Studied

A study of 123 newly diagnosed PML/RARα–positive patients

Efficacy (N = 123)

Hematologic CR was 89%
PML/RAR α RT-PCR tests were available in 99 cases at the end of induction and/or before consolidation. Fifty-one patients (51%) tested positive and 48 (49%) tested negative by PCR

Hematologic Recovery	Day to Recovery (Median [Range])
ANC >1000/mm^3	24 [5–57]
Platelets >50,000/mm^3	19 [6–45]

Toxicity (N = 123)

Adverse Event	% G3/G4
Fever	93
Bacteremia	22
Pulmonary	16
Oral	14
Cardiac	6
Hepatic	5
Hemorrhage	
Pulmonary	6
CNS	5
Neurologic	2
Renal	1
ATRA syndrome*	
Definitely present	6
Indeterminate	20
Definitely absent	74

There were 12 deaths: 1 due to ATRA syndrome, 3 due to infections, 8 due to intestinal, cerebral, or pulmonary hemorrhage

**Note:* Treatment with arsenic trioxide for remission induction is associated with symptoms identical with those of ATRA syndrome. Considering that this complex of symptoms is not specific to the use of retinoic acid, it is now referred to as the APL syndrome.

Therapy Monitoring

1. CBC with differential daily
2. Electrolytes, mineral panel, uric acid at least daily during active treatment until risk of tumor lysis is past
3. Bone marrow evaluation: after 5–6 weeks of induction chemotherapy

Notes

1. **ATRA or APL syndrome** occurs in about 25% of patients with APL within 2–21 days after treatment begins. It is characterized by fever, peripheral edema, pulmonary infiltrates, hypoxemia, respiratory distress, hypotension, renal and hepatic dysfunction, and serositis, resulting in pleural and pericardial effusions. Considering that this complex of symptoms is not specific to the use of retinoic acid but can occur during therapy with agents such as arsenic trioxide, it is now referred to as the APL syndrome. Early recognition and aggressive management with high-dose dexamethasone (10 mg IV every 12 hours for ≥3 days) has been effective in most patients. Temporary discontinuation of ATRA is indicated only in case of severe symptoms. Otherwise ATRA therapy is continued unless progression to an overt severe syndrome or lack of response to dexamethasone is observed. In patients with severe symptoms in whom tretinoin is discontinued, it can be restarted in most cases once the syndrome has resolved. In all patients dexamethasone should be maintained until symptoms disappear completely
2. **Hyperleukocytosis** occurs in up to 50% of patients treated with tretinoin alone for induction therapy and probably results from maturation of the leukemic cells. Most current remission induction regimens now combine tretinoin with cytotoxic chemotherapy as part of the initial treatment plan; this is likely to result in far fewer cases of hyperleukocytosis
3. Disseminated intravascular coagulation is frequently present at diagnosis in patients with APL, or it occurs soon after the initiation of cytotoxic chemotherapy. This complication constitutes a medical emergency because, if left untreated, it can cause pulmonary or cerebrovascular hemorrhage in up to 40% of patients with a 10–20% incidence of early hemorrhagic death. Tretinoin therapy appears to shorten the duration of the coagulopathy
4. In a randomized trial (Tallman MS et al. NEJM 1997;337:1021–1028) in patients with previously untreated APL, the use of ATRA in the induction or maintenance treatment improved disease-free survival and overall survival compared with chemotherapy alone
5. **Bone marrow evaluation:** Because tretinoin works slowly as a differentiating agent, marrow evaluation performed at the usual 7–10 days after completion of chemotherapy often appears cellular. This has often led to the erroneous conclusion that a patient requires additional chemotherapy. Bone marrow should be evaluated after 5–6 weeks of induction chemotherapy at hematopoietic recovery. Although PCR for the APL/RARα transcript will still be positive for most patients after induction, this result should become negative after completing consolidation treatment

REGIMEN

ARSENIC TRIOXIDE

Soignet SL et al. JCO 2001;19:3852–3860

Arsenic trioxide 0.15 mg/kg per day by intravenous infusion in 100–250 mL 5% dextrose injection (D5W) over 2 hours until bone marrow remission or up to a cumulative maximum of 60 doses (total dosage/week = 1.05 mg/kg), *or*
Arsenic trioxide 0.15 mg/kg per dose by intravenous infusion in 100–250 mL D5W over 2 hours for 5 days/week (eg, Monday through Friday) until bone marrow remission or up to a cumulative maximum of 60 doses (total dosage/week = 0.75 mg/kg)

Emetogenic potential: Moderate (Emetogenicity score = 3). See Chapter 39 for antiemetic regimens

Patient Population Studied

A study of 40 patients with either relapsed and/or refractory acute promyelocytic leukemia

Efficacy

Complete remission (CR)	85%
Median time to clinical CR	59 days

Toxicity (N = 40)

Adverse Event[a]	% All Grades	% G4
Nausea	75	
Vomiting	58	
Diarrhea	53	
Sore throat	40	
Abdominal pain	38	8
Cough	65	
Dyspnea	38	10
Headache	60	3
Insomnia	43	3
Dermatitis	43	
Hypokalemia	50	13
Hyperglycemia	45	13
Tachycardia	55	
Fatigue	63	
Fever	63	
QTc prolongation	40	
APL syndrome[b]	25	
Peripheral neuropathy	43	

[a] There were no treatment-related deaths
[b] Treatment with arsenic trioxide for remission induction is associated with symptoms identical with those of ATRA syndrome. Considering that this complex of symptoms is not specific to the use of retinoic acid, it is now referred as the APL syndrome

Therapy Monitoring

1. CBC twice weekly or more frequently, based on the transfusion requirement
2. LFTs, electrolytes, calcium, magnesium BUN, and serum creatinine twice weekly
3. Bone marrow biopsy
4. Electrocardiogram daily for 7 days to ensure QTc stability; then weekly

Treatment Modifications

Adverse Event	Dose Modification
APL syndrome	Hold arsenic trioxide and treat with dexamethasone 10 mg IV every 12 hours for ≥3–5 days, with subsequent taper over a week. Restart arsenic trioxide when symptoms and signs improve
Drug-related toxicity G ≥3, or nonhematologic toxicity G4	Hold therapy until toxicity is ≤G1or recovery to baseline. Restart treatment at 50% of the preceding dose on the same administration schedule. If the toxic event does not recur within 3 days after restarting at a reduced dosage, increase to the dose administered before symptoms began. If the same toxicity recurs, discontinue arsenic trioxide

Notes

1. Careful monitoring to maintain serum electrolytes in the upper range of normal reduces the risk of cardiac arrhythmias:

   Calcium ≥2.25 mmol/L (≥ 4.5 mEq/L, ≥9.00 mg/dL)

   Potassium ≥4.0 mmol/L

   Magnesium ≥0.9 mmol/L (≥1.8 mEq/L, ≥2.2 mg/dL)
2. **ATRA or APL syndrome** occurs in about 25% of patients with APL within 2–21 days after treatment begins. It is characterized by fever, peripheral edema, pulmonary infiltrates, hypoxemia, respiratory distress, hypotension, renal and hepatic dysfunction, and serositis, resulting in pleural and pericardial effusions. Considering that this complex of symptoms is not specific to the use of retinoic acid but can occur during therapy with agents such as arsenic trioxide, it is now referred as the APL syndrome. Early recognition and aggressive management with high-dose dexamethasone (10 mg IV every 12 hours for ≥3 days) has been effective in most patients. Therapy can be restarted in most cases once the syndrome has resolved.

20. Leukemia, Chronic Lymphocytic

Salah Abbasi, MD, and Bruce D. Cheson, MD

Epidemiology

Incidence: 10020 (estimated cases in the United States in 2006)
Deaths: 4660 (estimated cases in the United States in 2006)
Median age: 70 years
Female/male ratio: Approximately 1:2

Stage at Presentation (Rai)	
Stage 0:	31%
Stage I/II:	59%
Stage III/IV:	10%

Jemal A et al CA Cancer J Clin 2006;56:106–30

Diagnosis

NCI-working group diagnostic criteria

1. Absolute lymphocytosis in the peripheral blood with a count of $\geq$5000 /mm^3 and cells morphologically mature in appearance unexplained by other causes
2. At least 30% lymphocytes in a normocellular or hypercellular bone marrow
3. A monoclonal B-cell population with lymphocytes that express low levels of surface immunoglobulins, simultaneously with CD5, CD23, CD19 and CD20

Cheson BD et al. Blood 1996;87:4990–4997

Work-Up

Essential

1. Medical history and PE: Attention to node-bearing areas and to size of liver and spleen
2. Performance status
3. B-symptoms
4. Laboratory work-up: CBC with differential, serum LDH, BUN, creatinine, albumin, LFTs, calcium, and uric acid
5. Flow cytometry on the peripheral blood for CD5, CD19, CD20, and CD23 cells
6. Chest x-ray—PA and lateral
7. Unilateral bone marrow biopsy ± aspirate

Useful in certain circumstances

1. Quantitative immunoglobulins
2. β_2-Microglobulin
3. Reticulocyte count and direct Coombs' test, if anemic
4. Chest, abdomen, and pelvis CT scans, if adenopathy is present

Investigational

1. Cytogenetics/FISH analysis (eg, for −11q, +12q, −13q, and −17p)
2. CD38 expression
3. Zap-70 expression
4. IgVH gene mutation

NCCN Clinical Practice Guidelines in Oncology, V. 2. 2006

Staging and Survival

Rai	Lymphocytosis	Lymph Node Enlargement	Spleen/ Liver Enlargement	Hemoglobin <11 g/dL	Platelets <100,000/ mm^3	Survival Years
0	Yes	No	No	No	No	>13
I	Yes	Yes	No	No	No	8
II	Yes	±	Yes	No	No	6
III	Yes	±	±	Yes*	No	4
IV	Yes	±	±	±	Yes*	2

*Not immune-related

Kay NE et al. Chronic Lymphocytic Leukemia. Hematology. 2003(1):193–213

Prognosis

Poor risk factors

1. Advanced clinical stage
2. Rapid lymphocyte doubling time (<6 months)
3. Diffuse bone marrow involvement
4. High LDH, β_2-microglobulin

Investigational poor risk factors

1. 17p and 11q deletions. (Normal karyotype and trisomy 12 have an intermediate prognosis, whereas 13q deletion has a good prognosis)*
2. Expression of CD38 (>30%)
3. Unmutated IgVH genes
4. Zap-70 expression (>30%)

*Döhner H et al. NEJM 2000;43:1910–1916

Caveats

1. Indications for Therapy
    - Disease-related symptoms (eg, fever, chills, night sweats, weight loss)
    - Bone marrow involvement with progressive anemia and/or thrombocytopenia
    - Progressive or massive splenomegaly
    - Progressive or bulky lymphadenopathy
    - Autoimmune hemolytic anemia or thrombocytopenia
    - Recurrent bacterial infections
    - Rapidly increasing lymphocytosis (doubling in <6 months)

Cheson BD et al. Blood 1996;87:4990–4997

2. In the initial treatment of CLL, fludarabine is preferred because it yields a higher response rate, longer remission, and progression-free survival than chlorambucil, although it does not yield a difference in overall survival. As an oral agent, chlorambucil has some advantages
3. The combination of fludarabine and cyclophosphamide seems to have an advantage over single-agent fludarabine in the salvage setting, but it is not recommended for initial therapy. Similarly, single-agent alemtuzumab, fludarabine plus rituximab, and pentostatin plus cyclophosphamide can be considered as salvage regimens
4. Myelosuppression and infection remain the most significant complications of therapy in CLL
5. Prophylactic use of antibiotics during the course of fludarabine-based regimens is recommended only in some patients with high risk of infections (ie, hypogammaglobulinemia, prolonged steroid therapy, recurrent bacterial infections, or advanced disease)

REGIMEN

FLUDARABINE

Rai KR et al. NEJM 2000;343:1750–1757

Premedication:
Allopurinol 300 mg per day for 9 days orally. Begin the day before fludarabine treatment is started and continue until cycle day 8 every 28 days orally. Do this at least during the first 3 treatment cycles and for additional cycles if judged appropriate
Allopurinol is manufactured in the United States in tablets for oral administration containing either allopurinol 100 mg or 300 mg, and as an injectable product, Alloprim® (allopurinol sodium) for injection. Nabi®, Boca Raton, FL

Fludarabine 25 mg/m^2 per day for 5 days by intravenous infusion in 100–125 mL 5% dextrose injection (D5W) or 0.9% sodium chloride injection (0.9% NS) over 10–30 minutes, given on days 1–5 every 28 days for a maximum of 12 cycles (total dosage/cycle = 125 mg/m^2)

Emetogenic potential: Low (Emetogenicity score = 1). See Chapter 39

Patient Population Studied

A trial of 170 patients with previously untreated CLL (stages I–IV)

Efficacy (N = 170)

Complete response	20%
Partial response	43%
Stable or progressive disease	37%
Median duration of response	25 months
Median survival	66 months

Toxicity (N = 170)

	% Patients with G3/4
Thrombocytopenia	13
Neutropenia	27
Infection	16
Any G3/4 toxicity	55

Grade 3 = severe side effect
Grade 4 = life-threatening side effect
CALGB Expanded Common Toxicity Criteria

Treatment Modifications

Adverse Event	Dose Modification
G2 Toxicity	Reduce fludarabine dosage by 50%
G3/4 Toxicity	Suspend treatment. Make decisions about resumption at a reduced dose on a case-by-case basis
Major infection	Hold treatment until infection resolves, then resume with fludarabine dosage reduced by 50%

Therapy Monitoring

1. *Before each cycle:* CBC with differential, serum electrolytes, BUN, creatinine, and LFTs
2. *Response evaluation:* every 2–3 cycles

Notes

Active as a single agent. Recommended as an up-front regimen

REGIMEN

CHLORAMBUCIL

Rai KR et al. NEJM 2000;343:1750–1757

Premedication:
Allopurinol 300 mg per day for 9 days orally. Begin the day before chlorambucil treatment is started and continue until cycle day 8 every 28 days orally. Do this at least during the first 3 treatment cycles, and for additional cycles if judged appropriate
Allopurinol is manufactured in the United States in tablets for oral administration containing either allopurinol 100 mg or 300 mg, and as an injectable product, Alloprim® (allopurinol sodium) for injection. Nabi®, Boca Raton, FL

Chlorambucil 40 mg/m^2 single dose orally on day 1 every 28 days for a maximum of 12 cycles, (total dosage/cycle = 40 mg/m^2)

Alternative chlorambucil regimens:
(1) **Chlorambucil** 0.3 mg/kg per day orally for 5 consecutive days on days 1–5 every 28 days (total dosage/28-day cycle = 1.5 mg/kg)
(2) **Chlorambucil** 0.1 mg/kg per day orally (total dosage/28-day cycle = 2.8 mg/kg)
[Treat until clinical resistance develops]
Chlorambucil is manufactured in the United States in tablets for oral administration containing chlorambucil 2 mg. Leukeran® (chlorambucil), GlaxoSmithKline, Research Triangle Park, NC

Emetogenic potential: Low (Emetogenicity score = 1). See Chapter 39

Dighiero G et al. NEJM 1998;338:1506–1514

Patient Population Studied

A study pf 181 previously untreated patients with stages I–IV CLL

Efficacy (N = 181)

Complete response	4%
Partial response	33%
Stable or progressive disease	63%
Median duration of response	14 months
Median survival	56 months

Toxicity (N = 178)

	% Patients with G3/4
Thrombocytopenia	14
Neutropenia	19
Infection	9
Any G3/4 toxicity	44

Grade 3 = severe side effect
Grade 4 = life-threatening side effect
CALGB Expanded Common Toxicity Criteria

Treatment Modifications

Adverse Event	Dose Modification
G2 Toxicity	Reduce chlorambucil dosage by 50%
G3/4 Toxicity	Suspend treatment. Make decisions about resumption at a reduced dose on a case-by-case basis
Major infection	Hold treatment until infection resolves, then resume with chlorambucil dosage reduced 50%

Therapy Monitoring

1. *Before each cycle:* CBC with differential, serum electrolytes, BUN, creatinine, and LFTs
2. *Response evaluation:* Every 2–3 cycles

Notes

Active as a single agent. Chlorambucil is recommended as an up-front regimen in patients who cannot tolerate fludarabine-based regimens for any reason

REGIMEN

FLUDARABINE + CYCLOPHOSPHAMIDE

O'Brien SM et al. JCO 2001;19:1414–1420

Premedication:

Allopurinol 300 mg/day for 9 days orally. Begin the day before chlorambucil treatment is started and continue until cycle day 8 every 28 days. Use during at least the first 3 treatment cycles and for additional cycles if judged appropriate

Allopurinol is manufactured in the United States in tablets for oral administration containing either allopurinol 100 mg or 300 mg, and as an injectable product, Alloprim® (allopurinol sodium) for injection. Nabi®, Boca Raton, FL

Fludarabine 30 mg/m²/day by intravenous infusion in 100–125 mL 5% dextrose injection (D5W) or 0.9% sodium chloride injection (0.9% NS) over 10–30 minutes, given on days 1–3 every 28 days (total dosage/cycle = 90 mg/m²

Cyclophosphamide 300 mg/m²/day by intravenous infusion in 50–150 mL D5W or 0.9% NS over 10–30 minutes, given on days 1–3 every 28 days (total dosage/cycle = 900 mg/m²)

Antimicrobial prophylaxis for patients who receive steroids for any reason:

Cotrimoxazole (trimethoprim 160 mg + sulfamethoxazole 800 mg) orally twice weekly

Emetogenic potential: Low (Emetogenicity score = 1). See Chapter 39

Treatment Modifications

Adverse Event	Dose Modification
On cycle day 1, 4 weeks after last treatment, ANC ≤2000/mm³ or platelets ≤80,000/mm³	Delay treatment until ANC >2000/mm³ and platelets >80,000/mm³ (*Exception:* don't delay patients with baseline thrombocytopenia if platelet has recovered to pretherapy baseline)
5 weeks > last treatment ANC still ≤2000/mm³ and platelets ≤80,000/mm³	Reduce cyclophosphamide dosage to 250 mg/m²/day for 3 days
Pneumonia	
Septicemia	
Life-threatening infection	

Patient Population Studied

Patients with CLL

Previously untreated [n = 34]

Previously treated with alkylating agent [n = 20]

Previously treated with alkylating agent and fludarabine (sensitive to last treatment) [n = 46]

Previously treated with alkylating agent and fludarabine (refractory to last treatment) [n = 28]

Efficacy

Prior Therapy	CR	PR	Median Survival (months)
None	35%	24%	Not reached
Alkylating agent	15%	45%	38
Alkylating agent + fludarabine (sensitive to last treatment	12%	51%	21
Alkylating agent + fludarabine (refractory to last treatment)	3%	26%	12

Toxicity (N = 128)

Hematologic Toxicity During Any Cycle

	% G3	% G4
Neutropenia	75	48
Thrombocytopenia	13	16

Nonhematologic Toxicity During Any Cycle

	% G1/2	% G3/4
Fever or infection	37	40
Fatigue/aches	14	2
Nausea/vomiting	34	6
Diarrhea	5	0
Rash	10	2
Mental disorientation	0	2.7
Headache	8	0

Therapy Monitoring

1. *Before each cycle:* CBC with differential, serum electrolytes, BUN, creatinine, and LFTs
2. *Response evaluation:* Every 2–3 cycles

Notes

Recommended as salvage therapy. Remission rate is not higher than single-agent fludarabine, although duration of remissions may be longer

REGIMEN

ALEMTUZUMAB (CAMPATH-1H)

Keating MJ et al. Blood 2002;99:3554–3561

Premedication (30 minutes before alemtuzumab):
Diphenhydramine 50 m orally or by intravenous push 30 minutes before alemtuzumab, *and*
Acetaminophen 650 mg orally 30 minutes before alemtuzumab
Administer until maintenance dosing schedule is achieved and treatment is well tolerated
Level 1: Initial dose level—3 mg/dose
Alemtuzumab 3 mg daily by intravenous infusion in 100 mL 0.9% NaCl injection (0.9% NS) over 2 hours
Level 2: 10 mg/dose
Alemtuzumab 10 mg daily by intravenous infusion in 100 mL 0.9% NS over 2 hours
Level 3: Maintenance dose/schedule—30 mg/dose
Alemtuzumab 30 mg per dose, 3 doses per week (eg, Monday, Wednesday, and Friday) by intravenous infusion in 100 mL 0.9% NS over 2 hours for up to 12 weeks
Alemtuzumab dose escalation:
(1) Administer 3 mg intravenously on day 1. If tolerated, give 10 mg intravenously on day 2 or 3. If tolerated, give 30 mg intravenously on day 3 or 5. Then maintenance dose of 30 mg intravenous 3 times a week to allow the 30 mg dose to be reached in the first 3–5 days
(2) Based on patient tolerance
(3) Dose escalation proceeds if patient does not develop G ≥ 3 infusion-related adverse events
(4) If vascular access is temporarily lost, continue treatment with alemtuzumab subcutaneously in divided doses of no more than 1 mL (10 mg) per injection site

Antimicrobial primary prophylaxis:
Begin 8 days after starting alemtuzumab; continue a minimum of 2 months after alemtuzumab treatment is completed
(1) **Cotrimoxazole** (trimethoprim 160 mg + sulfamethoxazole 800 mg) orally, twice daily 3 times per week
(2) **Famciclovir** 250 mg orally, twice daily every day

Note: Famciclovir does not cover CMV. It is only for HSV and varicella prophylaxis

Famciclovir is manufactured in the United States in tablets for oral administration containing famciclovir 125 mg, 250 mg, and 500 mg. Famvir® (famciclovir). Novartis Pharmaceuticals Corporation, East Hanover, NJ

Emetogenic potential: Low (Emetogenicity score = 1). See Chapter 39

Patient Population Studied

A study of 93 patients with refractory B-cell CLL in whom an objective response to at least one fludarabine-containing therapy could not be achieved, or whose disease progressed while receiving or within 6 months after receiving a regimen containing fludarabine

Efficacy (N = 93)

Complete response	2%
Partial response	31%
Stable disease	54%
Median time to response	1.5 months
Median duration of response	8.7 months
Median survival	16 months
Median survival among responders	32 months

Treatment Modifications

Adverse Event	Dose Modification
G3/4 Infusion-related reactions	Continue daily treatment at previous dose level until administration is tolerated
Hematologic toxicities or G3/4 infection	Treatment postponed until toxicity or infection resolves. If delay >1 week; restart treatment at initial dose level
No change in disease status at 4 weeks	Continue treatment and reevaluate at 8 weeks
No change in disease status at 8 weeks	Discontinue therapy

Toxicity (N = 93)

Infusion-Related Events	% G1/2	% G3/4
Rigors	76	14
Fever	65	20
Nausea	53	0
Vomiting	37	1
Rash	33	0
Dyspnea	16	12
Hypotension	15	2
Hypoxia	1	2

Infusion-related toxicities decreased with time. Except for rashes, there was a substantial decrease in incidence from week 1 to weeks 2–4 and a further decrease beyond week 4

Other Treatment-Related events	% G1/2	% G3/4
Infections	28	27
Septicemia	4	11
CMV reactivation	3	4
Neutropenia	30% during week 5/6	
Thrombocytopenia	In first 2 weeks	

Therapy Monitoring

1. *Every week:* PE and CBC with differential
2. *Every month:* Serum electrolytes, creatinine, and LFTs
3. *Response evaluation*: Every 4 weeks
4. *After completing treatment:* PE, CBC with differential, serum electrolytes, creatinine, and LFTs every month for 6 months

Notes

Recommended as salvage therapy. Patients with bulky adenopathy, PS2 or lower, RAI stage IV with thrombocytopenia, and advanced age are less likely to respond. Active in fludarabine-refractory disease. Opportunistic infections are major complication, primarily bacterial but also CMV. Antibiotic prophylaxis is essential

REGIMEN

FLUDARABINE + RITUXIMAB

Byrd JC et al. Blood 2003;101:6–14

Premedication:
Allopurinol 300 mg/day orally, days 1–14
Allopurinol is manufactured in the United States in tablets for oral administration containing allopurinol 100 mg or 300 mg, and as an injectable product, Alloprim® (allopurinol sodium) for injection. Nabi®, Boca Raton, FL

Fludarabine 25 mg/m^2 by intravenous infusion in 100–125 mL 5% dextrose injection (D5W) or 0.9% NaCl injection (0.9% NS) over 20–30 minutes days 1–5 every 28 days for 6 cycles (total dosage/cycle = 125 mg/m^2)

Premedication for Rituximab (All Cycles):
Acetaminophen 650 mg orally 30 minutes before Rituximab
Diphenhydramine 50 mg by intravenous push 30 minutes before Rituximab

Cycle 1: **Rituximab** 375 mg/m^2 per dose by intravenous infusion in either D5W or 0.9% NS at a concentration of 1–4 mg/mL, days 1 and 4 (total dosage/cycle 1 = 750 mg/m2)
Cycles 2–6: **Rituximab** 375 mg/m^2 single dose by intravenous infusion in either D5W or 0.9% NS at a concentration of 1–4 mg/mL on day 1 every 28 days for 5 cycles (total dosage/cycle = 375 mg/m^2)

Emetogenic potential: Low (Emetogenicity score = 1). See Chapter 39

Treatment Modifications

Adverse Event	Dose Modification
Fludarabine-Related Toxicities	
G3 Neutropenia, thrombocytopenia, or anemia	Delay treatment until recovery to within 20% of baseline, then resume treatment with dosage of fludarabine reduced 25%
G4 Neutropenia, thrombocytopenia, or anemia	Delay treatment until recovery to within 20% of baseline, then resume treatment with dosage of fludarabine reduced 50%
Infection without G3/4 neutropenia	Hold treatment until infection resolves, then restart at the same dosage
Evidence of autoimmune hemolytic anemia or thrombocytopenia	Replace rituximab and fludarabine with alternative treatment as appropriate.
G ≥ 2 Nonhematologic adverse events attributable to fludarabine except nausea, vomiting, fatigue, diarrhea, infusion-related fever, or chills	Reduce fludarabine dosage by 50%
G3/4, or irreversible G2 nonhematologic toxicity	Reduce fludarabine dosage by 50%, or consider withdrawing fludarabine

Rituximab Infusion-Related Toxicities

Onset of infusion-related events (fevers, chills, rigors edema, congestion of the head and neck mucosa, hypotension):

1. Interrupt rituximab infusion
2. For fever, chills: Give additional dose of acetaminophen 650 mg orally and diphenhydramine 50 mg by intravenous push
3. For rigors: Give meperidine 12.5–25 mg by intravenous push ± promethazine 12.5–25 mg by intravenous infusion in at least 10 mL 0.9% NS or D5W over 5–15 minutes. If after 15–20 minutes the response to a single dose is considered inadequate, the dose may be repeated
4. After symptoms resolve, resume rituximab infusion at 50 mg/hour and increase by 50 mg/hour every 30 minutes as tolerated up to a maximum rate of 200 mg/hour

Dyspnea or wheezing, without allergic findings (urticaria, or tongue or laryngeal edema):

1. Interrupt rituximab infusion immediately
2. Give hydrocortisone 100 mg by intravenous push (or glucocorticoid equivalent)
3. Give a histamine H_2 antagonist (ranitidine 150 mg, cimetidine 300 mg, or famotidine 20 mg) by intravenous push
4. After symptoms resolve, resume rituximab infusion at 25 mg/hour with close monitoring. Do not increase rate

Patient Population Studied

A study of 51 previously untreated patients with CLL

Efficacy (N = 51)

Complete response	33%
Partial response	57%
Estimated 2-year progression-free survival	70%

Toxicity (N = 51)

Hematologic

Adverse Event	% G1/2	% G3/4
Neutropenia	8	76
Thrombocytopenia	47	20
Anemia	65	4
Infection	43	20

Modified NCI Criteria for CLL

Nonhematologic

Toxicity	% G1/2	% G3/4
Nausea	48	0
Vomiting	16	0
Myalgias	28	0
Fatigue/malaise	62	0
Dyspnea/hypoxemia*	12	14
Hypotension*	10	6
Fever*	32	0
Chills/rigors*	36	0
G3/4 pulmonary toxicity	3 cases	
Thrombocytopenic purpura	1 case	
Pure red cell aplasia	1 case	

*Infusion-related toxicities occur in 100% of patients—usually G1/2—although 20% experienced G3/4. Only 2 patients (4%) experienced infusion-related adverse events during a second administration
NCI CTC

Therapy Monitoring

1. *Before each cycle*: CBC with differential, serum electrolytes, creatinine, and LFTs
2. *Response evaluation:* Every 3 cycles

Notes

Recommended as salvage therapy, but increasingly used as initial therapy with or without cyclophosphamide

REGIMEN

PENTOSTATIN + CYCLOPHOSPHAMIDE

Weiss MA et al. JCO 2003;21:1278–1284

Hydration: ≥1500 mL 0.9% NaCl injection (0.9% NS) at ≥100 mL/hour before cyclophosphamide every 21 days

Premedication:
Allopurinol, 300 mg daily orally for 9 days. Begin the day before chemotherapy is started and continue until cycle day 8 every 21 days. Premedicate at least during the first 3 treatment cycles and for additional cycles if judged appropriate
Allopurinol is manufactured in the United States in tablets for oral administration containing allopurinol 100 mg or 300 mg, and as an injectable product, Aloprim® (allopurinol sodium) for injection. Nabi®, Boca Raton, FL

Cyclophosphamide 600 mg/m^2 by intravenous infusion in 50–150 mL 5% dextrose injection (D5W) or 0.9% NS over 15–60 minutes, given on day 1 every 3 weeks for up to 6 cycles (total dosage/cycle = 600 mg/m^2) *followed by:*

Pentostatin 4 mg/m^2 by intravenous infusion in 25–50 mL D5W or 0.9% NS, over 20–30 minutes, given on day 1 every 3 weeks for up to 6 cycles (total dosage/cycle = 4 mg/m^2)

Filgrastim daily subcutaneous injection, starting cycle day 3 and continuing until patient achieves a single post-nadir ANC > 5000/mm^3 or an ANC > 1500/mm^3 on 2 consecutive days
Dose is based on patients' body weight as follows:

Body Weight	Filgrastim Dose
≤70 kg	300 mcg/day
>70 kg	480 mcg/day

Antimicrobial primary prophylaxis:
Cotrimoxazole (trimethoprim 160 mg + sulfamethoxazole 800 mg) orally twice daily 3 times per week
Acyclovir 800 mg orally twice daily
Note: Acyclovir for herpes prophylaxis; does not cover CMV

Emetogenic potential: **Moderately high (Emetogenicity score = 4).** **See Chapter 39**

Patient Population Studied

A study of 23 previously-treated patients with CLL or small lymphocytic lymphoma (SLL). Patients had previously received from 3–5 regimens (median, 3). In 57%, disease was refractory to prior fludarabine

Efficacy (N = 23)

Complete response	17%
Partial response	57%
Stable disease	4.3%
Median response duration	7 months
Median survival	16 months

Treatment Modifications

Adverse Event	Dose Modification
Serum creatinine >2 mg/dL (>177 µmol/L) or increased by 20% above baseline	Hold treatment until serum creatinine ≤2 mg/dL (≤177 µmol/L) or is <20% greater than baseline result, or creatinine clearance ≥50 mL/min
G2 Toxicity	Hold drug until ≤G1, then restart at same dose
Repeated G2 toxicity	Hold drug until ≤G1, then restart at 25% dose reduction
G3/4 Toxicity	Hold drug until ≤G1, then restart at 25–50% dose reduction
Patient whose disease does not achieve at least a PR after 3 cycles	Therapy considered ineffective and discontinued

Toxicity (N = 17)

	% G1/2	% G3/4
Hematologic[a]		
Anemia	76	0
Thrombocytopenia	47	29
Neutropenia	18	41
Nonhematologic[b]		
Infection	41	12
Nausea	76	0
Vomiting	47	0
Constipation	47	0
Hepatic toxicity	24	0
Renal toxicity	47	0
Neurotoxicity	29	0

[a]NCI Working Group Guidelines
[b]NCI CTC

Therapy Monitoring

1. *Before each cycle:* CBC with differential, serum electrolytes, BUN, creatinine, and LFTs
2. *Response evaluation:* Every 3 cycles

REGIMEN

FLUDARABINE + CYCLOPHOSPHAMIDE + RITUXIMAB (FCR)

Keating MJ, et al. J Clin Oncol 2003;23:4079-88

Prophylaxis Against Tumor Lysis Syndrome (Cycle 1):
Allopurinol 300 mg/day, administer orally or intravenously for 7 consecutive days, days 1–7

Premedication for Rituximab (All Cycles):
Acetaminophen 650 mg, administer orally, *plus*
Diphenhydramine 25 mg, administer intravenously, 30–60 minutes before starting rituximab

Cycle 1	Cycles 2–6
Rituximab 375 mg/m², administer intravenously in 0.9% Sodium Chloride Injection (0.9%NS) or 5% Dextrose Injection (D5W), diluted to a concentration within the range of 1–4 mg/mL, on day 1 every 28 days (total dosage/cycle = 375 mg/m²)	**Rituximab** 500 mg/m², administer intravenously in 0.9%NS or D5W , diluted to a concentration within the range of 1–4 mg/mL, on day 1 every 28 days (total dosage/cycle = 500 mg/m²)

Notes on Rituximab administration

- Infuse initially at 50 mg/hour. If hypersensitivity or infusion reactions do not occur during the first 30 minutes, increase the rate by 50 mg/hour every 30 minutes as tolerated, to a maximum rate of 400 mg/hour. Subsequently, if previous administration was well tolerated, start at 100 mg/hour, and increase by 100 mg/hour every 30 minutes as tolerated, to a maximum rate of 400 mg/hour

Cycle 1	Cycles 2–6
Cyclophosphamide 250 mg/m² per day, administer intravenously in 25–250 mL 0.9%NS or D5W over 10–30 minutes, daily for 3 consecutive days, days 2–4 every 28 days (total dosage/cycle = 750 mg/m²)	**Cyclophosphamide** 250 mg/m² per day, administer intravenously in 25–250 mL 0.9%NS or D5W over 10–30 minutes, daily for 3 consecutive days, days 1–3 every 28 days (total dosage/cycle = 750 mg/m²)
Fludarabine 25 mg/m2 per day, administer by intravenous infusion in 100–125 mL 0.9%NS or D5W over 20–30 minutes, daily for 3 consecutive days, days 2–4 every 28 days (total dosage/cycle = 75 mg/m²)	**Fludarabine** 25 mg/m² per day, administer by intravenous infusion in 100 - 125 mL 0.9%NS or D5W over 20–30 minutes, daily for 3 consecutive days, days 1–3 every 28 days (total dosage/cycle = 75 mg/m²)

Supportive Care:
Valacyclovir 500 mg, administer orally, once daily for prophylaxis against herpes simplex and herpes zoster infections
Cotrimoxazole (trimethoprim 160 mg + sulfamethoxazole 800 mg), administer orally, twice weekly for PCP prophylaxis

Emetogenic Potential
Cycle 1, Day 1 = Low (Emetogenicity score = 2)
Cycle 1, Days 2–4 = Moderate–Moderately High (Emetogenicity score = 3–4)
Cycle 2 and subsequently, Days 1–3 = Moderate–Moderately High (Emetogenicity score = 3–4). (See Chapter 39)

Patient Population Studied

224 patients (median age 58 years) with CLL (Rai stage I–II, 67%; Rai stage III–IV, 33%)

Efficacy (N = 224)

Complete response:	70%
Nodular partial remission:	10%
Partial response:	15%
No response:	5%

Treatment Modifications

ANC ≤ 1000/mm³ or platelet ≤ 80,000/mm³ after the first treatment Cycle	Treatment postponed until ANC > 1000/mm³ and platelets >80,000/mm³. If delay > 1 week, restart treatment with reduction of the cyclophosphamide dosage to 200 mg/m² and fludarabine dosage to 20 mg/m². If further dose reduction is needed reduce the cyclophosphamide dosage to 150 mg/m² and fludarabine dosage to 15 mg/m². The rituximab dose is not reduced
Major infection	Reduce cyclophosphamide dosage to 200 mg/m² and fludarabine dosage to 20 mg/m². If further dose reduction is needed reduce the cyclophosphamide dosage to 150 mg/m² and fludarabine dosage to 15 mg/m² The rituximab dose is not reduced

Rituximab Infusion-Related Toxicities

Onset of infusion-related events (fevers, chills, rigors edema, congestion of the head and neck mucosa, hypotension):

1. Interrupt rituximab infusion
2. For fever, chills: Give additional dose of acetaminophen 650 mg orally and diphenhydramine 50 mg by intravenous push
3. For rigors: Give meperidine 12.5–25 mg by intravenous push ± promethazine 12.5–25 mg by intravenous infusion in at least 10 mL 0.9% NS or D5W over 5–15 minutes. If after 15–20 minutes the response to a single dose is considered inadequate, the dose may be repeated
4. After symptoms resolve, resume rituximab infusion at 50 mg/hour and increase by 50 mg/hour every 30 minutes as tolerated up to a maximum rate of 200 mg/hour

(continued)

Treatment Modifications
(Continued)

Dyspnea or wheezing, without allergic findings (urticaria, or tongue or laryngeal edema):

1. Interrupt rituximab infusion immediately
2. Give hydrocortisone 100 mg by intravenous push (or glucocorticoid equivalent)
3. Give a histamine H_2 antagonist (ranitidine 150 mg, cimetidine 300 mg, or famotidine 20 mg) by intravenous push
4. After symptoms resolve, resume rituximab infusion at 25 mg/hour with close monitoring. Do not increase rate

Toxicity (N = 224)

First Infusion of Rituximab

	% G1/2	% G3/4
Fever and chills	42	1
Hypotension	10	1
Dyspnea	13	—
Nausea	11	—
Vomiting	5	—
Back pain	3	—
Urrticaria	3	—
Headache	2	—

Fludarabine + Cyclophosphamide + Rituximab

	% G3	% G4
Neutropenia	24	28
Thrombocytopenia	4	<1
Infections		
Major	2.6 %	
Minor	10 %	

Therapy Monitoring

1. Prior to each cycle: CBC with differential, serum electrolytes, BUN, creatinine and LFTs
2. Response evaluation: every 2–3 cycles

Notes

Keating MJ et al. [abstract 2118] Proc Amer. Soc. Hem. (Blood) 2005;106:599a; Reported at the 2005 American Society of Hematology meeting. Three hundred previously untreated patients with CLL who received FCR had 83% 4-year survival, and 77% (CR+PR) 4-year remission duration. Autoimmune hemolytic anemia or red cell aplasia occurred in 25 and 6 cases, respectively. Three cases of acute myelogenous leukemia and 3 additional cases of myelodysplastic syndrome occurred.

21. Leukemia, Chronic Myelogenous

Michael M.W. Deininger, MD, and Brian J. Druker, MD

Epidemiology

Incidence: 1.6–2.1/10^5/year (United States 1998–2002)
The American Cancer Society estimates that 2640 men and 1960 women will be diagnosied with chronic myelogenous leukemia in 2005 (CML)

Deaths: 0.8/10^5/year (United States 1998–2002)

Median age: 66 years

Female/male ratio: ~1:1.7

Phases of Disease at Presentation
Chronic phase: 85–90%
Accelerated phase and blast crisis 10–15%

From SEER data (1998–2002) available at http://seer.cancer.gov
Cervantes F et al. Haematologica 1999;84:324–327
O'Brien SG et al. NEJM 2003;348:994–1004

Pathology

Peripheral blood findings at diagnosis: median (range)

1. *WBC:* 174,000/mm^3 (15,000–850,000/mm^3)
2. *Hemoglobin:* 10.3 g/dL (4.9–6.6 g/dL)
3. *Platelet count:* 430,000/mm^3 (17,000–3,182,000/mm^3)
4. Left-shifted white cell differential, basophilia, and eosinophilia
5. *Blasts:* <15%-chronic phase

Bone marrow findings at diagnosis

1. Increased cellularity
2. Increased myeloid:erythroid ratio with full myeloid maturation
3. Blasts <15%—chronic phase
4. Basophilia
5. Megakaryocyte hyperplasia
6. Reticulin fibrosis

Cytogenetics and molecular diagnostics

1. Philadelphia chromosome including variant translocations (90%)
2. *BCR-ABL* translocation by FISH (95%)
3. *BCR-ABL* transcripts by RT-PCR (95%)
4. Chromosomal abnormalities in addition to the Ph chromosome (clonal evolution):
   [Associated with disease progression, usually absent in the chronic phase at diagnosis]

Trisomy 8	52.9%
Second Ph chromosome	50.7%
Isochromosome 17	35.8%
Trisomy 19	24.3%

Note: Approximately 5% of patients with morphologically and clinically typical CML are negative for *BCR-ABL* by FISH and RT-PCR; these patients constitute a heterogeneous group with a poorer prognosis that is usually unresponsive to imatinib. The data given here do not apply to this group of patients

(*continued*)

Work-Up

1. H&P, CBC, platelet count, chemistry profile
2. Bone marrow aspirate and biopsy, morphologic review (percentage of blasts and basophils)
3. Bone marrow cytogenetics; FISH and RT-PCR for *BCR-ABL*
4. HLA-typing of patient and siblings if patient is considered a candidate for hematopoietic stem cell transplantation (HSCT)

NCCN Clinical Practice Guidelines in Oncology, V. 1. 2006

Pathology (*continued*)

Clonal evolution is associated with a less favorable response to standard drug therapy (imatinib), regardless of disease phase, but it is not an independent prognostic variable. In patients treated with non-imatinib therapies, isochromosome 17 is an adverse prognostic factor in multivariate analysis

Deininger MWN. Semin Hematol 2003;40(suppl 2):50–55
Johansson B et al. Acta Haematol 2002;107:76–94
Mitelman F. Leuk Lymphoma 1993;11(suppl 1):11–5
Savage DG et al. Br J Haematol 1997;96:111–116
Thiele J et al. Leuk Lymphoma 2000;36:295–308

Classification of Disease

Risk Stratification

1. *Primary risk stratification:* Disease phase
2. *Risk stratification in chronic phase on drug therapy other than imatinib or interferon alfa:*

   Sokal score with 4 parameters: age, spleen size (cm below costal margin), platelets, and peripheral blasts

$$RR = \exp[0.0116(\text{age} - 43.4) + 0.0345(\text{spleen size} - 7.51) + 0.188([\text{platelets}/700]^2 - 0.563) + 0.0887(\text{peripheral blasts} - 2.10)]$$

Low risk	< 0.8
Intermediate risk	0.8–1.2
High risk	> 1.2

3. *Risk stratification in chronic phase treated with interferon alfa:*

   European score with 6 parameters: age, spleen size (cm below costal margin), blasts, basophils, eosinophils, and platelets — calculator available at http://www.pharmacoepi.de/cgi-bin/pharmacoepi/cmlscore.cgi

Hasford J et al. J Natl Cancer Inst 1998;90:850–858
Sokal JE et al. Blood 1984;63:789–799

Phases of Disease

Chronic phase

1. Bone marrow and peripheral blood blasts <15%
2. Peripheral blood promyelocytes and blasts combined <30%
3. Peripheral blood basophils <20%
4. Platelets >100,000/mm^3

Accelerated phase

1. Bone marrow and peripheral blood blasts 15–30%
2. Peripheral blood promyelocytes + blasts ≥ 30% (but blasts alone < 30%)
3. Peripheral blood basophils ≥ 20%
4. Platelets ≤ 100,000/mm^3 (unless related to therapy)

Blast crisis

1. Bone marrow or peripheral blood blasts ≥ 30%
2. Myeloid immunophenotype: MPO-positive
3. Lymphoid immunophenotype: TdT-positive

Cytogenetic abnormalities in addition to the Philadelphia chromosome (typically isochromosome 17, trisomy 8, trisomy 19, second Ph chromosome) are considered indicative of accelerated phase by some authors, even without other defining criteria. Adverse prognostic significance is best documented for isochromosome 17

Johansson B et al. Acta Haematol 2002;107:76–94
Talpaz M et al. Blood 2002;99:1928–1937

Prognosis

Therapy with Imatinib

Chronic Phase—Newly Diagnosed (n = 553)	
Freedom from progression to advanced phase (12 months)	98.5%
Freedom from progression to advanced phase (18 months)	96.7%
Accelerated Phase (n = 119)	
Estimated overall survival at 12 months	78%
Myeloid Blast Crisis (n = 229)	
Estimated overall survival at 12 months	32%

Therapy with Interferon

Chronic Phase (n = 908)

European Score	Median Survival
Low risk	98 months
Intermediate risk	65 months
High risk	42 months

Bone Marrow Transplantation*

Classification	% 5-Year Survival
Chronic phase	58
Accelerated phase	34
Blast crisis	16

*10,206 patients reported to the European Blood and Marrow Transplantation Group

Important Note: Transplantation in second chronic phase is superior to transplantation in blast crisis (median time to progression 22.7 months in one study)

Gratwohl A. International Conference on Chronic Myelogenous Leukemia (Rapallo, 2003)
Visani G et al. Br J Haematol 2000;109:722–728

Caveats

1. The standard *nontransplant* regimen for the initial treatment of all phases of CML has recently changed to imatinib. Other regimens are considered second-line treatment and are reserved for patients who are intolerant or whose disease is resistant to imatinib
2. Interferon alfa is the nontransplant regimen of second choice and reserved for patients with intolerance to imatinib. Interferon alfa is generally not effective in patients with disease that is refractory or resistant to imatinib
3. Hydroxyurea is used for lowering excessively high white blood cell counts if the diagnosis is uncertain and in the case of intolerance or resistance to imatinib or interferon alfa. Hydroxyurea is considered a palliative regimen because it does not usually induce lasting remissions
4. Follow-up with imatinib is still limited
5. The Sokal score was validated in patients treated with drugs other than interferon alfa and imatinib. It does not separate intermediate from high risk in interferon-treated patients and may not apply to imatinib therapy
6. The European score was developed for patients treated with interferon and does not apply to patients treated with imatinib. An "imatinib score" is in development but not yet available
7. The definition of disease phases given above was used in the clinical trials of imatinib that led to regulatory approval. They are widely but not universally accepted
8. AML- or ALL-type chemotherapy is indicated for imatinib-resistant CML in myeloid and lymphoid blast crisis, respectively. No data from controlled trials are available that demonstrate superiority of one regimen over another. All efforts should be made to proceed to allogeneic stem cell transplantation as soon as possible. Complete hematologic remission is achieved in 40–60% of patients

Derderian PM et al. Am J Med 1993;94:69–74
Kantarjian HM et al. Am J Med 1987;83:445–454

REGIMEN

IMATINIB (Gleevec®, Glivec™)

Deininger MWN et al. JCO 2003;21:1637–1647

Chronic phase CML:
Initial dose:
Imatinib 400 mg/day orally with largest meal of the day
Dose escalation:
Escalate to 600 mg/day, if patient has not reached:
Complete hematologic response at 3 months
or
<65% Ph-negative metaphases at 6 months
or
<35% Ph-negative metaphases at 12 months
Recommendations are based on limited data and may change when more follow up becomes available

Accelerated phase and blast crisis CML:
Initial dose:
Imatinib 600 mg/day orally with largest meal of the day

Imatinib is marketed in the United States as tablets for oral administration containing either 100 mg or 400 mg imatinib base as the mesylate ester. Gleevec® (imatinib mesylate)

Emetogenic potential: Low (Emetogenicity score ≤2). See Chapter 39

Patient Population Studied

A study of 553 patients with newly diagnosed CML in chronic phase

Efficacy (Chronic Phase) (N = 553)

Complete hematologic response	95.3%
Complete cytogenetic response	73.8%
Partial cytogenetic response (1–35% Ph+ metaphases)	11.4%
Freedom from progression to accelerated phase or blast crisis for 12 months	98.5%
Freedom from progression to accelerated phase or blast crisis for 18 months	96.7%

Treatment Modifications

Hematologic Toxicity (no modifications for anemia)	
G1/2	No dose modifications
G3	Hold imatinib until toxicity resolves to G1[a], then restart at 400 mg/day
Recurrent G3	Hold imatinib until toxicity resolves to G1, then restart at 300 mg/day
G4	Withhold imatinib until toxicity resolves to G1, then restart at 300 mg/day
Recurrent G4	Hold imatinib until toxicity resolves to G1, then restart at 300 mg/day[b]
Nonhematologic Toxicity	
G1	No dose modifications
G2/3	Hold imatinib until toxicity resolves to G1, then restart at 400 mg/day
Recurrent G2/3	Hold imatinib until toxicity resolves to G1, then restart at 300 mg/day
G4	Hold imatinib until toxicity resolves to G1, then restart at 300 mg/day
Recurrent G4	Discontinue imatinib

[a]Consider filgrastim for persistent neutropenia
[b]No dose reduction to < 300 mg/day
Deininger MWN et al. JCO 2003;21:1637–1647

Therapy Monitoring

1. *CBC:* Weekly; every 2 weeks after achievement of complete hematologic response; every 4–6 weeks after achievement of complete cytogenetic response
2. *Blood chemistry:* Weekly; every 4–8 weeks after achievement of complete hematologic response
3. *Bone marrow cytogenetics:* Every 3 months; every 6–12 months after a complete cytogenetic response
4. *Quantitative RT-PCR for BCR-ABL from peripheral blood or bone marrow:* Every 3 months

Toxicity (N = 553) (>10% of Patients)

	% G1/2	% G3/4
Superficial edema	54.6	0.9
Thrombocytopenia	48.8	7.8
Neutropenia	46.5	14.3
Nausea	43	0.7
Anemia	41.5	3.1
Increased liver transaminases	38.1	5.1
Muscle cramps	37	1.3
Musculoskeletal pain	33.8	2.7
Rash	31.9	2.0
Fatigue	33.4	1.1
Diarrhea	31	1.8
Headache	30.8	0.4
Joint pain	25.9	2.4
Abdominal pain	24.6	2.4
Nasopharyngitis	22.0	—
Myalgia	19.9	1.5
Hemorrhage	20.2	0.7
Vomiting	15.4	1.5
Dyspepsia	16.2	—
Pharyngolaryngeal pain	15.8	0.2
Cough	14.3	0.2
Dizziness	13.6	0.9
Upper respiratory infection	14.3	0.2
Weight gain	12.5	0.9
Pyrexia	12.4	0.7
Insomnia	12.2	—

O'Brien SG et al. NEJM 2003;348:994–1004

Notes

In patients who develop disease progression while receiving imatinib, the option of allogeneic stem cell transplantation should be reevaluated

REGIMEN

HYDROXYUREA

Hehlmann R et al. Blood 1994;84:4064–4067

Starting dose: 40 mg/kg daily, continuously, orally after meals as single dose or divided into 2 doses

1. Optimal dose determined *empirically*, with frequent monitoring of CBC (eg, every 3 days)
2. A dosage of 1000–2000 mg/day is frequently sufficient for patients with WBC <100,000/mm^3. With higher WBCs and a need to rapidly lower WBC, 6000–8000 mg/day may be required initially
3. Total daily dose depends on disease activity and is extremely variable (range 500 mg–15,000 mg/day)
4. Therapeutic goal is normalization of the WBC (target: 5000–10,000/mm^3). This may require significantly higher or lower doses than the initial dose. If response is insufficient, aggressiveness of dose escalation must match aggressiveness of the disease. Frequent monitoring of WBC mandatory during changes to the regimen:
   (a) *Slowly rising WBC or failure to achieve therapeutic target:* Increase total daily dose 25–50%; assess effect after 5–7 days before further escalation
   (b) *Rapidly rising WBC:* Increase total daily dose by 50–100%; assess effect of dose increase for 3 days before further dose escalation
5. Very high doses carry risk of prolonged aplasia

Hydroxyurea is marketed in the United States as capsules for oral administration containing hydroxyurea 200, 300, or 400 mg, Droxia™ (hydroxyurea capsules); and as capsules for oral administration containing hydroxyurea 500 mg, Hydrea® (hydroxyurea capsules)

Emetogenic potential: Nonemetogenic (Emetogenicity score = 1). See Chapter 39

Patient Population Studied

A study of 194 patients with newly diagnosed CML in chronic phase

Efficacy (N = 194)

Five-year survival is 45%

Toxicity

Hematologic Side Effects

1. Neutropenia and anemia are common, whereas thrombocytopenia is rare
2. Cytopenias are usually rapidly reversible (within 3–4 days)
3. High doses and/or failure to interrupt treatment despite cytopenia may result in prolonged aplasia

Relatively Common Nonhematologic Side Effects

1. Gastrointestinal symptoms (stomatitis, anorexia, nausea, vomiting, diarrhea)
2. Acute skin reactions (rash, ulceration, dermatomyositis-like changes, erythema)

Rare Nonhematologic Side Effects

1. Chronic skin reactions (hyperpigmentation, atrophy of skin and nails, skin cancer, alopecia)
2. Headache, drowsiness, convulsions
3. Fever, chills, asthenia
4. Renal and hepatic impairment

Note: A comprehensive and detailed analysis of nonhematologic toxicity from a controlled trial is not available

Treatment Modifications

Hematologic Toxicity	
G1	No dose modifications. G1 WBC *or* ANC are acceptable or even desirable
G2 or G3	Hold hydroxyurea until toxicity resolves to G1, then restart at 75% of initial dose
Recurrent G2/3	Hold hydroxyurea until toxicity resolves to G1, then restart at 50% of initial dose
G4	Hold hydroxyurea until toxicity resolves to G1, then restart at 25% of initial dose
Recurrent G4	Hold hydroxyurea until toxicity resolves to G1, then restart at 50% previous dose
Nonhematologic Toxicity	
G1	No dose modifications
G2/3	Hold hydroxyurea until toxicity resolves to G1, then restart at initial dose
Recurrent G2/3	Hold hydroxyurea until toxicity resolves to G1, then restart at 75% of initial dose
G4	Hold hydroxyurea until toxicity resolves to G1, then restart at 50% maximal dose
Recurrent G4	Discontinue hydroxyurea

Therapy Monitoring

1. *CBC:* At least weekly at first, then every 2–4 weeks after achieving stable blood counts
2. *Blood chemistry profile:* Every 6 months
3. *Bone marrow morphology and cytogenetics:* Every 6 months

Notes

1. Hydroxyurea is the drug of choice when a rapid reduction of the white cell count is clinically mandated, but the diagnosis of *BCR-ABL*-positive CML has not been established
2. Hydroxyurea may be indicated in cases of imatinib intolerance or resistance

REGIMEN

INTERFERON ALFA

Baccarani M et al. Blood 2002;99:1527–1535
Hehlmann R et al. Blood 1994; 4:4064–4067

Premedication:
Acetaminophen 500–650 mg/dose orally every 4–6 hours as needed
Target dose of interferon alfa:
Interferon alfa-2a 5 million units/m^2 per day continuously, subcutaneously (preferably at bedtime)

or

Interferon alfa-2b 5 million units/m^2 per day continuously, subcutaneously (preferably at bedtime)
Typical dose of interferon alfa:
5 million units/m^2 per day. To increase tolerability, interferon alfa should be started at low doses (eg, 1.5 million units/m^2 per day) with gradual increases over several weeks until the target dose is achieved

Emetogenic potential: Nonemetogenic (Emetogenicity score = 1). See Chapter 39

Patient Population Studied

Patients with newly diagnosed CML in chronic phase
[n = 263 (Baccarani et al. Blood 2002;99:1527–1635)]
[n = 194 (Hehlmann et al. Blood 1994;84:4064-4077)]

Efficacy (N = 263)

Complete hematologic response	74%
Complete cytogenetic response	7.6%
Partial cytogenetic response	10.2%
5-year survival	65%

Baccarani M et al. Blood 2002;99:1527–1535

Treatment Modifications

Nonhematologic Toxicity	
G1	No dose reduction
G2	Reduce interferon alfa by 25%
G3/4	Stop interferon alfa. Restart at 50% of the previously administered dose after toxicity resolves. If resumption is tolerated, increase to 75% of the dose that produced G3/4 toxicity

Hematologic Toxicity	
G1/2	No dose reduction
G3	Reduce interferon alfa in 25% decrements until resolution to grade < 3
G4	Stop interferon alfa. Restart at 50% when toxicity resolves; increase to 75% if tolerated

The practical management of patients receiving interferon alfa is complex. The simplified dose modification schema shown here is only a minimal guideline
Modified from O'Brien S et al. Leuk Lymphoma 1996;23:247–252

Therapy Monitoring

1. *CBC:* Weekly; every 3–4 weeks after complete hematologic response, if counts are stable; every 4–6 weeks after complete cytogenetic response
2. *Blood chemistry:* Every 2 weeks; every 4–6 weeks after complete hematologic response
3. *Bone marrow cytogenetics:* Every 6 months; every 6–12 months after complete cytogenetic response
4. *Quantitative RT-PCR for BCR-ABL from peripheral blood or bone marrow:* Every 3 months

Toxicity

	% (All grades)
Fever	92
Asthenia or fatigue	88
Myalgia	68
Chills	63
Anorexia	48
Arthralgia/bone pain	47
Headache	44
Nausea, vomiting	37
Diarrhea	37
Depression	28
Cough	19
Hair changes	18
Skin rashes	18
Decreased mental status	16
Sweating	15
Dizziness	11
Sleep disturbances	11
Paresthesia	8
Dyspnea	8
Dysrhythmia	7
Involuntary movements	7
Dry skin	7
Pruritus	7
Visual disturbances	6

ROFERON®-A (interferon alfa-2a, recombinant) product label, April 2002. Hoffmann-La Roche Inc., Nutley, NJ

Notes

Interferon alfa is reserved for patients who are intolerant of imatinib. Patients whose disease is resistant to imatinib usually do not respond to interferon alfa

REGIMEN

DASATINIB (BMS-354825)

Sawyers et al, American Association for Cancer Research, 2006
Sawyers et al Blood, 2005; 106: Abstract #38
Talpaz et al, ASCO 2005 Annual Meeting, Abstract #6518

Dasatinib 70 mg administer orally twice per day, continuously
In the United States dasatinib is available in tablets for oral administration containing 20, 50 and 70 mg dasatinib
Emetogenic potential: Low (Emetogenicity score = 2). See Chapter 39 for antiemetic regimens

Patient Population Studied

CML patients whose disease proved to be imatinib-resistant (80%) and patients intolerant of imatinib (20%). Mutations were identified in 83% of patients (Sawyers et al, 2006).

Definitions of eligible patients.

1. *Primary resistance:* Lack of a complete hematologic response despite 400 mg/day imatinib for three months or rapid progression within less than 3 months of starting imatinib (including progression to accelerated phase or blast crisis)
2. *Acquired resistance:* Patient who achieved any hematologic response on imatinib but then had progressive disease including WBC > 10,000/mm^3 on 2 measurements 2 weeks apart or one measurement >15,000/mm^3 (including progression to accelerated phase or blast crisis)
3. *Imatinib intolerant:* Imatinib discontinued for any non-hematologic toxicity of any grade

Efficacy

All patients (N = 84)	MHR[1]	CHR[2]	MCyR[3]	CCyR[4]
Chronic phase CML (n = 40)		92.5%	45%	35%
Advanced Phase Disease (n = 11)	81%	45%	27%	18%
Myeloid Blast Crisis (n = 23)	61%	35%	35%	26%
Lymphoid Blast Crisis/Ph+ ALL (n = 10)	80%	70%	80%	30%

[1]Major hematologic response (<5% blasts)
[2]Complete hematologic response
[3]Major cytogenetic response
[4]Complete cytogenetic response

Sawyers et al Blood, 2005; 106:Abstract #38, November 16, 2005
Sawyers et al, American Association for Cancer Research, 2006

Dose Modification

Dosage Level	Dosage
Level +1	90–100 mg twice per day
Level 0 (Start)	70 mg twice per day
Level −1	50 mg twice per day
Level −2	40 mg twice per day

Adverse Event	Dose Modification
No hematologic response after one month	Increase dasatinib dosage one level
Persistent G4 thrombocytopenia	Reduce dasatinib dosage one level
G3/4 non-hematologic toxicity	Allow toxicity to resolve to G ≤ 1 then reduce dasatinib dosage one level
G1/2 pleural effusion	Monitor carefully; usually resolves without dose reduction

Toxicity

Toxicity	START A (N = 35)	START B (N = 34)	START C (N = 30)	START L (N = 28)
% Dose reductions	17	21[1]	20[1]	11
% Dose escalations	17	32	6.6	29
% G3/4 ANC	48	59	20	64
% G3/4 Platelets	57	56	20	71
% G1/2 Diarrhea	28.6	23.5	16.6[2]	NR
% G1/2 Nausea	14	5.9[2]	NR	NR
% G1/2 Peripheral edema	8.6	8.8	10	10.7
% G1/2 Pleural effusion	5.7	11.8	3.3	NR
% G1/2 Rash	NR	11.8	16.6	NR

[1]Mostly due to persistent thrombocytopenia
[2]Also one grade 3 toxicity

START A: Guilhot et al., Blood, 2005; 106:Abstract #39
START B: Talpaz et al., Blood, 2005; 106:Abstract #40
START C: Hochhaus et al., Blood, 2005; 106:Abstract #41
START L: Ottmann et al., Blood, 2005; 106:Abstract #42

Hematologic toxicity (N = 40)	% G3	% G4
Neutropenia	22.5	15
Anemia	25	7.5
Thrombocytopenia	17.5	10

Non-hematologic toxicity (N = 40)	% G1/2	% G3/4
Elevated ALT	27.5	—
Elevated creatinine	22.5	2.5
Diarrhea	17.5	—
Paresthesia	10	—
Headache	10	—
Nausea	5	—
Peripheral edema	5	—
Pleural effusion	2.5	2.5
Gastrointestinal hemorrhage	0	5

Talpaz et al, ASCO 2005 Annual Meeting, Abstract #6518

Hematologic toxicity (N = 84)*	% G3/4 ANC	% G3/4 Platelets
Chronic phase CML (n = 40)	45%	35%
Advanced Phase Disease (n = 11)	82%	82%
Myeloid Blast Crisis (n = 23)	96%	83%
Lymphoid Blast Crisis/Ph+ ALL (n = 10)	80%	70%

*Pre-treatment G3/4 myelosuppression existed in 2/3 of patients before starting dasatinib
Sawyers et al, American Association for Cancer Research, 2006

Non-hematologic toxicity (N = 84)	Chronic		Advanced	
	% G1-4	% G3/4	% G1-4	% G3/4
Diarrhea	18	—	27	2
Nausea	5	—	14	—
Vomiting	—	—	9	—
Peripheral edema	18	—	20	—
Pleural effusion	13	—	23	7
Generalized edema	5	—	5	—
Periorbital edema	5	—	9	—
Pericardial effusion	3	—	7	5
Dyspnea/ Pulmonary edema	10	—	14	5
Headache	10	—	7	—
Rash	3	—	18	—
Tumor lysis syndrome	—	—	5	5

Sawyers et al, American Association for Cancer Research, 2006

Therapy Monitoring

1. *Weekly:* CBC with differential
2. *Monthly (at least initially):* Bone marrow aspirate (with cytogenetics) in blast crisis

Notes

1. Dasatinib is a SRC/ABL kinase inhibitor that is active against all but one (T3151) of the known mutations in BCR/ABL that confer resistance to imatinib. Among patients in five phase II studies, the response rates have been as follows:

	Hematologic Response rate (%)	
CML stage	Mutation-Positive	All Patients
Chronic	90	90
Accelerated	62	59
Myeloid Blast	30	32
Ly/Ph+ALL	26	35

2. Imatinib binds the closed conformation of ABL. Imaitnib resistane mutations that impair kinase flexibility favor the open conformation. Dasatinib binds both the open and the closed conformations
3. Responses are durable in CP and AP patients, but relapses have occurred in the MBC and LBC/Ph+ ALL cohorts, often due to dasatinib-resistant BCR-ABL mutations

22. Leukemia, Hairy Cell

Martin S. Tallman, MD

Epidemiology

Incidence: Approximately 600–800 new patients per year in the United States
Median age: 52 years
Female/male ratio: ~4:1
Presentation: Typically, pancytopenia or suppression of only one or two cell lines, and splenomegaly
25% present with fatigue or weakness
25% present with infection

Bernstein L et al. Cancer Res 1990;50:3605–3609
Staines A et al. Br J Haematol 1993;85:714

Pathology

Peripheral blood findings at diagnosis

1. Pancytopenia: 50%
2. "Leukemic" phase with a WBC >1000/mm^3: 10–20%
3. Monocytopenia
4. Hairy cells identified in most patients, but the number is usually low

Bone marrow findings at diagnosis

1. Hypercellularity
2. Hairy cell infiltration: diffuse, patchy, or interstitial

   Diffuse infiltration—often results in complete effacement of bone marrow

   Patchy infiltration—subtle small clusters of hairy cells present focally or throughout the bone marrow

   Interstitial Infiltration—hairy cells do not form well-defined discrete aggregates, but merge almost imperceptibly with surrounding normal hematopoietic tissue
3. Hairy cell nuclei are usually round, oval, or indented and are widely separated from each other by abundant, clear or lightly eosinophilic cytoplasm. Rarely hairy cells can be convoluted or spindle-shaped
4. Extravasated blood cells create blood lakes in the bone marrow similar to those observed in the spleen
5. Mast cells are often numerous
6. Reticulin stain of the bone marrow almost always shows moderate to marked increase in reticulin fibers
7. Approximately 10–20% of patients show a hypocellular bone marrow

Immunophenotyping, cytogenetics and molecular diagnostic studies

1. *Cytochemical studies:* Tartrate-resistant acid phosphatase (TRAP) stain. However, TRAP is not specific for hairy cell leukemia (HCL)
2. *Hairy cell immunophenotype:* CD19(+), CD20(+), CD22(+), CD79B(+), CD5(−), CD10(−), CD11C(+), CD25 Sub(+), FMC(+), CD103(+), CD45(+)
3. *Clonal cytogenetics:* Abnormalities in approximately two-thirds of patients. Chromosome 1, 2, 5, 6, 11, 14, 19, and 20 are most frequently involved. Chromosome 5 is altered in approximately 40%, most commonly as a trisomy 5, pericentric inversion, and interstitial deletions involving band 5q13

(*continued*)

Work-Up

1. H&P
2. CBC with differential, serum electrolytes, BUN, creatinine, LFTs, and uric acid
3. Bone marrow aspirate and biopsy for TRAP and morphologic review; immunophenotyping by flow cytometry with B-cell associated antibodies including CD20, CD79A, or DBA.44

Tallman MS et al. Hairy cell leukemia. In: Hoffman, ed. Hematology: Basic Principles and Practice, 3rd ed. Churchill Livingstone, 2000:1363–1372

Pathology (*continued*)

Bartl R et al. Am J Clin Pathol 1983;79:531–545

Burke JS et al. Am J Clin Pathol 1978;70:876–884

Burke JS et al. Semin Oncol 1984;11:334–346

Brunning RD et al. Atlas of Tumor Pathology, 3rd Series, Fascicle 9. Washington DC, AFIP, 1994:277–278

Cornfield DB et al. Am J Hematol 2001;67:223–236

Ellison DJ et al. Blood 1994;84:4310–4315

Flandrin G et al. Semin Oncol 1984;11:458–471

Golomb HM et al. Ann Intern Med 1978; 89:677–683

Haglund U et al. Blood 1994;83:2637–2645

Hakimian D et al. Blood 1993;82:1798–802

Hanson CA et al. Am J Surg Pathol 1989;13:671–69

Hounieu H et al. Am J Clin Pathol 1992;98:26–33

Katayama I. Hematol Oncol Clin North Am 1988;2:585–602

Kluin-Nielmans HC et al. Blood 1994;84:3134–3441

Kroft SH et al. Blood Rev 1995;9:234–250

Lee WM et al. Cancer 1982;50:2207–2210

Robbins BA et al. Blood 1993;82:1277–1287

Sausville JE et al. Am J Clin Pathol 2003:119:213–217

Turner A et al. Medicine 1978;57:477–499

Wheaton S et al. Blood 1996;87:1556–1560

Yam LT et al. NEJM 1971;284:357–360

Differential Diagnosis

Other small B-cell lymphoproliferative disorders associated with splenomegaly:

1. Prolymphocytic leukemia
   a. Marked elevation in WBCs
   b. Characteristic morphology of the prolymphocytes
   c. Different immunophenotypic profile
2. Splenic marginal zone lymphoma (splenic lymphoma with villous lymphocytes)
   a. Cells are not usually TRAP-positive
   b. Bone marrow infiltrates are demarcated sharply
   c. Different immunophenotypic profile (−CD103)
3. HCL variant
   a. Morphologic features between hairy cells and prolymphocytes
   b. Usually associated with leukocytosis/lack of monocytopenia
   c. Absence of CD25 expression
4. Systemic mastocytosis
   a. Mast cells are negative for B-cell markers and positive for tryptase

Bartl R et al. Am J Clin Pathol 1983;79:531–545

Brunning RD et al. Atlas of Tumor Pathology, 3rd Series, Fascicle 9. Washington DC, AFIP, 1994:277–278

Burke JS et al. Am J Clin Pathol 1978;70:876–884

Burke JS et al. Semin Oncol 1984;11:334–346

Cornfield DB et al. Am J Hematol 2001;67:223–236

Ellison DJ et al. Blood 1994;84:4310–4315

Flandrin G et al. Semin Oncol 1984;11:458–471

Golomb HM et al. Ann Intern Med 1978; 89:677–683

Haglund U et al. Blood 1994;83:2637–2645

Hakimian D et al. Blood 1993;82:1798–802

Hanson CA et al. Am J Surg Pathol 1989;13:671–669

Hounieu H et al. Am J Clin Pathol 1992;98:26–33

Katayama I. Hematol Oncol Clin North Am 1988;2:585–602

Kluin-Nielmans HC et al. Blood 1994;84:3134–3441

Kroft SH et al. Blood Rev 1995;9:234–250

Lee WM et al. Cancer 1982;50:2207–2210

Robbins BA et al. Blood 1993;82:1277–1287

Sausville JE et al. Am J Clin Pathol 2003:119:213–217

Turner A et al. Medicine 1978;57:477–499

Wheaton S et al. Blood 1996;87:1556–1560

Yam LT et al. NEJM 1971;284:357–360

Prognosis

Therapy with purine analogues: Pentostatin (2′-deoxycoformycin) or cladribine (2-chlorodeoxyadenosine)

Complete remission	70–90%
Partial remission	10–20%
No response	5–10%
Relapse rate	5–25%
Estimated 5-year survival rate	85–90%
5–10-year survival rate	80–90%

Catovsky D et al. Leuk lymphoma 1994;14:109–113
Dearden CE et al. Br J Haematol 1999;106:515–519
Flinn IW et al. Blood 2000;96:2981–2986
Goodman GR et al. JCO 2003;21:891–896
Grever M et al. JCO 1995;13:974–982
Hoffman MA et al. JCO 1997;15:1138–1142
Jehn U et al. Ann Hematol 1999;78:139–144
Kraut EH et al. Blood 1994;84:4061–4063
Saven A et al. Blood 1998;92:1918–1926
Tallman MS et al. Blood 1996;88:1954–1959

Caveats

1. There is no clear advantage to either purine analogue as initial treatment for patients with previously untreated, relapsed, or refractory HCL. The ease of administration of cladribine, which requires only a single course of therapy, may offer some advantages
2. Fever is common with purine analogue therapy and usually occurs between days 5 and 7 of treatment with cladribine. It is rarely attributed to infection and may represent pyrogens released from lysed hairy cells
3. A diagnosis of HCL of itself is not necessarily an indication to initiate treatment. Treatment should be started when the patient has developed life-threatening cytopenias (absolute neutrophil count $<1000/mm^3$, hemoglobin <11 g/dL, or platelet count $<100,000/mm^3$) or in the presence of symptomatic splenomegaly or constitutional symptoms attributable to the disease

Estey EH et al. Blood 1992;79:882–887
Saven A et al. Blood 1998;92:1918–1926
Tallman MS et al. Blood 1992;80:2203–2209

REGIMEN

CLADRIBINE (2-CHLORODEOXYADENOSINE, 2-CDA)

Cheson BD et al. JCO 1998;16:3007–3015
Robak T et al. Leuk Lymphoma 1996;22:107–111
Tallman MS et al. Blood 1992;80:2203–2209
Tallman MS et al. Blood 1996;88:1954–1959

Cladribine 0.1 mg/kg per day by continuous intravenous infusion in 100–500 mL 0.9% NaCl injection (0.9% NS) over 24 hours for 7 consecutive days (total dosage/cycle = 0.7 mg/kg)

or

Cladribine 0.14 mg/kg per day intravenously in 100–500 mL of 0.9% NS over 2 hours for 5 consecutive days (total dosage/cycle = 0.7 mg/kg)

(Robak T et al. Leuk Lymphoma 1996;22:107–111)

or

Cladribine 0.15 mg/kg per dose intravenously in 100–500 mL 0.9% NS over 3 hours once a week for 6 consecutive weeks (total dosage/cycle = 0.9 mg/kg)

(Lauria F et al. Blood 1997;89:1838–1839; Chacko J et al. Br J Haematol 1999;105:1145–1146)

Optional: **Allopurinol** 300 mg/day orally, beginning on the first day of cladribine administration and continuing for 2 weeks. Tumor lysis is uncommon, and allopurinol need not be routinely administered

Emetogenic potential: Nonemetogenic (Emetogenicity score = 1). See Chapter 39

Treatment Modifications

Toxicity	Modification
Platelet count <15,000/mm^3	Administer platelets
Symptomatic anemia or hemoglobin <7 g/dL	Administer packed red blood cells

Toxicity (N = 895)

	% G1	% G2	% G3	% G4
All Toxicities				
Maximum grade	21	20	22	6
Nonhematologic Toxicities				
Maximum grade	14	18	17	4
Hemorrhage	2	2	0.6	0.6
Nausea/vomiting	14	4	0.5	0.3
Infection	1	13	13	3
Pulmonary	3	2	0.7	0.7
Skin	8	5	4	0.5
Fever >38.3°C (101°F)*				48%
Peripheral vein chemical phlebitis*				12%
Neurologic Toxicities				
Maximum grade	18	6	1	0.1
Motor	8	3	1	0
Headache	11	2	0.3	0
Constipation	5	1	0	0.1
Hematologic Toxicities				
ANC < 1000/mm^3 or >50% decrease from baseline or platelet count <100,000/mm^3 or >50% decrease from baseline*				66%

*Tallman MS et al. Blood 1992;80:2203–2209 (N = 26)
From Cheson BD et al. JCO 1998;16:3007–3015

Patient Population Studied

Patients with newly diagnosed as well as relapsed and refractory disease

Efficacy

Complete remission	75–90%
Partial remission	5–20%
Relapse rate	5–25%

Therapy Monitoring

1. *Every other day for the week of therapy, then weekly for the next 7 weeks:* CBC with differential, serum electrolytes, BUN, creatinine, LFTs, and uric acid
2. *Three months after completion of therapy:* Bone marrow aspirate and biopsy
3. *Long-term follow up:* CBC every 3–6 months for 2 years, then every 6 months for 3 years

Notes

Cladribine may be administered to patients with relapsed or refractory disease

REGIMEN

PENTOSTATIN (2′-DEOXYCOFORMYCIN, DCF)

Grever M et al. JCO 1995;13:974–982

Hydration: 5% dextrose/0.9% NaCl injection (D5W/0.9% NS) or 5% dextrose/0.45% NaCl injection (D5W/0.45% NS), 1000 mL before and at least 500 mL after pentostatin

Pentostatin 4 mg/m^2 by intravenous infusion over 20–30 min in 25–50 mL 0.9% NaCl injection (0.9% NS) or 5% dextrose injection (D5W) every 2 weeks until complete remission (total dosage/2-week course = 4 mg/m^2),

then

Pentostatin 4 mg/m^2 by intravenous infusion over 20–30 min in 25–50 mL 0.9%NS or D5W every 2 weeks for 2 courses (total dosage/2-week course = 4 mg/m^2)

Optional: **Allopurinol** 300 mg/day orally, beginning on the first day of pentostatin administration and continuing for 2 weeks. Tumor lysis is uncommon, and allopurinol need not be routinely administered

Emetogenic potential: Moderate (Emetogenicity score = 3). See Chapter 39

Patient Population Studied

A study of 154 patients with previously untreated HCL

Efficacy

Complete remission	70–80%
Partial remission	5–20%
Relapse rate	10–25%

Toxicity (N = 154)

	% G3	% G4
Allergy/rash	2.6	0
Nausea/vomiting/ anorexia	12	0
Chills/fever	1.3	0
Diarrhea	1.3	0
Neurologic	0.7	0
Hepatic	0.7	0
Renal	0.7	0
Anemia	0.7	0
Granulocytopenia (G4)	5.2	14
Thrombocytopenia	2.6	0
Suspected infection during induction		53%
Systemic antibiotics during induction		27%

Treatment Modifications

Toxicity	Dose Modification
Serum creatinine >20% over baseline	Hold pentostatin until serum creatinine returns to baseline or creatinine clearance on a 24-hour urine is >50 mL/min
New or suspected infection	Hold pentostatin until successful therapy being administered
G2 Nonhematologic toxicity	Reduce pentostatin by 33% after toxicity G ≤ 1
G3 Nonhematologic toxicity	Reduce pentostatin by 50% after toxicity G ≤ 1
G4 Nonhematologic toxicity	Discontinue pentostatin

Therapy Monitoring

1. *Two to 3 times per week during therapy:* CBC with differential, serum electrolytes, BUN, creatinine, LFTs, and uric acid
2. *Three months after completion of therapy:* Bone marrow aspirate and biopsy
3. *Long-term follow up:* CBC every 3–6 months for 2 years, then every 6 months for 3 years

REGIMEN

RITUXIMAB

Hagberg H et al. Br J Haematol 2001:115:609–611
Lauria F et al. Haematologica 2001;86:1046–1050
Nieva J et al. Blood 2003 102:810–813

Premedication:
(1) **Acetaminophen** 650–1000 mg orally 30 minutes before rituximab
(2) **Diphenhydramine** 25–50 mg orally or by intravenous push 30–60 minutes before rituximab

Rituximab 375 mg/m^2 per week intravenously in 0.9% NaCl injection (0.9% NS) or 5% dextrose injection (D5W) diluted to a concentration within the range of 1–4 mg/mL for 4 consecutive weeks (total dosage/4 week course = 1500 mg/m^2)

or

Rituximab 375 mg/m^2 per week intravenously in 0.9% NS or D5W diluted to a concentration of 1–4 mg/mL for 8 consecutive weeks with an additional 4 weekly doses (maximum of 12) if a patient does not achieve a complete remission but shows signs of continual improvement (total dosage/8-week and 12-week courses = 3000 mg/m^2 and 4500 mg/m^2, respectively)

Thomas DA et al. Blood 2003;102:3906–3911

Rituximab infusion rates:
First dose: 50 mg/hour. If hypersensitivity or infusion reactions do not occur during the first 30 minutes, increase the rate by 50 mg/hour every 30 minutes to a maximum of 400 mg/hour
Subsequent doses: If previous administration was well tolerated, start at 100 mg/hour and increase by 100 mg/hour every 30 minutes to a maximum of 400 mg/hour

Optional: **Allopurinol** 300 mg/day orally, beginning on the first day of rituximab administration and continuing for 2 weeks. Tumor lysis is uncommon and allopurinol need not be routinely administered

Emetogenic potential: Nonemetogenic (Emetogenicity score = 1). See Chapter 39

Patient Population Studied

Patients with relapsed or refractory HCL

Efficacy

Overall response	80%
Complete response	53%
Partial response	27%*
No response	20%

Includes 2 additional patients who achieved complete remission by hematologic parameters but had residual marrow disease (1–5% hairy cells)
Duration of response: With median follow-up of 32 months, 5 of 12 patients had progression of disease at 8, 12, 18, 23, and 39 months from the start of therapy

Thomas DA et al. Blood 2003;102:3906–3911

Toxicity (N = 15)

	No. of Patients	Grade	Dose No.
Fever and chills	9	1	1
Nausea and vomiting	4	1	1, 2
Hypotension*	1	1	1
Palpitations*	1	2	1, 2
Shortness of breath*	1	2	1
Myalgias	1	3	All 8
Fatigue	2	1, 2	1, 2
Back pain	1	1	1
Rash	1	1	1
Infection	0	—	—

*Infusional events associated with the first dose. Rapid resolution occurred with temporary cessation of infusion

Thomas DA et al. Blood 2003;102:3906–3911

Treatment Modifications

Rituximab Infusion-Related Toxicities

Onset of infusion-related events (fevers, chills, rigors edema, congestion of the head and neck mucosa, hypotension):
1. Interrupt rituximab infusion
2. For fever, chills: Give additional dose of acetaminophen 650 mg orally and diphenhydramine 25–50 mg by intravenous push
3. For rigors: Give meperidine 12.5–25 mg by intravenous push ± promethazine 12.5–25 mg by intravenous infusion in at least 10 mL 0.9% NS or D5W over 5–15 minutes. If after 15–20 minutes the response to a single dose is considered inadequate, the dose may be repeated
4. After symptoms resolve, resume rituximab infusion at 50 mg/hour and increase by 50 mg/hour every 30 minutes as tolerated up to a maximum rate of 200 mg/hour

Dyspnea or wheezing, without allergic findings (urticaria, or tongue or laryngeal edema):
1. Interrupt rituximab infusion immediately
2. Give hydrocortisone 100 mg by intravenous push (or glucocorticoid equivalent)
3. Give a histamine H_2 antagonist (ranitidine 150 mg, cimetidine 300 mg, or famotidine 20 mg) by intravenous push
4. After symptoms resolve, resume rituximab infusion at 25 mg/hour with close monitoring. Do not increase rate

Note: Medications for the treatment of hypersensitivity reactions should be available for immediate use in the event of a reaction during administration (eg intravenous fluids, epinephrine, antihistamines, glucocorticoids, and O_2)

Therapy Monitoring

1. *Weekly before each dose of rituximab:* CBC
2. *One to 3 months after the completion of therapy:* Bone marrow aspirate and biopsy with immunophenotyping
3. *Long-term follow up:* CBC every 3–6 months for 2 years, then every 6 months for 3 years

Notes

1. Patients requiring close monitoring during first and all subsequent infusions include those with preexisting cardiac and pulmonary conditions, prior clinically significant cardiopulmonary adverse events, or circulating malignant cells >25,000/mm^3 with or without evidence of high tumor burden
2. No clear benefit of 4 versus 12 doses

23. Lung Cancer

Enriqueta Felip, MD, and Rafael Rosell, MD

Epidemiology

Lung cancer is the leading cause of cancer death in both men and women in the United States. Approximately 85% of all lung cancers relate to cigarette smoking

Incidence:	174,470 (estimate for 2006 in the United States)
Deaths:	162,460 (estimate for 2006 in the United States)
Male:female ratio:	93,110:80,660

Jemal A et al. CA Cancer J Clin 2006;56:106–30
Weir HK et al. J Natl Cancer Inst 2003;95:1276–1299
For more information, see http://seer.cancer.gov

Pathology

Lung cancer is divided into two major classes:

1. Non–small cell lung cancer (NSCLC): 75–85%
   - Squamous cell carcinoma
   - Adenocarcinoma
   - Large-cell carcinoma
2. Small cell lung cancer (SCLC) 15–25%

Brambilla E et al. Eur Respir J 2001;18:1059–1068

Non–Small Cell Lung Cancer (NSCLC)

Work-Up

1. History and physical examination including performance status and weight loss
2. Chest x-ray, PA and lateral
3. CT scan of chest and upper abdomen including adrenals
4. CBC, serum electrolytes, BUN, creatinine, calcium, magnesium, and LFTs
5. CT scan and/or MRI of brain if neurologic history or examination is abnormal
6. Bone scan if there is bone pain, elevated calcium level, or elevated alkaline phosphatase level
7. Assessment of perioperative risks for potential candidates for surgery including pulmonary function tests (PFTs)

Stages I–II
- a. Bronchoscopy
- b. FDG-PET scan

Stage IIIA–IIIB
- a. Bronchoscopy
- b. FDG-PET scan
- c. MRI of the chest in superior sulcus tumors
- d. MRI of brain
- e. Bone scan
- f. Mediastinal lymph node biopsy if CT scan shows nodes >1 cm

Invasive tests: Mediastinoscopy, thoracoscopy, transbronchial needle aspiration, and endoscopic ultrasound and needle aspiration

Stage IV
- a. FDG-PET scan with no evidence of metastatic disease on CT scan
- b. Biopsy for otherwise potentially resectable patient with isolated adrenal mass or liver lesion

Diagnosis and Management of Lung Cancer: ACCP Evidence-Based Guidelines. Chest 2003;123(1 suppl):1S-337S
Pfister DG et al. J Clin Oncol 2004;22:330–353
More information in ESMO minimum clinical recommendations (www.esmo.org) and NCCN Clinical Practice Guidelines in Oncology, V. 2. 2006 (www.nccn.org)

Staging

Primary Tumor (T)

Tx	Primary tumor cannot be assessed, or tumor proven by the presence of malignant cells in sputum or bronchial washings but not visualized by imaging or bronchoscopy
T0	No evidence of primary tumor
Tis	Carcinoma in situ
T1	Tumor ≤3 cm in greatest dimension, surrounded by lung or visceral pleura, without bronchoscopic evidence of invasion more proximal than the lobar bronchus (ie, not in the main bronchus)
T2	Tumor with any of the following features of size extent: >3 cm in greatest dimension, involves main bronchus, ≥2 cm distal to the carina, invades the visceral pleura, associated with atelectasis or obstructive pneumonitis that extends to the hilar region but does not involve the entire lung
T3	Tumor of any size that directly invades any of the following: Chest wall (including superior sulcus tumor), diaphragm, mediastinal pleura, parietal pericardium; or tumor in the main bronchus <2 cm distal to the carina, but without involvement of the carina; or associated atelectasis or obstructive pneumonitis of the entire lung
T4	Tumor of any size that invades any of the following: Mediastinum, heart, great vessels, trachea, esophagus, vertebral body, carina; or separate tumor nodules in the same lobe; or tumor with a malignant pleural effusion

Regional Lymph Nodes (N)

NX	Regional lymph nodes cannot be assessed
N0	No regional lymph node metastasis
N1	Metastasis to ipsilateral peribronchial and/or ipsilateral hilar lymph nodes, and intrapulmonary nodes including involvement by direct extension of the primary tumor
N2	Metastasis to ipsilateral mediastinal and/or subcarinal lymph node(s)
N3	Metastasis to contralateral mediastinal, contralateral hilar, ipsilateral or contralateral scalene, or supraclavicular lymph node(s)

Distant Metastases (M)

MX	Distant metastasis cannot be assessed
M0	No distant metastasis
M1	Distant metastasis present

Note: M1 includes separate tumor nodule(s) in a different lobe (ipsilateral or contralateral)

Staging Groups

Occult carcinoma	TX	N0	M0
Stage 0	Tis	N0	M0
Stage IA	T1	N0	M0
Stage IB	T2	N0	M0
Stage IIA	T1	N1	M0
Stage IIB	T2	N1	M0
	T3	N0	M0
Stage IIIA	T3	N1	M0
	T1-3	N2	M0
Stage IIIB	Any T	N3	M0
	T4	Any N	M0
Stage IV	Any T	Any N	M1

Mountain CF. Chest 1997;111:1710–1177

5-Year Relative Survival Rates

All stages	15%
Stage I	56%
Stage II	32%
Stage III	9%
Stage IV	2%

More information in www.seer.cancer.gov

Caveats

1. Surgery is the standard treatment in stage I-II disease. Radiation therapy should be considered in medically inoperable stage I-II disease (inadequate pulmonary function tests or comorbid diseases)
2. Preoperative chemotherapy is the treatment of choice for resectable stage IIIA disease. Adjuvant chemotherapy is recommended for patients with stage IB–IIIA tumors who have a good performance status after surgery. Platinum-based chemotherapy and thoracic radiation therapy is the standard treatment for unresectable stage III. Concurrent chemoradiation appears to be better than sequential chemoradiation
3. Platinum-based chemotherapy prolongs survival, improves symptom control, and yields superior quality of life in stage IV disease. First-line chemotherapy should be a two-drug combination regimen. No specific new agent-platinum combination is clearly superior (cisplatin or carboplatin in combination with any of the following: paclitaxel, docetaxel, gemcitabine, vinorelbine). Non–platinum-containing regimens may be used as alternatives to platinum-based combinations
4. For elderly patients or patients with ECOG PS (performance status) 2, available data support the use of single-agent chemotherapy as first-line treatment
5. Docetaxel or pemetrexed are recommended as second-line therapy in advanced NSCLC patients with an adequate performance status (PS) who have had progression of their disease on a platinum-based therapy
6. Erlotinib is recommended in advanced NSCLC patients who have had disease progression after platinum and docetaxel

Pfister DG et al. JCO 2004;22:330–353
Winton TL et al. New Eng J Med 2005;352:2589–97

REGIMEN

PACLITAXEL + CARBOPLATIN

Kelly K et al. JCO 2001;19:3210–3218

Premedication (primary prophylaxis against hypersensitivity reactions from paclitaxel):
Dexamethasone 20 mg/dose for 2 doses orally the evening before and the morning of chemotherapy prior to paclitaxel, *plus*:
Diphenhydramine 50 mg for 1 dose by intravenous push 30 minutes before paclitaxel, *and*:
Ranitidine 50 mg or **cimetidine** 300 mg for 1 dose by intravenous infusion in 25–100 mL 0.9% NaCl injection (0.9% NS) or 5% dextrose injection (D5W) over 5–30 minutes, 30 minutes before paclitaxel
Paclitaxel 225 mg/m^2 by intravenous infusion in a volume of 0.9% NS or D5W sufficient to produce a solution with concentration within the range 0.3–1.2 mg/mL over 3 hours on day 1 every 3 weeks (total dosage/cycle = 225 mg/m^2)

Carboplatin [calculated dose] AUC = 6 by intravenous infusion in 50–150 mL D5W over 15–30 minutes, given on day 1 every 3 weeks (total dosage/cycle calculated to produce an AUC=6 mg/mL·min) (see equation below)

Filgrastim 5 mcg/kg per day subcutaneously may be used beginning 24 hours after chemotherapy and continued until ANC >10,000/mm^3 on two consecutive measurements
Dexamethasone 8 mg/dose for 6 doses after chemotherapy orally if G ≥ 2 arthralgias/myalgias occur

Emetogenic potential: High (Emetogenicity score = 5). See Chapter 39 for antiemetic regimens

Note: Carboplatin dose is based on Calvert's formula to achieve a target Area Under the plasma concentration versus time Curve (AUC) [AUC units=mg/mL·min]

$$\text{Total carboplatin dose (mg)} = (\text{Target AUC}) \times (\text{GFR} + 25)$$

In practice, creatinine clearance (Clcr) is used in place of glomerular filtration rate (GFR). Clcr can be calculated from the equation of Cockcroft and Gault:

$$\text{Males, Clcr} = \frac{(140 - \text{age [y]}) \times \text{body weight [kg]}}{72 \times (\text{Serum creatinine [mg/dL]})}$$

$$\text{Females, Clcr} = \frac{(140 - \text{age [y]}) \times \text{body weight [kg]}}{72 \times (\text{Serum creatinine [mg/dL]})} \times 0.85$$

Calvert AH et al. JCO 1989;7:1748–1756
Cockcroft DW, Gault MH. Nephron 1976;16:31–41
Jodrell DI et al. JCO 1992;10:520–528
Sorensen BT et al. Cancer Chemother Pharmacol 1991;28:397–401

Treatment Modifications

Adverse Event	Dose Modification
ANC nadir <500/mm^3, platelet nadir <50,000/mm^3, or febrile neutropenia	Reduce carboplatin dosage to AUC = 5 if previous cycle dose was AUC = 6; or to AUC = 4 if previous cycle dose was AUC = 5
ANC nadir <500/mm^3, platelet nadir <50,000/mm^3, or febrile neutropenia after 2 carboplatin dose reductions (AUC in previous cycle = 4)	Reduce paclitaxel dosage to 200 mg/m^2, and decrease carboplatin dosage to AUC = 3
Day 1 ANC <1500/mm^3 or platelets <100,000/mm^3	Delay chemotherapy until ANC >1500/mm^3 and platelets >100,000/mm^3, for maximum delay of 2 weeks
Delay of >2 weeks in reaching ANC >1500/mm^3 and platelet nadir >100,000/mm^3	Discontinue therapy
G2 neurotoxicity	Reduce paclitaxel dosage to 200 mg/m^2
G3 neurotoxicity	Reduce paclitaxel dosage to 175 mg/m^2
G2 arthralgia/myalgia despite dexamethasone prophylaxis	Reduce paclitaxel dosage to 200 mg/m^2
G3 arthralgia/myalgia despite dexamethasone prophylaxis	Reduce paclitaxel dosage to 175 mg/m^2
≥G2 AST or ≥G3 bilirubin	Hold paclitaxel
Moderate hypersensitivity	Patient may be retreated
Severe hypersensitivity	Discontinue therapy
Chest pain or arrhythmia during chemotherapy	Immediately stop chemotherapy and evaluate the patient
Symptomatic arrhythmias, or ≥2-degree AV block, or an ischemic event	Discontinue therapy

Patient Population Studied

A randomized comparison with vinorelbine + cisplatin in 206 patients with advanced, previously-untreated NSCLC

Efficacy (N = 203)

Response rate (CR + PR)	25%
Median progression-free survival	4 months
Median survival	8.6 months
1-year survival	38%
2-year survival	15%

WHO criteria

Toxicity (N = 203)

Adverse Event	% G3	% G4
Hematologic		
Leukopenia	26	5
Neutropenia	21	36
Thrombocytopenia	10	0
Anemia	11	2
Nonhematologic		
Nausea	7	0
Sensory neuropathy	13	0
Vomiting	4	0
Dehydration	4	0
Fatigue	8	0
Hyponatremia	3	0
Weakness (motor neuropathy)	8	0
Respiratory infection/neutropenia	1	0

NCI CTC criteria

Therapy Monitoring

1. *Before each cycle:* H&P, PS evaluation CBC with differential, LFTs, BUN and creatinine
2. *Every week:* CBC with differential and platelet count
3. *Response evaluation:* Every 2–3 cycles

REGIMEN

PACLITAXEL + CISPLATIN

Rosell R et al. Ann Oncol 2002;13:1539–1549

Premedication (primary prophylaxis against hypersensitivity reactions from paclitaxel):
Dexamethasone 20 mg/dose for 2 doses orally the evening before and the morning of chemotherapy before paclitaxel, *plus:*
Diphenhydramine 50 mg by intravenous push, 30 minutes before paclitaxel, *and:*
Ranitidine 50 mg or **cimetidine** 300 mg by intravenous infusion in 25–100 mL 0.9% NaCl injection (0.9% NS) or 5% dextrose injection (D5W) over 5–30 minutes, 30 minutes before paclitaxel
Paclitaxel 200 mg/m² intravenously in a volume of 0.9% NS or D5W sufficient to produce a solution with concentration within the range 0.3–1.2 mg/mL over 3 hours on day 1 every 21 days (total dosage/cycle = 200 mg/m²)

Hydration before cisplatin: Administer by intravenous infusion ≥1000 mL 0.9% NaCl injection (0.9% NS) over a minimum of 2–4 hours
Cisplatin 80 mg/m² by intravenous infusion in 100–250 mL 0.9% NS over 30 minutes, given on day 1 every 21 days (total dosage/cycle = 80 mg/m²)
Hydration after cisplatin: Administer by intravenous infusion ≥1000 mL 0.9% NS over a minimum of 2 to 4 hours. Also encourage high oral intake. Monitor and replace magnesium/electrolytes as needed

Dexamethasone 8 mg/dose for 6 doses after chemotherapy orally if G≥2 arthralgias/myalgias occur
Filgrastim 5 mcg/kg per day subcutaneously. May begin 24 hours after chemotherapy, and continue until ANC >10,000/mm³ on two consecutive measurements

Emetogenic potential: High (Emetogenicity score = 6). See Chapter 39 for antiemetic regimens

Patient Population Studied

A randomized comparison with paclitaxel + carboplatin in 309 patients with advanced (Stage III/IV) NSCLC not previously treated

Efficacy (N = 284)

Complete Response	1%
Partial Response	27%
Median progression-free survival*	4.2 months
Median survival*	9.8 months
Estimated 1-year survival	38%
2-year survival	15%

*Intention-to-treat analysis

WHO criteria

Toxicity (N = 302)

Hematologic

	% G3/4
Neutropenia	51
Leukopenia	16
Anemia	9
Infections	5
Febrile neutropenia	4
Thrombocytopenia	2

Nonhematologic

	% Severe
Nausea/vomiting	14
Asthenia	10
Arthralgia/myalgia	9
Peripheral neuropathy*	7
Diarrhea	2
Hypersensitivity	1
Renal*	1

*Grade 3

Treatment Modifications

Dose escalations not permitted. Dosage reductions based on toxicity encountered during a previous cycle

Adverse Event	Dose Modification
≥G2 arthralgias/myalgias	Add dexamethasone as secondary prophylaxis
Day 1 ANC <1500/mm³ or platelet count <100,000/mm³	Delay therapy until ANC >1500/mm³ and platelet count >100,000/mm³. If >2-week delay, the decision to retreat is based on caregiver's discretion
Febrile neutropenia	Reduce cisplatin and paclitaxel dosages by 25%
Bleeding associated with thrombocytopenia	Reduce cisplatin and paclitaxel dosages by 25%
Serum creatinine 1.6–2.0 mg/dL (141–177 μmol/L)	Reduce cisplatin dosage by 25%
Serum creatinine >2.0 mg/dL (177 μmol/L)	Hold cisplatin until serum creatinine ≤2.0 mg/dL (≤177 μmol/L)
G3/4 neurotoxicity	Delay therapy until ≤G2
Moderate hypersensitivity reactions	Decision to retreat based on severity and caregiver's discretion
Severe hypersensitivity reactions	Stop treatment
Symptomatic arrhythmias or AV block ≥second-degree, or documented ischemic event	Stop treatment
≥G2 AST (SGOT) or grade ≥3 bilirubin	Stop paclitaxel

Therapy Monitoring

1. *Before each cycle:* H&P, PS evaluation, CBC with differential, serum electrolytes, magnesium LFTs, BUN and creatinine
2. *Every week:* CBC with differential and platelet count
3. *Response evaluation:* Every 2–3 cycles

REGIMEN

GEMCITABINE + CISPLATIN

Sandler AB et al. JCO 2000;18:122–130

Gemcitabine 1000 mg/m² by intravenous infusion in 50–250 mL 0.9% NS over 30–60 minutes, given on days 1, 8, and 15, every 28 days (total dosage/cycle = 3000 mg/m²). On day 1 administer after or during hydration for cisplatin and follow with cisplatin

Hydration before cisplatin: ≥1000 mL 0.9% NaCl injection (0.9% NS) by intravenous infusion over a minimum of 2–4 hours

Cisplatin 100 mg/m² by intravenous infusion in 100–250 mL 0.9% NS over 30–120 minutes, given on day 1 every 28 days (total dosage/cycle=100 mg/m²)
Hydration after cisplatin: ≥1000 mL 0.9% NS by intravenous infusion over a minimum of 2–4 hours. Also encourage high oral intake. Monitor and replace magnesium/electrolytes as needed

Emetogenic potential:
Day 1: High (Emetogenicity score = 6)
Days 8 and 15: Low (Emetogenicity score = 2)
Potential for delayed symptoms after day 1. See Chapter 39 for antiemetic regimens

Patient Population Studied

A randomized comparison with single-agent cisplatin in 260 patients with advanced (Stage III/IV) previously untreated NSCLC

Efficacy (N = 260)

Complete response	1.2%
Partial response	29.2%
Est. median progression-free survival	5.6 months
Estimated median survival	9.1 months
Estimated 1-year survival	39%

Toxicity (N = 260)

	% G3	% G4
Hematologic		
Granulocytopenia	21.5	35.3
Thrombocytopenia	25	25.4
Anemia	21.9	3.1
Febrile neutropenia	4.6% of patients	
Platelet transfusions	20.4% of patients	
Erythrocyte transfusions	37.7% of patients	
Nonhematologic		
Nausea	25	2
Vomiting	11	12
Increased creatinine	4.4	0.4
Neurologic (hearing)	5.6	0.4
Neurologic (motor)	11.5	0
Dyspnea	4	3
Increased transaminases	2	1
Increased bilirubin	0.8	0.8

WHO criteria

Treatment Modifications

Adverse Event	Dose Modification
ANC <1500/mm³, or platelets <100,000/mm³	Hold chemotherapy until ANC >1500/mm³ and platelets >100,000/mm³
Febrile granulocytopenia that requires antibiotics	Reduce cisplatin and gemcitabine dosages by 25% in subsequent cycles
Bleeding associated with thrombocytopenia	
Intracycle: G1/2 nonhematologic toxicity or G1–3 nausea or vomiting	100% gemcitabine dosage on days 8 and 15
Intracycle: G3 nonhematologic toxicity, except nausea, vomiting, and alopecia	Reduce gemcitabine dosage by 25% on days 8 and 15, or hold treatment at clinician's discretion
Intracycle: G4 nonhematologic toxicity	Hold gemcitabine
Day 1 serum creatinine 1.6–2.0 mg/dL (141–177 μmol/L)	Reduce cisplatin dosage by 25%
Day 1 serum creatinine >2.0 mg/dL (>177 μmol/L)	Hold cisplatin until serum creatinine ≤2.0 mg/dL (≤177 μmol/L)
G3/4 neurotoxicity	Delay treatment until toxicity resolves to G1
Treatment delay >2 weeks	Discontinue therapy according to clinician's discretion

Therapy Monitoring

1. *Each cycle on day 1:* H&P, performance status reevaluation, CBC with differential and platelet count, serum electrolytes, magnesium serum creatinine, hepatic transaminases, bilirubin
2. *Cycle days 8 and 15*: CBC with differential and platelet count
3. *Response evaluation:* Every 2–3 cycles

REGIMEN

DOCETAXEL + CISPLATIN

Fossella F et al. JCO 2003;21:3016–3024

Prophylaxis for fluid retention and hypersensitivity reactions from docetaxel:
Dexamethasone 8 mg/dose for 6 doses orally as follows:

- One dose the evening before docetaxel
- Three doses the day of docetaxel (day 1):
  - First dose in the morning before docetaxel
  - Second dose 1 hour before docetaxel
  - Third dose in the evening after docetaxel
- Two doses the day after docetaxel (day 2)

Hydration before cisplatin: ≥1000 mL 0.9% NaCl injection (0.9% NS) by intravenous infusion over a minimum of 2–4 hours
Docetaxel 75 mg/m^2 by intravenous infusion in a volume of 0.9% NS or 5% dextrose injection (D5W) sufficient to produce a solution with concentration within the range 0.3–0.74 mg/mL over 1 hour on day 1 every 3 weeks (total dosage/cycle = 75 mg/m^2), *followed immediately by:*
Cisplatin 75 mg/m^2 by intravenous infusion in 100–250 mL 0.9% NS over 1 hour on day 1 every 3 weeks (total dosage/cycle = 75 mg/m^2)
Hydration after cisplatin: ≥1000 mL 0.9% NS by intravenous infusion over a minimum of 2–4 hours. Encourage oral intake. Monitor and replace magnesium/electrolytes as needed

Emetogenic potential: High (Emetogenicity score = 6). Potential for delayed symptoms. See Chapter 39 for antiemetic regimens

Patient Population Studied

A multicenter, international, prospective, open-label, randomized phase III comparison with vinorelbine + cisplatin in 408 patients with locally advanced or recurrent (Stage IIIB) or metastatic (Stage IV) NSCLC

Efficacy (N = 408)

Complete response	2.0%
Partial response	29.7%
Overall median survival	11.3 months
1-year survival	46%
2-year survival	21%

Toxicity (N = 406)

Toxicity*	% G3/4
Hematologic	
Leukopenia	42.8
Neutropenia	74.8
Thrombocytopenia	2.7
Anemia	6.9
Erythrocyte transfusions	10.3% of patients
Nonhematologic	
Infection	8.4
Asthenia	12.3
Nausea	9.9
Pulmonary	9.6
Pain	7.9
Vomiting	7.9
Diarrhea	6.7
Anorexia	5.4

*G3/4 adverse event in > 5% of patients
NCI CTC criteria

Treatment Modifications

Adverse Event	Dose Modification
ANC <1500/mm^3 or platelet count <100,000/mm^3	Hold chemotherapy until ANC >1500/mm^3 and platelets >100,000/mm^3
Febrile granulocytopenia that requires antibiotics	Reduce cisplatin and docetaxel dosages by 25% during subsequent cycles
Bleeding associated with thrombocytopenia	Reduce cisplatin and docetaxel dosages by 25% during subsequent cycles
Day 1 serum creatinine 1.6–2.0 mg/dL (141–177 μmol/L)	Reduce cisplatin dosage by 25%
Day 1 serum creatinine >2.0 mg/dL (>177 μmol/L)	Hold cisplatin until serum creatinine ≤2.0 mg/dL (≤177 μmol/L)
G3/4 neurotoxicity	Delay treatment
Treatment delay ≥2 weeks	Discontinue therapy or according to clinician's criteria

A maximum of 2 docetaxel or cisplatin dosage reductions are permitted

Therapy Monitoring

1. *Each cycle on day 1:* H&P, PS evaluation, CBC with differential, serum electrolytes, magnesium BUN, creatinine, and LFTs
2. *Every week:* CBC with differential and platelet count
3. *Response evaluation:* Every 2–3 cycles

REGIMEN

VINORELBINE + CISPLATIN

Wozniak AJ et al. JCO 1998;16:2459–2465

Vinorelbine 25 mg/m^2 by intravenous infusion in a volume of 0.9% NaCl injection (0.9% NS) or 5% dextrose injection (D5W) sufficient to produce a solution with concentration within the range 0.5–3 mg/mL over 6–10 minutes, given once weekly for 4 weeks (total dosage/cycle = 100 mg/m^2)

Hydration before cisplatin: ≥1000 mL 0.9% NS by intravenous infusion over a minimum of 2–4 hours
Cisplatin 100 mg/m^2 by intravenous infusion in 100–250 mL 0.9% NS over 1 hour on day 1 every 4 weeks (total dosage/cycle = 100 mg/m^2)
Hydration after cisplatin: ≥1000 mL 0.9% NS by intravenous infusion over a minimum of 2–4 hours. Encourage oral intake monitor and replace magnesium/electrolytes as needed

Emetogenic potential: High (Emetogenicity score = 5). Potential for delayed symptoms. See Chapter 39 for antiemetic regimens

Patient Population Studied

A randomized comparison with cisplatin of 206 patients with advanced previously untreated NSCLC

Efficacy

Complete response	2%
Partial response	24%
Median progression-free survival	4 months
Median survival	8 months
1-year survival	36%
2-year survival	12%

Toxicity (N = 204)

Hematologic

	% G3	% G4
Granulocytopenia	22	59
Thrombocytopenia	4	1
Anemia	21	3

Nonhematologic

	% G3/4
Fever/sepsis with granulocytopenia	10
Nausea/vomiting	20
Malaise/weakness	15
Constipation	3
Diarrhea	3
Electrolyte imbalance	6
Hearing	4
Vision	1
Neurologic (peripheral)	2
Neurologic (central)	2
Renal	5
Phlebitis/thrombosis	3

SWOG criteria

Treatment Modifications

Treatment day ANC must be ≥1500/mm^3 and platelets ≥100,000/mm^3 to treat on schedule at 100% dosages

Adverse Event	Dose Modification
Treatment day ANC 1000–1499/mm^3 or platelets 75,000–99,999/mm^3	Reduce cisplatin and vinorelbine dosages by 50%
Treatment day ANC <1000 or platelets <75,000/mm^3	Hold cisplatin and vinorelbine
Treatment delay >2 weeks but <3 weeks	Reduce subsequent cisplatin and vinorelbine dosages by 50%
Fever or sepsis with neutropenia in any cycle	Reduce subsequent cisplatin and vinorelbine dosages by 50%
ANC nadir <500/mm^3, or platelet nadir <50,000/mm^3	Reduce cisplatin dosage by 50% in subsequent cycles
Serum creatinine ≥1.6 mg/dL (≥141 µmol/L), but creatinine clearance ≥50 mL/min	Reduce cisplatin dosage by 50%
Creatinine clearance <50 mL/min	Hold cisplatin
Serum total bilirubin 2.1–3.0 mg/dL (35.9–51.3 µmol/L)	Reduce vinorelbine dosage by 50%
Serum total bilirubin >3.0 mg/dL (51.3 µmol/L)	Reduce vinorelbine dosage by 75%
Treatment delay >4 weeks	Discontinue therapy

If cisplatin treatment is held for any period of time, reduce cisplatin dosage 50% when treatment resumes

Therapy Monitoring

1. *Before repeated cycles:* H&P, PS evaluation, Serum creatinine and calculated creatinine clearance; serum electrolytes, magnesium, hepatic transaminases and bilirubin
2. *Weekly:* CBC with differential and platelet count
3. *Response evaluation:* Every 2–3 cycles

REGIMEN

VINORELBINE (ELDERLY PATIENTS)

Gridelli C et al. J Natl Cancer Inst 2003;95:362–372

Vinorelbine 30 mg/m^2 by intravenous infusion in a volume of 0.9% NaCl injection (0.9% NS) or 5% dextrose injection (D5W) sufficient to produce a solution with concentration within the range 0.5–3 mg/mL over 6–10 minutes, given on days 1 and 8 every 3 weeks for a maximum of 6 cycles (total dosage/cycle = 60 mg/m^2)

Emetogenic potential: Nonemetogenic (Emetogenicity score = 1). See Chapter 39 for antiemetic regimens

Patient Population Studied

A randomized comparison of gemcitabine + vinorelbine in 233 patients aged 70 years and older with advanced (Stage IIIB/IV) untreated NSCLC

Efficacy (Intent-to-Treat, N = 233)

Response rate	18%
Median survival	36 weeks
6-month survival	60%
Estimated 1-year survival	38%

Toxicity (N = 229)

	% G3	% G4
Hematologic		
Anemia	3	<1
Neutropenia	14	11
Thrombocytopenia	<1	—
Infection	3	—
Bleeding	1	—
Nonhematologic		
Nausea/vomiting	<1	—
Mucositis	1	—
Fatigue	7	—
Fever	2	—
Cardiac	1	<1
Pulmonary	1	—
Hepatic	<1	—
Constipation	3	<1
Peripheral neuropathy	1	—
Central neurotoxicity	—	<1

WHO criteria

Treatment Modifications

Adverse Event	Dose Modification
Days 1 and 8 ANC ≥1500/mm^3, platelet count ≥100,000/mm^3, and no organ toxicity (other than alopecia)	Vinorelbine given at 100% dosage
Days 1 and 8 ANC <1500/mm^3, platelet count <100,000/mm^3, or organ toxicity (other than alopecia)	Delay treatment for up to 2 weeks.
Serum total bilirubin 2.1–3.0 mg/dL (35.9–51.3 μmol/L)	Reduce vinorelbine dosage by 50%
Serum total bilirubin >3.0 mg/dL 51.3 μmol/L)	Reduce vinorelbine dosage by 75%

Therapy Monitoring

1. *Days 1* and *8:* CBC with differential and platelet count. Serum electrolytes, BUN, creatinine, and LFTs
2. *Weekly:* CBC with differential and platelet count
3. *Response evaluation:* Every 2–3 cycles

REGIMEN

DOCETAXEL

Shepherd FA et al. JCO 2000;18:2095–2103

Prophylaxis for fluid retention and hypersensitivity reactions from docetaxel:
Dexamethasone 8 mg/dose for 6 doses orally as follows:
- One dose the evening before docetaxel
- Three doses the day of docetaxel (day 1):
  - –First dose in the morning before docetaxel
  - –Second dose 1 hour before docetaxel
  - –Third dose in the evening after docetaxel
- Two doses the day after docetaxel (day 2)

Docetaxel 75 mg/m^2 by intravenous infusion in a volume of 0.9% NaCl injection (0.9% NS) or 5% dextrose injection (D5W) sufficient to produce a solution with concentration within the range 0.3–74 mg/mL over 1 hour on day 1 every 3 weeks (total dosage/cycle=75 mg/m^2)

Emetogenic potential: Low (Emetogenicity score=2). See Chapter 39 for antiemetic regimens

Treatment Modifications

Adverse Event	Dose Modification
G4 neutropenia for >7 days, alone, or accompanied by fever >38°C	Reduce docetaxel dosage by 25% in all subsequent treatments
G4 thrombocytopenia	Resume docetaxel after platelet count recovers with docetaxel dosage decreased by 25%
G4 vomiting not controlled by antiemetics	Reduce docetaxel dosage by 25%
≥G3 diarrhea	
≥G3 neuropathy	Discontinue therapy

Patient Population Studied

A randomized comparison with best supportive care of 55 patients with advanced (Stage III/IV) NSCLC previously treated with platinum-containing chemotherapy

Efficacy (N = 55)

Complete response	—
Partial response	7.1%
Median survival	7.5 months
1-year survival	37%

Toxicity (N = 55)

	% G3/4
Neutropenia	67.3
Anemia	5.5
Febrile neutropenia	1.8
Thrombocytopenia	0
Pulmonary	20
Asthenia	18.2
Infection	5.5
Nausea	3.6
Vomiting	3.6
Diarrhea	1.8
Neuromotor	1.8
Neurosensory	1.8

Therapy Monitoring

1. *Before treatment:* H&P, PS evaluation, CBC with differential, and LFTs
2. *Weekly:* CBC with differential and platelet count
3. *Response evaluation:* Every 2–3 cycles

REGIMEN

GEFITINIB

Kris MG et al. JAMA 2003;290:2149–2158

Gefitinib 250 mg per day orally for 28 days on days 1–28 (total dose/cycle = 7000 mg)
Gefitinib is manufactured in the United States in tablets for oral administration containing 250 mg gefitinib. IRESSA™ (gefitinib tablets) 250 mg. AstraZeneca Pharmaceuticals LP, Wilmington, DE

Emetogenic potential: Nonemetogenic (Emetogenicity score = 1). See Chapter 39 for antiemetic regimens

Treatment Modifications

For unacceptable toxicity, decrease gefitinib dosage to 100 mg per day orally

Patient Population Studied

A study of 106 patients with advanced NSCLC (Stage IIIB/IV) previously treated with two or more regimens containing cisplatin or carboplatin and docetaxel in a randomized comparison between orally administered gefitinib 250 mg daily and gefitinib 500 mg daily

Efficacy (N = 106)

Radiographic response rate	12%
Projected median survival	7 months
Estimated 1-year survival	27%
NSCLC symptoms improved	43%

Toxicity (N = 106)

	% G1	% G2	% G3	% G4
Cutaneous[a]	49	13	0	0
Diarrhea	47	9	1	0

Other Adverse Events[b]
G1/2 ocular itchiness or redness
G1/2 nausea or vomiting
G3 Thrombocytopenia
G3 Increase in ALT (SGPT) and AST (SGOT)

[a]Rash, pruritus, dry skin, or acne involving the face, neck, and trunk
[b]Observed in patients who received any study dose of gefitinib

NCI CTC criteria

Therapy Monitoring

1. *Before each 28-day cycle:* CBC with differential, LFTs, BUN and creatinine
2. *Response evaluation:* Every 2 cycles. Continue treatment until disease progression or unacceptable toxicity

REGIMEN

ERLOTINIB

Shepherd FA et al. NEJM 2005;353:123–132

Erlotinib 150 mg orally daily continually (total dose/week = 1050 mg)
Erlotinib is manufactured in the United States in film-coated tablets for oral administration containing 25 mg, 100 mg, and 150 mg erlotinib. Tarceva™ erlotinib tablets product label, November 2004. Manufactured by Schwarz Pharma Manufacturing, Seymour, IN. Manufactured by OSI Pharmaceuticals Inc, Melville, NY. Distributed by Genentech Inc., South San Francisco, CA

Emetogenic potential: Low (Emetogenicity score = 2). See Chapter 39 for antiemetic regimens

Patient Population Studied

A study of 485 patients with stage IIIB or stage IV NSCLC with performance status 1–3

Efficacy (N = 427)

Complete response	0.7%
Partial response	8.2%
Median overall survival	6.7 months
Median progression-free survival	2.2 months

Toxicity (N = 485)

	% All G	% G3–5
Rash	76	9
Anorexia	69	9
Nausea	40	3
Vomiting	25	3
Stomatitis	19	<1
Diarrhea	55	6
Dehydration	7	4
Ocular toxic effect	28	1
Fatigue	79	19
Infection	34	2
Pulmonary fibrosis	3	<1
Pneumonitis	3	<1
Death from pneumonitis		1 patient

Treatment Modifications

Adverse Event	Dose Modification
G2 Diarrhea	Loperamide, no dose reduction
G3 Diarrhea	Hold therapy until diarrhea is G ≤1, then restart erlotinib at 100 mg/day
G3 Diarrhea on 100 mg/day	Consider discontinuing erlotinib
G2 Skin rash	Hold erlotinib until toxicity G ≤ 1
Repeat G2 skin rash	Reduce erlotinib dose to 100 mg per day
G3 Rash	Hold therapy until rash is G ≤ 1, then restart erlotinib at 100 mg/day
G3 Rash on 100 mg/day	Consider discontinuing erlotinib
Other nonhematologic G2/3 toxicities	Hold erlotinib until toxicity G ≤ 1, then reduce erlotinib dose to 100 mg per day
G4 Toxicity	Discontinue erlotinib

Therapy Monitoring

1. *Before each 28-day cycle:* CBC with differential, LFTs, BUN and creatinine
2. *Response evaluation every 2 cycles:* Continue treatment until disease progression or unacceptable toxicity occurs

REGIMEN

PEMETREXED

Hanna N et al. JCO 2004;22:1589–15897

Folic acid 350–1000 mcg per day orally beginning 1–2 weeks before the first dose of pemetrexed and continuing until 3 weeks after the last dose of pemetrexed
Cyanocobalamin (vitamin B_{12}) 1000 mcg intramuscularly every 9 weeks, beginning 1–2 weeks before the first dose of pemetrexed
Dexamethasone 4 mg orally twice daily for 3 consecutive days, starting the day before pemetrexed administration to decrease the risk of severe skin rash associated with pemetrexed
Pemetrexed 500 mg/m^2 by intravenous infusion in 10 mL 0.9% NaCl injection (0.9% NS) over 10 minutes on day 1 every 21 days (total dosage/cycle = 500 mg/m^2)

Emetogenic potential: Low (Emetogenicity score = 2). See Chapter 39 for antiemetic regimens

Patient Population Studied

A study of 283 patients with stage III–IV NSCLC

Efficacy (N = 265)

Overall response rate	9.1%
1-year overall survival	29.7%
Median survival time	8.3 months
Median progression-free survival	2.9 months
Median time to progression	3.4 months
Median duration of response	4.6 months

Toxicity (N = 265)

	% Any G	% G3/4
Hematologic		
Neutropenia	Not given	5.3
Febrile neutropenia	Not given	1.9
Neutropenia with infection	Not given	0
Anemia	Not given	4.2
Thrombocytopenia	Not given	1.9
Nonhematologic		
Fatigue	34	5.3
Nausea	30.9	2.6
Vomiting	16.2	1.5
Pulmonary	0.8	0
Neurosensory	4.9	0
Stomatitis	14.7	1.1
Alopecia	6.4	0
Diarrhea	12.8	0.4
Rash	14	0.8
Weight loss	1.1	0
Edema	4.5	0

NCI CTC

Treatment Modifications

Adverse Event	Dose Modification
G3 Hematological toxicities	Hold therapy until toxicity returns to baseline, then reduce pemetrexed dosage by 25%
G4 Hematologic toxicities (thrombocytopenia)	Hold therapy until toxicity returns to baseline, then reduce pemetrexed dosage by 50%
Increased serum creatinine to 1.6–2 mg/dL (141–176 μmol/L)	Reduce pemetrexed dosage by 25%
Serum creatinine increased to ≥2 mg/dL (≥176 μmol/L)	Hold pemetrexed until serum creatinine <1.5 mg/dL (<133 μmol/L), then resume with pemetrexed dosage reduced by 25%
G ≥ 2 Diarrhea	Hold pemetrexed until toxicity resolves to G <2, then resume with pemetrexed dosage reduced by 25%
G3/4 Mucositis	Reduce pemetrexed dosage by 50%
Increased liver transaminases	Hold therapy until toxicity resolves, then resume with pemetrexed dosage reduced by 25%
Other G ≥ 3 nonhematologic toxicities (except nausea, vomiting, elevated transaminases and alopecia)	Delay treatment until toxicity resolves to baseline, then resume with pemetrexed dosage reduced by 25% from previous dose level

Note: If a patient requires 3 dose reductions, discontinue pemetrexed

Therapy Monitoring

1. *Before each 21-day cycle:* CBC with differential, LFTs, BUN, and creatinine
2. *Weekly:* CBC with differential
3. *Response evaluation every 2 cycles:* Continue treatment until disease progression or unacceptable toxicity
4. *Every 2–3 months:* Consider plasma homocysteine levels. (High homocysteine concentrations are a sensitive indicator of folate deficiency and may predict pemetrexed toxicity)

Notes

In the study reported by Hanna et al (JCO 2004;22:1589–97), 288 patients were treated with docetaxel 75 mg/m^2 by intravenous infusion every 21 days. Treatment with docetaxel resulted in clinically equivalent efficacy outcomes but had significantly higher side effects compared with pemetrexed

REGIMEN

PACLITAXEL + CARBOPLATIN + BEVACIZUMAB

Kelly K et al. JCO 2001;19:3210–3218
Sandler AB et al. ASCO 2005
http://www.asco.org/ac/1,1003,_12-002511-00_18-0034-00_19-004261,00.asp

Premedication (primary prophylaxis against hypersensitivity reactions from paclitaxel):
Dexamethasone 20 mg/dose for 2 doses orally the evening before and the morning of chemotherapy prior to paclitaxel, *plus:*
Diphenhydramine 50 mg for 1 dose by intravenous push 30 minutes before paclitaxel, *and:*
Ranitidine 50 mg or **cimetidine** 300 mg for 1 dose by intravenous infusion in 25–100 mL 0.9% NaCl injection (0.9% NS) or 5% dextrose injection (D5W) over 5–30 minutes, 30 minutes before paclitaxel
Paclitaxel 200 mg/m^2 by intravenous infusion in a volume of 0.9% NS or D5W sufficient to produce a solution with concentration within the range 0.3–1.2 mg/mL over 3 hours on day 1 every 3 weeks (total dosage/cycle=200 mg/m^2)

Carboplatin [calculated dose] AUC = 6 by intravenous infusion in 50–150 mL D5W over 15–30 minutes on day 1 every 3 weeks (total dosage/cycle calculated to produce an AUC = 6 mg/mL·min) (see equation below)

Bevacizumab 15 mg/kg intravenously in 100 mL 0.9% NS every 2 weeks (total dosage/3-week cycle = 15 mg/kg)

Note: Administration duration for the initial dose is 90 minutes. If administration is well tolerated, the administration duration may be decreased stepwise during subsequent administrations to 60 minutes and, finally, to a minimum duration of 30 minutes

Filgrastim 5 mcg/kg per day subcutaneously may be used beginning 24 hours after chemotherapy and continued until ANC >10,000/mm^3 on two consecutive measurements
Dexamethasone 8 mg/dose for 6 doses after chemotherapy orally if G ≥2 arthralgias/myalgias occur

Emetogenic potential: High (Emetogenicity score = 5). See Chapter 39

Note: Carboplatin dose is based on Calvert's formula to achieve a target Area Under the plasma concentration versus time Curve (AUC) [AUC units = mg/mL • min]

$$\text{Total carboplatin dose (mg)} = (\text{target AUC}) \times (\text{GFR} + 25)$$

In practice, creatinine clearance (Clcr) is used in place of glomerular filtration rate (GFR). Clcr can be calculated from the equation of Cockcroft and Gault:

$$\text{Males, Clcr} = \frac{(140 - \text{age [y]}) \times \text{body weight [kg]}}{72 \times (\text{Serum creatinine [mg/dL]})}$$

$$\text{Females, Clcr} = \frac{(140 - \text{age [y]}) \times \text{body weight [kg]}}{72 \times (\text{Serum creatinine [mg/dL]})} \times 0.85$$

Calvert AH et al. JCO 1989;7:1748–1756
Cockcroft DW, Gault MH. Nephron 1976;16:31–41
Jodrell DI et al. JCO 1992;10:520–528
Sorensen BT et al. Cancer Chemother Pharmacol 1991;28:397–401

Treatment Modifications

Adverse Event	Dose Modification
ANC nadir <500/mm^3, platelet nadir <50,000/mm^3, or febrile neutropenia	Reduce carboplatin dosage to AUC = 5 if previous cycle dose was AUC=6; or to AUC = 4 if previous cycle dose was AUC = 5
ANC nadir <500/mm^3, platelet nadir <50,000/mm^3, or febrile neutropenia after 2 carboplatin dose reductions (AUC in previous cycle = 4)	Reduce paclitaxel dosage to 200 mg/m^2, and decrease carboplatin dosage to AUC = 3
Day 1 ANC <1500/mm^3 or platelet <100,000/mm^3	Delay chemotherapy until ANC >1500/mm^3 and platelet >100,000/mm^3, for maximum delay of 2 weeks
Delay of >2 weeks in reaching ANC >1500/mm^3 and platelet >100,000/mm^3	Discontinue therapy
G2 Neurotoxicity	Reduce paclitaxel dosage to 200 mg/m^2
G3 Neurotoxicity	Reduce paclitaxel dosage to 175 mg/m^2
G2 Arthralgia/myalgia despite dexamethasone prophylaxis	Reduce paclitaxel dosage to 200 mg/m^2
G3 Arthralgia/myalgia despite dexamethasone prophylaxis	Reduce paclitaxel dosage to 175 mg/m^2
≥G2 AST or ≥G3 bilirubin	Hold paclitaxel
Moderate hypersensitivity	Patient may be retreated
Severe hypersensitivity	Discontinue therapy
Chest pain or arrhythmia during chemotherapy	Immediately stop chemotherapy and evaluate the patient
Symptomatic arrhythmias, or ≥2-degree AV block, or an ischemic event	Discontinue therapy

Patient Population Studied

A study of 855 patients with advanced, previously untreated stage IIIB (pleural or pericardial effusion only) NSCLC (non-squamous histologies). A randomized comparison with palcitael + carboplatin. ECOG PS 0 (40%) or 1 (60%). INR <1.5 and PTT no greater than upper limit normal. No history of thrombotic or hemorrhagic disorders. No gross hemoptysis defined as 1/2 teaspoon or more of bright red blood per day. Brain metastases were not allowed; 43% were age ≥65, and 28% had ≥5% weight loss

Efficacy (N = 357)

Overall response	27.2%
Complete response	1.4%
Partial response	25.8%
6-Month progression-free survival	55%
12-Month progression-free survival	14.6%
Median survival	12.5 months
1-Year survival	51.9%
2-Year survival	22.1%

Toxicity (N = 420)

Hematologic

Toxicity	% G4
Neutropenia	24[a]
Fever + neutropenia	3.3[a]
Thrombocytopenia	1.4
Anemia	0

Nonhematologic

	% ≥G3
Hemorrhage	4.5*
Hemoptysis	1.9*
CNS	1*
Gastrointestinal	1.2
Other	1
Hypertension	6*
Venous thrombosis	3.8
Areterial thrombosis	1.9

Treatment-Related Deaths

Hemoptysis	5 (1.2%)
Gastrointestinal bleeding	2 (0.5%)
Neutropenic fever	1 (0.25%)

*These values were statistically worse than those with paclitaxel + carboplatin alone

Therapy Monitoring

1. *Every week:* CBC with differential and platelet count
2. *Response evaluation:* Every 2–3 cycles

Notes

1. Compared with paclitaxel + carboplatin, overall survival advantage is confined to men; not seen in women ($P = .8$), despite statistically significant advantage for progression-free survival and response rate in women
2. Bevacizumab is associated with a small increase in serious bleeding, including hemoptysis. In a phase II trial, apparent risk factors for life-threatening hemorrhages included baseline hemoptysis brain metastases, anticoagulant therapy and squamous histology*
3. This therapy is the ECOG reference standard for first-line treatment of advanced NSCLC and is recommended by NCCN. Confirmatory trials have yet to be performed
4. Only patients with non-squamous histologies were included in this study

*Johnson DH et al. JCO 2004;22:2184–2191

Small Cell Lung Cancer (SCLC)

Work-Up

General work-up

1. History and physical examination
2. Complete blood count, liver and renal function tests, LDH, and serum electrolytes with special attention to serum sodium
3. Chest x-ray
4. CT scan of chest and upper abdomen including adrenals
5. Brain MRI (or CT scan)
6. Bone scan
7. FDG-PET scan (optional)

Individualized work-up

1. Bone marrow biopsy in selected patients
2. Pulmonary function tests and cardiac function assessment if thoracic radiation therapy is going to be performed
3. If a patient presents with pleural effusion, a diagnostic thoracocentesis is recommended. Consider thoracoscopy if thoracocentesis is inconclusive
4. Plain-film x-rays of bone scan abnormalities

Diagnosis and management of Lung Cancer: ACCP Evidence-Based Guidelines. Chest 2003;123 (1 Suppl):1S–337S
Pfister DG et al. J Clin Oncol 2004;22:330–353
More information in ESMO minimum clinical recommendations (www.esmo.org) and NCCN Practice Guidelines in Oncology V. 2. 2006 (www.nccn.org)

Staging

Limited disease	Disease confined to ipsilateral hemithorax within a single radiation port
Extensive disease	Disease beyond ipsilateral hemithorax or obvious metastatic disease

Østerlind K et al. Cancer Treat Rep 1983;67:3–9

Five-Year Survival for Each Stage

Limited Disease	
Median survival	14–20 months
2-year survival	40%
Extensive Disease	
Median survival	8–12 months
2-year survival	5%

More information in www.seer.cancer.gov

Caveats

Treatment of limited disease

1. Etoposide + cisplatin combination for 4–6 cycles is the regimen of choice to combine with concurrent chest radiation therapy
2. Chest radiation therapy increases local control and survival. Several studies suggest starting chest radiotherapy early
3. Prophylactic cranial irradiation is indicated in patients with complete remission; it reduces the risk of cerebral metastases and improves survival

Treatment of extensive disease

1. Etoposide + platinum or cyclophosphamide + doxorubicin regimens, for 4–6 cycles
2. Ongoing studies are evaluating the activity of an irinotecan + cisplatin combination

Second-line chemotherapy for both limited and extensive disease

1. Patients who relapse after a response to first-line chemotherapy should be considered for second-line chemotherapy with topotecan

REGIMEN

ETOPOSIDE + CISPLATIN WITH CONCURRENT THORACIC RADIATION THERAPY

Turrisi AT et al. NEJM 1999;340:265–271

Hydration before cisplatin: ≥1000 mL 0.9% NaCl injection (0.9% NS) by intravenous infusion over a minimum of 2–4 hours
Cisplatin 60 mg/m^2 by intravenous infusion in 50–150 mL 0.9% NS over 60 minutes, given on day 1 every 3 weeks for 4 cycles (total dosage/cycle = 60 mg/m^2)
Hydration after cisplatin: ≥1000 mL 0.9% NS by intravenous infusion over a minimum of 2–4 hours. Encourage oral intake. Monitor and replace magnesium/electrolytes as needed

Etoposide 120 mg/m^2 by intravenous infusion, diluted in 0.9% NS to a concentration within the range of 0.2–0.4 mg/mL over 60 minutes, given on days 1, 2, and 3 every 3 weeks for 4 cycles (total dosage/cycle = 360 mg/m^2)

Thoracic RT begins concurrently with the first cycle of chemotherapy to a total dose of 45 Gy delivered as:

[1] Once daily in 1.8-Gy fractions for 25 treatments over 5 weeks, *or*

[2] Twice daily in 1.5-Gy fractions for 30 treatments over 3 weeks

Prophylactic cranial RT is offered to patients who achieve a CR after completing systemic chemotherapy

Emetogenic potential:
Day 1: High (Emetogenicity score ≥6)
Days 2 and 3: Low (Emetogenicity score ~2). Potential for delayed symptoms after day 1. See Chapter 39 for antiemetic regimens

Patient Population Studied

A study of 417 patients with previously untreated limited SCLC. A randomized comparison between twice-daily and once-daily thoracic radiation therapy, both combined with etoposide and cisplatin given at fixed dosages

Treatment Modifications

Adverse Event	Dose Modification
G4 Toxicities, febrile neutropenia, documented infection, or thrombocytopenia with bleeding during cycles 3 and 4	Reduce etoposide dosage by 25%
Serum creatinine = 1.6–2.5 mg/dL (141–221 μmol/L) during cycles 3 and 4	Reduce cisplatin dosage by 25%
Platelets ≤50,000/mm^3	Interrupt radiation therapy
G2 Weight loss (≥4.5 kg or ≥10 pounds)	Interrupt radiation therapy
Hospitalization for febrile neutropenia or sepsis	Interrupt radiation therapy
Difficulty swallowing	Do not interrupt radiation therapy*
Fever with low ANC	Do not interrupt radiation therapy*

*In general, interruptions of thoracic radiation therapy are discouraged.
Note: Don't adjust chemotherapy during the first 2 cycles

Efficacy (N = 206/211)

	RT Fractionation	
	Once daily (N = 206)	Twice daily (N = 211)
Complete response	49%	56%
Partial response	38%	31%
Local failure	52%	36%
Median survival	19 months	23 months
2-year survival	41%	47%
5-year survival	16%	26%

Toxicity (N = 206/211)

Toxicity	% G3	% G4	% G5
Once-daily RT (N = 206)			
Overall toxicity	23	63	2
Esophagitis	11	5	0
Granulocytopenia	15	60	0
Thrombocytopenia	16	8	0
Anemia	23	3	0
Infection	6	1	1
Vomiting	8	2	0
Pulmonary effects	3	0.5	0.5
Weight loss	3	0	0
Twice-daily RT (N = 211)			
Overall toxicity	25	62	3
Esophagitis	27	5	0
Granulocytopenia	21	59	0
Thrombocytopenia	13	8	0
Anemia	23	5	0
Infection	6	2	1
Vomiting	8	1	0
Pulmonary effects	4	1	1
Weight loss	2	0	0

Therapy Monitoring

1. *Before each cycle:* H&P, CBC with differential, LFTs, BUN, creatinine, and serum electrolytes
2. *Response evaluation:* Evaluate therapy at the end of treatment

REGIMEN

IRINOTECAN + CISPLATIN

Noda K et al. NEJM 2002;346:85–91

Irinotecan 60 mg/m^2 by intravenous infusion in a volume of 5% dextrose injection (D5W) sufficient to produce a solution with concentration within the range of 0.12–2.8 mg/mL over 90 minutes, given on days 1, 8, and 15 every 4 weeks for 4 cycles (total dosage/cycle = 180 mg/m^2)

Hydration before cisplatin: ≥1000 mL 0.9% NaCl injection (0.9% NS) by intravenous infusion over a minimum of 2–4 hours
Cisplatin 60 mg/m^2 by intravenous infusion in 50–150 mL of 0.9% NS over 1 hour on day 1 every 4 weeks for 4 cycles (total dosage/cycle = 60 mg/m^2)
Hydration after cisplatin: ≥1000 mL 0.9% NS by intravenous infusion over a minimum of 2–4 hours. Encourage oral intake. Monitor and replace magnesium/electrolytes as needed

Emetogenic potential:
Day 1: High (Emetogenicity score = 6)
Days 8 and 15: Moderate (Emetogenicity score = 3). Potential for delayed symptoms after day 1. See Chapter 39 for antiemetic regimens

Patient Population Studied

A multicenter, prospective, randomized phase III comparison with etoposide + cisplatin in 77 patients with extensive-stage SCLC

Efficacy (N = 75)

Overall response rate	85%
Complete response	2.6%
Partial response	81.8%
Overall median survival	12.8 months
1-year overall survival	58.4%
2-year overall survival	19.5%
Complete response	2.6%
Partial response	82%

Toxicity (N = 75)

	G3/4
Hematologic	
Leukopenia	26.7%
Neutropenia	65.3%
Thrombocytopenia	5.3%
Anemia	26.7%
Nonhematologic	
Infection	5.3%
Nausea or vomiting	13.3%
Fever	1.3%
Diarrhea	16%

Japan Clinical Oncology Group Criteria

Treatment Modifications

Adverse Event	Dose Modification
On day 1, ANC <3500/mm^3 or platelet <100,000/mm^3	Hold irinotecan and cisplatin
ANC <2000/mm^3 or platelet count <50,000/mm^3 on day 8 or day 15	Hold irinotecan on day 8 and day 15. (If irinotecan is held on day 8, the day 15 dose is decided based on day 15 ANC and platelet counts)
G4 Diarrhea	Delay treatment until diarrhea resolves to G1, then resume with irinotecan dosage decreased by 10 mg/m^2
G4 Hematologic toxicity or G2/3 diarrhea	Reduce irinotecan dosage in subsequent cycles by 10 mg/m^2 per cycle for either or both events

Therapy Monitoring

1. *Weekly:* Assessment of symptoms, PE, CBC with differential, serum electrolytes, magnesium, BUN, creatinine, and LFTs
2. *Response evaluation:* Every 2 cycles

REGIMEN

TOPOTECAN

von Pawel J et al. JCO 1999;17:658–667

Topotecan HCl 1.5 mg/m^2 per day for 5 consecutive days intravenously in 50–250 mL 0.9% NaCl injection (0.9% NS) or 5% dextrose injection (D5W) over 30 minutes, given on days 1 through 5 every 21 days (total dosage/cycle = 7.5 mg/m^2)

Emetogenic potential: Low (Emetogenicity score = 2). See Chapter 39 for antiemetic regimens

Patient Population Studied

A study of 107 patients with SCLC and disease progression at least 60 days after having completed first-line chemotherapy. A randomized comparison with combination chemotherapy, including cyclophosphamide, doxorubicin, and vincristine

Efficacy (N = 107)

Intention-to-treat response rate	24.3%*
Median survival	25 weeks
6-month survival	46.7%
1-year survival	14.2%

*Partial responses

Toxicity (N = 107)

	% G3/4
Neutropenia	88
Thrombocytopenia	58
Anemia	42
Nausea	3.7
Fatigue	4.7
Vomiting	1.9
Stomatitis	1.9
Fever*	1.9
Diarrhea	0.9
Worsening LVEF: 2 of 26 patients (7.7%)	

*Excludes patients with febrile neutropenia
NCI CTC criteria

Treatment Modifications

Adverse Event	Dose Modification
Day 1 ANC <1000/mm^3, platelets <100,000/mm^3	Delay treatment until ANC > 1000/mm^3, platelets >100,000/mm^3
Toxicity G <2 during the previous cycle	Increase topotecan dosage to a maximum of 2 mg/m^2 per day in increments of 0.25 mg/m^2 per day
G4 Neutropenia with fever or infection, or of duration ≥7 days	Decrease topotecan dosage by 0.25 mg/m^2 per day*
G3 Neutropenia during the preceding cycle persisting after day 21	
G4 Thrombocytopenia	
G3/4 Nonhematologic toxicity, excluding grade 3 nausea	Decrease topotecan dosage by 0.25 mg/m^2 per day, or discontinue treatment*
Treatment delay >2 weeks	Discontinue treatment

*The minimum permissible daily topotecan dosage is 1 mg/m^2

Therapy Monitoring

1. *Before day 1 chemotherapy:* CBC with differential, LFTs and serum BUN and creatinine and electrolytes
2. *Weekly:* CBC with differential
3. *Day 15:* LFTs and serum BUN and creatinine
4. *Before starting and after completing treatment:* ECG and multiple-gated acquisition or echocardiogram assessment of left ventricular ejection fraction (LVEF)
5. *Response evaluation:* Every 2–3 cycles

Notes

Patients with objective responses continue treatment until disease progression or unacceptable toxicity, or for 6 additional cycles after maximal response

24. Lymphoma, Hodgkin

Christina M. Annunziata, MD, PhD, and Dan L. Longo, MD

Epidemiology

Incidence: 7800 estimated new cases in the United States in 2006
Deaths: 1490 estimated in the United States in 2006
Median age at diagnosis: Bimodal—larger peak of incidence in third decade of life; smaller peak in sixth decade
Male: female ratio: 1.2:1

Jemal A et al. CA Cancer J Clin 2006;56:106–130

Pathology

Since 1944, several classifications have been proposed for Hodgkin lymphoma (HL). Currently, the World Health Organization (WHO) Classification of Hematologic Malignancies is used:

1. Lymphocyte predominant, nodular (NLPHL) (5%)
2. Classic
   a. Lymphocyte-rich (LRCHL) (5%)
   b. Nodular sclerosis (NSHL) (60–80%)
   c. Mixed cellularity (MCHL) (15–30%)
   d. Lymphocyte depleted (LDHL) (1%)
   e. Unclassifiable (<1%)

Jaffe ES, Harris NL, Stein H, Vardiman JW , eds. World Health Organization Classification of Tumours. Pathology and Genetics of Tumours of Haematopoietic and Lymphoid Tissues. Lyon: IARC Press, 2001

Work-Up

1. History and physical exam
2. Laboratory tests: CBC with differential, ESR, electrolytes, albumin, liver function tests, mineral panel, LDH
3. HIV and hepatitis B and C serologies as clinically indicated
4. Chest x-ray (PA and lateral)
5. CT scan of chest, abdomen, and pelvis (and neck in selected cases)
6. Positron emission tomography (PET) scan if clinically indicated (equivocal CT)
7. Bone marrow aspirate and biopsy
8. Pulmonary function tests in selected cases
9. Echocardiogram or MUGA scan to determine cardiac ejection fraction as clinically indicated
10. Excisional lymph node biopsy to completely assess lymph node architecture is required at initial diagnosis. Fine-needle aspiration biopsy alone is not desirable for the initial diagnosis of lymphoma
11. Fertility counseling, if appropriate

NCCN Clinical Practice Guidelines in Oncology, vol.1, 2005, Non-Hodgkin Lymphoma © National Comprehensive Cancer Network, Inc, 2005 (www.nccn.org)

Five-Year Survival Rate

NLPHL	90% (10 years)
Classic HL	70–80%

Jaffe ES, Harris NL, Stein H, Vardiman JW, eds. World Health Organization Classification of Tumours. Pathology and Genetics of Tumours of Haematopoietic and Lymphoid Tissues. Lyon: IARC Press, 2001

Staging

Ann Arbor Staging Classification for Hodgkin and Non-Hodgkin Lymphomas

Stage	Description
I	Involvement of a single lymph node region (I) or involvement of a single extralymphatic organ or site (IE)
II	Involvement of 2 or more lymph node regions or lymphatic structures on the same side of the diaphragm alone (II) or with involvement of limited, contiguous extralymphatic organ or tissue (IIE)
III	Involvement of lymph node regions on both sides of the diaphragm (III), which may include the spleen (IIIS), or limited, contiguous extralymphatic organ or site (IIIE) or both (IIIES)
IV	Diffuse or disseminated foci of involvement of one or more extralymphatic organs or tissues with or without associated lymphatic involvement
	Abbreviations
A	Asymptomatic
B	Unexplained persistent or recurrent fever with temperature higher than 38°C or recurrent drenching night sweats within 1 month or unexplained loss of >10% body weight within 6 months
E	Limited direct extension into extralymphatic organ from adjacent lymph node
X	Bulky disease (mediastinal tumor width >one-third of the transthoracic diameter at T5/6, or a tumor diameter >10 cm)

Moormeier JA et al. Semin Oncol 1990;17:43–50

Caveats

For either limited-stage or advanced-stage disease, the following factors unfavorably affect prognosis:

Localized (Stage I/II)	Advanced (Stage III/IV)
• Bulky disease –Mediastinal mass >33% intrathoracic diameter –Any mass >10 cm • ESR >50 mm/hour • More than 3 sites • B symptoms	• Albumin <4 g/dL • Hemoglobin <10.5 g/dL • Male sex • Age >45 years • Stage IV • WBC >15,000/mm^3 • Lymphocyte count <8% of total WBC or <600/mm^3 absolute

1. Doxorubicin (Adriamycin®)/bleomycin/vinblastine/dacarbazine (ABVD) is the regimen of choice for primary therapy for all stages
2. Patients who do not achieve a complete response with initial combination chemotherapy should have involved-field radiation therapy to areas that are persistently positive on PET scans
3. If radiation therapy fails to produce a complete response or if disease recurs after a complete response is achieved, a salvage regimen should be used
4. Many salvage regimens exist. Response rates are similar and all possess positive attributes and drawbacks. A salvage regimen with an alkylating agent as a principal component is recommended for debulking in preparation for high-dose chemotherapy and autologous bone marrow transplantation (BMT). Examples include mechlorethamine, vincristine (Oncovin®), procarbazine, prednisone (MOPP), and chlorambucil/vinblastine/procarbazine/prednisolone (ChlVPP)
5. Although radiation is often used in the initial management of patients with HL, one cannot make an evidence-based recommendation for radiation therapy in the salvage setting. Anecdotally, radiation therapy can be considered in a patient who suffers a relapse in the mediastinum if the debulking conventional-dose salvage regimen fails to eradicate all PET-positive disease. This approach is based in part on the evidence that patients who undergo high-dose therapy and stem cell transplantation in clinical complete response do better than patients who enter that phase of treatment with residual disease
6. Once a maximum response has been obtained with conventional-dose salvage therapy, a patient undergoes high-dose chemotherapy with autologous BMT, regardless of how long the initial complete response lasted
7. Patients who suffer relapse after high-dose therapy may be significantly palliated by single agents
8. The long-term follow-up of patients who achieve a complete response to therapy has usually included careful radiographic monitoring. Before CT scans, follow-up consisted of serial lymphangiography of opacified lymph nodes; a practice that was subsequently replaced with CT scans every 3 months the first year, every 6 months the second year, and annually thereafter. This approach was based on two assumptions: (1) that asymptomatic relapses could be detected and (2) that asymptomatic relapses would have a better prognosis and respond better to salvage therapy than symptomatic relapses. However, data generated in lymphomas and some other cancers (although not specifically in Hodgkin lymphoma) indicate that routine careful surveillance does not usually detect asymptomatic relapses (>90% of relapses are detected by the patient, not by tests). Furthermore, the evidence does not support the argument that accidentally discovered relapses have a better prognosis. Consequently, one can recommend that patients undergo a careful history and physical (but no imaging tests) 3 times the first year, twice the second year, and annually thereafter, recognizing that 50% of all relapses happen in the first year and 85% before the end of the third year

General note: Bleomycin is a mixture of glycopeptide fractions (bleomycins A_1, A_2, A_3, A_4, A_5, A_6, B_1, B_2, B_3, B_4, B_5, and B_6). Although the primary constituent of commercial products (≥50%) is bleomycin A_2, the compound is nevertheless a mixture; potency is quantified in units of activity. Actual potency varies between 1.2 and 1.7 units/mg, but publications in which dosage and dose are reported in metric units of mass (and current usage) equate 1 mg with 1 unit

REGIMEN FOR NEWLY DIAGNOSED HL

DOXORUBICIN (Adriamycin®), BLEOMYCIN, VINBLASTINE, DACARBAZINE (ABVD)

Bonadonna G et al. Cancer 1975;36:252–259

Doxorubicin 25 mg/m² per dose by intravenous push over 3–5 minutes for 2 doses on days 1 and 15 every 28 days (total dosage/cycle = 50 mg/m²)
Bleomycin 10 units/m² per dose intravenously by slow push over 10 minutes for 2 doses on days 1 and 15 every 28 days (total dosage/cycle = 20 units/m²)
Vinblastine 6 mg/m² per dose by intravenous push over 1–2 minutes for 2 doses on days 1 and 15 every 28 days (total dosage/cycle = 12 mg/m²)
Dacarbazine 150 mg/m² per dose intravenously in 100–250 mL 0.9% NaCl injection (0.9% NS) or 5% dextrose injection (D5W) over 15–30 minutes for 5 consecutive days on days 1–5 every 28 days (total dosage/cycle = 750 mg/m²)

Emetogenic potential:
Day 1: Very high (Emetogenicity score = 6)
Days 2–5: High (Emetogenicity score = 5)
Day 14: Moderate (Emetogenicity score = 3). See Chapter 39 for antiemetic regimens

Patient Population Studied

Sixty patients were assigned to receive either ABVD or MOPP. Twenty patients treated with ABVD were evaluable for anlysis. No patient had previously received chemotherapy, but 4 patients in the ABVD arm had suffered relapse after primary radiation therapy

Efficacy (N = 20)

Stage	No. of Patients	% Complete Response	% Partial Response
IIB	1	100	0
III	11	73	9
IV	8	75	25
Total	20	75	15

Toxicity (N = 20)

	% of Patients
WBC <4000/mm³	45
Platelet count <130,000/mm³	15[a]
Alopecia	75
Skin changes[b]	40
Paresthesias	5
Amenorrhea	3/3[c]

[a]No platelet count <80,000/mm³
[b]Hyperpigmented striae and thickening from bleomycin
[c]In menstruating females

Therapy Monitoring

1. *Semiweekly and before each cycle:* CBC with differential
2. *Before each cycle:* Physical exam, chest x-ray
3. *After second and each subsequent cycle:* DLCO
4. *Response evaluation:* CT of chest, abdomen, and pelvis every 2 cycles starting after cycle 4. PET (or gallium scan if PET unavailable) at conclusion of therapy to document extent of remission. Bone marrow biopsy (if disease existed before therapy) performed 1 month after completing the sixth cycle

Notes

1. Regimen of choice for primary therapy for all stages of disease
2. If CT scan shows no change between cycles 4 and 6, obtain PET (or gallium) scan to confirm complete response. If PET/gallium is positive, consider radiation therapy to remaining site(s) of disease. If CT scan shows continued shrinkage of disease between cycles 4 and 6, continue treatment for an additional 2 cycles. If CT scan shows continued response between cycles 6 and 8, obtain PET scan and consider radiation therapy to any sites of active disease
3. If the WBC nadir is >2000/mm³, consider a 10% dose escalation of doxorubicin, vinblastine, and dacarbazine in the following cycle

Treatment Modifications

Adverse Event*	Dose Modification
WBC 3999–3000/mm³ or platelet count 129.000–100,000/mm³	Reduce doxorubicin and vinblastine dosages by 50%
WBC 2999–2000/mm³ or platelet count 99,000–80,000/mm³	Reduce dacarbazine dosage by 50%. Reduce doxorubicin and vinblastine dosages by 75%
WBC 1999–1500/mm³ or platelet count 79,000–50,000/mm³	Reduce dacarbazine dosage by 75%. Hold doxorubicin and vinblastine
WBC <1500/mm³ or platelet count <50,000/mm³	Hold doxorubicin, vinblastine, and dacarbazine
Clinical or radiologic evidence of pulmonary fibrosis or DLCO <50% pretreatment value	Discontinue bleomycin
Moderate to severe renal function impairment (creatinine clearance <50 mL/min)	Discontinue bleomycin until creatinine clearance improves to ≥50 mL/min

*Refers to values on days 1 or 15

SALVAGE REGIMEN FOR NEWLY DIAGNOSED HL

MECHLORETHAMINE, VINCRISTINE (Oncovin®), PROCARBAZINE, PREDNISONE (MOPP)

DeVita VT Jr et al. Ann Intern Med 1970;73:881–895
DeVita VT Jr et al. Ann Intern Med 1980;92:587–595

Mechlorethamine 6 mg/m² per dose by intravenous push over 1–3 minutes for 2 doses on days 1 and 8 every 28 days (total dosage/cycle = 12 mg/m²)
Vincristine 1.4 mg/m² per dose (the calculated dose is given; ie, doses *are not* "capped") by intravenous push over 1–3 minutes for 2 doses on days 1 and 8 every 28 days (total dosage/cycle = 2.8 mg/m²)
Procarbazine 100 mg/m² per day orally for 14 consecutive days on days 1–14 every 28 days (total dosage/cycle = 1400 mg/m²)
Prednisone 40 mg/m² per day orally for 14 consecutive days on days 1–14 every 28 days (total dosage/cycle = 560 mg/m²)

Note: In the original MOPP regimen, the investigators gave prednisone during cycles 1 and 4 only; subsequently, prednisone was administered with each cycle

Procarbazine is formulated for oral administration in the United States as capsules containing 50 mg as procarbazine HCl. Matulane® brand of procarbazine hydrochloride product label, February 2004. Sigma-Tau Pharmaceuticals, Inc
Prednisone is marketed in the United States in numerous solid formulations for oral administration, including prompt-release tablets containing 1 mg, 2.5 mg, 5 mg, 10 mg, 20 mg, and 50 mg prednisone, and in solutions and syrups

Special instructions:
Procarbazine is a weak monoamine oxidase inhibitor. Concurrent use of sympathomimetic or tricyclic antidepressant drugs and ingestion of tyramine-rich foods may produce severe hypertensive episodes in a patient receiving procarbazine.
McCabe BJ. J Am Diet Assoc 1986;86:1059–1064; Anonymous. Med Lett Drugs Ther 1989;31:11–12; and Da Prada M et al. J Neural Transm Suppl 1988;26:31–56

Supportive care:
Add a **proton pump inhibitor** during prednisone therapy to prevent peptic ulcer disease

Emetogenic potential:
Days 1 and 8: Very high (Emetogenicity score = 6)
Days 2–7, 9–14: Moderately high (Emetogenicity score = 4). See Chapter 39 for antiemetic regimens

Patient Population Studied

A total of 198 patients with all histologies of HL, and ranging from stage II to IV, were treated with MOPP chemotherapy. Of these, 32 had relapsed after primary radiation therapy, and 2 patients had received glucocorticoids for symptom control before entering the study

Treatment Modifications

Adverse Event*	Dose Modification*
WBC 3999–3000/mm³	Reduce procarbazine and mechlorethamine dosages by 50%
WBC 2999–2000/mm³ or platelet count 100,000–50,000/mm³	Reduce procarbazine and mechlorethamine dosages by 75%
WBC 1999–1000/mm³	Reduce procarbazine and mechlorethamine dosages by 75%, and reduce vincristine dosage by 50%
WBC <1000/mm³ or platelet count <50,000/mm³	Hold mechlorethamine, procarbazine, and vincristine

*Indicates counts on day 1; if counts expected to return to normal in 1 week, delay cycle 1 week, and treat based on counts at day 35

Efficacy (N = 198)

Stage	No. of Patients	% Complete Response	% Five-Year Disease-Free	% Alive 10 Years
II	14	93	84	78
III	70	84	75	65
IV	114	76	60	51

DeVita VT Jr et al. Ann Intern Med 1980;92:587–595

Efficacy (N = 43)

Stage	No. of Patients	% Complete Response
IIIA	3	100
IIIB	5	100
IVA	4	100
IVB	31	74
Total	43	81

DeVita VT Jr et al. Ann Intern Med 1970;73:881–895

Toxicity (N = 43)

	% of Patients
WBC <5000/mm^3	97
WBC <2000/mm^3	27
Platelet count <100,000/mm^3	22
Platelet count <50,000/mm^3	8

Toxicity	% Any G	G3/4/5
Nausea, vomiting	100	
Hyperesthesia	100	
Loss of deep tendon reflexes	100	
Alopecia	30	
Anemia	17	
Proteinuria	2	
Hemorrhagic cystitis	2	
Tumor lysis		2 deaths
Elevated transaminases	19	
Constipation	Encountered*	

*Alleviated with laxatives and stool softeners

DeVita VT Jr et al. Ann Intern Med 1970;73:881–895

Therapy Monitoring

1. *Weekly and before each cycle:* CBC with differential
2. *Before each cycle:* Physical exam, chest x-ray
3. *Response evaluation:* CT of chest, abdomen, and pelvis every 2 cycles starting after cycle 4. PET (or gallium scan if PET unavailable) at conclusion of therapy to document extent of remission. Bone marrow biopsy (if disease existed before therapy) performed 1 month after completing the sixth cycle

Notes

1. MOPP is most effective as a first-salvage regimen after ABVD relapse. It is more myelotoxic than ABVD, and more toxic to gonads, but has less lung toxicity. Prednisone is used during every cycle, and the vincristine dose *is not* capped at 2 mg per single dose. Vincristine dose is reduced in patients who develop a motor neuropathy (patient may have difficulty buttoning clothes), but not for sensory neuropathy
2. If CT scan shows no change between cycles 4 and 6, obtain PET (or gallium) scan to confirm complete response. If PET/gallium is positive, consider radiation therapy to remaining site(s) of disease. If CT scan shows continued shrinkage of disease between cycles 4 and 6, continue treatment for an additional 2 cycles. If CT scan shows continued response between cycles 6 and 8, obtain PET scan and consider radiation therapy to any sites of active disease
3. If the WBC nadir is >2000/mm^3, consider a 10% dose escalation of all four drugs in the following cycle

SALVAGE REGIMEN FOR NEWLY DIAGNOSED HL

CHLORAMBUCIL, VINBLASTINE, PROCARBAZINE, PREDNISOLONE (ChlVPP)

McElwain TJ et al. Br J Cancer 1977;36:276–380

Chlorambucil 6 mg/m² per day (maximum daily dose = 10 mg) orally for 14 consecutive days on days 1–14 every 28 days (total dosage/cycle = 84 mg/m²; maximum dose/cycle = 140 mg)
Vinblastine 6 mg/m² per dose (maximum single dose = 10 mg) by intravenous push over 1–2 minutes for 2 doses on days 1 and 8 every 28 days (total dosage/cycle = 12 mg/m²; maximum dose/cycle = 20 mg)
Procarbazine 100 mg/m² per day orally for 14 consecutive days on days 1–14 every 28 days (total dosage/cycle = 1400 mg/m²)
Prednisolone 40 mg per day orally for 14 consecutive days on days 1–14 every 28 days (total dose/cycle = 560 mg)

Chlorambucil is formulated in the United States for oral administration as tablets containing chlorambucil 2 mg. Leukeran® (chlorambucil) Tablets, product label, November 2004. GlaxoSmithKline Procarbazine is formulated in the United States for oral administration as capsules containing 50 mg as procarbazine HCl. Matulane® brand of procarbazine hydrochloride product label, February 2004. Sigma-Tau Pharmaceuticals, Inc
Prednisolone is marketed in the United States in numerous formulations for oral administration, including tablets containing 5 mg prednisolone, and in solutions and syrups in various concentrations

Special instructions:
Procarbazine is a weak monoamine oxidase inhibitor. Concurrent use of sympathomimetic or tricyclic antidepressant drugs and ingestion of tyramine-rich foods may produce severe hypertensive episodes in a patient receiving procarbazine.
McCabe BJ. J Am Diet Assoc 1986;86:1059–1064; Anonymous. Med Lett Drugs Ther 1989;31:11–12; Da Prada M et al. J Neural Transm Suppl 1988;26:31–56

Supportive care:
Add a **proton pump inhibitor** during prednisolone therapy to prevent peptic ulcer disease
Constipation prophylaxis is recommended

Emetogenic potential:
Days 1–14: Moderately high (Emetogenicity score = 4). See Chapter 39 for antiemetic regimens

Patient Population Studied

A group of 70 patients with advanced HL of all histologies completed therapy. Approximately 50% (n = 36) of the patients had received no prior treatment, one third (n = 22) had been treated with radiation therapy, and 12 had suffered relapse after chemotherapy and radiation

Therapy Monitoring

1. *Weekly and before every cycle:* CBC with differential
2. *Every cycle:* Physical exam, chest x-ray
3. *Response evaluation:* CT of chest, abdomen, and pelvis every 2 cycles starting after cycle 4. PET (or gallium scan if PET unavailable) at conclusion of therapy to document extent of remission. Bone marrow biopsy (if disease existed before therapy) performed 1 month after completing the sixth cycle

Toxicity (N = 70)

	% of Patients
G1/2 Paresthesias	7.1
G1/2 Constipation	7.1
G1 Alopecia	8.6
G1/2 Nausea	27
G1/2 Vomiting	8.6
Amenorrhea	2.8
Acne flare	2.8
Steroid myopathy	1.4
Leukopenia/thrombocytopenia	21.4

Treatment Modifications

Adverse Event	Dose Modification
WBC <3000/mm³ or platelet count <80,000/mm³	Delay treatment 1 week until WBC >3000/mm³ and platelet count >80,000/mm³

Efficacy (N = 70)

Prior Treatment	% Complete Response	% Partial Response
None (n = 36)	72	25
Radiation therapy (n = 22)	87	4.5
Chemotherapy + radiation therapy (n = 12)	58	17
Total (N = 70)	53	12

Notes

1. ChlVPP is probably as effective as MOPP and causes less nausea. Prednisone is used during every cycle, and the vincristine dose *is not* capped at 2 mg per single dose. Vincristine dose is reduced in patients who develop a motor neuropathy (patient may have difficulty buttoning clothes), but not for sensory neuropathy
2. If used in a newly diagnosed patient and CT scan shows no change between cycles 4 and 6, obtain PET (or gallium) scan to confirm complete response. If PET/gallium is positive, consider radiation therapy to remaining site(s) of disease. If CT scan shows continued shrinkage of disease between cycles 4 and 6, continue treatment for an additional 2 cycles. If CT scan shows continued response between cycles 6 and 8, obtain PET scan and consider radiation therapy to any sites of active disease
3. If the WBC nadir is >2000/mm³, consider a 10% dose escalation of all four drugs in the following cycle

REGIMEN FOR NEWLY DIAGNOSED HL

MECHLORETHAMINE, VINCRISTINE (Oncovin®), PROCARBAZINE, PREDNISONE (MOPP), DOXORUBICIN (Adriamycin®), BLEOMYCIN, VINBLASTINE, DACARBAZINE (ABVD)

Bonadonna G et al. Ann Intern Med 1986;104:739–746

MOPP

Mechlorethamine 6 mg/m² per dose by intravenous push over 1–3 minutes for 2 doses on days 1 and 8 every 56 days (total dosage/cycle = 12 mg/m²)
Vincristine 1.4 mg/m² per dose (the calculated dose is given; ie, doses *are not* capped) by intravenous push over 1–3 minutes for 2 doses on days 1 and 8 every 56 days (total dosage/cycle = 2.8 mg/m²; maximum dose/cycle = 4 mg/²)
Procarbazine 100 mg/m² per day orally for 14 consecutive days on days 1–14 every 56 days (total dosage/cycle = 1400 mg/m²)
Prednisone 40 mg/m² per day orally for 14 consecutive days on days 1–14 every 56 days (total dosage/cycle = 560 mg/²)

Note: In the MOPP/ABVD regimen reported by Bonadonna et al, the investigators gave prednisone only during cycles 1, 4, 7, and 10, emulating the every-third-cycle approach originally reported by DeVita et al

ABVD

Doxorubicin 25 mg/m² per dose by intravenous push over 3–5 minutes for 2 doses on days 29 and 43 every 56 days (total dosage/cycle = 50 mg/m²)
Bleomycin 10 units/m² per dose by slow intravenous push over 10 minutes for 2 doses on days 29 and 43 every 56 days (total dosage/cycle = 20 units/m²)
Vinblastine 6 mg/m² per dose by intravenous push over 1–2 minutes for 2 doses on days 29 and 43 every 56 days (total dosage/cycle = 12 mg/m²)
Dacarbazine 375 mg/m² per dose intravenously in 100–250 mL 0.9% NaCl injection (0.9% NS) or 5% dextrose injection (D5W) over 15–30 minutes for 2 doses on days 29 and 44 every 56 days (total dosage/cycle = 750 mg/m²)

Procarbazine is formulated in the United States for oral administration as capsules containing 50 mg as procarbazine HCl. Matulane® brand of procarbazine hydrochloride product label, February 2004. Sigma-Tau Pharmaceuticals, Inc
Prednisone is marketed in the United States in numerous solid formulations for oral administration, including prompt-release tablets containing 1 mg, 2.5 mg, 5 mg, 10 mg, 20 mg, and 50 mg prednisone, and in solutions and syrups

Special instructions:
Procarbazine is a weak monoamine oxidase inhibitor. Concurrent use of sympathomimetic or tricyclic antidepressant drugs and ingestion of tyramine-rich foods may produce severe hypertensive episodes in a patient receiving procarbazine.
McCabe BJ. J Am Diet Assoc 1986;86:1059–1064; Anonymous. Med Lett Drugs Ther 1989;31:11–122; Da Prada M et al. J Neural Transm Suppl 1988;26:31–56

Emetogenic potential:
MOPP regimen
Days 1 and 8: Very high (Emetogenicity score = 6)
Days 2–7, 9–14: Moderately high (Emetogenicity score = 4)
ABVD regimen
Days 29 and 43: Very high (Emetogenicity score = 6). See Chapter 39 for antiemetic regimens

Treatment Modifications

Adverse Event*	Dose Modification
WBC 3999–3000/mm³ or platelet count 129,000–100,000/mm³	*MOPP:* Reduce mechlorethamine and procarbazine dosages by 50% *ABVD:* Reduce doxorubicin and vinblastine dosages by 50%
WBC 2999–2000/mm³ or platelet count 99,000–80,000/mm³	*MOPP:* Reduce mechlorethamine and procarbazine dosages by 75%, and reduce vincristine dosage by 50% *ABVD:* Reduce dacarbazine dosage by 50% and doxorubicin and vinblastine dosages by 75%
WBC 1999–1500/mm³ or platelet count 79,000–50,000/mm³	*MOPP:* Reduce vincristine dosage by 75%. Hold mechlorethamine and procarbazine *ABVD:* Reduce dacarbazine dosage by 75%. Hold doxorubicin and vinblastine
WBC <1500/mm³ or platelet count <50,000/mm³	*MOPP:* Hold mechlorethamine, procarbazine, and vincristine *ABVD:* Hold doxorubicin, vinblastine, and dacarbazine
Clinical or radiologic evidence of pulmonary fibrosis, or DLCO <50% pretreatment value	Discontinue bleomycin
Chemical phlebitis from mechlorethamine	Substitute cyclophosphamide for mechlorethamine at a dosage of 650 mg/m²
Moderate to severe renal function impairment (creatinine clearance <50 mL/min)	Discontinue bleomycin until creatinine clearance improves to ≥50 mL/min

*Indicates counts on days 1, 15, 29 and 43. At days 1 and 29, a delay of 1 week is allowed if counts are expected to return to normal in 1 week; subsequent treatment is based on counts after 1 week delay

Patient Population Studied

Eighty-eight patients with all subtypes of HL were randomized to receive 12 cycles of MOPP (n = 45) versus 6 cycles of MOPP alternating with 6 cycles of ABVD (n = 43). No patient had previously received chemotherapy, but 12 patients (28%) in the MOPP arm and 13 patients (30%) in the MOPP/ABVD arm had undergone prior radiation therapy

Efficacy (N = 45)

	At 8 Years		
Complete Response	Progression-Free Survival	Alive	Alive After Complete Response
88.9%	64.6%	76.2%	85.9%

Toxicity (N = 45)

WBC <2500/mm^3	42%
WBC <1500/mm^3	22%
Platelet count <75,000/mm^3	16%
Platelet count <50,000/mm^3	7%
Alopecia	18%
Vincristine reduced 50% due to neuropathy	7%
Vincristine discontinued due to neuropathy	4%
Refusal to complete treatment	22%

Therapy Monitoring

1. *Weekly and before each cycle:* CBC with differential
2. *Before each cycle:* Physical exam, chest x-ray
3. *After second and each subsequent cycle:* DLCO
4. *Response evaluation:* CT of chest, abdomen, and pelvis every 2 MOPP and 2 ABVD cycles. PET (or gallium scan if PET unavailable) at conclusion of therapy to document extent of remission. Bone marrow biopsy (if disease existed before therapy) performed 1 month after completing therapy

Notes

1. If MOPP/ABVD (1 MOPP and 1 ABVD = 2 cycles) is used in a newly diagnosed patient and CT scan shows no change between cycles 4 and 6, obtain PET (or gallium) scan to confirm complete response. If PET/gallium is positive, consider radiation therapy to remaining site(s) of disease. If CT scan shows continued shrinkage of disease between cycles 4 and 6, continue treatment for an additional 2 cycles. If CT scan shows continued response between cycles 6 and 8, obtain PET scan and consider radiation therapy to any sites of active disease
2. If the WBC nadir is >2000/mm^3, consider a 10% dose escalation of all drugs except bleomycin in the following cycle

REGIMEN FOR NEWLY DIAGNOSED HL

STANFORD V

Bartlett NL et al. JCO 1995;13:1080–1088

Doxorubicin 25 mg/m² per dose by intravenous push over 3–5 minutes for 2 doses on days 1 and 15 every 28 days for 3 cycles (total dosage/cycle = 50 mg/m²)
Vinblastine 6 mg/m² per dose by intravenous push over 1–2 minutes for 2 doses on days 1 and 15 every 28 days for 3 cycles (total dosage/cycle = 12 mg/m²)
Note: For patients ≥50 years of age during the third cycle, decrease vinblastine dosage to 4 mg/m² per dose for 2 doses on days 1 and 15 (total dose during the third cycle = 8 mg/m²)
Mechlorethamine 6 mg/m² by intravenous push over 1–2 minutes on day 1 every 28 days for 3 cycles (total dosage/cycle = 6 mg/m²)
Vincristine 1.4 mg/m² per dose (maximum single dose = 2 mg) by intravenous push over 1–2 minutes for 2 doses on days 8 and 22 every 28 days for 3 cycles (total dosage/cycle = 2.8 mg/m²; maximum dose/cycle = 4 mg)
Note: For patients ≥50 years of age during the third cycle, decrease vincristine dosage to 1 mg/m² per dose (maximum single dose = 2 mg) for 2 doses on days 1 and 15 (total dosage during the third cycle = 2 mg/m²; maximum dose during the third cycle = 4 mg)
Bleomycin 5 units/m² per dose by slow intravenous push over 10 minutes for 2 doses on days 8 and 22 every 28 days for 3 cycles (total dosage/cycle = 10 units/m²)
Etoposide 60 mg/m² per day by intravenous infusion, diluted in 0.9% NaCl injection (0.9% NS) or 5% dextrose injection (D5W) to a concentration of 0.2–0.4 mg/mL over 1 hour for 2 doses on days 15 and 16 every 28 days for 3 cycles (total dosage/cycle = 120 mg/m²)
Prednisone 40 mg/m² per dose orally every other day (days 1, 3, 5, and so on) for 14 doses every 28 days
Note: Prednisone dosage is tapered by 10 mg/dose every other day starting on day 14 of the third cycle (total dosage/28-day cycle = 560 mg/m² until tapering begins)
Prednisone is marketed in the United States in numerous solid formulations for oral administration, including prompt-release tablets containing 1 mg, 2.5 mg, 5 mg, 10 mg, 20 mg, and 50 mg prednisone, and in solutions and syrups

Consolidative irradiation, starting 2 weeks after the completion of chemotherapy. Administer 36 Gy to sites of initial tumor bulk defined as disease ≥5 cm in horizontal diameter. The treatment port for patients with bulky mediastinal HL is referred to as a modified mantle and is restricted to the mediastinum and bilateral hilar and supraclavicular regions. Extension of HL to contiguous extralymphatic sites, usually associated with bulky disease is also included in the port. Limit doses to the lung and pleura to 16.5 Gy delivered in 0.75- to 0.9-Gy fractions; pericardial and subcarinal blocks should be placed at 15 Gy and 30 Gy, respectively

Supportive care:
Add a **proton pump inhibitor** to prevent glucocorticoid-induced gastritis/duodenitis
PCP prophylaxis: **Cotrimoxazole** (trimethoprim 160 mg + sulfamethoxazole 800 mg) orally twice daily on 3 days per week (eg, Monday, Wednesday, and Friday)
Antiviral prophylaxis: **Acyclovir** 200 mg orally 3 times daily
Antifungal prophylaxis: **Ketoconazole** 200 mg orally daily
Note: Although original regimen recommended daily ketoconazole, imidazole, and triazole antifungals are highly potent cytochrome P450 (CYP3A subfamily) inhibitors that may interfere with drug metabolism. It may be prudent to withhold these drugs the day before, the day of and the day after doxorubicin, vinblastine, vincristine, and etoposide are administered
To mitigate vinca alkaloid constipation: **Stool softeners** and/or laxatives daily

Emetogenic potential:
Day 1: Very high (Emetogenicity score = 6)
Days 8 and 22: Nonemetogenic (Emetogenicity score = 1)
Day 15: Moderately high (Emetogenicity score = 4)
Day 16: Low (Emetogenicity score = 2). See Chapter 39 for antiemetic regimens

Treatment Modifications

Adverse Event	Dose Modification
ANC < 1000/mm³	Reduce doxorubicin, vinblastine, mechlorethamine, and etoposide dosages by 35%
ANC < 500/mm³	Delay treatment 1 week then reduce doxorubicin, vinblastine, mechlorethamine, and etoposide dosages by 35%
Dose reduction or dose delay	Administer filgrastim 5 mcg/kg subcutaneously on days 3–13 and 16–26
Clinical or radiologic evidence of pulmonary fibrosis or DLCO <50% pretreatment value	Discontinue bleomycin
Moderate to severe renal function impairment (creatinine clearance <50 mL/min)	Discontinue bleomycin until creatinine clearance improves to ≥50 mL/min

Patient Population Studied

Patients between 15 and 60 years of age with either advanced-stage (III or IV) HL or stage II with bulky mediastinal involvement were treated with 3 cycles of chemotherapy followed by consolidative radiation to sites of initial bulky (>5 cm) disease

Efficacy (N = 65)

Stage at Diagnosis	Status at 3 Years	
	% Alive	% Disease-free
II (n = 21)		100
III (n = 20)		92
IV (n = 24)		76
All (n = 65)	96	87

Progression while on therapy	0
Relapse within 4–8 weeks after therapy	6.1% (IVB)

Four of 28 patients had positive gallium scans with mediastinal uptake. None had relapsed 6–42 months after consolidative mediastinal RT

Toxicity (N = 60)

Toxicities Requiring Hospitalization	
Fever/neutropenia	17%
Obstipation/ileus	11%
DVT	3%
Pneumonitis	2%
Palpitations	2%
Phlebitis	2%

Overall Toxicities

	% Any Grade	% G3/4
Neutropenia	82	45
Anemia	60	34
Nausea/vomiting	52	9
Sensory neuropathy	71	11
Motor neuropathy	34	8
Autonomic neuropathy	46	12
Phlebitis	38	
Myalgias/arthralgias	24	
Aseptic necrosis femoral head	2	

Therapy Monitoring

1. *Weekly:* CBC with differential
2. *Before every cycle:* CBC with differential, alkaline phosphatase and LDH, chest x-ray; DLCO after second and each subsequent cycle
3. *Response evaluation after completion of therapy:* CT of chest, abdomen, and pelvis after 2 cycles of chemotherapy and before the start of radiation therapy or after 3 cycles of chemotherapy. PET (or gallium scan if PET unavailable) at conclusion of therapy to document extent of remission. Bone marrow biopsy (if disease existed before therapy) performed 1 month after completing therapy

Notes

1. Stanford V is widely used, but requires radiation therapy in all patients with attendant late complications
2. If the WBC nadir is >2000/mm^3, consider 10% dose escalation of all drugs except bleomycin in the following cycle

REGIMEN FOR NEWLY DIAGNOSED HL

BLEOMYCIN, ETOPOSIDE, DOXORUBICIN (Adriamycin®), CYCLOPHOSPHAMIDE, VINCRISTINE (Oncovin®), PROCARBAZINE, PREDNISONE (BEACOPP)

Diehl V et al. JCO 1998;16:3810–3821

BEACOPP

Doxorubicin 25 mg/m² by intravenous push over 3–5 minutes on day 1 every 21 days (total dosage/cycle = 25 mg/m²)
Cyclophosphamide 650 mg/m² intravenously in 25–250 mL 0.9% NaCl injection (0.9% NS) or 5% dextrose injection (D5W) over 10–30 minutes on day 1 every 21 days (total dosage/cycle = 650 mg/m²)
Etoposide 100 mg/m² per day by intravenous infusion, diluted in 0.9% NS or D5W to a concentration of 0.2 to 0.4 mg/mL over 1 hour on days 1, 2, and 3 every 21 days (total dosage/cycle = 300 mg/m²)
Procarbazine 100 mg/m² per day orally for 7 consecutive days on days 1–7 every 21 days (total dosage/cycle = 700 mg/m²)
Prednisone 40 mg/m² per day orally for 14 consecutive days on days 1–14 every 21 days (total dosage/cycle = 560 mg/m²)
Bleomycin 10 units/m² by slow intravenous push over 10 minutes on day 8 every 21 days (total dosage/cycle = 10 units/m²)
Vincristine 1.4 mg/m² (maximum single dose = 2 mg) by intravenous push over 1–3 minutes on day 8 every 21 days (total dosage/cycle = 1.4 mg/m²; maximum dose/cycle = 2 mg)

Dose-Escalated BEACOPP

Doxorubicin 35 mg/m² by intravenous push over 3–5 minutes on day 1 every 21 days (total dosage/cycle = 35 mg/m²)
Cyclophosphamide 1200 mg/m² intravenously in 100–1000 mL 0.9% NS or D5W over 10–30 minutes on day 1 every 21 days (total dosage/cycle = 650 mg/m²)
Etoposide 200 mg/m² per day by intravenous infusion, diluted in 0.9% NS or D5W to a concentration of 0.2–0.4 mg/mL over 1 hour on days 1, 2, and 3 every 21 days (total dosage/cycle = 600 mg/m²)
Procarbazine 100 mg/² per day orally for 7 consecutive days on days 1–7 every 21 days (total dosage/cycle = 700 mg/m²)
Prednisone 40 mg/m² per day orally for 14 consecutive days on days 1–14 every 21 days (total dosage/cycle = 560 mg/m²)
Bleomycin 10 units/m² by slow intravenous push over 10 minutes on day 8 every 21 days (total dosage/cycle = 10 units/m²)
Vincristine 1.4 mg/m² (maximum single dose = 2 mg) by intravenous push over 1–3 minutes on day 8 every 21 days (total dosage/cycle = 1.4 mg/m²; maximum dose/cycle = 2 mg)
Filgrastim 300 mcg/day (patients with body weight <75 kg) or 400 mcg/day (body weight ≥75 kg) subcutaneously starting on day 8 and continuing until WBC ≥13,000/mm³ on 3 consecutive days

Procarbazine is formulated for oral administration in the United States as capsules containing 50 mg procarbazine HCl. Matulane® brand of procarbazine hydrochloride product label, February 2004. Sigma-Tau Pharmaceuticals, Inc
Prednisone is marketed in the United States in numerous solid formulations for oral administration including prompt-release tablets containing 1, 2.5, 5, 10, 20, and 50 mg prednisone, and in solutions and syrups

Special instructions:
Procarbazine is a weak monoamine oxidase inhibitor. Concurrent use of sympathomimetic or tricyclic antidepressant drugs and ingestion of tyramine-rich foods may produce severe hypertensive episodes in a patient receiving procarbazine.
McCabe BJ. J Am Diet Assoc 1986;86: 1059–64; Anonymous. Med Lett Drugs Ther 1989;31:11–12; Da Prada M et al. J Neural Transm Suppl 1988;26:31–56

(continued)

Treatment Modifications

Adverse Event	Dose Modification
BEACOPP and Dose-Escalated BEACOPP	
WBC <2500/mm³ or platelet count <80,000/mm³	Delay cycle until WBC >2500/mm³ and platelet count >80,000/mm³; if delayed >2 weeks, reduce dosage of doxorubicin, cyclophosphamide, etoposide, and procarbazine by 25%
Clinical or radiologic evidence of pulmonary fibrosis or DLCO <50% pretreatment value	Discontinue bleomycin
Moderate to severe impairment renal function (creatinine clearance <50 mL/min)	Discontinue bleomycin until creatinine clearance improves to ≥50 mL/min
Dose-Escalated BEACOPP	
Any G4 toxicity or a 2-week postponement in start of next cycle per above guidelines	Stepwise reduction of cyclophosphamide and etoposide dosages by 25% of the difference between the escalated dosage and standard BEACOPP; immediate reduction to standard BEACOPP dosages if G4 toxicity occurs in 2 successive cycles

(continued)

Supportive care:
Add a **proton pump inhibitor** during prednisone therapy

Emetogenic potential:
BEACOPP and dose-escalated BEACOPP:
Day 1: Very high (Emetogenicity score = 7). Potential for delayed symptoms
Days 2 and 3: High (Emetogenicity score = 5)
Days 4–7: Moderately high (Emetogenicity score = 4)
Day 8: Nonemetogenic (Emetogenicity score = 1). See Chapter 39 for antiemetic regimens

Patient Population Studied

Part of a phase III study of 909 patients, 16–65 years old, with advanced-stage (IIB and IIIA with at least one risk factor or IIIB and IV) HL. Patients were randomized to receive 8 cycles of BEACOPP or escalated BEACOPP. Radiation therapy was planned to sites of initial bulky disease (>5 cm)

Efficacy[a] (N = 323)

Complete response	92%
Partial response	1%
Relapse	6%
Death[b]	5.2%

[a]Results of a second interim analysis, not a final analysis
[b]HL 7 of 17; toxicity 6 of 17; leukemia 1 of 17; NHL 1 of 17

Toxicity (N = 1140; 854 Cycles)

	BEACOPP		Dose-Escalated BEACOPP	
	% Any Grade	% G3/4	% Any Grade	% G3/4
Leukopenia[a]	84	36	95	78
Thrombocytopenia[b]	8	2	65	36
Anemia[c]	56	6	90	27
Infection	12	3	3	3
Alopecia	73	52	83	64
Nausea	41	5	45	5
Neurologic	29	1	30	1
Mucositis	10	1	22	1
Pain	11	1	17	2
Digestive system	8	1	11	1
Respiratory	8	1	9	1
Skin	8	1	9	1
Medication fever	5	1	8	1
Cardiac	4	1	4	1
Allergy	5	1	2	1

[a]G3/4 = WBC <2000/mm^3
[b]G3/4 = platelets <50,000/mm^3
[c]G3/4 = Hgb <8 g/dL

Therapy Monitoring

1. *Weekly:* CBC with differential
2. *Before each cycle:* PE, CBC with differential, BUN, creatinine, LFTs, and LDH
3. *After the second and each subsequent cycle:* DLCO
4. *Response evaluation after completion of therapy:* CT of chest, abdomen, and pelvis every 2 cycles starting after cycle 4. PET (or gallium scan if PET unavailable) at conclusion of therapy to document extent of remission. Bone marrow biopsy (if disease existed before therapy) performed 1 month after completing the sixth cycle

Notes

Most patients reported to date also received involved-field radiation therapy. The use of radiation therapy together with the high doses of alkylating agents give this regimen an extremely high potential for late fatal complications

SALVAGE REGIMEN

LOMUSTINE (CCNU), BLEOMYCIN, VINBLASTINE, DEXAMETHASONE (CBVD)

Weiss J et al. Dtsch Med Wochenschr 1983;108:1428–1432 [in German with English abstract]

Lomustine 120 mg/m² orally as a single dose on day 1 every 42 days (total dosage/cycle = 120 mg/m²)
Bleomycin 15 units per slow intravenous push over 10 minutes for 2 doses on days 1 and 22 every 42 days (total dosage/cycle = 30 units)
Vinblastine 6 mg/m² per intravenous push over 1–2 minutes for 2 doses on days 1 and 22 every 42 days (total dosage/cycle = 12 mg/m²)
Dexamethasone 3 mg/m² per day orally for 21 consecutive days on days 1–21 every 42 days (total dosage/cycle = 63 mg/m²)

Lomustine (CCNU) is available in the United States as capsules for oral administration containing 10 mg, 40 mg, and 100 mg lomustine. CeeNU® (lomustine) Capsules product label, September 2004. Bristol-Myers Squibb Oncology, Bristol-Myers Squibb Company
Dexamethasone is marketed in the United States in numerous generic formulations for oral administration, including prompt-release tablets containing 0.25 mg, 0.5 mg, 0.75 mg, 1 mg, 2 mg, 4 mg, and 6 mg, and in elixirs (which contain alcohol) and solutions for oral administration

Supportive care:
Add a **proton pump inhibitor** during dexamethasone therapy

Emetogenic potential:
Day 1: High (Emetogenicity score = 5)
Day 22: Nonemetogenic (Emetogenicity score = 1). See Chapter 39 for antiemetic regimens

Patient Population Studied

A study of 20 patients with advanced HL whose disease had either not responded to prior regimens or had recurred within 1 year

Efficacy (N = 20)

Complete response	45%
Partial response	30%

Toxicity (N = 20)

WBC 1000–2000/mm³	55%
WBC ≤1000/mm³	20%
Platelet count ≤50,000/mm³	55%
Nausea and vomiting	95%
Alopecia	50%
Neurotoxicity	50%
Bleomycin reaction	40%
Gastroenteritis	10%
Herpes zoster	10%
Myalgias	10%
Orthostasis	10%
Duodenal ulcer	5%
Pneumonia	5%
Pulmonary fibrosis	5%

Treatment Modifications

Adverse Event	Dose Modification
WBC <4000/mm³ or platelet count <120,000/mm³	Reduce lomustine dosage by 20 mg/m²
WBC <3000/mm³ or platelet count <100,000/mm³	Delay cycle 1–2 weeks; then resume with lomustine dosage reduced by 20 mg/m²
Clinical or radiologic evidence of pulmonary fibrosis or DLCO <50% pretreatment value	Discontinue bleomycin
Moderate to severe impairment renal function (creatinine clearance <50 mL/min)	Discontinue bleomycin until creatinine clearance improves to ≥50 mL/min

Therapy Monitoring

1. *Weekly:* CBC with differential
2. *Before each cycle:* Physical exam, chest x-ray
3. *After second and each subsequent cycle:* DLCO
4. *Response evaluation:* Clinical examination, CT of the chest, abdomen, pelvis every 2 cycles starting after cycle 4. PET (or gallium scan if PET unavailable) at conclusion of therapy to document extent of remission. Bone marrow biopsy (if disease existed before therapy) performed 1 cycle after clinical complete response

Notes

1. If CT scan shows no change between cycles 4 and 6, obtain PET (or gallium) scan to confirm complete response. If CT scan shows continued shrinkage of disease between cycles 4 and 6, continue treatment for an additional 2 cycles
2. If the WBC nadir is >2000/mm³, consider a 10% dose escalation of all drugs except bleomycin in the following cycle

SALVAGE REGIMEN

PROCARBAZINE, CYCLOPHOSPHAMIDE, VINBLASTINE, PREDNISONE (PCVP)

Mandelli F et al. Haematologica 1986;71:205–208

Vinblastine 3 mg/m² by intravenous push over 1–2 minutes every 14 days (total dosage/14-day cycle = 3 mg/m²)
Procarbazine 70 mg/m² per dose orally every other day (days 1, 3, 5, and so on) for 7 doses every 14 days (total dosage/14-day cycle = 490 mg/m²)
Cyclophosphamide 70 mg/m² per dose orally every other day (days 1, 3, 5, and so on) for 7 doses every 14 days (total dosage/14-day cycle = 490 mg/m²)
Prednisone 8 mg/m² per dose orally every other day (days 1, 3, 5, and so on) for 7 doses every 14 days (total dosage/14-day cycle = 56 mg/m²)
Note: All 4 drugs are administered continually without interruption for at least 1 year if disease dose not progress

Procarbazine is formulated in the United States for oral administration as capsules containing 50 mg procarbazine HCl. Matulane® brand of procarbazine hydrochloride product label, February 2004. Sigma-Tau Pharmaceuticals, Inc
Cyclophosphamide is generically marketed in the United States as tablets for oral administration containing either 25 mg or 50 mg anhydrous cyclophosphamide
Prednisone is marketed in the United States in numerous solid formulations for oral administration, including: prompt-release tablets containing 1 mg, 2.5 mg, 5 mg, 10 mg, 20 mg, and 50 mg prednisone, and in solutions and syrups

Special instructions:
Procarbazine is a weak monoamine oxidase inhibitor. Concurrent use of sympathomimetic or tricyclic antidepressant drugs and ingestion of tyramine-rich foods may produce severe hypertensive episodes in a patient receiving procarbazine:
McCabe BJ. J Am Diet Assoc 1986;86:1059–64; Anonymous. Med Lett Drugs Ther 1989;31:11–12; Da Prada M et al. J Neural Transm Suppl 1988;26:31–56

Supportive care:
Add a **proton pump inhibitor** to prevent peptic ulcer disease.

Emetogenic potential on odd-numbered days (days 1, 3, 5, 7 and so on): Moderate to moderately high (Emetogenicity score ~4). See Chapter 39 for antiemetic regimens

Efficacy (N = 11)

	% Complete Remission
All patients	72
Complete response to previous therapy	100
Incomplete response to previous therapy	0
Continuous disease at presentation	0
More than 2 previous relapses	88.9

Toxicity (N = 11)

Treatment did not show hematologic toxicity and was well tolerated by patients

Treatment Modifications

Adverse Event	Dose Modification
ANC <1000/mm³ platelet count <50,000/mm³	Hold procarbazine and cyclophosphamide until ANC >1000/mm³ and platelet count >50,000/mm³; then restart therapy with procarbazine and cyclophosphamide dosages reduced to 50 mg/m²

Therapy Monitoring

1. *Weekly, then monthly:* CBC with differential
2. *Monthly to every other month:* Physical exam, LFTs, mineral panel, serum electrolytes, and chest x-ray
3. *Response evaluation:* CT of chest, abdomen, and pelvis every 2 cycles starting after cycle 4. PET (or gallium scan if PET unavailable) at conclusion of therapy to document extent of remission. Bone marrow biopsy (if disease existed before therapy) performed 1 cycle after clinical complete response

SALVAGE REGIMEN

LOMUSTINE (CCNU), ETOPOSIDE, VINDESINE, DEXAMETHASONE (CEVD)

Pfreundschuh MG et al. Cancer Treat Rep 1987;71:1203–1207

Lomustine 80 mg/m² orally on day 1 every 42 days (total dosage/cycle = 80 mg/m²)
Etoposide 60 mg/m² per dose by intravenous infusion, diluted in 0.9% NaCl injection (0.9% NS) to a concentration of 0.2–0.4 mg/mL, over 1 hour for 2 periods of 5 consecutive days/cycle (10 total doses) on days 1–5 and days 22–26 every 42 days (total dosage/cycle = 600 mg/m²), *or*
Etoposide 120 mg/m² per dose orally for 2 periods of 5 consecutive days/cycle (10 total doses) on days 1–5 and days 22–26 every 42 days (total dosage/cycle = 1200 mg/m²)
Vindesine 3 mg/m² per dose by intravenous push over 1–3 minutes for 2 doses on days 1 and 22 (total dosage/cycle = 6 mg/m²)
Note: Vindesine is no longer commercially available in the United States. Eli Lilly & Company, the only American manufacturer, withdrew on 06/23/05 its NDA for Eldisine®, its vindesine sulfate product
Dexamethasone 3 mg/m² per day orally for 8 consecutive days on days 1–8 every 42 days
followed by:
Dexamethasone 1.5 mg/m² per day orally for 18 consecutive days on days 9–26 every 42 days (total dosage/cycle = 51 mg/m²)

Lomustine (CCNU) is available in the United States as capsules for oral administration containing 10 mg, 40 mg, and 100 mg lomustine. CeeNU® (lomustine) Capsules product label, September 2004. Bristol-Myers Squibb Oncology, Bristol-Myers Squibb Company
Dexamethasone is marketed in the United States in numerous formulations for oral administration, such as 0.25-, 0.5-, 0.75-, 1-, 2-, 4-, and 6-mg tablets, and in elixirs (which contain alcohol) and solutions for oral administration
Etoposide is available in the United States as capsules containing 50 mg etoposide. VePesid® (etoposide) for Injection and Capsules, September 1998. Manufactured by R.P. Scherer GmbH Oncology Products, Eberback/Baden, Germany for Bristol Laboratories® Oncology products, A Bristol-Myers Squibb Company

Supportive care:
Add a **proton pump inhibitor** during dexamethasone therapy

Emetogenic potential:
Day 1: Very high (Emetogenicity score = 6). Potential for delayed symptoms
Days 2–5 and days 22–26 with intravenous etoposide: Low (Emetogenicity score = 2)
Days 2–5 and days 22–26 with oral etoposide: Moderate (Emetogenicity score = 3). See Chapter 39 for antiemetic regimens

Patient Population Studied

A study of 32 patients with advanced HL resistant to COPP/ABVD chemotherapy. Resistance defined as progressive or persistent disease after 6 cycles of COPP/ABVD, or relapse within 12 months after completing therapy

Efficacy (N = 32)

Response to COPP/ABVD	% Complete Response	% Partial Response
Complete response (n = 5)	80	20
Partial response (n = 12)	42	0
Progressive disease (n = 15)	33	20
Total (N = 32)	44	13

Treatment Modifications

Adverse Event	Dose Modification
WBC <3500/mm³ or platelet count <100,000/mm³	Delay treatment until WBC >3500/mm³ and platelet count >100,000/mm³

Toxicity (N = 32)

	% G1	% G2	% G3	% G4
Leukopenia	16	22	25	12
Thrombocytopenia	6	13	13	12
Nausea/vomiting	60	24	12	—
Neurotoxicity	11	6	—	—
Alopecia	11	29	60	—
Cushingoid features	48	24	12	—

WHO Criteria

Therapy Monitoring

1. *Weekly and before each cycle:* CBC with differential
2. *Before each cycle:* Physical exam, chest x-ray
3. *Response evaluation:* Clinical examination, CT of chest, abdomen, and pelvis. PET (or gallium scan if PET unavailable) at conclusion of therapy to document extent of remission. Bone marrow biopsy (if disease existed before therapy) performed 1 cycle after clinical complete response

SALVAGE REGIMEN

CYCLOPHOSPHAMIDE, DOXORUBICIN (Adriamycin®), PREDNISOLONE, ETOPOSIDE (CAPE)/PREDNISOLONE, DOXORUBICIN (Adriamycin®), LOMUSTINE, ETOPOSIDE (PALE)

Fairey AF et al. Ann Oncol 1993;4:857–860

Cyclophosphamide 600 mg/m² intravenously in 25–250 mL 0.9% NaCl injection (0.9% NS) or 5% dextrose injection (D5W) over 10–30 minutes on day 1 every 42 days (total dosage/cycle = 600 mg/m²)
Doxorubicin 50 mg/m² per dose per intravenous push over 3–5 minutes for 2 doses on days 1 and 22 every 42 days (total dosage/cycle = 100 mg/m²)
Prednisolone 50 mg/m² per day orally for 7 days on days 2, 3, 4, 5, 23, 24, and 25 every 42 days (total dosage/cycle = 350 mg/²)
Etoposide 250 mg/m² per dose by intravenous infusion, diluted in 0.9% NS to a concentration of 0.2–0.4 mg/mL over 1 hour for 2 doses on days 1 and 22 every 42 days (total dosage/cycle = 500 mg/m²)
Lomustine 80 mg/m² orally as a single dose on day 22 every 42 days (total dosage/cycle = 80 mg/m²)

In alternating 21-day cycles:
CAPE REGIMEN (odd-numbered cycles, 21-days in duration)
Cyclophosphamide 600 mg/m² on day 1; **doxorubicin** 50 mg/m² on day 1; **prednisolone** 50 mg/m² days 2–5; **etoposide** 250 mg/m² on day 1
PALE REGIMEN (even-numbered cycles, 21-days in duration)
Doxorubicin 50 mg/m² on day 1; **prednisolone** 50 mg/m² days 2–4; **etoposide** 250 mg/m² on day 1; **lomustine** 80 mg/m² on day 1

Notes: Administer CAPE followed by PALE for 3 or 4 cycles each
If counts are low but the clinical situation indicates, treat with vincristine and bleomycin weekly until counts recover (see Treatment Modifications)
Vincristine 2 mg per dose by intravenous push over 1–2 minutes weekly until counts recover (total dosage/week = 2 mg)
Bleomycin 15 units by slow intravenous push over 10 minutes weekly until counts recover (total dosage/week = 15 units)

Prednisolone is marketed in the United States in numerous formulations for oral administration, including tablets containing 5 mg prednisolone, and in solutions and syrups in various concentrations
Lomustine (CCNU) is available in the United States as capsules for oral administration containing 10 mg, 40 mg, and 100 mg lomustine. CeeNU® (lomustine) Capsules product label, September 2004. Bristol-Myers Squibb Oncology, Bristol-Myers Squibb Company

Supportive care:
Add a **proton pump inhibitor** during prednisolone therapy

Emetogenic potential:
CAPE, *day 1:* High (Emetogenicity score = 5)
PALE, *day 1:* Very high (Emetogenicity score = 6)
Weekly vincristine + bleomycin = Nonemetogenic (Emetogenicity score = 1). See Chapter 39 for antiemetic regimens

Patient Population Studied

A study of 25 patients with advanced HL who had not achieved complete response after 6 cycles of initial chemotherapy with ChIVPP regimen or its variants or who had relapsed within 1 year after treatment

Therapy Monitoring

1. *Weekly and before each cycle:* CBC with differential
2. *Before each cycle:* Physical exam, chest x-ray
3. *Response evaluation:* Every 2 cycles (1 CAPE/1 PALE) CT of chest, abdomen, and pelvis. PET (or gallium scan if PET unavailable) at conclusion of therapy to document extent of remission. Bone marrow biopsy (if disease existed before therapy) performed 1 cycle after clinical complete response

Treatment Modifications

Adverse Event[a]	Dose Modification
WBC 3000–3500/mm³ or platelet count 100,000–130,000/mm³	Reduce dosages of all drugs by 75% except prednisolone
WBC <3000/mm³ or platelet count <100,000/mm³	Postpone treatment for 1 week[b]
Moderate to severe renal function impairment (creatinine clearance <50 mL/min)	Discontinue bleomycin until creatinine clearance improves to ≥50 mL/min

[a]Based on day 22 and day 42 results
[b]If counts are low but clinical situation demands, treat with vincristine and bleomycin weekly until counts recover

Efficacy (N = 25)

Response to First-Line Treatment	% Complete Response	% Partial Response
Complete response (n = 13)	69	15
Partial response (n = 9)	33	33
Progressive disease (n = 3)	33	—
Total (N = 25)	52	20

Toxicity (N = 25 Patients; 132 Cycles)

Dose reductions	36% of cycles/76% of patients
Treatment delays	31% of cycles/68% of patients
Neutropenia + sepsis	9% of cycles/28% of patients
WHO G3 alopecia	100% of patients
WHO G3/4 nausea/vomiting	12% of patients

Notes

1. If CT scan shows no change between cycles 4 and 6, obtain a PET (or gallium) scan to confirm complete response. If CT scan shows continued shrinkage of disease between cycles 4 and 6, continue treatment for an additional 2 cycles
2. If the WBC nadir is >2000/mm³, consider a 10% dose escalation of all drugs except bleomycin in the following cycle

SALVAGE REGIMEN

DEXAMETHASONE, CARMUSTINE (BCNU), ETOPOSIDE, CYTARABINE (Ara-C), MELPHALAN (Alkeran®) (Dexa-BEAM)

Pfruendschuh MG et al. JCO 1994;12:580–586

Dexamethasone 8 mg orally every 8 hours for 10 consecutive days (30 doses) on days 1–10 every 28 days (total dose/cycle = 240 mg)
Carmustine 60 mg/m^2 intravenously in 100–250 mL 5% dextrose injection (D5W) over at least 60 minutes on day 2 every 28 days (total dosage/cycle = 60 mg/m^2)
Melphalan 20 mg/m^2 intravenously diluted in 0.9% NaCl injection (0.9% NS), to a concentration ≤0.45 mg/mL over 15–20 minutes on day 3 every 28 days (total dosage/cycle = 20 mg/m^2)
Etoposide 75 mg/m^2 per day by intravenous infusion diluted in 0.9% NS or D5W to a concentration of 0.2–0.4 mg/mL, over 1 hour for 4 doses on days 4–7 every 28 days (total dosage/cycle = 300 mg/m^2)
Cytarabine 100 mg/m^2 per dose by intravenous infusion in 25–500 mL 0.9% NS or D5W over 2 hours every 12 hours for 8 doses on days 4–7 every 28 days (total dosage/cycle = 800 mg/m^2)

Supportive care:
Add a **proton pump inhibitor** during prednisone therapy
PCP prophylaxis: **Cotrimoxazole** (trimethoprim 160 mg + sulfamethoxazole 800 mg) orally twice daily on 3 days per week (eg, Monday, Wednesday, and Friday)
Note: Consider antifungal prophylaxis

Emetogenic potential:
Day 2: Moderately high (Emetogenicity score = 4).
Day 3: Moderately high (Emetogenicity score = 4)
Days 4–7: Low–moderate (Emetogenicity score 2–3). See Chapter 39 for antiemetic regimens

Treatment Modifications

Adverse Event	Dose Modification
WBC <4000/mm^3 or platelet count <125,000/mm^3	Delay start of therapy 1 week, or reduce dosages of carmustine, melphalan, etoposide, and cytarabine by 20%

Toxicity (N = 54)

Toxicity	% Patients/ Cycles
G3/4 Granulocytopenia	92
G3/4 Thrombocytopenia	87
Mucositis	21
G3/4 Infection	10[a]
Nausea/vomiting	10
Cardiotoxicity	1.9
Psychosis	1.9
Death[b]	7.5

[a]10% of cycles
[b]Gram-negative sepsis during neutropenia
WHO Criteria

Patient Population Studied

A study of 55 patients with HL who had received prior therapy with COPP + ABVD or COPP + ABVD + IMEP. Forty-two patients had received radiation as well; 28 patients were at first relapse, 22 were on second salvage, and 5 patients had previously received 3 chemotherapy regimens

Efficacy (N = 54)

Response to Prior Therapy	% Complete Response	% Partial Response
Complete response; relapse >12 months (n = 12)	58	25
Complete response; relapse <12 months (n = 15)	27	33
Progressive disease (n = 27)	22	30
Total (N = 54)	31.5	29.6

Therapy Monitoring

1. *Weekly:* CBC with differential
2. *Before each cycle:* History and physical exam, CBC with differential, chest x-ray
3. *Response evaluation:* Clinical examination, CT of chest, abdomen, and pelvis. PET (or gallium scan if PET unavailable) at conclusion of therapy to document extent of remission. Bone marrow biopsy (if disease existed before therapy) performed 1 cycle after clinical complete response

Notes

If the WBC nadir is >2000/mm^3, consider a 10% dose escalation of all drugs except dexamethasone in the following cycle

SALVAGE REGIMEN

MITOXANTRONE, VINBLASTINE, LOMUSTINE (CCNU) (MVC)

Wiernik PH et al. Cancer J Sci Am 1998;4:254–260

Lomustine 100 mg/m^2 orally as a single dose on day 1 every 6–8 weeks (total dosage/cycle = 100 mg/m^2)
Mitoxantrone 8 mg/m^2 per day intravenously in 25–250 mL 0.9% NaCl injection (0.9% NS) or 5% dextrose injection (D5W) over 10–30 minutes for 3 consecutive days on days 1–3 every 6–8 weeks (total dosage/cycle = 24 mg/m^2)
Vinblastine 8 mg/m^2 per dose (maximum single dose = 10 mg) by intravenous push over 1–2 minutes on days 1 and 22 every 6–8 weeks (total dosage/cycle = 16 mg/m^2; maximum dose/cycle = 20 mg)
Note: Consider omitting vinblastine on day 22 to allow for more rapid completion of treatment cycles. Cycles are repeated every 6–8 weeks, depending on degree and duration of myelosuppression

Lomustine (CCNU) is available in the United States as capsules for oral administration containing 10 mg, 40 mg, and 100 mg lomustine. CeeNU® (lomustine) Capsules product label, September 2004. Bristol-Myers Squibb Oncology, Bristol-Myers Squibb Company

Supportive care:
Filgrastim 5 mcg/kg per day subcutaneously starting on day 4 and continuing beyond the ANC nadir until ANC exceeds 5000 cells/mm^3 on one reading. Consider interrupting filgrastim on days 21–23 if planning to administer vinblastine while still administering filgrastim

Emetogenic potential:
Day 1: Very high (Emetogenicity score = 6). Potential for delayed symptoms
Days 2 and 3: Moderate (Emetogenicity score = 3)
Day 22: Nonemetogenic (Emetogenicity score = 1). See Chapter 39 for antiemetic regimens

Patient Population Studied

A study of 36 patients with relapsed or refractory HL. Eighteen patients had received 1 prior regimen (including radiation therapy alone), 10 had received 2 prior regimens, and 8 had been treated with 3 chemotherapy regimens

Efficacy (N = 36)

No. of Prior Regimens	% Complete Response	% Partial Response
1 (n = 18)	44.4	39
2 (n = 10)	40	50
3 (n = 8)	25	75
Total (N = 36)	39	50

Toxicity (N = 53)

	% G3	% G4	% G5
Granulocytopenia	24.5	69.8	1.9
Thrombocytopenia	35.8	35.8	—
Infection	15	43.4	1.9
Bleeding	11.3	11.3	—
Nausea/vomiting	7.5	—	—
Constipation	7.5	1.9	—
Myelodysplasia	3.8		

Includes 17 patients with untreated poor-prognosis HL

Treatment Modifications

Adverse Event	Dose Modification
Day 1 WBC <3000/mm^3 or platelet count <75,000/mm^3	Reduce dosage of mitoxantrone, vinblastine, and lomustine by 25%
Nadir WBC <1000/mm^3 or nadir platelet count <50,000/mm^3	Reduce dosage of mitoxantrone, vinblastine, and lomustine by 50%[a]
Day 22 WBC <3000/mm^3	Hold vinblastine[b]

[a]Subsequent re-escalation allowed, depending on toxicity in cycle with reduced dosages
[b]Unless filgrastim is used, day 22 vinblastine dose will likely have to be withheld

Therapy Monitoring

1. *Weekly:* CBC with differential
2. *Before each cycle:* History and physical exam, CBC with differential, chest x-ray
3. *Response evaluation:* Clinical examination, CT of chest, abdomen, and pelvis. PET (or gallium scan if PET unavailable) at conclusion of therapy to document extent of remission. Bone marrow biopsy (if disease existed before therapy) performed 1 cycle after clinical complete response

Notes

1. If CT scan shows no change between cycles 4 and 6, obtain PET (or gallium) scan to confirm complete response. If CT scan shows continued shrinkage of disease between cycles 4 and 6, continue treatment for an additional 2 cycles
2. If the WBC nadir is >2000/mm^3, consider a 10% dose escalation of all drugs in the following cycle

PREPARATIVE SALVAGE REGIMEN (PRE-TRANSPLANTATION)

DOXORUBICIN (Adriamycin®), METHYLPREDNISOLONE (Solu-Medrol®), HIGH-DOSE CYTARABINE (Ara-C), CISPLATIN (ASHAP)

Rodriguez J et al. Blood 1999;93:3632–3636

Doxorubicin 10 mg/m^2 per day by continuous intravenous infusion via a central vascular access device in 100–1000 mL 0.9% NaCl injection (0.9% NS) or 5% dextrose injection (D5W) over 24 hours for 4 consecutive days on days 1–4 (days −5 to −2) every 28 days (total dosage/cycle = 40 mg/m^2)
Hydration before starting cisplatin:
1000 mL 0.9% NS by intravenous infusion over 6 hours
Cisplatin 25 mg/m^2 per day by continuous intravenous infusion via a central vascular access device in a volume equivalent to the dose, or diluted in 100 mL to ≥1000 mL 0.9% NS over 24 hours for 4 consecutive days on days 1–4 (days −5 to −2) every 28 days (total dosage/cycle = 80 mg/m^2)
Methylprednisolone 500 mg per day intravenously over 15 minutes for 5 consecutive days on days 1–5 (days −5 to −1) every 28 days (total dosage/cycle = 2500 mg)
Cytarabine 1500 mg/m^2 by intravenous infusion in 25–1000 mL 0.9% NS or D5W over 2 hours on day 5 (day −1) after completing day 4 (day −2) cisplatin administration every 28 days (total dosage/cycle = 1500 mg/m^2)
Note: Negative treatment days in parentheses are enumerated with respect to autologous hematopoietic stem cell transplant (HSCT) in which the autologous graft is readministered on day 0 (zero)

Emetogenic potential:
Days 1–4: High (Emetogenicity score ~5)
Day 5: Moderately high (Emetogenicity score = 4). See Chapter 39 for antiemetic regimens

Efficacy (N = 56)

Response to Last Therapy	% Complete Response	% Partial Response
Duration >6 months (n = 32)	34.3	31.2
Duration <6 months (n = 24)	33.3	41.7
Total (N = 56)	33.9	35.7

Toxicity (N = 56)

G3/4 Neutropenia	100%
G2/3 Thrombocytopenia	100%
G3/4 Nonhematologic	0
Cardiac	0
Renal	0

NCI CTC

Treatment Modifications

None specified as part of this brief tumor-reducing program before autologous BMT

Patient Population Studied

A study of 57 patients with relapsing HL. Patients had received MOPP and ABVD or comparable regimens. Patients received 2 cycles of ASHAP followed by assessment. Those with stable disease or any response then received a third cycle as they awaited autologous BMT

Therapy Monitoring

1. *Weekly:* CBC with differential
2. *Before each cycle:* History and physical exam, CBC with differential, chest x-ray, urinalysis, LFTs, BUN, creatinine, and mineral panel including magnesium
3. *Response evaluation:* Clinical examination, CT of chest, abdomen, and pelvis. PET at conclusion of therapy to document extent of remission

PREPARATIVE SALVAGE REGIMEN (PRE-TRANSPLANTATION)

CARMUSTINE (BCNU), ETOPOSIDE, CYTARABINE (Ara-C), MELPHALAN (Mini-BEAM)

Chopra R et al. Br J Haematol 1992;81:197–202
Martín A et al. Br J Haematol 2001;113:161–71

Carmustine 60 mg/m² intravenously in 100–500 mL 5% dextrose injection (D5W) over at least 60 minutes on day 1 (day −6) every 28 days (total dosage/cycle = 60 mg/m²)
Etoposide 75 mg/m² per day by intravenous infusion, diluted in 0.9% NaCl injection (0.9% NS) or D5W to a concentration of 0.2–0.4 mg/mL over 1 hour for 4 consecutive days on days 2–5 (days −5 to −2) every 28 days (total dosage/cycle = 300 mg/m²)
Cytarabine 100 mg/m² per dose by intravenous infusion in 25–1000 mL 0.9% NS or D5W over 15 minutes to 2 hours every 12 hours for 8 doses on days 2–5 (days −5 to −2) every 28 days (total dosage/cycle = 800 mg/m²)
Melphalan 30 mg/m² intravenously diluted in 0.9% NS, to a concentration ≤0.45 mg/mL, over 15–20 minutes on day 6 (day −1) every 28 days (total dosage/cycle = 30 mg/m²)
Note: Negative treatment days in parentheses are enumerated with respect to autologous hematopoietic stem cell transplant (HSCT) in which the autologous graft is readministered on day 0 (zero)

Emetogenic potential:
Day 1: Moderately high (Emetogenicity score = 4)
Days 2–5: Low (Emetogenicity score = 2)
Day 6: Moderately high (Emetogenicity score = 4). See Chapter 39 for antiemetic regimens

Toxicity (N = 23)

Toxicity	% G3/4
Neutropenia	100
Thrombocytopenia	100
Mucositis	4

Following First Course of Mini-BEAM (N = 23)	
Median time to ANC >500/mm³	15 days
Range of time to ANC >500/mm³	7–26 days
Median time to platelets >50,000/mm³	15 days
Range of time to platelets >50,000/mm³	0–26 days
Median period of hospitalization	23 days
Range of time of hospitalization	16–28 days
Febrile neutropenia	47%

Following Second Course of Mini-BEAM (n = 7)	
Median time to ANC >500/mm³	17 days
Range of time to ANC >500/mm³	0–22 days
Median time to platelets >50,000/mm³	21 days
Range of time to platelets >50,000/mm³	15–37 days
Median period of hospitalization	21 days
Range of time of hospitalization	15–37 days
Febrile neutropenia	71.5%

Following Third Course of Mini-BEAM (n = 3)*	
Febrile neutropenia	100%

*Values similar to second course
WHO Criteria
Chopra R et al. Br J Haematol 1992;81:197–202

Treatment Modifications

None specified as part of this tumor-reducing program before autologous BMT

Patient Population Studied

A study of 23 patients with relapsed advanced HL. Twenty-one patients had received at least 2 prior regimens or a hybrid-alternating regimen. Patients were sub-grouped according to intent of treatment: 13 were treated in an attempt to debulk lesions that were >10 cm before treatment with full-dose BEAM followed by autologous BMT. Seven patients were treated with the intention of eradicating disease from the bone marrow before autologous BMT, and 3 patients received mini-BEAM as salvage therapy

Efficacy (N = 23)

Intention of Treatment	% Complete Response	% Partial Response
Cytoreduction/ debulking (n = 13)	—	69
Clear disease from the bone marrow (n = 7)	14*	71.4*
Salvage (n = 3)	—	—
Total (N = 23)	4.3	60.9

*Patients without evidence of disease in bone marrow
Chopra R et al. Br J Haematol 1992;81:197–202

Therapy Monitoring

1. *Weekly:* CBC with differential
2. *Before each cycle:* History and physical exam, CBC with differential, chest x-ray
3. *Response evaluation:* Clinical examination, CT of chest, abdomen, and pelvis. PET at conclusion of therapy to document extent of remission

HIGH-DOSE SALVAGE REGIMEN (PRE-TRANSPLANTATION)

CYCLOPHOSPHAMIDE, CARMUSTINE (BCNU), ETOPOSIDE (VP-16) (CBV)

Jagannath S et al. JCO 1989;7:179–185

Note: Treatment days are enumerated with respect to autologous hematopoietic stem cell transplantation (HSCT), in which the autologous graft is readministered on day 0 (zero)
Carmustine 300 mg/m² intravenously in 100–500 mL 5% dextrose injection (D5W) over at least 60 minutes on day −6 (total dosage = 300 mg/m²)
Cyclophosphamide 1500 mg/m² per day intravenously in 100–1000 mL 0.9% NaCl injection (0.9% NS) or D5W over 10–30 minutes for 4 consecutive days on days −6, −5, −4, and −3 (total dosage = 6000 mg/m²)
Etoposide 125 mg/m² per dose by intravenous infusion, diluted in 0.9% NS to a concentration of 0.2–0.4 mg/mL over 1 hour every 12 hours for 6 doses on days −6, −5, and −4 (total dosage = 750 mg/m²)
Autologous BMT/HSCT is administered on day 0

Supportive care:
Bacterial prophylaxis: Oral antibiotics
Herpes simplex prophylaxis: **Ganciclovir** 5 mg/kg intravenously every 12 hours for 10 consecutive days (adjust dose for renal insufficiency) on days 1–10 after transplantation
See Chapter 50, Complications and Follow-up After Hematopoietic Stem Cell Transplantation, for additional information

Emetogenic potential:
Day −6: Very high (Emetogenicity score ≥6). Potential for delayed symptoms
Days −5 and −4: Very high (Emetogenicity score = 6). Potential for delayed symptoms
Day −3: High (Emetogenicity score = 5). Potential for delayed symptoms. See Chapter 39 for antiemetic regimens

Patient Population Studied

A study of 61 patients with relapsed HL. Median age 28 years (range 15–56 years). Median time from diagnosis to BMT 35 months (range 6–11 months). Marrow stored an average of 1 month (range 1 to 113 weeks) before transplantation. Zubrod performance status: 0 (n = 35), 1 (n = 18), 2 (n = 6), and 3 (n = 2). Disease staging: stage I (n = 5), stage II (n = 11), stage III (n = 6), and stage IV (n = 37), with 2 patients intensified in third complete response. Twenty-one patients had nodal disease only; 38 also had extranodal disease, including lung (n = 23), pleura (n = 7), bone (n = 5), and liver (n = 3)

Efficacy (N = 59)

	%	Median Survival
Complete response	46	>30 months
Partial response*	31	15 months
No response	23	2.7 months
All patients		30 months

*Six of 18 patients with partial response achieved complete response after radiation therapy to local sites

Treatment Modifications

None specified as part of this preparative regimen

Toxicity (N = 61)

	% of Patients
Nausea/vomiting	89
Severe mucositis	27
Hematuria	13.1
Seizures	3.3
Congestive heart failure	1.6
Febrile neutropenia	>90
Death*	6.6
Median time to ANC >500/mm³	22 days
Median time to platelets >50,000/mm³	26 days

*Candidemia in 2 patients; pulmonary fibrosis in 2 patients; all had received a cumulative etoposide dosage of 900 mg/m²

Therapy Monitoring

Intensive in-hospital monitoring. See Chapter 50, Complications and Follow-up After Hematopoietic Stem Cell Transplantation, for additional information

HIGH-DOSE SALVAGE REGIMEN (PRE-TRANSPLANTATION)

CARMUSTINE (BCNU), ETOPOSIDE, CYTARABINE (Ara-C), MELPHALAN (BEAM)

Chopra R et al. Blood 1993;81:1137–1145
Gribben JG et al. Blood 1989;73:340–344

Note: Treatment days are enumerated with respect to autologous hematopoietic stem cell transplant (HSCT) in which the autologous graft is readministered on day 0 (zero)
Carmustine 300 mg/m^2 intravenously in 100–500 mL 5% dextrose injection (D5W) over at least 60 minutes on day −6 (total dosage = 300 mg/m^2)
Etoposide 200 mg/m^2 per day by intravenous infusion, diluted in 0.9% NaCl injection (0.9% NS) to a concentration of 0.2–0.4 mg/mL over 1 hour for 4 consecutive days on days −5, −4, −3, and −2 (total dosage = 800 mg/m^2)
Cytarabine 200 mg/m^2 per dose by intravenous infusion in 25–1000 mL 0.9% NS or D5W over 15 minutes to 2 hours every 12 hours for 8 doses on days −5, −4, −3, and −2 (total dosage = 1600 mg/m^2)
Melphalan 140 mg/m^2 intravenously diluted in 0.9% NS to a concentration ≤0.45 mg/mL over 15–20 minutes on day −1 (total dosage = 140 mg/m^2)
Autologous BMT/HSCT is administered on day 0

Supportive care: See Chapter 50, Complications and Follow-up After Hematopoietic Stem Cell Transplantation, for additional information

Emetogenic potential:
Day −6: High (Emetogenicity score = 5). Potential for delayed symptoms
Days −5, −4, −3, and −2: Moderate (Emetogenicity score ~3)
Day −1: Moderately high (Emetogenicity score = 4). Potential for delayed symptoms.
See Chapter 39 for antiemetic regimens

Efficacy (N = 44)

	% of Patients	Median Survival[a]
Complete response	34	>50 months
Partial response[b]	52	
All patients		22 months

[a]After transplant
[b]Two patients with slowly resolving mediastinal masses achieved complete response without further therapy at 6 months; 5 of 7 patients achieved complete response after radiation to sites of residual disease

Gribben JG et al. Blood 1989;73:340–344

Toxicity (N = 44)

Severe mucositis	Frequent*
Febrile neutropenia	88%
Median time to ANC >500/mm^3	24 days
Range of time to ANC >500/mm^3	11–68 days
Median time to WBC >1000/mm^3	18 days
Range of time to WBC >1000/mm^3	9–48 days
Median time to platelets >50,000/mm^3	32 days
Range of time to platelets >50,000/mm^3	13–54 days
Death during aplastic phase	4.5%

*35% of patients required parenteral nutrition
Gribben JG et al. Blood 1989;73:340–344

Treatment Modifications

None specified as part of this preparative regimen

Patient Population Studied

A study of 44 patients with relapsed HL. All patients had active disease at time of transplantation. Twenty-two had never achieved a complete response with any prior therapy. Median age was 29 years (range 18–40 years). Median time from diagnosis to BMT was 20.5 months (range 7–195 months). Disease staging: stage I (n = 3), stage II (n = 16), stage III (n = 14), and stage IV (n = 11). All patients had nodal disease; 21 also had extranodal disease

Therapy Monitoring

Intensive in-hospital monitoring. See Chapter 50, Complications and Follow-up After Stem Cell Transplantation, for additional information

SALVAGE REGIMEN (PRE-TRANSPLANTATION)

HIGH-DOSE MELPHALAN

Stewart DA et al. Ann Oncol 1997;8:1277–1279

Melphalan 140 mg/m² intravenously diluted in 0.9% NS to a concentration ≤0.45 mg/mL, over 15–20 minutes on day −1, (total dosage = 140 mg/m²)
Autologous BMT/HSCT is administered on day 0

Supportive care: See Chapter 50, Complications and Follow-up After Hematopoietic Stem Cell Transplantation, for additional information

Emetogenic potential: Moderately high (Emetogenicity score = 4). Potential for delayed symptoms. See Chapter 39 for antiemetic regimens

Efficacy (N = 23)*

- Two of 8 patients (25%) with refractory disease and 9 of 15 (60%) with relapsed disease were free from progression 12–185 months (median 80 months) after transplantation
- Five-year overall survival was 52%
- Five-year progression-free survival rate was 50%

*After transplant

Toxicity (N = 23)

G3/4 Nonhematologic toxicity	0
Deaths	0
Median time to ANC >500/mm³	19 days*
Range of time to ANC >500/mm³	10–150 days
Median time to platelets >20,000/mm³	32 days*
Range of time to platelets >20,000/mm³	11–85 days

*Five patients who received stem cells had median times of 11 and 12 days for ANC and platelet recoveries, respectively

Treatment Modifications

None specified as part of this preparative regimen

Patient Population Studied

A study of 23 patients with relapsed (n = 15) or refractory (n = 8) HL. Median age was 29 years (range 17–45 years). Median time from diagnosis to BMT for relapsed patients was 59 months (range 14–144 months); for refractory patients, 12 months (range 7–55 months). Six patients had 1 prior regimen, 13 had 2 prior regimens, and 4 had 3 prior regimens. Seventeen patients had prior radiation therapy; 3 had a first relapse, 10 had a second relapse, 2 had a third relapse. Nine patients had progressive disease at time of transplantation

Therapy Monitoring

Intensive in-hospital monitoring. See Chapter 50, Complications and Follow-up After Hematopoietic Stem Cell Transplantation, for additional information

PALLIATIVE REGIMEN

VINBLASTINE

Little R et al. JCO 1998;16:584–588

Vinblastine 4–6 mg/m² by intravenous infusion in 25–250 mL 0.9% NaCl injection (0.9% NS) or 5% dextrose injection (D5W) over 15–30 minutes every 1–2 weeks (total dosage/cycle = 4–6 mg/m²)
Note: The average dose intensity for the first 26 weeks was 2.89 mg/m² consistent with administration of vinblastine 6 mg/m² every 2 weeks as the most commonly administered dosage and schedule

Emetogenic potential: Nonemetogenic (Emetogenicity score = 1). See Chapter 39 for antiemetic regimens

Efficacy (N = 16)

Complete response	12%[a]
Partial response	47%[a]
Stable disease	12%[b]
Median progression-free survival	8.3 months[c]
Median overall survival	38.8 months

[a]No correlation with prior vinblastine therapy
[b]Two patients with assessable disease had clinical benefit for 6 and 12 months, respectively
[c]14 months among responders, including 2 patients in complete remission 4.6+ and 9+ years, respectively

Toxicity (N = 16 Patients; 102 Cycles)

ANC <500/mm³	3% of cycles*
Platelets <50,000/mm³	1% of cycles
Fever/neutropenia	3% of cycles*
Vomiting	1% of cycles
Moderate constipation	1 patient
Mild paresthesias	2 patients
Pulmonary aspergillosis	1 patient
Pneumocystis carinii	1 patient

*Filgrastim was used in only 1 patient

Treatment Modifications

Adverse Event	Dose Modification
ANC <500/mm³ or platelet count <20,000/mm³	Reduce vinblastine dosage by 2 mg/m², or extend the cycle length to 2 weeks

Patient Population Studied

A study of 16 patients with HL who relapsed after autologous BMT with symptomatic disease, with an ANC >500/mm³, and platelets >20,000/mm³. Median age was 31 years; Eastern Cooperative Group (ECOG) performance status was 2. Seventy-one percent with stage III/IV disease, 6% with constitutional symptoms, and 59% with symptoms from their HL. Median number of prior regimens was 3 with a range of 2 to 5, and the median time to progression after transplantation was 8 months with a range of 2–47 months

Therapy Monitoring

1. *Weekly to every other week:* CBC with differential
2. *Every 4–12 weeks:* Physical exam, chest x-ray
3. *Response evaluation:* Every 4–12 weeks or as clinically indicated, CT of chest, abdomen, and pelvis. PET (or gallium scan if PET unavailable) at conclusion of therapy to document extent of remission

PALLIATIVE REGIMEN

GEMCITABINE

Venkatesh H et al. Clin Lymphoma 2004;5:110–115

Gemcitabine 1000 mg/m^2 per dose by intravenous infusion diluted with 0.9% NaCl injection (0.9% NS) to a concentration as low as 0.1 mg/mL over 30 minutes for 2 doses on days 1 and 8 every 21 days (total dosage/cycle = 2000 mg/m^2)

Emetogenic potential: Low (Emetogenicity score = 2). See Chapter 39 for antiemetic regimens

Efficacy (N = 27)

Complete response	0%
Partial response	22%
Median duration of partial response	5.1 months (range 2.3–19.3 months)

Toxicity (N = 27)

Toxicity	% G3	% G4
Hematologic (1000 mg/m^2; N = 19)		
Anemia	5.3	—
Leukopenia	10.5	—
Neutropenia	21.1	—
Thrombocytopenia	—	10.5
Neutropenia and fever	5.3	—
Hematologic (1250 mg/m2; N = 8)		
Anemia	12.5	—
Leukopenia	25	
Neutropenia	37.5	12.5
Thrombocytopenia	75	12.5
Neutropenia and fever	—	—

Treatment Modifications

Adverse Event	Dose Modification
WBC <3500/mm^3, ANC <1500/mm^3, or platelet count <100,000/mm^3	Delay treatment until WBC >3500/mm^3, ANC >1500/mm^3, and platelet count >100,000/mm^3

Patient Population Studied

A study of 29 patients with relapsed HL. All patients had received at least 2 (range 2–7) prior regimens for HL; 62% experienced a relapse after autologous BMT. Performance status among patients Eastern Cooperative Oncology Group (ECOG) was 0 (41.4%), 1 (48.3%), and 2 (10.3%)

Therapy Monitoring

1. *Weekly:* CBC with differential
2. *Every 2–3 cycles:* History and physical exam, chest x-ray
3. *Response evaluation:* Every 3 cycles, CT of chest, abdomen, and pelvis. PET (or gallium scan if PET unavailable) at conclusion of therapy to document extent of remission

PALLIATIVE REGIMEN

VINORELBINE

Devizzi L et al. Ann Oncol 1994;5:817–820

Vinorelbine 30 mg/m^2 per dose by intravenous infusion diluted in a volume of 0.9% NaCl injection or 5% dextrose injection sufficient to produce a solution with a concentration of 1.5–3 mg/mL over 6–10 minutes every week for 4 consecutive weeks (total dosage/cycle = 120 mg/m^2)

Emetogenic potential: Nonemetogenic (Emetogenicity score = 1). See Chapter 39 for antiemetic regimens

Toxicity (N = 23)

	% G1	% G2	% G3	% G4
Leukopenia	9	26	52	9
Granulocytopenia	13	30	44	9
Thrombocytopenia	4	0	0	4
Anemia	39	22	4	4
Alopecia	—	—	4	—
Injection site reaction	—	—	22	—
Stomatitis	—	9	—	—
Infection	—	9	13	—
Fever	9	39	—	—
Constipation	—	9	4	—
Peripheral neuropathy	48	13	—	—

NCI CTC

Treatment Modifications

Adverse Event	Dose Modification
WBC <3500/mm^3, ANC <1500/mm^3, or platelet count <100,000/mm^3	Delay treatment until WBC >3500/mm^3, ANC >1500/mm^3, and platelet count >100,000/mm^3

Efficacy (N = 22)

No. of Prior Regimens	% Complete Response	% Partial Response
<3 (n = 4)	25	—
≥3 (n = 18)	11	44
Total (N = 22)	14	36

Patient Population Studied

A study of 24 patients who had received at least 2 (range 2–7) prior regimens for HL, consisting of MOPP and ABVD given sequentially or in alternation, followed by various salvage regimens, including autologous BMT in 4 cases. All patients had been previously treated with at least 2 vinca alkaloids. Fifteen patients had undergone extensive radiation therapy

Therapy Monitoring

1. *Weekly:* CBC with differential
2. *Every 4 weeks:* Physical exam, chest x-ray
3. *Response evaluation:* Every 4–8 courses, CT of chest, abdomen, and pelvis. PET (or gallium scan if PET unavailable) at conclusion of therapy to document extent of remission. Bone marrow biopsy (if disease existed before therapy) performed 1 cycle after clinical complete response

25. Lymphoma, Non-Hodgkin

Kieron Dunleavy, MD, David R. Kohler, PharmD, and Wyndham H. Wilson, MD, PhD

Epidemiology

Estimated new cases in 2006 (United States): 58,870
Estimated deaths in 2006 (United States): 18,840
Median age at diagnosis: Sixth decade of life (Burkitt's lymphoma and lymphoblastic lymphoma typically occur in younger patients)
Male:female ratio: 1.1:1

Jemal A et al. CA Cancer J Clin 2006;56:106–30

Pathology

Over the past three decades, several classification schemes have been used for non-Hodgkin lymphoma (NHL). At the present time, the standard classification is the World Health Organization (WHO) Classification of Haematological Malignancies. This classification schema divides non-Hodgkin lymphoma into those of B-cell origin and those of T-cell and natural killer (NK)–cell origin

B-Cell Neoplasms

Precursor B-cell neoplasm
- Precursor B lymphoblastic leukemia/ lymphoma

Mature B-cell neoplasms
1. Diffuse large B-cell lymphoma (31%)*
2. Follicular lymphoma (22%)*
3. Chronic lymphocytic leukemia/small lymphocytic lymphoma (6%)*
4. Mantle cell lymphoma (6%)*
5. Extranodal marginal zone B-cell lymphoma of mucosa-associated lymphoid tissue (MALT-lymphoma) (5%)*
6. Lymphoplasmacytic lymphoma
7. Splenic marginal zone lymphoma
8. Nodal marginal zone B-cell lymphoma
9. Mediastinal (thymic) large B-cell lymphoma
10. Intravascular large B-cell lymphoma
11. Primary effusion lymphoma
12. Burkitt's lymphoma/leukemia

B-cell proliferations of uncertain malignant potential
1. Lymphomatoid granulomatosis
2. Post-transplantation lymphoproliferative disorder, polymorphic

*An asterisk denotes those that constitute a large enough percentage of all cases of NHL. The remaining B-cell lymphoma subtypes constitute <2% of all NHL

T-Cell and NK-Cell Neoplasms

Precursor T-cell neoplasms
1. Precursor T-lymphoblastic leukemia/lymphoma
2. Blastic NK-cell lymphoma

(*continued*)

Work-Up

1. H&P and performance status
2. *Laboratory tests:* CBC with differential, electrolytes, liver function tests, mineral panel, uric acid, LDH
3. HIV and hepatitis B and C serologies as clinically indicated
4. Chest x-ray (PA and lateral)
5. CT scan of chest, abdomen, and pelvis; neck CT as clinically indicated
6. CT or MRI brain scan if clinically indicated
7. Bone marrow aspirate and biopsy
8. Calculation of IPI (International Prognostic Index) or FLIPI (Follicular Lymphoma International Prognostic Index)
9. CSF evaluation (cytology and flow cytometry) in patients with high risk of CNS involvement (eg, those with Burkitt's lymphoma, AIDS-related lymphoma, lymphoblastic lymphoma, diffuse large B-cell lymphoma with multiple extranodal sites)
10. Echocardiogram or MUGA scan to determine cardiac ejection fraction as clinically indicated
11. Excisional lymph node biopsy to completely assess lymph node architecture is required at initial diagnosis. Fine-needle aspiration biopsy alone is not desirable for the initial diagnosis of lymphoma

NCCN Clinical Practice Guidelines in Oncology, V. 2. 2006

Pathology (*continued*)

Mature T-cell and NK-cell neoplasms

1. Peripheral T-cell lymphoma, unspecified (6%)*
2. Adult T-cell leukemia/lymphoma
3. Extranodal NK/T-cell lymphoma, nasal type
4. Enteropathy-type T-cell lymphoma
5. Hepatosplenic T-cell lymphoma
6. Mature T-cell and NK-cell neoplasms
7. Subcutaneous panniculitis-like T-cell lymphoma
8. Mycosis fungoides
9. Sézary syndrome
10. Primary cutaneous anaplastic large cell lymphoma
11. Angioimmunoblastic T-cell lymphoma
12. Anaplastic large cell lymphoma

T-cell proliferation of uncertain malignant potential

• Lymphomatoid papulosis

*The remaining T-cell and NK-cell sub-types constitute <2% of all NHL subtypes

Armitage JO et al. JCO 1998;16:2780–2795
Jaffe ES, Harris NL, Stein H, Vardiman JW, eds. World Health Organization Classification of Tumours. Pathology and Genetics of Tumours of Haematopoietic and Lymphoid Tissues. Lyon: IARC Press, 2001

5-Year Survival Rate

NHL Subtype	5-Year Survival Rates
Diffuse large B-cell lymphoma	Varies according to IPI and treatment
Follicular lymphoma	Varies according to FLIPI
Mantle cell lymphoma	≃30%

IPI, International Prognostic Index
FLIPI, Follicular Lymphoma International Prognostic Index
Fisher RI et al. Blood 1995;85:1075–1082

Staging

Ann Arbor Staging Classification for Hodgkin and Non-Hodgkin Lymphomas

Stage	Description
I	Involvement of a single lymph node region (I) or involvement of a single extralymphatic organ or site (IE)
II	Involvement of ≥2 lymph node regions or lymphatic structures on the same side of the diaphragm alone (II) or with involvement of limited, contiguous extralymphatic organ or tissue (IIE)
III	Involvement of lymph node regions on both sides of the diaphragm (III), which may include the spleen (IIIS) or limited, contiguous extralymphatic organ or site (IIIE) or both (IIIES)
IV	Diffuse or disseminated foci of involvement of one or more extralymphatic organs or tissues, with or without associated lymphatic involvement
Abbreviations	
A	Asymptomatic
B	Unexplained persistent or recurrent fever with temperature higher than 38°C, or recurrent drenching night sweats within 1 month, or unexplained loss of >10% body weight within 6 months
E	Limited direct extension into extralymphatic organ from adjacent lymph node
X	Bulky disease (mediastinal tumor width > one-third of the transthoracic diameter at T5/6, or a tumor diameter >10 cm)

Moormeier JA et al. Semin Oncol 1990;17:43–50

Caveats

International Prognostic Index (IPI)

A useful measure of clinical outcome for aggressive diffuse large B-cell lymphomas (DLBCL)
A point is given for the presence of each of the characteristics below. The maximum score is 5

1. Age >60 years
2. Serum lactate dehydrogenase concentration > upper limit of normal
3. ECOG performance status ≥2
4. Ann Arbor stages III or IV
5. Number of extranodal disease sites >1

The IPI scores were applied to a group of 2031 patients with aggressive NHL. The 5-year overall survival (OS) and complete response (CR) rates according to the score were as follows:

Score	Risk Group	% 5-Year OS	% CR
0–1	Low	73	87
2	Low-intermediate	51	67
3	High-intermediate	43	55
4–5	High	26	44

The International Non-Hodgkin's Lymphoma Prognostic Factors Project. NEJM 1993;329:987–994

Follicular Lymphoma International Prognostic Index (FLIPI)

A useful measure of clinical outcome for follicular (indolent) lymphomas
A point is given for the presence of each of the following characteristics:

1. Age ≥60 years
2. Ann Arbor stage III-IV
3. Hemoglobin level <12 g/dL
4. Serum LDH level >upper limit of normal
5. Number of nodal sites ≥5

Score	Risk Group	5-year OS
0–1	Low	90.6%
2	Intermediate	77.6%
≥3	High	52.5%

Solal-Céligny P et al. Blood 2004;104:1258–1265

Suggested Treatment Regimens

[NCCN Clinical Practice Guidelines in Oncology, V. 2. 2006, Non-Hodgkin's Lymphoma © National Comprehensive Cancer Network, Inc. 2005 (www.nccn.org)]

Note: The choice of initial therapy requires consideration of many factors, including age, comorbid pathologies, and future therapies (eg, stem cell transplantation). Therefore, treatment selection should be individualized

Diffuse Large B-cell Lymphoma

First-line therapy

- Rituximab-CHOP (cyclophosphamide, doxorubicin, vincristine, prednisone)
- Dose-adjusted EPOCH-R (etoposide, prednisone, vincristine, cyclophosphamide, doxorubicin, rituximab)

Second-line therapy

- ICE (ifosfamide, carboplatin, etoposide) ± rituximab
- ESHAP (etoposide, methylprednisolone, cytarabine, cisplatin)
- Dose-adjusted EPOCH ± rituximab
- Autologous or allogeneic (experimental) hematopoietic progenitor cell transplantation for sensitive diseases

Follicular Lymphoma

First-line therapy

- CVP (cyclophosphamide, vincristine, prednisone) ± rituximab
- Rituximab + CHOP (cyclophosphamide, doxorubicin, vincristine, prednisone)
- Fludarabine ± rituximab
- FND (fludarabine, mitoxantrone, dexamethasone) ± rituximab
- Alkylating agents (eg, chlorambucil or cyclophosphamide) ± prednisone ± rituximab
- Rituximab (selected circumstances)

Second-line therapy

- Rituximab
- Treatments listed under *First-line therapy*
- Radioimmunotherapy
- Allogeneic hematopoietic progenitor cell transplantation (experimental)

Small Lymphocytic Lymphoma

First-line therapy

- Fludarabine ± rituximab
- FC ± rituximab
- Alkylating agents (eg, chlorambucil or cyclophosphamide) ± prednisone ± rituximab
- CVP ± rituximab

Second-line therapy

- Alemtuzumab
- PC (pentostatin, cyclophosphamide) ± rituximab
- Treatments listed under *First-line therapy*
- Allogeneic hematopoietic progenitor cell transplantation (experimental)

Mantle Cell Lymphoma

First-line therapy

- Rituximab + CHOP
- Hyper-CVAD (cyclophosphamide, vincristine, doxorubicin, and dexamethasone, alternating with high-dose methotrexate and cytarabine) + rituximab
- Dose-adjusted EPOCH-R

Second-line therapy

- Treatments listed under *First-line therapy*
- FC (fludarabine + cyclophosphamide) ± rituximab
- PCR (pentostatin, cyclophosphamide, rituximab)
- Bortezomib
- Autologous or allogeneic hematopoietic progenitor cell transplantation (experimental)

REGIMEN

CYCLOPHOSPHAMIDE, DOXORUBICIN (HYDROXYLDAUNORUBICIN), VINCRISTINE (ONCOVIN®), PREDNISONE (CHOP)

Coiffier B et al. NEJM 2002;346:235–242
McKelvey EM et al. Cancer, 1976;38:1484–1493

Intravenous hydration before and after cyclophosphamide administration:
500–1000 mL 0.9% NaCl injection (0.9% NS)

Cyclophosphamide 750 mg/m^2 intravenously in 25–250 mL 0.9% NS or 5% dextrose injection (D5W) over 10–30 minutes, given on day 1 every 3 weeks (total dosage/cycle = 750 mg/m^2)
Doxorubicin 50 mg/m^2 by intravenous push over 3–5 minutes, given on day 1 every 3 weeks (total dosage/cycle = 50 mg/m^2)
Vincristine 1.4 mg/m^2 (maximum dose = 2 mg) by intravenous push over 1–3 minutes, given on day 1 every 3 weeks (total dosage/cycle = 1.4 mg/m^2; maximum dose/cycle = 2 mg)
Prednisone 40 mg/m^2 per day orally for 5 consecutive days on days 1–5 every 3 weeks (total dosage/cycle = 200 mg/m^2)
Prednisone is marketed in the United States in numerous solid formulations for oral administration, such as tablets containing 1, 2.5, 5, 10, 20, and 50 mg prednisone and in solutions and syrups

Supportive care:
Add a **proton pump inhibitor** during prednisone therapy

Emetogenic potential: Moderately high (Emetogenicity score = 4). See Chapter 39 for antiemetic regimens

Patient Population Studied

Previously untreated patients with diffuse large B-cell lymphoma 60–80 years of age were randomly assigned to receive 8 cycles of CHOP every 3 weeks (197 patients) or 8 cycles of CHOP plus rituximab given on day 1 of each cycle (202 patients). Patients who were serologically positive for HIV and patients with active hepatitis B infection were excluded

Efficacy (N = 197)

Complete response	37%
Unconfirmed complete response	26%
Partial response	6%
Stable disease	1%
Progressive disease	22%
Death without disease progression	6%
Could not be assessed	4%

Coiffier B et al. NEJM 2002;346:235–242

Toxicity (N = 197)

Adverse Event	% Any Grade*	% G3/4
Fever	59	5
Infection	65	20
Mucositis	31	2
Liver toxicity	46	5
Cardiac toxicity	35	8
Neurologic toxicity	54	9
Renal toxicity	14	2
Lung toxicity	30	11
Nausea or vomiting	48	8
Constipation	41	5
Alopecia	97	45
Other toxicities	80	25

*Percentage of patients with an event during at least 1 cycle

Coiffier B et al. NEJM 2002;346:235–242
NCI CTC

Treatment Modifications

Adverse Event	Dose Modification
G4 ANC or febrile neutropenia after any cycle	Administer filgrastim during subsequent cycles*
G4 Neutropenia during a cycle in which filgrastim was administered	Cyclophosphamide and doxorubicin dosages are reduced by 50% during subsequent cycles
G3/4 Thrombocytopenia	Cyclophosphamide and doxorubicin dosages are reduced by 50% during subsequent cycles
ANC < 1500/mm^3 or platelets <100,000/mm^3 before a scheduled cycle	The cycle is delayed for up to 2 weeks. Treatment is stopped if recovery has not occurred after a 2-week delay

***Filgrastim** 5 mcg/kg per day subcutaneously, starting in day 2 and continuing beyond ANC nadir until ANC exceeds 5000/mm^3 on one reading
Coiffier B et al. NEJM 2002;346:235–242

Therapy Monitoring

1. *Weekly:* CBC with differential
2. *Before each cycle:* Serum BUN, creatinine, LFTs, and PE

REGIMEN

CYCLOPHOSPHAMIDE, DOXORUBICIN (HYDROXYLDAUNORUBICIN), VINCRISTINE (ONCOVIN®), PREDNISONE (CHOP) + RITUXIMAB

Coiffier B et al. NEJM 2002;346:235–242

Premedication for rituximab:
Acetaminophen 650–1000 mg orally, *plus*
Diphenhydramine 25–50 mg orally or intravenously, 30–60 minutes before starting rituximab
Rituximab 375 mg/m^2 intravenously in 0.9% NaCl injection (0.9% NS) or 5% dextrose injection (D5W) diluted to a concentration of 1–4 mg/mL on day 1 every 21 days (total dosage/cycle=375 mg/m^2)

Notes on rituximab administration:

- Infuse initially at 50 mg/hour. If hypersensitivity or infusion reactions do not occur during the first 30 minutes, increase the rate by 50 mg/hour every 30 minutes as tolerated to a maximum rate of 400 mg/hour. Subsequently, if previous administration was well tolerated, start at 100 mg/hour and increase by 100 mg/hour every 30 minutes as tolerated, to a maximum rate of 400 mg/hour
- Interrupt rituximab administration for fever, chills, edema, congestion of the head and neck mucosa, hypotension, and other serious adverse events. Resume rituximab administration after adverse events abate

Intravenous hydration before and after cyclophosphamide administration:
500–1000 mL 0.9% NS

Cyclophosphamide 750 mg/m^2 intravenously in 25–250 mL 0.9% NS or D5W over 10–30 minutes, given on day 1 every 3 weeks (total dosage/cycle = 750 mg/m^2)
Doxorubicin 50 mg/m^2 by intravenous push over 3–5 minutes, given on day 1 every 3 weeks (total dosage/cycle = 50 mg/m^2)
Vincristine 1.4 mg/m^2 (maximum dose = 2 mg) by intravenous push over 1–3 minutes, given on day 1 every 3 weeks (total dosage/cycle = 1.4 mg/m^2; maximum dose/cycle = 2 mg)
Prednisone 40 mg/m^2 per day orally for 5 consecutive days, days 1–5 every 3 weeks (total dosage/cycle = 200 mg/m^2)
Prednisone is marketed in the United States in numerous solid formulations for oral administration, such as tablets containing 1, 2.5, 5, 10, 20, and 50 mg prednisone and in solutions and syrups

Supportive care:
Add a **proton pump inhibitor** during prednisone therapy

Emetogenic potential: Moderately high (Emetogenicity score = 4). See Chapter 39 for antiemetic regimens

Treatment Modifications

Adverse Event	Dose Modification
G4 ANC or febrile neutropenia after any cycle of chemotherapy	Filgrastim prophylaxis after chemotherapy during subsequent cycles*
G4 ANC during a cycle in which filgrastim was administered	Reduce cyclophosphamide and doxorubicin dosages 50% during subsequent cycles
G3/4 thrombocytopenia	
ANC <1500/mm^3 or platelet count <100,000/mm^3 on first day of a repeated cycle	Delay cycle for up to 2 weeks. Stop treatment if recovery has not occurred after a 2-week delay

***Filgrastim** 5 mcg/kg per day subcutaneously, starting on day 2 and continuing beyond ANC nadir until ANC exceeds 5000/mm^3 on one reading

Rituximab Infusion-Related Toxicities

Onset of infusion-related events (fevers, chills, rigors edema, congestion of the head and neck mucosa, hypotension):

1. Interrupt rituximab infusion
2. For fever, chills: Give additional dose of acetaminophen 650 mg orally and diphenhydramine 25–50 mg by intravenous push
3. For rigors: Give meperidine 12.5–25 mg by intravenous push ± promethazine 12.5–25 mg by intravenous infusion in at least 10 mL 0.9% NS or D5W over 5–15 minutes. If after 15–20 minutes the response to a single dose is considered inadequate, the dose may be repeated
4. After symptoms resolve, resume rituximab infusion at 50 mg/hour and increase by 50 mg/hour every 30 minutes as tolerated up to a maximum rate of 200 mg/hour

Dyspnea or wheezing, without allergic findings (urticaria, or tongue or laryngeal edema):

1. Interrupt rituximab infusion immediately
2. Give hydrocortisone 100 mg by intravenous push (or glucocorticoid equivalent)
3. Give a histamine H_2 antagonist (ranitidine 150 mg, cimetidine 300 mg, or famotidine 20 mg) by intravenous push
4. After symptoms resolve, resume rituximab infusion at 25 mg/hour with close monitoring. Do not increase rate

Note: Medications for the treatment of hypersensitivity reactions should be available for immediate use in the event of a reaction during administration (eg, intravenous fluids, epinephrine, antihistamines, glucocorticoids, and O_2)

Patient Population Studied

Previously untreated patients with diffuse large B-cell lymphoma 60–80 years of age were randomly assigned to receive 8 cycles of CHOP every 3 weeks (197 patients) or 8 cycles of CHOP plus rituximab given on the first day of each cycle (202 patients). Patients who were serologically positive for HIV and patients with active hepatitis B infection were excluded

Efficacy (N = 202)

Complete response	52%
Unconfirmed complete response	23%
Partial response	7%
Stable disease	1%
Progressive disease	9%
Death without disease progression	6%
Could not be assessed	1%

Coiffier B et al. NEJM 2002;346:235–242

Toxicity (N = 202)*

	% Any Grade	% G3/4
Fever	64	2
Infection	65	12
Mucositis	27	3
Liver toxicity	46	3
Cardiac toxicity	47	8
Neurologic toxicity	51	5
Renal toxicity	11	1
Lung toxicity	33	8
Nausea or vomiting	42	2
Constipation	38	2
Alopecia	97	39
Other toxicities	84	20

*Percentage of patients with event during at least 1 cycle

Coiffier B et al. NEJM 2002;346:235–242
NCI CTC

Therapy Monitoring

1. *Weekly:* CBC with differential
2. *Before each cycle:* LFTs, serum BUN, creatinine, PE

REGIMEN

DOSE-ADJUSTED ETOPOSIDE, PREDNISONE, VINCRISTINE (ONCOVIN®), CYCLOPHOSPHAMIDE, AND DOXORUBICIN (HYDROXYLDAUNORUBICIN) (DA-EPOCH)

Wilson WH et al. Blood 2002;99:2685–2693

Etoposide 50 mg/m² per day by continuous intravenous infusion over 24 hours for 4 consecutive days on days 1–4 every 21 days (total dosage/cycle = 200 mg/m²)
Doxorubicin 10 mg/m² per day by continuous intravenous infusion over 24 hours for 4 consecutive days on days 1–4 every 21 days (total dosage/cycle = 40 mg/m²)
Vincristine 0.4 mg/m² per day by continuous intravenous infusion over 24 hours for 4 consecutive days on days 1–4 every 21 days (total dosage/cycle = 1.6 mg/m²)

Intravenous hydration before and after cyclophosphamide administration:

Cyclophosphamide Dosage	Volume of 0.9% NS Before and After Dosage
≤900 mg/m²	500 mL
1080–1555 mg/m²	1000 mL
≥1866 mg/m²	1250 mL

Cyclophosphamide 750 mg/m² intravenously in 100 mL 0.9% NaCl injection (0.9% NS) or 5% dextrose injection (D5W) over 15–30 minutes, given on day 5 after completing etoposide + doxorubicin + vincristine infusion every 21 days (total dosage/cycle = 750 mg/m²)
Prednisone 60 mg/m² twice daily orally for 5 consecutive days on days 1–5 every 21 days (total dosage/cycle = 600 mg/m²)
Filgrastim 5 mcg/kg per day subcutaneously, starting on day 6 and continuing beyond ANC nadir until ANC exceeds 5000 cells/mm³ on one reading
Prednisone is marketed in the United States in numerous solid formulations for oral administration, such as tablets containing 1, 2.5, 5, 10, 20, and 50 mg prednisone and in solutions and syrups

Supportive care:

- Add a **proton pump inhibitor** during prednisone therapy
- **Stool softeners** and/or laxatives during infusional vincristine
- *PCP prophylaxis:* **Cotrimoxazole** (trimethoprim 160 mg + sulfamethoxazole 800 mg) orally twice daily on 3 days per week (eg, Monday, Wednesday, and Friday)

Notes:

- See instructions below for preparing a 3-in-1 admixture with etoposide, doxorubicin, and vincristine
- Etoposide + doxorubicin + vincristine admixtures are administered with an ambulatory (portable) infusion pump through a central venous access device
- Repeated cycles begin on day 22 if the ANC is ≥ 1000/mm³ and the platelet count is ≥ 100,000/mm³

Emetogenic potential:
Days 1–4: Low (Emetogenicity score = 2)
Day 5: Moderately high (Emetogenicity score = 4). See Chapter 39 for antiemetic regimens

(*continued*)

Treatment Modifications

<table>
<tr><th>Events[a]</th><th>Dose Modification[b]</th></tr>
<tr><td>Previous cycle ANC nadir count ≥500/mm³</td><td>Increase etoposide, doxorubicin, and cyclophosphamide dosages by 20% greater than the dosages given during the previous cycle</td></tr>
<tr><td>Previous cycle ANC nadir <500/mm³ on 1 or</td><td>Give the same dosages as last cycle</td></tr>
<tr><td>Previous cycle ANC nadir <500/mm³ on at least</td><td rowspan="2">Reduce etoposide, doxorubicin, and cyclophosphamide dosages by 20% less than the dosages given during the previous cycle</td></tr>
<tr><td>Previous cycle platelet nadir <25,000/mm³</td></tr>
<tr><td>Total bilirubin >4.0 mg/dL (>68.4 μmol/L)</td><td>Hold vincristine[c]</td></tr>
<tr><td>Total bilirubin >3.0 mg/dL, but <4.0 mg/dL (>51.3 μmol/L but <68.4 μmol/L)</td><td>Reduce vincristine dosage by 75%[c]</td></tr>
<tr><td>Total bilirubin >1.5 mg/dL but <3.0 mg/dL (>25.6 μmol/L but <51.3 μmol/L)</td><td>Reduce vincristine dosage by 50%[c]</td></tr>
<tr><td>G2 Neuropathy</td><td>Reduce vincristine dosage by 25%[c]</td></tr>
<tr><td>G3 Neuropathy</td><td>Reduce vincristine dosage by 50%[c]</td></tr>
</table>

[a]ANC and platelet nadir measurements are based on *twice-weekly* CBC with differential only
[b]Dosage adjustments *greater than the starting dose level* apply to only etoposide, doxorubicin, and cyclophosphamide. Dose adjustments *less than the starting dose level* apply to cyclophosphamide only
[c]Vincristine dosage is increased to 100% if neuropathy resolves to G ≤ 1 or bilirubin to <1.5 mg/dL (<88.5 μmol/L)

Patient Population Studied

A study of 50 patients with newly diagnosed diffuse large B-cell lymphoma. All patients were serologically negative for HIV

(continued)

Instructions for preparing a 3-in-1 admixture with etoposide, doxorubicin, and vincristine

Dilute the 3 drugs in 0.9% NS as follows:

Total Dose of Etoposide	Volume of 0.9% NS
≤ 62 mg	250 mL
62.1–125 mg	500 mL
> 125 mg	1000 mL

Etoposide (base) + doxorubicin + vincristine 3-in-1 admixtures:
Etoposide 50 mg/m^2, doxorubicin hydrochloride 10 mg/m^2, and vincristine sulfate 0.4 mg/m^2 admixtures diluted in 0.9% NS to produce a final etoposide concentration <250 mcg/mL in polyolefin-lined infusion bags were stable and compatible for 72 hours at 23°–25°C, and at 31°–33°C when protected from exposure to light

Wolfe JL et al. Am J Health Syst Pharm 1999;56:985–989

Etoposide (PHOSphate) + doxorubicin + vincristine 3-in-1 admixtures:
Etoposide PHOSphate, doxorubicin hydrochloride, and vincristine sulfate admixtures diluted in 0.9% NS to produce a final etoposide concentration <250 mcg/mL in polyolefin-lined infusion bags were stable and compatible for up to 124 hours at 2°–6°C and 35°–40°C in the dark and in regular fluorescent light. In admixtures stored at 35°–40°C and exposed to light, the initial drug concentrations decreased slightly, but remained within acceptable concentrations

Yuan P et al. Am J Health Syst Pharm 2001;58:594–598

The 3-in-1 admixtures described above do not prevent microbial growth after exposure to bacterial and fungal contamination. With respect to product sterility, expiration dating should be determined by the aseptic techniques used in preparation and local and national guidelines

Efficacy

	All Patients	IPI Score Low Risk (0–2)	IPI Score High Risk (3–5)
Response	N = 49	n = 27	n = 22
Complete	45 (92%)	26 (96%)	19 (86%)
Partial	4 (8%)	1 (4%)	3 (14%)
Overall	49 (100%)	27 (100%)	22 (100%)

Toxicity (N = 318 Cycles/50 Patients)

	% Cycles
Hospitalization	
Fever and neutropenia	8
Other reasons	5
Hematologic Toxicity	
ANC <100/mm^3	15
ANC 100–500/mm^3	34
Platelet count <25,000/mm^3	7
Platelet count 26,000–50,000/mm^3	13
Nonhematologic Toxicity: % G ≥ 2	
Nausea or vomiting	6
Stomatitis	12
Constipation	4
Toxicity	**% Patients**
Sensory effects	28
Motor effects	12
Fatigue G ≥ 2	26
Cardiac effects G ≥ 2	0
Treatment-related deaths	0

NCI CTC

Therapy Monitoring

1. *Twice weekly:* CBC with differential
2. *At the beginning of every cycle:* CBC with differential and LFTs

REGIMEN

DOSE-ADJUSTED ETOPOSIDE, PREDNISONE, VINCRISTINE (ONCOVIN®), CYCLOPHOSPHAMIDE, AND DOXORUBICIN (HYDROXYLDAUNORUBICIN) WITH RITUXIMAB (DA-EPOCH WITH RITUXIMAB)

Wilson WH et al. [Abstract #356] Blood 2003;102:105a

Premedication for rituximab:
Acetaminophen 650–1000 mg orally, *plus*
Diphenhydramine 25–50 mg orally or intravenously, 30–60 minutes before starting rituximab
Rituximab 375 mg/m^2 intravenously diluted to a concentration of 1–4 mg/mL in 0.9% NaCl injection (0.9% NS) or 5% dextrose injection (D5W) on day 1 every 21 days (total dosage/cycle = 375 mg/m^2)
Notes on rituximab administration:

- Infuse initially at 50 mg/hour. If hypersensitivity or infusion reactions do not occur during the first 30 minutes, increase the rate by 50 mg/hour every 30 minutes as tolerated, to a maximum rate of 400 mg/hour. Subsequently, if previous administration was well tolerated, start at 100 mg/hour, and increase by 100 mg/hour every 30 minutes as tolerated to a maximum rate of 400 mg/hour
- Interrupt rituximab administration for fever, chills, edema, congestion of the head and neck mucosa, hypotension and other serious adverse events. Resume rituximab administration after adverse events abate

Etoposide 50 mg/m^2 per day by continuous intravenous infusion over 24 hours for 4 consecutive days on days 1–4 every 21 days (total dosage/cycle = 200 mg/m^2)
Doxorubicin 10 mg/m^2 per day by continuous intravenous infusion over 24 hours for 4 consecutive days on days 1–4 every 21 days (total dosage/cycle = 40 mg/m^2)
Vincristine 0.4 mg/m^2 per day by continuous intravenous infusion over 24 hours for 4 consecutive days on days 1–4 every 21 days (total dosage/cycle = 1.6 mg/m^2)

Intravenous hydration before and after cyclophosphamide administration:

Cyclophosphamide Dosage	Volume of 0.9% NS Before and After Dosage
≤900 mg/m^2	500 mL
1080–1555 mg/m^2	1000 mL
≥1866 mg/mv	1250 mL

Cyclophosphamide 750 mg/m^2 intravenously in 100 mL 0.9% NS or D5W over 15–30 minutes, given on day 5 after completing etoposide + doxorubicin + vincristine infusion every 21 days (total dosage/cycle = 750 mg/m^2)
Prednisone 60 mg/m^2 twice daily orally for 5 consecutive days on days 1–5 every 21 days (total dosage/cycle = 600 mg/m^2)
Filgrastim 5 mcg/kg per day subcutaneously, starting on day 6 and continuing until ANC > 5000/mm^3
Prednisone is marketed in the United States in numerous solid formulations for oral administration, such as tablets containing 1, 2.5, 5, 10, 20, and 50 mg prednisone and in solutions and syrups

Supportive care:

- Add a **proton pump inhibitor** during prednisone therapy
- **Stool softeners** and/or laxatives during infusional vincristine
- *PCP prophylaxis:* **Cotrimoxazole** (trimethoprim 160 mg + sulfamethoxazole 800 mg) orally twice daily on 3 days per week (eg, Monday, Wednesday, and Friday)

(*continued*)

Treatment Modifications

Events[a]	Dose Modification[b]
Previous cycle ANC nadir count ≥500/mm^3	Increase etoposide, doxorubicin, and cyclophosphamide dosages by 20% greater than the dosages given during the previous cycle
Previous cycle ANC nadir <500/mm^3 on 1 or 2 measurements	Give the same dosages as last cycle
Previous cycle ANC nadir <500/mm^3 on at least 3 measurements	Reduce etoposide, doxorubicin, and cyclophosphamide dosages by 20% less than the dosages given during the previous cycle
Previous cycle platelet nadir <25,000/mm^3 on 1 measurement	Reduce etoposide, doxorubicin, and cyclophosphamide dosages by 20% less than the dosages given during the previous cycle
Total bilirubin >4.0 mg/dL (>68.4 μmol/L)	Hold vincristine[c]
Total bilirubin >3.0 mg/dL, but <4.0 mg/dL (>51.3 μmol/L but <68.4 μmol/L)	Reduce vincristine dosage by 75%[c]
Total bilirubin >1.5 mg/dL but <3.0 mg/dL (>25.6 μmol/L but <51.3 μmol/L)	Reduce vincristine dosage by 50%[c]
G2 Neuropathy	Reduce vincristine dosage by 25%[c]
G3 Neuropathy	Reduce vincristine dosage by 50%[c]

[a]ANC and platelet nadir measurements are based on *twice-weekly* CBC with differential only
[b]Dosage adjustments *greater than the starting dose level* apply to etoposide, doxorubicin, and cyclophosphamide only. Dose adjustments *less than the starting dose level* apply to cyclophosphamide only
[c]Vincristine dosage is increased to 100% if neuropathy resolves to G ≤ 1 or bilirubin to < 1.5 mg/dL (<88.5 μmol/L)

Rituximab Infusion-Related Toxicities

Onset of infusion-related events (fevers, chills, rigors edema, congestion of the head and neck mucosa, hypotension):

1. Interrupt rituximab infusion
2. For fever, chills: Give additional dose of acetaminophen 650 mg orally and diphenhydramine 25–50 mg by intravenous push

(*continued*)

(*continued*)

Notes:

- See instructions below for preparing a 3-in-1 admixture with etoposide, doxorubicin, and vincristine
- Etoposide + doxorubicin + vincristine admixtures are administered with an ambulatory (portable) infusion pump through a central venous access device
- Repeated cycles begin on day 22 if the ANC is ≥ 1000/mm^3 and the platelet count is ≥100,000/mm^3

Emetogenic potential:
Days 1–4: Low (Emetogenicity score = 2)
Day 5: Moderately high (Emetogenicity score = 4). See Chapter 39 for antiemetic regimens

Instructions for Preparing a 3-in-1 admixture with Etoposide, Doxorubicin, and Vincristine

Dilute the three drugs in 0.9% NS as follows:

Total Dose of Etoposide	Volume of 0.9% NS
≤62 mg	250 mL
62.1–125 mg	500 mL
>125 mg	1000 mL

Etoposide (base) + doxorubicin + vincristine 3-in-1 admixtures:
Etoposide 50 mg/m^2, doxorubicin hydrochloride 10 mg/m^2, and vincristine sulfate 0.4 mg/m^2 admixtures diluted in 0.9% NS to produce a final etoposide concentration <250 mcg/mL in polyolefin-lined infusion bags were stable and compatible for 72 hours at 23°–25°C, and at 31°–33°C when protected from exposure to light

Wolfe JL et al. Am J Health Syst Pharm 1999;56:985–989

Etoposide (PHOSphate) + doxorubicin + vincristine 3-in-1 admixtures:
Etoposide PHOSphate, doxorubicin hydrochloride, and vincristine sulfate admixtures diluted in 0.9% NS to produce a final etoposide concentration < 250 mcg/mL in polyolefin-lined infusion bags were stable and compatible for up to 124 hours at 2°–6°C and 35°–40°C in the dark and in regular fluorescent light. In admixtures stored at 35°–40°C and exposed to light, the initial drug concentrations decreased slightly, but remained within acceptable concentrations

Yuan P et al. Am J Health Syst Pharm 2001;58:594–598

The 3-in-1 admixtures described above do not prevent microbial growth after exposure to bacterial and fungal contamination. With respect to product sterility, expiration dating should be determined by the aseptic techniques used in preparation and local and national guidelines

Efficacy (N = 69)

	% Complete Response	% Progressive Disease	% Overall Response
All patients	92	5	95
Low risk IPI	100	0	100
High risk IPI	77	9	86

Treatment Modifications (*continued*)

3. For rigors: Give meperidine 12.5–25 mg by intravenous push ± promethazine 12.5–25 mg by intravenous infusion in at least 10 mL 0.9% NS or D5W over 5–15 minutes. If after 15–20 minutes the response to a single dose is considered inadequate, the dose may be repeated
4. After symptoms resolve, resume rituximab infusion at 50 mg/hour and increase by 50 mg/hour every 30 minutes as tolerated up to a maximum rate of 200 mg/hour

Dyspnea or wheezing, without allergic findings (urticaria, or tongue or laryngeal edema):

1. Interrupt rituximab infusion immediately
2. Give hydrocortisone 100 mg by intravenous push (or glucocorticoid equivalent)
3. Give a histamine H_2 antagonist (ranitidine 150 mg, cimetidine 300 mg, or famotidine 20 mg) by intravenous push
4. After symptoms resolve, resume rituximab infusion at 25 mg/hour with close monitoring. Do not increase rate

Note: Medications for the treatment of hypersensitivity reactions should be available for immediate use in the event of a reaction during administration (eg, intravenous fluids, epinephrine, antihistamines, glucocorticoids, and O_2)

Patient Population Studied

A study of 69 patients with newly diagnosed diffuse large B-cell lymphoma. All patients were serologically negative for HIV

Toxicity (N = 380 Cycles/69 Patients)

	Incidence
Platelets[a] <25,000/mm^3	9%
ANC[a] <500/mm^3	60%
Fever/neutropenia[a]	16%
GI toxicity > G2[a]	4%
Neurologic toxicity > G2[b]	11%
Treatment-related deaths[b]	3%

[a]Based on 380 total cycles
[b]Based on 69 total patients

NCI CTC

Therapy Monitoring

1. *Twice weekly:* CBC with differential
2. *At the beginning of every cycle:* CBC with differential and LFTs

REGIMEN

CYCLOPHOSPHAMIDE, MITOXANTRONE (NOVATRONE®), VINCRISTINE (ONCOVIN®), PREDNISONE (CNOP)

Pavlovsky S et al. Ann Oncol 1992;3:205–209

Intravenous hydration before and after cyclophosphamide administration:
500–1000 mL 0.9% NaCl injection (0.9% NS)

Cyclophosphamide 750 mg/m^2 intravenously in 25–250 mL 0.9% NS or 5% dextrose injection (D5W) over 10–30 minutes, given on day 1 every 21 days (total dosage/cycle = 750 mg/m^2)
Mitoxantrone 10 mg/m^2 intravenously in 25–250 mL 0.9% NS or D5W over 10–30 minutes, given on day 1 every 21 days (total dosage/cycle = 10 mg/m^2)
Vincristine 1.4 mg/m^2 (maximum dose = 2 mg) by intravenous push over 1–3 minutes, given on day 1 every 21 days (total dosage/cycle=1.4 mg/m^2; maximum dose/cycle = 2 mg)
Prednisone 50 mg/m^2 per day orally for 5 consecutive days on days 1–5 (total dosage/cycle=250 mg/m^2)
Prednisone is marketed in the United States in numerous solid formulations for oral administration, such as tablets containing 1, 2.5, 5, 10, 20, and 50 mg prednisone and in solutions and syrups

Supportive care:
Add a **proton pump inhibitor** during prednisone therapy

Emetogenic potential: Moderately high (Emetogenicity score = 4). See Chapter 39 for antiemetic regimens

Treatment Modifications

Adverse Event	Dose Modification
G4 ANC or febrile neutropenia during any cycle of chemotherapy	Administer secondary prophylaxis with filgrastim in subsequent cycles*
G4 Neutropenia during cycle in which filgrastim is given	Reduce mitoxantrone and cyclophosphamide dosages by 50%
G3/4 Thrombocytopenia	
Day 1 ANC <1500/mm^3 or platelets < 100,000/mm^3	Delayed treatment for up to 2 weeks
ANC < 1500/mm^3 or platelets <100,000/mm^3 >2-week treatment delay	Discontinue therapy

*__Filgrastim__ 5 mcg/kg per day subcutaneously, starting on day 2 and continuing beyond ANC nadir until ANC exceeds 5000/mm^3 on one reading

Patient Population Studied

Randomized, multicenter, phase III study comparing the efficacy and toxicity of CNOP with CHOP (cyclophosphamide, doxorubicin, vincristine, prednisone) in patients with intermediate and high-grade non-Hodgkin's lymphoma. Forty-five patients received CNOP and 44 patients received CHOP

Efficacy (N = 45)

Complete response	51%
Partial response	18%
Stable/progressive disease	24%
Death	7%

Toxicity (N = 45)

	% G1	% G2	% G3	% G4
Stomatitis	13.3	4.4	2.2	—
Nausea or vomiting	20	40	15.5	—
Alopecia	55.5	8.8	24.4	—
Cardiac	4.4	—	—	2.2
Infection	17.7	28.8	—	—
Renal	—	—	—	—
Neurologic	37.7	15.5	6.6	—
Diarrhea	11.1	11.1	2.2	—
Allergic	—	—	—	—
Cutaneous	15.5	6.6	2.2	—
Lung	6.6	2.2	—	—

Therapy Monitoring

1. *Weekly:* CBC with differential
2. *Before therapy on all cycles:* Serum BUN, creatinine, LFTs, and PE

Notes

The authors concluded that CHOP and CNOP have similar toxicities and are equivalent in previously untreated non-Hodgkin's lymphoma in terms of complete response rate, event-free survival and overall survival

REGIMEN

METHOTREXATE, CYTARABINE(ARA-C), CYCLOPHOSPHAMIDE, VINCRISTINE (ONCOVIN®), PREDNISONE, BLEOMYCIN (MACOP-B)

Klimo P, Connors JM. Ann Intern Med 1985;102:596–602

Odd-Numbered Weeks: 1, 3, 5, 7, 9, and 11

Doxorubicin 50 mg/m^2 per dose by intravenous push over 3–5 minutes for 6 doses on day 1 during weeks 1, 3, 5, 7, 9, and 11 (total dosage/12-week course = 300 mg/m^2)

Oral hydration before and after cyclophosphamide administration:
32–64 oz/day on the day cyclophosphamide is administered and for at least 1 day afterward

or

Intravenous hydration before and after cyclophosphamide administration:
500–1000 mL 0.9% NaCl injection (0.9% NS)

Cyclophosphamide 350 mg/m^2 per dose by intravenous infusion in 25–250 mL 0.9% NS or 5% dextrose injection (D5W) over 10–30 minutes for 6 doses on day 1 during weeks 1, 3, 5, 7, 9, and 11 (total dosage/12-week course = 2100 mg/m^2)

Even-Numbered Weeks: 2, 4, 6, 8, 10, and 12

Oral hydration with methotrexate:
100–128 oz/day

or

Intravenous hydration with methotrexate:
100–150 mL/hour 0.9% NS, D5W or 5% dextrose/0.45% NaCl (D5W/0.95% NS) injection, before, during, and after intravenous methotrexate administration

Sodium bicarbonate 500–2000 mg (sufficient to increase urine pH to 7.0) orally every 6 hours for 48–60 hours, starting 8–12 hours before starting methotrexate administration

Notes:

- Sodium bicarbonate may be administered parenterally to patients who require intravenous hydration (50–100 mEq sodium bicarbonate/1000 mL of parenteral fluid)
- In patients with measurable serum or plasma methotrexate concentrations ≥ 48 hours after methotrexate administration is completed, continue sodium bicarbonate administration and vigorous oral or parenteral hydration until methotrexate is no longer detectable

Methotrexate 100 mg/m^2 per dose by intravenous infusion in 10–50 mL 0.9% NS or D5W over 5–15 minutes or by intravenous push over 0.5–2 minutes, on day 1, *followed by*
Methotrexate 300 mg/m^2 per dose by intravenous infusion in 50–1000 mL 0.9% NS or D5W over 4 hours for 3 doses on day 1 during weeks 2, 6, and 10 (total intravenously-administered dosage/12-week course = 1300 mg/m^2)

Leucovorin rescue:
Leucovorin calcium 15 mg/dose orally every 6 hours for 6 doses, starting 28 hours after starting methotrexate during weeks 2, 6, and 10 (total dose during each week intravenous methotrexate is given = 90 mg)

Note: For patients with mucositis that precedes methotrexate administration and for those who develop mucositis during methotrexate or leucovorin administration, increase the total number of leucovorin doses from 6 to 12 doses

Vincristine 1.4 mg/m^2 per dose (maximum single dose = 2 mg) by intravenous push over 1–3 minutes for 6 doses on day 1 during weeks 2, 4, 6, 8, 10, and 12 (total dosage/12-week course = 8.4 mg/m^2; maximum dose/12-week course = 12 mg)

Bleomycin 10 units/m^2 per dose by intravenous push over 1–3 minutes for 3 doses on day 1 during weeks 4, 8, and 12 (total dosage/12-week course = 30 Units/m^2)

Prednisone 75 mg/day orally for 69 consecutive days, then taper the daily dose during the last 15 days of treatment (days 70–84)

(*continued*)

Treatment Modifications

Adverse Event	Dose Modification
ANC ≥ 1000/mm^3 on a day of treatment	Administer 100% of planned chemotherapy doses
ANC 100–999/mm^3 on a day of treatment	Administer 65% of planned chemotherapy doses
ANC < 100/mm^3 on a day of treatment	Delay treatment for 1 week
Thrombocytopenia (any severity)	Do not modify treatment, but give platelet transfusions for platelet count <10,000/mm^3
Creatinine clearance <60 mL/min (1.00 mL/s)	Give bleomycin 10 units/m^2 instead of methotrexate on weeks 2, 6, and 10*

*If low creatinine clearance is due to lymphoma and improves during treatment, reintroduce methotrexate

Patient Population Studied

A study of 61 patients with advanced newly diagnosed diffuse large B-cell lymphoma

Efficacy (N = 61)

Complete response	84%
Partial response	16%

(continued)

Leucovorin calcium is manufactured in the United States in tablets for oral administration containing 5, 15, or 25 mg leucovorin calcium
Prednisone is marketed in the United States in numerous solid formulations for oral administration, such as tablets containing 1, 2.5, 5, 10, 20, and 50 mg prednisone and in solutions and syrups

CNS prophylaxis:
For all patients with lymphoma involving bone marrow, starting after documented remission in bone marrow
Methotrexate 12 mg intrathecally via lumbar puncture twice weekly for 6 doses (total dose/week = 24 mg)
Cytarabine 30 mg/m^2 intrathecally via lumbar puncture twice weekly for 6 doses (total dose/week = 60 mg/m^2)

Supportive care:
- Add a **proton pump inhibitor** during prednisone therapy
- Primary prophylaxis with **stool softeners and/or laxatives** for vincristine-related constipation
- *PCP prophylaxis:* **Cotrimoxazole** (trimethoprim 160 mg + sulfamethoxazole 800 mg) orally twice daily on 3 days per week (eg, Monday, Wednesday, and Friday)

Emetogenic potential:
Cyclophosphamide + doxorubicin (weeks 1, 3, 5, 7, 9, and 11): Moderately high (Emetogenicity score = 4)
Methotrexate + vincristine (weeks 2, 6, and 10): Moderately high (Emetogenicity score = 4)
Vincristine + bleomycin (weeks 4, 8, and 12): Nonemetogenic (Emetogenicity score = 1)
Intrathecal methotrexate: Low (Emetogenicity score = 2). See Chapter 39 for antiemetic regimens

Toxicity (N = 61)

	% G1/2	% G3/4
Mucositis	56	26
Neurologic	92	8
Cutaneous	39	3
Hematologic		
Granulocytopenia (<500/mm^3)		21
Thrombocytopenia (<50,000/mm^3)		2
Anemia requiring red cell transfusion		20
Infection requiring hospitalization		11
Infection not requiring hospitalization		11
Endocrinologic		
Transient symptomatic hyperglycemia		3
Femoral osteonecrosis		2
Other Toxicities		
Disabling weakness		8
Hand and feet dermal blistering		
Overall		39
Severe		3

Therapy Monitoring

1. *Weekly:* CBC with differential, LFTs, serum BUN, and creatinine
2. *Daily following systemic methotrexate administration:* Methotrexate levels

REGIMEN

ETOPOSIDE, PREDNISONE, VINCRISTINE (ONCOVIN®), CYCLOPHOSPHAMIDE, AND DOXORUBICIN (HYDROXYLDAUNORUBICIN) (EPOCH)

Gutierrez M et al. JCO 2000;18:3633–3642

Etoposide 50 mg/m^2 per day by continuous intravenous infusion over 24 hours for 4 consecutive days on days 1–4 every 21 days (total dosage/cycle = 200 mg/m^2)
Doxorubicin 10 mg/m^2 per day by continuous intravenous infusion over 24 hours for 4 consecutive days on days 1–4 every 21 days (total dosage/cycle = 40 mg/m^2)
Vincristine 0.4 mg/m^2 per day by continuous intravenous infusion over 24 hours for 4 consecutive days on days 1–4 every 21 days (total dosage/cycle = 1.6 mg/m^2)

Intravenous hydration before and after cyclophosphamide administration:

Cyclophosphamide Dosage	Volume of 0.9% NS Before and After Dosage
≤900 mg/m^2	500 mL
1080–1555 mg/m^2	1000 mL
≥1866 mg/m^2	1250 mL

Cyclophosphamide 750 mg/m^2 intravenously in 100 mL 0.9% NaCl injection (0.9% NS) or 5% dextrose injection (D5W) over 15–30 minutes, given on day 5 after completing etoposide + doxorubicin + vincristine infusion every 21 days (total dosage/cycle = 750 mg/m^2)
Prednisone 60 mg/m^2 twice daily orally for 5 consecutive days on days 1–5 every 21 days (total dosage/cycle = 600 mg/m^2)
Filgrastim 5 mcg/kg per day subcutaneously starting on day 6 and continuing beyond ANC nadir until ANC exceeds 5000/mm^3 on one reading.

Supportive care
- Add a **proton pump inhibitor** during prednisone therapy
- **Stool softeners** and/or laxatives during infusional vincristine
- *PCP prophylaxis:* **Cotrimoxazole** (trimethoprim 160 mg + sulfamethoxazole 800 mg) orally twice daily on 3 days per week (eg, Monday, Wednesday, and Friday)

Notes:
- See instructions below for preparing a 3-in-1 admixture with etoposide, doxorubicin, and vincristine
- Etoposide + doxorubicin + vincristine admixtures are administered with an ambulatory (portable) infusion pump through a central venous access device
- Repeated cycles begin on day 22 if the ANC is ≥ 1000/mm^3 and the platelet count is ≥100,000/mm^3

Prednisone is marketed in the United States in numerous solid formulations for oral administration, such as tablets containing 1, 2.5, 5, 10, 20, and 50 mg prednisone and in solutions and syrups

Emetogenic potential:
Days 1–4: Low (Emetogenicity score = 2)
Day 5: Moderately high (Emetogenicity score = 4). See Chapter 39 for antiemetic regimens

(*continued*)

Treatment Modifications

Adverse Event[a]	Dose Modification
Day 1 ANC <1000/mm^3	Hold therapy until ANC > 1000/mm^3
Previous cycle ANC nadir count < 500/mm^3	Decrease cyclophosphamide dosage by 25% during the subsequent cycle
Previous cycle platelet nadir count <25,000/mm^3	Decrease cyclophosphamide dosage by 25% during the subsequent cycle
Previous cycle ANC nadir count >500/mm^3	Increase cyclophosphamide dosage by 25% to a maximum of 750 mg/m^2
G2 Neuropathy	Reduce vincristine dosage by 25%[b]
G3 Neuropathy	Reduce vincristine dosage by 50%[b]

[a]ANC and platelet nadir measurements are based on *twice-weekly* CBC with differential
[b]Vincristine dosage is increased to 100% if neuropathy resolves to G ≤ 1

Patient Population Studied

A study of 131 patients with relapsed or refractory NHL. All patients were serologically negative for HIV

Efficacy (N = 125)

Objective response	74%
Complete response	24%
Partial response	50%

(continued)

Instructions for Preparing a 3-in-1 Admixture with Etoposide, Doxorubicin, and Vincristine

Dilute the three drugs in 0.9% NS as follows:

Total Dose of Etoposide	Volume of 0.9% NS
≤62 mg	250 mL
62.1–125 mg	500 mL
>125 mg	1000 mL

Etoposide (base) + doxorubicin + vincristine 3-in-1 admixtures:
Etoposide 50 mg/m^2, doxorubicin hydrochloride 10 mg/m^2, and vincristine sulfate 0.4 mg/m^2 admixtures diluted in 0.9% NS to produce a final etoposide concentration <250 mcg/mL in polyolefin-lined infusion bags were stable and compatible for 72 hours at 23°–25°C, and at 31°–33°C when protected from exposure to light

Wolfe JL et al. Am J Health Syst Pharm 1999;56:985–989

Etoposide (PHOSphate) + doxorubicin + vincristine 3-in-1 admixtures:
Etoposide PHOSphate, doxorubicin hydrochloride, and vincristine sulfate admixtures diluted in 0.9% NS to produce a final etoposide concentration <250 mcg/mL in polyolefin-lined infusion bags were stable and compatible for up to 124 hours at 2°–6°C and 35°–40°C in the dark and in regular fluorescent light. In admixtures stored at 35°–40°C and exposed to light, the initial drug concentrations decreased slightly, but remained within acceptable concentrations

Yuan P et al. Am J Health Syst Pharm 2001;58:594–598

The 3-in-1 admixtures described above do not prevent microbial growth after exposure to bacterial and fungal contamination. With respect to product sterility, expiration dating should be determined by the aseptic techniques used in preparation and local and national guidelines

Toxicity (N = 535 Cycles/131 Patients)

	% of Cycles
Hematologic	
ANC <100/mm^3	18
ANC 100–500/mm^3	30
Platelet count <50,000/mm^3	24
Hospitalizations	
For fever/neutropenia	18
For other reasons	10
Nonhematologic	
G ≥ 2 Nausea or vomiting	5
G ≥ 2 Stomatitis	7
G ≥ 2 Constipation	2
	% of Patients
Neurologic toxicity	22
Cardiac adverse events	3
Treatment-related deaths	0

Therapy Monitoring

1. *Twice weekly*: CBC with differential
2. *At the beginning of every cycle:* CBC with differential, LFTs and PE

REGIMEN

ETOPOSIDE, METHYLPREDNISOLONE (SOLU-MEDROL), CYTARABINE (ARA-C), CISPLATIN (ESHAP)

Sweetenham JW, Johnson PWM. [Comment] JCO 1994;12:2766
Velasquez WS et al. JCO 1994;12:1169–1176

Hydration:
≥1000 mL 0.9% NaCl injection (0.9% NS) + 25–50 g mannitol daily intravenously, continuously throughout chemotherapy administration or longer if medically appropriate every 21–28 days for 6–8 cycles. Monitor and replace magnesium/electrolytes as needed
Cisplatin 25 mg/m^2 per day by continuous intravenous infusion in 100 mL to >1000 mL 0.9% NS over 24 hours for 4 consecutive days on days 1–4 every 21–28 days for 6–8 cycles (total dosage/cycle = 100 mg/m^2)
Etoposide 40 mg/m^2 per day by intravenous infusion, diluted in 0.9% NS to a concentration of 0.2–0.4 mg/mL over 1 hour for 4 consecutive days on days 1–4 every 21–28 days for 6–8 cycles (total dosage/cycle = 160 mg/m^2)
Methylprednisolone 250–500 mg/m^2 per day by intravenous infusion in 25–500 mL 0.9% NS over 15 minutes for 5 consecutive days on days 1–5 every 21–28 days for 6–8 cycles (total dosage/cycle = 1250–2500 mg/m^2)
Cytarabine 2000 mg/m^2 by intravenous infusion in 25–1000 mL 0.9% NS or 5% dextrose injection (D5W) over 2 hours on day 5 every 21–28 days for 6–8 cycles (total dosage/cycle = 2000 mg/m^2)

Supportive care:
Add a **proton pump inhibitor** during methylprednisolone therapy

Emetogenic potential:
Days 1–4: High (Emetogenicity score = 5)
Day 5: Moderately high (Emetogenicity score = 4). See Chapter 39 for antiemetic regimens

Patient Population Studied

A study of 122 patients with relapsed or refractory NHL

Efficacy (N = 122)

Complete response	37%
Partial response	27%
Overall response rate	64%

Toxicity (N = 122)

Median ANC nadir	500/mm^3
Median platelet nadir	70,000/mm^3
G1/2 Nausea/vomiting	49%
G3 Nausea/vomiting	6%
>2-fold increase in creatinine from baseline measurement	
Reversible	18%
Permanent	4%
Fever and neutropenia	30%
Treatment related death	5%

Treatment Modifications

Adverse Event*	Dose Modification
Previous cycle ANC nadir ≤ 200/mm^3	Reduce etoposide dosage by 20% and reduce cytarabine dosage by 50% during subsequent cycles
Previous cycle platelet count nadir ≤20,000/mm^3	
Documented sepsis during previous cycles	
Nonhematologic adverse events G3/4 in previous cycles	
Serum creatinine 1.5–2.0 mg/dL (133–177 μmol/L) immediately prior to a cycle	Reduce cisplatin dosage by 25% during subsequent cycles
Serum creatinine 2.1–3.0 mg/dL (186–265 μmol/L) immediately prior to a cycle	Reduce cisplatin dosage by 50% during subsequent cycles
Serum creatinine >3.0 mg/dL (>265 μmol/L) immediately before a cycle	Hold cisplatin

*For neutropenia consider Filgrastim 5 mcg/kg per day subcutaneously, starting on day 6 and continuing beyond ANC nadir until ANC exceeds 5000/mm3 on one reading

Therapy Monitoring

1. *Before each cycle:* PE, CBC with differential, serum electrolytes, BUN, creatinine and LFTs
2. *Daily on days of drug administration:* Serum electrolytes, magnesium, calcium and phosphorus. Cardiac, pulmonary, and renal status should be carefully monitored during administration of fluids
3. *Weekly:* CBC with differential

REGIMEN

DEXAMETHASONE, CYTARABINE (HIGH-DOSE ARA-C), CISPLATIN (DHAP)

Velasquez WS et al. Blood 1988;71:117–122

Hydration:
0.9% NaCl injection (0.9% NS) + 50 g mannitol/1000 mL at a rate of 250 mL/hour for 36 hours intravenously beginning at least 6 hours before starting cisplatin administration every 3–4 weeks for 6–10 cycles. Monitor and replace magnesium/electrolytes as needed
Cisplatin 100 mg/m^2 by continuous intravenous infusion over 24 hours in a volume equivalent to the dose, or diluted in 100 mL to ≥1000 mL 0.9% NS. Begin administration on day 1 after completing 6 hours of hydration every 3–4 weeks for 6–10 cycles (total dosage/cycle = 100 mg/m^2)
Cytarabine
Patients ≤ 70 years: **Cytarabine** 2000 mg/m^2 per dose by intravenous infusion over 3 hours in 50–500 mL 0.9% NS or 5% dextrose injection (D5W) every 12 hours for 2 doses, starting after the completion of cisplatin administration on day 2 every 3–4 weeks for 6–10 cycles (total dosage/cycle = 4000 mg/m^2)
Patients > 70 years: **Cytarabine** 1000 mg/m^2 per dose by intravenous infusion over 3 hours in 50–500 mL 0.9% NS or D5W every 12 hours for 2 doses, starting after the completion of cisplatin administration on day 2 every 3–4 weeks for 6–10 cycles (total dosage/cycle = 2000 mg/m^2)
Dexamethasone 40 mg/day orally or by intravenous infusion in 10–100 mL 0.9% NS or D5W over 10–30 minutes for 4 consecutive days on days 1–4 every 3–4 weeks for 6–10 cycles (total dosage/cycle = 160 mg)
Dexamethasone is marketed in the United States in numerous formulations for oral administration, such as 0.25-, 0.5-, 0.75-, 1-, 2-, 4-, and 6-mg tablets and in elixirs (which contain alcohol) and solutions

Supportive care:
Add a **proton pump inhibitor** during dexamethasone therapy

Emetogenic potential:
Day 1: High (Emetogenicity score = 5)
Day 2: Moderately high (Emetogenicity score = 4). See Chapter 39 for antiemetic regimens

Treatment Modifications

Adverse Event*	Dose Modification
ANC < 200/mm^3 during any cycle	Reduce cytarabine dosage to 1000 mg/m^2 per dose; maintain cisplatin dosage at 100 mg/m^2
Platelet count <20,000/mm^3 during any cycle	
Sepsis associated with neutropenia during any cycle	Reduce cytarabine dosage to 500 mg/m^2 per dose; maintain cisplatin dosage at 100 mg/m^2
Serum creatinine increase to 1.5–2.0 mg/mL (133–177 μmol/L)	Reduce cisplatin dosage to 75 mg/m^2
Serum creatinine increase to 2.1–3.0 mg/mL (186–265 μmol/L)	Reduce cisplatin dosage to 50 mg/m^2

*For neutropenia consider Filgrastim 5 mcg/kg per day subcutaneously, starting on day 6 and continuing beyond ANC nadir until ANC exceeds 5000/mm3 on one reading

Patient Population Studied

A study pf 90 patients with recurrent or refractory NHL

Efficacy (N = 90)

Complete response	31%
Partial response	24%
Overall response rate	55%
2 year survival	25%

Toxicity (N = 90)

	% of Patients
ANC nadir <300/mm^3	53
Platelet count nadir <20,000/mm^3	39
Gastrointestinal (severe)	20
Acute cerebellar syndrome	1
Acute tumor lysis syndrome	6
Early deaths	
Due to tumor lysis syndrome	3
Due to sepsis	2
Due to thromboembolism	1
Due to subdural hemorrhage	1
Reversible ↑ serum creatinine to >2 × baseline	16
Permanent ↑ serum creatinine to >2 × baseline	4
Chronic polyneuritis	4
Tinnitus	4
Severe hearing loss	3
Respiratory failure	6
Hospitalization for IV antibiotics	48
Documented sepsis	31
Death due to complications of sepsis	11

Therapy Monitoring

1. *Before each cycle:* PE, CBC with differential, serum electrolytes, BUN, creatinine, LFTs
2. *Daily on days of drug administration:* Serum electrolytes. Cardiac, pulmonary, and renal status are carefully monitored during administration of fluids
3. *Weekly:* CBC with differential

REGIMEN

IFOSFAMIDE/CARBOPLATIN/ETOPOSIDE (ICE)

Moskowitz CH et al. JCO 1999;17:3776–3785

Etoposide 100 mg/m^2 per day by intravenous infusion diluted in 0.9% NaCl injection (0.9% NS) to a concentration of 0.2–0.4 mg/mL over 1 hour for 3 consecutive days on days 1–3 every 2 weeks (total dosage/cycle = 300 mg/m^2)
Carboplatin [calculated dose] AUC = 5[a] (maximum absolute dose/cycle = 800 mg) by intravenous infusion in 100–500 mL 5% dextrose injection (D5W) or 0.9% NS over 15–30 minutes, given on day 2 every 2 weeks (total dosage/cycle calculated to produce an AUC = 5 mg/mL·min; maximum absolute dose/cycle = 800 mg)
Ifosfamide 5000 mg/m^2 with **mesna** 5000 mg/m^2 by continuous intravenous infusion diluted in 0.9% NS or D5W to a concentration of 0.6–20 mg/mL over 24 hours on day 2 every 2 weeks (total ifosfamide and mesna dosages/cycle = 5000 mg/m^2)
Note: Ifosfamide and mesna may be administered separately or may be combined in a single container
Filgrastim 5 mcg/kg per day subcutaneously for 8 consecutive days on days 5–12

[a]Carboplatin dose is derived from a formula described by Calvert et al. as a function of a targeted area under the plasma concentration versus time curve (AUC) and estimates of renal and nonrenal drug clearance:

$$\text{Total carboplatin dose (mg)} = (\text{target AUC}) \times (\text{GFR} + 25)$$

In application, creatinine clearance (Clcr) is used in place of glomerular filtration rate (GFR). Clcr can be calculated from the equation of Cockcroft and Gault, thus:

$$\text{Males, Clcr} = \frac{(140 - \text{age [y]}) \times \text{body weight [kg]}}{72 \times (\text{Serum creatinine [mg/dL]})}$$

$$\text{Females, Clcr} = \frac{(140 - \text{age [y]}) \times \text{body weight [kg]}}{72 \times (\text{Serum creatinine [mg/dL]})} \times 0.85$$

Calvert AH et al. JCO 1989;7:1748–1756
Cockcroft DW, Gault MH. Nephron 1976;16:31–41
Jodrell DI et al. JCO 1992;10:520–528
Sorensen BT et al. Cancer Chemother Pharmacol 1991;28:397–401

Emetogenic potential:
Days 1 and 3: Low (Emetogenicity score = 2)
Day 2: Very high (Emetogenicity score = 6). See Chapter 39 for antiemetic regimens

Patient Population Studied

A study of 163 patients with relapsed or primary refractory NHL. All patients in this study were eligible for autologous transplantation and proceeded to transplantation if they achieved a PR or CR

Efficacy (N = 163 patients)

Complete response	24%
Partial response	42.3%
Overall response rate	66.3%

Treatment Modifications

Adverse Event	Dose Modification
ANC <1000/mm^3 and platelet count <50,000/mm^3.	Delay start of treatment until ANC is >1000/mm^3 and platelet count is > 50,000/mm^3

Toxicity (N = 163 Patients; 381 Cycles)

	% of Cycles
G3/4 Thrombocytopenia	29.4
G4 Neutropenia with hospitalization	12.9
Gross hematuria*	1
	% of Patients
Neurologic toxicity	3
Cardiac toxicity	1

*Seen in 4 cycles. Self-limiting. All patients received additional cycles without incident

Therapy Monitoring

Before each cycle: CBC with differential, serum BUN, and creatinine

Notes

1. Used for cytoreduction and stem-cell mobilization in transplant-eligible patients. There were no dose reductions. Sixty six of 381 cycles were delayed because of hematologic toxicity
2. Four patients developed confusion that resolved without intervention. These patients were not re-treated.

REGIMEN

CYCLOPHOSPHAMIDE, VINCRISTINE, PREDNISONE (CVP)

Bagley CM Jr et al. Ann Intern Med 1972;76:227–234
Flinn IW et al. Ann Oncol 2000;11:691–695

Cyclophosphamide 400 mg/m² per day orally for 5 consecutive days on days 1–5 every 3 weeks for at least 4 cycles + 2 additional cycles after complete response (total dosage/cycle = 2000 mg/m²)

or

Cyclophosphamide 1000 mg/m² by intravenous infusion as either undiluted cyclophosphamide (20 mg/mL) or diluted in 150–1000 mL 0.9% NaCl injection (0.9% NS) or 5% dextrose injection (D5W) over 15–60 minutes, given on day 1 every 3 weeks for at least 4 cycles + 2 additional cycles after complete response (total dosage/cycle = 1000 mg/m²)
Vincristine 1.4 mg/m² by intravenous push over 1–3 minutes, given on day 1 every 3 weeks for at least 4 cycles + 2 additional cycles after complete response (total dosage/cycle = 1.4 mg/m²)
Prednisone 100 mg/m² per day orally for 5 consecutive days on days 1–5 every 3 weeks for at least 4 cycles + 2 additional cycles after complete response (total dosage/cycle = 500 mg/m²)

Cyclophosphamide is manufactured in the United States in tablets for oral administration containing cyclophosphamide 25 mg and 50 mg
Prednisone is marketed in the United States in numerous solid formulations for oral administration, such as tablets containing 1, 2.5, 5, 10, 20, and 50 mg prednisone, and in solutions and syrups

Emetogenic potential:
Days 1–5 (with orally administered cyclophosphamide): Moderate (Emetogenicity score = 3)
Day 1 (with intravenously administered cyclophosphamide: Moderately high (Emetogenicity score = 4). See Chapter 39 for antiemetic regimens

Treatment Modifications

At the start of a treatment cycle:

		% of Planned Dosages		
ANC	Platelet Count	C	V	P
> 4000/mm³	≥100,000/mm³	100	100	100
3–4000/mm³	50–100,000/mm³	75	100	100
2–3000/mm³	50–100,000/mm³	50	100	100
1–2000/mm³	<50,000/mm³	25	50	100
0–1000/mm³	<50,000/mm³	0	0	0

Note: Repeated cycles may be delayed for up to 1 week for incomplete hematologic recovery (ie, day 1 ANC must be > 1000/mm³ from prior treatment)

C, cyclophosphamide; V, vincristine; P, prednisone

Patient Population Studied

A study of 35 patients with advanced NHL, among whom 32 previously had not received antineoplastic therapy

Efficacy (N = 35)

Complete response	57%
Partial response	34%
Overall response rate	91%

Toxicity (N = 35)

Severe infections	14%
Mild cystitis without bleeding	8.6%

Hematologic Nadirs During 6 Consecutive Cycles

Cycle	WBC Count	Platelet Count
1	2400/mm³	220,000/mm³
2	2300/mm³	204,000/mm³
3	3100/mm³	192,000/mm³
4	2000/mm³	200,000/mm³
5	3200/mm³	224,000/mm³
6	2800/mm³	213,000/mm³

Therapy Monitoring

1. *Prior to each cycle:* PE, CBC, differential, LFTs, serum BUN and creatinine
2. *Weekly:* CBC with differential and LFTs

REGIMEN

FLUDARABINE

Solal-Céligny P et al. JCO 1996;14:514–519

Prophylaxis against tumor lysis:
See also Chapter 39
Allopurinol 300 mg per day orally for 9 consecutive days, beginning the day before fludarabine treatment starts. Repeat a course of prophylaxis during at least the first 2 treatment cycles and for additional cycles if judged appropriate

Fludarabine 25 mg/m^2 per day by intravenous infusion in 100–125 mL 0.9% NaCl injection (0.9% NS) or 5% dextrose injection (D5W) over 30 minutes for 5 consecutive days on days 1–5 every 4 weeks for up to 9 cycles (total dosage/cycle = 125 mg/m^2)
Note: The maximum planned treatment duration is 9 cycles. Treatment is discontinued in the event of disease progression or after 6 cycles for patients who achieve a CR after 3 cycles and for those whose disease does not respond during the first 6 cycles

Allopurinol is manufactured in the United States in tablets for oral administration containing either allopurinol 100 mg or 300 mg, and as an injectable product, Aloprim® (allopurinol sodium) for injection (Nabi®, Boca Raton, FL)

Emetogenic potential: Nonemetogenic (Emetogenicity score = 1). See Chapter 39 for antiemetic regimens

Treatment Modifications

Adverse Event	Dose Modification
ANC <1500/mm^3 or platelet count <100,000/mm^3	Delay treatment until ANC is ≥ 1500/mm^3, and platelet count ≥100,000/mm^3 then resume treatment but reduce fludarabine dosage to 20 mg/m^2 per day for 5 days
Treatment delay >2 weeks	Discontinue fludarabine treatment

Therapy Monitoring

Before each cycle: CBC with differential, LFTs, serum BUN, and creatinine

Patient Population Studied

A study of 54 untreated patients with advanced follicular lymphoma. All patients were serologically negative for HIV

Efficacy (N = 49)

Overall response	65%
Complete response	37%
Partial response	28%

Toxicity (N = 53 Patients; 336 Cycles)

Toxicity	% of Patients	% of Cycles
G ≥ 3 Neutropenia	41	14.4
G ≥ 3 Thrombocytopenia	5.7	1.2
Toxicity	**% of Patients**	
G1 Infections	15	
G2 Infections	9	
G ≥ 3 Infections	0	
Neurologic toxicity	3.8	
Interstitial pneumonitis	1.9	
Hepatitis	1.9	

WHO Criteria

REGIMEN

RITUXIMAB

Davis TA et al. JCO 1999;17:1851–1857

Premedication for rituximab:
Acetaminophen 650–1000 mg orally, *plus*
Diphenhydramine 25–50 mg orally or intravenously 30–60 minutes before starting rituximab

Rituximab 375 mg/m^2 intravenously diluted to a concentration of 1–4 mg/mL in 0.9% NaCl injection or 5% dextrose injection, weekly for 4 consecutive weeks (days 1, 8, 15, and 22) (total dosage/course = 1500 mg/m^2)

Notes on rituximab administration:

- Infuse initially at 50 mg/hour. If hypersensitivity or infusion reactions do not occur during the first 30 minutes, increase the rate by 50 mg/hour every 30 minutes as tolerated, to a maximum rate of 400 mg/hour. Subsequently, if previous administration was well tolerated, start at 100 mg/hour, and increase by 100 mg/hour every 30 minutes as tolerated to a maximum rate of 400 mg/hour
- Interrupt rituximab administration for fever, chills, edema, congestion of the head and neck mucosa, hypotension, and other serious adverse events. Resume rituximab administration after adverse events abate

Emetogenic potential: Low (Emetogenicity score = 2). See Chapter X

Patient Population Studied

A study of 31 patients who had either low-grade or follicular B-cell NHL with either relapsed disease or primary therapy failure and progressive disease that required further treatment. Additional requirements included a demonstrable monoclonal CD2O-positive B-cell population in a pathologic lymphnode or bone marrow specimen and a WHO PS of 0, 1, or 2. Concurrent steroid use was not permitted.

Efficacy (N = 28)

Complete response	4%
Partial response	39%
Overall response rate	43%

Toxicity

	% of Patients
Transient fever	61
Leukopenia	23
Nausea	19
Dizziness	19
Throat irritation	19
G1/2 Chills	36
G3/4 Chills	3
G3/4 Pulmonary disorders	6
G3/4 Infusion-related hypotension	3

NCI Adult Toxicity Criteria (February 1988 guidelines)

Treatment Modifications

Treatment prerequisites: Within 2 weeks before starting rituximab, study patients were required to have a hemoglobin ≥ 8.0 g/dL, ANC ≥ 1500/mm^3, platelet count ≥ 75,000/mm^3, serum creatinine concentration ≤ 2 mg/dL (177 μmol/L), total bilirubin level ≤ 2 mg/dL (34.2 μmol/L), and alkaline phosphatase and AST ≤ 2 times the upper limit of normal.

Rituximab Infusion-Related Toxicities

Onset of infusion-related events (fevers, chills, rigors edema, congestion of the head and neck mucosa, hypotension):

1. Interrupt rituximab infusion
2. For fever, chills: Give additional dose of acetaminophen 650 mg orally and diphenhydramine 25–50 mg by intravenous push
3. For rigors: Give meperidine 12.5–25 mg by intravenous push ± promethazine 12.5–25 mg by intravenous infusion in at least 10 mL 0.9% NS or D5W over 5–15 minutes. If after 15–20 minutes the response to a single dose is considered inadequate, the dose may be repeated
4. After symptoms resolve, resume rituximab infusion at 50 mg/hour and increase by 50 mg/hour every 30 minutes as tolerated up to a maximum rate of 200 mg/hour

Dyspnea or wheezing, without allergic findings (urticaria, or tongue or laryngeal edema):

1. Interrupt rituximab infusion immediately
2. Give hydrocortisone 100 mg by intravenous push (or glucocorticoid equivalent)
3. Give a histamine H_2 antagonist (ranitidine 150 mg, cimetidine 300 mg, or famotidine 20 mg) by intravenous push
4. After symptoms resolve, resume rituximab infusion at 25 mg/hour with close monitoring. Do not increase rate

Note: Medications for the treatment of hypersensitivity reactions should be available for immediate use in the event of a reaction during administration (eg, intravenous fluids, epinephrine, antihistamines, glucocorticoids, and O_2)

Therapy Monitoring

Weekly: CBC with differential, LFTs, serum BUN, and creatinine

REGIMEN

FLUDARABINE, MITOXANTRONE (NOVANTRONE), DEXAMETHASONE (FN-D)

McLaughlin P et al. JCO 1996;14:1262–1268

Fludarabine 25 mg/m^2 per day by intravenous infusion in 100–125 mL 0.9% NaCl injection (0.9% NS) or 5% dextrose injection (D5W) over 30 minutes for 3 consecutive days on days 1–3 every 4 weeks for up to 8 cycles (total dosage/cycle = 75 mg/m^2)
Mitoxantrone 10 mg/m^2 by intravenous infusion in 50–150 mL 0.9% NS or D5W over 5–30 minutes, given on day 1 every 4 weeks for up to 8 cycles (total dosage/cycle = 10 mg/m^2)
Dexamethasone 20 mg/day orally or by intravenous infusion in 10–100 mL 0.9% NS or D5W over 10–30 minutes for 5 consecutive days on days 1–5 every 4 weeks for up to 8 cycles (total dosage/cycle = 100 mg)

Supportive care:
- PCP prophylaxis with **cotrimoxazole** (trimethoprim 160 mg + sulfamethoxazole 800 mg) orally, one dose 3 times per week (eg, Monday, Wednesday, and Friday)
- Add a **proton pump inhibitor** during dexamethasone therapy

Dexamethasone is marketed in the United States in numerous solid formulations for oral administration, such as 0.25-, 0.5-, 0.75-, 1-, 2-, 4-, and 6-mg tablets, and in elixirs (which contain alcohol) and solutions

Emetogenic potential:
Day 1: Moderate (Emetogenicity score = 3)
Days 2–5: Nonemetogenic (Emetogenicity score = 1). See Chapter 39 for antiemetic regimens

Patient Population Studied

A study of 51 patients with recurrent or refractory indolent lymphoma. Patients were excluded who were serologically positive for HIV

Efficacy (N = 51)

Complete response	47%
Partial response	47%
Overall response rate	94%
Median survival	34 months
Median progression free survival	14 months

Toxicity (N = 51 Patients; 182 Cycles)

Adverse Event	% of Cycles
ANC < 500/mm^3	20
Platelet count <100,000/mm^3	31
Platelet count <50,000/mm^3	8
Infectious complications	**12**
Toxicity	**% of Patients**
Nausea	20
Vomiting	6
Stomatitis	12
Neurologic toxicities	8
Congestive heart failure	4
Diarrhea	4

Treatment Modifications

Adverse Event	Dose Modification
Sepsis during any cycle	Reduce fludarabine and mitoxantrone dosages by 20% during subsequent cycles
ANC < 100/mm^3 or platelet count <20,000/mm^3 during any cycle	

Therapy Monitoring

1. *On days of drug administration:* CBC with differential, LFTs, serum BUN, and creatinine
2. Cardiac status was monitored every 2 to 3 cycles with a cardiac scan or echo cardiogram

Notes

In monitoring cardiac status and deciding whether to continue mitoxantrone the authors used the following approach: Monitoring of cardiac status was performed after every two to three courses with cardiac scan or echocardiogram. For patients who had received prior anthracyclines, a potential cumulative cardiotoxic dose was estimated by assuming that a full cardiotoxic dose of mitoxantrone was 160 mg/m^2, and that of doxorubicin by bolus, 450 mg/m^2. (For doxorubicin by continuous infusion, the thresholds used were 675 mg/m^2 for 48-hour infusion and 800 mg/m^2 for 96-hour infusion). The following calculation was used: if the total doses of mitoxantrome and doxorubicin per square meter are "m" and "d" respectively, then m/160 + d/450 must be less than 1. If this potential cardiotoxic threshold was exceeded, or if cardiac symptoms occurred, discontinuation of mitoxantrone was advised.

REGIMEN

CYCLOPHOSPHAMIDE, VINCRISTINE (ONCOVIN®), DOXORUBICIN, METHOTREXATE (CODOX-M) + IFOSFAMIDE, ETOPOSIDE (VP-16), CYTARABINE (ARA-C) (I-VAC)

Magrath I et al. JCO 1996;14:925–934

Patients are stratified into high-risk and low-risk groups according to extent of disease and LDH at presentation

Findings at Presentation	Treatment Regimen
Low Risk	
A single extra-abdominal mass or completely resected abdominal disease, *and* serum LDH <350 units/L or a concentration within institutional normal range	3 Cycles A → A → A
High Risk	
All other patients	4 Cycles A → B → A → B

High- and Low-Risk Patients

Preparation for definitive therapy:

Allopurinol orally or intravenously
- *Initial dosage:* **Allopurinol** 3.3 mg/kg per dose, 3 times daily (daily dosage = 10 mg/kg)
- *Three days after induction treatment commences:* Allopurinol dosage may be decreased to 1.7 mg/kg per dose, 3 times daily (daily dosage = 5 mg/kg)
- *Two weeks after beginning induction treatment:* Allopurinol may be discontinued

Hydration with allopurinol:
3000–4500 mL/m^2 per day as tolerated by intravenous infusion with a solution containing at least 75 mEq sodium/1000 mL
- **Sodium bicarbonate** is added to parenteral hydration solutions in the presence of plasma uric acid ≥9 mg/dL to maintain urine pH ≥ 7.0

  Notes:
  - Discontinue urinary alkalinization after serum uric acid decreases to <8 mg/dL and before starting chemotherapy
  - **Potassium** is not added to parenteral hydration solutions during the first few days of induction therapy unless serum potassium decreases to <3.0 mEq/dL

Furosemide 20–40 mg, orally or intravenously, is used to ensure that fluid output is consistent with intake
- Diuresis is maintained for at least the first 72 hours after starting chemotherapy in the absence of metabolic aberrations or after metabolic complications have normalized

Allopurinol is manufactured in the United States in tablets for oral administration containing either allopurinol 100 mg or 300 mg and as an injectable product, Alloprim® (allopurinol sodium) for injection (Nabi®, Boca Raton, FL)

High-Risk Patients

4 Cycles A → B → A → B

Regimen A: CODOX-M
Cyclophosphamide 800 mg/m^2 by intravenous infusion in 50–100 mL 0.9% NaCl (0.9% NS) or 5% dextrose injection (D5W) over 30 minutes, given on day 1, *followed by:*
Cyclophosphamide 200 mg/m^2 per day by intravenous infusion in 50–100 mL 0.9% NS D5W over 15 minutes for 4 consecutive days on days 2–5 (total dosage/cycle = 1600 mg/m^2)
Doxorubicin 40 mg/m^2 by intravenous injection over 3–5 minutes, given on day 1 (total dosage/ cycle = 40 mg/m^2)
Vincristine 1.5 mg/m^2 per dose (maximum single dose is 2.5 mg) by intravenous injection over 1–3 minutes, as follows:
- During cycle 1, for 2 doses on days 1 and 8 (total dosage/cycle = 3 mg/m^2; maximum dose/cycle = 5 mg)
- During cycle 3, for 3 doses on days 1, 8, and 15 (total dosage/cycle = 4.5 mg/m^2; maximum dose/cycle = 7.5 mg)

Hydration with methotrexate:
3000 mL/m^2 per day with a solution containing at least 75 mEq sodium/1000 mL by intravenous infusion during methotrexate administration (day 10) and for at least 24 hours afterward. **Sodium bicarbonate** 50–100 mEq/1000 mL is added to the parenteral solution to maintain urine pH ≥ 7.0
Methotrexate 1200 mg/m^2 by intravenous infusion in 25–250 mL dextrose or saline fluids ± 50–100 mEq sodium bicarbonate over 1 hour on day 10, *followed immediately by:*
Methotrexate 240 mg/m^2 per hour by continuous intravenous infusion in 250–6000 mL dextrose or saline fluids ± sodium bicarbonate 50–100 mEq/1000 mL over 23 hours on day 10 (total dosage/cycle [not including intrathecal methotrexate] = 6720 mg/m^2)

(continued)

(continued)

Notes:

- For logistical practicality and efficiency, parenteral admixtures containing methotrexate may include a portion or all of the fluid and sodium bicarbonate needed to meet hydration and urinary alkalinization requirements during methotrexate administration
- Methotrexate administration is discontinued after a total duration of 24 hours without regard for any portion not administered

Calcium leucovorin 192 mg/m^2 by intravenous infusion in 25–250 mL 0.9% NS or D5W over 1 hour at 36 hours after methotrexate administration began, *followed 6 hours later by:*
Calcium leucovorin 12 mg/m^2 per dose by intravenous infusion in 25–250 mL 0.9% NS or D5W over 15 minutes every 6 hours until serum methotrexate concentration is <0.05 micromol/L

Note:

- Calcium leucovorin may be administered orally after completing 1 day of parenteral administration if patients are compliant, not vomiting, and without other potentially mitigating complications

Filgrastim 5 mcg/kg per day subcutaneously starting on day 13 and continuing until the next treatment cycle (ie, when ANC recovers to ≥ 1000/mm^3)

Emetogenic potential:
Day 1: High (Emetogenicity score = 5)
Days 2–5: Moderate (Emetogenicity score = 3)
Days 8 and 15: Nonemetogenic (Emetogenicity score = 1)
Day 10: Moderately high (Emetogenicity score = 4). See Chapter 39 for antiemetic regimens

Regimen B: IVAC
Ifosfamide 1500 mg/m^2 + **mesna** 360 mg/m^2 per day by intravenous infusion in 100–250 mL 0.9% NS or D5W over 1 hour for 5 consecutive days on days 1–5 (total ifosfamide dosage/cycle = 7500 mg/m^2)
Mesna 360 mg/m^2 per dose by intravenous infusion in 25–150 mL 0.9% NS or D5W over 15 minutes every 3 hours for 6 doses, starting 3 hours after each ifosfamide + mesna administration is completed (total mesna dosage/day [7 doses/24 hours] = 2520 mg/m^2; total mesna dosage/cycle = 12,600 mg/m^2)
Etoposide 60 mg/m^2 per day by intravenous infusion in 150 mL 0.9% NS or D5W over 1 hour for 5 consecutive days on days 1–5 (total dosage/cycle = 300 mg/m^2)
Cytarabine 2000 mg/m^2 per dose by intravenous infusion in 150 mL D5W over 3 hours every 12 hours for 4 doses on days 1 and 2 (total dosage/cycle = 8000 mg/m^2)
Filgrastim 5 mcg/kg per day subcutaneously starting on day 13 and continuing until the next treatment cycle (i.e., when ANC recovers to ≥ 1000/mm^3)

Emetogenic potential:
Days 1 and 2: Very high (Emetogenicity score = 6)
Days 3–5: Moderately high (Emetogenicity score = 4). See Chapter 39

Intrathecal Medications for Prophylaxis of High-Risk Patients and Treatment of Patients with CNS Disease

Dose in Milligrams Adjusted to Patient's Age in Years (y)			Days of Administration			
			Prophylaxis		Treatment	
≥3 y	2 y	1 y	A[a]	B[b]	A[a]	B[b]
Cytarabine by Lumbar Puncture						
70	50	35	1, 3	—	1, 3, 5	7, 9
Cytarabine by Intraventricular Route						
15	12	9	1, 3	—	1, 3, 5	7, 9
Methotrexate by Lumbar Puncture[c]						
12	10	8	15	5	15, 17	5
Methotrexate by Intraventricular Route[c]						
2	1.5	1	15	5	15, 17	5

[a]A, CODOX-M: Cycles 1 and 3
[b]B, IVAC: Cycles 2 and 4
[c]**Calcium leucovorin** 12 mg/m^2 orally for one dose at 24 hours after each intrathecal dose of methotrexate

(continued)

(continued)

Low-Risk Patients

3 Cycles: A → A → A

Modified Regimen A: (modified) CODOX-M

Cyclophosphamide 800 mg/m^2 by intravenous infusion in 50–100 mL 0.9% NS or D5W over 30 minutes, given on day 1, *followed by:*

Cyclophosphamide 200 mg/m^2 per day by intravenous infusion in 50–100 mL 0.9% NS D5W over 15 minutes, for 4 consecutive days on days 2–5 (total dosage/cycle = 1600 mg/m^2)

Doxorubicin 40 mg/m^2 by intravenous injection over 3–5 minutes, given on day 1 (total dosage/ cycle = 40 mg/m^2)

Vincristine 1.5 mg/m^2 per dose (maximum single dose is 2.5 mg) by intravenous injection over 1–3 minutes for 2 doses on days 1 and 8 (total dosage/cycle = 3 mg/m^2; maximum dose/cycle = 5 mg)

Hydration with methotrexate:

3000 mL/m^2 per day with a solution containing at least 75 mEq sodium/1000 mL by intravenous infusion during methotrexate administration (day 10) and for at least 24 hours afterward. **Sodium bicarbonate** 50–100 mEq/1000 mL is added to the parenteral solution to maintain urine pH ≥ 7.0

Methotrexate 1200 mg/m^2 by intravenous infusion in 25–250 mL dextrose or saline fluids ± 50–100 mEq sodium bicarbonate over 1 hour on day 10, *followed immediately by:*

Methotrexate 240 mg/m^2 per hour by continuous intravenous infusion in 250–6000 mL dextrose or saline fluids ± sodium bicarbonate 50–100 mEq/1000 mL, over 23 hours on day 10 (total dosage/cycle [not including intrathecal methotrexate] = 6720 mg/m^2)

Notes:

- For logistical practicality and efficiency, parenteral admixtures containing methotrexate may include a portion or all of the fluid and sodium bicarbonate needed to meet hydration and urinary alkalinization requirements during methotrexate administration
- Methotrexate administration is discontinued after a total duration of 24 hours without regard for any portion not administered

Calcium leucovorin 192 mg/m^2 by intravenous infusion in 25–250 mL 0.9% NS or D5W over 1 hour at 36 hours after methotrexate administration began, *followed 6 hours later by:*

Calcium leucovorin 12 mg/m^2 per dose by intravenous infusion in 25–250 mL 0.9% NS or D5W over 15 minutes every 6 hours until serum methotrexate concentration is <0.05 micromol/L

Note:

- Calcium leucovorin may be administered orally after completing 1 day of parenteral administration if patients are compliant, are not vomiting, and have no other potentially mitigating complications

Filgrastim 5 mcg/kg per day subcutaneously starting on day 13 and continuing until the next treatment cycle (ie, when ANC recovers to ≥ 1000/mm^3)

CNS Prophylaxis

Cytarabine on day 1/methotrexate on day 3		
Patient's Age	**Cytarabine**	**Methotrexate**
1 year	35 mg	8 mg
2 years	50 mg	10 mg
≥3 years	70 mg	12 mg

Administer intrathecally by lumbar puncture

Emetogenic potential:

Day 1: High (Emetogenicity score = 5)

Days 2–5: Moderate (Emetogenicity score = 3)

Days 8 and 15: Nonemetogenic (Emetogenicity score = 1)

Day 10: Moderately high (Emetogenicity score = 4). See Chapter 39 for antiemetic regimens

Efficacy

Complete response	95%
Partial response	5%
Event-free survival	92% at 2 years

Patient Population Studied

A study of 41 previously untreated patients with small noncleaved (Burkitt's or Burkitts-like) lymphoma. Thirty-four patients (15 adults + 19 children) were considered to be at high risk by the criteria stated above. Seven patients (5 adults + 2 children) were considered low risk

Therapy Monitoring

1. *Before each cycle:* PE, CBC with differential, LFTs, serum BUN, creatinine, creatinine clearance, urinalysis
2. *During the first 3–5 days of induction therapy:*
   - Every 4–6 hours: Serum creatinine and electrolytes, calcium, and phosphorus
   - Daily until normal levels are achieved: LDH
   - On days of chemotherapy: CBC with differential, serum creatinine, electrolytes, calcium, and phosphorus
3. *Weekly during the intervals between treatments:* CBC with differential, serum creatinine and electrolytes, calcium, and phosphorus
4. *After high-dose systemic methotrexate administration:* Daily methotrexate levels

Toxicity (N = 41)

	Regimen	Patient's Ages (years)	% of Cycles G3	% of Cycles G4
Neutropenia	A	<18	0	97.6
		≥18	2.2	97.8
	B	<18	0	100
		≥18	0	100
Leukopenia	A	<18	0	97.6
		≥18	4.4	95.6
	B	<18	0	100
		≥18	0	100
Thrombocytopenia	A	<18	17.1	53.7
		≥18	9.3	39.5
	B	<18	14.3	82.9
		≥18	3.7	96.3
Liver function abnormalities	A	<18	24.4	2.4
		≥18	24.4	2.4
	B	<18	5.9	0
		≥18	0	0
Stomatitis	A	<18	26.8	41.5
		≥18	28.9	20
	B	<18	5.7	2.9
		≥18	3.4	0
Documented infection	A	All ages	46.6	
	B		54.5	
Fever of unknown origin	A + B	<18	46.3	
		≥18	32.4	
Septicemia	A + B	<18	22.5	
		≥18	21.6	

Neurologic Adverse Events (N = 41 Patients)

Toxicity	% of Patients
Painful disabling neuropathy	26.8
Marked motor/severe sensory neuropathy	19.5
Severe motor weakness	7.3
Mild-moderate neuropathy	29.3

A, CODOX-M; B, IVAC
Magrath I et al. JCO 1996;14:925–934
Weintraub M et al. JCO 1996;14:935–940

Treatment Modifications

Treatment prerequisites:

- Cycles 2, 3, and 4 are started, when possible, on the day that the ANC recovers to ≥1000/mm³ after prior treatment
- A platelet count ≥50,000/mm³ without platelet transfusion support is required before starting repeated cycles. If a patient's ANC recovers to ≥1000/mm³, but the platelet count has not recovered to ≥50,000/mm³ without platelet transfusion, the patient should continue to receive daily filgrastim until the platelet count recovers to ≥50,000/mm³
- For CODOX-M, methotrexate is given without regard for blood counts
- Intravenously administered methotrexate is given only if creatinine clearance is >50 mL/min (0.83 mL/sec)

Adverse Event	Dose Modification
Motor weakness or unremitting obstipation	Continue treatment, but hold vincristine. When symptoms resolve, reintroduce vincristine at 50% dosage during subseqeuent treatments
Severe sensory symptoms	Reduce vincristine dosage by 50% during subsequent treatment
Serum sodium <130 mmol/L	Hold cyclophosphamide. Resume cyclophosphamide after serum sodium recovers to ≥130 mmol/L and change hydration fluid and diluent fluids to 0.9% NS
Hemorrhagic cystitis	Hold cyclophosphamide
Total bilirubin >2.5 mg/dL (42.8 μmol/L)	Reduce doxorubicin dosage by 50%
Total bilirubin >3.0 mg/dL (51.3 μmol/L)	Hold doxorubicin
Cerebellar toxicity	Hold cytarabine
Acute renal failure	Hold ifosfamide

NCI CTC

REGIMEN

NHL-BFM 86 (BERLIN-FRANKFURT-MÜNSTER 86)

Reiter A et al. JCO 1995;13:359–372

Group B Regimen: Treatment was stratified by stage into three arms of different intensity. All patients received a cytoreductive prephase followed by two alternating courses of chemotherapy as follows:

B-SRG: Stage I and Completely Resected Stage II	
3 cycles	A→ B → A
B-RG: Stage II Nonresected and Stage III	
6 cycles	A → B → A → B → A → B
B-IV/ALL: Stage IV and B-ALL	
6 cycles	AA → BB → AA → BB → AA → BB

Prophylaxis against tumor lysis syndrome during the first cycle:
Hydration with 2400–3000 mL/day as tolerated, 5% dextrose/0.45% NaCl injection (D5W/0.45% NS) with sodium bicarbonate injection 100 mEq/1000 mL intravenously at 100–125 mL/hour (2400–3000 mL/day)

Notes:
- **Sodium bicarbonate** is added to parenteral hydration solutions in the presence of plasma uric acid ≥9 mg/dL to maintain urine pH ≥7.0
- **Potassium** is not added to parenteral hydration solutions during the first few days of induction therapy unless serum potassium decreases to <3.0 mEq/L

Furosemide 20–40 mg intravenously every 12–24 hours to maintain fluid balance

Note: Diuresis is maintained for at least the first 72 hours after starting chemotherapy in the absence of metabolic aberrations or after metabolic complications normalize

Allopurinol orally or intravenously
- *Initial dosage:* **Allopurinol** 3.3 mg/kg per dose 3 times daily (daily dosage = 10 mg/kg)
- *Three days after induction treatment commences:* Allopurinol dosage may be decreased to 1.7 mg/kg per dose 3 times daily (daily dosage = 5 mg/kg)
- *Two weeks after beginning induction treatment:* Allopurinol may be discontinued

Cytoreductive prephase:
Prednisone 30 mg/m^2 per day orally for 5 consecutive days on days 1–5 (total dosage = 150 mg/m^2)
Cyclophosphamide 200 mg/m^2 per day by intravenous infusion in 50–1000 mL 0.9% NaCl injection (0.9% NS) or 5% dextrose injection (D5W) over 15–60 minutes for 5 consecutive days on days 1–5 (total dosage = 1000 mg/m^2)

Emetogenic potential: Days 1–5: Moderate (Emetogenicity score = 3)

Course A:
Dexamethasone 10 mg/m^2 per day orally for 5 consecutive days on days 1–5 (total dosage/course = 50 mg/m^2)
Ifosfamide 800 mg/m^2 per day by intravenous infusion in 100–250 mL 0.9% NS or D5W over 1 hour for 5 consecutive days on days 1–5 (total dosage/course = 4000 mg/m^2)
Methotrexate 50 mg/m^2 by intravenous infusion in 25–250 mL 0.9% NS or D5W over 30 minutes, given on day 1, *followed immediately by:*
Methotrexate 450 mg/m^2 by continuous intravenous infusion in 250 mL to ≥1000 mL 0.9% NS or D5W (or saline and dextrose combinations) over 23.5 hours on day 1 (total dosage/course [not including intrathecal methotrexate] = 500 mg/m^2)
Methotrexate 12 mg* intrathecally on day 1, two hours after systemic methotrexate began (total dose/course [not including systemic methotrexate] = 12 mg)
Cytarabine 30 mg* intrathecally on day 1, two hours after systemic methotrexate began (total dose/course [not including systemic cytarabine] = 30 mg)
Prednisolone 10 mg intrathecally on day 1, two hours after systemic methotrexate began (total dose/course = 10 mg)
Leucovorin calcium 15 mg/m^2 per dose by intravenous infusion in 10–250 mL 0.9% NS or D5W over 15–30 minutes for 3 doses at hours 48, 51, and 54 after systemic methotrexate began (total dosage/course = 45 mg/m^2)
Cytarabine 150 mg/m^2 per dose by intravenous infusion in 25–500 mL 0.9% NS or D5W over 1 hour every 12 hours for 4 doses on days 4 and 5 (total dosage/course [not including intrathecal cytarabine] = 600 mg/m^2)

(*continued*)

(continued)

Teniposide 100 mg/m^2 per day by intravenous infusion, diluted in 0.9% NS or D5W to a concentration of 0.1, 0.2, or 0.4 mg/mL, over 1 hour for 2 consecutive days on days 4 and 5 (total dosage/course = 200 mg/m^2)

Course B:
Dexamethasone 10 mg/m^2 per day orally for 5 consecutive days on days 1–5 (total dosage/course = 50 mg/m^2)
Cyclophosphamide 200 mg/m^2 per day by intravenous infusion in 50–1000 mL 0.9% NS or D5W over 1 hour for 5 consecutive days on days 1–5 (total dosage/course = 1000 mg/m^2)
Methotrexate 50 mg/m^2 by intravenous infusion in 25–250 mL 0.9% NS or D5W over 30 minutes, given on day 1, *followed immediately by:*
Methotrexate 450 mg/m^2 by continuous intravenous infusion in 250 mL to ≥1000 mL 0.9% NS or D5W (or saline and dextrose combinations) over 23.5 hours on day 1 (total dosage/course [not including intrathecal methotrexate] = 500 mg/m^2)
Methotrexate 12 mg* intrathecally on day 1, two hours after systemic methotrexate began (total dose/course [not including systemic methotrexate] = 12 mg)
Cytarabine 30 mg* intrathecally on day 1, two hours after systemic methotrexate began (total dose/course = 30 mg)
Prednisolone 10 mg intrathecally on day 1, two hours after systemic methotrexate began (total dose/course = 10 mg)
Leucovorin calcium 15 mg/m^2 per dose by intravenous infusion in 10–250 mL 0.9% NS or D5W over 15–30 minutes for 3 doses at hours 48, 51, and 54 after systemic methotrexate began (total dosage/course = 45 mg/m^2)
Doxorubicin 25 mg/m^2 per day by intravenous infusion in 25–250 mL 0.9% NS or D5W over 1 hour for 2 consecutive days on days 4 and 5 (total dosage/course = 50 mg/m^2)

Course AA:
Dexamethasone 10 mg/m^2 per day orally for 5 consecutive days on days 1–5 (total dosage/course = 50 mg/m^2)
Ifosfamide 800 mg/m^2 per day by intravenous infusion in 100–250 mL 0.9% NS or D5W over 1 hour, for 5 consecutive days on days 1–5 (total dosage/course = 4000 mg/m^2)
Vincristine 1.5 mg/m^2 (maximum 2 mg/dose) by intravenous injection over 1–3 minutes, given on day 1 (total dosage/course = 1.5 mg/m^2; maximum 2 mg/dose)
Methotrexate 500 mg/m^2 by intravenous infusion in 50–250 mL 0.9% NS or D5W over 30 minutes, given on day 1, *followed immediately by:*
Methotrexate 4500 mg/m^2 by continuous intravenous infusion in 250 mL to ≥1000 mL 0.9% NS or D5W over 23.5 hours on day 1 (total dosage/course [not including intrathecal methotrexate] = 5000 mg/m^2)
Methotrexate 6 mg/dose* intrathecally for 2 doses on days 1 and 5, two hours after systemic methotrexate began on day 1 and then again on day 5 (total dose/course [not including systemic methotrexate] = 12 mg)
Cytarabine 15 mg/dose* intrathecally for 2 doses on days 1 and 5, two hours after systemic methotrexate began on day 1 and then again on day 5 (total dose/course [not including systemic cytarabine] = 30 mg)
Prednisolone 5 mg/dose intrathecally for 2 doses on days 1 and 5, two hours after systemic methotrexate began on day 1 and then again on day 5 (total dose/course=10 mg)
Leucovorin calcium 15 mg/m^2 per dose by intravenous infusion in 10–250 mL 0.9% NS or D5W over 15–30 minutes every 6 hours for 6 doses, starting 36 hours after systemic methotrexate began (total dosage/course = 90 mg/m^2)
Cytarabine 150 mg/m^2 per dose by intravenous infusion in 25–500 mL 0.9% NS or D5W over 1 hour every 12 hours for 4 doses on days 4 and 5 (total dosage/course [not including intrathecal cytarabine] = 600 mg/m^2)
Teniposide 100 mg/m^2 per day by intravenous infusion, diluted in 0.9% NS or D5W to a concentration of 0.1, 0.2, or 0.4 mg/mL, over 1 hour, for 2 consecutive days on days 4 and 5 (total dosage/course = 200 mg/m^2)

Course BB:
Dexamethasone 10 mg/m^2 per day orally for 5 consecutive days on days 1–5 (total dosage/course = 50 mg/m^2)
Cyclophosphamide 200 mg/m^2 per day by intravenous infusion in 50–1000 mL 0.9% NS or D5W over 1 hour for 5 consecutive days on days 1–5 (total dosage/course = 1000 mg/m^2)
Vincristine 1.5 mg/m^2 (maximum 2 mg/dose) by intravenous injection over 1–3 minutes, given on day 1 (total dosage/course = 1.5 mg/m^2; maximum 2 mg/dose)
Methotrexate 500 mg/m^2 by intravenous infusion in 50–250 mL 0.9% NS or D5W over 30 minutes, given on day 1, *followed immediately by:*
Methotrexate 4500 mg/m^2 by continuous intravenous infusion in 250 mL to ≥1000 mL 0.9% NS or D5W over 23.5 hours on day 1 (total dosage/course [not including intrathecal methotrexate] = 5000 mg/m^2)
Methotrexate 6 mg/dose* intrathecally for 2 doses on days 1 and 5, two hours after systemic methotrexate began on day 1 and then again on day 5 (total dose/course [not including systemic methotrexate] = 12 mg)
Cytarabine 15 mg/dose* intrathecally for 2 doses on days 1 and 5, two hours after systemic methotrexate began on day 1 and then again on day 5 (total dose/course = 30 mg)
Prednisolone 5 mg/dose intrathecally for 2 doses on days 1 and 5, two hours after systemic methotrexate began on day 1 and then again on day 5 (total dose/course = 10 mg)
Leucovorin calcium 15 mg/m^2 per dose by intravenous infusion in 10–250 mL 0.9% NS or D5W over 15–30 minutes every 6 hours for 6 doses, starting 36 hours after systemic methotrexate began (total dosage/course = 90 mg/m^2)
Doxorubicin 25 mg/m^2 per day by intravenous infusion in 25–250 mL 0.9% NS or D5W over 1 hour for 2 consecutive days on days 4 and 5 (total dosage/course = 50 mg/m^2)

(continued)

(continued)

*Doses are adjusted for patients <3 years of age. See following table

CNS Prophylaxis (Intrathecal)

A and B: Cytarabine/methotrexate on day 1 (AA and BB: Cytarabine/methotrexate on days 1 + 5)		
Patient's Age	Cytarabine (Dose/day)	Methotrexate (Dose/day)
1 year	18 mg (9 + 9)	8 mg (4 + 4)
2 years	24 mg (12 + 12)	10 mg (5 + 5)
≥3 years	30 mg (15 + 15)	12 mg (6 + 6)

Prednisone is marketed in the United States in numerous formulations for oral administration, such as 1-, 2.5-, 5-, 10-, 20-, and 50-mg tablets, and in solutions and syrups
Dexamethasone is marketed in the United States in numerous formulations for oral administration, such as 0.25-, 0.5-, 0.75-, 1-, 2-, 4-, and 6-mg tablets, and in elixirs (which contain alcohol) and solutions for oral administration
Allopurinol is manufactured in tablets for oral administration containing either allopurinol 100 mg or 300 mg and as an injectable product, Alloprim® (allopurinol sodium) for injection (Nabi®, Boca Raton, FL)

Emetogenic potential:
Courses A, B, AA, and BB
Days 1, 4, and 5: Moderately high (Emetogenicity score = 4)
Days 2 and 3: Moderate (Emetogenicity score = 3). See Chapter 39 for antiemetic regimens

Treatment Modifications

Treatment prerequisites

1. *Conditions for starting treatment courses 2, 3, and 4:* Platelet count >50,000/mm³; WBC count >1000/mm³; ANC >200/mm³
2. *Conditions for starting treatment courses 5 and 6:* WBC count >2000/mm³; ANC >500/mm³
3. Minimally, a 2-week interval must elapse between the first days of 2 courses in succession

Treatment notes

1. All treatments were completed within 2–3 months for the B-SRG arm, and within 4–5 months for the B-RG and B-IV/B-ALL arms
2. Cranial irradiation was optional for patients with overt CNS disease
3. Patients without CNS disease did not receive cranial radiation
4. Males with testicular involvement were to receive radiation to the testes
5. Local radiation therapy was limited to patients with residual unresectable active disease

Patient Population Studied

A study of 319 pediatric patients (ages ≤18 years), among whom 111 patients had a diagnosis of Burkitt's lymphoma. Group B included Burkitt's-type lymphomas, B-ALL, and most large cell lymphomas including Ki-1 anaplastic large-cell lymphoma.

Efficacy

For 152 patients with Burkitt's lymphoma or B-ALL, the probability of event-free survival at 7 years was 79% ±3%

Treatment Group	Probability of Event Free Survival at 7 years
SRG (N = 42)	98 ± 2%
RG (N = 117)	79 ± 4%
IV/B-ALL (N = 66)	75 ± 5%

Toxicity

Not described

Therapy Monitoring

1. *After the first 2 treatment courses, and then before each subsequent treatment course:* Evaluation of tumor response
2. *Daily methotrexate levels:* Following high-dose systemic methotrexate administration
3. In patients with proven bone marrow or CNS involvement, bone marrow biopsies and CSF sampling, respectively, were repeated only until there was no more evidence of disease

Notes

1. Second-look surgery was projected for patients who had residual tumors by physical examination or imaging modalities after completing 2 treatment courses.
2. Most patients were treated before the widespread use of filgrastim.

REGIMEN

HYPERFRACTIONATED CYCLOPHOSPHAMIDE, VINCRISTINE, DOXORUBICIN (ADRIAMYCIN), DEXAMETHASONE (HYPER-CVAD)

Thomas DA et al. JCO 1999;17:2461–2470

Prophylaxis against tumor lysis syndrome during the first cycle:
Hydration with 2400–3000 mL/day as tolerated, 5% dextrose/0.45% NaCl injection (D5W/0.45% NS), with sodium bicarbonate injection 100 mEq/1000 mL intravenously at 100–125 mL/hour (2400–3000 mL/day)

Notes:

- **Sodium bicarbonate** is added to parenteral hydration solutions in the presence of plasma uric acid ≥9 mg/dL to maintain urine pH ≥7.0
- **Potassium** is not added to parenteral hydration solutions during the first few days of induction therapy unless serum potassium decreases to <3.0 mEq/L

Furosemide 20–40 mg intravenously every 12–24 hours to maintain fluid balance

Note: Diuresis is maintained for at least the first 72 hours after starting chemotherapy in the absence of metabolic aberrations, or after metabolic complications normalize

Allopurinol 300 mg/day orally for 7 consecutive days on days 1–7 [Longer treatment may be needed]

Hyper-CVAD (cycles 1, 3, 5, and 7):
Cyclophosphamide 300 mg/m^2 per dose intravenously over 2 hours in 500 mL 0.9% NaCl injection (0.9% NS) every 12 hours for 6 doses (days 1, 2, and 3) for 4 cycles, cycles 1, 3, 5, and 7 (total dosage/cycle = 1800 mg/m^2)
Mesna 600 mg/m^2 per day (25 mg/m^2 per hour) by continuous intravenous infusion over 24 hours in 2000 mL 0.9% NS, starting 1 hour before cyclophosphamide and continuing until 12 hours after the last dose of cyclophosphamide (total duration approximately 75 hours/cycle) for 4 cycles, cycles 1, 3, 5, and 7 (total dosage/cycle = 1875 mg/m^2)
Vincristine 2 mg/dose by intravenous push over 1–3 minutes for 2 doses on days 4 and 11 (total dose/cycle = 4 mg)
Doxorubicin 50 mg/m^2 by intravenous infusion via central venous access in 25–250 mL 0.9% NS or 5% dextrose injection (D5W) over 2 hours on day 4 (total dosage/cycle = 50 mg/m^2)
Dexamethasone 40 mg/day orally or by intravenous infusion in 25–150 mL 0.9% NS or D5W over 15–30 minutes for 8 doses on days 1–4 and days 11–14 (total dosage/cycle = 320 mg)
Filgrastim 10 mcg/kg per day subcutaneously, starting 24 hours after the last dose of chemotherapy, and continuing until post-nadir WBC count ≥3000/mm^3

High-dose methotrexate and cytarabine (cycles 2, 4, 6, and 8)
Hydration with D5W/0.45% NS with sodium bicarbonate injection 100 mEq/1000 mL intravenously at 100–125 mL/hour (2400–3000 mL/day)
Methotrexate 1000 mg/m^2 by continuous intravenous infusion in 250 mL to ≥1000 mL 0.9% NS or D5W (or saline and dextrose combinations) over 24 hours on day 1 (total dosage/cycle [not including intrathecal methotrexate] = 1000 mg/m^2)
Cytarabine 3000 mg/m^2 per dose intravenously in 50–500 mL 0.9% NS or D5W over 2 hours every 12 hours for 4 doses on days 2 and 3 (total dosage/cycle [not including intrathecal cytarabine] = 12,000 mg/m^2)
Calcium leucovorin 50 mg intravenously in 10–100 mL 0.9% NS or D5W over 10–20 minutes for one dose, 12 hours after methotrexate administration is completed (36 hours after starting methotrexate), followed 6 hours later by:
Calcium leucovorin 15 mg intravenously in 10–100 mL 0.9% NS or D5W over 10–20 minutes every 6 hours for 8 doses, or until blood methotrexate concentrations is <0.1 micromol/L

- Calcium leucovorin doses are escalated to 50 mg intravenously every 6 hours if serum methotrexate concentrations are:
  - >20 micromol/L at the end of methotrexate administration (hour 24)
  - >1 micromol/L at 24 hours after the end of methotrexate administration (hour 48), or
  - >0.1 micromol/L at 48 hours after the end of methotrexate administration (hour 72)

(continued)

Treatment Modifications

Treatment prerequisites

- Second and subsequent cycles are implemented when WBC count ≥3000/mm^3 and platelet count ≥60,000/mm^3 at least 24 hours after a filgrastim dose was administered
- Subsequent cycles may be repeated at intervals less than every 21 days, but not more frequently than 14 days after the previous cycle

Adverse Event	Dose Modification
On day 21 of a treatment cycle, if WBC count ≥3000/mm^3, but platelet count <60,000/mm^3	Re-evaluate hematologic laboratories every 3 days until platelet count ≥60,000/mm^3
On day 21 of a treatment cycle, if WBC count ≥30,000/mm^3, but platelet count <60,000/mm^3	Hold filgrastim and reevaluate hematologic laboratories every 3 days until platelet count ≥ 60,000/mm^3
Patient age ≥60 years	Reduce cytarabine dosage to 1000 mg/m^2 per dose
Blood methotrexate concentration >20 micromol/L at the start of treatment	Reduce cytarabine dosage to 2000 mg/m^2 per dose and reduce methotrexate dosage by 50%
Serum creatinine >2 mg/dL (>177 micromol/L)	
Serum creatinine >3 mg/dL (>265 micromol/L)	Reduce methotrexate dosage by 75%
Delayed methotrexate excretion or nephrotoxicity attributable to previous methotrexate treatment	Reduce methotrexate dosage by 50–75% (commensurate with the severity of nephrotoxicity)
Total bilirubin >2 g/dL (34.2 μmol/L)	Reduce vincristine dose to 1 mg
Total bilirubin 2–3g/dL (34.2–51.3 μmol/L)	Reduce doxorubicin dosage by 25%
Total bilirubin 3–4g/dL (51.3–68.4 μmol/L)	Reduce doxorubicin dosage by 50%
Total bilirubin >4g/dL (68.4 μmol/L)	Reduce doxorubicin dosage by 75%

(continued)

(continued)

Filgrastim 10 mcg/kg per day subcutaneously, starting 24 hours after the last dose of chemotherapy; and continuing until post-nadir WBC count ≥ 3000/mm^3

Allopurinol is manufactured in the United States in tablets for oral administration containing either allopurinol 100 mg or 300 mg and as an injectable product, Alloprim® (allopurinol sodium) for injection (Nabi®, Boca Raton, FL)
Dexamethasone is marketed in the United States in numerous formulations for oral administration, such as 0.25-, 0.5-, 0.75-, 1-, 2-, 4-, and 6-mg tablets, and in elixirs (which contain alcohol) and solutions for oral administration

CNS prophylaxis (all patients):
Methotrexate intrathecally on day 2 for 8 cycles (8 doses): 12 mg/dose via lumbar puncture or 6 mg/dose via intraventricular route (eg, Ommaya reservoir). Total dose throughout 8 cycles [not including systemic methotrexate] = 96 mg via lumbar puncture or 48 mg intraventricularly
Cytarabine 100 mg intrathecally via lumbar puncture or via intraventricular route on day 7 for 8 cycles (total of dose 8 doses throughout 8 cycles [not including systemic cytarabine] = 800 mg)

CNS treatment:
Methotrexate 12 mg/dose intrathecally via lumbar puncture or 6 mg/dose via intraventricular route twice weekly until CSF cell count normalizes and cytology becomes negative for malignant disease; then administer intrathecally during subsequent cycles on day 2
Cytarabine 100 mg intrathecally via lumbar puncture or intraventricular route twice weekly until CSF cell count normalizes and cytology becomes negative for malignant disease; then administer intrathecally during subsequent cycles on day 2

Supportive care:
- PCP prophylaxis with **cotrimoxazole** (trimethoprim 160 mg + sulfamethoxazole 800 mg) orally twice daily
- Fever/neutropenia prophylaxis with **ciprofloxacin** 500 mg orally twice daily, *or* **Levofloxacin** 500 mg orally daily
- Antifungal prophylaxis with **fluconazole** 200 mg orally daily except on the days of vincristine administration
- Antiviral prophylaxis with **acyclovir** 200 mg orally twice daily, *or* **Valacyclovir** 500 mg orally daily

Emetogenic potential:
With Hyper-CVAD (cycles 1, 3, 5, and 7)
Days 1–4: Moderate (Emetogenicity score = 3)
With high-dose methotrexate and cytarabine (cycles 2, 4, 6, and 8)
Day 1: Moderate (Emetogenicity score = 3)
Days 2 and 3: Moderately high (Emetogenicity score = 4). See Chapter 39 for antiemetic regimens

Treatment Modifications (*continued*)

Disease involving the stomach or small bowel	Eliminate doxorubicin during the first Hyper-CVAD cycle
If high-dose cytarabine is eliminated due to adverse effects	Omit the high-dose methotrexate + cytarabine regimen, replacing it with repeated cycles of Hyper-CVAD
Peripheral neuropathy	Discontinue vincristine
Proximal myopathy	Discontinue dexamethasone
Cerebellar neurotoxicity	Reduce cytarabine dosage or omit cytarabine during subsequent treatments
Tumor lysis syndrome during induction with renal failure requiring hemodialysis	Reduce methotrexate dosage
G3 Mucositis	

Patient Population Studied

A study of 26 consecutive adult patients with newly diagnosed, untreated Burkitt's-type acute lymphoblastic leukemia (23 patients with FAB L3 subtype; 3 patients classified L1 or L2)

Efficacy (N = 26/21)

N = 26	
Complete response	81%
Progression during treatment	15%
Estimated median survival	16 months
N=21	
Relapse after CR	43%
Median time to relapse	7 months
3 year continuous CR	61%

Toxicity

Toxicities in Patients with CR (N = 21)

	Age <60 (n = 13)	Age ≥60 (n = 8)
G3/4 Neurotoxicity	15%	29%
Tumor lysis in first cycle	8%	25%
Creatinine increased more than 2-fold after methotrexate	23%	12%
Infection with cycle 2	54%	38%

Infectious Complications During First Cycle (N = 37)

Febrile neutropenia	86%
Fever of unknown origin	38%
Pneumonia	32%
Sepsis	11%
Bacterial meningitis	3%
Herpes simplex virus infections	3%

Infectious Complications in Cycles After First (N = 152)

Febrile neutropenia during high-dose methotrexate/cytarabine	47–55%
Febrile neutropenia during Hyper-CVAD	30–39%
Herpes simplex virus infections	8%

Events Concurrent with Thrombocytopenia (N = 152)

Hemorrhage with thrombocytopenia (all)	12%
Severe epistaxis	4%
Retinal	2%
Gastrointestinal	2%
CNS	2%
Pulmonary	1%
Antecubital hematoma	1%

Other Toxicities

Deaths during induction	19%
Cerebellar neurotoxicity	3.8%

NCI CTC

Therapy Monitoring

1. *Before each cycle:* PE, CBC with differential, LFTs, serum BUN, creatinine and urinalysis
2. *Daily during treatment:* Serum electrolytes, glucose, BUN, creatinine, total bilirubin, LFTs, LDH, uric acid, albumin, alkaline phosphatase, and CBC with differential
3. *Daily following high-dose systemic methotrexate administration:* Methotrexate levels

REGIMEN

THE BONN PROTOCOL

Pels H et al. JCO 2003;21:4489–4495

Sequence of cycles (periods of drug administration are separated by a 2-week interval)

A1 →	B1 →	C1 →	A2 →	B2 →	C2
D1–5	D22–26	D43–49	D64–68	D85–89	D106–112

Cycle A:
Hydration with 5% dextrose/0.45% NaCl injection (D5W/0.45% NS) with sodium bicarbonate injection 100 mEq/1000 mL intravenously at 100–125 mL/hour (2400–3000 mL/day). Monitor fluid status carefully
Patients ≤64 years:
Methotrexate loading dose 500 mg/m^2 by intravenous infusion in 25–500 mL 0.9% NaCl injection (0.9% NS) or 5% dextrose injection (D5W) over 30 minutes, given on day 1, *followed immediately by:*
Methotrexate continuous infusion 4500 mg/m^2 by continuous intravenous infusion in 250–3000 mL 0.9% NS or D5W over 23.5 hours on day 1 (total dosage/ cycle [not including intrathecal methotrexate] = 5000 mg/m^2)
Patients >64 years:
Methotrexate loading dose 500 mg/m^2 by intravenous infusion in 25–500 mL 0.9% NaCl injection (0.9% NS) or 5% dextrose injection (D5W) over 30 minutes, given on day 1, *followed immediately by:*
Methotrexate continuous infusion 2500 mg/m^2 by continuous intravenous infusion in 250–3000 mL 0.9% NS or D5W over 23.5 hours on day 1 (total dosage/ cycle [not including intrathecal methotrexate] = 3000 mg/m^2)
All patients:
Leucovorin calcium 30 mg/m^2 intravenously in 5–50 mL D5W or 0.9% NS over 10–30 minutes

Leucovorin Administration Schedule

Normal Methotrexate Clearance Anticipated	Delayed Methotrexate Clearance
At 10, 18, 24, 30, and 42 hours after methotrexate administration concludes	Every 4 hours until serum methotrexate is <0.2 micromol/L

Vincristine 2 mg by intravenous injection over 1–3 minutes, given on day 1 (total dose/cycle = 2 mg)
Ifosfamide 800 mg/m^2 per day by intravenous infusion in 100–250 mL 0.9% NS or D5W over 1 hour for 4 consecutive days on days 2–5 (total dosage/cycle = 3200 mg/m^2)
Mesna 800 mg/m^2 per day by continuous intravenous infusion in 250–1000 mL 0.9% NS or D5W over 24 hours for 4 consecutive days on days 2–5 (total dosage/cycle = 3200 mg/m^2)
Dexamethasone 10 mg/m^2 per day orally for 4 consecutive days on days 2–5, *only during the A2 cycle* (total dosage/cycle = 40 mg/m^2)
Prednisolone 2.5 mg per day intrathecally for 3 consecutive days on days 1–4 (total dose/cycle = 10 mg)
Methotrexate 3 mg per day intrathecally for 3 consecutive days on days 1–4 (total dose/cycle [not including systemic methotrexate] = 12 mg)
Cytarabine 30 mg intrathecally on day 5 (total dose/cycle = 30 mg)

Cycle B:
Hydration with D5W/0.45% NS with sodium bicarbonate injection 100 mEq/1000 mL intravenously at 100–125 mL/hour (2400–3000 mL/day). Monitor fluid status carefully
Patient ≤64 years:
Methotrexate loading dose 500 mg/m^2 by intravenous infusion in 25–500 mL 0.9% NaCl injection (0.9% NS) or 5% dextrose injection (D5W) over 30 minutes, given on day 1, *followed immediately by:*

(*continued*)

Treatment Modifications

Adverse Event	Dose Modification
Creatinine clearance (Clcr) <100 mL/min	Decrease methotrexate dosage by a percentage equivalent to the percentage decrease from creatinine clearance of 100 mL/min (eg, for Clcr = 90 mL/min, decrease methotrexate dosage by 10%)
G ≥3 Peripheral neuropathy	Omit vincristine and vindesine from subsequent cycles. Can re-institute at reduced dosage (50%) if neuropathy improves to ≤G2

Patient Population Studied

A study of 65 consecutive patients with newly diagnosed primary central nervous system lymphoma. Radiation therapy was deferred

Efficacy (N = 61)

Complete response	61%
Partial response	10%
Progressive disease	20%
Not evaluated	9%
Estimated time to treatment failure*	21 months
Estimated median overall survival*	50 months
Estimated 2-year survival	69% (57–80%)
Estimated 5-year survival	43% (26–60%)

*Kaplan-Meser estimate

(continued)

Methotrexate continuous infusion 4500 mg/m² by continuous intravenous infusion in 250–3000 mL 0.9% NS or D5W over 23.5 hours on day 1 (total dosage/ cycle [not including intrathecal methotrexate] = 5000 mg/m²)
Patient >64 years:
Methotrexate loading dose 500 mg/m² by intravenous infusion in 25–500 mL 0.9% NaCl injection (0.9% NS) or 5% dextrose injection (D5W) over 30 minutes, given on day 1, *followed immediately by:*
Methotrexate continuous infusion 2500 mg/m² by continuous intravenous infusion in 250–3000 mL 0.9% NS or D5W over 23.5 hours on day 1 (total dosage/ cycle [not including intrathecal methotrexate] = 3000 mg/m²)
All patients:
Leucovorin calcium 30 mg/m² intravenously in 5–50 mL D5W or 0.9% NS over 10–30 minutes

Leucovorin Administration Schedule

Normal Methotrexate Clearance Anticipated	Delayed Methotrexate Clearance
At 10, 18, 24, 30, and 42 hours after methotrexate administration concludes	Every 4 hours until serum methotrexate is <0.2 micromol/L

Vincristine 2 mg by intravenous injection over 1–3 minutes, given on day 1 (total dose/cycle = 2 mg)
Cyclophosphamide 200 mg/m² per day by intravenous infusion in 25–1000 mL 0.9% NS over 1 hour for 4 consecutive days on days 2–5 (total dosage/cycle = 800 mg/m²)
Mesna 200 mg/m² per day by continuous intravenous infusion in 250–1000 mL 0.9% NS or D5W over 24 hours for 4 consecutive days on days 2–5 (total dosage/cycle = 800 mg/m²)
Dexamethasone 10 mg/m² per day orally for 4 consecutive days on days 2–5, *only during the B2 cycle* (total dosage/cycle = 40 mg/m²)
Prednisolone 2.5 mg per day intrathecally for 3 consecutive days on days 1–4 (total dose/cycle = 10 mg)
Methotrexate 3 mg per day intrathecally for 3 consecutive days on days 1–4 (total dose/cycle [not including systemic methotrexate] = 12 mg)
Cytarabine 30 mg intrathecally on day 5 (total dose/cycle = 30 mg)

Cycle C:
Cytarabine 3000 mg/m² per day by intravenous infusion in 50–500 mL 0.9% NS or D5W over 3 hours for 2 doses on days 1 and 2 (total dosage/cycle [not including intrathecal cytarabine] = 6000 mg/m²)
Vindesine* 5 mg by intravenous injection over 1–3 minutes, given on day 1 (total dose/cycle = 5 mg)
Dexamethasone 10 mg/m² per day orally for 5 consecutive days on days 3–7 (total dosage/cycle = 50 mg/m²)
Prednisolone 2.5 mg per day intrathecally for 4 consecutive days on days 3–6 (total dose/cycle = 10 mg)
Methotrexate 3 mg per day intrathecally for 4 consecutive days on days 3–6 (total dose/cycle = 12 mg)
Cytarabine 30 mg intrathecally on day 7 (total dose/cycle [not including systemic cytarabine] = 30 mg)

*Although vindesine had once received FDA approval for commercial use, it is not currently marketed in the United States

Dexamethasone is marketed in the United States in numerous formulations for oral administration, such as 0.25-, 0.5-, 0.75-, 1-, 2-, 4-, and 6-mg tablets, and in elixirs (which contain alcohol) and solutions for oral administration

Emetogenic potential:
During A and B cycles
Day 1: Moderately high (Emetogenicity score = 4)
Days 2–5: Moderate (Emetogenicity score = 3)
During C cycles
Days 1 and 2: Moderately High (Emetogenicity score = 4). See Chapter 39

Toxicity (N = 65)

Toxicity	% Patients
G3/4 Leukopenia	94
G3/4 Thrombocytopenia	89
Febrile neutropenia	17
G4 Infection	9
G3 Infection	9
Sepsis	8
Treatment-related death	9
Ommaya reservoir-associated infections	19
G2 nephrotoxicity (transient)	14
G ≥3 Mucositis	12
Deep venous thrombosis	5
Transient vasculitis	3
Transient encephalopathy [a]	9
Clinical peripheral neuropathy	2
White matter changes on MRI	35[b]

[a]With methotrexate and ifosfamide
[b]20 of 57 patients
WHO Toxicity Scale

Therapy Monitoring

1. *Daily on days of chemotherapy:* CBC with differential, serum electrolytes, BUN, creatinine, and LFTs
2. *Weekly:* CBC with differential, serum electrolytes, BUN, creatinine and LFTs
3. *Following methotrexate administration:* Daily methotrexate levels

REGIMEN

NEW APPROACHES TO BRAIN TUMOR THERAPY (NABTT) CNS CONSORTIUM 96-07

Batchelor T et al. JCO 2003;21:1044–1049
Herrlinger U et al. Ann Neurol 2002;51:247–252

Hydration with each cycle:
5% Dextrose/0.45% NaCl injection with sodium bicarbonate 50–75 mEq/1000 mL, *or* 5% Dextrose/0.2% NaCl injection with sodium bicarbonate 100–125 mEq/1000 mL intravenously at a rate sufficient to produce a urine output >100 mL/hour and urine pH ≥7.0. Continue until serum methotrexate concentration is <0.1 micromol/L. Begin methotrexate administration after urine output >100 mL/hour and urine pH ≥7.0 for ≥4 hours

Induction
Methotrexate 8000 mg/m^2 by continuous intravenous infusion in 100 mL to ≥1000 mL 0.9% NaCl injection (0.9% NS) or 5% dextrose injection (D5W) over 4 hours every 14 days until complete response or a maximum of 8 cycles (total dosage/cycle = 8000 mg/m^2)
Calcium leucovorin 25 mg by intravenous infusion in 25–250 mL 0.9% NS or D5W over 5–30 minutes every 6 hours, starting 24 hours after methotrexate began, continuing until serum methotrexate <0.10 micromol/L
Consolidation (after CR):
Methotrexate 8000 mg/m^2 by continuous intravenous infusion in 100 mL to ≥1000 mL 0.9% NS or D5W over 4 hours every 14 days for 2 cycles (total dosage/cycle = 8000 mg/m^2), *then*:
Calcium leucovorin 25 mg by intravenous infusion in 25–250 mL 0.9% NS or D5W over 5–30 minutes every 6 hours, starting 24 hours after methotrexate began, continuing until serum methotrexate <0.10 micromol/L
Maintenance:
Methotrexate 8000 mg/m^2 by continuous intravenous infusion in 100 mL to ≥1000 mL 0.9% NS or D5W over 4 hours every 28 days for 11 cycles (total dosage/cycle = 8000 mg/m^2)
Calcium leucovorin 25 mg by intravenous infusion in 25–250 mL 0.9% NS or D5W over 5–30 minutes every 6 hours, starting 24 hours after methotrexate began, continuing until serum methotrexate <0.10 micromol/L

Emetogenic potential: Moderately high (Emetogenicity score = 4). See Chapter 39 for antiemetic regimens

Toxicity

1. After 287 cycles of high-dose methotrexate, 12 patients experienced 18 episodes of G3/4 adverse events (unspecified)
2. Mini-Mental State Evaluation score declined from 29 at baseline to 27 at follow-up in 1 of 19 patients

Therapy Monitoring

1. *Daily during hospital admission for high-dose methotrexate:* Serum BUN, creatinine, WBC, hemoglobin, platelet count, and methotrexate level
2. *Before each repeated cycle:* 24-hour urine collection for creatinine clearance, CBC with differential, ophthalmologic examination, and CSF cytopathology if it was originally positive before repeated cycles

Treatment Modification

Adverse Event	Dose Modification
Creatinine clearance (Clcr) <100 mL/	Decrease methotrexate dosage by a percentage equivalent to the percentage decrease from creatinine clearance of 100 mL/min (eg, for Clcr = 90 mL/min, decrease methotrexate dosage by 10%)

Patient Population Studied

A study of 25 patients with primary CNS lymphoma, among whom 5 patients had evidence of ocular lymphoma

Efficacy (N = 23)

Radiographic complete response	52%
Radiographic partial response	22%
Disease progression during treatment	22%
Among 5 patients with ocular involvement	
Radiographic complete response in brain	80%
Radiographic partial response in brain	20%
Resolution of ocular signs	80%

REGIMEN

MEMORIAL SLOAN-KETTERING REGIMEN (RTOG 93-10)

DeAngelis LM et al. JCO 2002;20:4643–4648

Induction (pre-irradiation) chemotherapy
Methotrexate 2500 mg/m^2 per dose by intravenous infusion in 250 mL to ≥1000 mL 0.9% NaCl injection (0.9% NS) or 5% dextrose injection (D5W) (or saline and dextrose combinations) over 2–3 hours every second week for 5 doses on day 1 during weeks 1, 3, 5, 7, and 9 (total dosage/10-week course [not including intrathecal methotrexate] = 12,500 mg/m^2)
Leucovorin calcium 20 mg/dose orally every 6 hours for 12 doses, starting 24 hours after methotrexate administration on days 2–4
Hydration after methotrexate:
D5W , 5% dextrose/0.2% NaCl injection (D5W/0.2% NS), or 5% dextrose/0.45% NaCl injection (D5W/0.45% NS), with sodium bicarbonate injection 50–125 mEq/1000 mL intravenously at 1500–1800 mL/m^2 for 24 hours, then 1000 mL/m^2 per day for the next 48 hours
Vincristine 1.4 mg/m^2 per dose (maximum single dose = 2.8 mg) by intravenous injection over 1–3 minutes every second week for 5 doses on day 1 during weeks 1, 3, 5, 7, and 9 (total dosage/10-week course = 7 mg/m^2; maximum dose/10-week course = 14 mg)
Procarbazine 100 mg/m^2 per day orally for 7 consecutive days every 28 days for 3 cycles on days 1–7 during weeks 1, 5, and 9 (total dosage/cycle = 700 mg/m^2; total dosage/10 week course = 2100 mg/m^2)
Methotrexate 12 mg/dose intrathecally via intraventricular catheter or reservoir (eg, Ommaya) every second week for 5 doses, weeks 2, 4, 6, 8, and 10 (total dosage/10-week course [not including systemic methotrexate] = 60 mg)
Leucovorin calcium 10 mg/dose orally every 6 hours for 8 doses, starting the evening after each intrathecal methotrexate administration
Dexamethasone orally every day on a de-escalating dose sequence during weeks 1–6, as follows:

Dexamethasone Dose*

Week	Daily	Total per week
1	16 mg	112 mg
2	12 mg	84 mg
3	8 mg	56 mg
4	6 mg	42 mg
5	4 mg	28 mg
6	2 mg	14 mg

*Dexamethasone dose can be adjusted based on a patient's neurologic condition; can discontinue after week 6.

Procarbazine is manufactured in the United States in capsules for oral administration containing 50 mg procarbazine HCl
Dexamethasone is marketed in the United States in numerous formulations for oral administration, such as 0.25-, 0.5-, 0.75-, 1-, 2-, 4-, and 6-mg tablets, and in elixirs (which contain alcohol) and solutions for oral administration
Leucovorin calcium is manufactured in the United States in tablets for oral administration containing 5, 15, and 25 mg leucovorin calcium

Whole-brain radiation therapy
1.8 Gy/fraction per day for 5 days/week for 5 weeks, weeks 11–15 (ie, "standard radiation therapy"; total dose/course=45 Gy)

Notes:

- For ocular lymphoma, both eyes are included in the irradiated field at 1.8 Gy/fraction to a total dose of 36 Gy in 20 fractions
- Dose rate is modified for patients who achieve a CR at the end of the initial 10 weeks of chemotherapy to 1.2 Gy/fraction, 2 fractions/day separated by ≥6 hours, for 15 days (total dose/course = 36 Gy)

(*continued*)

Treatment Modifications

None described

Patient Population Studied

A study of 102 patients with primary CNS lymphoma

Efficacy (N = 50*)

Response after pre-irradiation chemotherapy	
Complete response	58%
Partial response	36%

*Patients in whom tumors had not been completely resected prior to study treatment

Toxicity

Induction Therapy (N = 98 patients)	
Any G3/4 adverse event	53%
G3/4 Myelosuppression	28%
G3/4 Nephrotoxicity	3%
G3/4 Acute CNS symptoms	9%
Radiation Therapy (N = 82 patients)	
Any G3/4/5 adverse event	73%
G3/4 Myelosuppression*	46%
Severe delayed neurologic toxicities	15%
Leukoencephalopathy	16%
Death due to neurologic toxicity	10%
Patients with a CR after chemotherapy and standard radiation therapy (N = 27)	
G3 Neurotoxicity	3.7%
Patients with a CR after chemotherapy and hyperfractionated radiation therapy (N = 13)	
G 4/5 Neurotoxicity	23%

*The final chemotherapy cycle may have contributed to this toxicity
NCI CTC

(continued)

Postirradiation chemotherapy
Cytarabine 3000 mg/m^2 per day by intravenous infusion in 50–500 mL 0.9% NS over 3 hours for 2 consecutive days, weeks 16 and 19 (total dosage/course = 6000 mg/m^2)

Supportive care
- *PCP prophylaxis*: **Cotrimoxazole** (trimethoprim 160 mg + sulfamethoxazole 800 mg) orally, one dose, 3 times per week (eg, Monday, Wednesday, and Friday)
- *Oropharyngeal antifungal prophylaxis:* **Clotrimazole** 10-mg troche one troche 5 times daily

Emetogenic potential:
During induction chemotherapy (weeks 1, 5, and 9)
Day 1: High (Emetogenicity score = 5)
Days 2–7: Moderately high (Emetogenicity score = 4)
During induction chemotherapy (weeks 3 and 7)
Day 1: Moderately high (Emetogenicity score = 4)
During postirradiation chemotherapy (weeks 16 and 19)
Days 1 and 2: Moderately high (Emetogenicity score = 4). See Chapter 39 for antiemetic regimens

Therapy Monitoring

1. *Before each cycle:* PE, CBC with differential, LFTs, BUN and creatinine
2. *Daily during hospital admission for high-dose methotrexate:* Serum BUN, creatinine, WBC count, hemoglobin, platelet count, and methotrexate level
3. *Before each repeated cycle*: 24-hour urine collection for creatinine clearance, CBC with differential, ophthalmologic examination, and CSF cytopathology if it was originally positive before repeated cycles

26. Melanoma

Michael M. Boyiadzis, MD, MHSc, and Barry Gause, MD

Epidemiology

Incidence: 62,190 new cases in 2006
Estimated deaths: 7910 in 2006
Median age: 45–55 years
Male/female ratio: 1.1:1

Stage at Presentation	
Stage 0:	49.3%
Stage I:	36.3%
Stage II:	7.3%
Stage III:	3.7%
Stage IV:	3.4%

Jemal A et al. CA Cancer J Clin 2006;56:106–30
Koh HK. NEJM 1991;325:171–182
National Cancer Institute, Surveillance, Epidemiology and End Results (SEER) Program

Work-Up

Stage IB Stage II	Chest x-ray (optional), LDH (optional) Further imaging as clinically indicated for stage IIB, IIC patients (CT scan ± PET/MRI)
Stage IIIA	Chest x-ray, LDH. Further imaging if clinically indicated (CT scan ± PET, and/or MRI)
Stage IIIB Stage IIIC	FNA preferred, if feasible, otherwise lymph node biopsy Chest x-ray, LDH, pelvic CT and if inguinofemoral nodes positive Further imaging if clinically indicated (CT scan ± PET, or MRI)
Stage IV	FNA preferred, if feasible, otherwise lymph node biopsy Chest x-ray and/or chest CT, LDH; consider abdomen/pelvic CT, head MRI and/or PET Further imaging if clinically indicated

National Comprehensive Cancer Network. Version 1.2004

Pathology

Melanoma types

1. Superficial spreading melanoma	60–70 %
2. Nodular melanoma	15–30%
3. Lentigo maligna melanoma	5%
4. Acral lentiginous melanoma	2–8%

Lotze MT, Dollard RM, Kirkwood JM, Flickinger JC. Cutaneous melanoma. In: DeVita VT et al: Cancer: Principles & Practice of Oncology, 6th ed. Lippincott Williams & Wilkins, 2001

Staging

Primary Tumor

Tx	Primary tumor cannot be assessed
T0	No evidence of primary tumor
Tis	M in situ
T1	M ≤ 1.0 mm in thickness with or without ulceration
T1a	M ≤ 1.0 mm in thickness and level II or III, no ulceration
T1b	M ≤ 1.0 mm in thickness and level IV or V or with ulceration
T2	M 1.01–2.0 mm in thickness with or without ulceration
T2a	M 1.01–2.0 mm in thickness, no ulceration
T2b	M 1.01–2.0 mm in thickness with ulceration
T3	M 2.01–4.0 mm in thickness with or without ulceration
T3a	M 2.01–4.0 mm in thickness, no ulceration
T3b	M 2.01–4.0 mm in thickness with ulceration
T4	M > 4.0 mm in thickness with or without ulceration
T4 a	M > 4.0 mm in thickness, no ulceration
T4b	M > 4.0 mm in thickness, with ulceration

M, melanoma
AJCC Cancer Staging Manual, 6th ed. New York: Springer-Verlag, 2002

Distant Metastasis (M)

MX	Distant metastasis cannot be assessed
M0	No distant metastasis
M1	Distant metastasis
M1a	Metastasis to skin or subcutaneous tissues or distant lymph nodes
M1b	Metastasis to lung
M1c	Metastasis to all other visceral sites or distant metastasis at any site associated with elevated serum LDH

Reproduced, with permission, of the American Joint Committee on Cancer (AJCC), Chicago, Illinois. The original source for this material is the AJCC Cancer Staging Manual, 6th edition (2002) published by Springer-Verlag, New York, www.springeronline.com.

Clinical Staging

Stage 0	Tis, N0, M0
Stage IA	T1a, N0, M0
Stage IB	T1b, N0, M0 T2a, N0, M0
Stage IIA	T2b, N0, M0 T3a, N0, M0
Stage IIB	T3b, N0, M0 T4a, N0, M0
Stage IIC	T4b, N0, M0
Stage III	Any T, N1, M0 Any T, N2, M0 Any T, N3, M0
Stage IV	Any T, any N, M1

Clinical staging includes microstaging of the primary melanoma and clinical/radiologic evaluations for metastases. By convention, it should be used after complete excision of the primary melanoma with clinical assessment for regional and distant metastases
AJCC Cancer Staging Manual, 6th ed. New York: Springer-Verlag, 2002

Pathologic Staging

Stage 0	Tis, N0, M0
Stage IA	T1a, N0, M0
Stage IB	T1b, N0, M0 T2a, N0, M0
Stage IIA	T2b, N0, M0 T3a, N0, M0
Stage IIB	T3b, N0, M0 T4a, N0, M0
Stage IIC	T4b, N0, M0
Stage III A	T1-4a, N1a, M0
Stage IIIB	T1-4a, N2a, M0 T1-4b, N1a, M0 T1-4b, N2a, M0 T1-4a, N1b, M0 T1-4a, N2b, M0 T1-4a/b, N2c, M0
Stage IIIC	T1-4b, N1b, M0 T1-4b, N2b, M0 Any T, N3, M0
Stage IV	Any T, any N, M1

Pathologic staging includes microstaging of the primary melanoma and pathologic information about the regional lymph nodes after partial or complete lymphadenopathy. PS0 or PSIA patients are exception; they do not require pathologic evaluation of their lymph nodes
Reproduced, with permission, of the American Joint Committee on Cancer (AJCC), Chicago, Illinois. The original source for this material is the AJCC Cancer Staging Manual, 6th edition (2002) published by Springer-Verlag, New York, www.springeronline.com.

Five-Year Relative Survival

Stage I:	97%
Stage II:	75%
Stage III:	48%
Stage IV:	13%

NCI, Surveillance, Epidemiology and End Results (SEER) Program

Caveats

Tumor Thickness	Recommended Margins
In situ	0.5 cm
≤1.0 mm	1.0 cm
1.01–2.0 mm	1–2 cm
2.01–4.0 mm	2.0 cm
>4.0 mm	2.0 cm

The recommended surgical margin in the treatment of melanoma depends on the tumor thickness
National Comprehensive Cancer Network: Version 1 (2004)

1. Interferon is recommended as adjuvant therapy for patients with stage III or lesions >4.0 mm thickness (T4)
2. In other than the adjuvant setting, although a higher response rate can be achieved with CDB ± TAM compared with single-agent dacarbazine or single-agent temozolomide, the overwhelming majority of responses are partial responses, so that overall survival appears to be similar. Thus, the available evidence indicates single-agent therapy may be as effective as a combination regimen
3. The advantage of adding thalidomide to temozolomide is uncertain; a direct comparison with single-agent temozolomide has not been performed, precluding definite conclusions as to whether it results in a significantly longer prolongation of survival with tolerable side effects
4. For many patients, single-agent chemotherapy may be considered the optimal first choice especially in the elderly and in patients with comorbid conditions and poor performance status
5. When possible, patients with metastatic melanoma should be referred for clinical trials

REGIMEN

INTERFERON ALFA-2B

Kirkwood JM et al. JCO 1996;14:7–17 [Trial E1684]

Interferon alfa-2b 20 million units/m^2 per dose intravenously over 20 minutes in 0.9% NaCl injection (0.9% NS), sufficient to produce a solution with an interferon concentration ≥10 million units/100 mL, 5 consecutive days/week for 4 weeks (total dosage/week = 100 million units /m^2), *then:*
Interferon alfa-2b 10 million units /m^2 per dose subcutaneously 3 days/week for 48 weeks (total dosage/week = 30 million units /m^2)

Emetogenic potential: Nonemetogenic (Emetogenicity score = 1). See Chapter 39 for antiemetic regimens

Patient Population Studied

A study of 143 patients with deep primary (T4) or regionally metastatic (N1) cutaneous melanoma who had no evidence of distant metastatic disease or significant medical or psychiatric comorbidity and had not previously received systemic adjuvant therapy

Efficacy (N = 143)

Median relapse-free survival	1.72 years
Overall median survival	3.8 years
5-year relapse-free survival rate	37%

Toxicity (N = 143)

	% G1/2	% G3/4
Constitutional*	50	48
Myelosuppression	66	24
Neutropenia		26
Neurologic	55	28
Depression		10
Hepatotoxicity	48	14

*Fever, chills, fatigue, malaise, diaphoresis

(1) Other adverse effects of IFN alfa-2b: anorexia, weight loss, alopecia, transient mild rashlike erythema, exacerbation of psoriasis, erythema or induration at the site of injection, impaired cognitive function, alternating episodes of manic depression
(2) Rare adverse effects of IFN alfa-2b: rhabdomyolysis, delirium, cutaneous necrosis at the site of injection
(3) Thyroid dysfunction (hypothyroidism or hyperthyroidism) occurs in 8–20% of patients

Kirkwood JM et al. JCO 2002;20:3703–3718
Kirkwood JM et al. JCO 1996;14:7–17

Therapy Monitoring

1. *WBC, LFTs, electrolytes, and mineral panel:* Weekly during induction, monthly during maintenance therapy for at least 3 months, then no less frequently than every 3 months in patients who are stable with no new complaints
2. *Other standard tests (e.g., serum electrolytes, thyroid stimulating hormone (TSH) levels):* Recommended at baseline and at least every 3 months during treatment

Treatment Modifications

Adverse Event	Dose Modification
First occurrence of a DLT*	Hold dose until resolution, then reduce interferon alfa dosage by 33%
Second occurrence of a DLT*	Hold dose until resolution, then decrease interferon alfa dosage by 66%
Third occurrence of a DLT*	Discontinue interferon alfa therapy

(1) Dose reductions or delays are usually required at least once for 50% of patients during the IV treatment phase and for 48% during the subcutaneous treatment phase
(2) 74% of patients with appropriate dose reductions continue treatment on protocol for 1 year or until relapse
(3) Most treatment withdrawals occur in the first 4 months of treatment, after which, discontinuation of therapy due to toxicity is unusual
(4) A response to other adverse events is determined largely by the patient and treating physician. Side effects are rarely life threatening and should not lead to discontinuation if appropriate and proactive supportive care is provided

*Definitions of dose-limiting toxicities (DLTs): hematologic DLT, granulocyte count <500/mm^3; hepatic DLT, SGPT (ALT) or SGOT (AST) >5 times ULN (upper limit of normal)

Buzaid AC et al. Cancer Ther 1998;1:178–183
Kirkwood JM et al. JCO 2002;20:3703–3718

Notes

Developed as an adjuvant regimen

REGIMEN

CISPLATIN, DACARBAZINE (DTIC), CARMUSTINE (BCNU) + TAMOXIFEN (CDB + TAM)

Creagan ET et al. JCO 1999;17:1884–1890

Cisplatin 25 mg/m^2 per day intravenously in 500 mL 5% dextrose and 0.45% NaCl injection (D5W/0.45% NS) over 30–45 minutes for 3 consecutive days on days 1–3 every 21 days (total dosage/cycle = 75 mg/m^2)
Hydration: Encourage high oral intake. Monitor and replace magnesium/electrolytes as needed
Dacarbazine 220 mg/m^2 per day intravenously in 500 mL D5W/0.45% NS over 60 minutes for 3 consecutive days on days 1–3 every 21 days (total dosage/cycle = 660 mg/m^2)
Carmustine 150 mg/m^2 single dose intravenously over 2–3 hours in 750–1000 mL 5% dextrose injection (D5W) on day 1 every 42 days (total dosage/2 consecutive cycles = 150 mg/m^2)
Note: Carmustine treatment is repeated only during odd-numbered cycles (ie, during cycles 1, 3, 5, 7, etc)

Tamoxifen 20 mg orally daily (total dose/cycle = 420 mg)

Tamoxifen citrate is available in the United States in tablet formulations containing either 10 mg or 20 mg of tamoxifen base. Nolvadex® (tamoxifen citrate) AstraZeneca Pharmaceuticals LP, Wilmington, DE

Emetogenic potential:
Day 1: Very high (Emetogenicity score = 7 with carmustine; 6 without carmustine)
Days 2 and 3: Very high (Emetogenicity score = 6)
High potential for delayed symptoms. See Chapter 39 for antiemetic regimens

Patient Population Studied

A study of 92 patients with advanced malignant melanoma with no CNS metastasis and no prior chemotherapy

Efficacy (N = 92 CDB + TAM)

Measurable Disease (n = 72)	
Complete response	0%
Partial responses	32%
Assessable Disease (n = 20)	
Regression	10%
Measurable and Assessable Disease (N = 92)	
Objective response rate	27%
Mean duration of response	6.6 months
Median time to progression	3.1 months
Median survival	6.9 months

Toxicity (N = 86 CDB + TAM)

	% G3/4
Nonhematologic	
Lethargy	12
Nausea	10
Vomiting	9
Neuromotor	5
Hematologic	
Leukopenia (<2000 WBC/mm^3)	~40
Thrombocytopenia (<50,000 platelets/mm^3)	65

Treatment Modifications

Adverse Event	Dose Modification
Nadir ANC <1500/mm^3	Reduce cisplatin, carmustine, and dacarbazine dosages by 33%
Nadir platelet count <50,000/mm^3	Reduce cisplatin, carmustine, and dacarbazine dosages by 33%
Creatinine clearance <50% baseline value	Hold chemotherapy until creatinine clearance >50% baseline

In the referenced study, dose reductions were required frequently. After 2 cycles, at least 45% of patients were receiving less than 95% of the original dose. By the fifth cycle at least two-thirds of patients were receiving reduced doses

Therapy Monitoring

1. *Before each cycle:* CBC with differential, serum creatinine, LFTs, mineral panel, and electrolytes. Creatinine clearance is measured if serum creatinine increases by >25% from pretreatment values
2. *Response evaluation every 2 cycles:* PE, chest x-ray, and CT scans

REGIMEN

CISPLATIN, DACARBAZINE (DTIC), CARMUSTINE (BCNU) [CDB]

Creagan ET et al. JCO 1999;17:1884–1890

Cisplatin 25 mg/m^2 per day intravenously in 500 mL 5% dextrose and 0.45% NaCl injection (D5W/0.45% NS) over 30–45 minutes for 3 consecutive days on days 1–3 every 21 days (total dosage/cycle = 75 mg/m^2)
Hydration: Encourage high oral intake. Monitor and replace magnesium/electrolytes as needed
Dacarbazine 220 mg/m^2 per day intravenously in 500 mL D5W/0.45% NS over 60 minutes for 3 consecutive days on days 1–3 every 21 days (total dosage/cycle = 660 mg/m^2)
Carmustine 150 mg/m^2 single dose intravenously over 2–3 hours in 750–1000 mL 5% dextrose injection (D5W) on day 1 every 42 days (total dosage/2 consecutive cycles = 150 mg/m^2)

Note: Carmustine treatment is repeated only during odd-numbered cycles (ie, during cycles 1, 3, 5, 7, etc)

Emetogenic potential:
Day 1: Very high (Emetogenicity score = 7 with carmustine; 6 without carmustine)
Days 2 and 3: Very high (Emetogenicity score = 6)
High potential for delayed symptoms. See Chapter 39 for antiemetic regimens

Treatment Modifications

Adverse Event	Dose Modification
Nadir ANC <1500/mm^3	Reduce cisplatin, carmustine, and dacarbazine dosages by 33%
Nadir platelet count <50,000/mm^3	Reduce cisplatin, carmustine, and dacarbazine dosages by 33%
Creatinine clearance <50% baseline value	Hold chemotherapy until creatinine clearance >50% baseline

In the referenced study, dose reductions were required frequently. After 2 cycles, at least 45% of patients were receiving less than 95% of the original dose. By the fifth cycle at least two-thirds of patients were receiving reduced doses

Patient Population Studied

A study of 92 patients with advanced malignant melanoma with no CNS metastasis and no prior chemotherapy

Efficacy (N = 92)

Measurable Disease (n = 72)	
Complete response	13%
Partial responses	24%
Assessable Disease (n = 20)	
Regression	20%
Measurable and Assessable Disease (N = 92)	
Objective response rate	33%
Mean duration of response	4.4 months
Median time to progression	3.4 months
Median survival	6.8 months

Toxicity (N = 90)

	% G3/4
Nonhematologic	
Lethargy	9
Nausea	9
Vomiting	3
Neuromotor	4
Hematologic	
Leukopenia (<2000 WBC/mm^3)	~40
Thrombocytopenia (<50,000 platelets/mm^3)	85

Therapy Monitoring

1. *Before each cycle:* CBC with differential, serum creatinine, LFTs, mineral panel, and electrolytes. Creatinine clearance is measured if serum creatinine increases by >25% from pretreatment values
2. *Response evaluation every 2 cycles:* PE, chest x-ray, and CT scans

REGIMEN

DACARBAZINE (DTIC)

Middleton MR et al. JCO 2000;18:158–166

Dacarbazine 250 mg/m^2 (initial dosage) per day intravenously in 50–250 mL of either 5% dextrose injection (D5W) or 0.9% NaCl injection (0.9% NS) over 30 minutes for 5 consecutive days on days 1–5 every 21 days (total dosage/cycle = 1250 mg/m^2)

Emetogenic potential:
Days 1–5: High (Emetogenicity score = 5)
Potential for delayed symptoms. See Chapter 39 for antiemetic regimens

Treatment Modifications

Retreatment allowed if ANC ≥ 1500/mm^3 and platelet count ≥100,000/mm^3

Adverse Event	Dose Modification
Retreatment delayed by ≥2 weeks	Reduce dacarbazine dosage by 25%
G3/4 Nonhematologic toxicity	Reduce dacarbazine dosage by 50%
>2 dosage reductions	Discontinue therapy

Patient Population Studied

A study of 136 patients with histologically confirmed incurable or unresectable advanced metastatic melanoma. Patients with nonmeasurable disease, ocular melanoma, or CNS metastases were excluded

Efficacy (N = 136)

Complete response	2.9%
Partial response	10.3%
Stable disease	17.7%
Progressive disease	69.1%
Median overall survival	6.4 months

Toxicity (N = 136)

	% All G	% G3	% G4
Hematologic			
Anemia	11	0	1
Neutropenia	3	1	1
Thrombocytopenia	9	4	4
Nonhematologic			
Asthenia	14	1	0
Fatigue	18	2	0
Fever	18	2	0
Headache	12	1	0
Pain	39	13	0
Anorexia	20	2	0
Constipation	29	3	0
Nausea	38	4	0
Vomiting	24	4	0
Somnolence	13	1	0

Therapy Monitoring

1. *Before each cycle:* CBC with differential, LFTs, mineral panel, and electrolytes
2. *Response evaluation every 2 cycles:* PE, chest x-ray, and CT scans

REGIMEN

TEMOZOLOMIDE

Middleton MR et al. JCO 2000;18:158–166

Temozolomide 200 mg/m² per day orally for 5 consecutive days on days 1–5 every 28 days (total dosage/cycle = 1000 mg/m²)

Temozolomide is manufactured in the United States in capsules for oral administration in the following product strengths: 5 mg, 20 mg, 100 mg, and 250 mg. TEMODAR® (temozolomide) CAPSULES. Schering Corporation, Kenilworth, NJ

Emetogenic potential:
Days 1–5: Low (Emetogenicity score = 1). See Chapter 39 for antiemetic regimens

Patient Population Studied

A study of 144 patients with histologically confirmed incurable or unresectable advanced metastatic melanoma. Patients with nonmeasurable disease, ocular melanoma, or CNS metastases were excluded

Efficacy (N = 144)

Complete response	2.8%
Partial response	11.8%
Stable disease	19.4%
Progressive disease	66%
Median overall survival	7.7 months

Toxicity (N = 144)

	% All G	% G3	% G4
Asthenia	12	3	0
Fatigue	20	3	0
Fever	11	1	1
Headache	22	5	1
Pain	34	7	0
Anorexia	15	0	0
Constipation	30	3	0
Nausea	52	4	0
Vomiting	34	4	1
Somnolence	12	0	0
Anemia	8	1	1
Neutropenia	5	1	2
Thrombocytopenia	9	2	5

Treatment Modifications

Retreatment allowed if ANC ≥1500/mm³ and platelet count ≥100,000/mm³

Adverse Event	Dose Modification
Retreatment delayed by ≥2 weeks	Reduce temozolomide dosage by 25%
G3/4 Hematologic toxicity	Reduce temozolomide dosage by 25%
G3/4 Nonhematologic toxicity	Reduce temozolomide dosage by 50%
>2 dosage reductions	Discontinue therapy

Therapy Monitoring

1. *Before each cycle:* CBC with differential, LFTs, mineral panel, and electrolytes
2. *Response evaluation every 2 cycles:* PE, chest x-ray, and CT scans

REGIMEN

TEMOZOLOMIDE + THALIDOMIDE

Hwu WJ et al. JCO 2003;21:3351–3356

Temozolomide 75 mg/m^2 per day orally for 6 consecutive weeks every 8 weeks (2 weeks rest between cycles; total dosage/cycle = 3150 mg/m^2)
Patients <*70 years:* **Thalidomide** 200 mg per day orally for 6 weeks every 8 weeks (2 weeks rest between cycles) with dose escalation to 400 mg/day
Patients ≥*70 years of age:* **Thalidomide** 100 mg per day orally for 6 weeks every 8 weeks (2 weeks rest between cycles) with dose escalation to 250 mg/day

Temozolomide is manufactured in the United States in capsules for oral administration in the following product strengths: 5 mg, 20 mg, 100 mg, and 250 mg. TEMODAR® (temozolomide) CAPSULES. Schering Corporation, Kenilworth, NJ
Thalidomide is manufactured in the United States in capsules for oral administration in the following product strengths: 50 mg, 100 mg, and 200 mg. THALOMID® (thalidomide) CAPSULES. Celgene Corporation, Warren, NJ

Emetogenic potential: Low (Emetogenicity score = 2). See Chapter 39 for antiemetic regimens

Treatment Modifications

Thalidomide Dose Modification

Thalidomide dose escalation: Increase 50 mg/day every 2 weeks to allow adjustment for sedative effects

G3/G4 Neurotoxicity	Withhold thalidomide until toxicity is ≤1, then reduce thalidomide dose by 50 mg/day to a minimum of 50 mg/day. Continue with temozolomide at the same dose
G3/G4 Neurotoxicity at 50 mg/day	Discontinue therapy

Temozolomide Dose Modification

Retreatment allowed if ANC ≥1500/mm^3 and platelet count ≥100,000/mm^3

Retreatment delayed by ≥2 weeks	Reduce temozolomide dosage by 25%
Grades 3/4 Hematologic toxicity	Reduce temozolomide dosage by 25%
Grades 3/4 Nonhematologic toxicity	Reduce temozolomide dosage by 50%
>2 dosage reductions	Discontinue therapy

Most side effects/dose modifications are due to thalidomide
If a lower dose of thalidomide is tolerated, attempt to reescalate the dose every 2 weeks

Patient Population Studied

A study of 38 patients with unresectable stage III or IV melanoma. Patients with brain metastasis were excluded

Efficacy (N = 38)

Complete response	3%
Partial response*	29%
Minor response	18%
Stable disease	18%
Mixed response	5%
Progressive disease	26%
Overall median survival	9.5 months

*Five patients with >90% PR, surgical CR after resection

Toxicity (N = 38)

	% G2	% G3	% G4
Hematologic			
Lymphopenia	0	37	0
Leukopenia	13	8	3
Neutropenia	11	0	5
Anemia	11	3	0
Thrombocytopenia	0	0	3
Nonhematologic			
Rash	34	8	0
Constipation	29	11	0
Vomiting	29	5	0
Fatigue	21	11	0
Dizziness	24	3	0
Dyspnea	21	3	3
Nausea	16	8	0
Headache	13	3	0
Diarrhea	13	0	0
Edema	13	0	0
Infection	8	5	0
Drowsiness	11	0	0
Tremor	11	0	0
Abdominal cramps	8	0	0
Ataxia	8	0	0
Blurred vision	8	0	0
Neurosensory	8	0	0
Tumor pain	5	3	0
Tachycardia (SVT)	0	5	0
Laboratory Abnormalities			
Hyperglycemia	5	0	0
ALT	5	3	0
AST	3	3	0

Therapy Monitoring

1. *Before each cycle:* CBC with differential, LFTs, mineral panel, and electrolytes.
2. *Response evaluation after each 8-week cycle:* PE, chest x-ray, and CT scan.

27. Mesothelioma

Verna Vanderpuye, MD, and Nicholas J. Vogelzang, MD

Pleural Mesothelioma

Epidemiology

Incidence: 3000 new cases per year

Median age: 60 years

Male:female ratio: 3:1

Mortality rate: >10,000 deaths per year worldwide

Overall survival: 6–18 months

Peto J et al. Lancet 1995;345:535–539
Vogelzang NJ et al. Cancer 1984 53:377–383

Etiology

Causative factors

1. Asbestos exposure (~80% of cases, occur 30–40 years after exposure):
   a. Serpentine (Chrysolite) fibers
   b. Amphibole (Crocidolite, amosite) fibers
2. Others (~20% of cases):
   a. Therapeutic irradiation/Thorotrast™ (ThO_2 contrast medium)
   b. Chronic pleuritis
   c. Fibrous silicates, erionate, zeolite
   d. Viral oncogenes: Simian virus 40 (SV40) ~20–40% of cases
   e. Familial (Turkish families)
   f. Idiopathic/unknown

Carbone M et al. Semin Oncol 2002;29:2–17

Pathology

H & E staining

1. Epithelioid: 60% of cases = tubopapillary, granular, solid (occasional 5-year survival)
2. Sarcomatoid/mixed: 40% of cases (0% 5-year survival)

Immunohistochemical staining: Keratin positive, CEA negative, Leu M negative, calretinin positive
Cytogenetics: Deletion of short arm of chromosome 1 and 3 and long arm of chromosome 22

Chaihinan AP et al. In: Holland JC, Frei E, eds. Cancer Medicine, 5th ed. 2000:1293–1312
Corson SM. Semin Thorac Cardiovasc Surg 1997;9:347–355

Work-Up

1. *Chest x-ray:* Initial tool in diagnosing pleural plaques and effusion
2. *CT scan or MRI:* CT scan or MRI can be used to assess extent of disease. Calcifications are not generally visible on CT scan. Furthermore, the CT scan is less sensitive than the MRI in depicting diaphragmatic, pericardial and chest wall involvement
3. *PET scan:* Has shown benefit in assessing lymph node involvement but is useful in only 50–70% of cases
4. *Thoracentesis:* Used when there is a pleural effusion (30% diagnostic yield)
5. *CT-guided biopsy:* Depends on CT findings. If tumor is thick and easily biopsied, do a CT-directed biopsy
6. *Video-assisted thorascopic (VAT) surgery:* Do if on CT scan disease is thin or minimal or in a difficult location and thoracentesis is negative (90% diagnostic yield)

Flores RM et al. Proc Am Soc Clin Oncol 2003;22:620 [Abstract 2495]
Patz EF Jr et al. AJR Am J Roentgenol 1992;159:961–966
Schneider DB et al. J Thorac Cardiovasc Surg 2000;120:128–133
Steel JPC. Semin Oncol 2000;29:36–40

Staging

No defined universal staging system

Rusch VW. Chest 1995;108:1122–1128

Additional information

1. *Thoracic lymph node involvement:* 20% at presentation/70% at autopsy
2. *Hematogenous metastases:* Liver, lung, and bone: usually late in disease course

Adverse Prognostic Factors

1. Age
2. Performance status ≥2 (ECOG scale)
3. Nonepithelioid pathology
4. Low hemoglobin
5. Increased platelets
6. Increased WBC
7. Increased lactate dehydrogenase

Other factors

1. Increased cystathionine—vitamin B_6 deficiency
2. Tumor volume/chest plain
3. Low albumin/weight loss

Curran D et al. JCO 1998;16:145–52
Herndon JE et al. Chest 1998;113:723–731
Symanowski JT et al. Proc Am Soc Clin Oncol 2003;22:647 [Abstract 2602]

Caveats

Basic management issues

A. Surgical management

1. *Radical resection:* Role is controversial, especially in advanced disease because of the high morbidity and mortality rate as well as the high incidence of local recurrence
2. *Pleurectomy and decortication:* Indicated for minimal bulky disease associated with massive or recurrent pleural effusions
3. *Extrapleural pneumonectomy:* Indicated for early-stage epithelioid type with extensive involvement of the diaphragm and visceral pleural surfaces

B. Radiation therapy

Because of the large volume of lung in the radiation field, radiation is not usually recommended as single-modality treatment. It is, however, recommended for palliating pain and to prevent or treat chest wall masses that are the result of seeding from sites of invasive procedures, such as prior thoracocentesis or thorascopic surgery

C. Chemotherapy

Although there is no standard chemotherapy regimen, a two-drug regimen is recommended by most investigators. See text

Antman KH et al. In: DeVita VT Jr, Hellman S, Rosenberg SA, eds. Cancer: Principles & Practice of Oncology, 5th ed. Philadelphia: Lippincott, 1997:1856–1865
van Ruth S et al. Chest 2003;123:551–561

REGIMEN

GEMCITABINE + CISPLATIN

Byrne MJ et al. JCO 1999;17:25–30
van Haarst JW et al. Lung Cancer 2000;29(1 suppl 1):18 [Abstract 56]

Hydration: 0.9% NaCl injection (0.9% NS) ≥1000 mL before and after cisplatin by intravenous infusion over a minimum of 2–4 hours. Monitor and replace magnesium/electrolytes as needed

Cisplatin 100 mg/m² single dose by intravenous infusion in 100–250 mL 0.9% NS over 60 minutes, given on day 1 every 28 days for 6 cycles (total dosage/cycle = 100 mg/m²), *plus*
Gemcitabine 1000 mg/m² per dose by intravenous infusion in 50–250 mL 0.9% NS over 30 minutes, given on days 1, 8, and 15 every 28 days for 6 cycles (total dosage/cycle = 3000 mg/m²),

or

Cisplatin 80 mg/m² single dose by intravenous infusion in 100–250 mL 0.9% NS over 60 minutes, given on day 1 every 3 weeks for a maximum of 6 cycles (total dosage/cycle = 80 mg/m²), *plus*
Gemcitabine 1250 mg/m² per dose by intravenous infusion in 50–250 mL 0.9% NS over 30 minutes, given on days 1 and 8 every 3 weeks for a maximum of 6 cycles (total dosage/cycle = 2500 mg/m²)

Emetogenic potential:
Day 1: High (Emetogenicity score = 6). Potential for delayed symptoms after day 1
Days 8 and 15: Low (Emetogenicity score = 2). See Chapter 39 for antiemetic regimens

Treatment Modifications

Serum creatinine >1.4 mg/dL (>124 μmol/L), but <1.7 mg/dL (<150 μmol/L)	Decrease cisplatin by 50% and gemcitabine by 25%
Serum creatinine >1.7 mg/dL (>150 μmol/L)	Withhold cisplatin and gemcitabine until serum creatinine <1.7 mg/dL (<150 μmol/L), then administer 50% of the previous cisplatin dosage and 75% of the previous gemcitabine dosage
WBC <3000/mm³ or platelet <100,000/mm³ on days 1, 8, or 15	Decrease gemcitabine by 25%
WBC <2000/mm³ or platelet <75,000/mm³ on days 8 or 15	Omit gemcitabine

Byrne MJ et al. JCO 1999;17:25–30

Patient Population Studied

A study of 21 patients with advanced measurable pleural mesothelioma (Byrne MJ et al.)
A study of 25 patients with advanced measurable pleural mesothelioma (van Haarst JW et al.)

Efficacy (N = 46)

Response rate	18–47%
Duration of response	5–7 months
Estimated median survival	9.5–12 months
Estimated 1-year survival	41%

Nine of 10 responding patients achieved substantial or complete symptomatic improvement. Symptoms decreased significantly in three additional patients who achieved disease stabilization
From Byrne MJ et al. JCO 1999;17:25–30; and van Haarst JW et al. Lung Cancer 2000;29(1 suppl 1):18 [Abstract 56]

Toxicity (N = 21)

	Worst Toxicity Grade (%)				
	0	1	2	3	4
Hematologic					
Leukopenia	29	10	24	38	0
Thrombocytopenia[a]	24	14	29	14	19
Anemia	14	29	57	0	0
Nonhematologic					
Nausea/vomiting[b]	0	14	52	33	0
Stomatitis	62	38	0	0	0
Alopecia	71	24	5	0	0
Hearing loss	57	33	5	5	0
Neurologic	90	10	0	0	0

[a]Thrombocytopenia on days 8 or 15 was the major cause of dose modification
[b]One-third of patients had ≥ 1 episodes of severe nausea and vomiting, and symptoms were worse >24 hours after treatment

From Byrne MJ et al. JCO 1999;17:25–30

Therapy Monitoring

1. *Before chemotherapy on cycle days 1, 8, and 15:* CBC with differential, serum electrolytes, creatinine, bilirubin, ALT, and alkaline phosphatase
2. *Treatment evaluation:* Every 2 cycles

Byrne MJ et al. JCO 1999;17:25–30

REGIMEN

PEMETREXED + CISPLATIN

Vogelzang NJ et al. JCO 2003;21:2636–2644

Folic acid 350–1000 mcg daily orally, beginning 1–3 weeks before chemotherapy and continuing throughout treatment with pemetrexed + cisplatin, *and*
Cyanocobalamin (vitamin B_{12}) 1000 mcg intramuscularly every 9 weeks, beginning 1–3 weeks before chemotherapy and continuing throughout treatment with pemetrexed + cisplatin
Dexamethasone 8 mg intravenously or orally daily for 3 consecutive days, starting the day before pemetrexed administration to decrease the risk of severe skin rash associated with pemetrexed
Hydration: 0.9% NaCl injection (0.9% NS), ≥1000 mL before and after cisplatin by intravenous infusion over a minimum of 2–4 hours. Monitor and replace magnesium/electrolytes as needed
Pemetrexed 500 mg/m^2 by intravenous infusion in 10 mL 0.9% NS over 10 minutes, given on day 1 every 21 days (total dosage/cycle = 500 mg/m^2)
Cisplatin 75 mg/m^2 single dose by intravenous infusion in 1000 mL 0.9% NS over 2 hours on day 1, beginning 30 minutes after pemetrexed has been administered every 21 days (total dosage/cycle = 75 mg/m^2)

Emetogenic potential: High (Emetogenicity score = 6). Potential for delayed symptoms. See Chapter 39 for antiemetic regimens

Patient Population Studied

A study of 456 patients with advanced measurable pleural mesothelioma

Efficacy

Response rate	40–45%
Median time to progression	5–6 months
1-year survival	50%
Median survival	12–13 months

Therapy Monitoring

1. *Before initial and repeated treatments:* H&P, CBC with differential, calculated creatinine clearance, serum electrolytes glucose, calcium, LFTs, and vitamin metabolites
2. *Treatment evaluation*: Every 2 cycles

Toxicity

(N = 168 Fully Supplemented With Vitamins)

	% CTC G3/4
Hematologic	
Hemoglobin	4.2
Leukocytes	14.9
Neutrophils	23.2
Platelets	5.4
Febrile neutropenia	0.6
Nonhematologic	
Nausea	11.9
Fatigue	10.1
Vomiting	10.7
Diarrhea	3.6
Dehydration	4.2
Stomatitis	3
Anorexia	1.2
Rash	0.6

Three deaths thought possibly related to pemetrexed + cisplatin occurred before folic acid and vitamin B_{12} supplementation was added; none occurred thereafter

Treatment Modifications

Delay cycle until ANC is >1500/mm^3 and platelet >100,000/mm^3

Adverse Event	Dose Modification
G3 Hematologic toxicities	Hold therapy until returns to baseline. Then decrease both drug dosages by 25%
G4 Hematologic toxicities (thrombocytopenia)	Hold therapy until returns to baseline. Then decrease both drug dosages by 50%
Serum creatinine 1.6–2 mg/dL (140–176 μmol/L)	Decrease cisplatin dosage 25%
Serum creatinine ≥2 mg/dL (≥176 μmol/L)	Hold therapy until serum creatinine <2 mg/dL (<176 μmol/L), then decrease cisplatin dosage 25%
G ≥ 2 Diarrhea	Hold chemotherapy until toxicity resolves to grade <2, then decrease both drug dosages 25%
G3/4 Mucositis	Decrease pemetrexed dosage 50%
Increased liver transaminases	Hold therapy until toxicity resolves, then decrease pemetrexed dosage by 25%
Other G ≥ 3 nonhematologic toxicities (except N/V, elevated transaminases and alopecia)	Delay treatment until toxicity resolves to baseline, then, decrease both drug dosages by 25% from previous dose levels

Delays of ≤42 days are permitted for recovery from pemetrexed- and cisplatin-related toxicities

Patients requiring 3 dose reductions: discontinue therapy

Notes

1. G2 neutropenia and anemia secondary to pemetrexed are brief and not cumulative
2. Anemia is cumulative with cisplatin. Consider using erythropoietin therapy if anemia >G1 occurs
3. Folate deficiency is best measured with homocysteine levels
4. Vitamin B_{12} deficiency can be tested most readily with methylmalonic acid (MMA) levels

Peritoneal Mesothelioma

Epidemiology

Incidence: 10% of all mesothelioma (200–400 new cases per year)
Median age: 53 years
Median survival: <1 year
Male: female ratio: 1:1

Etiology

Causative factors

1. Asbestos exposure-related—in men only
2. Non–asbestos-related—mostly in women (considered to be a primary peritoneal carcinoma and behaves like papillary serous ovarian cancers)

Cocco P, Dosemeci M. Am J Ind Med 1999;35:9–14
Heller DS et al. Int J Gynecol Cancer 1999;9:452–455
Smith DD. Chest 2002;122:1885 [Comment on: Chest 2002;122:2224–2229
Sridhar KS et al. Cancer 1992;70:2969–2979

Clinical Presentation

1. Malignant ascites
2. Intra-abdominal mass

Prognostic Factors

Outcome more favorable than pleural mesothelioma:

1. Female sex (survive longer/not asbestos-related)
2. Complete cytoreduction
3. Use of intraperitoneal chemotherapy
4. Second-look surgery

Mikulski SM et al. JCO 2002;20:274–281
Sugarbaker PH et al. Semin Oncol 2002;29:51–61

Caveats

1. No standard treatment
2. Resectable disease
   a. *In women:* Treatment is the same as for ovarian cancer because these tumors behave and respond similarly to cytoreduction followed by cisplatin-based chemotherapy. Intraperitoneal (IP) chemotherapy has shown superiority over intravenous chemotherapy for advanced ovarian cancer
   b. *In men:* Treatment is the same as for pleural mesothelioma, or if disease is not related to asbestos exposure, it can be treated with IP chemotherapy
3. Locally advanced or recurrent disease: Give systemic chemotherapy as for pleural mesothelioma

Alberts DS et al. [Editorial] JCO 2002;20:3944–3949
Eltabbakh GH et al. J Surg Oncol 1999;70:6–12
Markman M, Kelsen D. J Cancer Res Clin Oncol 1992;118:547–550
Markman M et al. JCO 2001;19:1001–1007

REGIMEN

INTRAPERITONEAL (IP) CISPLATIN + PACLITAXEL

Rothenberg ML et al. JCO 2003;21:1313–1319

Dexamethasone 20 mg/dose orally for 2 doses, 12 hours and 6 hours before paclitaxel on days 1 and 8, *plus*
Diphenhydramine 50 mg by intravenous push, 30–60 minutes before paclitaxel on days 1 and 8, *plus*
Ranitidine 50 mg or **cimetidine** 300 mg intravenously in 25–100 mL 0.9% NaCl injection (0.9% NS) or 5% dextrose injection (D5W), over 5–30 minutes beginning 30–60 minutes before paclitaxel on days 1 and 8
Paclitaxel 135 mg/m^2 single dose by intravenous infusion in a volume of 0.9% NS or D5W sufficient to produce a solution with concentration within the range 0.3–1.2 mg/mL over 24 hours on day 1 every 21 days for 6 cycles (total paclitaxel dosage/cycle given intravenously = 135 mg/m^2)
Cisplatin 100 mg/m^2 IP in 2000 mL 0.9% NS warmed to body temperature on day 2 every 21 days for 6 cycles (total dosage/cycle = 100 mg/m^2)
Paclitaxel 60 mg/m^2 IP in 2000 mL 0.9% NS, warmed to body temperature on day 8 every 21 days for 6 cycles (total paclitaxel dosage/cycle from IP route = 60 mg/m^2)
Additional information: Drug distribution facilitated by placing patients R side down, L side down, in Trendelenberg and in reverse Trendelenberg position for 15 minutes each after drugs are instilled IP. Cisplatin- and paclitaxel-containing fluids are not drained after instillation
Emetogenic potential:
Days 1 and 8: Low (Emetogenicity score = 2)
Day 2: High (Emetogenicity score = 5). See Chapter 39

Patient Population Studied

A study of 68 patients with FIGO stage III epithelial ovarian cancer (tumor extending outside the pelvis and/or positive retroperitoneal or inguinal lymph nodes) with residual peritoneal disease ≤1 cm in largest dimension after surgical staging by GOG standards

Efficacy (N = 68)

Median disease-free survival	33 months
Median survival	51 months
2-year survival rate	91%

Toxicity (N = 68)

	% G3	% G4
Hematologic		
Neutropenia	21	59
Anemia	15	4
Thrombocytopenia	9	0
Infection with neutropenia	12	0
Nonhematologic		
Nausea	50	0
Vomiting	29	4
Abdominal pain	12	1
Diarrhea	4	1
Fatigue/malaise/lethargy	24	0
Sensory neuropathy	3	0
Catheter-related infection	10	0
	% G1	**% G2**
Alopecia	10	66

96% of patients experienced ≥1 G3/4 toxicity

Treatment Modifications

ANC ≥ 3000/mm^3 and platelet ≥100,000/mm^3 required to start cycle. Delay therapy up to 2 weeks to allow hematologic recovery

Adverse Event	Dose Modification
Hematologic toxicity	No dose modifications. Day 8 paclitaxel given without regard for CBC
G > 2 Peripheral neuropathy	Delay therapy until toxicity grade ≤2, then decrease all drug dosages by 20%
G2 Abdominal pain	Decrease IP drug dosage by 20%
G3/4 Abdominal pain	Decrease IP drug dosages by 40%
CrCl <50 mL/min	Hold cisplatin until CrCl > 50 mL/min, then decrease cisplatin dosage to 75 mg/m^2 during all subsequent cycles
Peritoneal catheter dysfunction or inability to administer therapy IP	Modify regimen schedule and route of administration for all remaining cycles: Paclitaxel 135 mg/m^2 intravenously over 24 hours on day 1 every 21 days Cisplatin 100 mg/m^2 intravenously on day 2, every 21 days

Therapy Monitoring

1. *Before each treatment cycle:* PE, CBC with differential, serum creatinine, and serum bilirubin
2. *Weekly:* CBC, serum electrolytes, serum creatinine, calcium, magnesium, and LFTs

28. Multiple Myeloma

Robert Dean, MD, and Cynthia E. Dunbar, MD

Epidemiology

Incidence: 16,570 (estimated cases in the United States in 2006)
Deaths: 11,310 (estimated in the United States in 2006)
Median age: 71 years
Male/female: 53%/47%

Durie-Salmon Stage at Presentation
Stage I: 6%
Stage II: 21%
Stage III: 73%

Durie GM, Salmon SF. Cancer 1975;36:842–854
Jacobson JL et al. Br J Haematol 2003;122:441–450
Jemal A et al. CA Cancer J Clin 2006;56:106–30
National Cancer Institute, SEER database; http://seer.cancer.gov/ 2004

Pathology

Monoclonal gammopathy of uncertain significance (MGUS)
- Stable serum M-protein level < 3 g/dL *and* bone marrow clonal plasma cells < 10%
- Urine Bence Jones protein absent or minimal
- No related organ/tissue impairment (ROTI)*
- No evidence of other B-lymphoproliferative disorders
- Progression to multiple myeloma (MM) in ~1% per year (median 10 years)

Asymptomatic ("smoldering") myeloma
- Serum M-protein level ≥ 3 g/dL *and/or* bone marrow plasma cells ≥ 10%
- No ROTI or symptoms

Multiple myeloma (symptomatic)
- Detectable M protein in serum or urine
- Clonal bone marrow plasma cells, or plasmacytoma
- Presence of ROTI

Note: Minimum levels of M protein and bone marrow plasma cells are not required for the diagnosis of MM when symptoms (ie, ROTI) are present

Extramedullary plasmacytoma
- Extramedullary tumor of clonal plasma cells
- Normal bone marrow
- Normal skeletal survey
- M protein absent or disappears from blood/urine after excision or irradiation of solitary lesion
- Absence of ROTI
- Progression to MM in ~15%

Solitary plasmacytoma of bone
- 3–5% of plasma cell dyscrasias
- Isolated bone tumor consisting of monoclonal plasma cells
- Normal bone marrow
- M protein absent or disappears from blood/urine after excision or irradiation of solitary lesion
- Absence of other ROTI
- Multiple or recurrent in up to 5% of patients
- Progression to MM in ~50%

(*continued*)

Work-Up

All patients
1. H&P
2. CBC with differential; serum, electrolytes, BUN, creatinine, calcium and albumin, LDH
3. Quantitative immunoglobulins, serum protein electrophoresis, and immunofixation
4. 24-hour urine protein electrophoresis, immunofixation, and Bence Jones quantitation
5. Skeletal survey
6. Unilateral bone marrow aspirate and biopsy
7. Bone marrow cytogenetics (chromosome 13 deletion in 50% of cases; associated with worse survival)
8. β_2-Microglobulin (abnormally high result is associated with poor prognosis)

Selected patients
1. MRI of the spine (evaluate for solitary plasmacytoma of bone or suspected cord compression)
2. Tissue biopsy (evaluate for solitary plasmacytoma)
3. Serum viscosity (if M-protein level is markedly elevated or symptoms of hyperviscosity are present)
4. Erythropoietin level

Additional tests (prognostic markers)
1. Plasma cell labeling index (abnormally high result associated with poor prognosis)
2. C-reactive protein (abnormally high result associated with poor prognosis)

Pathology (*continued*)

Plasma Cell Leukemia

- 5% of newly presenting MM patients
- Peripheral blood absolute plasma cell count 2000/mm^3
- More than 20% plasma cells in differential count of peripheral blood leukocytes

*ROTI: Myeloma-Related Organ/Tissue Impairment:
1. Hypercalcemia
2. Renal insufficiency
3. Recurrent bacterial infections (>2 episodes in 12 months)
4. Bone lesions (lytic, or osteoporotic with compression fractures)
5. Symptomatic hyperviscosity
6. Amyloidosis
7. Anemia

The International Myeloma Working Group. Br J Haematol 2003;121:749–57

Staging

Durie-Salmon Staging System

	Stage I	Stage II[a]	Stage III[b]
Myeloma cell mass	Low	Intermediate	High
Hemoglobin	>10 g/dL	8.5–10	<8.5 g/dL
Serum calcium	≤12 mg/dL	≤12 mg/dL	>12 mg/dL
Skeletal survey	Normal[c]	Normal	Lytic bone lesions
Serum M-protein levels: IgG	<5 g/dL	5–7	>7 g/dL
Serum M-protein levels: IgA	<3 g/dL	3–5	>5 g/dL
24-hour urinary light-chain excretion	<4 g	4–12 g	>12 g

[a]Not meeting criteria for either stage I or stage III
[b]Need to meet one or more of the criteria listed
[c]Or solitary plasmacytoma

Note: Subclassification: For each stage, "A" denotes serum creatinine < 2 mg/dL (<177 μmol/L), whereas "B" denotes serum creatinine ≥ 2 mg/dL (≥177 μmol/L)

International Staging System

	Stage I	Stage II		Stage III
Serum β_2-microglobulin	<3.5 μg/mL	<3.5 μg/mL	≥3.5 μg/mL, <5.5 μg/mL	≥5.5 μg/mL
Albumin	≥3.5 g/dL	<3.5 g/dL	—	—

Durie GM, Salmon SF. Cancer 1975;36:842–854
Greipp PR et al. JCO 2005;23:3412–120

Median Survival by Stage

	Durie-Salmon	International Staging System
Stage I	57 months	62 months
Stage II	40 months	44 months
Stage III	IIIA, 35 months IIIB, 21 months	29 months

Greipp PR et al. JCO 2005;23:3412–3420
Jacobson JL et al. Br J Haematol 2003;122:441–450

Caveats

1. Determine whether patient is a candidate for high-dose therapy with autologous peripheral blood stem cell (PBSC) transplantation before initiating chemotherapy. Avoid alkylating agents in such patients before autologous PBSCs are collected, because exposure to alkylating agents may prevent the collection of an adequate number of PBSCs for autologous transplantation. For induction therapy in transplant candidates, preferred regimens include dexamethasone, thalidomide/dexamethasone, and vincristine/doxorubicin/dexamethasone (VAD). Note that dexamethasone is the most active agent in the VAD regimen, and the inconvenience and potential complications associated with VAD therapy (eg, prolonged infusions, indwelling catheter-related complications, alopecia) lead many clinicians and patients to prefer alternatives such as dexamethasone or thalidomide/dexamethasone.

   Patients with responsive disease are eligible to undergo autologous PBSC transplantation, typically after 3–4 cycles of induction therapy. After autologous transplantation, investigational approaches for further consolidation include a second autologous PBSC transplantation or nonmyeloablative allogeneic PBSC transplantation.

   Patients who are ineligible for autologous PBSC transplantation at diagnosis generally undergo primary therapy with melphalan/prednisone or another alkylating agent-based regimen. Note that intensive alkylating agent combinations are associated with significantly more toxicity than melphalan/prednisone and have not consistently shown an improvement in treatment outcomes over the latter. Induction therapy in this setting is usually continued for a minimum of 12 months until a plateau is reached.

   Similarly, patients who are ineligible for autologous PBSC transplantation after primary induction therapy may be treated with melphalan/prednisone or another regimen until a plateau is achieved after 12 months of treatment.

Durie BG et al. Hematol J 2003;4:379–398
Kyle RA, Rajkumar SV. NEJM 2004;351:1860–1873

2. Treatment with a bisphosphonate is recommended to reduce skeletal complications for all myeloma patients with skeletal lesions. Pamidronate, zolendronic acid, and clodronate have demonstrated efficacy in this setting. Because renal toxicity can result from bisphosphonate therapy, renal function should be monitored closely, since the dose of the bisphosphonate may require dose adjustment or discontinuation. See Chapter 44 for specific dosage and monitoring guidelines.
3. Anemia is present in most patients with MM. Reversible causes of anemia should be evaluated and treated. Patients with symptomatic anemia may benefit from therapy with recombinant erythropoietin (see Chapter 43).
4. Waldenström's macroglobulinemia presents with lymphoplasmacytic bone marrow infiltration and IgM paraproteinemia. Therapy usually consists of an alkylating agent (eg, chlorambucil) with or without steroids, or a purine analogue such as fludarabine or cladribine. Other management considerations focus on complications caused by the macroglobulin, such as hyperviscosity, cryoglobulinemia, and hemolytic anemia.
5. Primary amyloidosis is characterized by organ dysfunction resulting from monoclonal light-chain production and tissue deposition. Carefully selected patients may benefit from high-dose melphalan with autologous PBSC support, which can result in hematologic remission, regression of light chain deposition, and improvement in organ function. Melphalan and prednisone may also be used as palliative treatment.
6. Maintenance interferon provides little, if any, incremental benefit following other therapy. See meta-analysis by Myeloma Trialists' Collaborative Group (Br J Haematol 2001;113:1020–1031).

REGIMEN

HIGH-DOSE MELPHALAN (CONDITIONING REGIMEN BEFORE AUTOLOGOUS PERIPHERAL BLOOD STEM CELL TRANSPLANTATION)

Moreau P et al. Blood 2002;99:731–735

Conditioning for autologous PBSC transplantation:
Melphalan 200 mg/m^2 intravenously, diluted in sufficient 0.9% NaCl injection (0.9% NS) to produce a concentration ≤ 0.45 mg/mL, over 30 minutes, 2 days before PBSC reinfusion (on day −2; total dosage = 200 mg/m^2). PBSC reinfusion on day 0, *or*
Melphalan 100 mg/m^2 per day intravenously, diluted in sufficient 0.9% NS to produce a concentration ≤ 0.45 mg/mL over 30 minutes for 2 consecutive days, 3 and 2 days before PBSC reinfusion (on days −3 and −2; total dosage = 200 mg/m^2). PBSC reinfusion on day 0

Supportive care:
Growth factor support:
Filgrastim (G-CSF), 5–10 mcg/kg per day subcutaneously starting on day +7 after PBSC reinfusion and continuing until granulocyte counts recover, *or*
Sargramostim (GM-CSF) 5–10 mcg/kg per day subcutaneously starting on day +7 after PBSC reinfusion and continuing until granulocyte counts recover
Antibacterial prophylaxis (PCP prophylaxis):
Trimethoprim + sulfamethoxazole (TMP + SMZ) 160 mg/800 mg orally, daily, for 3 months, *or*
TMP + SMZ 80 mg/400 mg orally daily for 3 months, *or*
TMP + SMZ 160 mg/800 mg orally 3 days per week for 3 months
Antifungal prophylaxis:
Fluconazole 200–400 mg orally or intravenously, daily for 30 days > PBSC or until neutrophil engraftment occurs (ANC > 500/mm^3)
Acyclovir or valacyclovir prophylaxis to HSV seropositive recipients to prevent reactivation of HSV during the early post-transplantation period:
Acyclovir 200 mg orally every 8 hours for 30 days, *or*
Acyclovir 250 mg/m^2 per dose intravenously every 12 hours for 30 days, *or*
Valacyclovir 500 mg orally daily for 30 days
Note: Routine acyclovir prophylaxis for > 30 days after hematopoietic stem cell transplantation is not recommended

Fluconazole is available in the United States in various formulations for oral administration, including immediate-release tablets containing 50-mg, 100-mg, 150-mg, and 200-mg powdered fluconazole for preparing liquid suspensions
Acyclovir is available in the United States generically in formulations for oral administration, including immediate-release tablets (400 and 800 mg per tablet), immediate-release capsules (200 mg/capsule), and a powdered product for preparing a liquid suspension (200 mg/5 mL)
Valacyclovir is available in the United States as tablets for oral administration containing either 500 or 1000 mg valacyclovir HCl (Valtrex® caplets. GlaxoSmithKline, Research Triangle Park, NC)

Emetogenic potential: Moderately high (Emetogenicity score = 4). See Chapter 39 for antiemetic regimens

Treatment Modifications

1. PBSCs were collected and reinfused, provided there was no evidence of tumor progression (> 25% increase in tumor mass) and if cardiopulmonary, hepatic, and renal function (serum creatinine less than 150 μmoles/liter = 1.7 mg/dL, but otherwise not specified) remained adequate after the third course of VAD
2. Patients with renal failure (serum creatinine > 2 mg/dL, >177 μmol/L) may be considered for high-dose therapy and peripheral blood stem cell and PBSCT. Reduction of the melphalan dose to 140 mg/m^2 is recommended for such patients

Badros A et al. Br J Haematol 2001;114:822–829

Patient Population Studied

A study of 142 patients ≤65 years old with symptomatic MM responding to primary chemotherapy with VAD
Exclusions:
1. Stable stage 1 MM deemed not to require therapy (Durie-Salmon classification)
2. Previous cytotoxic chemotherapy other than VAD in preparation for transplantation*
3. Previous radiation therapy
4. Severe abnormalities of cardiac, pulmonary and hepatic functions (not specified)
5. Serum creatinine level above 500 μmoles/L (5.66 mg/dL)

*VAD was chosen as the regimen because of its "speedy tumor cell reduction without induction of hematopoietic stem cell compromise" (Moreau et al)

Efficacy (N = 142)

Response to HDT

Complete response	35%
Very good partial response*	20%
Partial response	39%
Stable or progressive disease	6%
Toxic death	0%
Median event-free survival	20.5 months

*90% decrease in serum paraprotein level

Toxicity (N = 142)

	Median Values in Days (Range)
Hematopoietic growth factor	7 (0–23)
Neutropenia	8 (4–34)
Thrombocytopenia	7 (0–30)
IV antibiotics	8 (0–30)
Length of hospital stay	19 (11–47)
Supportive Measure	**Median Values in Days (Range)**
Platelet transfusions	1 (0–18)
RBC transfusions	2 (0–9)
G3/4 Toxicity	**WHO Criteria**
Cardiac	0.7%
Mucositis	30%
Pulmonary	1.4%
Renal	2.1%
Liver	0.7%
Toxic death	0%

Therapy Monitoring

CBC with differential, daily to every third day as recovery occurs

Notes

This conditioning regimen was part of a more comprehensive therapy for MM that included the following:

1. Before PBSC harvest, patients received 3 cycles of VAD
2. In the absence of tumor progression (>25% increase in tumor mass) and if cardiopulmonary, hepatic, and renal functions (serum creatinine 150 μmoles/liter = 1.7 mg/dL, but otherwise not specified) remained adequate after the third course of VAD, PBSCs were collected
3. After PBSC collection, patients received a fourth course of VAD

Response to VAD Regimen After Stem Cell Collection

Complete response	5%
Very good partial response*	12%
Partial response	61%
Stable disease	22%
Stem Cell Collection	
G-CSF priming	75%
Stem cell factor + G-CSF	4%
Cyclophosphamide + G-CSF	21%
Number of CD34 infused	1.2–132 × 10^6/kg
Median number of CD34	5 × 10^6/kg infused

*90% decrease in serum paraprotein level

4. After completion of high-dose therapy and PBSCT treatment with recombinant interferon alfa (3 × 10^6 units subcutaneously 3 times weekly) was given when granulocytes exceeded 1500/mm^3 and platelets exceeded 100,000/mm^3 during the first year after transplantation. Interferon was continued at the physician's discretion, in case of disease progression, or when it induced severe and persistent adverse effects. The value of maintenance interferon in this or any setting is uncertain

REGIMEN

MELPHALAN + PREDNISONE

Oken MM et al. Cancer 1997;79:1561–1567

Melphalan 8 mg/m² per day orally for 4 consecutive days on days 1–4 every 28 days for 1 year, then continue every 6 weeks as maintenance therapy (total dosage/cycle = 32 mg/m²)
Prednisone 60 mg/m² per day orally for 4 consecutive days on days 1–4 every 28 days for 1 year, then continue every 6 weeks as maintenance therapy (total dosage/cycle = 240 mg/m²)
Note: After an induction period of approximately 1 year (13 cycles of MP), patients with continuing objective responses enter the maintenance phase, which consists of treatment with their induction regimens at a frequency of every 6 weeks times 3 followed by every 8 weeks until relapse

Alternative dose schedules:
Melphalan 0.15 mg/kg per day orally for 7 consecutive days on days 1–7 every 6 weeks (total dosage/cycle = 1.05 mg/kg)
Prednisone 20 mg 3 times daily orally for 7 consecutive days on days 1–7 every 6 weeks (total dose/cycle = 420 mg/kg),

or

Melphalan 0.25 mg/kg per day orally for 4 consecutive days on days 1–4 every 4–6 weeks (total dosage/cycle = 1 mg/kg)
Prednisone 20 mg 3 times daily orally for 4 consecutive days on days 1–4 every 4–6 weeks (total dose/cycle = 240 mg)

Melphalan is available in the United States as immediate-release tablets for oral administration containing 2 mg melphalan. ALKERAN® (melphalan) Tablets product label, November 2004. Celgene Corporation, Warren, NJ
Prednisone is marketed in the United States in numerous generic formulations for oral administration, including immediate-release tablets containing 1, 2.5, 5, 10, 20, and 50 mg, and in solutions and syrups for oral administration

Emetogenic potential: Nonemetogenic (Emetogenicity score = 1). See Chapter 39 for antiemetic regimens

Patient Population Studied

A study of 221 patients with previously untreated MM. Patients with prior chemotherapy, hyperbilirubinemia (2 mg/dL = 34.2 μmol/L), smoldering MM, localized plasmacytoma or monoclonal gammopathy of undetermined significance without further evidence of MM were excluded

Efficacy (N = 221)

Objective response[a]	51%
Stable disease	25%
Progressive disease	24%
Median response duration	18 months
SWOG-OR[b]	38%
SWOG-OR + I[c]	

[a]Minimum 50% decrease in serum paraprotein
[b]75% decrease in M-protein synthetic index
[c]50% decrease in M-protein synthetic index

Treatment Modifications

Adverse Event	Dose Modification
Patient ages ≥70 years	Reduce initial melphalan dose by 25%
If on day 1 of cycle ≥2, ANC >2000/mm³ and platelets >100,000/mm³	100% doses
If on day 1 of cycle ≥2, ANC <2000/mm³ but >1000/mm³ or platelets <100,000/mm³ but >75,000/mm³	Continue treatment, but reduce melphalan dosage by 25%
If on day 1 of cycle ≥2, ANC 751–1000/mm³ and platelets >75,000/mm³	Continue treatment, but reduce melphalan dosage by 50%
If on day 1 of cycle ≥2, ANC 751–1000/mm³ and platelets ≤75,000/mm³	Delay treatment until platelets >75,000/mm³, then continue treatment, but reduce melphalan dosage by 50%
If on day 1 of cycle ≥2, ANC ≤750/mm³ or platelets ≤50,000/mm³	Delay treatment until ANC ≥751/mm³ and platelets >75,000/mm³, then continue treatment, but reduce melphalan dosage by 50%
If ANC nadir ≤1000/mm³ or platelets nadir ≤50,000/mm³	Continue treatment, but reduce melphalan dosage by 25%
Severe manifestations of hypercorticism, including severe hyperglycemia, irritability and insomnia or oral candidiasis	Reduce daily prednisone dosage by 20% for G3 toxicity and 40% for G4 or recurrent G3

Toxicity (N = 221)

Adverse Effect	Incidence
Any toxicity ≥ G3	54%
Hematologic	
Neutropenia ≥ G3	37%
Thrombocytopenia ≥ G3	23%
Nonhematologic	
Infection ≥ G3	14%
Nausea/vomiting ≥ G2	10%
Peripheral neuropathy ≥ G2	2%
Alopecia ≥ G1	7%
Secondary Malignancies (Time Unspecified)	
Hematologic malignancies	13 patients
Solid tumors	12 patients
Myelodysplatic syndrome	10 patients

ECOG Toxicity Criteria

Therapy Monitoring

1. *Before each cycle:* CBC with differential and blood chemistries (including BUN, creatinine, and calcium)
2. *Every 2–3 months:* Quantitation of immunoglobulin and M-protein levels

REGIMEN

INFUSIONAL VINCRISTINE, DOXORUBICIN, AND DEXAMETHASONE (VAD)

Anderson H et al. Br J Cancer 1995;71:326–330

Vincristine 0.4 mg/day by continuous intravenous infusion in a convenient volume of 0.9% NaCl injection (0.9% NS) or 5% dextrose injection (D5W) over 24 hours, daily for 4 consecutive days on days 1–4 every 21 days (total dose/cycle = 1.6 mg)
Doxorubicin 9 mg/m^2 per day continuous intravenous infusion in a convenient volume of 0.9% NS or D5W over 24 hours, daily for 4 consecutive days on days 1–4 every 21 days (total dosage/cycle = 36 mg/m^2)
Dexamethasone 40 mg/day orally for 4 consecutive days on days 1–4 every 21 days (total dose/cycle = 160 mg)

Dexamethasone is marketed in the United States in numerous generic formulations for oral administration, including immediate-release tablets containing 0.25, 0.5, 0.75, 1, 2, 4, and 6 mg, and in elixirs (which contain alcohol) and solutions for oral administration

Supportive care:
Hyperuricemia prophylaxis during the initial cycle, particularly for patients with renal insufficiency:
Urine alkalinization
Sodium bicarbonate 1000–2000 mg (50–100 mEq) orally 4 times daily for 14 days *and/or*
Allopurinol 300 mg per day orally for 14 days
Infection prophylaxis:
Cotrimoxazole (sulfamethoxazole 800 mg + trimethoprim 160 mg) orally, twice daily, *and*
Fluconazole 200–400 mg per day orally, *or*
Ketoconazole 400 mg per day orally
Optional prophylaxis for steroid-induced dyspepsia:
Ranitidine 150 mg per day orally for 7 days when a patient commences prednisone, *or*
Cimetidine 400 mg orally twice daily for 7 days when a patient commences prednisone

Allopurinol is manufactured in the United States in tablets for oral administration containing either allopurinol 100 mg or 300 mg, and as an injectable product, Alloprim® (allopurinol sodium) for injection. Nabi®, Boca Raton, FL
Cotrimoxazole is generically available in the United States in a variety of formulations and product strengths, including tablets containing sulfamethoxazole 800 mg + trimethoprim 160 mg or tablets containing sulfamethoxazole 400 mg + trimethoprim 80 mg
Fluconazole is available in the United States in various formulations for oral administration, including immediate-release tablets containing 50 mg, 100 mg, 150 mg, or 200 mg powdered fluconazole for preparing liquid suspensions
Ketoconazole is available in the United States generically as tablets for oral administration containing 200 mg of ketoconazole

Emetogenic potential: *Days 1–4:* Low (Emetogenicity score = 2). See Chapter 39 for antiemetic regimens

Treatment Modifications

Adverse Event	Dose Modification
Severe manifestations of hypercorticism including severe hyperglycemia, irritability and insomnia or oral candidiasis	Reduce daily dexamethasone dosage by 20% for G3 toxicity and 40% for G4 or recurrent G3

Patient Population Studied

A study of 142 patients with either untreated (n = 75) or relapsed/refractory MM (n = 67). All patients treated except those with a serious concurrent medical condition that precluded high-dose dexamethasone (uncontrolled cardiac failure, unstable diabetes, or chronic chest infection, eg, bronchiectasis)

Efficacy (N = 142)

	Untreated (n = 75)	Relapsed or Refractory (n = 67)
Complete response	27%	3%
Partial response	57%	58%
Stable disease	9%	22%
Progressive disease	1%	6%
Deaths	5%	10%
Median survival*	36 months	10 months

*After VAD, some patients received maintenance therapy or bone marrow/stem cell transplants

Toxicity (N = 142)

Nonhematologic	
Alopecia	84%
Infection requiring antibiotics	54%
Documented bacteremia	14%
Dyspepsia	37%
Constipation	30%
Paresthesia	28%
Steroid associated edema	27%
Mild heart failure treated with diuretics	5%
Cathether complications	24%
Nausea and vomiting (WHO grades ≤2)	21%
Central nervous system	13%
Oral candida infection[a]	13%
Deaths[b]	6%

[a]Despite ketoconazole prophylaxis
[b]Nine deaths (6%) occurred within 30 days after VAD. Causes: MM (n = 5), infection/MM (n = 3), progressive multifocal leukoencephalopathy (n = 1)

Hematologic	
Infection with ANC < 1000/mm^3	15.4%
Grade ≥ 1 thrombocytopenia	11%

Alexanian R et al. Am J Hematol 1990;33:86–89
WHO criteria

Therapy Monitoring

1. *Every week:* CBC with differential
2. *Every month:* Serum electrolytes, BUN, creatinine, and calcium. Serum for quantitative immunoglobulins and serum protein electrophoresis (SPEP); 24-hour urine for quantification of light chains, total protein excretion, and creatinine clearance; serum/urine M protein

REGIMEN

BOLUS VINCRISTINE, DOXORUBICIN, AND DEXAMETHASONE (BOLUS VAD)

Segeren CM et al. Br J Haematol 1999;105:127–130

Vincristine 0.4 mg/day intravenously in 100 mL 0.9% NaCl injection (0.9% NS) over 30 minutes daily for 4 consecutive days on days 1–4 every 4 weeks for up to 4 cycles (total dose/cycle = 1.6 mg)
Doxorubicin 9 mg/m^2 per day intravenously in 100 mL 0.9% NS over 30 minutes daily for 4 consecutive days on days 1–4 every 4 weeks for up to 4 cycles (total dosage/cycle = 36 mg/m^2)
Cycles 1 and 3 only:
Dexamethasone 40 mg/day orally for 4 consecutive days on days 1–4, 9–12, and 17–20 (total dose/cycle = 480 mg)
Note: Dexamethasone is not given during cycles 2 and 4

Dexamethasone is marketed in the United States in numerous generic formulations for oral administration, including immediate-release tablets containing 0.25, 0.5, 0.75, 1, 2, 4, and 6 mg, and in elixirs (which contain alcohol) and solutions for oral administration

Infection prophylaxis:
Cotrimoxazole (sulfamethoxazole 800 mg + trimethoprim 160 mg) orally twice daily, *and*
Fluconazole 200–400 mg per day orally

Cotrimoxazole is generically available in the United States in a variety of formulations and product strengths, including tablets containing sulfamethoxazole 800 mg + trimethoprim 160 mg and tablets containing sulfamethoxazole 400 mg + trimethoprim 80 mg
Fluconazole is available in the United States in various formulations for oral administration, including immediate-release tablets containing 50 mg, 100 mg, 150 mg, and 200 mg powdered fluconazole for preparing liquid suspensions

Emetogenic potential: Days 1–4: Low (Emetogenicity score = 2). See Chapter 39

Patient Population Studied

A prospective multicenter study of 134 patients with previously untreated stages II or III MM, ages ≤65 years. Patients received 3 or 4 cycles of bolus VAD as a remission induction treatment before randomization to further intensified therapy. Patients were followed up for at least 1 year after bolus VAD

Efficacy (N = 139)

	All	Stage II	Stage III
Number of patients	139	43	96
Complete response	5%	9%	3%
Partial response	62%	56%	65%
No response (SD)	27%	30%	26%
Progressive disease	2%	2.5%	4%
Early death	4%	2.5%	2%

Note: Duration of response was not evaluable owing to therapy administered subsequent to VAD

ECOG criteria

Treatment Modifications

Adverse Event	Dose Modification
Severe manifestations of hypercorticism including severe hyperglycemia, irritability and insomnia or oral candidiasis	Reduce daily dexamethasone dosage by 20% for G3 toxicity and 40% for G4 or recurrent G3
G3/4 Nonhematologic toxicity	Hold treatment until toxicity resolves to ≤ G1, then resume with a 25% dose reduction for vincristine and doxorubicin

Toxicity (N = 416 Cycles/139 Patients)

WHO Toxicity Grades ≥ 2	% Cycles
Nausea and vomiting	2
G2/3 mucositis	2
Liver	2
Renal function	1
Cardiac	0.5

Toxicity	% G1	% G2	% G3
Neurotoxicity	4	9	9
Infections		27	

Five deaths occurred during bolus VAD treatment, which were attributed to progressive disease (n = 1) septic shock (n = 1) septic shock and acute tubular necrosis (n = 1) congestive heart failure (n = 1) and myocardial infarction (n = 1)
WHO criteria

Therapy Monitoring

1. *Twice a week during therapy:* CBC with differential
2. *3–4 weeks after last cycle of VAD:* Bone marrow sample, measurement of serum and urine M protein

REGIMEN

THALIDOMIDE

Singhal S et al. NEJM 1999;341:1565–1571

Initial dose:
Thalidomide 200 mg/day orally at bedtime
Dose escalation:
If the previously administered dose is tolerated, the thalidomide dose is escalated by 200 mg/day every 2 weeks for 6 weeks, eg,
Weeks 3 and 4: **Thalidomide** 400 mg/day orally at bedtime
Weeks 5 and 6: **Thalidomide** 600 mg/day orally at bedtime
Week ≥ 7: **Thalidomide** 800 mg/day orally at bedtime

	% Patients	
Dose	On-time Escalation	Reaching This Dose
400 mg	83	86
600 mg	62	68
800 mg	47	55

Thalidomide is marketed in the United States in immediate-release capsules for oral administration containing 50 mg, 100 mg, or 200 mg. THALOMID® (thalidomide) CAPSULES product label, February 2004. Celgene Corporation, Warren, NJ

Emetogenic potential: Nonemetogenic (Emetogenicity score = 1). See Chapter 39

Treatment Modifications

Adverse Event	Dose Modification
G ≥ 3 Hematologic and nonhematologic toxicities (ie, somnolence and constipation)	Hold thalidomide until symptoms resolve to G ≤ 1, then resume thalidomide at dose previously tolerated. Attempt to advance dose again after 2 weeks
Peripheral neuropathy	Discontinue thalidomide, since it may be irreversible. If symptoms return to baseline, then resume thalidomide at dose previously tolerated*

*Physicians' Desk Reference 1999;53:3457–3462

Patient Population Studied

A study of 84 patients with previously treated refractory MM, including 76 with relapse after high-dose chemotherapy

Efficacy (N = 84)

	Paraprotein	Bone Marrow
Complete remission	2%	2/2
≥90% decrease	7%	5/6
≥75% decrease	7%	3/5
≥50% decrease:	8%	4/4
≥25% decrease	7%	3/4
No response	68%	4/27
Median event-free survival (all patients)		3 months
Median TTP (patients with response)		>14.5 months

Toxicity

	% Patients with G1/2 Toxicity*			
	Daily Thalidomide Dose			
	200 mg (n = 83)	400 mg (n = 72)	600 mg (n = 57)	800 mg (n = 46)
Nonhematologic				
Constipation	35	44	44	59
Weakness or fatigue	29	31	39	48
Somnolence	34	43	40	43
Tingling or numbness	12	14	19	28
Dizziness	17	25	23	28
Rash	16	18	21	26
Mood changes or depression	16	24	23	22
Incoordination	16	17	14	22
Tremors	10	13	19	22
Edema	6	10	12	22
Nausea	12	15	23	11
Headache	12	10	14	11

Hematologic

G1/2 leukopenia	<5%
G3/4 thrombocytopenia	3.5%

*Grades 3/4 adverse events in < 10% of patients

WHO criteria

Therapy Monitoring

1. *Weekly:* CBC with differential
2. *Weekly for first two months then monthly:* M-protein measurements (myeloma protein in serum, Bence Jones protein in urine)

REGIMEN

THALIDOMIDE + DEXAMETHASONE

Rajkumar SV et al. JCO 2002;20:4319–4323

Thalidomide 200 mg/day orally, continually for a minimum of 4 cycles (total dose/30-day cycle = 6000 mg)
Odd-numbered monthly cycles (1, 3, etc):
Dexamethasone 40 mg/day orally for 4 consecutive days on days 1–4, 8–11, and 16–19 (total dose/cycle = 480 mg)
Even-numbered monthly cycles (2, 4, etc):
Dexamethasone 40 mg/day orally for 4 days on days 1–4 (total dose/cycle = 160 mg)

Thalidomide is marketed in the United States in immediate-release capsules for oral administration containing 50 mg, 100 mg, and 200 mg. THALOMID® (thalidomide) CAPSULES product label, February 2004. Celgene Corporation, Warren, NJ
Dexamethasone is marketed in the United States in numerous generic formulations for oral administration, including immediate-release tablets containing 0.25, 0.5, 0.75, 1, 2, 4, and 6 mg, and in elixirs (which contain alcohol) and solutions for oral administration

Infection prophylaxis:
Cotrimoxazole (sulfamethoxazole 800 mg + trimethoprim 160 mg) orally, twice daily, *and*
Fluconazole 200–400 mg per day orally

Cotrimoxazole is generically available in the United States in a variety of formulations and product strengths, including tablets containing sulfamethoxazole 800 mg + trimethoprim 160 mg and tablets containing sulfamethoxazole 400 mg + trimethoprim 80 mg
Fluconazole is available in the United States in various formulations for oral administration, including immediate-release tablets containing 50 mg, 100 mg, 150 mg, and 200 mg powdered fluconazole for preparing liquid suspensions

Emetogenic potential: Nonemetogenic (Emetogenicity score = 1). See Chapter 39

Treatment Modifications

Adverse Event	Dose Modification
G ≥ 2 Hematologic and nonhematologic toxicities (ie, somnolence and constipation)	Decrease daily thalidomide dose to 50–100 mg
Peripheral neuropathy	Discontinue thalidomide, since it may be irreversible. If symptoms return to baseline, resume thalidomide at dose previously tolerated*
Severe manifestations of hypercorticism including severe hyperglycemia, irritability and insomnia or oral candidiasis	Reduce daily dexamethasone dosage by 20% for G3 toxicity and by 40% for G4 or recurrent G3

*Physicians' Desk Reference 1999;53:3457–3462

Patient Population Studied

A study of 50 patients with previously untreated symptomatic MM

Efficacy (N = 42–50)

Response Level[a]	% Monoclonal Protein[b]	% Bone Marrow[c]
≥90%	30	24
75–90%	22	29
50–75%	16	14
25–50%	24	10
10–25%	—	10
No response or progression	8	14

[a]Decrements from baseline measurements
[b]N = 50 patients. Measurements in serum, or in urine, when serum protein was </dL
[c]n = 42 patients

ECOG criteria

Toxicity (N = 50)

	% G1/2	% G3/4
Thrombosis	NR	12
Constipation	72	8
Rash	38	6
Dyspnea	NR	4
Neuropathy	58	2
Fatigue	50	NR
Sedation	46	2
Tremor	30	NR
Depression	NR	2
Edema	28	2
Arrhythmia	NR	2
Rash	NR	2
Inner ear	NR	2
Syncope	NR	2
Increased alkaline phosphatase	22	NR
Treatment-related deaths*	6%	

*One each pancreatitis, pulmonary embolism, infection

NCI CTC

Therapy Monitoring

Monthly: Measure serum and urine M protein

Notes

1. After 4 cycles, eligible patients were permitted to pursue stem cell collection and transplantation
2. Thalidomide dose escalation was discontinued after serious skin toxicity occurred in 2 of the first 7 patients

REGIMEN

DEXAMETHASONE

Alexanian R et al. Blood 1992;80:887–890

Dexamethasone 20 mg/m^2 per dose orally for 4 consecutive days, on days 1–4, 9–12, and 17–20, every 35 days (total dosage/cycle = 240 mg/m^2 per 12 doses)
Alternatively:
Dexamethasone 40 mg per dose orally for 4 consecutive days, on days 1–4, 9–12, and 17–20, every 35 days (total dose/cycle = 480 mg/12 doses)

Dexamethasone is marketed in the United States in numerous generic formulations for oral administration, including immediate-release tablets containing 0.25, 0.5, 0.75, 1, 2, 4, and 6 mg, and in elixirs (which contain alcohol) and solutions for oral administration

Infection prophylaxis:
Cotrimoxazole (sulfamethoxazole 800 mg + trimethoprim 160 mg) orally twice daily *and*
Fluconazole 200–400 mg per day orally

Cotrimoxazole is generically available in the United States in a variety of formulations and product strengths, including tablets containing sulfamethoxazole 800 mg + trimethoprim 160 mg or tablets containing sulfamethoxazole 400 mg + trimethoprim 80 mg
Fluconazole is available in the United States in various formulations for oral administration, including: immediate-release tablets containing 50 mg, 100 mg, 150 mg, and 200 mg powdered fluconazole for preparing liquid suspensions

Emetogenic potential: Nonemetogenic (Emetogenicity score = 1). See Chapter 39

Patient Population Studied

A study of 112 patients with previously untreated symptomatic MM

Efficacy (N = 112)

	Stage I	Stage II/III
Overall response	51%	37%

Toxicity (N = 112)

No myelosuppression. Most patients develop cushingoid features and/or insomnia. Other complications occurring at < 5% frequency:

- Oral candidiasis
- Herpesvirus infection
- Diabetes
- Peptic ulcer
- Hiccoughs
- Quadriceps weakness

Two deaths reported within first 4 weeks of treatment.
Four patients were hospitalized during treatment. Reasons for hospitalization: perforated diverticulum (n = 2), pancreatitis (n = 1) pneumonia (n = 1)

Treatment Modifications

Adverse Event	Dose Modification
Severe manifestations of hypercorticism, including severe hyperglycemia, irritability, and insomnia or oral candidiasis	Reduce daily dexamethasone dosage by 20% for G3 toxicity and 40% for G4 or recurrent G3 toxicity

Therapy Monitoring

After each cycle: Measure serum and urine M protein

Notes

In this study, the authors noted that: "No more than three cycles of DEX were required to confirm a response. Furthermore, "All responding patients were maintained on α interferon 2 × 10^6 U/m^2 subcutaneously every Monday, Wednesday and Friday." The value of maintenance interferon in this setting is uncertain

(Alexanian R et al. Blood 1992;80:887)

REGIMEN

BORTEZOMIB

Richardson PG et al. NEJM 2003;348:2609–2617

Bortezomib 1.3 mg/m^2 per dose by rapid intravenous injection over 3–5 seconds for 4 doses on days 1, 4, 8, and 11 every 21 days (total dosage/cycle = 5.2 mg/m^2)
In patients with disease progression after 2 cycles, or with stable disease after 4 cycles, add:
Dexamethasone 20 mg per dose orally for 8 doses on days 1, 2, 4, 5, 8, 9, 11, and 12 (total dose per cycle: 160 mg)

Infection prophylaxis:
Cotrimoxazole (sulfamethoxazole 800 mg + trimethoprim 160 mg) orally, twice daily, *and*
Fluconazole 200–400 mg per day orally

Cotrimoxazole is generically available in the United States in a variety of formulations and product strengths, including tablets containing sulfamethoxazole 800 mg + trimethoprim 160 mg or tablets containing sulfamethoxazole 400 mg + trimethoprim 80 mg
Fluconazole is available in the United States in various formulations for oral administration, including immediate-release tablets containing 50 mg, 100 mg, 150 mg, and 200 mg powdered fluconazole for preparing liquid suspensions

Emetogenic potential: Low (Emetogenicity score = 2). See Chapter 39 for antiemetic regimens

Treatment Modifications

Adverse Event	Dose Modification
G3 Nonhematologic toxicity or G4 hematologic toxicity	Hold treatment until toxicity resolves to ≤G1, then resume at a reduced dose with bortezomib 1 mg/m^2
G3 Nonhematologic toxicity or G4 hematologic toxicity in a patient receiving bortezomib 1 mg/m^2	Hold treatment until toxicity resolves to ≤G1, then resume at a reduced dose with bortezomib 0.7 mg/m^2
Severe manifestations of hypercorticism including severe hyperglycemia, irritability and insomnia or oral candidiasis	Reduce daily dexamethasone dosage by 20% for G3 toxicity and by 40% for G4 or recurrent G3 toxicity

Patient Population Studied

A multicenter, open-label, nonrandomized, phase II trial of 202 patients with relapsed MM, refractory to the therapy they had received most recently

Efficacy (N = 193)

Complete response	10%
Partial response	18%
Minimal response	7%
No change	24%
Progressive disease	41%
Median time to first response	1.3 months
Median response duration*	12 months

*In the 67 patients with a complete, partial, or minimal response to bortezomib alone

European Group for Blood and Marrow Transplantation Criteria

Toxicity (N = 202)

	% All G	% G3/4
Nonhematologic		
Nausea	55	6
Diarrhea	44	8
Fatigue	41	12
Peripheral neuropathy	31	12
Vomiting	27	9
Anorexia	25	2
Fever	22	4
Headache	19	3
Constipation	16	2
Rash	15	<1
Limb pain	13	7
Dizziness, not vertigo	12	1
Weakness	11	6
Dehydration	10	7
Hematologic		
Thrombocytopenia	40	31
Anemia	21	8
Neutropenia	19	14

Note: Ten deaths occurred within 20 days after last bortezomib dose. Most attributed to progressive disease. Two deaths were possibly related to treatment

NCI Common Toxicity Criteria

Therapy Monitoring

1. *Weekly:* CBC with differential
2. *Every 2 cycles:* Serum BUN, creatinine and LFTs, and serum and urine M protein

REGIMEN

LIPOSOMAL DOXORUBICIN HCL, VINCRISTINE, DEXAMETHASONE (DVD)

Hussein MA et al. Cancer 2002;95:2160–2168

Doxorubicin HCl liposome injection (Doxil®) 40 mg/m² intravenously in 250 mL (doses ≤90 mg) to 500 mL (doses >90 mg) 5% dextrose injection (D5W) over 30 minutes, given on day 1 every 4 weeks
Vincristine 2 mg intravenously in 100 mL 0.9% NaCl injection (0.9% NS) over 30 minutes, given on day 1 every 4 weeks
Dexamethasone 40 mg orally or intravenously in 10–100 mL 0.9% NS or D5W over 10–30 minutes, given on days 1, 2, 3, and 4

Note: Repeat cycle every 4 weeks for a minimum of 6 cycles and for 2 cycles after the maximum response is achieved

Dexamethasone is marketed in the United States in numerous generic formulations for oral administration, including immediate-release tablets containing 0.25, 0.5, 0.75, 1, 2, 4, and 6 mg, and in elixirs (which contain alcohol) and solutions for oral administration

Supportive care:
Management of acute infusion-related reactions:
If an acute infusion-related reaction occurs, interrupt liposomal doxorubicin HCl infusion and *administer:*
Diphenhydramine 25–50 mg intravenously per push, *and*
Hydrocortisone 100 mg intravenously per push. After symptoms resolve, resume liposomal doxorubicin HCl infusion at 50% of the previous rate

Management of palmar-plantar erythrodysesthesia (PPE):
Pyridoxine 200 mg orally should be administered daily to patients who develop grade 1 or 2 PPE

Growth factor support:
May be used in patients who experience prolonged neutropenia or febrile neutropenia during a previous cycle of treatment
Filgrastim (G-CSF) 5–10 mcg/kg per day subcutaneously, starting on day 5 and continuing until ANC ≥5000/mm³ on two successive determinations, *or*
Sargramostim (GM-CSF) 5–10 mcg/kg per day, starting on day 5 and continuing until ANC ≥5000/mm³ on two successive determinations

Emetogenic potential: Low (Emetogenicity score = 2). See Chapter 39 for antiemetic regimens

Treatment Modifications

Pegylated Liposomal Doxorubicin

Modification Guidelines for Hematologic Toxicity on Day 1 of Planned Therapy

Grade	Cell Count	Dose Modification
G1	ANC 1000–1500/mm³, platelets 75–100,000/mm³	Resume treatment with no dose reduction
G2	ANC 500–999/mm³, platelets 50–75,000/mm³	Hold treatment until toxicity resolves to ≤G1 or 75% of the level at the start of the previous cycle then resume without dose reduction
G3/4	ANC <500/mm³, platelets <25,000/mm³	First episode: Hold treatment until toxicity resolves to ≤G1, then resume with a 25% dose reduction or continue at full dose with cytokine support. Reduce dose by 25% if neutropenia occurs despite growth factor use

Dose Modification Guidelines for Cardiac Toxicity

Toxicity	Dose Modification
LVEF decreases by ≥15% from baseline, or to <45%	Discontinue pegylated liposomal doxorubicin

Dose Modification Guidelines for Palmar-Plantar Erythrodysesthesia

Grade	4 Weeks After Dose	5 Weeks After Dose	6 Weeks After Dose
G1: Mild erythema, swelling, or desquamation not interfering with daily activities	Re-dose unless patient has experienced previous G3/4 skin toxicity. If so, delay an additional week	Re-dose unless patient has experienced previous G3/4 skin toxicity. If so, delay an additional week	Re-dose at 25% dose reduction; return to 4-week interval or discontinue therapy
G2: Erythema, desquamation, or swelling interfering with, but not precluding, normal physical activities; small blisters or ulcerations <2 cm in diameter	Delay treatment 1 week	Delay treatment 1 week	Re-dose at 25% dose reduction; return to 4-week interval or discontinue therapy
G3: Blistering, ulceration, or swelling interfering with walking or normal daily activities; cannot wear regular clothing	Delay treatment 1 week	Delay treatment 1 week	Discontinue therapy
G4: Diffuse or local process causing infectious complications, a bedridden state, or hospitalization	Delay treatment 1 week	Delay treatment 1 week	Discontinue therapy

Patient Population Studied

A single-center, open-label, phase II trial of 33 patients with newly diagnosed, symptomatic MM

Efficacy (N = 33)

Complete response	12%
Major response	55%
Minor response	21%
Stable disease	9%
Progressive disease	3%
Median time to first response	1.1 months
Median time to maximum response	4.6 months
Median time to progression	23.1 months

Toxicity (N = 33)

	% G3	% G4
Nonhematologic		
Palmar-plantar erythrodysesthesia	18	3
Mucositis	12	0
Deep vein thrombosis	3	0
Dehydration	3	0
Hematologic		
Anemia	12	9
Neutropenia	21	9
Thrombocytopenia	9	0

NCI Common Toxicity Criteria

Therapy Monitoring

1. *Weekly:* CBC with differential
2. *After each cycle:* Serum electrolytes, creatinine, BUN, and LFTs. Serum and urine protein electrophoresis with immunofixation. Serum β_2-microglobulin
3. *After 6 cycles or as soon as there is no peripheral evidence of disease:* Bone marrow biopsy. Repeat every other cycle until maximum response is achieved
4. Complete bone survey every 6 months
5. *After a cumulative dose of 500 mg/m² pegylated liposomal doxorubicin:* Reevaluate LVEF by MUGA. Subsequently, reevaluate LVEF before every other cycle

REGIMEN

DEXAMETHASONE, THALIDOMIDE, CISPLATIN, DOXORUBICIN, CYCLOPHOSPHAMIDE, ETOPOSIDE (DTPACE)

Lee CK et al. JCO 2003;21:2732–2739

Dexamethasone 40 mg orally daily on days 1, 2, 3, and 4 (total dose per cycle = 160 mg)
Thalidomide 400 mg orally daily throughout the cycle (total dose per cycle = 11,200 mg for 28-day cycle to 16,800 mg for 42-day cycle)
Cisplatin 10 mg/m^2 per day in 1000 mL 0.9% NaCl injection (0.9% NS) containing the daily dose of cisplatin, cyclophosphamide, and etoposide as a continuous IV infusion over 24 hours daily for 4 doses on days 1, 2, 3, and 4 (total dosage/cycle = 40 mg/m^2)
Cyclophosphamide 400 mg/m^2 per day in 1000 mL 0.9% NS containing the daily dose of cisplatin, cyclophosphamide, and etoposide as a continuous IV infusion over 24 hours daily for 4 doses on days 1, 2, 3, and 4 (total dosage/cycle = 1600 mg/m^2)
Etoposide 40 mg/m^2 per day in 1000 mL 0.9% NS containing the daily dose of cisplatin, cyclophosphamide, and etoposide as a continuous IV infusion over 24 hours daily for 4 doses on days 1, 2, 3, and 4 (total dosage/cycle = 160 mg/m^2)
Doxorubicin 10 mg/m^2 daily for 4 doses in a minimum volume of 50 mL of 5% dextrose injection (D5W) as a continuous IV infusion over 24 hours daily on days 1, 2, 3, and 4 (total dosage/cycle = 40 mg/m^2)

Notes:

- Repeat cycle every 4–6 weeks that provided the ANC has recovered to > 1000/mm^3 and the platelet count is > 100,00/mm^3
- Administer infusions through a central venous catheter using a portable infusion pump
- If patient is to undergo autologous PBSC transplantation, administer **filgrastim (G-CSF)** 10 mcg/kg per day subcutaneously every day, starting on day 5 of the first cycle and continuing until stem cell collection is complete
- Administer up to 6 cycles in patients not undergoing PBSC transplantation

Maintenance therapy:
Dexamethasone 20 mg orally daily on days 1, 2, 3, and 4 every 28 days (total dose per 28 days = 80 mg), *and*
Thalidomide 50–200 mg orally daily throughout the cycle (total dose per 28 days = 1400–5600 mg). Initiate after completion of DTPACE or autologous PBSC transplantation

Dexamethasone is marketed in the United States in numerous generic formulations for oral administration, including immediate-release tablets containing 0.25, 0.5, 0.75, 1, 2, 4, and 6 mg, and in elixirs (which contain alcohol) and solutions for oral administration
Thalidomide is marketed in the United States in immediate-release capsules for oral administration containing 50 mg, 100 mg, or 200 mg. THALOMID® (thalidomide) CAPSULES product label, February 2004. Celgene Corporation, Warren, NJ

Supportive care:
Filgrastim (G-CSF), 300 mcg/day, beginning on day 5 of the cycle and continuing until ANC >1000/mm^3 for 2 consecutive days.
Consider H_2 antagonist or proton pump inhibitor
Consider venous thromboembolism prophylaxis

Infection prophylaxis:
Cotrimoxazole (sulfamethoxazole 800 mg + trimethoprim 160 mg) orally twice daily for 2 days per week
Fluconazole 200 mg orally 4 times per day, beginning on day 1 of the cycle and continuing until ANC >1000/mm^3 for 2 consecutive days
Levofloxacin 250 mg orally 4 times per day, beginning on day 1 of the cycle and continuing until ANC >1000/mm^3 for 2 consecutive days
Acyclovir 400 mg orally twice a day, beginning on day 1 of the cycle and continuing until ANC >1000/mm^3 for 2 consecutive days

Cotrimoxazole is generically available in the United States in a variety of formulations and product strengths, including tablets containing sulfamethoxazole 800 mg + trimethoprim 160 mg and tablets containing sulfamethoxazole 400 mg + trimethoprim 80 mg

(*continued*)

Treatment Modifications

Adverse Event	Dose Modification
G3/4 nonhematologic toxicity	Hold treatment until toxicity resolves to ≤G2, then resume with a 25–50% dose reduction
Hematologic toxicity: ANC ≤1000/mm^3, *or* platelets ≤100,000/mm^3	Hold treatment until recovery, then resume with a dose reduction

Patient Population Studied

A single-center, open-label, phase III trial of 236 patients with previously treated MM and with no prior autologous or allogeneic transplantation. Patients received 2 cycles of DTPACE before randomization to either tandem autologous transplantation or up to 4 more cycles of DTPACE

Efficacy (N = 236)

Complete remission or near-CR	21%
Partial response	19%
Improvement*	58%
No improvement or progressive disease	2%

*Minimum 50% reduction in serum paraprotein or 75% reduction in Bence Jones protein excretion, or a 50% reduction in bone marrow plasmacytosis from pretreatment values, without meeting criteria for PR, near-CR, or CR

(continued)

Fluconazole is available in the United States in various formulations for oral administration, including immediate-release tablets containing 50 mg, 100 mg, 150 mg, and 200 mg powdered fluconazole for preparing liquid suspensions

Levofloxacin is available in the United States in three formulations for oral administration, including immediate-release tablets (250, 500, and 750 mg/tablet) and an oral solution (25 mg/mL). Levaquin® (levofloxacin) Tablets, Levaquin® (levofloxacin) Oral Solution product label, October 2004. Ortho-McNeil Pharmaceutical, Inc, Raritan, NJ

Acyclovir is available generically in the United States in formulations for oral administration, including immediate-release tablets (400 and 800 mg per tablet), immediate-release capsules (200 mg/capsule), and a powdered product for preparing a liquid suspension (200 mg/5 mL)

Emetogenic potential:

Days 1–4: Very high. (Emetogenicity score = 6). See Chapter 39 for antiemetic regimens

Therapy Monitoring

1. *Weekly:* CBC with differential, serum electrolytes, BUN, creatinine, and LFTs
2. *After every 2 cycles:* Serum and urine M protein. Bone marrow biopsy and aspiration

Toxicity (N = 435 cycles)

	% Cycles	
	G1/2/3/4	G3/4
Hematologic		
Neutropenia (ANC <500/mm^3)		39
Thrombocytopenia (<75,000/mm^3)		11
Nonhematologic		
Nausea/vomiting	21	6
Stomatitis/pharyngitis	19	4
Thromboembolism	15	5
Sensory neuropathy	13	4
Documented infection	4	4
Neutropenic fever	12	9
Hypophosphatemia	17	4

Other G3/4 toxicities occurring in <3% of cycles: Esophagitis/gastritis, colitis, diarrhea, hyperbilirubinemia, hypoalbuminemia, sinus bradycardia, supraventricular arrhythmia, hypotension, congestive heart failure, pulmonary infiltrates, pulmonary edema, seizure, syncope, ataxia, erythema or rash, hypocalcemia, hypomagnesemia, hypokalemia, hyponatremia, and decrease in bicarbonate

Treatment-related mortality was 4% at 3 months after 2 cycles of treatment

NCI Common Toxicity Criteria

29. Ovarian Cancer

Eddie Reed, MD

Epidemiology

Incidence: 20,180 cases (estimated in 2006)
Mortality: 15,310 (estimated in 2006)

5-Year Survival
(Trends in 5-year survival, all races, all stages)

1974–1976:	37%
1983–1985:	41%
1992–1999:	53%
Stages I and II*:	95%
Stages III and IV:	31%

*Percentage of patients diagnosed in good prognosis stages I and II = 29%
Jemal A et al. CA Cancer J Clin 2006;56:106–30

Pathology

WHO classification of malignant ovarian tumors

1. Common epithelial tumors (60% of all neoplasms of ovary; 90% of all malignant neoplasm of ovary)
2. Sex cord–stromal tumor (5% of malignant neoplasms of ovary)
3. Lipid (lipoid) cell tumors (rare)
4. Gonadoblastoma (rare)

Tumor Grade

- Grade 1—Well differentiated
- Grade 2—Moderately-well differentiated
- Grade 3—Poorly-differentiated

Note: Alternately ovarian carcinoma can be classified into either low grade and high grade

A detailed WHO classification is critical to the ovarian cancer specialist. However, to the general oncologist, a more simplified approach can be taken

Histology	Response to Cytotoxic Chemotherapy	Comment
Epithelial cell	Respond well	Debulking surgery recommended
Germ cell	Respond well (regimens similar to testicular cancer)	
Stromal cell	Generally do not respond well	

Ozols RF, Schwartz PE, Eifel PJ. In: DeVita VT Jr, Hellman S, Rosenberg SA, eds. Cancer: Principles & Practice of Oncology, 6th ed. Philadelphia: Lippincott Williams & Wilkins, 2001:1596–1632

Work-Up

1. Personal and family history, physical examination
2. Liver function tests, BUN, creatinine, LDH
3. CBC with platelets, PT, PTT, INR
4. Tumor markers (CA 125, alpha fetoprotein (AFP), β-HCG)
5. CT scan of abdomen and pelvis, and chest x-ray. CT of chest if chest x-ray is abnormal
6. Radiographic tests of unclear utility: MRI of abdomen and pelvis, PET scan

Notes:

- Consider possible abnormal hormone secretion syndromes
- Consider possible concurrent malignancies elsewhere
- Consider possible metastases to the ovary from elsewhere (eg, breast, colon)
- Consider GI evaluation if clinically indicated

Staging

Stage	Description
Stage I	**Growth limited to one or both ovaries**
IA	Growth limited to one ovary. No ascites. No tumor on the external surfaces. Capsule intact
IB	Growth limited to both ovaries. No ascites. No tumor on the external surfaces. Capsule intact
IC	Tumor either stage IA or IB but with tumor on the surface of one or both ovaries; capsule ruptured; ascites present containing malignant cells; or positive peritoneal washings
Stage II	**Growth involving one or both ovaries with pelvic extension**
IIA	Extension and/or metastases to the uterus and/or fallopian tubes
IIB	Extension to other pelvic organs
IIC	Tumor either stage IIA or IIB but with tumor on the surface of one or both ovaries; capsule(s) ruptured; ascites present containing malignant cells; or positive peritoneal washings
Stage III	**Tumor involving one or both ovaries with peritoneal implants outside the pelvis and/or positive retroperitoneal or inguinal nodes: metastases to the surface of the liver equals stage III; tumor is limited to the true pelvis but with histologically verified malignant extension to the small bowel or omentum**
IIIA	Tumor grossly limited to the true pelvis with negative nodes but with histologically confirmed microscopic seeding of abdominal peritoneal surfaces
IIIB	Tumor of one or both ovaries; histologically confirmed implants of abdominal peritoneal surfaces, none >2 cm in diameter; node-negative
IIIC	Abdominal implants >2 cm in diameter and/or positive retroperitoneal or inguinal nodes
Stage IV	**Growth involving one or both ovaries with distant metastases. If pleural effusion is present, there must be positive cytologic test results to designate a case as stage IV. Parenchymal liver metastasis equals stage IV**

AJCC Cancer Staging Manual, 6th ed

Treatment and Survival by Stage

Treatment and survival by stage cannot be summarized simply for ovarian cancer. Each stage is strongly influenced by whether the disease is amenable to surgery, by the histologic type and grade, by the bulk of residual disease after the completion of surgery, and by other factors

There are situations in early-stage disease, for example, in which one can reasonably treat the patient with surgery or with external-beam radiation therapy. Within a stage, the choice of therapy depends on disease residua. Furthermore, the management of recurrent disease is an evolving art form that requires a detailed knowledge of the disease, knowledge of the treatment options available, and an understanding of what the patient wants

Caveats

Chemotherapy

Early-Stage Disease

1. In good-prognosis, early-stage disease, surgery alone is adequate therapy: there is a 95% 10-year survival rate (Ia or Ib)
2. In early-stage patients who have an increased risk for recurrence (poorly differentiated histologies):
   - Three cycles of cisplatin + cyclophosphamide, reduced the risk of recurrence and improve survival
   - A comparable European study gives similar data for cisplatin alone versus ^{32}P
   - Three cycles of paclitaxel and carboplatin may offer as much benefit, but the data are not yet conclusive

Bolis G et al. Ann Oncol 1995;6:887–893
Young RC et al. JCO 2003;21:4350–4355
Young RC. Semin Oncol 2000;27(3 suppl 7):8–10

Advanced-Stage Disease (≥IIc)

1. Standard of care for advanced-stage disease: depends in part on the amount of residual disease
   - Pts with stage III disease that is optimally debulked with no residual mass greater than 1 cm in diameter after surgery should be treated, if possible, with intraperitoneal cisplatin and paclitaxel
   - Six cycles of paclitaxel + carboplatin, are used if debulking surgery was not optimal
2. Benefit of 3-drug combinations in this setting is uncertain:
   - Paclitaxel + carboplatin, + topotecan
   - Paclitaxel + carboplatin + gemcitabine
   - Paclitaxel + cisplatin + cyclophosphamide (most effective 3-drug regimen)
3. Generally, dose-intense approaches requiring stem cell of support are ill advised
4. Benefit of "consolidation" therapy, after an initial 6 cycles of systemic treatment is uncertain
   - Consolidation regimens: Several additional cycles of single-agent paclitaxel or a paclitaxel combination

Kohn EC et al. Gynecol Oncol 1996;62:181–191
McGuire WP et al. NEJM 1996;334:1–6
Ozols RF et al. JCO 2003;21:3194–200
Sarosy GA, Reed E. [Editorial] Ann Intern Med 2000;133:555–556

Recurrent Disease

1. Treatment of recurrent disease is complex. Decisions should be based on:
   - Likelihood of sensitivity/resistance to agents given in the past: Platinum-sensitive or platinum-resistant disease
   - Residual toxicity from prior treatments
   - Comorbid illnesses, including renal, hepatic, and cardiac function
   - Desires of the patient
2. *Platinum-sensitive disease*
   - Epithelial ovarian cancer that recurs ≥1–2 years after platinum-based chemotherapy
   - Response rate to re-treatment with another platinum agent-based regimen tends to be high (<70%)
3. *Platinum-resistant disease*
   - Disease progression in the face of appropriate initial platinum-based treatment
   - Disease recurrence within the first 6 months after an initial response to platinum-based therapy
   - Poor prognosis, especially if disease progresses during their initial 6 cycles of therapy with platinum agents
   - Use of non–cross-resistant agents in the second-line and third-line setting is critically important

Leitao MM Jr et al. Gynecol Oncol 2003;91:123–129
Markman M et al. J Cancer Res Clin Oncol 2004;130:25–28
Markman M et al. Gynecol Oncol 2004;93:699–701
Reed E et al. Gynecol Oncol 1992;46:326–329

Platinum Hypersensitivity

1. Platinum hypersensitivity can develop in patients who have received ≥6 cycles of cisplatin or carboplatin
2. A desensitization regimen should be used
3. Rarely desensitization is not successful. In this situation, consider doxorubicin with cyclophosphamide

Surgery

1. Ideally, a gynecologic oncologist should perform all surgical procedures for ovarian cancer including:
   - Initial staging and debulking surgery
   - Second-look procedure (if done)
   - Any interval surgical debulking procedure
2. Goals of initial surgical procedure:
   - Stage disease
   - Remove all visible disease from the abdominopelvic cavity; or, if surgeon cannot remove all visible disease, remove all disease possible (debulking surgery)
3. Debulking important because subsequent survival and response to chemotherapy are linked to:
   - Dimension of the largest remaining tumor lesion after completion of surgery
   - Possibly, the overall volume of residual disease
4. Surgery alone is the preferred approach to patients with good-prognosis, early-stage epithelial ovarian cancer:
   - Stages: Ia or Ib
   - Any epithelial histology other than clear cell
   - Well differentiated or moderately well differentiated histologic grade (low grade). [Any early-stage patient other than the latter should have postsurgery chemotherapy]
5. Neoadjuvant chemotherapy (has not received widespread acceptance):
   - Two to three cycles of chemotherapy before an initial staging and debulking procedure
   - Data suggest a less morbid operation with reduced blood loss and a shorter operative procedure

Hoskins WJ et al. Am J Obstet Gynecol 1994;170:974–979; discussion 979–980
Schwartz PE, Zheng W. Gynecol Oncol 2003;90:644–650
Schwartz PE et al. Gynecol Oncol 1999;72:93–99

Germ Cell Tumors

The recommended laboratory evaluation for germ cell tumors should include:

1. A comprehensive metabolic panel, CBC with platelets, magnesium level, LDH, AFP, and β-HCG levels
2. Pulmonary function studies may be obtained
3. Complete surgical staging surgery is recommended as initial surgery, with fertility-sparing surgery considered in those desiring fertility

Stage I dysgerminoma or immature teratoma

1. Patients who have had complete surgical staging and no evidence of disease is found outside the ovary should be observed
2. Patients who have had incomplete surgical staging for whom observation without chemotherapy is being considered, should undergo a complete staging procedure. If no evidence of disease is found outside the ovary these patients may be observed. If, at the time of a complete surgical staging, tumor is found outside the ovary, patients should receive bleomycin + etoposide + cisplatinum (BEP) in the postoperative period

Stages II–IV dysgerminoma or stage I, grade 2-3 immature teratoma or embryonal tumors or endodermal sinus tumors

1. These patients should receive chemotherapy for 3–4 cycles with bleomycin + etoposide + cisplatinum (BEP)
2. Patients achieving a complete clinical response should be observed clinically every 2–4 months with AFP and β-HCG levels (if initially elevated) for 2 years
3. Patients with radiographic evidence of residual tumor but with normal AFP and β-HCG levels should be considered for surgical resection of the tumor; observation can be considered
4. Patients with persistently elevated AFP and/or β-HCG after chemotherapy, or with clinically or radiographically evident disease, should receive chemotherapy or radiation or supportive care. Acceptable regimens for recurrent disease include:
   - Cisplatin + etoposide
   - VIP (etoposide + ifosfamide + cisplatin)
   - VeIP (vinblastine + ifosfamide + cisplatin)
   - VAC (vincristine + dactinomycin + cyclophosphamide)

Radiation

1. External-beam radiation therapy:
   - Very useful in the treatment of some subsets of patients with early-stage disease
   - Has fallen out of favor in the United States
   - Commonly used in some academic centers in Canada and Europe
   - Major drawback is the reduction in reserve function of organs within the radiation field, such as the bone marrow
   - Useful in the management of tumor masses that might cause extreme pain, bleeding, or other medical problems and in cases in which surgery is not a good option
   - On occasion, large lesions in the pelvis or metastases to bone (unusual) respond readily to radiation
2. Intraperitoneal colloidal ^{32}P:
   - Useful in the treatment of early-stage disease
   - Can be of palliative value in other settings
   - Has fallen out of favor in the United States
3. Gamma-knife, intensity-modulated radiation therapy (IMRT), and standard whole-brain radiation:
   - Metastases to the brain occur uncommonly but are no longer considered rare
   - Several approaches are effective in controlling CNS disease
   - Use of these approaches depends on the clinical setting and the technology available

Ovarian Stromal Tumors

1. Patients with stage IA–C ovarian stromal tumors desiring fertility should be treated with fertility-sparing surgery. Otherwise, complete staging is recommended to all other patients
2. Those with surgical findings of stage I tumor should be observed
3. Patients having high-risk stage I (tumor rupture, poorly differentiated tumor, tumor size >10–15 cm) or stages II–IV tumors can be observed or can receive radiation therapy or undergo cisplatin-based chemotherapy with germ cell regimens preferred
4. Patients subsequently having a clinical relapse may consider secondary cytoreductive surgery, enter a clinical trial, or be offered supportive care

NCCN® Practice Guidelines in Oncology. vol. 1, 2005

Toxicities: Ovarian Cancer Chemotherapy

1. **Myelosuppression**

   Associated with all the agents listed in this chapter except tamoxifen. All three lineages are affected. Persistent thrombocytopenia is associated with the platinum compounds

2. **Nausea and vomiting**

   Preventive treatment is very important. Delayed nausea and vomiting is very common. Steroids, serotonin (HT_3)-receptor antagonists, and tachykinin (NK_1)-receptor antagonists are recommended for routine use with platinum-containing regimens

3. **Renal dysfunction**

   Seen with cisplatin and with carboplatin, but usually more clinically significant with cisplatin. Serum creatinine may be normal in the face of a markedly reduced creatinine clearance. This is important because other drugs that are eliminated by the kidney may be needed (eg, antibiotics). Platinum-related renal insufficiency is nonoliguric: be vigilant

4. **Neurotoxicity**

   Clinically occurs before detectable changes on EMG/NCTs. Bilateral paresthesias in stocking-and-glove distribution usually are progressive with repeated platinum doses and can become severe. Cisplatin is more likely to cause this problem than carboplatin

5. **Fatigue/weakness**

   May be related to anemia, but is a common side effect of several newer agents, including gemcitabine and topotecan

6. **Altered sexual function**

   A common side effect, but is seldom discussed spontaneously by a patient. It can be an underlying contributing factor to family disruption and clinical reactive depression; usually is a combined function of surgery and effect of neuroactive anticancer agent (platinum agents)

7. **Clinical depression**

   A common side effect. Many patients request medication for this. Sometimes may be a severe problem

8. **Rare toxicities**

   Acute hypersensitivity to paclitaxel. Acute hypersensitivity to cisplatin/carboplatin (usually occurs after 6–8 cycles of therapy). Desensitization is occasionally appropriate and can be successful. On most occasions, switch to another agent right away

REGIMEN

CISPLATIN AND CYCLOPHOSPHAMIDE

Young RC et al. JCO 2003;23:4350–4355

Cyclophosphamide 1000 mg/m^2 intravenously in 1000 mL 0.9% NaCl injection (0.9% NS) over 30–60 minutes, given on day 1 every 21 days for 3 cycles (total dosage/cycle = 1000 mg/m^2)
Cisplatin 100 mg/m^2 intravenously in 250 mL 0.9% NS over 30–60 minutes, given on day 1 every 21 days for 3 cycles (total dosage/cycle = 100 mg/m^2)
Emetogenic potential: Very high (Emetogenicity score = 6). See Chapter 39 for antiemetic regimens

Patient Population Studied

Prospective randomized clinical trial conducted by the GOG of 251 patients: 124 patients randomized to ^{32}P and 127 randomized to chemotherapy. Eligible patients were either FIGO stage Ia or Ib (grade 3), or stage Ic or II (any grade). In addition, all stages I and II patients with clear cell histology (any grade) were eligible

Efficacy

10-Year Cumulative Incidence of Recurrence	
All patients	28%
Stage I	24%
Stage II	39%

Toxicity

	% G3/4
Hematologic	
Leukopenia	69.5
Granulocytopenia	68
Thrombocytopenia	8.5
Nonhematologic	
Gastrointestinal	11.9
Renal	1.7
Ototoxicity	0.8
Bowel perforation	0

Therapy Monitoring

Before repeated cycles: PE, CBC with differential, and serum electrolytes, magnesium, calcium, BUN, and creatinine

Notes

Although compared with intraperitoneal ^{32}P, there were no statistically significant differences in survival, the authors concluded: "the lower cumulative recurrence seen with CP (cisplatin + cyclophosphamide) and complications of ^{32}P administration make platinum-based combinations the preferred adjuvant therapy for early ovarian cancer patients at high-risk for recurrence"

Treatment Modifications

(Specific recommendations not provided by authors)

Adverse Event	Dose Modification
Creatinine clearance[a] 30–60 mL/min	Reduce cisplatin so that dose in milligrams equals the creatinine clearance value in mL/min[b]
Creatinine clearance[a] <30 mL/minute	Hold cisplatin
If on day 1 of a cycle, leukocyte count <3000/mm^3, ANC <1000/mm^3, or platelets <100,000/mm^3	Hold chemotherapy for 1 week, then resume treatment if leukocytes ≥3000/mm^3, ANC ≥1000/mm^3, platelets >100,000/mm^3
If on day 1 of a cycle, G ≥2 nonhematologic adverse event or serum creatinine ≥1.8 mg/dL (≥160 µmol/L)	Hold chemotherapy for 1 week, then resume with chemotherapy dose reduced by 20–30% if nonhematologic toxicity resolved to G ≤1 and creatinine ≤1.5 mg/dL (≤133 µmol/L)
G4 Neutropenia (with or without fever)	Add primary prophylaxis with filgrastim 5 mcg/kg per day subcutaneously for 14 days with same chemotherapy doses during all subsequent cycles
Febrile neutropenia despite filgrastim support	Hold treatment until adverse event resolves, then resume chemotherapy with chemotherapy dosage reduced by 20–30%

[a]Creatinine clearance used as a measure of glomerular filtration rate (GFR)
[b]Also applies to patients with creatinine clearance (GFR) of 30–60 mL/min at outset of treatment

EPITHELIAL OVARIAN CANCER REGIMEN ADVANCED STAGE DISEASE

INTRAPERITONEAL CISPLATIN AND PACLITAXEL

Armstrong DK, et al. NEJM 2006; 354:34–43
Walker JL, et al. Gynecol Oncol 2006; 100:27–32
GOG Protocol #0172

Note: Regimen for stage III epithelial ovarian or peritoneal carcinoma optimally debulked with no residual mass greater than 1 cm in diameter after surgery. Sub-optimally debulked disease should not be treated with this regimen

Premedication for paclitaxel:
Dexamethasone 20 mg/dose, administer orally or intravenously per push, at 12–14 hours and 6–7 hours (2 doses) before starting paclitaxel or
Dexamethasone 20 mg, administer intravenously per push, 30 minutes before administering paclitaxel plus
Diphenhydramine 50 mg, administer intravenously per push, 30 minutes before administering paclitaxel
Cimetidine 300 mg, administer intravenously in 20–50 mL 0.9% Sodium Chloride Injection (0.9%NS) or 5% Dextrose Injection (D5W), USP, over 5–20 minutes 30 minutes before administering paclitaxel

Paclitaxel 135 mg/m^2, administer by intravenous infusion in a volume of 0.9%NS or D5W sufficient to produce a concentration within the range 0.3–1.2 mg/mL over 24 hours on day 1 every 21 days for 6 cycles (total dosage/cycle = 135 mg/m^2)

Intraperitoneal cisplatin
Hydration before cisplatin: ≥1000 mL 0.9%NS, administer by intravenous infusion over a minimum of 2 to 4 hours.
Note: If a large amount of ascites is present it should be drained prior to the instillation of cisplatin.
Cisplatin 100 mg/m^2, administer intraperitoneally as rapidly as possible in warmed (37°C) 0.9%NS 2000 mL through an implanted peritoneal catheter on day 2, every 21 days for 6 cycles (total dosage/21-day cycle = 100 mg/m^2). Following the infusion, patients alternate position from prone, supine, and left and right lateral decubitus every 15 minutes over 2 hours to maximize drug distribution throughout the peritoneal cavity
Note: Do not attempt to retrieve the infusate
Hydration after cisplatin: ≥1000 mL 0.9%NS, administer by intravenous infusion over a minimum of 3 to 4 hours. Also encourage high oral fluid intake. Goal is to achieve a urine output of ≥100 mL/hour

Intraperitoneal paclitaxel
Note: If a large amount of ascites is present it should be drained prior to the instillation of paclitaxel.
Paclitaxel 60 mg/m^2, administer intraperitoneally as rapidly as possible in warmed (37°C) 0.9%NS or D5W 1000 mL through an implanted peritoneal catheter, followed by an additional 1000 mL of 0.9%NS or D5W on day 8, every 21 days for 6 cycles (total dosage/21-day cycle = 60 mg/m^2)
Note: Do not attempt to retrieve the infusate

Systemic cisplatin
If intraperitoneal therapy is discontinued substitute:
Cisplatin 75 mg/m^2, administer intravenously in 250 mL 0.9%NS over 30–60 minutes on day 2, every 21 days for 3 cycles (total dosage/cycle = 75 mg/m^2)

Supportive care
Dexamethasone, 8 mg/dose × 6 doses after chemotherapy, administer orally, if G ≥ 2 arthralgias/myalgias occur

Emetogenic potential
Day 1: Low (Emetogenicity score = 2)
Day 2: High (Emetogenicity score = 5). Potential for delayed symptoms
Day 8: Low (Emetogenicity score approximately 2).
See Chapter 39 for antiemetic regimens

Treatment Modifications

Dose Modification Levels for Treatment

	IV Paclitaxel	IP Cisplatin	IP Paclitaxel
Starting dose	135 mg/m^2	100 mg/m^2	60 mg/m^2
Level −1	110 mg/m^2	75 mg/m^2	45 mg/m^2

Note: No dose escalations performed

Dose escalations for hematologic toxicity

Adverse Event	Treatment Modification
ANC <1500/mm^3 or platelet count <100,000/mm^3 on day 1 of a cycle	Delay start of next cycle until ANC ≥1500/mm^3 or platelet count ≥100,000/mm^3. Do not adjust dosages nor add filgrastim if the delay is less than 2 weeks
>2 weeks, but ≤3 weeks delay to start next cycle because ANC <1500/mm^3 or platelet count <100,000/mm^3 on day 1	Reduce intravenous paclitaxel dosage one level
>2 weeks ANC delay in start of a cycle because <1500/mm^3 or platelet count <100,000/mm^3 on day 1 despite one dose reduction	Add filgrastim 5 micrograms/kg/day beginning 24 hours after completion of intravenous chemotherapy and continuing for 14 days
>3 weeks delay to start next cycle because ANC <1500/mm^3 or platelet count <100,000/mm^3 on day 1 regardless of whether filgrastim was or was not used	Discontinue therapy
ANC <1500/mm^3 or platelet count <100,000/mm^3 on day 8 of a cycle	Do not delay nor adjust intraperitoneal paclitaxel dosage
Uncomplicated WBC or ANC nadirs	Do not modify dosages

(*continued*)

Treatment Modifications (continued)

Adverse Event	Treatment Modification
ANC <500/mm³ on day 8	Add filgrastim 5 micrograms/kg/day until ANC >5000–10,000/mm³
Nadir platelet count <25,000/mm³	Reduce intravenous paclitaxel dosage one dose level.
First episode of febrile neutropenia or sepsis requiring intravenous antibiotics	Reduce intravenous paclitaxel dosage one dose level. Do not add filgrastim
Febrile neutropenia or sepsis requiring intravenous antibiotics despite reduction of paclitaxel one dosage level	Add filgrastim beginning 24 hours after completion of IV chemotherapy and continuing for 14 days without additional dosage modification

Abdominal Pain Score

G0	No pain
G1	Mild pain. Narcotic analgesia not required; pain causes minimal interference with daily activities and lasts for less than 72 hours
G2	Moderate pain. Narcotic analgesia required; pain causes moderate interference with daily activities and lasts longer than 72 hours
G3	Severe pain. Narcotic analgesia required; pain confines patient to bed and causes sever interference with daily activities

(continued)

Patient Population Studied

205 women with stage III epithelial ovarian or peritoneal carcinoma optimally debulked with no residual mass greater than 1 cm in diameter after surgery. All patients had a Gynecologic Oncology Group (GOG) performance status of 0 to 2.

Efficacy (N = 205)

Variable	Months
Median progression-free survival (PFS)	23.8
PFS in pts with gross residual disease	18.3
PFS in pts without visible residual disease	37.6
Median overall survival	65.6

Toxicity (N = 201)

Toxicity	% G3/4
Hematologic Toxicities	
WBC <1000/mm³	76
Platelet count <25,000/mm³	12
Other hematologic event	94
Non-hematologic Toxicities	
Gastrointestinal event	46
Metabolic event	27
Neurologic event	19
Fatigue	18
Infection	16
Pain	11
Cardiovascular event	9
Fever	9
Renal or genitourinary event	7
Pulmonary event	3
Hepatic event	3
Other	3
Cutaneous change	1
Event involving lymphatic system	1
Complications of IP access devices	
Port complications	19.5%
Inflow obstruction	8.8%
Infection	10.2%
Bowel Injury	2%

Armstrong DK, et al. NEJM 2006; 354:34–43
Walker JL, et al. Gynecol Oncol 2006; 100:27–32

(continued)

Treatment Modifications (*continued*)

Adverse Event	Treatment Modification
G2 abdominal pain	Reduce intraperitoneal cisplatin or paclitaxel, whichever is causing symptoms, by one dose level
Recurrent G2 abdominal pain after a dose reduction or G3 abdominal pain or complications involving the intraperitoneal catheter prohibiting further intraperitoneal therapy	Discontinue intraperitoneal therapy and administer intravenous cisplatin instead
Any grade gastrointestinal toxicity	Hospitalize patient if necessary but do not adjust dosages
G2 peripheral neuropathy	Reduce cisplatin dosage by one dose level
G3/4 peripheral neuropathy	Hold therapy until peripheral neuropathy G ≤ 1 then restart therapy with cisplatin dosage reduced by one dose level. Consider discontinuing therapy if not recovered to baseline by 2–3 weeks
Increase in serum creatinine >0.7–1.0 mg/dL (62–88 μmol/L) above baseline	Hold therapy until serum creatinine returns to baseline and reduce intraperitoneal cisplatin one dosage level. Consider discontinuing therapy if not recovered to baseline by 2–3 weeks

Toxicity (N = 201) (*continued*)

Discontinuation of IP therapy (N = 119)		
Reason	Primary	Contributing
Catheter-related	**40**	**10**
IP catheter infection	21	4
IP catheter blocked	10	0
IP catheter leak	3	2
Access problem	5	3
Fluid leak out vagina	1	1
Not IP catheter related	**34**	**28**
Nausea/Vomiting/Dehydration	16	16
Renal/Metabolic	15	12
Disease Progression	3	0
Possibly IP treatment-related	**45**	**42**
Other infection (not catheter)	7	5
Abdominal pain	4	16
Patient refusal	19	8
Bowel complication	4	4
Other	11	9

Walker JL, et al. Gynecol Oncol 2006; 100:27–32

Notes

1. Among all randomized phase 3 trials conducted by the GOG among patients with advanced ovarian cancer, this therapy yielded the longest median survival (65.6 months)
2. Only 42% of patients received all six cycles of intraperitoneal therapy
3. The primary reason for discontinuation of intraperitoneal therapy was catheter-related complications
4. Among 205 patients randomly allocated to the intraperitoneal arm, 58% (119) did not complete all six cycles of intraperitoneal therapy. Of these 119 patients, 34% (40/119 = 34%) discontinued intraperitoneal therapy primarily due to catheter complications, while 29% (34/119 = 29%) discontinued for unrelated reasons. 37% (45/119 = 37%) discontinued for reasons that were possibly related to the intraperitoneal treatment (see table under toxicities)
5. Hysterectomy, appendectomy, small bowel resection and ileocecal resection were not associated with failure to complete six cycles
6. There appears to be an association between rectosigmoid colon resection and the ability to initiate intraperitoneal therapy. Intraperitoneal therapy was not initiated 16% of patients who had a left colon or rectosigmoid colon resection versus 5% of those who did not have such a resection ($p = 0.015$)
7. Intraperitoneal therapy should begin as soon as possible after surgery. A delay of intraperitoneal therapy allows opportunity for adhesions to develop and may limit access of the IP fluid
8. The 2 liters of intraperitoneal fluid administered with the intraperitoneal therapy does not replace the need for intravascular saline administration and adequate urine output. Administration of at least one liter of saline both prior to and after cisplatin is essential

Armstrong DK, et al. NEJM 2006; 354:34–43
Walker JL, et al. Gynecol Oncol 2006; 100:27–32

Therapy Monitoring

1. *Prior to start of therapy:* PE, CBC with differential, electrolytes, serum creatinine, BUN, mineral panel, LFTs, CA-125, audiogram only in patients with a history of hearing loss, and chest-X-ray
2. *Weekly:* CBC with differential
3. *Prior to each cycle:* PE, CBC with differential, electrolytes, serum creatinine, BUN, mineral panel, LFTs

REGIMEN

CARBOPLATIN + PACLITAXEL

Ozols RF et al. JCO 2003;21:3194–3200

Note: Regimen for optimally debulked ovarian cancer and suboptimally debulked disease as well

Premedication for paclitaxel:
Dexamethasone 20 mg/dose orally for 2 doses at 12 hours and 6 hours before administering paclitaxel or
Dexamethasone 20 mg intravenously per push or in 10–50 mL 0.9% NaCl injection (0.9% NS) or 5% dextrose injection (D5W) 30 minutes before paclitaxel plus
Diphenhydramine 50 mg intravenously per push 30 minutes before paclitaxel
Cimetidine 300 mg intravenously in 20–50 mL 0.9% NS or D5W over 5–20 minutes 30 minutes before paclitaxel

Paclitaxel 175 mg/m^2 by intravenous infusion in a volume of 0.9% NS or D5W sufficient to produce a concentration of 0.3–1.2 mg/mL over 3 hours on day 1 every 3 weeks (total dosage/cycle = 175 mg/m^2)
Carboplatin [calculated dose] AUC = 7.5, intravenously in 0.9% NS or D5W 100–500 mL over 1 hour on day 1 after completing paclitaxel, every 3 weeks (total dosage/cycle calculated to produce an AUC = 7.5 mg/mL·min)

Carboplatin dose is based on Calvert's formula to achieve a target area under the plasma concentration versus time curve (AUC) [AUC units = mg/mL·min]

$$\text{Total carboplatin dose (mg)} = (\text{Target AUC}) \times (\text{GFR} + 25)$$

In practice, creatinine clearance (Clcr) is used in place of glomerular filtration rate (GFR). Clcr can be calculated from the equation of Cockcroft and Gault:

$$\text{Males, Clcr} = \frac{(140 - \text{age [y]}) \times \text{body weight [kg]}}{72 \times (\text{Serum creatinine [mg/dL]})}$$

$$\text{Females, Clcr} = \frac{(140 - \text{age [y]}) \times \text{body weight [kg]}}{72 \times (\text{Serum creatinine [mg/dL]})} \times 0.85$$

Calvert AH et al. JCO 1989;7:1748–1756
Cockcroft DW, Gault MH. Nephron 1976;16:31–41
Jodrell DI et al. JCO 1992;10:520–528
Sorensen BT et al. Cancer Chemother Pharmacol 1991;28:397–401

Emetogenic potential: High (Emetogenicity score = 5). See Chapter 39 for antiemetic regimens

Treatment Modifications

Adverse Event	Dose Modification
At start of a cycle, ANC ≤1000/mm^3 or platelets ≤100,000/mm^3	Delay start of cycle up to 2 weeks until ANC >1000/mm^3 and platelets >100,000/mm^3
ANC ≤1000/mm^3 or platelets ≤100,000/mm^3 for more than 2 but less than 3 weeks after scheduled start of next cycle	Reduce paclitaxel and carboplatin dosages by 20% (140 mg/m^2 and AUC = 6, respectively)
At start pf a cycle ANC ≤1000/mm^3 and platelets ≤100,000/mm^3 despite dose reduction	Delay start of cycle until ANC >1000/mm^3 and platelets >1000/mm^3; then administer filgrastim 5 mcg/kg/day subcutaneously for 14 days with same chemotherapy dosages
Serum creatinine >2 mg/dL (>177 micromol/L) or G ≥3 peripheral neuropathy	Delay start of cycle up to 2 weeks; if serum creatinine not ≤2 mg/dL (≤177 micromol/L) or G <3 peripheral neuropathy, discontinue therapy

Toxicity (Carboplatin: N = 392)

	% G3	% G4
Hematologic		
Leukopenia	53	6
Granulocytopenia	17	72
Thrombocytopenia	19	20
Nonhematologic		
Gastrointestinal	5	5
Neurologic*	7	0
Alopecia	0	0
Metabolic	2	1
Genitourinary	1	0
Pain	1	0

*Primarily peripheral neuropathy
GOG toxicity criteria

Patient Population Studied

A randomized study of 792 women with pathologically verified stage III epithelial ovarian cancer who were left with no residual disease >1 cm in diameter; 400 cisplatin arm and 392 carboplatin arm. McGuire et al (NEJM 1996;334:1–6) had shown that cisplatin plus paclitaxel was superior to cisplatin plus cyclophosphamide in advanced-stage epithelial ovarian cancer. This study was a **noninferiority trial** of cisplatin and paclitaxel versus carboplatin and paclitaxel to show equivalence of the two regimens

Efficacy (Carboplatin: N = 392)

Median progression-free survival	20.7 months
Median overall survival	57.4 months

Therapy Monitoring

Before repeated cycles: PE, CBC with differential, and serum electrolytes, magnesium, calcium, BUN, and creatinine

REGIMEN

CISPLATIN + PACLITAXEL

Ozols RF et al. JCO 2003;21:3194–3200

Paclitaxel 135 mg/m^2 by continuous intravenous infusion in a volume of 0.9% NaCl injection (0.9% NS) or 5% dextrose injection (D5W) sufficient to produce a concentration within the range 0.3–1.2 mg/mL over 24 hours on day 1 every 3 weeks for 6 cycles (total dosage/cycle = 135 mg/m^2)
Cisplatin 75 mg/m^2 intravenously in 0.9% NS 100–250 mL over 1 hour after completing paclitaxel on day 2, every 3 weeks for 6 cycles (total dosage/cycle = 75 mg/m^2)
Emetogenic potential:
Day 1: Low (Emetogenicity score = 2)
Day 2: High (Emetogenicity score = 5). See Chapter 39 for antiemetic regimens

Efficacy (Comparison of Regimens)

	Cisplatin (N = 400)	Carboplatin (N = 392)
Median progression-free survival (months)	19.4	20.7
Median overall survival (months)	48.7	57.4

Toxicity

	Cisplatin (N = 400)		Carboplatin (N = 392)	
	% G3	% G4	% G3	% G4
Hematologic				
Leukopenia*	51	12	53	6
Granulocytopenia	15	78	17	72
Thrombocytopenia*	3	2	19	20
Nonhematologic				
Gastrointestinal*	14	9	5	5
Neurologic	8	0	7	0
Alopecia	0	0	0	0
Metabolic*	6	2	2	1
Genitourinary*	3	0	1	0
Pain	1	0	1	0
	% G1/2		% G1/2	
Pain	15		26	

*Statistically significant difference at the .05 level

Treatment Modifications

Adverse Event	Dose Modification
Delay in achieving ANC ≥1000/mm^3 and platelets ≥100,000/mm^3 <2 weeks	No dose adjustment; no filgrastim
Delay in achieving ANC ≥1000/mm^3 and platelets ≥100,000/mm^3 ≥2 weeks but ≤3 weeks	Reduce carboplatin dosage by 20%
Recurrent delays in achieving ANC ≥1000/mm^3 and platelets ≥100,000/mm^3 ≥2 weeks but ≤3 weeks	Add filgrastim 5 mcg/kg per day subcutaneously. Start 24 hours after completing chemotherapy, and continue for 14 days without further dosage modification
Episode of febrile neutropenia after earlier delay in achieving ANC and platelets led to a reduction in carboplatin dosage	Add filgrastim 5 mcg/kg/day subcutaneously. Start 24 hours after completing chemotherapy, and continue for 14 days without further dosage modification
G3/4 Neurologic toxicity that has not resolved even after a 3-week delay	Discontinue therapy
Creatinine clearance <30 mL/min	Discontinue therapy

*Creatinine clearance used as a measure of glomerular filtration rate (GFR)

Notes

There were no differences in efficacy between the cisplatin + paclitaxel and the carboplatin + paclitaxel treatment regimens. However, there were differences with respect to toxicities. The authors interpreted the data as showing that the carboplatin + paclitaxel regimen was equally efficacious and significantly less toxic than the cisplatin + paclitaxel regimen

REGIMEN

CYCLOPHOSPHAMIDE + PACLITAXEL + CISPLATIN

[>2- to 3-cm residual after surgery, or stage IV disease]

Kohn EC et al. Gynecol Oncol 1996;62:181–191

Premedication for paclitaxel:
Dexamethasone 20 mg/dose orally or intravenously for 2 doses at 12–14 hours and 6–7 hours before starting paclitaxel, *or*
Dexamethasone 20 mg intravenously per push 30 minutes before paclitaxel, *plus*
Diphenhydramine 50 mg intravenously per push 30 minutes before paclitaxel
Cimetidine 300 mg intravenously in 20–50 mL 0.9% NaCl injection (0.9% NS) or 5% dextrose injection (D5W) over 5–20 minutes 30 minutes before paclitaxel
Hydration:
5% Dextrose/0.9% NaCl injection (D5W/0.9% NS) intravenously at 100 mL/hour, starting 3 hours before cyclophosphamide until paclitaxel administration is completed. *Then*
D5W/0.9% NS with 20 mEq potassium chloride/1000 mL intravenously at 150 mL/hour, continuously until 8 hours after cisplatin administration is completed. Monitor and replace magnesium/electrolytes as needed
Cyclophosphamide 750 mg/m^2 intravenously in 100 mL 0.9% NS or D5W over 15 minutes every 21 days (total dosage/cycle = 750 mg/m^2)
Paclitaxel 250 mg/m^2 by continuous intravenous infusion in a volume of 0.9% NS or D5W sufficient to produce a concentration of 0.3–1.2 mg/mL over 24 hours every 21 days (total dosage/cycle = 250 mg/m^2)

Premedication for cisplatin:
Dexamethasone 20 mg orally or intravenously 6 hours before starting cisplatin, *plus*
Diphenhydramine 50 mg intravenously per push 30 minutes before cisplatin
Cimetidine 300 mg intravenously in 20–50 mL 0.9% NS or D5W over 5–20 minutes 30 minutes before cisplatin
Mannitol before cisplatin:
Mannitol 12.5 g intravenously per push 60 minutes before starting cisplatin, *followed immediately by:*
Mannitol 40 g (20% solution) intravenously at 50 mL (10 g)/hour for 4 hours
Cisplatin 75 mg/m^2 intravenously in 250 mL 0.9% NS over 60 minutes every 21 days for up to 6 cycles (total dosage/cycle = 75 mg/m^2)

(continued)

Treatment Modifications

Dose Level	Cyclophosphamide mg/m^2	Paclitaxel mg/m^2	Cisplatin mg/m^2
−3	750	135	75
−2	750	175	75
−1	750	200	75
0	750	250	75
+1	750	250	100
+2	750	250	125

Adverse Event	Dose Modification
G3 Nonhematologic toxicity (neuropathy, ototoxicity, mucositis)	Reduce dosage by one dose level
Fever + neutropenia (ANC ≤ 500/mm^3)	Increase filgrastim to 20 mcg/kg per day
ANC ≤ 500/mm^3) for ≥ 5 days despite filgrastim	Reduce dosage by one dose level
Fever + neutropenia (ANC ≤ 500/mm^3) despite filgrastim 20 mcg/kg per day	Reduce dosage by one dose level
Requirement for platelet transfusion	Reduce dosage by one dose level
Myalgias/arthralgias requiring narcotics	Reduce, filgrastim by 2.5–5 mcg/kg per day

Patient Population Studied

This is a report of 36 patients: 80% with grade III histology; 23 patients with stage IIIC; 12 patients with stage IV disease; 31 patients with > 2-cm residual disease; 25 patients with > 3-cm disease after initial surgery

(*continued*)

Filgrastim 10 mcg/kg per day subcutaneously for at least 9 days (days 3–11) or until WBC count recovers to ≥30,000/mm^3

Emetogenic potential:
Day 1: Moderately high (Emetogenicity score ~4)
Day 2: High (Emetogenicity score = 5). See Chapter 39 for antiemetic regimens

Individualized Chemotherapy Administration

[A minimum of 6 cycles before surgical evaluation]

Radiographic assessment	⇒	Every 2 cycles
Complete resolution of disease by PE, CA 125, and radiographic studies	⇒	Peritoneoscopy for biopsies and peritoneal washings
Negative peritoneoscopy results	⇒	Second-look laparotomy
Negative second-look laparotomy	⇒	2 Additional cycles of paclitaxel + cyclophosphamide
Microscopic disease on second-look laparotomy	⇒	2–4 Additional cycles of paclitaxel + cyclophosphamide, depending on therapy toxicity

Therapy Monitoring

1. *Before repeated cycles:* History, PE, CBC with differential, serum electrolytes, magnesium, calcium, BUN, serum creatinine, and CA 125 measurement
2. *Every two cycles:* Radiographic assessment with measurements

Efficacy (N = 36)

(Median progression-free survival: >22 months)

Clinical Response

Level	Patients	CR	PR	SD	PD
−3	4	2	1	1	
−2	3	1	1	1	
−1	5	5	0	0	
0	13	11	1		1
+1	7	5	2		
+2	4	2	1		1
Total	36	27	5	2	2
Percentage		75%	14%	5%	5%

Pathologic Response After Surgery

Level	Patients	CR	Microscopic	PR
−3	2	1	0	1
−2	2	1	0	1
−1	4	1	1	2
0	12	5	6	1
+1	6	4	1	1
+2	3	1	1	1
Total	29	13	9	7
Percentage		36%	25%	19%

Notes

Promising results in pathologic response rates, progression-free survival and overall survival most apparent in subgroup with ≥3-cm residual tumor. Further investigation of this regimen in a prospective randomized trial is needed to characterize its response and survival benefits

Toxicity

	% G1	% G2	% G3	% G4
Hematologic				
Thrombocytopenia	17	25	22	36
Anemia	3	14	78	6
Nonhematologic				
Allergic episodes	14	0	6	3
Diarrhea	50	36	11	3
Nausea	55	42	3	0
Vomiting	58	36	3	0
Mucositis	0	8	0	0
Myalgia/arthralgia	—	3	3	0
Peripheral neuropathy	—	36	28	0
Ototoxicity	25	3	0	0
Hypomagnesemia	—	14	14	64
Renal insufficiency	—	0	0	6[a]
Elevated transaminases	—	14	0	0
Hyperbilirubinemia	—	8	6	8[b]

[a]Acute renal failure at the time of sepsis
[b]Cause in 3 patients: Following RBC transfusion; Gilbert's syndrome; multiorgan failure

NCI CTC

REGIMEN

PLATINUM RETREATMENT (CISPLATIN OR CARBOPLATIN)

Leitao M et al. Gynecol Oncol 2003;91:123–129

Hydration before cisplatin: ≥1000 mL 0.9% NaCl injection (0.9% NS) by intravenous infusion over a minimum of 3–4 hours. Monitor and replace magnesium/electrolytes as needed
Cisplatin 80–100 mg/m² by intravenous infusion in 100–500 mL 0.9% NS over 30–60 minutes, given on day 1 every 3 weeks for a maximum of 8 cycles (total dosage/3-week cycle = 80–100 mg/m²)
Hydration after cisplatin: ≥1000 mL 0.9% NS by intravenous infusion over a minimum of 3–4 hours. Also encourage high oral fluid intake. Goal is to achieve a urine output of ≥100 mL/hour, *or*

Carboplatin [calculated dose] AUC = 6 by intravenous infusion in 50–150 mL D5W over 15–30 minutes, given on day 1 every 3 weeks (total dosage/cycle calculated to produce an AUC = 6 mg/mL·min)
Carboplatin dose is based on Calvert's formula to achieve a target area under the plasma concentration versus time curve (AUC) [AUC units = mg/mL·min]

$$\text{Total carboplatin dose (mg)} = (\text{Target AUC}) \times (\text{GFR} + 25)$$

In practice, creatinine clearance (Clcr) is used in place of glomerular filtration rate (GFR). Clcr can be calculated from the equation of Cockcroft and Gault:

$$\text{Males, Clcr} = \frac{(140 - \text{age [y]}) \times \text{body weight [kg]}}{72 \times (\text{Serum creatinine [mg/dL]})}$$

$$\text{Females, Clcr} = \frac{(140 - \text{age [y]}) \times \text{body weight [kg]}}{72 \times (\text{Serum creatinine [mg/dL]})} \times 0.85$$

Calvert AH et al. JCO 1989;7:1748–1756
Cockcroft DW, Gault MH. Nephron 1976;16:31–41
Jodrell DI et al. JCO 1992;10:520–528
Sorensen BT et al. Cancer Chemother Pharmacol 1991;28:397–401

With either regimen:
Filgrastim 5 mcg/kg per day subcutaneously. May be used beginning 24 hours after chemotherapy and continued until ANC > 10,000/mm³ on two consecutive measurements
Dexamethasone 8 mg/dose orally for 6 doses after chemotherapy if G ≥2 arthralgias/myalgias occur

Emetogenic potential: High (Emetogenicity score = 5). See Chapter 39 for antiemetic regimens

Treatment Modifications

Adverse Event	Dose Modification
Cisplatin	
Creatinine clearance 40–60 mL/min	Reduce cisplatin so that dose in milligrams equals the creatinine clearance[a] value in mL/min[b]
Creatinine clearance <40 mL/min	Hold cisplatin
On treatment day 1, serum creatinine 1.6–2.0 mg/dL (141–177 μmol/L)	Reduce cisplatin dosage by 25%
On treatment day 1, serum creatinine >2.0 mg/dL (177 μmol/L)	Hold cisplatin until serum creatinine ≤2.0 mg/dL (≤177 μmol/L)
Day 1 WBC <2000/mm³ or platelet count <100,000/mm³	Delay cisplatin for 1 week, or until myelosuppression resolves
Second treatment delay due to myelosuppression	Delay cisplatin for 1 week, or until myelosuppression resolves, then decrease dosage to 60–80 mg/m² during subsequent treatments
Sepsis during an episode of neutropenia	
Bleeding associated with thrombocytopenia	Reduce cisplatin to 60–80 mg/m²
Carboplatin	
ANC nadir <500/mm³, platelet nadir <50,000/mm³ or febrile neutropenia	Reduce carboplatin dosage to AUC = 5 mg/mL·min if previous cycle dose was AUC = 6; or to AUC = 4 if previous cycle dose was AUC = 5
ANC nadir <500/mm³, platelet nadir <50,000/mm³, or febrile neutropenia after 2 carboplatin dose reductions (AUC in previous cycle = 4 mg/mL·min)	Decrease carboplatin dosage to AUC = 3 mg/mL·min

(continued)

Patient Population Studied

A study of 30 patients with platinum-resistant ovarian cancer, who received nonplatinum chemotherapy for recurrent epithelial ovarian cancer before additional platinum therapy. Platinum resistance was defined as less than a partial response to platinum therapy or progression within 6 months of the last platinum therapy

Efficacy (N = 30)

Variable	No. of Patients	% PR
Best Response to Last Platinum Regimen		
Complete or partial response	14	43
Stable or progressive disease	16	6
Platinum-Free Interval		
≤6 months	2	0
6–12 months	8	63
>12 months	20	10
Number of Intervening Nonplatinum Agents		
≤3	20	35
>3	10	0
Time to Progression After Last Platinum Regimen		
≤6 months	23	17
>6 months	6	50
Number of Prior Platinum Regimens		
1 prior regimen	9	33
2 or 3 prior regimens	21	19

Treatment Modifications (*continued*)

Adverse Event	Dose Modification
Day 1 ANC <1500/mm³ or platelets <100,000/mm³	Delay chemotherapy until ANC >1500/mm³ and platelets >100,000/mm³, for maximum delay of 2 weeks
Delay of >2 weeks in reaching ANC >1500/mm³ and platelets >100,000/mm³	Discontinue therapy
Bleeding associated with thrombocytopenia	Reduce carboplatin dosages to AUC 4–5 mg/mL·min

[a]Creatinine clearance used as a measure of glomerular filtration rate

[b]This also applies to patients with creatinine clearance (GFR) of 40–60 mL/min at the outset of treatment

Toxicity

Cisplatin

(PLATINOL®-AQ [cisplatin injection] product label, November 2002. Bristol-Myers Squibb)

Toxicity	Incidence
Individual and cumulative dose-related renal toxicity: Increased serum creatinine, uric acid, and BUN *Renal tubular damage with electrolyte wasting:* Hypomagnesemia, hypocalcemia, hyponatremia, hypokalemia, and hypophosphatemia	28–36%[a]
Dose-related, cumulative peripheral neuropathies: Bilateral paresthesias, areflexia, loss of proprioception and vibratory sensation, motor neuropathies	30–100% depending on cumulative doses
Optic neuritis, papilledema, and cerebral blindness	rare
Cumulative ototoxicity: With tinnitus or high frequency hearing loss. Vestibular toxicity	31%[a]
Nausea and vomiting at any dose: Severe and delayed emesis at dosages $\geq$ 50 mg/m^2	Varies (moderate to severe in virtually all without antiemetics)
Transiently increased liver transaminases	rare
Hypersensitivity reactions: Anaphylactoid reactions, facial edema, wheezing, tachycardia, and hypotension	1–20%
Coombs'-positive hemolytic anemia	rare
Dose-related leukopenia, thrombocytopenia, anemia	25–30%[a]

Carboplatin

(PARAPLATIN® [carboplatin aqueous solution] Injection product label, January 2004. Bristol-Myers Squibb)

Toxicity	Incidence
Nausea and vomiting	92%[b]
Diarrhea, constipation, other GI side effects	21%
Thrombocytopenia: < 100,000/mm^3 < 50,000/mm^3	62% 35%
Neutropenia: < 1000/mm^3	21%
Anemia: < 11 g/dL < 8 g/dL	90% 21%
Nephrotoxicity: Increased serum creatinine Increased BUN	10% 22%
Hyponatremia, hypomagnesemia, hypocalcemia, hypokalemia	47%, 43%, 31%, 28%
Peripheral neuropathies: Paresthesias, ataxia, distal motor deficits; decreased vibratory sense, light touch, pinprick, and joint position; areflexia	
Cumulative ototoxicity: Tinnitus, high-frequencies hearing loss, audiogram deficits	1.1%
Increased alkaline phosphatase, AST, total bilirubin	37%
Alopecia	19%
Hypersensitivity reactions: Facial flushing, generalized urticaria, hypotension, rash, pruritus, bronchospasm, shortness of breath	5%

[a]Incidence after a single treatment with cisplatin 50 mg/m^2
[b]All data are based on the experience of 553 patients with previously treated ovarian carcinoma who received single-agent carboplatin, without regard for their baseline status

Therapy Monitoring

1. *Before repeated cycles:* PE, CBC with differential, serum electrolytes, magnesium, calcium, BUN, and creatinine
2. *Every month:* Serum CA 125 level
3. *Every 2–3 months:* Restaging radiographic studies

REGIMEN

FLUOROURACIL + LEUCOVORIN

Reed E et al. Gynecol Oncol 1992;46:326–329

Leucovorin 500 mg/m² per dose by intravenous infusion in 25–100 mL 0.9% NaCl injection (0.9% NS) or 5% dextrose injection (D5W), over 30 minutes daily for 5 consecutive days on days 1–5 every 21 days (total dosage/cycle = 2500 mg/m²). Each leucovorin dose is *followed after 1 hour by:*
Fluorouracil 375 mg/m² per dose by intravenous push over 3–5 minutes, daily for 5 consecutive days, days 1–5 every 21 days (total dosage/cycle = 1875 mg/m²)

Emetogenic potential: Low (Emetogenicity score = 2). See Chapter 39 for antiemetic regimens

Treatment Modifications

Adverse Event	Dose Modification
G2 Nonhematologic toxicity	Reduce fluorouracil dose by 25%
WBC <3000/mm³ or platelet count <75,000/mm³ on treatment day	Delay cycle 1 week until WBC >3000/mm³ or platelet count >75,000/mm³

If no toxicity >G1 is documented in a cycle, then increase fluorouracil dose by 25%

Patient Population Studied

A study of 29 patients with recurrent advanced-stage ovarian cancer of epithelial histology who had progressive disease while receiving or had suffered relapse after high-dose cisplatin therapy

Efficacy (N = 29)

	Relapsed After Response to Platinum-Based Therapy (n = 8)	Progressive Disease on Platinum-Based Therapy (n = 21)
CR	13%	5%
PR	—	5%
SD*	38%	38%
PD	50%	52%

*SD: 5, 5, 7, 8, 8, 8, 10, 13, 14, 21, and 27 months

Toxicity (N = 29/204 Cycles)

	Number of Cycles			
	G1	G2	G3	G4
Hematologic				
Neutropenia	1	5	7	4
Thrombocytopenia	7	2	4	4
Anemia	4	6	5	1
Nonhematologic				
Nausea/vomiting	9	3	2	0
Stomatitis	9	5	4	2
Diarrhea	11	3	3	0

NCI CTC

Therapy Monitoring

Before repeated cycles: PE, CBC with differential, and serum electrolytes

Notes

Since this regimen is well tolerated, it represents an option for patients when more attractive options have been exhausted

REGIMEN

GEMCITABINE

Markman M et al. Gynecol Oncol 2003;90:593–596

Gemcitabine 1000 mg/m^2 per dose intravenously diluted to a concentration ≥0.1 mg/mL in 0.9% NaCl injection (0.9% NS) over 30 minutes for 3 doses on days 1, 8, and 15 every 28 days (total dosage/cycle = 3000 mg/m^2)

Emetogenic potential: Low (Emetogenicity score = 2). See Chapter 39 for antiemetic regimens

Patient Population Studied

A study of 51 patients with ovarian (41), fallopian tube (1), and primary peritoneal cancer (9) and prior chemotherapy with a platinum agent (cisplatin or carboplatin) and a taxane (paclitaxel or docetaxel). If a patient had previously responded to such therapy, and the treatment-free interval had been 3 months, the patient had to be retreated with a platinum agent or a taxane to confirm clinical resistance

Efficacy (N = 51)

Partial response	8%
≥75% decrease in CA 125	8%
Median duration of response	4 months
Survival (all patients)	7 months
Survival (patients with response)	15 months

Toxicity (N = 51)

	% Patients
Hematologic	
Grade 4 neutropenia	24
Grade 3 thrombocytopenia	7
Nonhematologic	
Grade 3 fatigue	10
Fever/chills (no neutropenia)	15
Rash	4
Conjunctivitis	4

Treatment Modifications

Adverse Event	Dose Modification
ANC nadir <1000/mm^3 or platelet count nadir ≤100,000/mm^3	Hold treatment until ANC recovers to 1000/mm^3 and platelets to 100,000/mm^3, then resume with gemcitabine dosage decreased by 200 mg/m^2 per dose
Second occurrence of ANC nadir ≤1000/mm^3 or platelet count nadir ≤100,000/mm^3	Hold treatment until ANC recovers to 1000/mm^3 and platelets to 100,000/mm^3, then resume with gemcitabine dosage decreased by an additional 200 mg/m^2 per dose
Third occurrence of ANC nadir ≤1000/mm^3 or platelet count nadir ≤100,000/mm^3	Discontinue gemcitabine therapy
G3 Nonhematologic toxicity	Hold treatment until toxicities resolve to G <1, then resume with gemcitabine dosage decreased by an additional 200 mg/m^2 per week
Second occurrence of G3 nonhematologic toxicity	Hold treatment until toxicities resolve to G ≤1, then resume with gemcitabine dosage decreased by an additional 200 mg/m^2 per dose

Therapy Monitoring

Before repeated cycles: PE, CBC with differential, and serum electrolytes, magnesium, calcium, BUN, creatinine, and LFTs

Notes

A dose of 1250 mg/m^2 resulted in excessive toxicity

REGIMEN

ORAL ALTRETAMINE (HEXAMETHYLMELAMINE)

Chan JK et al. Gynecol Oncol 2004;92:368–371

Altretamine 65 mg/m^2 per dose orally 4 times daily, after meals and at bedtime, for 14 consecutive days on days 1–14 every 28 days (total dosage/cycle = 3640 mg/m^2) *or*
Altretamine 65 mg/m^2 per dose orally 4 times daily, after meals and at bedtime, for 21 consecutive days on days 1–21 every 28 days (total dosage/cycle = 5460 mg/m^2)

Altretamine (HEXALEN®) is available in the United States as capsules for oral administration containing 50 mg

Emetogenic potential: Moderate (Emetogenicity score = 3). See Chapter 39 for antiemetic regimens

Patient Population Studied

A study of 2 women with recurrent ovarian cancer. Includes review of the literature

Efficacy

Response to altretamine appears to be:

1. Correlated with response to initial platinum therapy: Higher in patients whose disease responded to initial therapy
2. Correlated with treatment-free interval after an initial response to platinum therapy: The longer the interval, the higher the response
3. Higher in platinum-sensitive (PS) disease than in platinum-resistant (PR) disease: Response rates for PS disease in several studies range from 17% to 50%, whereas response rates for PR disease range from 0% to 35%

Toxicity

Hematologic	
Moderate to severe anemia	13%
Platelet counts <50,000/mm^3	≤10%
WBC counts <2000/mm^3	≤1%
Nonhematologic	
Nausea and vomiting	33%*
Severe nausea and vomiting	1%*
Moderate to severe peripheral sensory neuropathy	9%*
Mild sensory neuropathy	22%
Increased alkaline phosphatase	9%
Mood disorders*: Depression, insomnia, confusion, personality changes, anxiety	≤1%
Movement and coordination disorders*	1%
Fatigue, malaise, lethargy	1%

*Symptoms are more likely to occur in patients who receive continuous daily treatment with high doses of altretamine than with moderate doses administered on an intermittent schedule

Treatment Modifications

Adverse Event	Dose Modification
GI intolerance unresponsive to symptomatic measures	Discontinue altretamine for ≥14 days, then resume at 50 mg/m^2 per dose 4 times daily
WBC <2000/mm^3 or ANC <1000/mm^3	
Platelet count <75,000/mm^3	
Progressive neurotoxicity	
Progressive neurotoxicity that does not stabilize on a reduced altretamine dosage	Discontinue altretamine indefinitely

Therapy Monitoring

Before repeated cycles: PE, CBC with differential, and serum electrolytes, magnesium, calcium, BUN, and creatinine

REGIMEN

DOXORUBICIN HCl LIPOSOME INJECTION (LIPOSOMAL DOXORUBICIN)

Thigpen JT et al. Gynecol Oncol 2005;96:10–18
Lorusso D et al. Oncology 2004;67:243–249

Doxorubicin HCl liposome injection 40–50 mg/m² by intravenous infusion diluted in 250 mL 5% dextrose injection (D5W) for doses ≤90 mg and in 500 mL D5W for doses >90 mg every 3–4 weeks (total dosage/cycle = 40–50 mg/m²)
Note: Administer at an initial rate of 1 mg/minute for 10–15 minutes. If infusion reactions are not observed, the rate may be increased to complete drug administration over 60 minutes

Emetogenic potential: Low (Emetogenicity score = 2). See Chapter 39 for antiemetic regimens

Treatment Modifications

Adverse Event	Dose Modification
Hand-foot syndrome	Reduce dosage to 40 mg/m²
G3/4 Nonhematologic toxicity	
Stomatitis G ≥2	
Persistent (>3 weeks) G1/2 toxicity	Increase dosing interval to 4 weeks
Persistent (>4 weeks) G3/4 toxicity	Discontinue therapy

Patient Population Studied

A study of 37 patients with advanced ovarian cancer in whom first-line therapy had failed to provide benefit

Efficacy

Response rates of 7.7–26% have been reported in several studies with a median progression-free survival of 4–6 months

Therapy Monitoring

Before repeated cycles: PE, CBC with differential, and serum electrolytes, magnesium, calcium, BUN, and creatinine

Toxicity (N = 37)

	% G1	% G2	% G3	% G4
Hematologic				
Neutropenia	—	—	—	—
Thrombocytopenia	3	—	—	—
Anemia	24	—	—	—
Febrile neutropenia	—	—	—	—
Nonhematologic				
PPE	11	8	3	—
Stomatitis/mucositis	8	—	—	—
Nausea/vomiting	14	—	—	—
Asthenia	24	—	—	—
Hair loss	16	—	—	—
Anaphylactic reactions	5	—	—	—
Liver toxicity	—	—	—	—
Cardiac toxicity	—	—	—	—

Note: Toxicity grades for palmar plantar erythrodysesthesia (PPE):
G1 Mild erythema, swelling or desquamation not interfering with daily activities
G2 Erythema, swelling or desquamation interfering with daily activities; small blisters or ulcerations <2 cm
G3 Blistering, ulcerations or swelling interfering with daily activities; patient cannot wear regular clothing
G4 Diffuse or local process causing infectious complications, a bedridden state, or hospitalization

Lorusso D et al. Oncology 2004;67:243–249

Notes

Conclusions from reports of the opinion of a panel of experts in the management of ovarian carcinoma:

1. Based on survival and toxicity advantages and a once-monthly administration schedule, liposomal doxorubicin is considered by some to be the first-choice nonplatinum agent for relapsed ovarian cancer
2. Tolerability is improved with the use of liposomal doxorubicin 40 mg/m² on an every-4-week schedule. Hand-foot syndrome (PPE) is the most commonly reported adverse event associated with liposomal doxorubicin. Avoid this toxicity by using lower dosages of liposomal doxorubicin [40 mg/m² every 4 weeks, or 10 mg/m² weekly], rather than omitting or decreasing doses as a consequence of adverse events

Thigpen JT et al. Gynecol Oncol 2005;96:10–18

REGIMEN

VINORELBINE

Rothenberg ML et al. Gynecol Oncol 2004;95:506–512

Vinorelbine 30 mg/m² per dose by intravenous push over 1–2 minutes for 2 doses on days 1 and 8 every 21 days (total dosage/cycle = 60 mg/m²)

Emetogenic potential: Nonemetogenic (Emetogenicity score = 1). See Chapter 39 for antiemetic regimens

Treatment Modifications

Adverse Event	Dose Modification
ANC <1000/mm³ or platelet count <75,000/mm³ on the day before or the day of vinorelbine administration	Hold vinorelbine dose on this day
ANC 1000–1499/mm³ or platelet count 75,000–99,999/mm³ on the day before or the day of vinorelbine administration	Administer vinorelbine, but reduce vinorelbine dosage by 7.5 mg/m²
On the day before or the day of repeated vinorelbine administration, ANC 1000–1499/mm³ or platelet count 75,000–99,999/mm³ after vinorelbine 15 mg/m²	Discontinue therapy

Toxicity (N = 79)

	% G0	% G1	% G2	% G3	% G4
Hematologic					
Anemia	27	23	38	13	0
Granulocytopenia	24	4	16	28	28
Leukopenia	11	19	23	39	8
Thrombocytopenia	78	19	3	0	0
Nonhematologic					
Abdominal pain	72	10	13	5	0
Alopecia	71	16	13	0	0
Anorexia	76	24	0	0	0
Constipation	51	28	15	6	0
Dyspnea	78	0	18	3	1
Fever without infection	79	13	8	0	0
Insomnia	89	11	0	0	0
Malaise/fatigue/lethargy	34	27	28	11	0
Nausea	42	39	11	8	0
Numbness/other symptoms of peripheral neuropathy	75	0	25	0	0
Pain	69	15	11	5	0
Paresthesia	89	5	6	0	0
Vomiting	71	14	13	1	0
Weakness	86	8	3	3	0

NCI CTC

Patient Population Studied

A study of 79 patients with recurrent or resistant epithelial ovarian cancer after treatment with platinum and paclitaxel

Efficacy (N = 79)

Partial response (n = 71)	3%
Median time to progression	3 months
6-month survival rate	65%
Median Survival	
All patients (N = 79)	10.1 months
Chemotherapy-resistant (n = 52)	8 months
Chemotherapy-sensitive (n = 27)	16 months

Therapy Monitoring

Before repeated cycles: CBC with differential

Notes

During the initial 10 weeks of treatment, vinorelbine did not appear to be effective in relieving the symptom-related distress or progressive impairment of physical functioning associated with refractory ovarian cancer

REGIMEN

PACLITAXEL (24-HOUR PACLITAXEL INFUSION EVERY 3 WEEKS; WEEKLY PACLITAXEL)

24 Hour Paclitaxel

Omura GA et al. JCO 2003;21:2843–2848

Premedication for paclitaxel:

Dexamethasone 20 mg/dose orally or intravenously per push for 2 doses 12–14 hours and 6–7 hours before starting paclitaxel *or*

Dexamethasone 20 mg intravenously per push 30 minutes before administering paclitaxel

Diphenhydramine 50 mg intravenously per push 30 minutes before administering paclitaxel

Cimetidine 300 mg intravenously in 20–50 mL 0.9% NaCl injection (0.9% NS) or 5% dextrose injection (D5W) over 5–20 minutes 30 minutes before administering paclitaxel

Paclitaxel 175 mg/m^2 by intravenous infusion in a volume of 0.9% NS or D5W sufficient to produce a concentration of 0.3–1.2 mg/mL over 24 hours on day 1 every 3 weeks (total dosage/cycle = 175 mg/m^2)

Filgrastim 5 mcg/kg per day subcutaneously; may be used beginning 72 hours after chemotherapy and continued until ANC >10,000/mm^3 on two consecutive measurements

Emetogenic potential: Low (Emetogenicity score = 2). See Chapter 39 for antiemetic regimens

or

Weekly Paclitaxel

Ghamande S et al. Int J Gynecol Cancer 2003;13:142–147

Premedication for paclitaxel:

Dexamethasone 20 mg intravenously per push 30 minutes before paclitaxel

Diphenhydramine 50 mg intravenously per push 30 minutes before paclitaxel

Ranitidine 50 mg intravenously in 20–100 mL of 0.9% NS or D5W over 5–20 minutes, 30 minutes before administering paclitaxel

Paclitaxel 70–80 mg/m^2 per dose by intravenous infusion in a volume of 0.9% NS or D5W sufficient to produce a concentration of 0.3–1.2 mg/mL over 60 minutes, weekly for a minimum of 6 consecutive weeks or days 1, 8, and 15 every 28 days (total dosage/cycle = 210–240 mg/m^2)

Emetogenic potential: Low (Emetogenicity score = 2). See Chapter 39 for antiemetic regimens

Treatment Modifications

Adverse Event	Dose Modification
24-Hour Paclitaxel Infusion Every 3 Weeks	
G ≥ 3 Nonhematologic toxicity	Reduce paclitaxel dose to 135 mg/m^2
Delay in achieving ANC ≥1000/mm^3 and platelets ≥100,000/mm^3 <2 weeks	No dose adjustment; no filgrastim
Recurrent delays in achieving ANC ≥1000/mm^3 and platelets ≥100,000/mm^3 ≥2 weeks but ≤3 weeks	Add filgrastim 5 mcg/kg per day without further dosage modification
G3/4 Neurologic toxicity that has not resolved even after a 3-week delay	Discontinue therapy
Weekly Paclitaxel Regimen	
WBC < 2500/mm^3	Hold chemotherapy until WBC >2500/mm^3
ANC < 1500/mm^3	Hold chemotherapy until ANC >1500/mm^3
Platelets < 75,000/mm^3	Hold chemotherapy until Platelets >75,000/mm^3
G3/4 Neurologic toxicity that has not resolved even after a 3-week delay	Discontinue therapy

Patient Population Studied

A study of 164 patients with epithelial ovarian cancer who had been treated with not more than one platinum-based regimen and no prior taxane

Omura GA et al. JCO 2003;21:2843–2848

A study of 23 patients with advanced recurrent ovarian cancer with disease deemed resistant to platinum agents and paclitaxel (defined as either progression of disease while on therapy or progression within 12 months of prior paclitaxel therapy)

Ghamande S et al. Int J Gynecol Cancer 2003;13:142–147

Efficacy

24-Hour Paclitaxel Infusion Every 3 Weeks (N = 164)

Median time to death	13.1 months
Platinum-Resistant Disease	
Complete response	5%
Partial response	17%
No response	78%
Platinum-Sensitive Disease	
Complete response	15%
Partial response	33%
No response	52%

Omura GA et al. JCO 2003;21:2843–2848

Weekly Paclitaxel (N = 23)

	Paclitaxel-Free Interval	
	<12 months (n = 10)	>12 months (n = 13)
Partial response*	0	70%
Stable disease	30%	15%
Progressive disease	70%	15%

*Partial response based on Rustin's criteria with more than 50% reduction in CA 125 levels

Ghamande S et al. Int J Gynecol Cancer 2003;13:142–147

Toxicity (N = 164)

24-Hour Paclitaxel Infusion Every 3 Weeks

	% G3/4
Anemia	7
Thrombocytopenia	5
Nausea/vomiting	5
Neuropathy	7
Myalgia/arthralgia	3
G4 neutropenia	22 [First cycle without filgrastim]

Omura GA et al. JCO 2003;21:2843–2848

Weekly Paclitaxel (N = 28)

	% Patients
G2 neutropenia	10.7
G3 neutropenia	21.4
G1 thrombocytopenia	3.6
G2 anemia	32.1
G2 neuropathy	7.1
G >2 neuropathy	3.6

Ghamande S et al. Int J Gynecol Cancer 2003;13:142–147

Therapy Monitoring

1. *Before repeated cycles:* CBC with differential
2. *Twice per week:* Obtain CBC with differential in patients treated with the weekly regimen

REGIMEN

TOPOTECAN HCl

Bhoola SM et al. Gynecol Oncol 2004;95:564–569

Topotecan HCl 2.25–4 mg/m² (median, 3.7 mg/m²) per dose by intravenous infusion in 50–250 mL 0.9% NaCl injection (0.9% NS) or 5% dextrose injection (D5W) over 30 minutes weekly, continually (total dosage/week = 2.25–4 mg/m²)

Emetogenic potential: Low (Emetogenicity score = 2). See Chapter 39 for antiemetic regimens

or

Topotecan HCl 1.5 mg/m² per dose by intravenous infusion in 50–250 mL 0.9% NS or D5W over 30 minutes for 5 days on days 1–5 every 21 days (total dosage/cycle = 7.5 mg/m²)

Emetogenic potential: Low (Emetogenicity score = 2). See Chapter 39 for antiemetic regimens

Efficacy: Weekly Regimen (N = 42[a])

Measurable Disease (n = 35)	
Partial response	31%
Stable disease	43%
Progressive disease	26%

↑ CA 125[b]

	All with ↑ CA 125 (n = 41)	↑ CA 125[b] only (n = 7)
Partial response	27	29
Stable disease	24	29
Progressive disease	49	42

Platinum-Sensitive Disease	
Partial response	39
Stable disease	43
Progressive disease	18

Platinum-Resistant or Platinum-Refractory Disease	
Partial response	21
Stable disease	37
Progressive disease	42

[a]Includes only patients who received ≥2 cycles

[b]Partial response defined as a 50% reduction in CA 125 levels maintained for ≥1 month. Progressive disease defined as a 25% increase in CA 125 levels

Toxicity: Weekly Regimen (N = 50)

	% G2	% G3	% G4
Hematologic			
Anemia	42	24	0
Leukopenia	38	2	2
Neutropenia	24	14	4
Thrombocytopenia	4	10	0

	% G1/2	% G3/4
Nonhematologic		
Fatigue	14	4
Neuropathy	6	0
Nausea	2	0
Dehydration	2	0
Diarrhea	2	0
Alopecia	2	0

Patient Population Studied

A study of 50 patients with ovarian cancer who had received multiple prior regimens

Treatment Modifications

Adverse Event	Dose Modification
G3/4 Neutropenia on treatment day 1 (every 21 day regimen)	Hold topotecan until ANC ≥1000/mm³ ± Reduce topotecan dose 10–20% ± Administer filgrastim in subsequent cycles*
G3/4 Neutropenia on treatment day 1 (weekly regimen)	Hold topotecan until ANC ≥1000/mm³ ± Reduce topotecan dose 10–20% ± Administer filgrastim in subsequent cycles* ± Change schedule to 2 weeks on/1 week off
≥G2 Anemia	Administer erythropoietin
≥G2 Fatigue	Administer erythropoietin

*With every 21 day administration schedule administer filgrastim 5 mcg/kg per day subcutaneously beginning 24 hours after the day 5 dose and continuing until ANC > 10,000/mm³ on two consecutive measurements

Therapy Monitoring

Before repeated cycles: CBC with differential

Notes

A retrospective chart study of patients with rapidly progressive disease or clinical deterioration excluded from analysis. Efficacy of both regimens are comparable; toxicity of weekly regimen tolerable

REGIMEN

ORAL ETOPOSIDE

Moosavi AS et al. J Obstet Gynaecol 24:292–293

Etoposide 50 mg/day orally once daily for 21 consecutive days, days 1–21 every 4 weeks (total dose/cycle = 1050 mg)

Etoposide is available in the United States as capsules containing 50 mg etoposide (VePesid®)

Emetogenic potential: Low (Emetogenicity score = 2). See Chapter 39 for antiemetic regimens

Patient Population Studied

Ten patients with epithelial ovarian cancer and evidence of disease progression; GOG performance status ≤2

Efficacy (N = 10)

Partial response rate	20%*
Response duration	3.5 and 6 months
Median progression-free interval	7.5 months
Median survival time	8.5 months

*Both patients who responded were deemed to have platinum-sensitive disease

Toxicity (N = 10)

	% Patients
Hematologic	
G1 ANC	50%
G2 ANC	30%
Nonhematologic	
Nausea/vomiting	40%
Mild mucositis	10%
Alopecia	100%

Treatment Modifications

Adverse Event	Dose Modification
Nausea and vomiting[a] or after eating	Ingest doses with food
G3/4 ANC	Hold therapy. Resume treatment when ANC ≥1500/mm^3 using alternative schedule[b] (every other day, MWF, 2 of every 3 days, M–F)

[a]Nausea and vomiting are more common after oral administration than after parenteral administration with bioequivalent doses. Food ingestion does not affect absorption of etoposide doses <200 mg

[b]The 50-mg etoposide capsules cannot be opened or broken because they contain a liquid product

Therapy Monitoring

Every week: CBC with differential and platelet count

Notes

Although oral etoposide has activity in recurrent ovarian cancer, response and survival durations are short with a high rate of complications

REGIMEN

TAMOXIFEN

Markman M et al. Gynecol Oncol 2004;93:390–393

Tamoxifen 10 mg/dose orally twice daily, continually (total dose/week = 140 mg)

Tamoxifen citrate is available in the United States in tablet formulations containing either 10 mg or 20 mg of tamoxifen base. [Nolvadex® (tamoxifen citrate)]

Emetogenic potential: Nonemetogenic (Emetogenicity score = 1). See Chapter 39 for antiemetic regimens

Patient Population Studied

A study of 56 patients with recurrent ovarian (n = 44), fallopian tube (n = 3), or primary peritoneal carcinoma (n = 9). All patients had a prior response to primary platinum/taxane–based therapy or a platinum therapy used in the second-line setting and a treatment-free interval of ≥3 months. *Patients had no symptoms believed to be due to recurrent cancer*

Efficacy (N = 57 Episodes)

Median duration of treatment	3 months
Tamoxifen ≥6 months	42%
Tamoxifen ≥12 months	19%
Tamoxifen ≥12 months (1 prior therapy)	18%
Tamoxifen ≥12 months (2 prior therapies)	25%

Treatment Modifications

Grade 3 toxicities with this dose of tamoxifen are very uncommon and usually do not require dose reductions

Toxicity

No patient discontinued tamoxifen due to unacceptable side effects. This is a very well-tolerated dose schedule. The most common toxicities in females are hot flashes and some degree of vaginal discharge and, in premenopausal females, menstrual irregularities, such as irregular menses or amenorrhea. The risk for thromboembolic events increases with tamoxifen treatment, but is very low at this dose and usually administered for a short period of time. Neuropsychiatric (depression and other mood disorders) toxicities are uncommon. Liver and dermatologic toxicities can be very serious, but are rare

Therapy Monitoring

1. *Every month:* Serum CA 125 level
2. *Every 2–3 months*: Restaging radiographic studies

Notes

Best used in asymptomatic cases with a rising CA 125; or in cases in which comorbid illnesses argue against more aggressive therapy

30. Pancreatic Cancer

Michael M. Boyiadzis, MD, MHSc, and Daniel D. Von Hoff, MD

Epidemiology

Incidence: 32,180 (estimated new cases in the United States in 2005)
Mortality: 31,800 (estimated deaths in the United States in 2005)
Median age at diagnosis: 69 years
Male/female ratio: 1.2-1.5 to 1

Stage at Presentation

Stage	
Stage I:	20%
Stage II:	40%
Stage III–IV:	40%

Jemal A et al. CA Cancer J Clin 2006;56:106–30
Takhar AS et al. Br Med J 2004;329:668–673

Pathology

Most cancers of the pancreas arise in the head of the pancreas (60–70%), 15% in the body, and 5% in the tail; in 20%, the neoplasm diffusely involves the entire gland

Malignant Tumors of Pancreatic Origin

Ductal adenocarcinoma	85–90%
Acinar cell carcinoma	1–2%
Undifferentiated carcinoma (anaplastic giant cell, osteoclastic giant cell)	<1%
Sarcomatoid carcinoma/carcinosarcoma	<1%

Braud F et al. Crit Rev Oncol/Hematol 2004;50:147–155
Solcia E et al: Tumors of the pancreas. In: Atlas of Tumor Pathology, 3rd series. Washington DC: Armed Forces Institute, 1997
Clark MA et al. Lancet Oncology 2004;5:149–157
Ryan DP et al. NEJM 2000;342:792–800

Work-Up

The diagnosis of pancreatic cancer is based on imaging studies and histologic confirmation performed under CT or ultrasound guidance or during laparatomy

1. H&P
2. CBC, serum electrolytes, creatinine, mineral panel, LFTs, PT, PTT
3. Imaging:
   - Spiral CT provides localization, size of the primary tumor, and evidence of metastasis, and it evaluates major vessels adjacent to the pancreas for neoplastic invasion or thrombosis. CT is almost 100% accurate in predicting unresectable disease. However, the positive predictive value of the test is low, and approximately 25–50% of patients predicted to have resectable disease on CT turn out to have unresectable lesions at laparotomy
   - Endoscopic retrograde cholangiopancreatography can also be useful in patients in whom the CT scan is equivocal, because less than 3% of patients with pancreatic carcinoma have normal pancreatograms
   - Endoscopic ultrasonography is a relatively new technique. It role in diagnosis and staging is under investigation

Takhar AS et al. Br Med J 2004;329:668–673
Von Hoff DD, Evans DB, Hruban RH, eds. Pancreatic Cancer. Jones & Bartlett Publishers, 2005:165–180

Staging

Primary Tumor (T)

TX	Primary tumor cannot be assessed
T0	No evidence of primary tumor
Tis	Carcinoma in situ
T1	Tumor limited to the pancreas, ≤2 cm in greatest dimension
T2	Tumor limited to the pancreas, >2 cm in greatest dimension
T3	Tumor extends beyond the pancreas but without involvement of the celiac axis or the superior mesenteric artery
T4	Tumor involves the celiac axis or the superior mesenteric artery (unresectable primary tumor)

Regional Lymph Nodes (N)

NX	Regional lymph nodes cannot be assessed
N0	No regional lymph node metastasis
N1	Regional lymph node metastasis

Distant Metastasis (M)

MX	Distant metastasis cannot be assessed
M0	No distant metastasis
M1	Distant metastasis

Staging Groups

Stage 0	Tis	N0	M0
Stage IA	T1	N0	M0
Stage IB	T2	N0	M0
Stage IIA	T3	N0	M0
Stage IIB	T1-3	N1	M0
Stage III	T4	Any N	M0
Stage IV	Any T	Any N	M1

AJCC Cancer Staging Manual, 6th ed

Survival

1-year survival for all stages	19%
5-year survival for all stages	4%
5-year survival in resected patients	20%

American Cancer Society, 2002 Facts & Figures
Jemal A et al. CA Cancer J Clin 2005;55:10–30
Li D et al. Lancet 2004;363:1049–1057

Caveats

Surgery

- The only curative therapy for pancreatic cancer is resection of the tumor and surrounding tissues. Patients with resectable disease make up the smallest group (~15%)
- Criteria for unresectable tumors include:
  - –Distant metastases
  - –Superior mesenteric artery, celiac encasement
  - –Superior mesenteric vein, portal vein occlusion
  - –Aortic or inferior vena cava invasion, or encasement
  - –Invasion of superior mesenteric vein below the transverse mesocolon

Adjuvant Therapy

- Patients should be encouraged to enroll in clinical trials evaluating the potential benefits of chemotherapy or chemoradiation as well as new therapies
- The NCCN Panel recommends that postoperative RT should be administered at a dose of 45–54 Gy with concurrent fluorouracil, regardless of the margin or nodal status
- The efficacy of combined radiation and fluorouracil as **adjuvant therapy** for pancreatic cancer was demonstrated by a small prospective randomized study conducted by the Gastrointestinal Tumor Study Group (GITSG). Twenty-two patients were randomized to no adjuvant treatment, and 21 patients assigned to receive combined-modality therapy (radiation therapy; two courses of 2000 Gy, each given for 5 days separated by an interval of 2 weeks + fluorouracil 500 mg/m^2 intravenously on each of the first 3 days of each 2000 Gy segment of radiation). Subsequently, treatment continued 1 month after completion of radiation with fluorouracil 500 mg/m^2 per dose intravenously, 3 doses/week on days 1–3 for 2 years of therapy. The median survival for the treatment group was 20 months compared with 11 months for the control group, and the median disease-free survival was 11 months for the treated group compared with 9 months for the control group. This study and a later confirmatory study of an additional 30 patients treated with radiation + fluorouracil, provided evidence for the role of adjuvant combined modality therapy in combination with surgery.
  Gastrointestinal Tumor Study Group. Cancer 1987;59:2006–2010
  Kalser MH et al. Arch Surg 1985;120:899–903
- The European Study Group for Pancreatic Cancer 1 Trial randomly assigned patients with **resected** pancreatic ductal adenocarcinoma to treatment with chemoradiation (73 patients received a 2000 Gy dose given in 10 daily fractions over a 2-week period + fluorouracil 500 mg/m^2 intravenously on each of the first 3 days of RT, and fluorouracil 500 mg/m^2 repeated once, 4 weeks after the initial cycle), chemotherapy alone (75 patients received leucovorin 20 mg/m^2 intravenously followed by fluorouracil 425 mg/m^2 per day intravenously on 5 consecutive days every 28 days for 6 cycles), chemoradiation followed by chemotherapy (72 patients), and observation (69 patients). The estimated 5-year survival rate was 10% among patients assigned to receive chemoradiation and 20% among patients who did not receive chemoradiation (P = .05). The 5-year survival rate was 21% among patients who received chemotherapy and 8% among patients who did not receive chemotherapy (P = .009). The authors concluded that **adjuvant** chemotherapy has a significant survival benefit in patients with resected pancreatic cancer, whereas **adjuvant** chemoradiation has a deleterious effect on survival
  Neoptolemos JP et al. NEJM 2004;350:1200–1210
- Preliminary results presented at the 2005 ASCO meeting described the administration of gemcitabine 1000 mg/m^2 per dose intravenously for 3 doses on days 1, 8, and 15 every 4 weeks for 6 months (total dosage/cycle = 3000 mg/m^2) as **adjuvant therapy** starting 6 weeks **after surgical resection.** This treatment was associated with a median disease-free survival of 14.2 months compared with that of an observation arm (7.5 months, P = .05)
  Neuhaus P et al. [Abstract] Proc Am Soc Clin Oncol 2005;23:311s
- Chemoradiation is a conventional option for the management of **unresectable** locoregional pancreatic cancer. The recommended doses are 50–60 Gy with concomitant fluorouracil. Gemcitabine may be considered an alterative to fluorouracil-based chemoradiation in patients with **unresectable** locoregional pancreatic cancer

Treatment for Metastatic Disease

- Gemcitabine has been established as standard first-line therapy for patients with metastatic disease
- Gemcitabine can be administered over 30 minutes or in a fixed-dose rate (10 mg/m^2/min)
- The addition of erlotinib to gemcitabine has been demonstrated in a randomized phase III trial to improve survival and progression-free survival in advanced pancreatic cancer. Patients were randomized to receive either erlotinib 100 mg orally once daily (total dose/week = 700 mg) *or* placebo + gemcitabine 1000 mg/m^2 per dose intravenously weekly for 7 consecutive weeks, followed by 1 week without treatment (total dosage/8-week cycle = 7000 mg/m^2) *followed by* gemcitabine 1000 mg/m^2 per dose intravenously weekly for 3 consecutive weeks, followed by 1 week without treatment (total dosage/4-week cycle = 3000 mg/m^2). There was a difference in overall survival [P = .025; log-rank test] that favored the erlotinib arm with a hazard ratio of 0.81 [95% CI 0.67–0.97]. The corresponding 1-year survival rates were 24% versus 17%. Progression-free survival was also significantly improved in the gemcitabine + erlotinib treatment group, with a hazard ratio of 0.76, P = .003. The tumor control rates [CR/PR/SD] were 57% [CR/ PR = 9%] and 49% [CR/PR = 8%] for the erlotinib and placebo groups, respectively

Lockhart CA et al. Gastroenterology 2005;128:1642–1654
Moore MJ et al. [Abstract] Proc Am Soc Clin Oncol 2005;23:1s
National Comprehensive Cancer Network, vol. 1,2004

METASTATIC DISEASE REGIMEN

GEMCITABINE

Burris HA et al. JCO 1997;15:2403–2413*

Gemcitabine 1000 mg/m^2 per dose by intravenous infusion in 50–250 mL 0.9% NaCl injection (0.9% NS) over 30 minutes on days 1, 8, and 15 every 28 days (total dosage/cycle = 3000 mg/m^2)

Emetogenic potential: Low (Emetogenicity score = 2). See Chapter 39 for antiemetic regimens

*In the referenced trial, for the first cycle patients received gemcitabine 1000 mg/m^2 once weekly for up to 7 weeks. Thereafter, gemcitabine was administered once weekly for 3 consecutive weeks out of every 4 weeks

Patient Population Studied

A study of 63 patients with locally advanced or metastatic pancreatic cancer not amenable to curative surgical resection. Patients who had received previous chemotherapy were not eligible

Efficacy (N = 63)

Median survival	5.65 months
Survival rate at 12 months	18%
Clinical benefit response*	23.8%

*Clinical benefit response was a composite of measurements of pain, performance status, and weight that was sustained more than 4 weeks in at least one parameter without worsening in any others

Note: In this pivotal clinical trial, gemcitabine was compared in a randomized fashion with fluorouracil (600 mg/m^2/week). The median survival in the fluorouracil arm was 4.41 months, survival rate at 12 months was 2%, and clinical benefit response 4.8%

Toxicity (N = 63)

	% Who Grade			
	Grade I	Grade II	Grade III	Grade IV
WBC	26	36	10	0
Platelets	16	21	10	0
Hemoglobin	31	24	7	3
Bilirubin	3	10	2	2
Alkaline phosphatase	33	22	16	0
Aspartate transaminase	41	20	10	1.6
BUN	8	0	0	0
Creatinine	2	0	0	0
Diarrhea	18	5	2	0
Constipation	5	2	3	0
Pain	2	6	2	0
Fever	22	8	0	0
Infection	5	3	0	0
Pulmonary	3	3	0	0
Hair	16	2	0	0
Proteinuria	10	0	0	0
Hematuria	12.7	0	0	0
Nausea/vomiting	29	22	10	3

WHO Toxicity

Treatment Modifications

Adverse Event	Dose Modification
WBC 500 to 1000/mm^3 or platelets 50,000–99,000/mm^3 on day of treatment	Reduce gemcitabine dosages by 25%
G ≥ 3 nonhematologic adverse event during the previous treatment cycle	
WBC < 500/mm^3 or platelets <50,000/mm^3 on day of treatment	Delay chemotherapy for up to 2 weeks
Treatment delay >2 weeks for recovery from hematologic adverse event	Discontinue treatment

Therapy Monitoring

1. *Every week:* CBC with differential
2. *Before each cycle:* CBC with differential, serum electrolytes, creatinine, mineral panel, and LFTs
3. *Response assessment:* Every 2 months

METASTATIC DISEASE REGIMEN

GEMCITABINE FIXED DOSE-RATE INFUSION (10 mg/m² per minute)

Tempero M et al. JCO 2003;21:3402–3408

Gemcitabine 1500 mg/m² per dose by intravenous infusion in 50–250 mL 0.9% NaCl injection (0.9% NS) at an infusion rate of 10 mg/m² per minute (150 min) on days 1, 8, and 15 every 4 weeks (total dosage/cycle = 4500 mg/m²)

Emetogenic potential: Low (Emetogenicity score = 2). See Chapter 39 for antiemetic regimens

Patient Population Studied

A study of 43 patients with locally advanced (n = 5) and metastatic (n = 38) pancreatic adenocarcinoma

Efficacy (N = 43)

Median survival time	8 months
1-year survival	28.8%
2-year survival	18.3%

Note: In this phase II randomized trial (JCO 2003;21:3402–408), patients were treated with 2200 mg/m² intravenous gemcitabine over 30 minutes *or* 1500 mg/m² intravenous gemcitabine over 150 minutes on days 1, 8, and 15 of every 4-week cycle
The median time to treatment failure was comparable to both arms (1.8 months versus 2.1 months), but in the 30-minute infusion arm the median survival was 5 months; 1-year survival rate 9%; 2-year survival rate 2.2%, compared with the median survival of 8 months (P = .013); 1-year survival rate 28.8% (P = .014); 2-year survival rate 18.3% (P = .07) in the fixed dose-rate infusion arm

Toxicity (N = 43)

G3/4	%
Anemia	23.3
Nausea/vomiting	20.9
Thrombocytopenia	37.2
Neutropenia	48.8
Leukopenia	39.5
ALT	7.3
Diarrhea	4.7

Treatment Modifications

Adverse Event	Dose Modification
WBC 500–1000/mm³ or platelets 50,000–99,000/mm³ on day of treatment	Reduce gemcitabine dosages by 50%
WBC <500/mm³ or platelets <50,000/mm³ on day of treatment	Delay chemotherapy for up to 2 weeks
Patients with G4 granulocytopenia, thrombocytopenia, or nonhematologic toxicity during the previous treatment cycle	Reduce gemcitabine dosages by 25%

Therapy Monitoring

1. *Every week:* CBC with differentia
2. *Before each cycle:* CBC with differential, serum electrolytes, creatinine, mineral panel, and LFTs
3. *Response assessment:* Every 2 months

31. Pheochromocytoma

Michael M. Boyiadzis, MD, MHSc, Karel Pacak, MD, PhD Sc, and Tito Fojo, MD, PhD

Epidemiology

Annual incidence*:	3–8 per million
Hereditary contribution:	>20%
Average age at diagnosis:	42 years

*The annual incidence of pheochromocytoma in the United States is not precisely known, but the high prevalence (0.05%) of pheochromocytomas found in autopsy series indicates that the tumor is underdiagnosed and that the annual incidence is likely to be higher than indicated

Eisenhofer G et al. Endocr Related Cancer 2004;11:423–436

Pathology

- Approximately 80–85% of pheochromocytomas are located in the adrenal gland. The remaining 15–20% are located along the para-aortic sympathetic chain, aortic bifurcation, and urinary bladder
- Bilateral tumors occur in ~10% of patients and are much more common in familial pheochromocytomas
- 5–36% of pheochromocytomas are malignant, but no widely accepted pathologic criteria exist for differentiating between benign and malignant pheochromocytoma
- A diagnosis of malignancy requires evidence of metastases at non–chromaffin sites distant from that of the primary tumor
- Although most cases of pheochromocytomas are sporadic, a significant proportion occur secondary to several hereditary syndromes. The propensity of malignancy in hereditary pheochromocytoma syndromes is highly variable

Pheochromocytoma in Hereditary Syndromes

Hereditary Syndrome	Gene	Frequency*	Predisposition to Malignancy	Adrenal Disease	Extra-adrenal Disease
Von Hippel-Lindau disease (VHL)	*VHL*	6–20%	3%	++	+
Multiple endocrine neoplasia types IIA and IIB (MEN IIA, MEN IIB)	*RET*	30–50%	<3%	++	–
Neurofibromatosis type 1 (NF1)	*NF*	1–5%	<3%	++	+
Familial paraganglioma and/or pheochromocytoma syndromes caused by mutation of succinate dehydrogenase gene family members	*SDHB*	4–9%	66–83%	+	++
	SDHD	2–8%	<2%	+	++

++, very common; +, common; –, rare
*Frequency in sporadic tumors

Eisenhofer G et al. Endocr Related Cancer 2004;11:423–436
John H et al. Urology 1999;53:679–683
O'Riordain DS et al. World J Surg 1996;20:916–921; discussion 922
Pacak K et al. Ann Intern Med 2001;134:315–329

Evaluation

The diagnosis of pheochromocytoma is confirmed by biochemical evidence of elevated catecholamine production (preferably with measurement of plasma metanephrines) and by radiologic studies (Figure 31–1)

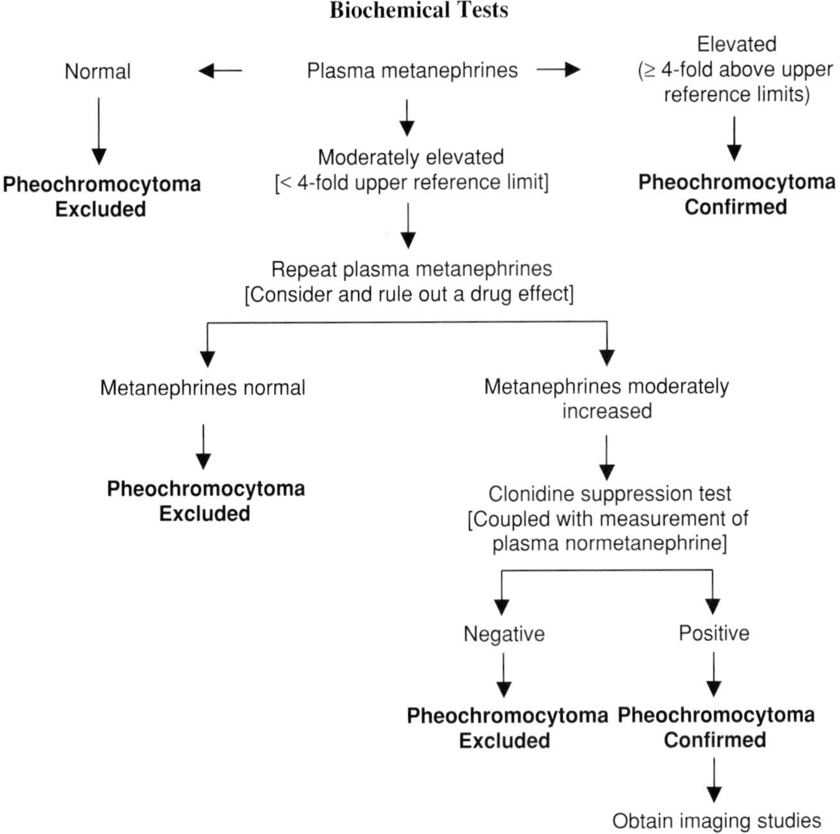

Figure 31–1. Biochemical tests.

Acetaminophen may interfere with measurement of plasma metanephrines. Other drugs including benzodiazepines, buspirone, diuretics, levodopa, tricyclic antidepressants, and sympathomimetics (α- and β-adrenergic blockers) may cause false-positive elevations of plasma or urine catecholamines or metanephrines

Imaging Studies

- *CT or MRI of abdomen (90–100% sensitivity):* Because of inadequate specificity, detection of a mass by these tests does not justify a diagnosis. ^{123}I Metaiodobenzylguanidine (MIBG) scanning is needed for confirmation
- *MIBG scan:* Used to confirm diagnosis when CT or MRI detects a tumor mass. In addition, if abdominal imaging is negative, whole-body evaluation by CT or MRI and MIBG scan are indicated to investigate for extra-adrenal pheochromocytoma. Drugs that may interfere with MIBG study include labetelol, calcium channel blockers, guanethidine, reserpine, sympathomimetics, tricyclic antidepressants
- *6-[^{18}F] Fluorodopamine positron emission tomography:* This is used when the biochemical tests are positive, but conventional studies cannot locate the tumor

Eisenhofer G et al. J Clin Endocrinol Metab 2003;88:2656–2666
Ilias I, Pacak K. J Clin Endocrinol Metab 2004;89:479–491
Pacak K et al. Ann Intern Med 2001;134:315–329

Staging

There is no accepted staging system for pheochromocytoma

Survival

For patients with resectable pheochromocytoma, the overall survival is equal to that of the age-matched normal population. Although the 5-year survival of malignant pheochromocytomas is less than 50%, malignant pheochromocytomas can be slow-growing, and patients may have minimal morbidity and survive as long as 20 years

Bravo EL et al. Endocr Rev 2003;24:539–553
John H et al. Urology 1999;53:679–683
Remine WH et al. Ann Surg 1974;179:740–748
van Heerden JA et al. Surgery 1982;91:367–373

Treatment Notes

Surgery

- The definite treatment for pheochromocytoma is surgical excision of the tumor. Surgical removal can cure pheochromocytoma in up to 90% of cases, whereas, if left untreated, the tumor can prove fatal. Laparoscopic adrenalectomy is now considered the standard approach for excision of most pheochromocytomas with the exception of very large (>10 cm) tumors. The survival rates after surgery are 97.7–100%
- Surgery for **malignant** pheochromocytoma is rarely curative, but resection of the primary mass or metastases can reduce exposure of the cardiovascular system and organs to toxic levels of circulating catecholamines. Consequently, aggressive surgical resection of accessible primary or recurrent disease or metastases should be attempted if the surgery renders the patient free of gross disease with the potential for normal biochemical determinations
- Surgery for **malignant** pheochromocytoma may be indicated for lesions in life-threatening or debilitating anatomic locations
- The value of surgical debulking for **malignant** pheochromocytoma before chemotherapy or radiation therapy is not proved
- The median time for recurrence of pheochromocytoma after initial resection is approximately 6 years and may be as long as 20 years
- Alternatives to surgical resection include external-beam radiation, cryoablation, radiofrequency ablation, transcatheter arterial embolization, chemotherapy, and radiopharmaceutical therapy
- Biochemical testing should always be repeated after recovery from surgical resection of a primary mass to exclude any remaining disease or metastasis
- Postoperative follow-up of patients includes evaluation of plasma metaneprine levels 6 weeks and 6 and 12 months after surgery, then yearly. Imaging studies should be performed on the basis of follow-up test results. Exceptions: (1) Patients with SDHB because they have a higher risk of malignancy and (2) those with an extra-adrenal tumor or a primary >5 cm who should be followed up more frequently (every 6 months for the first 5 years)
- Before surgery, patients with pheochromocytoma must undergo pharmacologic blockage of catecholamine synthesis and activity as well as volume expansion because they have reduced intravascular volume due to a persistent vasoconstricted state. The combination of phenoxybenzamine (α-blocker), atenolol (β-blocker) and metyrosine (tyrosine hydroxylase inhibitor), and liberal salt intake starting 2–3 weeks before surgery leads to better control of blood pressure and decreases surgical risks
  - Routine preoperative use of phenoxybenzamine opposes catecholamine-induced vasoconstriction. A β-adrenoceptor blocker (atenolol) is added to prevent the reflex tachycardia associated with α-blockade. The pressor effects of a pheochromocytoma must be controlled by α-blockade before β-blockers are initiated

    Note: β-Blockade **alone** can be dangerous in patients with pheochromocytoma and is contraindicated because it does not prevent and can actually augment effects of cathecholamines at α-adrenoceptors
  - Metyrosine is used to reduce the synthesis of new catecholamines by the tumor
  - The liberal salt intake should lead to an increase in weight of at most 1 kg per day

Drug	Mechanism	Oral Dose	Side Effects
Phenoxybenzamine	Long-acting nonselective α-adrenergic antagonist	Initial dose: 10 mg twice daily, gradually increased to 20 and 40 mg 2 or 3 times daily (approximately 1–2 mg/kg/day). Final dose is determined by the patient's blood pressure	Tachycardia, orthostatic hypotension, nausea, abdominal pain, nasal congestion, fatigue, and retrograde or difficulty in ejaculation
Atenolol	Long-acting β_1-selective (cardioselective) β-adrenergic antagonist	Initial dose: 25 mg once a day. This can be increased to 25 mg twice daily and 50 mg twice daily if needed	Hypotension, bradycardia, postural hypotension, cardiac failure, dizziness, tiredness, fatigue, and depression
Metyrosine	Competitively inhibits tyrosine hydroxylase, the rate-limiting enzyme in catecholamine synthesis	Initially, 250 mg 3 times a day. This may be increased by 250–500 mg daily to a maximum of 4 g/day in divided doses	Extrapyramidal neurologic symptoms, crystalluria, diarrhea, anxiety, depression, headache, fatigue, and xerostomia

(*continued*)

Treatment Notes (*continued*)

Phenoxybenzamine is available in the United States as capsules for oral administration containing phenoxybenzamine HCl 10 mg [DIBENZYLINE® Capsules brand of phenoxybenzamine hydrochloride]
In the United States, **atenolol** is available as tablets for oral administration containing 25 mg, 50 mg, and 100 mg atenolol
Metyrosine is available in the United States as capsules for oral administration containing 250 mg [DEMSER® (METYROSINE) Capsules]

Important note:
Several drugs (including some commonly used by oncologists) may lead to a hypertensive crisis in a patient with a diagnosis of pheochromocytoma, and should be avoided. These include:

- ACTH
- Amphetamine
- Cocaine
- Droperidol*
- Glucagon*
- Histamine*
- **Morphine**
- **Metoclopramide***
- Saralasin
- **Tricyclic antidepressants**
- Tyramine

*Has been used as a provocative test for pheochromocytoma

Eigelberger MS, et al. Curr Treat Options Oncol 2001;2:321-329
Eisenhofer G et al. Endocr Relat Cancer 2004;11:423–436
Pacak K et al. Ann Intern Med 2001;134:315–329
Westphal SA. Am J Med Sci 2005;329:18–21

REGIMEN

CYCLOPHOSPHAMIDE, VINCRISTINE, DACARBAZINE (CVD)

Averbuch SD et al. Ann Intern Med 1988;109:267–273

Recommendation: Hospitalization while first cycle is administered
Cyclophosphamide 750 mg/m^2 intravenously in 100–250 mL 0.9% NaCl injection (0.9% NS) or 5% dextrose injection (D5W) over 15–30 minutes on day 1 every 21 days (total dosage/cycle = 750 mg/m^2)
Vincristine 1.4 mg/m^2 intravenously per push over 1–2 minutes on day 1 every 21 days (total dosage/cycle = 1.4 mg/m^2)
Dacarbazine 600 mg/m^2 per dose intravenously in 100–250 mL 0.9% NS or D5W over 15–30 minutes for 2 doses on days 1 and 2 every 21 days (total dosage/cycle = 1200 mg/m^2)

Emetogenic potential:
Day 1: Very high (Emetogenicity score = 6)
Day 2: High (Emetogenicity score = 5). See Chapter 39 for antiemetic regimens

Patient Population

A study of 14 patients with advanced malignant pheochromocytoma

Efficacy (N = 14)

Tumor Response	
Complete response	2 (14%)
Partial response	6 (43%)
Overall response	57%
Median duration	21 months
Biochemical Response	
Complete response	3 (21%)
Partial response	8 (57%)
Overall response	78%
Median duration	22 months

Toxicity (N = 14)

Hematologic	
WBC nadir <1000/mm^3	21% (3/14)
Mean nadir WBC	2100/mm^3
Platelet count nadir <50,000/mm^3	29% (4/14)
Mean nadir platelet count	144,000/mm^3
Nonhematologic	
Mild sensory impairment	Mean grade 0.9/4
Paresthesias	Mean grade 0.9/4
Nausea and vomiting	Mean grade 1.6/4
Hypotension	4 episodes

Therapy Monitoring

1. *During initial treatment cycles:* Careful hemodynamic monitoring
2. *Before each cycle:* Plasma/serum metanephrines and catecholamines, CBC with differential, LFTs, and neurologic exam

Treatment Modifications

Counts on Day 1 of Repeated Cycles	
WBC 3000–3999/mm^3 or platelets 75,000–100,000/mm^3	Vincristine 100%. Reduce cyclophosphamide and dacarbazine dosages by 25%
WBC 2000–2999/mm^3 or platelets 50,000–75,000/mm^3	Vincristine 100%. Reduce cyclophosphamide and dacarbazine dosages by 50%
WBC 1000–1999/mm^3 or platelets 25,000–50,000/mm^3	Vincristine 100%. Hold cyclophosphamide and dacarbazine
Total bilirubin 1.5–2 mg/dL (132–177 µmol/L) or serum AST 75–150 units/L	Reduce vincristine dosage by 50%
Total bilirubin 3–5.9 mg/dL (264–519 µmol/L) or serum AST 151–300 units/L	Reduce vincristine dosage by 75%
Total bilirubin >6 mg/dL (>528 µmol/L) or serum AST >300 units/L	Hold vincristine
G1/2 Neuropathy	Decrease vincristine dosage by 50%
G3/4 Neuropathy	Hold vincristine
Nadir Counts During the Previous Cycle	
WBC 1000–1999/mm^3 or platelets 50,000–75,000/mm^3	Vincristine 100%. Reduce cyclophosphamide and dacarbazine dosages by 50%
WBC <1000/mm^3 or platelets <50,000/mm^3	Vincristine 100%. Reduce cyclophosphamide and dacarbazine dosages by 75%

Notes

Several drugs (including some commonly used by oncologists) may lead to a hypertensive crisis in a patient with a diagnosis of pheochromocytoma, and should be avoided:

1. ACTH
2. Amphetamine
3. Cocaine
4. Droperidol
5. Glucagon*
6. Histamine*
7. **Morphine**
8. **Metoclopramide***
9. Saralasin
10. **Tricyclic antidepressants**
11. Tyramine

*Used as a provocative test for pheochromocytoma

32. Prostate Cancer

Peter F. Lebowitz, MD, PhD, and William L. Dahut, MD

Epidemiology

Incidence: 234,460 (estimated new cases in the United States in 2006)

Deaths: 27,350 (estimated deaths in the United States in 2006)

Stage at Presentation	
Stage I:	50%
Stage II:	20%
Stage III:	17%
Stage IV:	13%

Greenlee RT et al. CA Cancer J Clin 2000;50:7–33
Jemal A et al. CA Cancer J Clin 2006;56:106–30
http://seer.cancer.gov

Pathology

Adenocarcinoma (acinar):	>95%
Ductal adenocarcinoma*:	<1%
Mucinous*:	<1%
Small cell*:	<1%
Transitional cell*:	<1%
Small cell*:	<1%

Gleason Score at Presentation
(Radical prostatectomy specimens)

2–4:	6%
5–6:	54%
7:	30%
8–9:	10%

*:Poor prognosis

Kantoff PW et al. Prostate Cancer: Principles & Practice. Philadelphia: Lippincott

Work-Up

T1, T2	Pelvic CT or MRI if nomogram indicates probability of lymph node involvement >20% Bone scan (if Gleason score ≥8 or PSA >20 ng/mL or T3, T4 or symptomatic) Positive lymph node on imaging (any T) → fine-needle aspiration (FNA) of node
T3, T4	Pelvic CT or MRI Bone scan Positive lymph node on imaging (any T); obtain a fine-needle aspiration (FNA) of node

NCCN Clinical Practice Guidelines in Oncology, V. 2. 2006
http://urology.jhu.edu/Partin_tables/

Staging

Primary Tumor (T)

TX	Primary tumor cannot be assessed
T0	No evidence of primary tumor
T1	Clinically unapparent tumor Neither palpable nor visible by imaging a) incidental finding in ≤5% of tissue b) incidental finding in >5% of tissue c) identified by needle biopsy for elevated PSA
T2	Tumor confined within prostate a) involves ≤half of one lobe b) involves >half of one lobe c) involves both lobes
T3	Tumor extends through the prostate capsule a) extracapsular extension b) invades seminal vesicles
T4	Tumor fixed or invading adjacent structures

Regional Lymph Nodes (N) Clinical

NX	Regional lymph nodes cannot be assessed
N0	No regional lymph node metastases
N1	Metastasis to regional lymph nodes

Distant Metastasis (M)

MX	Distant metastasis cannot be assessed
M0	No distant metastasis
M1	Distant metastasis a) non-regional lymph nodes b) bone c) other sites with or without bone disease

Staging Groups

Stage I	T1a N0 M0 (Gleason score 2–4)
Stage II	T1a N0 M0 (Gleason score >4)
	T1b - T2 N0 M0
Stage III	T3 N0 M0
Stage IV	T4 N0 M0 Any T N1 M0 Any T any N M1

AJCC Cancer Staging Manual, Sixth Edition

Epstein JI, et al. Am J Surg Pathol 1996; 20:286–92
Johansson JE, et al. JAMA 1997; 277:467–71

15-Year Relative Survival

Stage I–II	81%
Stage III	57%
Stage IV	6%

10-Year Free Disease Survival

(After radical prostatectomy for localized disease)

Gleason score 2–4	96%
Gleason score 5–6	82%
Gleason score 7	52%
Gleason score 8–9	35%

Caveats

Localized prostate cancer

Primary treatment options for initial therapy include surgery, radiation (external beam and/or brachytherapy), or expectant management depending on risk of spread and comorbid illnesses. Optimal treatment requires assessment of risk (refer to Partin tables). In general, with high risk of extracapsular spread or seminal vesicle involvement, external-beam radiation is preferable to surgery or brachytherapy alone

Locally advanced prostate cancer

Optimal approach involves neoadjuvant hormonal therapy, which is used before, during, and after external-beam radiation therapy

Lymph node involvement

Hormonal therapy is used early. Radiation therapy to nodes is controversial

Metastatic prostate cancer

Hormonal therapy with LHRH agonist (with an androgen receptor antagonist at the start of therapy to prevent flare) or orchiectomy is used initially. Combined androgen blockade can be used initially; however, the benefits are not clear and side effects are increased. With disease progression, second-line hormonal therapy is used. With further disease progression, docetaxel-based chemotherapy is most active

Partin tables

Predict pathologic stage based on PSA, Gleason Score, and clinical stage: http://urology.jhu.edu/Partin_tables/

Bolla M et al. Lancet 2002;360:103–108
Prostate Cancer. In: NCCN Clinical Practice Guidelines in Oncology, V. 2. 2005. © National Comprehensive Cancer Network, Inc., 2001, 2002, 2003

REGIMEN

DOCETAXEL + PREDNISONE

Sinibaldi VJ et al. Cancer 2002;94:1457–1465
Tannock I et al. NEJM 2004;351:1502–1512

Premedication:
Dexamethasone 8 mg orally twice daily for 3 days (starting 24 hours before docetaxel)
Docetaxel 75 mg/m² by intravenous infusion in a volume of 0.9% NaCl injection (0.9% NS) or 5% dextrose injection (D5W) sufficient to produce a solution with concentration within the range 0.3–0.74 mg/mL over 1 hour on day 1 every 21 days (total dosage/cycle = 75 mg/m²)
Prednisone 5 mg/dose orally twice daily continuously for 21 days (total dosage/21-day cycle = 210 mg)

Prednisone is marketed in the United States in numerous generic formulations for oral administration including immediate-release tablets containing 1, 2.5, 5, 10, 20 and 50 mg, and in solutions and syrups for oral administration

Emetogenic potential:
Day 1: Low (Emetogenicity score = 2)
Days 2–21: Nonemetogenic (Emetogenicity score = 1). See Chapter 39 for antiemetic regimens

Patient Population Studied

A study of 335 patients with hormone-refractory metastatic prostate cancer and no prior chemotherapy other than estramustine

Efficacy

	Docetaxel + Prednisone	Mitoxantrone + Prednisone
Median survival	18.9 months (n = 335)	16.5 months (n = 357)
Pain response	35% (n = 153)	22% (n = 157)
50% ↓ PSA	45% (n = 291)	32% (n = 300)

Toxicity (N = 332)

	% All Grades	% G3/4
Hematologic		
Neutropenia	—	32
Anemia	—	5
Thrombocytopenia	—	1
Febrile neutropenia	3	—
Infection	—	6
Nonhematologic		
Fatigue	53	5
Nausea/vomiting	42	—
Diarrhea	32	2
Sensory neuropathy	30	—
Stomatitis	20	—
Dyspnea	15	—
Peripheral edema	15	—
Myalgias	14	—

Treatment Modifications

Adverse Event	Dose Modification
G4 Neutropenia ≥7 days duration, febrile neutropenia, infection, or ANC <1500/mm³ on day of therapy	Delay therapy until ANC >1500/mm³ *or* reduce dose of docetaxel by 25%
G3/4 thrombocytopenia	Delay therapy until Thrombocytopenia G ≤2, or reduce dosage of docetaxel by 25%
G3/4 toxicities other than those listed above	Wait for toxicity to recover to G ≤1, then reduce docetaxel dosage to 60 mg/m²
G3/4 Neurotoxicity	Stop therapy
G4 Nonhematologic toxicity that occurs with 60 mg/m² docetaxel	
Aspartate/alanine aminotransferase (AST/ALT) >1.5 × upper limits of normal (ULN) and alkaline phosphatase >2.5 × ULN Bilirubin >ULN	Hold docetaxel until resolved

Therapy Monitoring

Before each cycle: CBC with differential, liver function tests, PSA if indicated

REGIMEN

MITOXANTRONE + PREDNISONE (M + P)*

Tannock IF et al. JCO 1996;14:1756–1764
Hussain M et al. Semin Oncol 1999;26(5 suppl 17):55–60

Mitoxantrone 12 mg/m^2 intravenously in 50 mL 0.9% NaCl injection (0.9% NS) or 5% dextrose injection (D5W) over 5–30 minutes, given on day 1 every 21 days (total dosage/cycle = 12 mg/m^2)
Prednisone 5 mg/dose orally twice daily continuously for 21 days (total dosage per cycle = 210 mg)

Prednisone is marketed in the United States in numerous generic formulations for oral administration including immediate-release tablets containing 1, 2.5, 5, 10, 20 and 50 mg, and in solutions and syrups for oral administration

Emetogenic potential:
Day 1: Moderate (Emetogenicity score = 3)
Days 2–21: Nonemetogenic (Emetogenicity score = 1). See Chapter 39 for antiemetic regimens

*Usually administered for a total of 6 cycles

Patient Population Studied

Patients with metastatic prostate cancer with symptoms (including pain) and disease progression despite standard hormonal therapy. Randomized comparison with prednisone alone

Efficacy (N = 80)

Palliative response*	29–38%
Palliative response duration	43 weeks

*Defined as a decrease in pain parameters

Efficacy: PSA Response (N = 57)

≥50% decrease	33%
≥75% decrease	23%

Toxicity (N = 654 and 796 cycles)

	% Cycles	
	% G1/2	% G3/4
Hematologic (N = 796 cycles)		
Neutropenia	NA	45
Febrile neutropenia	NA	7
Thrombocytopenia	4.2	0.6
Nonhematologic (N = 654 cycles)		
Nausea/vomiting	29	0.5
Alopecia	24	—
Cardiac dysfunction	2.5	1.7

WHO criteria

Treatment Modifications

Adverse Event	Dose Modification
WBC <3000/mm^3, ANC <1500/mm^3, or platelet <100,000/mm^3	Delay therapy until WBC >3000/mm^3, ANC >1500/mm^3, or platelet >100,000/mm^3
Nadir ANC <500/mm^3, or nadir platelet <50,000/mm^3	Reduce mitoxantrone dosage by 2 mg/m^2 per dose
Nadir ANC >1000/mm^3, and nadir platelet >100,000/mm^3, and minimal nonhematologic toxicity	May increase mitoxantrone dosage to 14 mg/m^2 per dose
Patients who received a total cumulative lifetime mitoxantrone dosage of 140 mg/m^2	Stop mitoxantrone, but continue prednisone

Therapy Monitoring

1. *Before starting therapy:* Echocardiogram
2. *Before each cycle:* CBC with differential, LFTs, PSA if indicated

REGIMEN

KETOCONAZOLE + HYDROCORTISONE

Bok RA, Small EJ. Drug Saf 1999;20:451–458
Small EJ et al. J Urol 1997;157:1204–1207

Ketoconazole 400 mg orally every 8 hours, continuously
Hydrocortisone 20 mg orally every morning, continuously
Hydrocortisone 10 mg orally every evening, continuously

Notes

1. Ketoconazole absorption can be decreased with concurrent use of antacids, H_2-antagonist antihistamines, and proton pump inhibitors (PPI). Avoid H_2- antagonists and PPI. If antacid treatment is needed, ketoconazole should be taken at least 2 hours before antacids
2. To avoid nausea, start ketoconazole at a low dose (eg, 200 mg 3 times daily) and gradually increase to full doses after several days

Ketoconazole is available in the United States generically as tablets for oral administration containing 200 mg of ketoconazole
Hydrocortisone is available in the United States in many solid and liquid formulations, including tablets for oral administration containing 2.5, 5, 10, and 20 mg hydrocortisone

Emetogenic potential: Nonemetogenic (Emetogenicity score = 1). See Chapter 39 for antiemetic regimens

Patient Population Studied

A study of 48 patients with hormone-refractory metastatic prostate cancer with progression after antiandrogen withdrawal

Efficacy

>50% PSA decline (≥8 weeks)	62.5%
Median change in PSA	79.5% decline
Mean duration of response	3.5 months

Small EJ et al. J Urol 1997;157:1204–1207

Toxicity (N = Varies)

	% Patients	
	Mild (G1/2)	Moderate/Severe
Nausea/vomiting	10	—
LFT abnormalities[a]	4–20	—
Fulminant hepatitis	—	0.1–1
Fatigue	6	—
Edema	6	—
"Sticky-skin"[b,c]	10	—
Rash[c]	4	—
Nail dystrophy[c]	Common	—
Dry mouth[c]	Often	—
Gynecomastia[d]	10–15	—
Adrenal insufficiency[e]	Varies	
Impotence	Anticipated	

[a]Asymptomatic increases; usually resolve with discontinuation of treatment
[b]Subjective sensation of stickiness to the skin, usually noted in axillary area
[c]Cutaneous and mucosal effects probably related to inhibitory effect on retinoic acid metabolism
[d]Not observed with ketoconazole 200–400 mg/day, but may occur with higher doses
[e]Steroid replacement recommended
From Bok RA, Small EJ. Drug Saf 1999;20:451–458

Treatment Modifications

Adverse Event	Dose Modification
Toxicity G ≥ 2	Hold ketoconazole until adverse events have resolved

Note: Ketoconazole is a potent inhibitor of the cytochrome P450 enzyme, CYP3A4. It has been reported to inhibit the metabolism of many drugs and drug metabolites that are metabolized by CYP3A-subfamily enzymes, resulting in elevated concentrations of the drugs. Affected drugs include (but are not limited to):

1. Warfarin (enhances anticoagulant effect)
2. Dihydropyridine calcium channel antagonists (eg, amlodipine, felodipine, nifedipine)
3. Loratadine
4. Some HIV protease inhibitors (saquinavir, indinavir and nelfinavir)
5. Statin hypolipidemic drugs (HMG-CoA reductase inhibitors)
6. Many other drugs and natural products

Drugs that are susceptible to pharmacokinetic interactions because of concomitant use with ketoconazole may require dose or schedule adjustments. It may be prudent to consider alternative treatment options, or if clinically appropriate, discontinue drugs that are known to interact with ketoconazole

Therapy Monitoring

Monthly: LFTs including AST, ALT, bilirubin, alkaline phosphatase, PSA if indicated

Notes

1. Liver transaminases may be transiently increased. Therapy can be continued in a setting of a grade 1 increase in transaminases with close monitoring, but there is a small risk (0.1–1%) of idiosyncratic hepatitis, which can be fatal
2. Some clinicians administer higher doses of hydrocortisone (30 mg in the morning and 20 mg in the evening)
3. In addition to corticosteroid replacement, some patients require mineralocorticoid supplementation with fludrocortisone 100–200 mcg daily orally in the morning

Fludrocortisone acetate is available in the United States as tablets for oral administration containing 100 mcg of fludrocortisone acetate. Florinef® Acetate (fludrocortisone acetate tablets). Monarch Pharmaceuticals, Inc, Bristol, TN

REGIMEN

HORMONAL AGENTS

Bolla M et al. Lancet 2002;360:103–108
Delaere KPJ, Van Thilo EL. Semin Oncol 1991;18(5 suppl 6):13–8
Iversen P et al. J Urol 2000;164:1579–1582
Janknegt RA. Cancer 1993;72(12 suppl):3874–3877
Janknegt RA. J Urol 1993;149:77–83
Periti P et al. Clin Pharmacokinet 2002;41:485–504
Tyrrell CJ. Eur Urol 1994;26(suppl 1):15–19

Treatment options:

1. Surgical castration: Orchiectomy
2. Medical castration: LHRH agonists
3. Nonsteroidal antiandrogens
4. Combined androgen blockade (CAB):
   - Orchiectomy + antiandrogen
   - LHRH agonist + antiandrogen

LHRH agonists:

1. **Leuprolide depot** 7.5 mg intramuscularly every month
2. **Leuprolide depot** 22.5 mg intramuscularly every 3 months
3. **Leuprolide depot** 30 mg intramuscularly every 4 months
4. **Goserelin implant** 3.6 mg, insert subcutaneously every 4 weeks
5. **Goserelin implant** 10.8 mg, insert subcutaneously every 3 months

Nonsteroidal antiandrogens:

1. **Flutamide** 250 mg/dose orally 3 times per day, continuously
2. **Bicalutamide** 50 mg orally daily, continuously; or 150 mg/day if given as monotherapy orally, continuously
3. **Nilutamide** 300 mg/day orally for 1 month with castration, followed by nilutamide 150 mg/day orally, continuously

Flutamide is available in the United States generically as capsules for oral administration containing 125 mg of flutamide
Bicalutamide is available in the United States as tablets for oral administration containing 50 mg of bicalutamide. Casodex® bicalutamide tablets product label. AstraZeneca Pharmaceuticals, LP, Wilmington, DE
Nilutamide is available in the United States as tablets for oral administration containing 150 mg of nilutamide. NILANDRON® (nilutamide). Aventis Pharmaceuticals, Inc, Kansas City, MO

Emetogenic potential: Nonemetogenic (Emetogenicity score = 1). See Chapter 39 for antiemetic regimens

Patient Population Studied

Patients with metastatic and locally advanced prostate cancer treated with hormonal therapy

Efficacy

Metastatic disease

1. LHRH agonists >85% response rate
2. No significant differences among LHRH agonists
3. Single-agent antiandrogen therapy may be inferior to medical (LHRH agonist) or surgical castration
4. Use of combined androgen blockade (CAB) as front-line therapy is controversial with limited evidence of clinical benefit

Locally advanced disease

Concurrent radiation and hormonal therapy in locally advanced disease appears to have a survival benefit. LHRH agonist + an antiandrogen are used for up to 3 months before, during, and for 3 years after radiation treatment

Bolla M et al. Lancet 2002;360:103–108
Laverdière J et al. Int J Radiat Oncol Biol Phys 1997;37:247–252
Prostate Cancer Trialists' Collaborative Group. Lancet 2000;355:1491–1498
Seidenfeld J et al. Ann Intern Med 2000;132:566–577

Toxicity

Common Toxicities of Androgen Deprivation

Hot flashes	LHRH Ag > AA
Loss of libido, impotence	LHRH Ag >> AA
Bone and muscle loss	LHRH Ag >> AA
Breast tenderness	AA >> LHRH Ag
Gynecomastia	AA >> LHRH Ag
Skin and hair changes	N/A
Weight gain	N/A
Asthenia	N/A

AA, antiandrogens; LHRH Ag, LHRH agonists

Toxicities of Individual Androgen Therapies

	% Patients
LHRH Agonists	
Tumor flare	Variable
Injection site reactions	Variable
Flutamide	
Gynecomastia	45–50
Diarrhea	20
Nausea/vomiting	5
Hepatitis	2.5
Vertigo	2.5
Hot flashes	2.5
Bicalutamide	
Gynecomastia	49
Breast tenderness	40
Constipation	14
Aggravation reaction	13
Hot flashes	13
Asthenia	12
Urinary retention	10
Diarrhea	6
Nausea/vomiting	5
Nilutamide	
Hot flashes	28
Visual disturbance[a]	27–50
Nausea	10 (7–20)
Dyspnea	6
Interstitial pneumonitis	1–2
Gynecomastia	4
Alcohol intolerance	5–19
Increased LFTs[b]	4–8
Anemia	4

[a]Includes decreased adaptation to darkness, blurred vision
[b]Transient in a majority of patients

Therapy Monitoring

All antiandrogens

1. *Monthly for the first 4 months:* LFTs
2. *Every 2–3 months after the first 4 months:* LFTs

Nilutamide

1. Baseline chest x-ray before therapy
2. *For respiratory symptoms:* Discontinue therapy pending evaluation

Wysowski DK, Fourcroy JL. J Urol 1996;155:209–212

Notes

1. For patients with metastatic prostate cancer being treated with an LHRH agonist alone, a testosterone level should be checked at 1 month. If it is >20 ng/dL, consider orchiectomy or adding antiandrogen
2. Concurrent antiandrogen therapy can be used with LHRH agonist for the first 2–4 weeks of treatment to avoid tumor flare
3. Antiandrogen withdrawal should be considered the first therapeutic maneuver in men whose disease has progressed after treatment with combined androgen blockade. Approximately 20% of patients have a significant decrease in serum PSA when antiandrogen is withdrawn
4. With acute cord compression or other oncologic emergency caused by a growing prostate tumor, ketoconazole and/or orchiectomy is the preferred treatment because of the rapidity of action

Kelly WK et al. J Urol 1993;149:607–609
Pont A. J Urol 1987;137:902–904

33. Renal Cell Carcinoma

Michael M. Boyiadzis, MD, MHSc, and Susan Bates, MD

Epidemiology

Incidence: 38,890 new cases in 2006
Estimated deaths: 12,840 in 2006
Median age: Seventh and eight decades
Male/female ratio: 1.6:1

Stage at Presentation
Stage I: 50.4%
Stage II: 14.6%
Stage III: 20.7%
Stage IV: 14.3%

Jemal A et al. CA Cancer J Clin 2006;56:106–30
National Cancer Institute, Surveillance, Epidemiology and End Results (SEER) Program

Pathology

Clear cell	70–80%
Papillary	10–15%
Chromophobe	5%
Collecting duct	0.4–2.6%

Zambrano NR et al. J Urol 1999;162:1246–1258

Work-Up (For Suspicious Renal Mass)

1. H&P
2. CBC, chemistry profile
3. Urinalysis
4. Chest x-ray
5. Abdominal and pelvic CT with contrast
6. Chest CT if abnormal chest x-ray or advanced lesion
7. MRI if CT suggests caval thrombosis or renal insufficiency
8. Bone scan or brain MRI if clinically indicated

National Comprehensive Cancer Network. V. 2. 2005

Staging

Primary Tumor (T)

TX	Primary tumor cannot be assessed
T0	No evidence of primary tumor
T1	Tumor 7 cm or less in greatest dimension, limited to the kidney
T1a	Tumor 4 cm or less in greatest dimension, limited to the kidney
T1b	Tumor more than 4 cm but not more than 7 cm in greatest dimension, limited to the kidney
T2	Tumor more than 7 cm in greatest dimension, limited to the kidney
T3	Tumor extends into major veins or invades adrenal gland or perinephric tissues but not beyond Gerota's fascia
T3a	Tumor directly invades the adrenal gland or perirenal and or renal sinus fat but not beyond Gerota's fascia
T3b	Tumor grossly extends into the renal vein or its segmental (muscle-containing) branches or vena cava below the diaphragm
T3c	Tumor grossly extends into vena cava above diaphragm or invades the wall of the vena cava
T4	Tumor invades beyond the Gerota's fascia

Regional Lymph Nodes (N)

NX	Regional lymph nodes cannot be assessed
N0	No regional lymph node metastases
N1	Metastases in a single regional lymph node
N2	Metastases in more than one regional lymph node

Distant Metastasis

MX	Distant metastasis cannot be assessed
M0	No distant metastasis
M1	Distant metastasis

Staging Groups

Stage I	T1 N0 M0
Stage II	T2 N0 M0
Stage III	T1 N1 M0 T2 N1 M0 T3 N0 M0 T3 N1 M0
Stage IV	T4 N0 M0 T4 N1 M0 Any T N2 M0 Any T Any N M1

Relative 5-Year Survival

Stage I	91%
Stage II	86%
Stage III	67%
Stage IV	17%

National Cancer Institute, Surveillance, Epidemiology and End Results (SEER) Program

Caveats

1. Patients with metastatic RCC should be referred for clinical trials
2. Incidentally discovered small renal mass (<3 cm) should be considered for surgical resection in the patient with no comorbid conditions
3. Nephrectomy in patients with metastatic disease is recommended before immunotherapy or chemotherapy
4. Five percent of RCCs are hereditary

Adverse prognostic factors in patients with metastatic RCC

1. Karnofsky performance status <80%
2. LDH >1.5 × upper limit of normal
3. Hemoglobin < lower limit of normal
4. Corrected serum calcium >10 mg/dL
5. Absence of prior nephrectomy

Risk Groups Based on Prognostic Factors

Risk Group	No. of Risk Factors	Median Survival
Favorable	0	20 months
Intermediate	1 or 2	10 months
Poor	3 or more	4 months

Linehan WM et al. Cancer of the kidney. In: DeVita VT, Hellman S, Rosenberg SA, eds. Cancer: Principles & Practice of Oncology, 7th ed. Philadelphia: Lippincott Williams & Wilkins; 2004:1139–1157
Motzer RJ et al. JCO 1999;17:2530–2540

REGIMEN

HIGH-DOSE ALDESLEUKIN (INTERLEUKIN-2; IL-2)

Yang JC et al. JCO 2003;21:3127–3132

Aldesleukin 720,000 units/kg per dose intravenously in 50 mL of albumin (human) 5% over 15 minutes every 8 hours for a maximum of 15 doses/cycle, if tolerated, for 2 cycles (after treatment commences the administration schedule is preserved; treatment is not extended to replace doses that were omitted owing to adverse events). Each cycle is separated by 7–10 days of rest. Treatment is repeated every 2 months

Emetogenic potential: Moderate (Emetogenicity score = 3). See Chapter 39 for antiemetic regimens

Ancillary Medications: See special section below

Patient Population Studied

A study of 156 patients with metastatic RCC without prior IL-2 therapy. Patients with brain metastases, coronary artery disease, active autoimmune disorder, or significant renal, pulmonary, or hepatic insufficiency were excluded

Efficacy (N = 155)

Complete response	6%
Partial response	15%

Treatment Modifications: Guidelines for Delay or Discontinuation of Aldesleukin and for Treatment of Adverse Events

Relative Criteria	Absolute Criteria
Cardiac	
Sinus tachycardia (120–130 beats/min)	Sustained sinus tachycardia (>130 beats/min) despite correcting hypotension, fever, and tachycardia and stopping dopamine) *ECG changes:* Atrial fibrillation Supraventricular tachycardia Ventricular arrhythmias (frequent PVCs, bigeminy, tachycardia) Changes suggestive of ischemia *Laboratory:* Elevated CPK isoenzymes or troponin
Dermatologic	
	Moist desquamation
Gastrointestinal	
Diarrhea, 1000 mL/8 hours Ileus/abdominal distention *Laboratory:* Bilirubin >7 mg/dL (120 μmol/L)	Diarrhea, 1000 mL/8 hours × 2 Vomiting not responsive to medication Severe abdominal distention affecting breathing Severe abdominal pain, unrelenting
Hemodynamic	
Maximum phenylephrine 1–1.5 μg/kg/min	Maximum phenylephrine 1.5–2 μg/kg/min
Minimum phenylephrine >0.5 μg/kg/min	Minimum phenylephrine >0.8 μg/kg/min
Hemorrhagic	
Guaiac-positive sputum, emesis, or stool *Laboratory:* Platelets 30,000–50,000/mm^3	Frank blood in sputum, emesis, or stool *Laboratory:* Platelets <30,000/mm^3
Infectious	
	Strong clinical suspicion or documented infection
Musculoskeletal	
Weight gain >15%	
Extremity tightness	Extremity paresthesias
Neurologic	
Vivid dreams	Hallucinations
Emotional lability	Persistent crying Mental status changes not reversible in 2 hours Inability to subtract serial 7s or spell words backwards Disorientation
Pulmonary	
Resting shortness of breath	
3–4 L O_2 by nasal cannula for saturation ≥95%	>4 L O_2 by nasal cannula for saturation ≥95% *or* 40% O_2 mask for saturation ≥95%
Rales one-third up lower chest	Endotracheal intubation Moist rales halfway up chest Pleural effusion requiring thoracentesis or chest tube while on therapy

(*continued*)

Treatment Modifications: Guidelines for Delay or Discontinuation of Aldesleukin and for Treatment of Adverse Events (*continued*)

Renal	
Urine 80–160 mL/shift Urine 10–20 mL/hour *Laboratory:* Creatinine 2.5–2.9 mg/dL	Urine <80 mL/shift Urine <10 mL/hour *Laboratory:* Creatinine >3 mg/dL (>264 μmol/L)

When to Delay or Discontinue Aldesleukin

Observation	Action
Any relative criteria	Initiate corrective measure ± delay aldesleukin
>3 relative criteria	Initiate corrective measure, delay aldesleukin Stop aldesleukin if not easily reversible
Any absolute criteria	Initiate corrective measures, delay aldesleukin Stop aldesleukin if not easily reversible

Adapted from Schwartzentruber DJ. J Immunother 2001;24:287–293

Corrective Measures for Aldesleukin Symptoms/Findings

Symptom	Corrective Measure
Cardiac	
Tachycardia (sinus)	Correct fever, hypotension, hypoxia, anemia; consider discontinuation of dopamine if used
Arrhythmia (other than sinus tachycardia)	Stop aldesleukin (most arrhythmias); correct electrolytes, minerals, anemia, hypoxia; use medications as indicated
Creatine kinase elevation	Measure isoenzymes or troponin, and obtain ECG; if evidence of myocarditis, stop aldesleukin; will need exercise ECHO before next cycle of aldesleukin to rule out myocardial dysfunction; future aldesleukin may be considered if ECHO is normal
Troponin elevation	Must stop aldesleukin; will need exercise ECHO before next cycle of aldesleukin to rule out myocardial dysfunction; future aldesleukin may be considered if the ECHO is normal
Constitutional	
Chills (generally after first or second aldesleukin dose)	Warm blankets as first measure; intravenous meperidine if chills persist
Fever breakthrough	Increase indomethacin to every 6 hours; consider septic work-up if happens after first 24 hours of therapy (ie, high spike above baseline during therapy)
Nasal congestion	Room humidifier, decongestant (no aerosolized steroids)
Dermatologic	
Moist desquamation	Oatmeal baths, lotions (no steroid- or alcohol-containing lotions)
Pruritus	Oatmeal baths, lotions, antipruritics
Gastrointestinal	
Diarrhea	Antidiarrheals (alternate medications); avoid overuse because of complicating ileus and distention

(*continued*)

Toxicity (N = 156)

Adverse Event	% G3/4
Hypotension	36
Malaise	21
Nausea or vomiting	13
Oliguria (<80 mL/8 hours)	12
CNS: Orientation	10
Thrombocytopenia	9
Diarrhea	9
Arrhythmia, atrial	4
Hyperbilirubinemia	3
Elevated ALT	3
CNS: Level of consciousness	3
Infection	3
Peripheral edema	0.4

All toxicities were reversible and no deaths occurred

Treatment Modifications: Guidelines for Delay or Discontinuation of Aldesleukin and for Treatment of Adverse Events *(continued)*

Nausea/vomiting	Antiemetics (alternate medications and routes if any medication is not effective)
Abdominal pain	Evaluate cause; give indomethacin rectally; consider antacids
Mucositis/stomatitis	Frequent oral care, mouthwashes, topical anesthetics, room humidifier
Hemodynamic	
Hypotension	Initially fluids; add phenylephrine after 1–1.5 L of fluid boluses
Acidosis: CO_2 <20 mmol/L	Give 50 mEq sodium bicarbonate intravenously
Acidosis: CO_2 <18 mmol/L	Give 100 mEq sodium bicarbonate intravenously
Hemorrhagic	
Anemia	Transfuse packed red blood cells to maintain hematocrit above 28% during aldesleukin dosing
Thrombocytopenia	Consider transfusion if platelet count <20,000/mm^3
Infectious	
Infection	Stop aldesleukin and treat infection as indicated
Laboratory	
Hypoalbuminemia	Observe
Hypocalcemia	Maintain above lowest normal value
Hypokalemia	Maintain potassium above 3.6 mmol/L
Hypomagnesemia	Maintain above lowest normal value
Musculoskeletal	
Weight gain >15%	Use fluids judiciously
Pulmonary	
Shortness of breath	Check transcutaneous O_2 saturation; if <95%, use O_2; use fluids judiciously; do not use aerosolized steroids
Renal	
Edema	Elevate symptomatic extremity; use fluids judiciously
Oliguria	Initially fluids; add dopamine after 1–1.5 L of fluid boluses

Adapted from Schwartzentruber DJ. J Immunother 2001;24:287–293

(*continued*)

Treatment Modifications: Guidelines for Delay or Discontinuation of Aldesleukin and for Treatment of Adverse Events (*continued*)

Ancillary Medications for Adverse Events Associated with High-Dose Aldesleukin Therapies

Adverse Event	Medication	Dose, Schedule, and Route of Administration
	Scheduled Medications	
Fever/myalgia	Acetaminophen	650 mg/4 hours PO/PR
	Indomethacin	50–75 mg/6–8 hours PO/PR
Gastritis	Ranitidine HCl	50 mg/8 hours IV
Nausea	Granisetron HCl	0.01 mg/kg daily
Prevent central line sepsis	Cefazolin Clindamycin	1000–2000 mg/6 hours, IV or 900 mg every 8 hours, IV
	As Needed (PRN) Medications	
Agitation/combativeness	Haloperidol	1–5 mg/ 1 hour IV/IM
Anxiety	Lorazepam	0.5–1 mg/6 hours PO/IV
Chills	Meperidine HCl	25–50 mg/1 hour IV
Diarrhea	Loperamide	2 mg/3 hours PO
	Diphenoxylate HCl/ atropine sulfate	2.5 mg/0.025 mg/3 hour PO
	Codeine sulfate	30–60 mg/4 hours PO
Gastric upset	$Al_2(OH)_3/Mg_2(OH)_3/$ simethicone	200 mg/200 mg/20 mg every 3 hours PO
Hypocalcemia	Calcium gluconate 10%	1000 mg over 1 hour IV
Hypokalemia	Potassium chloride	10 mEq over 1 hour IV
Hypomagnesemia	Magnesium sulfate	1000 mg (8.12 mEq) over 1 hour IV
Hypophosphatemia	Potassium phosphate	10–15 mmol over 6 hours IV
Hypotension	0.9% NaCl injection	250–500 mL IV
	Phenylephrine	0.1–2 mcg/kg/min IV
Insomnia	Temazepam	15–30 mg at bedtime PO
	Zolpidem	5–10 mg at bedtime PO
Mucositis	Sodium bicarbonate	30 g (~6 tsp)/1500 mL, swish and swallow
Nausea	Prochlorperazine	25 mg/4 hour PR; or 10 mg/6 hours IV
	Ondansetron HCl	10 mg/8 hours IV
	Lorazepam	0.5–1 mg/6 hours PO/IV
Oliguria	0.9% NS	250–500 mL IV
	Dopamine HCl	2–5 mcg/kg/min IV
Perianal discomfort	Tucks®	Apply locally

(*continued*)

Treatment Modifications: Guidelines for Delay or Discontinuation of Aldesleukin and for Treatment of Adverse Events (*continued*)

Pruritus	Hydroxyzine HCl	10–25 mg/6 hours PO
	Diphenhydramine HCl	25–50 mg/4 hours PO/IV
	Oatmeal powder/baths	Apply locally
	Lubriderm/camphor/menthol	Apply locally
Sinus congestion	Pseudoephedrine HCl	30 mg/6 hours PO

Adapted from Schwartzentruber DJ. J Immunother 2001;24:287–293

Therapy Monitoring (In-Patient Il-2 Administration)

Parameter to Monitor	Not Requiring Vasopressors	Requiring ICU/ Vasopressors
1. *Monitoring during therapy*		
Vital signs	Every 4 hours	Every 1 hour
Intake and output	Every 8 hours	Every 1 hour
Weight	Daily	Daily
Mental status	Every 8 hours	Every 8 hours
IV site/injection site*	Every 8 hours	Every 8 hours
CBC and leukocyte differential count	Daily	Twice daily
Electrolytes, glucose, BUN, creatinine	Daily	Twice daily
AST, ALT, alk phosphatase, total bilirubin	Daily	Daily
Albumin, calcium, magnesium, phosphorus	Daily	Daily
Creatine phosphokinase	Daily	Daily
PTT, PT	Every 3 days	Every 3 days
Thyroid stimulating hormone and free T_4	Each cycle	Each cycle
Urinalysis	Each cycle	Each cycle
ECG	Each cycle	Each cycle
Chest x-ray	Each cycle	Each cycle

*Monitor for extravasation or irritation. Change peripheral IV site every 3 days

2. *Response evaluation*

Radiologic evaluation or physical measurement of all sites of disease	Every 2 months

Rosenberg SA. Principles and Practice of the Biologic Therapy of Cancer, 3rd ed. Philadelphia: Lippincott Williams & Wilkins; 2000

Notes

1. Patients are re-treated with another course of IL-2 if disease is stable or regressing
2. Therapy is stopped and patients observed if they have two consecutive post-treatment evaluations that are unchanged
3. In a two-arm comparison with low-dose IL-2 (72,000 units/kg), there was no overall survival difference

REGIMEN

SUBCUTANEOUS LOW-DOSE ALDESLEUKIN (INTERLEUKIN-2; IL-2)

Yang JC et al. JCO 2003;21:3127–3132

Aldesleukin 250,000 units/kg subcutaneously 5 days per week during the first week, *followed by:*
Aldesleukin 125,000 units/kg subcutaneously 5 days per week during the next 5 weeks, followed by 2 weeks without aldesleukin (total dosage/cycle = 4,375,000 units/kg)
Eight-week treatment cycle = 6 consecutive weeks of treatment followed by 2 weeks without aldesleukin

Emetogenic potential: Nonemetogenic (Emetogenic score = 1). See Chapter 39 for antiemetic regimens

Patient Population Studied

A study of 94 patients with metastatic RCC who had not previously received aldesleukin. Patients with brain metastases, coronary artery disease, active autoimmune disorder, or significant renal, pulmonary, or hepatic insufficiency were excluded

Efficacy (N = 93)

Complete response	2%
Partial response	8%

Therapy Monitoring (Outpatient IL-2 Administration)

Parameter to Monitor Outpatient	Frequency
1. *Monitoring during therapy*	
Vital signs	As needed
Intake and output	Not strictly measured
Weight	Daily
Mental status	Daily
IV site/injection site*	Daily
CBC and leukocyte differential counts	Weekly
Electrolytes, glucose, BUN, creatinine	Weekly
AST, ALT, alkaline phosphatase, bilirubin	Weekly
Albumin, calcium, magnesium, phosphorus	Each course
Creatine phosphokinase	Weekly
PTT, PT	Weekly
Thyroid stimulating hormone and free T_4	Each course
Urinalysis	Each course
ECG	Each course
Chest x-ray	Each course

*Monitor for extravasation or irritation. Change peripheral IV site every 3 days

2. *Response evaluation*

Radiologic evaluation or physical measurements of all sites of disease	Every 2 months

Rosenberg SA. Principles and Practice of the Biologic Therapy of Cancer, 3rd ed. Philadelphia: Lippincott Williams & Wilkins, 2000

Treatment Modifications

Adverse Event	Dose Modification
G3/4 Toxicities except reversible G3 toxicities commonly seen with low-dose IL-2 (see Toxicity)	Skip doses until toxicity resolves
G3/4 Toxicities easily reversed by supportive measures	No dose adjustment or delay
Local inflammation at the injection site with or without nodular induration	No dose adjustment or delay. Apply local measures

Toxicity (N = 94)

	% G3/4
Malaise	9*
Nausea or vomiting	4*
Diarrhea	2*
CNS: Orientation	2
Oliguria (<80 mL/8 hours)	1
Infection	1*
Increased ALT	0.6
Hyperbilirubinemia	0
Peripheral edema	0
Thrombocytopenia	0
Hypotension	0
CNS: Level of consciousness	0

*All toxicities were reversible and no deaths occurred

Notes

1. Doses may be skipped, depending on patient tolerance
2. Patients are retreated with another course of IL-2 if disease is stable or regressing
3. Therapy is stopped and patients observed if they have two consecutive post-treatment evaluations that are unchanged
4. Patients without evidence of disease receive one additional consolidation cycle
5. Comparison of objective responses achieved with high-dose intravenous aldesleukin and subcutaneous aldesleukin demonstrated a small but statistically significant difference that favored high-dose treatment

REGIMEN

INTERFERON ALFA-2A

Negrier S et al. NEJM 1998;338:1272–1278

Induction:
Interferon alfa-2a 18 million units subcutaneously, 3 doses per week for 10 weeks (total dose/10-week induction = 540 million units)
Maintenance:
Interferon alfa-2a 18 million units subcutaneously, 3 doses per week for 13 weeks (total dose/13-week maintenance = 702 million units)
Note: Patients should take interferon doses around bedtime, allowing them to sleep through a period of most severe symptoms

Ancillary medications:

1. *Primary antipyretic prophylaxis:*
   Acetaminophen 650–1000 mg orally *or*
   Ibuprofen 400–600 mg orally starting 1 hour before interferon, then every 4 hours as needed
2. *Secondary antiemetic prophylaxis:*
   If required as secondary prophylaxis, then use as primary prophylaxis with subsequent doses

Emetogenic potential: Nonemetogenic (Emetogenicity score = 1). See Chapter 39 for antiemetic regimens

Treatment Modifications

Adverse Event	Dose Modification
Hypotension resistant to intravenous vasopressors	Stop treatment. Resume cautiously if blood pressure recovers
Life-threatening or persistent, severe toxic reactions	Discontinue therapy
WHO G ≥ 3 toxicity	Stop treatment. Resume when toxicity G ≤ 1 at original dose
Recurrent WHO G ≥ 3 toxicity	Stop treatment. Resume when toxicity G ≤ 1 with interferon alfa-2a dose decreased by 50%

Patient Population Studied

A study of 147 patients with RCC and progressive metastasis. Patients were excluded if they had brain metastases, cardiac dysfunction, any contraindications to the use of vasopressor agents, active infection, previous aldesleukin or interferon alfa treatment, chemotherapy or radiation therapy within 6 weeks before enrollment, or current treatment with steroids

Efficacy (N = 147)

Week 10	
Complete response	0%
Partial response	7%
Disease stabilization	31%
Disease progression	Not evaluated
Week 25	
Complete response	1%
Partial response	5%
Disease stabilization	13%
Disease progression	Not evaluated

Toxicity (N = 147)

	% G3/4
Impaired performance status	16
Anemia	6
Nausea or vomiting	5
Fever	5
Weight loss	4
Increased ALT or AST	3
Pulmonary symptoms	3
Diarrhea	1
Hypotension resistant to pressors	1
Neurologic symptom	1
Cardiac signs	1
Leukopenia	1
Infection	1
Cutaneous signs	0
Thrombocytopenia	0
Increased creatinine	0
Renal symptoms	0
Hyperbilirubinemia	0

WHO criteria

Therapy Monitoring

1. *Before each cycle:* CBC with differential, serum electrolytes, BUN, creatinine, LFTs, and mineral panel
2. *Response evaluation:* After each maintenance cycle

Notes

Interferon alfa-2a has been used in the treatment of metastatic RCC at different doses (3–18 million units) and modes of administration with a median overall survival of 13 months

Motzer RJ et al. JCO 2002;20:289–296

REGIMEN

FLUOROURACIL + GEMCITABINE

Rini BI et al. JCO 2000;18:2419–2426

Gemcitabine 600 mg/m^2 as an intravenous infusion in 50–250 mL 0.9% NaCl injection (0.9% NS), over 30 minutes, given on days 1, 8, and 15 every 28 days (total dosage/cycle = 1800 mg/m^2)
Fluorouracil 150 mg/m^2 by continuous intravenous infusion in 500–1000 mL 0.9% NS or 5% dextrose injection (D5W) over 24 hours for 21 days on days 1–21 every 28 days (total dosage/cycle = 3150 mg/m^2)

Emetogenic potential: Low (Emetogenicity score = 2). See Chapter 39

Patient Population Studied

A study of 41 patients with unresectable or metastatic RCC. Patients were excluded if they had active CNS metastasis or prior treatment with fluorouracil or gemcitabine for metastatic RCC

Efficacy (N = 39)

Complete response	0%
Partial response	18%
Median progression-free survival	28.7 weeks

Toxicity (N = 41)

	% G2	% G3	% G4
Hematologic			
Anemia	41	5	0
Neutropenia	32	12	2
Thrombocytopenia	15	2	2
Nonhematologic			
Fatigue	22	7	0
Mucositis	12	10	0
Nausea/Vomiting	12	2	0
Diarrhea	7	0	0
Rash	7	0	0
Renal	5	0	0
Cardiac toxicity	Complete heart block (1 patient) Atrial flutter (1 patient)		

Treatment Modifications

Adverse Event	Dose Modification
CALGB G3/4 toxicity	No further therapy in ongoing cycle. Begin subsequent cycle on schedule or when toxicity resolves to ≤G2 with gemcitabine and fluorouracil doses decreased by 50%*
Second episode of CALGB G3/4 toxicity	No further therapy in ongoing cycle. Begin subsequent cycle on schedule or when toxicity resolves to ≤G2 with gemcitabine and fluorouracil doses decreased by 50% from current doses*
Third episode of CALGB G3/4 toxicity	Discontinue therapy
CALGB G3/4 toxicity not resolved to ≤G2 after 4 weeks	Discontinue therapy

*If a patient whose doses had been decreased experiences no more than grade 1 toxicity in a cycle in which reduced doses are administered, then both gemcitabine and fluorouracil dosages can be increased by 25% in the subsequent cycle

Therapy Monitoring

1. *Before each cycle:* CBC with differential, serum electrolytes, BUN, creatinine, LFTs, and mineral panel
2. *Response evaluation:* CT and/or bone scan after every 2 cycles

Notes

Two subsequent regimens that added agents to fluorouracil + gemcitabine reported a lower efficacy

Desai AA et al. Cancer 2002;15:1829–1836
George CM et al. Ann Oncol 2002;13:116–120

REGIMEN

SORAFENIB (NEXAVAR; BAY 43-9006)

Escudier B et al. [abstract LBA4510] Proc Am Soc Clin Oncol 2005;23(16S, Part 1)380S
Ratain MJ et al. [abstract 4544] Proc Am Soc Clin Oncol 2005;23(16S, Part 1)388S
May 2005 Annual Meeting http://www.asco.org/ac (Escudier et al)

Sorafenib 400 mg orally every 12 hours (eg, morning and evening) continually in 28-day cycles

Notes:

- Patients should swallow tablets whole with approximately 250 mL (8 oz.) of water. Tablets may be taken with or without food
- *Special precautions:* Sorafenib is metabolized by the cytochrome P450 CYP3A subfamily enzymes and has been shown in preclinical studies to inhibit multiple CYP isoforms. Therefore, all patients who are taking concomitant medications that are metabolized by the liver should be closely observed for side effects of these concomitant medications. Special caution should be use with any of the following medications: ketoconazole, itraconazole, ritonavir, cyclosporine, carbamazepine, phenytoin, and phenobarbital. Furthermore, patients taking narrow therapeutic index medications (warfarin, quinidine, digoxin) should be monitored proactively. *Patients should also be advised to avoid consuming grapefruit and grapefruit juice for as long as they continue to use sorafenib*

Supportive care:

- For patients who develop a hand-foot reaction, use topical emollients (such as Aquaphor®), topical and/or oral steroids, antihistamine agents, or vitamin B_6 (pyridoxine: 50 – 150 mg, orally, each day)
- If diarrhea develops and does not have an identifiable cause other than sorafenib therapy, administer loperamide 2 mg orally every 2 hours while awake and loperamide 4 mg orally every 4 hours during hours of sleep until the patient is free of diarrhea for 12 hours, at which time loperamide can be discontinued. This regimen can be repeated for each diarrheal episode

Note: Although this dosage regimen may exceed the usual loperamide dosage recommendations (16 mg/day), it is similar to the dosing regimen recommended for diarrhea associated with irinotecan administration and has been successfully and safely used

- If a patient develops blood or mucus in the stool, dehydration, or hemodynamic instability or if diarrhea persists >48 hours despite loperamide, hospitalize the patient for treatment with intravenous fluids as needed. For persistent diarrhea, other potentially helpful treatments may also be administered, such as somatostatin analogues or propantheline bromide

Sorafenib tosylate (Nexavar®;Onyx Pharmaceuticals, Emeryville, CA) is available in the United States in a film-coated, 10-mm, round, salmon-colored biconvex tablet containing 200 mg of sorafenib base as the tosylate salt

***Emetogenic potential*:** Low (Emetogenicity score = 2). See Chapter 39 for antiemetic regimens

Treatment Modifications

Dose Levels

Starting dose level	400 mg every morning; 400 mg every evening
Dose level −1	200 mg every morning; 400 mg every evening
Dose level −2	200 mg every morning; 200 mg every evening
Dose level −3	200 mg once daily

Adverse Event	Dose Modification
G1 Toxicity	Continue therapy
G2 Nausea/ vomiting/diarrhea	Institute symptomatic treatment and continue therapy
G2 Nausea/ vomiting/diarrhea despite symptomatic treatment	Reduce to dose level −1
First occurrence of G2 toxicity other than nausea/ vomiting/diarrhea excluding easily correctable toxicities[b]	Hold therapy until toxicity G ≤ 1 or pretreatment baseline then continue starting dose level
Second occurrence of G2 toxicity other than nausea/ vomiting/diarrhea excluding easily correctable toxicities[b]	Hold therapy until toxicity G ≤ 1, or pretreatment baseline. If <3 weeks to achieve toxicity G ≤1, reduce dose by 1 level; if >3 weeks to achieve toxicity G ≤ 1, reduce dose by 2levels
G3 Nausea/ vomiting/diarrhea and tumor pain	Institute maximal symptomatic treatment. If improvement to G ≤ 2 occurs within 48 hours, hold until toxicity G ≤ 1 or pretreatment baseline and reduce by 1 dose level. If Improvement to G ≤ 2 does not occur within 48 hours, hold until toxicity G ≤ 1 or pretreatment baseline and reduce dose by 2 levels

(*continued*)

Treatment Modifications (*continued*)

Adverse Event	Dose Modification
G3 Nonhematologic toxicity (excluding nausea/vomiting/diarrhea tumor pain without maximal symptomatic treatment and easily correctable toxicities[a] *or* G3 Hematologic toxicity	Hold therapy until toxicity improves to G ≤ 1 or pretreatment baseline. If < 3 weeks to achieve toxicity G ≤ 1 then reduce by 2 dose levels. If >3 weeks to achieve toxicity G ≤ 1, then discontinue therapy
G4 Hematologic toxicity	Hold sorafenib until toxicity improves to G ≤ 1 or pretreatment baseline. If <3 weeks to achieve toxicity G ≤ 1, then reduce by 2 dose levels or to dose level −3 if already receiving dose level −2. If >3 weeks to achieve toxicity G ≤1, then discontinue therapy
G4 Hematologic toxicity on level −3	Discontinue therapy
G4 Nonhematologic toxicity[b]	Discontinue therapy
G2 Toxicity other than nausea/vomiting/diarrhea on dose level −3	Discontinue therapy

[a]Easily correctable toxicities: Those that can be corrected within 24 hours, including metabolic toxicities such as abnormalities in glucose, potassium, magnesium, phosphorus, and sodium

[b]Except pulmonary embolism without significant hypoxia and hemodynamic instability, G4 hyperuricemia and easily correctable toxicities

Dose Modification Guidelines for Sorafenib-Induced Hypertension

Toxicity Grade for Hypertension

G1	Asymptomatic, transient (<24 hours) increase by >20 mm Hg (diastolic) or to >150/100 if previously within normal limits; intervention not indicated
G2	Recurrent or persistent (>24 hours) or symptomatic increase by >20 mm Hg (diastolic) or to >150/100 if previously within normal limits; monotherapy may be indicated
G3	Requiring more than one drug or more intensive therapy than previously
G4	Life-threatening (eg, hypertensive crisis)

Adverse Event	Dose Modification
G1	Continue sorafenib at same dose and schedule
G2 Asymptomatic	Treat with antihypertensives and continue sorafenib at same dose and schedule
G2 Symptomatic or persistent G2 despite anti-hypertensives *or* Diastolic BP >110 mm/Hg *or* G3 Hypertension	Treat with antihypertensives. Hold sorafenib (maximum 2 weeks until symptoms resolve and diastolic BP <100 mm Hg); then continue sorafenib at 1 dose level lower *Note:* If sorafenib is held more than 2 weeks. discontinue therapy
G4	Discontinue therapy

Patient Population Studied

Randomized trial of sorafenib versus placebo; 385 patients assigned to placebo; 384 patients assigned to sorafenib arm. Poor-risk Motzer group was excluded

Median age	59 years (19–86 years)
Median time from diagnosis	2 years (<1–19 years)
Characteristic	
Clear cell	100%
ECOG PS 0/1/2	48%/49%/2%
Low Motzer criteria	52%
Intermediate Motzer criteria	48%
Prior nephrectomy	93%
Prior radiation	28%
Prior cytokine-based therapy	83%
Metastatic sites: 1/2/≥2	15%/27%/57%
Lung metastases	75%
Liver metastases	26%

Efficacy (N = 335–384)

	Sorafenib	Placebo
Partial response	2%	0
Stable disease at 12 weeks	78%	55%
Progressive disease at 12 weeks	9%	30%
Median progression-free survival	24 weeks	12 weeks

Toxicity (N = 384)

	% Any G	% G3/4
Cardiac, general		
Hypertension	8	1
Constitutional symptoms		
Fatigue	18	2
Gastrointestinal		
Diarrhea	30	1
Nausea	14	<1
Anorexia	9	1
Vomiting	8	—
Constipation	6	—
Mucositis	7	1
Dermatologic/skin		
Rash/desquamation	31	1
Hand-foot skin reaction	26	5
Alopecia	23	—
Pruritus	14	<1
Dry skin	7	—
Flushing	6	<1
Neurology		
Neuropathy–sensory	9	<1

Therapy Monitoring

1. *During treatment cycles:* CBC with differential weekly
2. *Before each cycle:* CBC with differential, serum electrolytes, BUN, and creatinine
3. *Weekly for the first 4 weeks of cycle 1 of therapy and as needed subsequently:* Blood pressure

REGIMEN

SUNITINIB (SUTENT®; SU11248)

Motzer RJ et al. [abstract 4508] Proc Am Soc Clin Oncol 2005; 23(16S, Part 1)380S
May 2005 Annual Meeting http://www.asco.org/ac (Motzer et al)
Motzer RJ et al. Phase 2 trials of SU11248 show antitumor activity in second-line therapy for patients with metastatic renal cell carcinoma (RCC). May 2005 ASCO Annual Meeting (cited 2005 Nov 14]:[1 screen]. Available from: URL: http://www.asco.org/ac/1 ,1003,_12-002640-00_18-0034-00_19-0030432,00.asp

Sunitinib 50 mg orally daily for 28 consecutive days on days 1–28, followed by a 14-day hiatus (4 weeks on, followed by 2 weeks off), every 6 weeks (total dose/6-week cycle = 2400 mg)

Emetogenic potential: Low (Emetogenicity score = 2). See Chapter 39 for antiemetic regimens

Patient Population Studied

Two consecutive studies in 63 patients (Trial 1) and 106 patients (Trial 2) with renal cell cancer; second-line therapy after prior cytokine therapy

	Trial 1	Trial 2
Number of patients	N = 63	N = 106
Median age	60 years	56 years
Characteristic	**% of Patients**	
Clear cell/Other histologies	87/13	100/0
MSKCC Risk Factors 0/≥1	54/46	58/42
ECOG PS 0/1	54/46	55/45
Prior nephrectomy	92	100
Prior radiation	40	19
Prior interferon	57	44
Prior aldesleukin	30	47
Prior interferon + aldesleukin	13	9
Metastatic sites: 1/≥2	13/87	12/88
Lung metastases	81	81
Bone metastases	51	26
Liver metastases	16	27

Efficacy (N = 63 and 106)

	Trial 1 (N = 63)	Trial 2 (N = 106)
Complete response	0	1%
Partial response (PR)	40%	39%
Stable disease >12 weeks	28%	23%
Progressive disease at 12 weeks	9%	30%
Overall survival	16.4	Ongoing
Median time to PR (n = 25)		2.3 months
Median duration of PR (n = 25)		12.5 months
Median time to progression		8.7 months*

*In Trial 1; 95% CI: 5.5, 10.7

RECIST Criteria

Treatment Modifications

		% with Dose Reductions to −1/−2*	
		Trial 1	Trial 2
Dosage level +3	87.5 mg/day		
Dosage level +2	75 mg/day		
Dosage level +1	62.5 mg/day		
Starting dosage level	50 mg/day	—	—
Dosage level −1	37.5 mg/day	32	16
Dosage level −2	25 mg/day	3	6

*Primary reason for dose reductions: Fatigue, stomatitis and increased amylase/lipase

Adverse Events	Treatment Modifications
G ≥ 3 hematologic or nonhematologic toxicity	Reduce by one dose level or, if administering 25 mg/day, discontinue therapy
G ≥ 3 fatigue	
G ≥ 3 stomatitis	
Clinical manifestations of congestive heart failure (CHF)	Discontinue sunitinib
Decreased ejection fraction by 20–50% less than baseline without clinical evidence of congestive heart failure (CHF)	Interrupt sunitinib treatment and/or reduce the dose or, if administering 25 mg/day, discontinue therapy
Grade 2/3/4 serum lipase or serum amylase	Hold therapy until level G1, then resume therapy. Reduce by one dose level or, if administering 25 mg/day, discontinue therapy

(*continued*)

Treatment Modifications (*continued*)

Adverse Events	Treatment Modifications
Co-administration of potent CYP3A4 inhibitors (e.g., ketoconazole, itraconazole, clarithromycin, atazanavir, ritonavir, telithromycin)[1]	Reduce sunitinib dose to a minimum of 37.5 mg daily
Co-administration of potent CYP3A4 inducers (e.g., rifampin, phenytoin, phenobarbital, dexamethasone, carbamazepine, St. John's, wort)[1]	Increase sunitinib dose one level to a maximum of 87.5 mg daily

[1]If a medication with no effect on enzyme activity cannot be substituted

Toxicity (Trial 1, N = 63; Trial 2, N = 106)

Nonhematologic toxicity

	% Grade 2		% Grade 3	
	Trial 1	Trial 2	Trial 1	Trial 2
Fatigue	27	14	11	8
Diarrhea	21	13	3	3
Nausea	16	13	3	0
Stomatitis	17	9	2	5
Dermatitis	6	6	2	5
LVEF decline	9	3	2	2
Hypertension	3	8	2	6

Laboratory Abnormalities

	% Grade 2		% Grade 3/4	
	Trial 1	Trial 2	Trial 1	Trial 2
Neutropenia	32	26	13	13
Anemia	27	19	10	6
↓ Platelets	18	13	0	6
↑ Lipase	3	13	21	15
↑ Amylase	2	5	8	3

Therapy Monitoring

1. *During treatment cycles:* CBC with differential weekly
2. *Before each cycle:* Blood pressure, CBC with differential, serum electrolytes, BUN, serum amylase, lipase, and creatinine
3. Because patients receiving sunitinib who have a history of "cardiac events" may be at increased risk for developing left ventricular dysfunction they should be monitored for clinical signs and symptoms of congestive heart failure. Baseline and periodic evaluations of left ventricular ejection fraction should be considered. A baseline evaluation of ejection fraction should be considered in patients without cardiac risk factors
4. *Patients who experience stress such as surgery, trauma or severe infection:* Monitor for adrenal insufficiency

Notes

1. In its approval the FDA noted: "Decreases in left ventricular ejection fraction (LVEF) have been noted with sunitinib. Dose reduction and/or addition of antihypertensive or diuretic medications may be required; spontaneous recovery has also been observed. Patients should be monitored for signs and symptoms of congestive heart failure and sunitinib should be discontinued if these are observed"
2. Blood pressure monitoring is also recommended during treatment with sunitinib. Hypertension should be treated with standard therapies. Temporary suspension of sunitninb is recommended in severe cases until hypertension is controlled
3. Monitoring for adrenal insufficiency is also advised in patients who experience stress such as surgery, trauma, or severe infection

34. Sarcomas

Janice Walshe, MD, Tito Fojo, MD, PhD, and Lee Helman, MD

Sarcomas: Primary Malignant Bone Tumors

Epidemiology

Incidence: 2760 estimated cases in the United States in 2006
Mortality: 1260 estimated deaths in 2006

Gurney JG et al. Malignant bone tumors. In: Reis LAG, Smith MA, Gurney JG et al, eds. Cancer incidence and survival among children and adolescents: United States SEER program, 1975–1995. Bethesda, MD: National Cancer Institute SEER Program. NIH Pub. No. 99-4649, 1999:99–110
Jemal A et al. CA Cancer J Clin 2006;56:106–30

Work-Up

1. History and physical examination
2. *Laboratory tests*: CBC with differential; electrolytes; liver function tests; mineral panel, including alkaline phosphatase; lactate dehydrogenase
3. Plain films of affected bone
4. Chest x-ray (PA and lateral)
5. CT scan of chest, abdomen, and pelvis (particularly chest because 80% of metastatic lesions occur here)
6. MRI to ascertain extent of the tumor, involvement of surrounding neurovascular structures, invasion of the adjacent joint, and the presence of skip metastases
7. Bone scan to identify skip lesions within affected bones or distant metastatic disease
8. Bone marrow aspirate for light microscopy examination in the case of Ewing's sarcoma
9. No radiologic studies are pathognomonic, so bone biopsy remains essential to diagnosis
10. Echocardiogram or MUGA scan to determine cardiac ejection fraction as clinically indicated
11. Audiogram before cisplatin chemotherapy

NCCN Clinical Practice Guidelines in Oncology, vol. 1, 2006, Bone tumors

Classification

1. **Osteosarcoma**
   a. Conventional (intramedullary) high-grade:
      (1) Osteoblastic
      (2) Chondroblastic
      (3) Fibroblastic
      (4) Mixed
      (5) Small cell
      (6) Other: telangiectactic, epithelioid, giant cell
   b. Intramedullary low-grade
   c. Periosteal
   d. Parosteal
2. **Chondrosarcoma**
   a. Intramedullary
      (1) Conventional
      (2) Clear cell
      (3) Dedifferentiated
      (4) Mesenchymal
   b. Juxtacortical
3. **Ewing's sarcoma/primitive neuroectodermal tumor**
4. **Angiosarcoma**
5. **Fibrosarcoma/malignant fibrous histiocytoma**

AJCC Cancer Staging Manual, 6th ed. New York: Springer-Verlag, 2002:187–192
Dahlin DC, Unni KK. Am J Surg Pathol 1977;1:61–72

Surgical Staging

The surgical system as described by Enneking et al is based on the GTM classification: grade (G), location or site (T), and lymph node involvement and metastases (M)

Grade [G]	
G1	Any low-grade tumor
G2	Any high-grade tumor
Site [T]	
T1	Intracompartmental location of the tumor
T2	Extracompartmental location of the tumor
Lymph Node Involvement and Metastases [M]	
M0	No metastases
M1	Regional or distal metastases

Staging Groups

Stage	Grade	Site	Metastases
IA	Low (G1)	T1	M0
IB	Low (G1)	T2	M0
IIA	High (G2)	T1	M0
IIB	High (G2)	T2	M0
IIIA	Any G	T1	M1
IIIB	Any G	T2	M1

Enneking WF et al. Clin Orthop 1980;153:106–120

Clinical Staging

IUCC and TNM Staging

Primary Tumor	
TX	Primary tumor cannot be assessed
T0	No evidence of primary tumor
T1	Tumor ≤8 cm in greatest dimension
T2	Tumor >8 cm in greatest dimension
T3	Discontinuous tumors in the primary bone site

Grade	
GX	Grade cannot be assessed
G1	Well differentiated–low grade
G2	Moderately differentiated–low grade
G3	Poorly differentiated–high grade
G4	Undifferentiated–high grade

Nodal Status	
NX	Regional lymph nodes cannot be assessed
N0	No regional metastasis
N1	Regional lymph nodes metastasis

Metastases	
MX	Distant metastasis cannot be assessed
M0	No distant metastases
M1	Distant metastases M1a Lung M1b Other distant sites, including lymph nodes

Stage Grouping

IA	G1,2	T1	N0	M0
IB	G1,2	T2	N0	M0
IIA	G3,4	T1	N0	M0
IIB	G3,4	T2	N0	M0
III	Any G	T3	N0	M0
IVA	Any G	Any T	N0	M0
IVB	Any G	Any T	Any N	M0
	M0	Any T	N1	M1

International Union Against Cancer (IUCC) and American Joint Committee on Cancer (AJCC) TNM Staging, 6th ed. System for Bone Sarcomas

Primary Malignant Bone Tumors: Osteosarcoma

Epidemiology

Incidence: 400 estimated cases of osteosarcoma per year in the United States
Male:female ratio: 1.5:1

American Cancer Society: Cancer Facts and Figures 2005 http://cancer.org
Gurney JG, Swensen AR, Bulterys M. Malignant bone tumors. In: Reis LAG, Smith MA, Gurney JG et al, eds. Cancer incidence and survival among children and adolescents: United States SEER program, 1975–1995. Bethesda, MD: National Cancer Institute SEER Program. NIH Pub. No. 99-4649, 1999:99–110

Caveats

Neoadjuvant chemotherapy

1. Neoadjuvant therapy has a recognized role in the treatment of high-grade osteosarcoma with long-term survival rate of >60% using current treatment regimens (neoadjuvant therapy followed by surgery followed by adjuvant therapy).[5] This is considerable when compared with a long-term survival rate of 20% in patients treated with surgery alone[2]
2. The benefits of presurgical chemotherapy include the ability to assess the in vivo activity of the chemotherapeutics and facilitate easier surgery[1]
3. The degree of tumor necrosis after neoadjuvant therapy is a powerful independent predictor of both event-free and overall survival. Patients whose tumors exhibit a good response (usually defined as ≥90% necrosis) consistently have superior local tumor control as well as disease-free and overall survival compared with patients who have a poor response[3]
4. It is now widely accepted that the four most important drugs in the treatment of osteosarcoma include high-dose methotrexate, doxorubicin, cisplatin, and ifosfamide. However, the optimal use of these in 2-, 3-, or 4-drug combinations remains controversial[4]

Surgery

1. Limb-sparing surgery is presently performed on 80% of patients. Contraindication to limb-sparing surgery includes:
   - Pathologic fracture
   - Major neurovascular involvement
   - Inappropriate biopsy sites before definitive surgery
   - Extensive muscle involvement
2. Low-grade osteosarcomas have little propensity for metastatic spread, and surgical resection alone is usually curative

Note: Because inappropriate biopsies can compromise future surgery, it is recommended that a biopsy should be undertaken only by an experienced surgeon in a center familiar with bone sarcoma

Adverse prognostic factors

1. Large tumors
2. Axial tumor position, as opposed to appendicular lesions
3. Increased levels of lactate dehydrogenase or alkaline phosphatase

References

1. Eilber FR, Rosen G. Semin Oncol 1989;16:312–322
2. Link MP et al. NEJM 1986;314:1600–1606
3. Meyers PA et al. JCO 1992;10:5–15
4. Meyers PA et al. JCO 2005;23:2004–2011
5. Provisor AJ et al. JCO 1997;15:76–84

Histologic Grading Systems for Assessing Response to Induction Chemotherapy in Osteosarcoma

Salzer-Kuntschik	
I:	No viable cells
II:	Single viable tumor cells or cluster <0.5 cm
III:	Viable tumor <10%
IV:	Viable tumor 10–50%
V:	Viable tumor >50%
VI:	No effect on chemotherapy

Picci	
Total response:	No viable tumor
Good response:	90–99% necrosis
Fair response:	60–89% necrosis
Poor response:	<60% necrosis

Huvos	
IV:	No histologic evidence of viable tumor
III:	Only scattered foci of viable tumor cells
II:	Areas of necrosis with areas of viable tumor
I:	Little or no chemotherapy effect

Picci P et al. Cancer 1985;56:15151521
Salzer-Kuntschik M et al. Pathologe 1983;4:135141
Wunder JS et al. J Bone Joint Surg Am 1998;80:10201033

Five-Year Survival

Nonmetastatic (80% of patients at diagnosis)	
Good histologic response (>90% necrosis)	75%
Poor histologic response (<90% necrosis)	55%
Metastatic (20% of patients at diagnosis)	20%

REGIMEN

HIGH-DOSE METHOTREXATE, CISPLATIN, AND DOXORUBICIN

Meyers PA et al. JCO 2005;23:2004–2011

Regimen consists of 10 weeks of induction chemotherapy followed by surgery (limb-sparing surgery or amputation), which is followed by adjuvant maintenance chemotherapy beginning in week 12 and continuing until week 31

Note: Maintenance should begin at week 12, provided that wound healing is adequate

Hydration before and after cisplatin: ≥1000 mL 0.45% NaCl injection (0.45% NS) by intravenous infusion over a minimum of 2–4 hours. Monitor and replace magnesium/electrolytes as needed

Cisplatin 120 mg/m² intravenously in 150–1000 mL 0.9% NaCl injection (0.9% NS) over 4 hours every 5 weeks for 4 cycles during weeks 0 and 5 in the induction phase and weeks 12 and 17 in the maintenance phase (total dosage/cycle = 120 mg/m²)

Doxorubicin 25 mg/m² per day by continuous intravenous infusion in 50–1000 mL 0.9% NS or 5% dextrose injection (D5W) over 24 hours for 3 consecutive days on days 1–3 every 5 weeks for 6 cycles during weeks 0 and 5 in the induction phase and weeks 12, 17, 22, and 27 in the maintenance phase (total dosage/cycle = 75 mg/m²)

Hydration with methotrexate: 1500–3000 mL/m² per day. Use a solution containing a total amount of sodium not >0.9% NaCl injection (ie, 154 mEq/1000 mL) by intravenous infusion during methotrexate administration and for at least 24 hours afterward

- Fluid administration may commence 2–12 hours before starting methotrexate, depending on patient's fluid status
- Urine output should be at least 100 mL/hour before starting methotrexate infusion
- Maintain hydration at a rate that maintains urine output of at least 100 mL/hour until the serum methotrexate concentration is <0.1 micromol/L

Sodium bicarbonate 50–150 mEq/1000 mL is added to the parenteral solution to maintain urine pH ≥7.0

Base Solution Sodium Content	Sodium Bicarbonate Additive	Total Sodium Content
0.45% NaCl injection (0.45% NS)		
77 mEq/L	50–75 mEq	127–152 mEq/L
0.2% NaCl injection (0.2% NS)		
34 mEq/L	100–125 mEq	134–159 mEq/L
5% Dextrose injection (D5W)		
0 mEq/L	125–150 mEq	125–150 mEq/L
D5W/0.45% NS		
77 mEq/L	50–75 mEq	127–152 mEq/L
D5W/0.2% NS		
34 mEq/L	100–125 mEq	134–159 mEq/L

Methotrexate 12,000 mg/m² (maximum dose = 20,000 mg) intravenously in 500–2000 mL 0.9% NS or D5W (or saline + dextrose combinations) over 4 hours for 12 cycles during weeks 3, 4, 8, and 9 in the induction phase and weeks 15, 16, 20, 21, 25, 26, 30, and 31 in the maintenance phase (total dosage/cycle = 12,000 mg/m²; maximum dose/cycle = 20,000 mg)

Note: For logistical practicality and efficiency, parenteral admixtures containing methotrexate may include a portion or all of the fluid and sodium bicarbonate needed to meet hydration and urinary alkalinization requirements during methotrexate administration

(*continued*)

Treatment Modifications

Adverse Event	Dose Modification
Delayed methotrexate clearance during weeks 3, 15, 20, and 25	Do not administer the scheduled course of methotrexate during the ensuing weeks (4, 16, 21, and 26) to ensure that doxorubicin is administered on schedule

Patient Population Studied

A prospective randomized intergroup phase III study of newly diagnosed patients with histologically confirmed high-grade, intramedullary osteosarcoma who were 30 years of age or younger. There were 677 patients enrolled without clinically detectable metastases; 340 received this regimen, including 168 who also received liposomal muramyl tripeptide

Efficacy (N = 172)

Event free-survival at 3 years	71%
Event free-survival at 5 years	64%
Second malignant neoplasm	3 occurrences
Favorable necrosis (Huvos III/ IV)	43%

Toxicity (N = 172)

	Frequency
Elevations in ALT after methotrexate	Common
Stomatitis	Common
Infections	Common
Objective hearing loss	11%
Renal dysfunction	Rare

(*continued*)

Leucovorin 10 mg (an absolute dose) by intravenous infusion in 25–250 mL 0.9% NS or D5W over 15 minutes every 6 hours, starting 24 hours after methotrexate administration *began* and continuing until the serum methotrexate concentration is <0.1 micromol/L (ie, $<1 \times 10^{-7}$ mol/L, or <100 nmol/L)

Note: Leucovorin may be administered orally after completing 1 day of parenteral administration if patients are compliant, are not vomiting, and have no other potentially mitigating complications

Leucovorin 10 mg (absolute dose) orally every 6 hours continuing until the serum methotrexate concentration is <0.1 micromol/L (ie, $<1 \times 10^{-7}$ mol/L, or <100 nmol/L)

Leucovorin rescue for delayed methotrexate excretion:

- Hydration, urinary alkalinization, and a more intensive leucovorin regimen are required if methotrexate excretion is delayed (eg, worsening renal function, effusions present)
- If 24 hours after the completion of methotrexate administration a patient's serum creatinine is increased by $\geq 50\%$ above the baseline value or if serum methotrexate concentration is ≥ 5 micromol/L ($\geq 5 \times 10^{-6}$ mol/L), increase the leucovorin dosage and schedule to 100 mg/m^2 per dose intravenously every 3 hours until serum methotrexate level is <0.1 micromol/L ($<1 \times 10^{-7}$ mol/L, <100 nmol/L); then resume leucovorin 10 mg/dose every 6 hours until serum methotrexate concentrations is <0.05 micromol/L ($<5 \times 10^{-8}$ mol/L, or <50 nmol /L) or until undetectable (if the lower limit of assay sensitivity is ≥ 0.05 micromol/L [≥ 50 nmol/L])

Emetogenic potential:

During cycles with cisplatin + doxorubicin:
- *Day 1:* Very high (Emetogenicity score = 6). Potential for delayed symptoms
- *Days 2–3:* Moderate (Emetogenicity score = 3)

During cycles with doxorubicin alone:
- *Days 1–3:* Moderate (Emetogenicity score = 3)

During methotrexate:
- *Day 14:* Moderately high (Emetogenicity score = 4). See Chapter 39 for antiemetic regimens

Therapy Monitoring

1. *During treatment cycles:* Daily renal function
2. *After high-dose systemic methotrexate administration:* Daily methotrexate levels
3. *Before each cycle:* CBC with differential, serum electrolytes, BUN, and creatinine

REGIMEN

ETOPOSIDE + HIGH-DOSE IFOSFAMIDE + MESNA

Goorin AM et al. JCO 2002;20:426–433

This regimen was initially developed for newly diagnosed osteosarcoma and included high-dose methotrexate, cisplatin, and doxorubicin as part of the continuation therapy. The protocol summarized here assumes that patients previously received high-dose methotrexate, cisplatin, and doxorubicin as part of their up-front therapy

	Induction Chemotherapy
Start: Hour 0 End: Hour 1	**Etoposide** 100 mg/m² per day intravenously in 250 mL/m² 5% dextrose and 0.20% NaCl injection (D5W/0.2% NS) over 1 hour for 5 consecutive days on days 1–5 every 21 days (total dosage/cycle = 500 mg/m²)
Start: Hour 1 End: Hour 5	An admixture containing **ifosfamide** 3500 mg/m² + **mesna** 700 mg/m² per day intravenously in 800 mL/m² D5W/0.2% NS over 4 hours, starting immediately after etoposide administration is completed, for 5 consecutive days on days 1–5 every 21 days (total ifosfamide dosage/cycle = 17,500 mg/m²)
Start: Hour 5 End: Hour 8	**Mesna** 700 mg/m² per day by continuous intravenous infusion in 600 mL/m² D5W/0.2% NS over 3 hours, starting after ifosfamide administration is completed, for 5 consecutive days on days 1–5 every 21 days
Start: Hour 5 End: Hour 14	**Hydration** with D5W/0.2% NS at 150 mL/m² per hour by continuous intravenous infusion for 9 hours for 5 consecutive days on days 1–5 every 21 days
Start: Hours 8, 11, and 14 End: Hours 8:15, 11:15, 14:15	**Mesna** 700 mg/m² per dose intravenously diluted with 0.9% NaCl injection (0.9% NS) or 5% dextrose injection (D5W) to a concentration of 1–20 mg/mL, over 15 minutes every 3 hours for 3 doses/day, starting 3 hours after ifosfamide administration is completed, for 5 consecutive days on days 1–5 every 21 days (total mesna dosage/cycle = 17,500 mg/m²)
Start: Hour 14 End: Hour 24	**Hydration** with D5W/0.2% NS at 100 mL/m² per hour by continuous intravenous infusion for 10 hours for 5 consecutive days on days 1–5 every 21 days

Note: After 2 cycles of treatment, radiologic evaluation is completed and patients should have surgery for any metastatic sites of disease. Surgical removal of all metastatic sites is recommended when feasible

	Continuation Chemotherapy
Start: Hour 0 End: Hour 1	**Etoposide** 100 mg/m² per day intravenously in 250 mL/m² D5W/0.2% NS over 1 hour for 5 consecutive days on day 15 every 21 days (total dosage/cycle = 500 mg/m²)
Start: Hour 1 End: Hour 5	An admixture containing **ifosfamide** 2400 mg/m² + **mesna** 480 mg/m² per day intravenously in 800 mL/m² D5W/0.2% NS over 4 hours, starting immediately after etoposide administration is completed, for 5 consecutive days on days 1–5 every 21 days (total ifosfamide dosage/cycle = 12,000 mg/m²)
Start: Hour 5 End: Hour 8	**Mesna** 480 mg/m² per day by continuous intravenous infusion in 600 mL/m² D5W/0.2% NS over 3 hours, starting after ifosfamide administration is completed, for 5 consecutive days on days 1–5 every 21 days; which is *followed by:*

(continued)

Treatment Modifications

None specified

Patient Population Studied

A prospective phase II/III trial in 41 evaluable patients of ages ≤30 years with measurable, newly diagnosed, biopsy-proven, high-grade, metastatic osteosarcoma with normal renal, hepatic, and bone marrow profile and ECOG performance status ≤2

Efficacy (N = 23–41)

Response Rate[a]	
Combined pathologic + radiologic response (n = 39)	59% ± 8%
Pathologic response alone[b] (n = 23)	65% ± 10%
Radiologic response alone (n = 27)	52% ± 9%

[a]Assessed after 2 cycles of etoposide + ifosfamide with mesna

[b]As measured by necrosis of the primary tumor

(continued)

Start: Hour 5 End: Hour 14	**Hydration** with D5W/0.2% NS at 150 mL/m^2 per hour by continuous intravenous infusion for 6 hours for 5 consecutive days on days 1–5 every 21 days
Start: Hours 8, 11, and 14 End: Hours 8:15, 11:15, 14:15	**Mesna** 480 mg/m^2 per dose intravenously diluted with 0.9% NS or D5W to a concentration of 1–20 mg/mL over 15 minutes every 3 hours for 3 doses/day, starting 3 hours after ifosfamide administration is completed, for 5 consecutive days on days 1–5 every 21 days (total mesna dosage/cycle = 12,000 mg/m^2)
Start: Hour 14 End: Hour 24	**Hydration** with D5W/0.2% NS at 100 mL/m^2 per hour by continuous intravenous infusion for 10 hours for 5 consecutive days on days 1–5 every 21 days

Supportive care after induction and continuation regimens:
Filgrastim 5 mcg/kg per day subcutaneously, starting on day 6 and continuing until the ANC recovers to ≥5000/mm^3 on two successive postnadir determinations

Emetogenic potential:
Days 1–5: Moderately high (Emetogenicity score = 4). Potential for delayed symptoms. See Chapter 39 for antiemetic regimens

Toxicity (N = 41)

	% G3	% G4
Hematopoietic		
WBC count	2	83
ANC	2	29
Platelets	17	27
Hemoglobin	5	5
Nonhematopoietic		
Sepsis	10	—
Bacterial infection	7	—
Viral infection	2	—
Fanconi's syndrome	7	—
Stomatitis	7	—
Sodium	2	—
Creatinine	2	—
Hematuria	2	—
Poor Karnofsky score	2	—
Vomiting	2	—
Potassium	2	

Toxicities listed are those pertaining only to the 2 cycles of induction chemotherapy using ifosfamide and etoposide

Therapy Monitoring

1. *Before each cycle:* CBC with differential, serum electrolytes, BUN, and creatinine
2. *During treatment cycles:* Daily serum electrolytes, BUN, and creatinine; CBC with differential at least twice weekly

Notes

1. Although few patients were treated, the response to ifosfamide and etoposide seemed to be dose-dependent
2. This combination may be more active against bony metastases than other regimens

Primary Malignant Bone Tumors: Ewing's Sarcoma

Epidemiology

Incidence: Estimated 0.1/100,000; 5% of all childhood bone tumors in 2005
Median age at diagnosis: 14 years; 90% of patients, ages <20 years
Mortality rate: 0.05/100,000
Male:female ratio: Slightly more prevalent in males

American Cancer Society: Cancer Facts and Figures 2005 http://cancer.org
Gurney JG et al. Malignant bone tumors. In: Reis LAG, Smith MA, Gurney JG et al, eds. Cancer incidence and survival among children and adolescents: United States SEER program, 1975–1995. Bethesda, MD: National Cancer Institute SEER Program. NIH Pub. No. 99-4649, 1999:99–110

Stage at Diagnosis

Nonmetastatic	80%
Metastatic	20%

Five-Year Survival

Localized	60–70%
Metastatic	20%

Treatment Notes

Treatment of Ewing's sarcoma is similar to that of osteosarcoma because it involves the use of neoadjuvant chemotherapy followed by local therapy (surgery or radiation), which is then followed by adjuvant chemotherapy

Chemotherapy
1. The most commonly used drugs are doxorubicin, vincristine, ifosfamide, etoposide, dactinomycin, and cyclophosphamide
2. The use of combination chemotherapy as part of a multidisciplinary approach has increased 5-year survival rates from <10% to approximately 60%

Local therapy
1. Local therapy in the treatment of Ewing's sarcoma varies from surgery alone, to radiation alone, to a combination of both modalities, depending on where disease is located
2. Surgery remains the preferred route of local control. A wide surgical margin should be attempted
3. In contrast to osteosarcoma and the soft tissue sarcomas, Ewing's tumors are radiosensitive. Therefore, in patients in whom surgery is not possible or for those patients with marginal and intralesional surgery, radiation is an effective therapeutic option

Adverse prognostic factors
1. Metastatic disease
2. Pelvic localization
3. Tumor diameter >8–10 cm
4. Age >15 years
5. Elevated LDH
6. Poor histologic response to preoperative chemotherapy
7. Radiation therapy as the only local treatment

Grier HE et al. NEJM 2005;348:694–701

Pathology

Ewing's sarcoma are rare tumors arising in the bone marrow from primitive neural elements and constitute approximately 10% of bone sarcomas. Subtypes include:

1. Classic Ewing's sarcoma
2. Primitive neuroectodermal tumor

Note: They are distinguished immunohistochemically from other pediatric tumors by expression of the MIC2 gene. The most commonly detected translocation is the t(11;22) (q24;q12)

REGIMEN

Newly Diagnosed—Ewing's Sarcoma, Primitive Neuroectodermal Tumor Of Bone, Primitive Sarcoma Of Bone

VINCRISTINE, CYCLOPHOSPHAMIDE, AND DOXORUBICIN OR DACTINOMYCIN ALTERNATING WITH IFOSFAMIDE AND ETOPOSIDE

Grier HE et al. NEJM 2003;348:694–701

Patients receive 2 complete courses of alternating induction chemotherapy (1 course comprises 1 cycle with vincristine, doxorubicin, and cyclophosphamide followed by 1 cycle with ifosfamide and etoposide). Local therapy (surgery or radiation) occurs at week 12 and, after recovery, adjuvant chemotherapy with the same chemotherapy regimens ensues in alternation for a further 7 cycles of vincristine, doxorubicin, and cyclophosphamide and 6 cycles of ifosfamide and etoposide (total: 17 cycles of chemotherapy)

Cycles of vincristine, doxorubicin (or dactinomycin) and cyclophosphamide + mesna:
Vincristine 2 mg/m^2 (maximum single dose "capped" at 2 mg) by intravenous push over 1–3 minutes on day 1 every 42 days (total dosage/cycle = 2 mg/m^2; maximum dose/cycle = 2 mg)
Doxorubicin 75 mg/m^2 intravenously per push over 3–5 minutes on day 1 every 42 days (total dosage/cycle = 75 mg/m^2; total cumulative dosage permitted = 375 mg/m^2)
When a total doxorubicin dosage of 375 mg/m^2 has been administered, no additional doxorubicin is given. Instead, doxorubicin is *replaced by:*
Dactinomycin 1.25 mg/m^2 intravenously per push over 3–5 minutes on day 1 every 42 days (total dosage/cycle = 1.25 mg/m^2). Dactinomycin is used only after doxorubicin is discontinued from the regimen
An admixture containing **cyclophosphamide** 1200 mg/m^2 + **mesna** 240 mg/m^2 intravenously in 100–250 mL 0.9% NaCl injection (0.9% NS) or 5% dextrose injection (D5W) over 15–30 minutes on day 1 every 42 days (total cyclophosphamide dosage/cycle = 1200 mg/m^2)
Then, either:
Mesna 240 mg/m^2 per dose intravenously diluted with 0.9% NS or D5W to a concentration of 1–20 mg/mL, over 15 minutes for 2 doses at 4 hours and 8 hours after cyclophosphamide administration is completed on day 1 every 42 days (total mesna dosage/cycle = 720 mg/m^2), *or*
Mesna 480 mg/m^2 per dose orally for 2 doses at 2 hours and 6 hours after cyclophosphamide administration is completed on day 1 every 42 days (total mesna dosage/cycle = 1200 mg/m^2)

Cycles of ifosfamide + mesna and etoposide:
An admixture containing **ifosfamide** 1800 mg/m^2 + **mesna** 360 mg/m^2 per day intravenously in a volume of 0.9% NS or D5W sufficient to produce ifosfamide concentrations between 0.6 and 20 mg/mL over 60 minutes for 5 consecutive days on days 22–26 every 42 days (total ifosfamide dosage/cycle = 9000 mg/m^2)
Then, either:
Mesna 360 mg/m^2 per dose intravenously diluted with 0.9% NS or D5W to a concentration of 1–20 mg/mL, over 15 minutes for 2 doses per day at 4 hours and 8 hours after ifosfamide administration is completed for 5 consecutive days on days 22–26 every 42 days (total mesna dosage/cycle = 5400 mg/m^2), *or*
Mesna 720 mg/m^2 per dose orally for 2 doses per day at 2 hours and 6 hours after ifosfamide administration is completed for 5 consecutive days on days 22–26 every 42 days (total mesna dosage/cycle = 9000 mg/m^2)
Etoposide 100 mg/m^2 per day by intravenous infusion, diluted in 0.9% NS to a concentration of 0.2–0.4 mg/mL over 60 minutes for 5 consecutive days on days 22–26 every 42 days (total dosage/cycle = 500 mg/m^2)

Supportive care:
Hematopoietic support with *either:*
Filgrastim 5 mcg/kg per day subcutaneously once daily, starting at least 24 hours after chemotherapy administration is completed and continuing until the ANC recovers to ≥5000/mm^3, *or*

(continued)

Treatment Modifications

None specified

Patient Population Studied

This was a prospective randomized intergroup phase III study in newly diagnosed patients with primary bone tumors who were 30 years of age or younger. Patients had adequate renal, liver, and cardiac function; 300 patients were enrolled and 198 received this regimen

Efficacy (N = 198)

5-year event-free survival	69%
5-year overall survival	72%
Pattern of Treatment Failure	
Local progression	4.5%
Systemic progression	22.2%
Local and systemic progression	2%
Progression at unknown site	0.5%
Death	3.5%
Infection	3%
Hemorrhage	0.5%
Second malignant neoplasms	2%

Therapy Monitoring

1. *Weekly:* CBC with differential
2. *Before each cycle:* CBC with differential, serum creatinine, liver function tests, and urinalysis
3. *Response evaluation:* At conclusion of first 4 cycles of chemotherapy

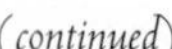

Sargramostim 250 mcg/kg per day subcutaneously once daily starting at least 24 hours after chemotherapy administration is completed and continuing until the ANC recovers to $\geq$5000/mm^3

After the first 4 cycles of chemotherapy (2 complete courses, 12 weeks), local control is planned to consist of radiation therapy, surgery, or both

Radiation alone

Treat the extent of the initial soft tissue and osseous involvement with a 3-cm margin to a dose 4500 cGy. Then treat with an additional 1080 cGy the postchemotherapy, preradiation therapy tumor volume

Surgery without residual disease

No radiation therapy is administered

Gross residual tumor after surgery

Treat as if treating with radiation alone

Microscopic residual disease after surgery

Treat the extent of the initial soft tissue and osseous involvement with a 1-cm margin to a dose 4500 cGy

Emetogenic potential:

During cycles with vincristine, doxorubicin or dactinomycin, and cyclophosphamide

Day 1: High (Emetogenicity score = 5). Potential for delayed symptoms

During cycles with ifosfamide and etoposide

Days 1–5: Moderately high (Emetogenicity score = 4). See Chapter 39 for antiemetic regimens

REGIMEN

CYCLOPHOSPHAMIDE + TOPOTECAN

Saylors RL III et al. JCO 2001;19:3463–3469

Pretreatment hydration: 500 mL/m^2 of appropriate fluids [0.9% NaCl injection (0.9% NS), 0.45% NaCl injection (0.45% NS), or 5% dextrose injection/0.45% NaCl injection (D5W/0.45% NS)] orally or intravenously for 2–4 hours before starting chemotherapy

Cyclophosphamide 250 mg/m^2 per day intravenously in 25–250 mL 0.9% NS or 5% dextrose injection (D5W) over 30 minutes for 5 consecutive days on days 1–5 every 21 days (total dosage/cycle = 1250 mg/m^2)

Topotecan HCl 0.75 mg/m^2 per day by intravenous infusion in 50–250 mL 0.9% NS or D5W over 30 minutes after cyclophosphamide for 5 consecutive days on days 1–5 every 21 days (total dosage/cycle = 3.75 mg/m^2)

Post-treatment hydration: Hydration continues orally or intravenously at a rate of 3000 mL/m^2 per 24 hours until 24 hours after the last dose of chemotherapy

Filgrastim 5 mcg/kg per day subcutaneously once daily, starting 24 hours after chemotherapy is completed (day 6) and continuing until the ANC recovers to ≥1500/mm^3 after the time of the expected nadir

Emetogenic potential:

Days 1–5: Moderately high (Emetogenicity score = 4). See Chapter 39 for antiemetic regimens

Toxicity (N = 307 Cycles)

	% of Cycles with G3/4
Neutropenia	53
Thrombocytopenia	44
Anemia	27
Infection[a]	11
Nausea/vomiting	0.65
Hematuria[b]	0.65
Perirectal mucositis	0.33
Transaminase elevation	0.33

[a]Includes admissions for fever/neutropenia: 5 bacteremia or fungemia, 1 herpes zoster, 1 infectious cystitis

[b]In 2 patients with history of hematuria on ifosfamide

NCI CTC

Therapy Monitoring

1. *Daily during therapy:* Urinalysis
2. *Twice weekly:* CBC with differential until recovery from hematopoietic toxicity
3. *Weekly:* Physical examination
4. *Before each cycle:* Serum creatinine, LFTs with bilirubin, serum electrolytes, including calcium, magnesium, and phosphorus
5. *Response evaluation:* After the first and second cycles, then after every 2 cycles

Treatment Modifications

None specified

Patient Population Studied

A study of 91 pediatric patients with recurrent or refractory solid tumors, including Ewing's sarcoma (n = 17), rhabdomyosarcoma (n = 15), and neuroblastoma (n = 13)

Efficacy

Ewing's Sarcoma (n = 17)	
Complete response	12%
Partial response	24%
Rhabdomyosarcoma (n = 15)	
Complete response	0
Partial response	67%

Notes

Responses were observed in patients who had received >1 year of intensive alkylating agent therapy and/or ablative therapy with autologous stem cell rescue

Sarcomas: Soft Tissue Sarcomas

Epidemiology

Incidence: 9530 estimated cases in the United States for 2006
Mortality: 3500 estimated deaths for 2006
Male:female ratio: 1.2:1

Most Common Subtypes

Malignant fibrous histiocytoma	28%
Liposarcoma	15%
Leiomyosarcoma	12%
Synovial sarcoma	10%
Malignant peripheral nerve sheath tumors	6%
Rhabdomyosarcoma	5%
All others	≤3%

Disease Distribution

Extremity	43%
Lower	30%
Upper	13%
Intra-abdominal	34%
Visceral	19%
Retroperitoneal	15%
Trunk	10%
Other	13%

Jemal A et al. CA Cancer J Clin 2006;56:106–30
Brennan MF et al. Sarcomas of the soft tissues and bone. In: DeVita, VT, Jr, Hellman S, Rosenberg SA, ed. Cancer: Principles & Practice of Oncology, 7th ed. Philadelphia: Lippincott Williams & Wilkins, 2005:1581–1637

Work-Up

1. History and physical examination
2. *Laboratory tests:* CBC with differential; electrolytes; liver function tests; mineral panel, including alkaline phosphatase and lactate dehydrogenase
3. Radiologic imaging modality is variable and dictated by the site of disease. This involves a combination of plain x-rays, CT, MRI, and PET imaging. Although CT remains the imaging modality of choice in the staging of retroperitoneal soft tissue sarcoma, MRI is used more frequently to stage soft tissue sarcoma of the extremity
4. Bone marrow aspirate for light microscopy examination in Ewing's sarcoma
5. No radiologic studies are pathognomonic, so biopsy remains essential to diagnosis. Carefully plan biopsy to establish grade and histologic subtype and if needed molecular & cytogenetic studies
6. Echocardiogram or MUGA scan to determine cardiac ejection fraction as clinically indicated

NCCN Clinical Practice Guidelines in Oncology, V. 2. 2006, Soft Tissue Sarcoma © National Comprehensive Cancer Network, Inc. 2006 (www.nccn.org)

Staging

UICC and TNM Staging (AJCC) TNM

Primary Tumor

TX	Primary tumor cannot be assessed
T0	No evidence of primary tumor
T1	Tumor ≤5 cm in greatest dimension
T1a	Tumor above superficial fascia
T1b	Deep tumor*
T2	Tumor >5 cm in greatest dimension
T2a	Tumor above superficial fascia
T2b	Deep tumor

Nodal Status

NX	Regional lymph nodes cannot be assessed
N0	No regional lymph node metastasis
N1	Regional lymph nodes metastasis

Metastases

MX	Distant metastasis cannot be assessed
M0	No distant metastases
M1	Distant metastases
M1a	Lung
M1b	Other distant sites, including lymph nodes
GX	Grade cannot be assessed
G1	Well differentiated–low grade
G2	Moderately differentiated–low grade
G3	Poorly differentiated–high grade
G4	Undifferentiated–high grade

Stage Grouping

IA	G1-2	Low grade	T1a-b	N0	M0
IB	G1-2	Low grade	T2a-b	N0	M0
IIA	G3-4	High grade	T1a-b	N0	M0
IIB	G3-4	High grade	T2a	N0	M0
III	G3-4	High grade	T2b	N0	M0
IV	Any G	Any grade	Any T	N1	M0
	Any G	Any grade	Any T	N0	M1

*Deep tumors are tumors deep to the superficial fascia or those that have invaded through the fascia

International Union Against Cancer (UICC) and American Joint Committee on Cancer (AJCC) TNM Staging, 6th ed. System for Bone Sarcomas Reproduced, with permission, of the American Joint Committee on Cancer (AJCC), Chicago, Illinois. The original source for this material is the AJCC Cancer Staging Manual, 6th edition (2002) published by Springer-Verlag, New York, www.springeronline.com.

Caveats

Prognostic factors

1. In multivariate analyses, tumors of high histologic grade, large tumor size (>5 cm), positive surgical margins, or intraoperative violation of the tumor capsule have been associated with a high local recurrence rate
2. Histologic grade and tumor size are the most significant risk factors for distant metastasis and tumor-related mortality

Grading systems

There is no universally accepted grading system. Several systems have been generated to grade soft tissue sarcomas. The most frequently used are the National Cancer Institute system developed by Costa et al and the FNCLCC system (Federation Nationale des Centres de Lutte Contre le Cancer) developed by the French Federation of Cancer Centres Sarcoma Group

- The NCI system is based on the evaluation of tumor histologic type or subtype, location, and the amount of tumor necrosis, cellularity, nuclear pleomorphism, and the mitosis count
- The FNCLCC system is based on a score generated by the evaluation of three parameters: tumor differentiation, mitotic rate, and the amount of tumor necrosis

French Histologic Grading System

Grade 1 = Score 2–3
Grade 2 = Score 4–5
Grade 3 = Score 6–8

Score	Tumor Differentiation	Mitotic Index*	Necrosis*
0	—	—	None
1	Resembles normal adult tissue	0–9	≤50%
2	Histologic typing certain	10–19	≥50%
3	Biphasic sarcomas Monophasic sarcomas Ewing's—extraskeletal Primitive neuroectodermal tumor Undifferentiated sarcoma	≥20	—

*Number of mitoses per 10 HPF

Surgery

1. Surgery is the mainstay of treatment
2. The type of surgical resection selected is determined by the tumor location, tumor size, depth of invasion, involvement of nearby structures, necessity for skin graft, and the patient' performance status

Costa J et al. Cancer 1984;53:530–541
Trojani M et al. Int J Cancer 1984;33:37–42

Five-Year Survival

Nonmetastatic (80% of patients at diagnosis)	
Stage II	70%
Stage III	25%
Metastatic (20% of patients at diagnosis)	20%

Soft Tissue Sarcomas: Rhabdomyosarcoma

Epidemiology

Incidence: 350 estimated new cases in the United States per year; rhabdomyosarcoma represents 50% of all diagnosed soft tissue sarcomas

Staging

For protocol purposes, patients are classified according to their risk of recurrence as low risk, intermediate risk, or high risk. The assignment proceeds as follows:

1. Determine the group (I, II, III or IV)
2. Determine the stage (1, 2, 3, or 4)
3. Use the group and stage assignment together with histology to assign a risk category

Group classification system: A surgicopathologic grouping system with groups defined by the extent of disease and by the extent of initial surgical resection after pathologic review of the tumor specimens
Staging classification system: Classifies tumors based on primary site and size
Risk classification system: Used to assess the risk of recurrence as low, intermediate, and high risk; combines the clinical group and stage information

Group Classification System

Group	Extent of Disease and Initial Surgical Resection After Pathologic Review of Specimen	%*
I	Localized disease that is completely resected with no regional nodal involvement	14
IIA	Localized, grossly resected tumor with microscopic residual disease but no regional node involvement	20
IIB	Locoregional disease with tumor-involved lymph nodes with complete resection and no residual disease	
IIC	Locoregional disease with tumor-involved lymph nodes, grossly resected, but with evidence of microscopic residual tumor at the primary site and/or histologic involvement of the regional node (from the primary site)	
III	Localized, gross residual disease including incomplete resection, or biopsy primary site	48
IV	Distant metastatic disease present at the time of diagnosis	18

*Percentage of all rhabdomyosarcomas

Staging Classification System

Stage	Description
1	Localized disease involving the orbit or head and neck (excluding parameningeal sites) or genitourinary region (excluding bladder/prostate sites) or biliary tract **(favorable sites)**
2	Localized disease of any other primary site not included in stage 1 **(unfavorable sites)**. Primary tumor must be ≤5 cm in diameter with no clinical regional lymph node involvement by tumor
3	Localized disease of any other primary site not included in stage 1 **(unfavorable sites)**. These patients differ from stage 2 patients by having primary tumors >5 cm in diameter and/or regional node involvement
4	Metastatic disease at diagnosis

Lawrence W Jr et al. JCO 1987;5:46–54

Pathology

Embryonal Embryonal Botryoid* Spindle*	60–70%	Higher incidence in the 0- to 4-year age group
Alveolar	20%	Similar incidence throughout childhood
Pleomorphic	10–20%	

*These subtypes are associated with more favorable outcomes

Disease Sites at Diagnosis

Site	%
Parameningeal[a]	23
Nonparameningeal	8
Bladder and prostate	11
Non–bladder and prostate[b]	16
Limbs	16
Orbit	9
Other	17

[a]Sites in anatomic proximity to the base of the skull and adjacent meninges; eg, nasopharynx and middle ear
[b]Genitourinary other than bladder and prostate that include para-testicular, vagina, and uterus

Stevens MCG. Lancet Oncol 2005;6:77–84

Five-Year Survival

Low risk	>90%
Intermediate risk	55–70%
High risk	20–25%

Staging *(continued)*

Risk Classification System

Risk	Histology	Stage	Group
Low	All	1	I, II, III
	Embryonal	2, 3	I, II
Intermediate	Embryonal	2, 3	III
	Embryonal[a]	4	IV
	Alveolar	1, 2, 3	I, II, III
	Undifferentiated	1, 2, 3	I, II, III
High	All[b]	4	IV
	Undifferentiated	4	IV

[a]<10 years

[b]Exception: Embryonal in children <10 years

Raney RB et al. J Pediatr Hematol Oncol 2001;23:215–220

Caveats

1. Disease prognosis is related to the age of the adolescent, site of origin, resectability, presence of metastases, number of metastatic sites, and the unique biological characteristics of the rhabdomyosarcoma tumor cells[1,2]
2. Distinctive molecular characteristics can be used to confirm alveolar and embryonal subtypes:

   Alveolar rhabdomyosarcoma: Unique translocation between the *FKHR* gene on chromosome 13 and either the *PAX3* gene on chromosome 2 (55% cases) or the *PAX7* gene on chromosome 1 (20% cases)

   Embryonal tumors: Often show loss of specific genomic material from the short arm of chromosome 11. The consistent loss of genomic material from the chromosome 11p15 region in embryonal tumors suggests the presence of a tumor suppressor gene. No such gene has yet been identified[3]
3. The variability with which rhabdomyosarcoma presents at different anatomic sites has a strong effect on treatment strategies

References

1. Breneman JC et al. JCO 2003;21:78–84
2. Breneman J et al. [abstract 210] Int J Radiat Oncol Biol Phys 2001;51(3 suppl 1):118
3. Barr FG. J Pediatr Hematol Oncol 1997;19:483–491

REGIMEN

VINCRISTINE + DACTINOMYCIN (ACTINOMYCIN D) + CYCLOPHOSPHAMIDE (VAC)

Crist WM et al. JCO 2001;19:3091–3102

Treatment Schedule

Drugs	Induction (Weeks 0–16)																
	0	1	2	3	4	5	6	7	8	9	10	11	12	13	14	15	16
Vincristine (V)	V	V	V	V	V	V	V	V	V	V	V	V	V				V
Dactinomycin (A)	A			A			A										A
Cyclophosphamide (C)	C			C			C			C			C				C
										Radiation therapy							

Drugs				Continuation (Weeks 20–28)								
	17	18	19	20	21	22	23	24	25	26	27	28
Vincristine (V)				V	V	V	V	V	V			
Dactinomycin (A)				A			A					
Cyclophosphamide (C)				C			C					

Vincristine 1.5 mg/m^2 per dose (maximum single dose = 2 mg) intravenously per push over 1–2 minutes (total dosage during the weeks in which vincristine is administered = 1.5 mg/m^2; maximum dose/treatment = 2 mg). The administration schedule for vincristine appears in the preceding table
Dactinomycin 0.015 mg/kg per day (maximum single dose = 0.5 mg) intravenously per push over 1–2 minutes for 5 consecutive days on days 1–5 (total dosage during the weeks in which dactinomycin is administered = 0.075 mg/kg; maximum dose/cycle = 2.5 mg). The week on which each 5-day course of dactinomycin administered is indicated in the preceding table
An admixture containing **cyclophosphamide** 2200 mg/m^2 + **mesna** 120 mg/m^2 administered intravenously in 100–1000 mL 0.9% NaCl injection (0.9% NS) or 5% dextrose injection (D5W) over 10–30 minutes (total dosage during the weeks in which cyclophosphamide is administered = 2200 mg/m^2). The administration schedule for cyclophosphamide appears in the preceding table, *then*

Mesna 1200 mg/m^2 by continuous intravenous infusion in 250–1000 mL of 0.9% NS or D5W over 24 hours (rate of 50 mg/m^2 per hour), starting immediately after each dose of cyclophosphamide (total dosage during the weeks in which cyclophosphamide is administered = 1320 mg/m^2)

To ameliorate dose-limiting hematopoietic toxicity:
Filgrastim 5 mcg/kg per day subcutaneously, starting at least 24 hours after completing chemotherapy (day 6 during VAC cycles and day 2 during vincristine and cyclophosphamide (VC) cycles; administration may continue throughout the weeks when vincristine is administered alone) and continue until the ANC recovers to ≥1500/mm^3 after the time of the expected nadir
Note: Filgrastim use concurrently with weekly vincristine is possible because vincristine's myelotoxicity is limited

Emetogenic potential:
During treatment with VAC:
Day 1: Very high (Emetogenicity score = 6). Potential for delayed symptoms
Days 2–5: Moderate (Emetogenicity score = 3)
During treatment with VC:
Day 1: High (Emetogenicity score = 5). Potential for delayed symptoms
During treatment with vincristine alone: Nonemetogenic (Emetogenicity score = 1). See Chapter 39 for antiemetic regimens

Treatment Modifications

Percentage of Courses in Which ≥75% of Protocol-Specified Drugs Were Delivered	
Vincristine	81%
Dactinomycin	81%
Cyclophosphamide	86%

Patients with severe toxicity attributed to VAC (eg, veno-occlusive disease of the liver) were switched to VIE (vincristine, ifosfamide and etoposide) therapy

Patient Population Studied

A study of 884 patients with previously untreated nonmetastatic rhabdomyosarcoma who had undergone surgery. Randomization to 1 of 4 study arms: VA (vincristine + dactinomycin, n = 134), VAC (n = 291), VAI (vincristine + dactinomycin + ifosfamide, n = 223), and VIE (vincristine, ifosfamide, and etoposide, n = 236). Patients with preexisting renal abnormalities predisposing to nephrotoxicity were assigned to VAC

Efficacy (N = 134)

	Failure-Free Survival (3-year)	Overall Survival (3-year)
Patients with preexisting renal abnormalities (n = 56)	75%*	80%*
All VAC patients (n = 134)	75%	84%

*Estimated

Toxicity (N = 884[a])

	% of Patients
Myelosuppression	>90
Severe infections	55
Severe renal toxicity	2
Second cancer[b]	1.1
Death[c]	0.9

[a]Combined data for patients receiving either VA (vincristine + dactinomycin, n = 134) ,VAC (n = 291), VAI (vincristine + dactinomycin + ifosfamide, n = 223), or VIE (vincristine, ifosfamide, and etoposide, n = 236). There were no statistically significant differences in toxicities among the different regimens

[b]Among 10 patients who developed a secondary malignancy, 6 were treated with VAC; 3-year estimated cumulative incidence of secondary malignancy was 2%

[c]Fatality rate (5%) was highest in patients with preexisting renal abnormalities who were treated with VAC

NCI CTC

Therapy Monitoring

1. *Daily during therapy:* Urinalysis
2. *Twice per week:* CBC with differential until recovery from hematopoietic toxicity
3. *Weekly:* Physical examination
4. *Before each cycle:* Serum creatinine, LFTs with bilirubin, serum electrolytes, including calcium, magnesium, and phosphorus
5. *Response evaluation:* After the third, sixth, and eighth cycles

REGIMEN

IRINOTECAN

Cosetti M et al. J Pediatr Hematol Oncol 2002;24:101–105

Irinotecan 20 mg/m^2 per dose intravenously diluted in a volume of 5% dextrose injection (D5W) or 0.9% NaCl injection (0.9% NS) sufficient to produce a concentration of 0.12–2.8 mg/mL over 60 minutes for 10 doses on days 1–5 and days 8–12 every 21–28 days (total dosage/cycle = 200 mg/m^2)

Regimen for delayed diarrhea (adult patients):
Loperamide 4 mg orally after first loose stool, *then:*
Loperamide 2 mg orally with each loose stool to a maximum daily dose of 24 mg until 12 hours after the last loose stool or for a maximum of 48 hours, whichever condition occurs first
If diarrhea persists >24 hours despite loperamide: Add oral prophylactic broad-spectrum antibiotic.
Ciprofloxacin 500 mg orally twice daily, if absolute neutrophil count <500/mm^3 (even with no fever or diarrhea) or if patient is febrile in association with diarrhea. Antibiotics should also be administered if patient is hospitalized with prolonged diarrhea and should be continued until resolution of diarrhea
If diarrhea persists >48 hours despite loperamide: Stop loperamide and hospitalize patient for IV hydration. Consider an alternative antidiarrheal treatment: **Octreotide** 100–150 mcg subcutaneously 3 times daily. Maximum total daily dose = 1500 mcg
Regimen for acute cholinergic syndrome:
Atropine sulfate 0.25–1 mg subcutaneously. If symptoms are severe, add prophylaxis during subsequent cycles

Emetogenic potential: Moderate (Emetogenicity score = 3). See Chapter 39 for antiemetic regimens

Patient Population Studied

A study of 22 heavily pretreated children with multiply relapsed tumors

Efficacy (N = 4)

Complete response	50%
Partial response	25%

Toxicity (N = 22*)

	% G1	% G2	% G3	% G4
Hematologic				
Anemia	9.1	13.6	0	0
Leukopenia	18.2	22.7	18.2	0
Neutropenia	4.5	13.6	9.1	18.2
Thrombocytopenia	18.2	9.1	13.6	13.6
Nonhematologic				
SGOT	13.6	0	0	0
SGPT	4.5	4.5	0	0
Diarrhea	40.9	13.6	13.6	4.5
Pneumonitis/pulmonary infiltrates				4.5

*Four patients with rhabdomyosarcoma; the rest had other diagnoses, but clinically very similar
SGOT, serum glutamic oxaloacetic transaminase (AST); SGPT, serum glutamic pyruvic transaminase (ALT)

NCI CTC

Treatment Modifications

None specified; the following are suggested

Adverse Event	Dose Modification
WBC <4000/mm^3, platelet count <100,000/mm^3, or diarrhea	Delay start of cycle by 1 week until WBC >4000/mm^3, platelet count >100,000/mm^3, and no diarrhea
Day 8 or 15 WBC <3000/mm^3 or platelet count <100,000/mm^3	Hold irinotecan
>G1 Diarrhea	Hold irinotecan
If WBC <1000/mm^3, platelet count <50,000/mm^3, or diarrhea >G2 at any time in cycle	Reduce subsequent irinotecan dosage by 50%

Therapy Monitoring

1. *Weekly:* CBC with differential
2. *Before each cycle:* CBC with differential, LFTs with bilirubin
3. *Response evaluation:* After every 2 cycles

Soft Tissue Sarcomas: Adult Soft Tissue Sarcomas, other than Rhabdomyosarcomas or GIST

Classification of Malignant Adult Soft Tissue Sarcomas

1. Fibrous tumors
   a. Fibrosarcoma:
      (1) Adult fibrosarcoma
      (2) Inflammatory fibrosarcoma
2. Fibrohistiocytic tumors
   a. Malignant fibrous histiocytoma
      (1) Storiform-pleomorphic
      (2) Myxoid (myxofibrosarcoma)
      (3) Giant cell (malignant giant cell tumor of the soft parts)
      (4) Inflammatory
3. Lipomatous
   a. Liposarcoma
      (1) Well-differentiated liposarcoma
         (a) Lipoma-like liposarcomas
         (b) Sclerosing liposarcoma
         (c) Inflammatory liposarcoma
      (2) Dedifferentiated liposarcoma
      (3) Myxoid or round cell liposarcoma
      (4) Pleomorphic liposarcoma
4. Smooth muscle tumors
   a. Leiomyosarcoma
   b. Epithelioid leiomyosarcoma
5. Skeletal muscle tumors
   a. Rhabdomyosarcoma
      (1) Embryonal rhabdomyosarcoma
      (2) Botryoid rhabdomyosarcoma
      (3) Spindle cell rhabdomyosarcoma
      (4) Alveolar rhabdomyosarcoma
      (5) Pleomorphic rhabdomyosarcoma
   b. Rhabdomyosarcoma with ganglionic differentiation (ectomesenchymoma)
6. Tumors of the blood and lymph nodes
   a. Epithelioid hemangioendothelioma
   b. Angiosarcoma and lymphangiosarcoma
   c. Kaposi's sarcoma
7. Perivascular tumors
   a. Malignant glomus tumor (glomangiosarcoma)
   b. Malignant hemangiopericytoma
8. Synovial tumors
   a. Malignant giant cell tumor of tendon sheath
9. Neural tumors
   a. Malignant peripheral nerve sheath tumor (MPNST)
      (1) Malignant Triton tumor (MPSNT with rhabdomyosarcoma)
      (2) Glandular MPNST
      (3) Epithelioid MPNST
   b. Malignant granular cell tumor
   c. Primitive neuroectodermal tumor
      (1) Neuroblastoma
      (2) Ganglioneuroblastoma
      (3) Neuroepithelioma (peripheral neuroectodermal tumor)
10. Paraganglionic tumors
    a. Malignant paraganglioma
11. Extraskeletal cartilaginous and osseous tumors
    a. Extraskeletal chondrosarcoma
       (1) Myxoid chondrosarcoma
       (2) Mesenchymal chondrosarcoma
    b. Extraskeletal osteosarcoma
12. Pluripotential mesenchymal tumors
    a. Malignant mesenchyma
13. Miscellaneous tumors
    a. Alveolar soft part sarcoma
    b. Epithelioid sarcoma
    c. Malignant extrarenal rhabdoid tumor
    d. Desmoplastic small cell tumor
    e. Ewing's sarcoma—extraskeletal
    f. Clear cell sarcoma
    g. Gastrointestinal stromal tumors
    h. Synovial sarcoma

Brennan MF et al. Sarcomas of the soft tissues and bone. In: DeVita VT Jr, Hellman S, Rosenberg SA, eds. Cancer: Principles & Practice of Oncology, 7th ed. Philadelphia: Lippincott Williams & Wilkins, 2005:1581–1637

Caveats

1. Surgery with wide margins is the first line of treatment for adult soft tissue sarcomas
2. In adults with extremity soft tissue sarcomas, radical or limb-sparing surgery with wide margins plus radiation therapy dramatically improves the local control.[1–4] Radiation alone is used only in patients with lesions not amenable to surgery because of size or proximity to vital structures. However, despite the improvement in local control rates, many patients still die from metastatic disease, highlighting the need for effective systemic therapies
3. For most adults with unresectable or metastatic soft tissue sarcoma, chemotherapy is palliative
4. Doxorubicin and ifosfamide are routinely used in adults with unresectable or metastatic soft tissue sarcoma
5. Single-agent doxorubicin is considered by many to be the drug of choice
6. Single-agent ifosfamide also has activity, although it may be less when used as second-line therapy in patients previously treated with doxorubicin. The value of dose intensity has not been proved[5,6]
7. The value of combination therapy has not been proved. Although some studies have suggested that combination chemotherapy has a higher response rate than does doxorubicin (although no benefit in terms of survival), the largest study performed by the EORTC Soft Tissue and Bone Sarcoma Group showed significantly more myelosuppression with the combination of ifosfamide and doxorubicin. However, response rates that were not significantly different[7]
8. Some have suggested using (high-dose) ifosfamide with doxorubicin for younger patients with aggressive tumors; however, whether this approach provides a survival advantage is uncertain[8,9]

References

1. Brennan MF et al. Sarcomas of the soft tissues and bone. In: DeVita VT Jr, Hellman S, Rosenberg SA, eds. Cancer: Principles & Practice of Oncology, 7th ed. Philadelphia: Lippincott Williams & Wilkins, 2005:1581–1637
2. Flugstad DL et al. Arch Surg 1999;134:856–861
3. O'Sullivan B et al. Semin Radiat Oncol 1999;9:328–348
4. Dirix LY, van Oosterom AT. Curr Opin Oncol 1999;11:285–295
5. van Oosterom AT et al. Eur J Cancer 2002;38:2397–2406
6. Yalcin B et al. Exp Oncol 2004;26:320–325
7. Santoro A edt al JCO 1995;13:1537–1545
8. Worden FP et al. JCO 2005;23:105–112
9. Maurel J et al et al, J Surg Oncol 2004;88:44–49

REGIMEN

DOXORUBICIN

O'Bryan RM et al. Cancer 1973;32:1–8
O'Bryan RM et al. Cancer 1977;39:1940–1948

Doxorubicin 60 mg/m^2 intravenously per push over 3–5 minutes on day 1 every 21 days (total dosage per cycle = 60 mg/m^2)

Emetogenic potential: Moderately high (Emetogenicity score = 4). See Chapter 39 for antiemetic regimens

Patient Population Studied

Patients with metastatic or unresectable locoregional recurrent soft tissue sarcoma

Efficacy (N = 64; N = 98)

	Partial Response*
All histologies (N = 64)	21 (32.8%)
Fibrosarcomas (n = 14)	2 (14.3%)
Leiomyosarcoma (n = 8)	3 (37.5%)
Hemangiosarcoma (n = 3)	2 (66.7%)
Other (n = 12)	4 (33.3%)
Rhabdomyosarcomas (n = 11)	3 (27.3%)
Osteogenic sarcoma (n = 9)	5 (55.5%)
Ewing's sarcoma (n = 7)	2 (28.6%)

*Includes only patients who received 2 courses of doxorubicin
O'Bryan RM et al. Cancer 1973;32:1–8 (N = 64)

Risk Category and Dose (N = 98)*	Partial Response
Good risk; 75 mg/m^2 (n = 41)	15 (37%)
Good risk; 60 mg/m^2 (n = 10)	2 (20%)
Good risk; 45 mg/m^2 (n = 28)	5 (18%)
Poor risk; 50 mg/m^2 (n = 9)	1 (11%)
Poor risk; 25 mg/m^2 (n = 10)	0

*Patients were classified as "good risk" if in the opinion of the investigator they were able to tolerate 75 mg/m^2 for 3 doses. Poor-risk patients were expected to tolerate 50 mg/m^2 for 3 doses. The latter included those older than 65, those with prior radiation therapy or chemotherapy, and those with poor tolerance of myelosuppressive terapy.
O'Bryan RM et al. Cancer 1977;39:1940–1948 (N = 98)

Treatment Modifications

Adverse Event	Dose Modification
WBC <3000/mm^3 or platelets <100,000/mm^3	Delay treatment 1 week until WBC ≥3000/mm^3 and platelets ≥100,000/mm^3
>2-Week delay in start of cycle	Reduce doxorubicin dose by 15 mg/m^2
WBC nadir <1000/mm^3 or platelet nadir <29,500/mm^3	Reduce doxorubicin dosage by 15 mg/m^2
WBC nadir 1000–1499/mm^3 or platelet nadir 30,000–49,500/mm^3	Reduce doxorubicin dosage by 30 mg/m^2
G ≥3 Mucositis	Reduce doxorubicin dosage 10–15 mg/m^2
Doxorubicin total cumulative lifetime dosage ≥400 to 450 mg/m^2	Obtain frequent MUGA scans to monitor cardiac function
A fall in ejection fraction (Possible guidelines: Resting cardiac ejection fraction decreased ≥10–15% below baseline, or to <35–40%)	Discontinue therapy

Toxicity (N = 472; N = 818)

Toxicity			No. of Patients (%)
Hematologic			
WBC/mm^3	or	Platelets/mm^3	
3000–4000	or	75,000–100,000	91 (19.3)
2000–2999	or	50,000–74,500	113 (23.9)
1000–1999	or	25,000–49,500	91(19.3)
<1000	or	<25,000	52 (11)
Nonhematologic			
Mild gastrointestinal toxicity			40 (8.5)
Moderate gastrointestinal toxicity			152 (32.2)
Severe gastrointestinal toxicity			10 (2.1)

O'Bryan RM et al. Cancer 1973;32:1–8 (N = 472)

Hematologic Toxicity			% of Patients		
Dosage (mg/m^2)			75	60	45
WBC/mm^3	or	Platelets/mm^3			
3000–4000	or	75,000–100,000	3	13	19
2000–2999	or	50,000–74,500	28	31	6
1000–1999	or	25,000–49,500	27	23	31
<1000	or	<25,000	14	15	13

O'Bryan RM et al. Cancer 1977;39:1940–1948 (N = 818)

(*continued*)

Toxicity (*continued*)

Congestive Heart Failure: According to Cumulative Dosage

Cumulative Dosage	No. of Patients (%)
<200 mg/m^2 (n = 491)	1 (0.2)
201–300 mg/m^2 (n = 145)	2 (1.4)
301–400 mg/m^2 (n = 84)	5 (5.9)
401–550 mg/m^2 (n = 98)	5 (5.1)
Total (N = 818)	13 (1.6)

O'Bryan RM et al. Cancer 1977;39:1940–1948 (N = 818)

General Summary of Toxicities

Myelosuppression	Dose-limiting toxicity. Leukopenia more common than thrombocytopenia or anemia; nadir usually on days 10–14 with recovery by day 21 after treatment
Nausea and vomiting	Moderate severity on the day of treatment; delayed symptoms (>24 hours after treatment) uncommon.
Mucositis and diarrhea	Common, but not dose limiting
Cardiotoxicity (acute)	Incidence not related to dosage. Presents within 3 days after treatment as arrhythmias, conduction abnormalities, ECG changes, pericarditis, and/or myocarditis. Usually transient and asymptomatic.
Cardiotoxicity (chronic)	Dosage-dependent dilated cardiomyopathy associated with congestive heart failure. Risk increases with increasing cumulative doses
Strong vesicant	Avoid extravasation
Skin	Hand-foot syndrome, with skin rash, swelling, erythema, pain, and desquamation. Onset at 5–6 weeks after starting treatment. Hyperpigmentation of nails, rarely skin rash, urticaria. Potential for radiation recall
Alopecia	Common, but generally reversible within 3 months after discontinuing doxorubicin
Infusion reactions	Signs and symptoms include flushing, dyspnea, facial swelling, headache, back pain, chest and/or throat tightness, and hypotension May occur with a first treatment. Symptoms resolve within several hours to a day after discontinuing doxorubicin
Urine discoloration	Red-orange discoloration usually within 1–2 days after drug administration

Therapy Monitoring

1. *During treatment cycles:* CBC with differential weekly
2. *Before each cycle after a cumulative doxorubicin dosage of 400 to 450 mg/m^2:* Cardiac ejection fraction

Notes

1. Single-agent doxorubicin remains the standard therapy for palliation of metastatic disease
2. Although some advocate higher dosages up to 70–75 mg/m^2 per dose, the accumulated evidence does not convincingly support the use of these higher doses

REGIMEN

IFOSFAMIDE

van Oosterom AT et al. Eur J Cancer 2002;38:2397–2406

Hydration and mannitol diuresis: Administer 1000 mL 5% dextrose and 0.9% NaCl injection (D5W/0.9% NS) over 2 hours, beginning 2 hours before the start of chemotherapy **Mannitol** is given to patients who have received adequate hydration. Administer **mannitol** 20% 200 mL over 30 minutes, starting 1 hour before the start of chemotherapy. Continued hydration is essential

Mesna 600 mg/m^2 intravenously diluted with 0.9% NaCl injection (0.9% NS) or 5% dextrose injection (D5W) to a concentration of 1–20 mg/mL over 15 minutes just before the start of the ifosfamide + mesna admixture, *plus*
An admixture containing **ifosfamide** 5000 mg/m^2 + **mesna** 2500 mg/m^2 intravenously diluted in a volume of D5W/0.9% NS sufficient to produce an ifosfamide concentration between 0.6 and 20 mg/mL over 24 hours on day 1 every 21 days (total ifosfamide dosage/cycle = 5000 mg/m^2), *followed by:*
Mesna 1250 mg/m^2 intravenously in 2000 mL D5W/0.9% NS over 12 hours on day 2 after completing ifosfamide administration every 21 days (total mesna dosage per cycle = 4350 mg/m^2)

or

Mesna 600 mg/m^2 intravenously diluted with 0.9% NS or D5W to a concentration within the range of 1–20 mg/mL over 15 minutes for 3 consecutive days on days 1–3 just before the start of the ifosfamide + mesna admixture, *plus*
An admixture containing **ifosfamide** 3000 mg/m^2 + **mesna** 1500 mg/m^2 per dose intravenously diluted in a volume of D5W/0.9% NS sufficient to produce an ifosfamide concentration between 0.6 and 20 mg/mL over 4 hours daily for 3 consecutive days on days 1–3 every 21 days (total ifosfamide dosage/cycle = 9000 mg/m^2), *followed by:*
Mesna 500 mg/m^2 per dose orally, or intravenously diluted with 0.9% NS or D5W to a concentration of 1–20 mg/mL over 15 minutes at 4 and 8 hours after the completion of the ifosfamide infusion daily for 3 consecutive days on days 1–3 every 21 days (total mesna dosage/cycle = 9300 mg/m^2)

Note: Although the use of mesna before ifosfamide administration was reported by these authors with both of these regimens, ifosfamide, like cyclophosphamide, has to be metabolized to active (and toxic) metabolites before there is a need to protect the uroepithelium. Consequently, pretreating with mesna may be of little value

Emetogenic potential:
1-Day schedule: Moderately high (Emetogenicity score = 4)
3-Day schedule: Moderate (Emetogenicity score = 3). See Chapter 39 for antiemetic regimens

Patient Population Studied

A study of 182 adult patients with metastatic or unresectable locoregional recurrent soft tissue sarcoma

Treatment Modifications

Adverse Event	Dose Modification
WHO G1 WBC or platelets	Reduce dosage by 10%
WHO G2 WBC or platelets	Delay start of therapy until WBC or platelets G1 or better, then reduce dosage by 10%
3-Week delay in start of cycle because WBC or platelets have not reached WHO G1 toxicity	Discontinue therapy
WBC nadir <500/mm^3 or platelet nadir <50,000/mm^3	Reduce dosage by 20%, regardless of WBC or platelet count on day 1
Resting cardiac ejection fraction <40%	Discontinue therapy

Efficacy (N = 174)

	5000 mg/m^2	3000 mg/m^2/day × 3 days
First-Line Therapy		
	n = 49	n = 49
Partial response	10%	24.5%
Median*	52 weeks	44 weeks
2-year survival	25%	25%
Second-Line Therapy		
	n = 36	n = 40
Complete response	3%	3%
Partial response	3%	5%
Median survival*	45 weeks	36 weeks

*Estimated median survival
WHO Criteria

Toxicity (N = 182)

Toxicity*	5000 mg/m²	3000 mg/m²/ day × 3 days
	First-Line Therapy: Hematologic	
	n ≤ 48	n ≤ 47
WBC G3/4	4%/15%	23%/34%
Nadir median	3050/mm³	1500/mm³
Nadir range	100–10,600/mm³	200–8900/mm³
ANC G3/4	7%/13%	12%/44%
Nadir median	1990/mm³	600/mm³
Nadir range	10–14,600/mm³	0.0–6520/mm³
Platelets G3/4	2%/2%	2%/2%
Nadir median	218,000/mm³	203,000/mm³
Nadir range	12,000–571,000/mm³	16,000–415,000/mm³
Hgb G3/4	6%/0	13%/2%
Nadir median	6.8 mmol/L 11 g/dL	6.5 mmol/L 10.5 g/dL
Nadir range	4.3–12.2 mmol/L 6.9–19.6 g/dL	0.7-8.3 mmol/L 1.1-13.4 g/dL
	First-Line Therapy: Nonhematologic	
Alopecia	13%	30%
G3/G4 Nausea/ vomiting	10%/0	10%/0
G3/4 Neurotoxicity	6%/0	11%/0
G3/4 Infection	2%/2%	4%/6%
	Second-Line Therapy: Hematologic	
	n ≤ 37	n ≤ 41
WBC G3/4	27%/5%	24%/39%
Nadir median	3200/mm³	1500/mm³
Nadir range	200–7700/mm³	0.0–10,000/mm³
ANC G3/4	19%/12%	31%/46%
Nadir median	1780/mm³	520/mm³
Nadir range	50–7810/mm³	0.0–5250/mm³
Platelets G3/4	3%/0	7%/7%
Nadir median	212,000/mm³	175,000/mm³
Nadir range	38,000–439,000/ mm³	14,000–482,000/ mm³

(*continued*)

Toxicity (N = 182) (*continued*)

Second-Line Therapy: Hematologic		
Hgb G3/4	3%/3%	15%/5%
Nadir median	6.5 mmol/L 10.5 g/dL	6 mmol/L 9.6 g/dL
Nadir range	2.8–9.2 mmol/L 4.5–14.8 g/dL	2.8–8.2 mmol/L 4.5–13.2 g/dL
Second-Line Therapy: Nonhematologic		
Alopecia	50%	65%
G3/G4 Nausea/vomiting	9%/0	15%/2%
G3/4 Neurotoxicity	3%/0	2%/2%
G3/4 Infection	0/0	10%/0

*Worst WHO grade per patient
WHO Criteria

Therapy Monitoring

During treatment cycles: CBC with differential twice weekly

Notes

Despite differences in response rates in first-line therapy, there were no differences in survival between the two regimens

REGIMEN

DOXORUBICIN + IFOSFAMIDE

Le Cesne A et al. JCO 2000;18:2676–2684

Hydration and mannitol diuresis:
Administer 1000 mL 5% dextrose and 0.9% NaCl injection (D5W/0.9% NS) over 2 hours, starting 2 hours before the start of chemotherapy
Mannitol may be given to patients that have received adequate hydration. Administer **mannitol** 20% 200 mL over 30 minutes, starting 1 hour before the start of chemotherapy. Continued hydration is essential

Doxorubicin 50 mg/m^2 intravenously per push over 3–5 minutes on day 1 every 21 days (total dosage/cycle = 50 mg/m^2), *followed immediately afterward by:*
Mesna 600 mg/m^2 intravenously diluted with 0.9% NaCl injection (0.9% NS) or 5% dextrose injection (D5W) to a concentration within the range of 1–20 mg/mL over 15 minutes just before the start of the ifosfamide + mesna admixture, *plus*
An admixture containing **ifosfamide** 5000 mg/m^2 + **mesna** 2500 mg/m^2 by continuous intravenous infusion in 3000 mL D5W/0.9% NS over 24 hours on day 1 every 21 days (total ifosfamide dosage/cycle = 5000 mg/m^2), *followed by:*
Mesna 1250 mg/m^2 intravenously in 2000 mL D5W/0.9% NS over 12 hours on day 2 every 21 days (total mesna dosage/cycle = 4350 mg/m^2)

Emetogenic potential: Moderately high (Emetogenicity score = 4). See Chapter 39 for antiemetic regimens

Patient Population Studied

A study of 294 adult patients with metastatic or unresectable locoregional recurrent soft tissue sarcoma randomly assigned to receive ifosfamide with either standard-dose doxorubicin (50 mg/m^2; n = 147) or intensified doxorubicin (75 mg/m^2; n = 133) with sargramostim support

Treatment Modifications

Adverse Event	Dose Modification
WBC <3000/mm^3 or platelets <100,000/mm^3	Delay treatment 1 week until WBC ≥3000/mm^3 and platelets ≥100,000/mm^3
Treatment delay 3 times (3 weeks) without achieving a WBC ≥3000/mm^3 and platelets ≥100,000/mm^3	Discontinue therapy
Serum creatinine >1.7 mg/dL (>150 μmol/L) or creatinine clearance <50 mL/min (<0.83 mL/s)	Delay treatment until serum creatinine <1.7 mg/dL (<150 μmol/L) or creatinine clearance >50 mL/min (>0.83 mL/s)
Nonhematologic life-threatening toxicity	Discontinue therapy
Resting cardiac ejection fraction below 40%	Discontinue therapy

Efficacy (N = 147)

Complete response	3.4%
Partial response	17.7%
Early death due to toxicity	1 patient
Median duration of response	47 weeks

Therapy Monitoring

1. *During treatment cycles:* CBC with differential twice weekly
2. *Before each cycle:* CBC with differential, serum electrolytes, BUN, and creatinine (creatinine clearance if serum creatinine >1.7 mg/dL (>150 μmol/L)
3. *Before each cycle after a cumulative doxorubicin dosage of 400–450 mg/m^2:* Cardiac ejection fraction

Toxicity (N = 147)

Toxicity	% of Patients or Levels
Hematologic	
G3/4 WBC	86
G3/4 ANC	92
Median ANC nadir (all cycles):	200/mm^3
Range of ANC nadir (all cycles):	0–5500/mm^3
Infection	4.6
G3/4 Platelets	8
Median platelet nadir (all cycles):	141,000/mm^3
Range of platelet nadir (all cycles):	5–323,000/mm^3
Nonhematologic	
G3/4 Asthenia	4.5
G3/4 Stomatitis	3.9
G3/4 Vomiting	10
G2/3 Myocardial insufficiency	1.3
G ≥ 2 Diarrhea	6.5
G3/4 Fever	2.6
G ≥ 2 Flulike syndrome	1
G ≥ 2 Bone pain/myalgia	6

NCI CTC

Notes

Combination chemotherapy may produce a higher response rate than single-agent therapy, but toxicity is greater and survival advantages for the more aggressive regimens have not been reproducibly reported

Soft Tissue Sarcomas: GI Stromal Tumors (GIST)

Epidemiology

Incidence: 2000–5000 estimated cases in the United States annually
Male:female ratio: 1:1
Gastrointestinal stromal tumors (GIST) account for <1% of all primary tumors of the gastrointestinal tract

Site of Disease	% of Patients
Stomach	60–70
Small bowel	20–30
Other*	10

*Large bowel, esophagus, rectum, mesentery, and omentun

Risk Factors Used to Assess Localized GIST

Risk	Tumor Size (cm)	Mitotic Rate
Very low	<2	<5/50 HPF
Low	2–5	<5/50 HPF
Intermediate	<5	6–10/50 HPF
	5–10	<5/50 HPF
High	>5 cm	>5/50 HPF
	>10 cm	Any mitotic rate
	Any size	>10/50 HPF

Fletcher CD et al. Hum Pathol 2002;33:459–465

Work-Up

1. History and physical examination
2. *Laboratory tests:* CBC with differential, electrolytes, LFTs
3. PA and lateral chest x-ray
4. Contrast-enhanced CT scan of chest, abdomen, and pelvis
5. PET scan can complement conventional CT helping to differentiate benign from malignant tissue (Van den Abbeele)
6. Upper endoscopy or endoscopic ultrasound-guided (EUS) fine-needle biopsy to obtain a tissue diagnosis. EUS can usually accurately differentiate leiomyoma and leiomyosarcoma

Van den Abbeele A, Badawi R. Eur J Cancer 2002;38 (suppl 5):S60–S65

Histologic Classification

Cell Type	% of Tumors
Spindle	70
Epithelioid	20
Mixed	10

KIT Mutations

Mutation	Site	% Incidence
Exon 11	Juxtamembrane domain	67
Exon 9	External domain	17
Exon 13	TK1	2
Exon 17	TK2	2
None*		13

*Wild-type *KIT*, although some have mutant *PDGFRA*
Heinrich MC et al. JCO 2002;21:4342–4349

Caveats

1. GIST consist of mesenchymal tumors that arise from the interstitial cells of Cajal (ICC) in the myenteric plexus
2. The true incidence of these tumors remains unknown because until relatively recently they were classified as tumors either of smooth muscle (eg, leiomyosarcomas) or of neural crest origin (eg, schwannomas)
3. Because nearly all GIST express the cell surface tyrosine kinase receptor, c-*KIT*, immunohistochemical staining facilitates the diagnosis
4. More than 90% of patients with GIST have activating *KIT* or *PDGFR-α* mutations (platelet-derived growth factor receptor-α)
5. Oncogenic mutations result in activation of *KIT* and its downstream pathways leading to uncontrolled cell division and resistance to apoptosis
6. Complete surgical resection remains the gold standard in the treatment of localized GIST. The goal of surgery is to remove all disease with negative resection margins. This is accomplished in up to 60% of GIST. Because nodal metastases are rare, lymphadenectomy is unnecessary. However, peritoneal surfaces and liver should be closely examined at laparotomy for evidence of metastatic spread
7. Despite curative resection, most patients subsequently have recurrence: the median time to recurrence is 1.5–2 years. The most acceptable and easily applied morphologic criteria for predicting tumor behavior are tumor size and mitotic rate
8. GIST is considered resistant to standard chemotherapy regimens for sarcoma such as doxorubicin and ifosfamide
9. Imatinib (STI571/Glivec/Gleevec) is an orally administered small-molecule selective tyrosine kinase inhibitor that is active in GIST (Demetri et al). Imatinib inhibits the activity of tyrosine kinases such as Bcr-Abl, PDGFR-α and the stem cell factor receptor c-*KIT*. As a competitive antagonist of ATP binding, imatinib blocks the ability of the kinases to transfer phosphate groups from ATP to tyrosine residues on substrate proteins, interrupting signal transduction
10. Clinical response to imatinib and survival rates seem to correlate with the presence or absence of certain *KIT* mutations: Mutations in exon 11 that encodes the intracellular juxtamembrane domain account for ≈70% of cases and are associated with an 85% response rate to imatinib
11. Imatinib is less effective in tumors without *KIT* mutations and in those with *KIT* mutations other than exon 11
12. The mutational status of *KIT* also seems to influence the progression-free survival, with longer survival in patients who harbor exon 11 mutations compared with those lacking an exon 11 mutation (Singer et al)
13. Because PDGFR-α is also an imatinib substrate, some tumors without *KIT* mutations respond to imatinib. However, unlike *KIT* mutations, most *PDGFR-α* mutations occur in the kinase domain and are unresponsive to imatinib
14. Over time, acquired resistance to imatinib is seen in approximately 20% of patients. In view of the high likelihood of tumor recurrence in these patients, imatinib is currently being investigated in the adjuvant setting. It is possible that it will have its maximal effect in the setting of minimal disease

Demetri GD et al. NEJM 2002;347:472–480
Singer S et al. JCO 2002;20:3898–3905

REGIMEN

IMATINIB MESYLATE

Demetri GD et al. NEJM 2002;347:472–280

Imatinib 400–600 mg/day orally with largest meal of the day

Imatinib is marketed in the United States as tablets for oral administration containing either 100 mg or 400 mg imatinib base as the mesylate ester. Gleevec® (imatinib mesylate)

Emetogenic potential: Low (Emetogenicity score ≤2). See Chapter 39 for antiemetic regimens

Patient Population Studied

A randomized open-label, multicenter phase II trial in 147 adults with histologically confirmed, heavily pretreated, unresectable or metastatic GIST that express CD117 (a marker of *KIT*-receptor tyrosine kinase); ECOG ≤3. Patients were randomized to imatinib mesylate 400 mg or 600 mg daily. Seventy-three patients were assigned to the 400-mg dose arm, and 74 patients were assigned to the 600-mg dose arm. Patients whose tumors progressed on 400 mg were permitted a dose increase to 600 mg daily. Patients whose tumors progressed on 600 mg daily were discontinued from the study

Efficacy[a] (N = 73; 400-mg dose)

Complete response	0%
Partial response	49.3%
Stable disease	31.5%
Progressive disease	16.4%
Could not be evaluated	2.7%
Median time to an objective response[b]	13 weeks
Median response duration weeks	>24

[a]There was no significant difference in the rate or duration of response between the two doses
[b]Combining both arms

Treatment Modifications

Not specified

Dosage Levels[a]	
600 mg	
400 mg	
300 mg	
Hematologic (No Modifications for Anemia)	
G1/2	No dose modifications
G3	Hold imatinib until toxicity resolves to G1; then restart at same dose
Recurrent G3	Hold imatinib until toxicity resolves to G1; then restart at 1 lower dose
G4	Hold imatinib until toxicity resolves to G1; then restart at 1 lower dose
Recurrent G4	Hold imatinib until toxicity resolves to G1; then restart at 1 lower dose[b]
Nonhematologic	
G1	No dose modifications
G2/3	Hold imatinib until toxicity resolves to G1; then restart at same dose
Recurrent G2/3	Hold imatinib until toxicity resolves to G1; then restart at 1 lower dose
G4	Hold imatinib until toxicity resolves to G1; then restart at 1 lower
Recurrent G4	Discontinue imatinib

[a]No dose reduction to <300 mg/day
[b]Consider filgrastim for persistent neutropenia

Recommendations are adapted from CML studies, Deininger MWN et al. JCO 2003;21:1637–1647

Therapy Monitoring

During treatment cycles: CBC with differential and serum electrolytes weekly at first, moving gradually to monthly over time

Toxicity (N = 73; 400-mg dose)

Adverse Event	% Any G	% G3/4
Nonhematologic		
Any event[a]	97.3	20.5
Edema or fluid retention[b]	71.2	1.4
Diarrhea	39.7	1.4
Myalgia	37	0
Fatigue	30.1	0
Nausea	29	1.4
Abdominal pain	26	1.4
Dermatitis/rash	24.7	2.7
Headache	19.2	0
Flatulence	19.2	0
Vomiting	13.7	0
Hemorrhage	11.0	4.1[c]
Dyspepsia	9.6	0
Increased lacrimation	6.8	0
Loose stools	6.8	0
Abdominal distention	5.5	0
Abnormal LFTs	5.5	2.7
Pain (in an extremity)	5.5	0
Blurred vision	5.5	0
Taste disturbance	2.7	0
Pruritus	2.7	0
Arthalgia	1.4	0
Paresthesia	1.4	0
Esophageal reflux	1.4	0
Hematologic		
Neutropenia	8.2	6.8
Anemia	5.5	1.4
Leukopenia	5.5	2.7

[a]Any event suspected to be related to study drug
[b]Mostly preorbital
[c]The most serious adverse events were gastrointestinal or intra-abdominal hemorrhages in patients with large bulky tumors

Notes

1. This phase II trial was not powered to distinguish between the efficacy of the 400-mg dose and that of the 600-mg dose. However, based on these data, 400 mg daily of imatinib was approved by the FDA for the treatment of advanced GIST. At the time of printing, this remains the recommended dose
2. The optimal dose of imatinib remains to be determined. A trial by the EORTC Soft Tissue and Bone Sarcoma Group, the Italian Sarcoma Group, and the Australasian Gastrointestinal Trials Group randomly allocated 946 patients to receive 400 mg imatinib either once or twice daily (total dose 800 mg/day) (Verveij). The primary endpoint was progression-free survival. The results of this study can be summarized as follows:
   - Treatment in both arms was reported to be "fairly-well tolerated," although more dose-reductions (60% versus 16%) and treatment interruptions (64% versus 40%) were recorded in patients allocated to the twice-daily regimen
   - Five percent of patients achieved a complete response and 47% a partial response with no difference between the two groups
   - At a median follow-up of 760 days, 56% of patients allocated to imatinib once daily had progressed compared with 50% of those assigned to twice-daily therapy (estimated hazard ratio of 0.82, P = .026)
   - The authors concluded: "if response induction is the only aim of treatment, a daily dose of 400 mg imatinib (given for 4–6 months) is sufficient; however, a dose of 400 mg achieves a significantly longer progression-free survival. In patients with widespread metastatic disease, the prolonged progression-free survival achieved with 400 mg twice daily might lead one to favour this regimen"

Note: The results do not allow one to decide whether an intermediate dose of 600 mg might be more active but less toxic or whether a similar outcome with fewer side effects could be achieved by starting with a dose of 400 mg and proceeding with stepwise dose escalations to 400 mg twice a day

Additional information:

1. At the time of the report, progression-free survival did not differ between patients with a complete or a partial response
2. Most responses happened in the first 9 months of treatment, but occasional best responses were reported after as long as 2 years of treatment
3. Dose reductions were made only after "extensive efforts" to keep the original dose with other supportive measures. Consequently, less than 20% of patients in the two treatment arms were treated with a daily dose of 300 mg or less. The authors noted "although no published data lend support to clinical activity at these doses," progression-free survival in patients treated at 300 mg did not seem to differ from that seen in patients receiving higher doses. However, they did notice a worse progression-free survival in patients who needed a dose reduction to 200 mg

Verweij J et al. Lancet 2004;364:1127–1134

ADVANCED GASTROINTESTINAL STROMAL TUMORS

SUNITINIB (SUTENT®; SU11248)

Demetri GD, et al.
Demetri GD, et al. ASCO/ASTRO Gastrointestinal Cancer Symposium abstract #8, January 2006
<http://www.asco.org/portal/site/ASCO/menuitem.c543a013502b2a89de912310320041a0/?v gnextoid=db5ac54f6a0 49010Vgn VCM100000ed730ad1RCRD>

Sunitinib 50 mg/day, administer orally, for 28 consecutive days, days 1–28, followed by a 14-day hiatus (4 weeks 'on', followed by 2 weeks 'off'), every 6 weeks (total dose/6-week cycle = 1400 mg)
Sunitinib malate is marketed in the United States as hard gelatin capsules for oral administration containing the equivalent of 12.5 mg, 25 mg, or 50 mg sunitinib, Sutent® Capsules. Pfizer Labs, Division of Pfizer Inc., New York, NY
Note: Strong CYP3A4 inhibitors may increase sunitinib plasma concentrations. The FDA recommends the concomitant use of medications without or with only minimal enzyme inhibition potential. If co-administration of potent CYP3A4 inhibitors (e.g., ketoconazole, itraconazole, clarithromycin, atazanavir, ritonavir, telithromycin) is required, a dose reduction to a minimum of 37.5 mg sunitinib per day should be considered

Emetogenic Potential: Low–Moderate (Emetogenicity score ≥ 2). See Chapter 39 for antiemetic regimens

Patient Population Studied

207 patients with GIST whose tumor has stopped responding to Gleevec® (imatinib mesylate) or who could not tolerate the administration of Gleevec®. Median age: 58 y (23–84 y). ECOG PS of 0/1 in 99%

Efficacy[a] (N = 207)

Complete response	0
Partial response (PR)	7%
Stable disease ≥ 22 wk	17%
Median time to progression	27.3 weeks
6-month survival	79.4%
Imatinib-intolerant patients	
Partial response (PR)	44% (4/9)
Stable disease	44% (4/9)

[a]There was consistent evidence of sunitinib activity across all pre-defined patient subsets including: Age < 65 years, Age ≥ 65 years, initial diagnosis < 6 months, initial diagnosis ≥ 6 months, imatinib treatment ≤ 6 months, imatinib treatment > 6 months, maximum imatinib dose ≤ 400 mg/day, imatinib treatment > 400 mg/day

RECIST Criteria

Toxicity (N = 202)

Toxicity	% All grades	% G3/4
Diarrhea	40	4
Skin discoloration	30	0
Mucositis/Stomatitis	29	1
Asthenia	22	5
Altered taste	21	0
Other toxicities without specific percentages		
↓ LVEF		
Hypertension		
Hypothyroidism		
↑ Lipase		
↑ Amylase		

Treatment Modifications

	mg/day
Dosage level +3	87.5
Dosage level +2	75
Dosage level +1	62.5
Starting dosage level	**50**
Dosage level −1	37.5
Dosage level −2	25

Adverse Events	Treatment Modifications
G ≥ 3 hematologic or non-hematologic toxicity	Reduce by one dose level or, if administering 25 mg/day, discontinue therapy
G ≥ 3 fatigue	
G ≥ 3 stomatitis	
Clinical manifestations of congestive heart failure (CHF)	Discontinue sunitinib
Decreased ejection fraction by 20–50% less than baseline without clinical evidence of congestive heart failure (CHF)	Interrupt sunitinib treatment and/or reduce the dose or, if administering 25 mg/day, discontinue therapy
Grade 2/3/4 serum lipase or serum amylase	Hold therapy until level GI, then resume therapy. Reduce by one dose level or, if administering 25 mg/day, discontinue therapy
Co-administration of potent CYP3A4 inhibitors (e.g., ketoconazole, itraconazole, clarithromycin, atazanavir, ritonavir, telithromycin)[1]	Reduce sunitinib dose to a minimum of 37.5 mg daily
Co-administration of potent CYP3A4 inducers (e.g., rifampin, phenytoin, phenobarbital, dexamethasone, carbamazepine, St. John's, wort)[1]	Increase sunitinib dose one level to a maximum of 87.5 mg daily

[1]If a medication with no effect on enzyme activity cannot be substituted

Therapy Monitoring

1. *During treatment cycles:* CBC with differential weekly
2. *Before each cycle:* Blood pressure, CBC with differential, serum electrolytes, BUN, serum amylase, lipase, and creatinine
3. Because patients receiving sunitinib who have a history of "cardiac events" may be at increased risk for developing left ventricular dysfunction they should be monitored for clinical signs and symptoms of congestive heart failure. Baseline and periodic evaluations of left ventricular ejection fraction should be considered. A baseline evaluation of ejection fraction should be considered in patients without cardiac risk factors
4. *Patients who experience stress such as surgery, trauma or severe infection:* Monitor for adrenal insufficiency

Notes

1. In its approval the FDA noted: "Decreases in left ventricular ejection fraction (LVEF) have been noted with sunitinib. Dose reduction and/or addition of antihypertensive or diuretic medications may be required; spontaneous recovery has also been observed. Patients should be monitored for signs and symptoms of congestive heart failure and sunitinib should be discontinued if these are observed"
2. Blood pressure monitoring is also recommended during treatment with sunitinib. Hypertension should be treated with standard therapies. Temporary suspension of sunitninb is recommended in severe cases until hypertension is controlled
3. Monitoring for adrenal insufficiency is also advised in patients who experience stress such as surgery, trauma, or severe infection

35. Testicular Cancer

Michael M. Boyiadzis, MD, MHSc, and Scott Saxman, MD

Epidemiology

Incidence: 8250 (United States, 2006)
Median age: 20–40 years
Estimated deaths: 370 (United States, 2006)

	Stage at Presentation			
	Seminoma	*Nonseminoma*	*Risk Groups*	
Stage I	81.4%	54.2%	Good risk	60%
Stage II	10.1%	23.3%	Intermediate risk	26%
Stage III	8.5 %	22.7%	Poor risk	14%

Jemal A et al. CA Cancer J Clin 2006;56:106–30
National Cancer Institute, Surveillance, Epidemiology and End Results (SEER) Program
International Germ Cell Cancer Collaborative Group. JCO 1997;15:594–603

Work-Up

Suspicious Testicular Mass	Seminomas	Nonseminoma Germ Cell Tumors
Alpha fetoprotein (AFP), β-HCG	Abdominopelvic CT	Abdominopelvic CT
Serum electrolytes, creatinine, mineral panel, and LDH	Chest CT, if abdominal CT positive or chest x-ray abnormal	Chest CT, if abdominal CT is positive or chest x-ray abnormal
Chest x-ray	Repeat β-HCG, LDH, AFP, if elevated preoperatively	Repeat β-HCG, LDH, AFP
Testicular ultrasound	Brain MRI; bone scan, if clinically indicated	Brain MRI; bone scan, if clinically indicated

National Comprehensive Cancer Network. V. 1. 2006

Pathology

A. Germ cell tumors (95%)
   1. Seminoma (50%)
      a. Classic (85%)
      b. Anaplastic (5–10%)
   2. Nonseminoma
      a. Embryonal carcinoma
      b. Teratoma (2–3%)
         (1) Mature
         (2) Immature
         (3) Mature or immature teratoma with malignant transformation
      c. Choriocarcinoma (<1%)
      d. Yolk sac tumor

B. Sex cord-stromal (gonadal stromal) tumors
   1. Leydig cell tumor (2%)
   2. Sertoli cell tumor (<1%)
   3. Granulosa cell tumor

C. Both germ cell and gonadal stromal elements
   1. Gonadoblastoma

D. Adnexal and paratesticular tumors
   1. Mesothelioma
   2. Adnexal of rete testis

E. Miscellaneous neoplasms
   1. Carcinoid
   2. Lymphoma

Note:
Sixty percent of testicular tumors are composed of more than one of the "pure" patterns

Bosl GJ, Motzer RJ. NEJM 1997;337:242–253. Erratum in: NEJM 1997;337:1404
Epstein JI. In: Kumar V, Abbas A, Fausto N, eds. Robbins & Cotran Pathologic Basis of Disease, 7th ed, WB Saunders, 2005:1040–1047

Staging

Serum Tumor Markers (S)

Sx	Markers not available or not performed
S0	Marker study levels within normal limits
S1	LDH <1.5 × normal and β-hCG <5000 IU/L (mIU/mL) and AFP <1000 ng/mL
S2	LDH 1.5–10 × normal or β-hCG 5000–50,000 IU/L (mIU/mL) or AFP 1000–10,000 ng/mL
S3	LDH >10 × normal or β-hCG >50,000 IU/L (mIU/mL) or AFP >10,000 ng/mL

Regional Lymph Nodes (N) Clinical Classification

NX	Regional lymph nodes cannot be assessed
N0	No regional lymph node metastasis
N1	Metastasis with a lymph node mass 2 cm or less in greatest dimension; or multiple lymph nodes, none more than 2 cm in greatest dimension
N2	Metastasis with a lymph node mass more than 2 cm but not more than 5 cm in greatest dimension; or multiple lymph nodes, any one mass greater than 2 cm but not more than 5 cm in greatest dimension
N3	Metastasis with a lymph node mass more than 5 cm in greatest dimension

Primary Tumor (T)

Pathologic stage after radical orchiectomy

pTX	Primary tumor cannot be assessed
pT0	No evidence of primary tumor
pTis	Intratubular germ cell neoplasia (carcinoma in situ)
pT1	Tumor limited to the testis and epididymis without vascular or lymphatic invasion; tumor may invade into the tunica albuginea but not the tunica vaginalis
pT2	Tumor limited to the testis and epididymis with vascular and lymphatic invasion or tumor extending through the tunica albuginea with involvement of the tunica vaginalis
pT3	Tumor invades the spermatic cord with or without vascular/lymphatic invasion
pT4	Tumor invades the scrotum with or without vascular/lymphatic invasion

Except for pTis and pT4, the extent of primary tumor is classified by radical orchiectomy. TX may be used for other categories in the absence of radical orchiectomy

Metastasis (M)

MX	Distant metastasis cannot be assessed
M0	No distant metastasis
M1	Distant metastasis
M1a	Nonregional nodal or pulmonary metastasis
M1b	Distant metastasis other than to nonregional lymph nodes and lungs

Staging Groups

Stage 0	pTis, N0, M0, S0
Stage I	pT1-4, N0, M0, SX
Stage IA	pT1, N0, M0, S0
Stage IB	pT2, N0, M0, S0
	pT3, N0, M0, S0
	pT4, N0, M0
Stage IS	Any pT/Tx, N0, M0, S1-3
Stage II	Any pT/Tx, N1-3, M0, Sx
Stage IIA	Any pT/Tx, N1, M0, S0
	Any pT/Tx, N1, M0, S1
Stage IIB	Any pT/Tx, N2, S0, M0
	Any pT/Tx , N2, MO, S1
Stage IIC	Any pT/Tx , N3, M0, S0
	Any pT/Tx, N3, M0, S1
Stage III	Any pT/Tx, any N, M1, SX
Stage IIIA	Any pT/Tx, any N, M1a, S0
	Any pT/Tx, any N, M1a, S1
Stage IIIB	Any pT/Tx, N1-3, M0, S2
	Any pT/Tx, any N, M1a, S2
Stage IIIC	A any pT/Tx, N1-3, M0, S3
	Any pT/Tx, any N, M1a, S3
	Any pT/Tx, any N, M1b, any S

Risk Classification

Nonseminoma

Good risk
Testicular or retroperitoneal primary tumor and no nonpulmonary visceral metastases and good markers—all of the following:

AFP <1000 ng/mL
β-hCG <5000 units/L (mIU/mL)
LDH <1.5 × upper limit of normal

Intermediate risk
Testicular or retroperitoneal primary tumor and no nonpulmonary visceral metastases and intermediate markers—any of the following:

AFP 1000–10,000 ng/mL
β-hCG 5000–50,000 units/L (mIU/mL)
LDH 1.5–10 × upper limit of normal

Poor risk
Mediastinal primary tumors or nonpulmonary visceral metastases or poor markers—any of the following:

AFP >10,000 ng/mL
β-hCG >50,000 units/L (mIU/mL)
LDH >10 × upper limit of normal

Seminoma

Good Risk
Any primary site and no nonpulmonary visceral metastases plus:

Normal AFP
Any β-HCG
Any LDH

Intermediate risk
Any primary site and nonpulmonary visceral metastases plus:

Normal AFP
Any β-HCG
Any LDH

Poor Risk
No patients classified as poor prognosis

International Germ Cell Cancer Collaborative Group. JCO 1997;15:594–603

5-Year Survival

Good risk	91%
Intermediate risk	79%
Poor risk	48%

Caveats

1. Ninety-five percent of patients with a mass within the testicle have malignancy. Orchiectomy is the preferred treatment for patients with a testicular mass; testicular biopsy is not recommended for a testicular mass. Radical inguinal orchiectomy is the surgical procedure of choice for a testicular mass
2. The tumor of a patient with a seminoma who has an elevated AFP level or any focus of nonseminomatous germ cell tumor should be considered and treated as a nonseminomatous germ cell tumor
3. Sperm banking should be discussed with patients before initiation of therapy

Nonseminomas

Stage I

- In patients with clinical stage I disease, surveillance is a reasonable option. The risk of recurrence is approximately 20–30%, and if the disease recurs, >95% of the patients are curable with BEP (bleomycin, etoposide, cisplatin) chemotherapy.
- Retroperitoneal lymph node dissection (RPLND) can also be considered, especially in patients for whom close surveillance is not possible. In patients found to have positive lymph nodes, observation or BEP for 2 cycles are treatment options that can be considered.

Stage II

- In general, patients with adenopathy >3 cm should receive BEP chemotherapy. Residual mass after chemotherapy should be resected.
- In patients with adenopathy <3 cm, either retroperitoneal lymphadenectomy or BEP for 3 cycles can be considered depending on the clinical circumstances. Following RPLND, patients with complete resection can be considered candidates for adjuvant chemotherapy (BEP for 2 cycles) or surveillance

Stage III

- Patients in good risk category should be given BEP chemotherapy for 3 cycles
- Patients in intermediate or poor-risk category should be given BEP chemotherapy for 4 cycles.
- Four cycles of VIP (etoposide, ifosfamide, cisplatin) is as effective as 4 cycles of BEP in patients with poor-risk germ cell tumors, but VIP is associated with greater toxicity
- VIP can be considered for patients in whom bleomycin is contraindicated
- With few exceptions, any residual mass after chemotherapy should be resected.

Seminomas

Stage I: surveillance, radiation therapy, or single-dose carboplatin
Stage II: adenopathy >5 cm—BEP for 3 cycles; adenopathy <5 cm—radiation therapy or BEP for 3 cycles.
Stage III: BEP chemotherapy for 3–4 cycles

Saxman SB et al. JCO 1998;16:702–706
Vaughn DJ et al. Ann Intern Med 2002;136:463–470

REGIMEN

BLEOMYCIN, ETOPOSIDE, CISPLATIN (BEP × 3–4 CYCLES)

de Wit R et al. JCO 2001;19:1629–1640
Nichols CR et al. JCO 1998;16:1287–1293

Hydration for cisplatin: Hydrate using 0.9% NaCl Injection (0.9% NS) to insure a urine output of at least 100 cc/hour prior to each dose of cisplatin. Hydration should be continued until the patient has completed chemotherapy and is able to take adequate oral liquids to prevent dehydration. Monitor and replace electrolytes/magnesium as needed
Etoposide 100 mg/m^2 intravenously in 500 mL 0.9% NS over 60 minutes, given on days 1–5 and repeated every 21 days for 3–4 cycles (total dosage/cycle = 500 mg/m^2)
Cisplatin 20 mg/m^2/day intravenously in 25–250 mL 0.9% NS over 30–60 minutes, given on days 1–5 and repeated every 21 days for 3–4 cycles (total dosage/cycle = 100 mg/m^2)
Bleomycin 30 units/week as a single intravenous injection, weekly for 9–12 weeks (total dosage/9-week course = 270 units; total dosage/12-week course = 360 units)

Emetogenic potential:
Days 1–5: High (Emetogenicity score = 6). Potential for delayed symptoms. See Chapter 39 for antiemetic regimens

Treatment Modifications

Adverse Event	Dose Modification
Myelosuppression not improving during the first 4 days of therapy	Omit day 5 etoposide. Administer full-dose cisplatin
Febrile neutropenia	Add filgrastim during ongoing cycle and subsequent cycles to administer full-dose chemotherapy
Febrile neutropenia while receiving filgrastim	Reduce etoposide dosage by 25%
Clinical (rales or inspiratory lag) or radiographic evidence of pulmonary toxicity or fibrosis	Discontinue bleomycin

Repeated treatment cycles should begin on schedule without regard for the degree of myelosuppression noted on the day of scheduled treatment. Daily CBC is obtained to document marrow recovery

Patient Population Studied

Patients with good-prognosis germ cell cancer treated with 3 cycles of BEP. Patients with disseminated germ cell cancer of advanced stage treated with 4 cycles of BEP

Efficacy
BEP × 3 Cycles (N = 397)

CR after chemotherapy	70.8%
CR after chemotherapy and surgery	2.3%
Incomplete response/progression	2.3%
Insufficient data to evaluate response*	24.7%
2-year overall survival	97%

*Most cases were residual masses in patients with pure seminoma

de Wit R et al. JCO 2001;19:1629–1640

Efficacy
BEP × 4 Cycles (N = 141)

Complete response	30%
Partial response	30%
NED + teratoma[a]	11%
Favorable response[b]	59%
2-year overall survival	71%

[a]Patients who had complete resection of only mature or immature teratoma after chemotherapy
[b]Complete response, NED with surgery, and patients with stable or improving partial remission with complete serologic remission for ≥2 years

Nichols CR et al. JCO 1998;16:1287–1293

Toxicity
BEP × 3 Cycles (N = 406)

Hematologic

Neutrophils <1000/mm^3	9%
Platelets <25,000/mm^3	3%
Febrile neutropenia (<2000/mm^3)	15%

Nonhematologic

	% G1	% G2	% G3	% G4
Sensory neuropathy	20	4		—
Ototoxicity	10	13*	—	—
Fatigue	39	21		—
Pulmonary	13		1	

*Tinnitus

de Wit R et al. JCO 2001;19:1629–1640

Therapy Monitoring

1. *Every cycle:* Chest x-ray, serum electrolytes, creatinine and mineral panel, CBC with differential and serum markers (β-HCG, AFP, and LDH)
2. *Response evaluation:* Restage with CT scan after completion of the final course of chemotherapy

Toxicity
BEP × 4 Cycles (N = 148)

	% G3	% G4
Hematologic toxicity	39	34
Nonhematologic		
Nausea/vomiting	7	
Infection	5	
Neurologic toxicity	7	
Hepatic toxicity	3	
Renal (creatinine >3 × normal)	1	
Respiratory*	5	

Therapy-Related Deaths

Respiratory failure	1% (2 patients)
Sepsis	2% (3 patients)
Pulmonary hemorrhage	1% (1 patient)

*Four patients experienced adverse events characteristic of bleomycin toxicity

Nichols CR et al. JCO 1998;16:1287–1293

REGIMEN

ETOPOSIDE, IFOSFAMIDE, CISPLATIN (VIP)

Nichols CR et al. JCO 1998;16:1287–1293

Hydration for cisplatin and ifosfamide: Hydrate using 0.9% NaCl Injection (0.9% NS) to insure a urine output of at least 100 cc/hour prior to each dose of cisplatin. Hydration should be continued until the patient has completed chemotherapy and is able to take adequate oral liquids to prevent dehydration. Monitor and replace electrolytes/magnesium as needed

Etoposide 75 mg/m^2 intravenously in 500 mL 0.9% NaCl injection (0.9% NS) over 60 minutes, given on days 1–5 and repeated every 21 days for 4 cycles (total dosage/cycle = 375 mg/m^2)

Mesna 500 mg/m^2 intravenously starting simultaneously with ifosfamide, then 500 mg/m^2 4 and 8 hours after the first dose for a total of three doses for each day ifosfamide is given. Alternatively, the first dosage of 500 mg/m^2 IV may be followed by 1000 mg/m^2 orally. 2 and 6 hours later. Oral doses of mesna should be rounded to the nearest 200 mg. Patients who vomit within 2 hours of taking oral mesna should repeat the dose or receive IV mesna. Total dosage per cycle = 7500 mg/m^2 intravenously, or 12,500 mg/m^2 intravenously (2500 mg/m^2) and orally (10,000 mg/m^2)

Ifosfamide 1200 mg/m^2 intravenously in 0.9% NS or D5W to produce a concentration between 0.6 and 20 mg/mL over 30–60 minutes, given on days 1–5 and repeated every 21 days for 4 cycles (total dosage/cycle = 6000 mg/m^2)

Cisplatin 20 mg/m^2 per day intravenously in 25–250 mL of 0.9% NS over 30–60 min on days 1–5, repeated every 21 days for 4 cycles (total dosage/cycle = 100 mg/m^2)

Filgrastim 5 mcg/kg per day subcutaneously for 10 days on days 6–15

Emetogenic potential:
Days 1–5: High (Emetogenicity score = 6). Potential for delayed symptoms. See Chapter 39 for antiemetic regimens

Treatment Modifications

Adverse Event	Dose Modification
Febrile neutropenia	Reduce etoposide and ifosfamide dosages by 25% in subsequent cycles
Thrombocytopenia with bleeding	Reduce etoposide and ifosfamide dosages by 25% in subsequent cycles
Serum creatinine >3 mg/dL (>264 μmol/L)	Delay cisplatin until serum creatinine <3 mg/dL (<264 μmol/L); continue etoposide and ifosfamide on schedule

Treatment cycles are repeated every 3 weeks without regard for the degree of myelosuppression on the day of scheduled treatment

Patient Population Studied

At least 151 men with disseminated germ cell cancer of advanced stage without prior chemotherapy

Efficacy (N = 151)

Complete response	36%
Partial response	21%
NED + teratoma[a]	10%
Favorable response[b]	59%
2-year overall survival	70%

Includes all patients evaluable for toxicity
[a]Patients who had complete resection of only mature or immature teratoma after chemotherapy
[b]Complete response, NED with surgery, and patients with stable or improving partial remission with complete serologic remission for ≥2 years

Toxicity (N = 151)

	% G3	% G4	% G5
Hematologic	28	60	1
Nonhematologic			
Nausea/vomiting	9		
Infection	6		
Neurologic	8		
Hepatic	3		
Renal (serum creatinine >3 × upper limit of normal)	4		
Respiratory	4		
Therapy-Related Deaths			
Sepsis	3% (4 patients)		
Cerebral hemorrhage	1% (1 patient)		

Therapy Monitoring

1. *Every cycle:* Chest x-ray, serum electrolytes, creatinine, mineral panel, CBC with differential and serum markers (β-HCG, AFP, and LDH)
2. *Response evaluation:* Restage with CT scan after completion of the final course of chemotherapy

REGIMEN

VINBLASTINE, IFOSFAMIDE, CISPLATIN (VeIP)

Loehrer PJ Sr et al. JCO 1998;16:2500–2504

Hydration for cisplatin and ifosfamide: Hydrate using 0.9 NaCl Injection (0.9% NS) to insure a urine output of at least 100 cc/hour prior to each dose of cisplatin. Hydration should be continued until the patient has completed chemotherapy and is able to take adequate oral liquids to prevent dehydration. Monitor and replace electrolytes/magnesium as needed
Mesna 500 mg/m^2 intravenously starting simultaneously with ifosfamide, then 500 mg/m^2 4 and 8 hours after the first dose for a total of three doses for each day ifosfamide is given. Alternatively, the first dosage of 500 mg/m^2 IV may be followed by 1000 mg/m^2 orally. 2 and 6 hours later. Oral doses of mesna should be rounded to the nearest 200 mg. Patients who vomit within 2 hours of taking oral mesna should repeat the dose or receive IV mesna. Total dosage per cycle = 7500 mg/m^2 intravenously, or 12,500 mg/m^2 intravenously (2500 mg/m^2) and orally (10,000 mg/m^2)
Vinblastine 0.11 mg/kg by intravenous push over 1–2 minutes, given on days 1 and 2 and repeated every 3 weeks for 4 cycles (total dosage/cycle = 0.22 mg/kg)
Ifosfamide 1200 mg/m^2 intravenously in 0.9% NS or 5% dextrose injection (D5W) to produce a concentration between 0.6 and 20 mg/mL over 30–60 minutes, given on days 1–5 and repeated every 3 weeks for 4 cycles (total dosage/cycle = 6000 mg/m^2)
Cisplatin 20 mg/m^2 intravenously in 25–250 mL of 0.9% NS over 30–60 minutes, given on days 1–5 and repeated every 3 weeks for 4 cycles (total dosage/cycle = 100 mg/m^2)

Growth factors: **Filgrastim** 5 mcg/kg per day subcutaneously on days 6–15

Emetogenic potential:
Days 1–5: High (Emetogenicity score = 6). Potential for delayed symptoms. See Chapter 39 for antiemetic regimens

Patient Population Studied

A study of 135 patients with progressive disseminated recurrent germ cell tumors treated as second-line therapy after induction chemotherapy with a cisplatin-etoposide–based combination chemotherapy. Patients who progressed within 3 weeks after previous cisplatin were not eligible

Efficacy (N = 135)

All Patients	
Disease-free status	49.6%
NED (teratoma)	11.1%
NED (carcinoma)	7.4%
Other	31.1%
Relapse from disease-free status*	49%
Median time to relapse*	18 months
Median progression-free survival	4.7 years

Patients Never Free of Disease After Induction Therapy	
Disease-free status	24.7%
Relapse from disease-free status*	42%

*Patients who achieved disease-free status with VeIP therapy

Toxicity (N = 135)

Hospitalization for fever and neutropenia	71%
Requirement for platelet transfusion	27%
Requirement for RBC transfusion	49%
Reversible renal insufficiency [Serum creatinine <4 mg/dL (<354 μmol/L)]	4.5%
Irreversible renal insufficiency [Serum creatinine >4 mg/dL (>354 μmol/L)]	1.5%

Treatment Modifications

Adverse Event	Dose Modification
Serum creatinine >2 mg/dL (>177 μmol/L)	Reduce ifosfamide dosage by 25%
Febrile neutropenia, or thrombocytopenia requiring platelet transfusion	Reduce ifosfamide and vinblastine dosages by 25%
Myelosuppression on day 1 of second and subsequent cycles	Administer full doses of chemotherapy; monitor daily WBC and platelets
WBC <2500/mm^3 or platelets <100,000/mm^3 on day 5	Omit day 5 ifosfamide
≥10 erythrocytes/HPF on daily urinalysis during therapy	Hold ifosfamide; continue hydration and intravenous mesna

Therapy Monitoring

1. *Every cycle:* Chest x-ray, serum electrolytes, creatinine, mineral panel, CBC with differential and serum markers (β-HCG, AFP, and LDH)
2. *Response evaluation:* Restage with CT scan after completion of the final course of chemotherapy

36. Thymic Carcinoma

Hanneke Wilmink, MD, and Guisseppe Giaconne, MD

Epidemiology

Incidence: 0.13 cases per 100,000 (0.2–1.5% of all malignancies)
Median age: 40–60 years
Male/female: No predisposition

Stage at Presentation (Masaoka Staging System)

Stage I:	32%
Stage II:	23%
Stage III:	34%
Stage IV:	11%

Engels EA, Pfeiffer RM. Int J Cancer 2003;105:546–551
Schmidt-Wolf IGH et al. Ann Hematol 2003;82:69–76
Tomiak EM, Evans WK. Crit Rev Oncol Hematol 1993;15:113–124

Pathology

Several histologic classifications of thymomas have been proposed. There is general agreement that the epithelial cells represent the malignant cells in this tumor type and the lymphocytic cells are considered benign

Classification of Thymic Epithelial Tumors

Muller-Hermelink	WHO Type	Levine and Rosai
Thymoma	Thymoma	Thymoma
Medullary type	Type A	Encapsulated
Mixed type	Type AB	—
Predominantly cortical	Type B1	Malignant type I (invasive)
Cortical type	Type B2	—
Well differentiated carcinoma	Type B3	—
Thymic carcinoma	Type C	Malignant type II

Müller-Hermelink HK, Marx A. Curr Opin Oncol 2000;12:426–433
Okumura M et al. Cancer 2002;94:624–632
Levine GD, Rosai J. Hum Pathol 1978;9:495–515

Work-Up

1. Radiologic staging should include a CT scan of the thorax
2. Extrathoracic disease such as metastases to the kidney, bone, liver, and brain are rare. Consequently, an extensive work-up for disease outside the thorax is not indicated in the absence of symptoms
3. Pleural or pericardial effusion represents the most common form of metastatic involvement
4. Proper intrathoracic staging is surgical

Ströbel P et al. Blood 2002;100:159–166
Thomas CR Jr et al. JCO 1999;17:2280–2289

Clinical Staging of Thymic Epithelial Tumors

Masaoka's Clinical Staging System of Thymoma

Stage I	Macroscopically encapsulated and microscopically no capsular invasion
Stage II	Macroscopic invasion into surrounding fatty tissue or mediastinal pleura, or microscopic invasion into capsule
Stage III	Macroscopic invasion into neighboring organs, i.e. pericardium, great vessels, lung
Stage IVa	Pleural or pericardial dissemination
Stage IVb	Lymphogenous or hematogenous metastasis

Masaoka A et al. Cancer 1981;48:2485–2492

Five-Year Survival

Stage I:	96–100%
Stage II:	86–96%
Stage III:	56–69%
Stage IV:	11–50%

Schneider PM et al. Ann Surg Oncol 1997;4:46–56

Caveats

Surgical excision is the treatment of choice for nonmetastatic thymoma and thymic carcinoma, even if locally advanced. Radiation therapy and chemotherapy may have adjunctive roles. Patients with locally advanced or bulky lesions may benefit from preoperative chemotherapy. Chemotherapy is used in patients with unresectable or metastatic thymoma and for thymic carcinoma. There is no single regimen that is considered standard for this disease

Syndromes and Diseases Associated with Thymoma

Symptoms	%
Asymptomatic	30
Myasthenia gravis	35
Pure red cell anemia	5
Hypogammaglobulinemia	5
Rheumatoid disease	10
Other diseases	15

Schmidt-Wolf IGH et al. Ann Hematol 2003;82:69–76

REGIMEN

DOXORUBICIN + CISPLATIN + VINCRISTINE + CYCLOPHOSPHAMIDE (ADOC)

Berruti A et al. Br J Cancer 1999;81:841–845

Hydration: ≥1000 mL 0.9% NaCL injection (0.9% NS) over 2 to 4 hours before chemotherapy commences. Monitor and replace electrolytes/magnesium as needed
Doxorubicin 40 mg/m² by intravenous push over 3–5 minutes, given on day 1 every 3 weeks (total dosage/cycle = 40 mg/m²)
Cisplatin 50 mg/m² intravenously in 50–250 mL 0.9% NS over 1 hour on day 1 every 3 weeks (total dosage/cycle = 50 mg/m²)
Vincristine 0.6 mg/m² by intravenous push over 1–2 minutes, given on day 2 every 3 weeks (total dosage/cycle = 0.6 mg/m²)
Cyclophosphamide 700 mg/m² intravenously, in 50–150 mL 0.9% NS or 5% dextrose injection (D5W) over 15 minutes, given on day 4 every 3 weeks (total dosage/cycle = 700 mg/m²)

Emetogenic potential:
Day 1: High (Emetogenicity score 6)
Day 2: Low (Emetogenicity score 1)
Day 4: Moderate (Emetogenicity score 3). Potential for delayed symptoms > day 1. See Chapter 39 for antiemetic regimens

Note: Use of steroids is discouraged, except for patients with myasthenia gravis previously receiving a stable dose of steroids

Patient Population Studied

A study of 16 patients with unresectable locally advanced nonmetastatic thymomas and locally advanced disease after radical surgery. Ten patients with stage III disease, and 6 patients with stage IVa disease. Three patients had recurrent disease after previous surgery

Efficacy (N = 16)

Complete response	6.25%
Partial response	75%
Stable disease	12.5%
Progressive disease	6.25%

WHO criteria

Toxicity (N = 16 patients/68 Cycles)

	% G3/4
Neutropenia	12.5
Anemia	—
Nausea/vomiting	6.25
Nephrotoxicity	—

WHO criteria

Treatment Modifications

Adverse Event	Dose Modification
ANC <1500/mm³ or platelet count <100,000/mm³	Delay therapy a maximum of 2 weeks until ANC >1500/mm³ or platelet count >100,000/mm³
2-week delay	Decrease dosage of all 4 drugs
Serum creatinine 1.6–2 mg/dL (141–177 μmol/L)	Hold therapy until serum creatinine <1.6 mg/dL (<141 μmol/L), then reduce cisplatin dosage 25%
Serum creatinine ≥2 mg/dL (≥177 μmol/L)	Hold therapy until serum creatinine <1.6 mg/dL (<141 μmol/L), then reduce cisplatin dosage 50%

Therapy Monitoring

1. *Pretreatment evaluation:* H&P, chest x-ray, CBC with differential, serum electrolytes, creatinine, LFTs, ECG, CT chest and abdomen, and anterior mediastinotomy with mediastinal biopsy
2. *Before each treatment cycle:* CBC with differential, and serum creatinine
3. *Response evaluation*: Chest x-ray after 2 cycles. Complete restaging including CT of chest and abdomen after 4 cycles

Notes

1. Patients who achieve a CR or PR are referred for surgery after 4 cycles of ADOC chemotherapy
2. Additional ADOC is administered to patients with residual disease that is not surgically resectable for a maximum of 6 cycles
3. Patients with histologic evidence of malignancy at surgery receive fractionated RT (total dose = 45 Gy) followed by 2 additional cycles of ADOC

REGIMEN

ETOPOSIDE + IFOSFAMIDE + CISPLATIN (VIP)

Loehrer PJ Sr et al. Cancer 2001;91:2010–2015

Hydration: Daily hydration with ≥1000 mL 0.9% NaCl injection (0.9% NS) before administering chemotherapy. Administer fluids over a minimum of 2–4 hours. Monitor and replace electrolytes/magnesium as needed
Cisplatin 20 mg/m² per day intravenously in 50–150 mL of 0.9% NS over 15–30 minutes, given on days 1–4 every 3 weeks (total dosage/cycle = 80 mg/m²)
Ifosfamide 1200 mg/m² per day intravenously, diluted to a concentration of 0.6–20 mg/mL with 0.9% NS or 5% dextrose injection (D5W) over 60 minutes, given on days 1–4 every 3 weeks (total dosage/cycle = 4800 mg/m²)
Mesna 240 mg/m² per dose by intravenous push, 3 doses/day [15 minutes before and 4 and 8 hours after ifosfamide] on days 1–4 every 3 weeks (total dosage/cycle = 2880 mg/m²)
Etoposide 75 mg/m² per day intravenously in 0.9% NS or D5W over 60–90 minutes, given on days 1–4 every 3 weeks (total dosage/cycle = 300 mg/m²)

Filgrastim 5 mcg/kg per day subcutaneously for 11 days on days 5–15 (or until WBC count ≥10,000/mm³ after WBC nadir)
Treatment is repeated for a total of 4–6 cycles

Emetogenic potential:
Days 1–4: High (Emetogenicity score 6). See Chapter 39 for antiemetic regimens

Note: Use of steroids is discouraged, except for patients with myasthenia gravis previously receiving a stable dose of steroids

Treatment Modifications

Adverse Event	Dose Modification
ANC <1500/mm³ or platelet count <100,000/mm³	Delay therapy a maximum of 2 weeks until ANC >1500/mm³ *or* platelet count >100,000/mm³
2-week delay	Decrease dosage of all 3 drugs
Serum creatinine 1.6–2 mg/dL (141–177 μmol/L)	Hold therapy until serum creatinine <1.6 mg/dL (<141 μmol/L), then reduce cisplatin dosage 25%
Serum creatinine ≥2 mg/dL (≥177 μmol/L)	Hold therapy until serum creatinine <1.6 mg/dL (<141 μmol/L), then reduce cisplatin dosage 50%

Patient Population Studied

A study of 28 patients with extensive advanced thymoma or thymic carcinoma (distant disease and pleural/pulmonary metastases with/without mediastinal disease). Patients with disease confined to mediastinum and ipsilateral supraclavicular nodes eligible if not candidates for primary surgical resection or definitive radiation therapy. Patients who previously received RT eligible if distant metastases are present or documented disease progression is at site of previous radiation therapy

Efficacy (N = 28)

Complete response	0%
Partial response	32%
Stable disease	61%
Progressive disease	7%
Median survival	31.6 months

Toxicity (N = 28)

	% G3	% G4
Worst toxicity	35.2	47
Hematologic		
Granulocytopenia	—	17.6
Leukopenia	23.5	23.5
Thrombocytopenia	11.8	41.2
Anemia	41.2	2.9
Hemorrhage	2.9	2.9
Nonhematologic		
Infection	8.8	—
Nausea	26.5	—
Emesis	2.9	5.9
Diarrhea	2.9	—
Pulmonary	8.8	2.9
Cardiac	—	2.9
Hypotension	5.9	—
Phlebitis	2.9	—
Neuromotor	2.9	—
Neuropsychiatric	2.9	—
Neuroclinical	2.9	—
Abdominal cramps	2.9	—

CTC

Therapy Monitoring

1. *Pretreatment evaluation:* H&P, CBC with differential, serum creatinine, LFTs, electrolytes, chest s-ray; creatinine clearance if adequacy of renal function is in doubt
2. *Before each treatment cycle:* H&P, chest x-ray, CBC with differential, serum creatinine, LFTs, and electrolytes
3. *Response evaluation every 2 cycles:* CT scans of chest/abdomen

REGIMEN

CISPLATIN + DOXORUBICIN + CYCLOPHOSPHAMIDE (PAC)

Loehrer PJ Sr et al. JCO 1997;15:3093–3099

Prechemotherapy hydration: ≥1000 mL 0.9% NaCl injection (0.9% NS) intravenously over a minimum of 2 to 4 hours. Monitor and replace electrolytes/magnesium as needed
Cisplatin 50 mg/m^2 intravenously in 50–150 mL of 0.9% NS over 15–30 minutes, given on day 1 every 3 weeks (total dosage/cycle = 50 mg/m^2)
Doxorubicin 50 mg/m^2 by intravenous push over 3–5 minutes, given on day 1 every 3 weeks (total dosage/cycle = 50 mg/m^2)
Cyclophosphamide 500 mg/m^2 intravenously in 50–150 mL of 0.9% NS over 15–60 minutes, given on day 1 every 3 weeks (total dosage/cycle = 500 mg/m^2)
Postchemotherapy hydration: ≥1000 mL 0.9% NS intravenously over a minimum of 2 to 4 hours after chemotherapy is completed

Emetogenic potential:
Day 1: Very high (Emetogenicity score 7). See Chapter 39 for antiemetic regimens

Note: Use of steroids is discouraged, except for patients with myasthenia gravis previously receiving a stable dose of steroids

Treatment Modifications

Adverse Event	Dose Modification
ANC <1500/mm^3 or platelet count <100,000/mm^3	Delay therapy a maximum of 2 weeks until ANC >1500/mm^3 or platelet count >100,000/mm^3
2-week delay	Decrease dosage of all 3 drugs
Serum creatinine 1.6–2 mg/dL (141–177 μmol/L)	Hold therapy until serum creatinine <1.6 mg/dL (<141 μmol/L) then reduce cisplatin dosage 25%
Serum creatinine ≥2 mg/dL (≥177 μmol/L)	Hold therapy until serum creatinine <1.6 mg/dL (<141 μmol/L), then reduce cisplatin dosage 50%

Patient Population Studied

A study of 23 patients with limited-stage, unresectable thymoma or thymic carcinoma. Patients with limited-stage disease were defined as those patients with disease that could be encompassed by a single radiation therapy portal

Efficacy (N = 23)

Complete response	21.7%
Partial response	47.8%
Progressive disease	4.3%
Median survival	93 months

Toxicity (N = 26)

	% G1	% G2	% G3	% G4
Hematologic				
Worst hematologic	19	23	12	42
Nonhematologic				
Emesis	15	23	15	—
Diarrhea	8	8	—	—
Infection	12	12	—	—
Cardiac	—	—	4	—
Mucositis	19	—	—	—
Neurologic/clinical	19	—	4	—
Genitourinary	23	4	—	—
Hepatic	19	—	—	—
Worst nonhematologic	23	42	23	8

ECOG grade

Therapy Monitoring

1. *Pretreatment evaluation:* H&P, CBC with differential, serum creatinine, LFTs, electrolytes, chest x-ray; creatinine clearance if adequacy of renal function is in doubt
2. *Before each treatment cycle:* H&P, CBC with differential, serum creatinine, LFTs, and electrolytes
3. *Disease evaluation every 2 cycles*: Response evaluated before starting RT

Notes

1. Patients who achieve a CR or PR after 2 or 4 cycles of chemotherapy are referred for RT (total dose = 54 Gy) to primary tumor and mediastinal and bilateral hilar lymph nodes
2. A maximum of 6 additional cycles of PAC chemotherapy can be administered after completing RT

37. Thyroid Cancer

Kenneth B. Ain, MD

Epidemiology

Incidence:	30,180 (estimated new cases in the United States, 2006)
Male/female ratio:	25/75
Mortality:	1500 (Estimated United States, 2006) (male/female 42/58)
Median age:	50 years

Jemal A et al. CA Cancer J Clin 2006; 56:106–30

Pathology

Epithelial Carcinomas	Incidence	Other Cell Types	Incidence
Papillary carcinomas	75%	Medullary carcinoma	<8%
Usual papillary	(75)	Anaplastic carcinomas*	2%
Follicular variant	(15)	Lymphoma	Very rare
Tall cell variant	(4)	Angiomatoid neoplasms	Very rare
Columnar cell variant	(<1)	Mucoepidermoid carcinomas	Very rare
Diffuse sclerosing variant	(3)	Malignant adult thyroid teratomas	Very rare
Oxyphilic (Hürthle cell) variant	(2)	Carcinomas with thymic features	Very rare
Follicular carcinomas	10%	Paragangliomas	Very rare
Usual follicular	(76)		
Oxyphilic (Hürthle cell) variant	(20)		
Insular carcinoma	(4)		

*Evolved from papillary or follicular

LiVolsi VA. Surgical Pathology of the Thyroid. Philadelphia: WB Saunders, 1990

Ain KB. Unusual types of thyroid cancer. Rev Endocr Metab Disord 2000;1:225

Work-Up

Thyroid nodule

1. TSH level
2. Fine-needle aspiration (FNA) biopsy
3. No role for thyroid scanning unless thyrotoxic (TSH suppressed): If thyrotoxic and palpated nodule is "hot" on scan, it is likely benign and biopsy is unnecessary

Neck node

1. FNA biopsy is appropriate

Mass at site distant from neck

1. Biopsy (resection) and immunohistochemistry for thyroglobulin; calcitonin

Initial Work-up (Histologic Diagnosis Established)

Papillary or follicular carcinomas (usually iodine avid)

1. *Do not use iodinated contrast for radiography of any type of papillary or follicular carcinomas.* This stable iodine can interfere with ^{131}I scans/therapy for up to 10 months
2. *Preop (if needed):* Neck ultrasound or neck MRI, noncontrast chest CT
3. *Postop:* ^{131}I scanning (see below) for papillary or follicular carcinomas and thyroglobulin (TG) level

Dedifferentiated papillary/follicular cancers (iodine non-avid, often not apparent initially)

1. *CT scans (may use contrast if known to be nonavid for iodine):* Often "fused" with PET scans
2. *PET scans (^{18}F-deoxyglucose):* Sensitivity enhanced with recombinant human TSH pretreatment
3. TG level
4. Radiographic bone surveys

(*continued*)

Work-Up *(continued)*

Anaplastic carcinoma

1. Complete CT survey (with contrast)
2. May need re-staging at 2- to 4-week intervals because of rapid rate of tumor progression

Medullary carcinoma

1. Complete CT survey (with contrast)
2. Whole-body nuclear scanning (scanning agents: SESTAMIBI, radiolabeled octreotide)
3. Calcitonin level
4. CEA level

Follow-up (Histologic Diagnosis Established)

Papillary or follicular carcinomas (and their subtypes)

In patients who have had thyroidectomy and are receiving suppressive doses of levothyroxine (maintain TSH $\leq$ 0.1):

1. Serial TG levels every 6 months (monitor for presence of interfering anti-TG antibodies).

Note: The "normal range" for TG in this situation is "undetectable"

2. Physical exams, patient neck self-exams
3. ^{131}I whole-body scans (WBS) every 6 months until scan and TG are negative ^{131}I therapy is administered if WBS is positive (see Initial ^{131}I WBS below)
4. CT of chest (noncontrast only) (interval defined by disease status)
5. PET scans if ^{131}I WBS is negative but TG is positive. Sensitivity correlates with tumor dedifferentiation and hexokinase I expression (interval defined by disease status)
6. Radiographic bone survey (interval defined by disease status)
7. Neck ultrasonography (interval defined by disease status)

Initial ^{131}I whole body scans (WBS): Prepare with hypothyroid protocol:

- *≈6 weeks before scan*: Stop levothyroxine therapy. Continue without levothyroxine >6 weeks if needed until TSH >30 mIU/L (first 4 weeks on **cytomel [liothyronine]** 25 mcg orally twice per day)
- *2 weeks before and during scan*: Institute low-iodine diet

If the ^{131}I WBS is positive or if the TG level is above the lowest detectable limit*	Treat with ^{131}I. Obtain ^{131}I whole-body scan (post-treatment WBS) 48–72 hours after ^{131}I therapy. Value of subsequent treatments is based on verifying uptake on post-treatment WBS and/or significant decrease of stimulated TG
If the ^{131}I WBS is negative *despite* hypothyroid protocol *and* if TG level is undetectable	Resume levothyroxine therapy and confirm absence of de-differentiated disease (see No. 4–7). If still negative, in subsequent studies use recombinant human TSH preparation protocol (below)

*The lowest detectable limit differs considerably from one TG assay to another. Check with laboratory

Follow-up ^{131}I WBS: Prepare with recombinant human TSH (Thyrogen) protocol:

- *2 weeks before and during scan:* Institute low-iodine diet
- *Days 1 and 2:* Administer **recombinant human TSH** 0.9 mg intramuscularly on days 1 and 2
- *Day 3:* Administer 4–5 mCi ^{131}I orally
- *Day 5:* Perform ^{131}I WBS (≥30 minutes/view; ≥140,000 counts)
- *Day 5:* Obtain serum TG, antithyroglobulin autoantibody, and TSH levels

Note: Frequency of follow-up ^{131}I WBS and TG levels: Every 6 months until both ^{131}I WBS and TG levels are negative, then double the time interval between each negative study. Follow-up is life-long, considering current diagnostic modalities. Maximum interval between negative studies is 5 years
A TG level > the lowest detectable limit is sufficient evidence for persistent/recurrent disease, even in the absence of positive ^{131}I WBS.
Antithyroglobulin autoantibodies occur in 20% of patients and interfere with the TG assay, making it insensitive. Can sometimes be a surrogate marker for persistent disease

Medullary carcinoma

1. Complete CT survey (with contrast)
2. SESTAMIBI and/or octreotide whole-body nuclear scan
3. Calcitonin and CEA levels

Staging

Primary Tumor (T)

TX	Primary tumor cannot be assessed
T0	No evidence of primary tumor
T1	Tumor ≤2 cm, intrathyroidal [*Note:* All previous AJCC editions considered T1 as tumors ≤1 cm]
T2	Tumor >2 cm but 4 cm or less in size, intrathyroidal
T3	Tumor >4 cm ± minimal extrathyroidal invasion Any size tumor with extrathyroidal invasion to trachea, nerve, esophagus, larynx, or subcutaneous tissues
T4a	Tumor invades prevertebral fascia or encases carotid artery or mediastinal vessels
T4b	Anaplastic cancer, surgically resectable
	Anaplastic cancer, not surgically resectable

Regional Nodes (N)

NX	Regional nodes cannot be assessed
N0	No regional lymph node metastasis
N1	Regional lymph node metastasis
N1a	Metastasis to level VI
N1b	Metastasis to unilateral, bilateral, contralateral, or superior mediastinal nodes

Distant Metastasis (M)

MX	Distant metastasis cannot be assessed
M0	No distant metastasis
M1	Distant metastasis

Papillary or Follicular: Age <45 years

Stage I	Any T, any N, M0
Stage II	Any T, any N, M1

Papillary or Follicular: Age ≥45 years

Stage I	T1, N0, M0
Stage II	T2, N0, M0
Stage III	T3, N0, M0 or T1-3, N1a, M0
Stage IVA	T4a, N0-1a, M0 or T1-3, N1a-b, M0
Stage IVB	T4b, any N, M0
Stage IVC	Any T, any N, M1

Medullary Carcinoma

Stage I	T1, N0, M0
Stage II	T2, N0, M0
Stage III	T3, N0, M0 or T1-3, N1a, M0
Stage IVA	T4a, N0-1a, M0 or T1-4a, N1b, M0
Stage IVB	T4b, any N, M0
Stage IVC	Any T, any N, M1

Anaplastic Carcinoma

Stage IVA	T4a, any N, M0
Stage IVB	T4b, any N, M0
Stage IVC	Any T, any N, M1

Note: Relative survival statistics worsen as clinical stage advances. However, there is sufficient variation in biological behavior of histologic subtypes and rate of tumor progression to make specific numbers based on clinical stage to be clinically meaningless. Even for low-stage tumors, recurrences may be seen for several decades after initial therapy, necessitating long-term vigilance

Caveats

Surgical Approach

1. *Cytologically (or clinically) suspicious or indeterminate:* Ipsilateral complete lobectomy and isthmusectomy followed by completion (during initial or subsequent procedure) of total thyroidectomy if malignancy confirmed, unless there is solitary intrathyroidal papillary microcarcinoma with no lymphadenopathy
2. *Thyroid biopsy or extrathyroidal site biopsy positive for cancer:* Total thyroidectomy with ipsilateral and central modified node dissection unless it is a solitary intrathyroidal papillary microcarcinoma (≤ 1.0 cm) with no lymphadenopathy (in which case perform a lobectomy only)
3. *Grossly invasive tumor or bilateral disease:* Total thyroidectomy with bilateral and central modified node dissection (exception: thyroidectomy not necessary for lymphomas)
4. Medullary thyroid carcinoma requires total thyroidectomy with bilateral and central neck dissections, since treatment is primarily surgical. There are no known effective systemic agents for medullary thyroid cancer
5. Anaplastic carcinoma requires as complete a local resection as possible, often despite grossly invasive disease. Initially unresectable tumor might be resected after a partial course of external-beam radiation therapy

Radioactive Iodine (^{131}I)

(Prepare with **hypothyroid protocol** [see WORK-UP, Initial ^{131}I WBS])

Initial ablation for papillary and follicular carcinomas

1. *Intrathyroidal disease with no metastases:* 100 mCi empiric dosing
2. *N1M0 disease:* 140–200 mCi empiric dosing
3. *T3-4 or M1 disease:* 200 mCi empiric dosing or treat to maximal red marrow tolerance (200 REM, ascertain with whole body/blood dosimetry analysis)

Follow-up treatments for positive ^{131}I WBS or TG level > lowest detection limit

1. 150–200 mCi empiric dosing

Follow-up treatments for M1 disease

1. Single dose to maximal red marrow tolerance (200 REM; ascertain with whole body/blood dosimetry analysis)
2. Adjuvant **lithium carbonate** to enhance ^{131}I tumor retention: **Lithium carbonate** 600 mg as loading dose orally, followed by **lithium carbonate** 300 mg orally every 8 hours. Begin lithium carbonate 2 days before the administration of ^{131}I and continue for an additional 5 days after ^{131}I (total 7 days).

Note: On the morning of ^{131}I therapy, obtain stat trough lithium level. Titrate dose to a trough level of 0.6–1.2 mEq/L

Repeat Surgery

Indications:

1. Resection of macroscopic residual disease before ^{131}I
2. Localized non–iodine-avid tumor
3. Distant critical sites (eg, spinal cord, brain)
4. Bone metastases
5. Isolated distant metastases and palliation of recurrent disease

Suppression of TSH with Levothyroxine

Indication: Chronic (lifelong) tumoristatic therapy in all cases of papillary and follicular carcinomas
Goal: TSH ≤ 0.1 mIU/L, using minimal suppressive daily levothyroxine dosage
Note: May use a beta-adrenergic blocker to mitigate tachycardia and risk of late left ventricular hypertrophy

External-Beam Radiation Therapy

Indications:

1. Localized non–iodine-avid disease (after surgical resection)
2. Protection of thoracic inlet after resection of anaplastic carcinoma (use hyperfractionation, if tolerated)
3. Palliation of distant sites of disease

Selected Multimodal Approaches

Anaplastic carcinoma: Complete primary resection followed by local external-beam radiation. Restage to detect early recurrence or distant disease, then treat with chemotherapy using these sites to assess response

Systemic Chemotherapy

Aside from a clearly effective role in thyroid lymphoma, as well as a necessary (although usually futile) use in anaplastic thyroid cancer, there is no clinically relevant role for systemic chemotherapy. Nonetheless, in patients with distant metastases that are unresponsive to ^{131}I, and "sufficiently progressive," the physician may administer systemic chemotherapy. Taxanes generally prove most likely to evoke a clinical response

REGIMEN

NEOADJUVANT + ADJUVANT DOXORUBICIN AND RADIATION WITH DEBULKING SURGERY

Tennvall J et al. Cancer 1994;74:1348–1354
Reviewed: Nilsson O et al. World J Surg 1998;22:25–30

TREATMENT A

Preoperative treatment:
Doxorubicin 20 mg by intravenous injection over 3–5 minutes starting 1–2 hours before radiation therapy weekly for 3 weeks (total dose/3-week course = 60 mg)
Radiation 1 Gy per fraction twice daily for 30 fractions with a minimum of 6 hours between fractions 5 days/week to a target dose of 30 Gy in 3 weeks
Debulking surgery:
Around week 5 approximately 10–14 days after completing preoperative radiation therapy
Postoperative treatment:
Doxorubicin 20 mg by intravenous injection over 3–5 minutes weekly starting 1–2 hours before radiation therapy (total dose/week = 20 mg)
Radiation 1 Gy per fraction twice daily for 16 fractions with a minimum of 6 hours between fractions 5 days/week to a target dose of 16 Gy (total cumulative radiation including preoperative dose = 46 Gy over approximately 70 days)
Additional doxorubicin:
Doxorubicin 20 mg by intravenous injection over 3–5 minutes weekly in patients considered to be in "reasonably good condition" (maximum dosage/complete treatment = 750 mg/m^2)
Note: Doxorubicin is administered as a fixed dose (20 mg), but cumulative dose is calculated as mg/m^2

Emetogenic potential (doxorubicin + radiation treatment): Moderate (Emetogenicity score ≥3). See Chapter 39 for antiemetic regimens

TREATMENT B

Preoperative treatment:
Doxorubicin 20 mg by intravenous injection over 3–5 minutes weekly, starting 1–2 hours before radiation therapy for 3 weeks (total dose/3 week course = 60 mg)
Radiation 1.3 Gy/per fraction twice daily for 23 fractions with a minimum of 6 hours between fractions, 5 days/week to a target dosage of 30 Gy
Debulking surgery:
Around week 4 (approximately 2 weeks after completing preoperative radiation therapy)
Postoperative treatment:
Doxorubicin 20 mg by intravenous injection over 3–5 minutes weekly, starting 1 hour before radiation therapy (total dose/week = 20 mg)
Radiation 1.3 Gy/per fraction twice daily for 12 fractions with a minimum of 6 hours between fractions 5 days/week to a target dosage of 16 Gy (total cumulative radiation dose including preoperative dose = 46 Gy over approximately 50 days)
Additional doxorubicin:
Doxorubicin 20 mg by intravenous injection over 3–5 minutes weekly in patients considered to be in "reasonably good condition" (maximum dosage/complete treatment = 400–440 mg)

Emetogenic potential (doxorubicin + radiation treatment): Moderate (Emetogenicity score ≥3). See Chapter 39 for antiemetic regimens

Treatment Modifications

Postoperative doxorubicin was administered to patients with good performance status and in the absence of disease progression

Patient Population Studied

A study of 33 patients with anaplastic thyroid carcinoma treated with combined radiation, chemotherapy, and surgery. 160 patients in later review

Efficacy (N = 33)

	Treatment	
	A (n = 16)	B (n = 17)
Median survival	3.5 months	4.5 months
Local control	5 patients	11 patients
Local failure*	6 patients	2 patients
Persistent local disease*	5 patients	3 patients

*Cause of death.

1. 24% of patient deaths attributed to local failure
2. 48% of patients had no signs of local recurrence
3. Preoperative doxorubicin and concomitant hyperfractionated radiation therapy converted unresectable tumors into a resectable state in 23 patients

Toxicity (N = 33)

1. WHO grades I and II mucosal and skin toxicity
2. Hematologic toxicity not observed
3. Treatment-related toxicities did not prevent any patient from completing planned treatment

Therapy Monitoring

1. *Weekly:* CBC with differential
2. *Before each treatment:* CBC with differential
3. *Every 2 to 3 cycles:* Imaging studies to evaluate response

Notes

Doxorubicin has been used historically; however, as a single agent it is not considered an effective chemotherapeutic drug for anaplastic carcinoma

REGIMEN

96-HOUR CONTINUOUS-INFUSION PACLITAXEL [WEEKLY PACLITAXEL]

Ain KB et al. Thyroid 2000;10:587–594

Optional premedication (Primary prophylaxis against hypersensitivity reactions from paclitaxel):*
Dexamethasone 20 mg/dose orally for 2 doses on the evening before and the morning of chemotherapy before paclitaxel *plus*:
Diphenhydramine 50 mg for 1 dose by intravenous push 30 minutes before paclitaxel *and*:
Ranitidine 50 mg or **cimetidine** 300 mg for 1 dose by intravenous infusion in 25–100 mL 0.9% NaCl injection (0.9% NS) or 5% dextrose injection (D5W) over 5–30 minutes given 30 minutes before paclitaxel

**Note:* The incidence of hypersensitivity reactions with 96-hour continuous infusion of paclitaxel is much lower than with other paclitaxel regimens, and in most patients premedication is not required. If a premedication regimen is not used, observe the patient carefully for at least 1 hour in the first cycle to ensure that no reaction occurs. If a reaction occurs, immediately stop the infusion and administer the suggested regimen, substituting intravenous dexamethasone
Paclitaxel 30–35 mg/m² per day by continuous intravenous infusion in a volume of 0.9% NaCl injection (0.9% NS) or 5% dextrose injection (D5W) sufficient to produce a solution with concentration within the range 0.3–1.2 mg/mL over 24 hours for 4 consecutive days on days 1–4 every 3 weeks for up to 6 cycles (total dosage/cycle for 30 mg/m² per day = 120 mg/m² for 35 mg/m² per day = 140 mg/m²)

Emetogenic potential: Low to nonemetogenic (Emetogenicity score ≤ 2). See Chapter 39 for antiemetic regimens

Note: Subsequent clinical experience suggests that optimal use of paclitaxel uses a 1-hour infusion of 175 mg/m² given weekly for 3 weeks every month, with restaging each month, and continuing until there is progressive disease or limiting toxicity. *This dose must be administered carefully and with growth factor support assessing patient before each dose with attention to occurrence of mucositis and neutropenia*
Paclitaxel 175 mg/m² by intravenous infusion in a volume of 0.9% NS or D5W sufficient to produce a solution with concentration of 0.3–1.2 mg/mL over 3 hours on day 1 every week for 3 weeks of every month (total dosage/cycle = 525 mg/m²)

Treatment Modifications

Adverse Event	Dose Modification
96-Hour Continuous Infusion Paclitaxel	
G2 Hematologic adverse events	Hold paclitaxel until adverse events resolve to G1 or disappear, then resume paclitaxel with dosage reduced by 25%
G2/3 Gastrointestinal, neurologic, cardiac, musculoskeletal toxicities or mucositis	
G4 or unremitting G3 adverse events	Discontinue paclitaxel
ANC nadir <500/mm³, platelet nadir <50,000/mm³, or febrile neutropenia	Reduce paclitaxel dosage by 25%
Day 1 ANC <1500/mm³ or platelets <100,000/mm³	Delay chemotherapy until ANC >1500/mm³ and platelets >100,000/mm³ for maximum delay of 2 weeks
Weekly Paclitaxel	
Day 1 ANC <1500/mm³ or platelets <100,000/mm³	Delay chemotherapy until ANC >1500/mm³ and platelets >100,000/mm³ for maximum delay of 2 weeks
Delay of >2 weeks in reaching ANC >1500/mm³ and platelets >100,000/mm³	Discontinue therapy
G2 neurotoxicity	Reduce paclitaxel dosage to 135 mg/m²
G3 Neurotoxicity	Discontinue paclitaxel
G2 Arthralgia/myalgia despite dexamethasone prophylaxis	Reduce paclitaxel dosage to 135 mg/m²
G3 Arthralgia/myalgia despite dexamethasone prophylaxis	Discontinue paclitaxel
Moderate hypersensitivity	Patient may be retreated
Severe hypersensitivity	Discontinue therapy

Patient Population Studied

A study of 20 patients with metastatic anaplastic thyroid cancer

Efficacy (N = 19)

Partial responses	47%
Complete responses	5%
Disease stabilization	5%
Progressive disease	42%
Therapeutic response	Median survival: 32 weeks
No therapeutic response	Median survival: 10 weeks

From WHO criteria

Toxicity (N = 11/8)

(140 mg/m², n = 11[a])

	G1	G2
Nausea	6	1
Alopecia	3	
Vomiting	2	
Diarrhea	3	
Fever	1	2

(120 mg/m², n = 8[b])

	G1	G2
Nausea	1	
Alopecia	1	
Stomatitis	1	
Fatigue	1	
Neutropenia		1

[a]Patients who received paclitaxel 35 mg/m² per day for 4 days (total dosage/cycle = 140 mg/m²)
[b]Patients who received paclitaxel 30 mg/m² per day for 4 days (total dosage/cycle = 120 mg/m²)

CTC criteria

Therapy Monitoring

1. *Before every cycle:* CBC with differential, platelet count, and LFTs
2. *Radiologic studies:* Every 2 cycles

38. Vaginal Cancer

Thomas Chen, MD, and Franco Muggia, MD

Epidemiology

Incidence: Estimated 2420 new cases for year 2006 in United States
Incidence of clear cell adenocarcinoma due to in utero diethylstilbestrol exposure estimated at 1/1000

Mortality: 820 deaths estimated for year 2006 in United States

Mean age: Squamous cell cancer (60–65 years); adenocarcinoma/clear cell (19 years)

Stage at Presentation	
Stage I:	28%
Stage II:	43%
Stage III:	16%
Stage IV:	13%

http://SEER.cancer.gov. 2006
Detailed guide: Vaginal Cancers. American Cancer Society. www.cancer.org
Daling JR et al. Gynecol Oncol 2002 84:263–270
Eddy GL et al. Am J Obstet Gynecol 1991;165:292–296; discussion 296–298
Jemal A et al. CA Cancer J Clin 2006;56:106–30

Pathology

Histologic Classification of Vaginal Neoplasia

VAIN (vaginal intraepithelial neoplasia): Vaginal cancer precursors
Squamous intraepithelial tumors: VAIN I/II/III (mild/moderate/severe dysplasia/carcinoma in situ)
Hallmark of VAIN: Cytologicatypia, pleomorphism, irregular nuclear contours, chromatin clumping, abnormal maturation, nuclear enlargement

Invasive carcinoma

1. Invasive squamous cell carcinoma	85%
2. Glandular lesions (mullerian papilloma, adenosis, adenocarcinoma)	10%
3. Other invasive tumors (adenosquamous, adenoid cystic, carcinoid, small cell, undifferentiated)	1–2%
4. Mesenchymal tumors (leiomyosarcoma, sarcoma botryoides, endometrioid sarcoma)	2%
5. Mixed epithelial and mesenchymal tumors	<1%
6. Other primary vaginal tumors (melanoma, sarcoma, yolk sac tumors, lymphoma)	3–4%

Histological Classification of Tumors of the Female Genital Tract. WHO/ISGYP (in press)
Data available at http://www.
http://www/vh/prg/adult/provider/pathology/OBGYNOncology/PathologyManualHome.html
Proportion of all vaginal neoplasms. In: Hoskins WJ, Perez CA, Young RC, eds. Principles and Practice of Gynecologic Oncology, 3rd ed. Philadelphia: Lippincott-Raven, 2000
Higinia R et al. Vagina. In: Hoskins WJ, Perez CA, Young RC, eds. Principles and Practice of Gynecologic Oncology, 4th ed. Philadelphia: Lippincott Williams & Wilkins, 2000:707–742

Work-Up

VAIN (Vaginal Intraepithelial Neoplasia)

1. H&P, including bimanual examination and palpation of vagina
2. Multiple site-directed biopsies, including cervical biopsies to rule out invasive disease and primary cervical cancer

Invasive carcinoma

1. H&P, including bimanual examination and palpation of vagina
2. Multiple site-directed biopsies, including cervical biopsies to rule out invasive disease and primary cervical cancer
3. Metastatic work up: Chest x-ray, cystoscopy, proctosigmoidoscopy, and intravenous pyelogram
4. If clinically warranted, barium enema and CT scan or MRI

Staging is best performed by gynecologic and radiation oncologists with the patient under general anesthesia. Additional biopsies of the vagina should be done to determine the limits of abnormal vaginal mucosa

Hoskins WJ, eds. Principles and Practice of Gynecologic Oncology, 2nd ed. Philadelphia: Lippincott-Raven, 1997

Staging

Primary Tumor (T)/FIGO Stages

TX	Primary tumor cannot be assessed
T0	No evidence of primary tumor
Tis/0	Carcinoma in situ
T1/I	Tumor confined to vagina
T2/II	Tumor invades paravaginal tissues but not to pelvic wall
T3/III	Tumor extends to pelvic wall
T4/IVA	Tumor invades bladder mucosa or rectum and/or extends beyond the true pelvis

Regional Lymph Nodes (N)

NX	Regional nodes cannot be assessed
N0	No regional lymph node metastasis
N1/IVB	Pelvic or inguinal lymph node metastasis

Distant Metastasis (M)

MX	Distant metastasis cannot be assessed
M0	No distant metastasis
M1/IVB	Distant metastasis

AJCC Staging Groups

Stage 0	Tis, N0, M0
Stage I	T1, N0, M0
Stage II	T2, N0, M0
Stage III	T1, N1, M0
	T2, N1, M0 T3, N0, M0 T3, N1, M0
Stage IVA	T4, any N, M0
Stage IVB	Any T, any N, M1

Relative Survival: 5-Year

Stage 0	100%
Stage I	72%
Stage II	70%
Stage III	53%
Stage IV	42%

Kirkbride P et al. Gynecol Oncol 1995;56:435–443

Caveats

General:

1. Vaginal neoplasms are rare and are considered primary only if neither the vulva nor the cervix is involved at time of diagnosis[a]
2. A carcinoma involving the upper vagina and cervix should be considered a cervical primary and managed accordingly[a,b]
3. Histologically, most vaginal carcinomas are squamous, and chemotherapeutic management is usually based on extrapolation from experience with cervical carcinoma, given similarities in location, pattern of spread, histologic appearance, relation to HPV, and response to radiation therapy

Therapeutic principles:

1. *Vaginal intraepithelial neoplasia:* Treated with local modalities such as CO_2 laser ablation, topical fluorouracil, local radiation therapy, or surgical excision. Regression rates are excellent. Close cytologic surveillance is warranted[c]
2. *Stages I and II:* Standard treatment by gynecologic or radiation oncologists is highly effective[d]
3. *Stages III and IVA:* Radiation therapy alone has yielded suboptimal results.[e,f] Reports of combined chemoradiation have been more encouraging,[g] and, bcause of similarities with cervical cancer, cisplatin-based chemoradiation has been advocated as standard therapy[h]
4. *Stage IVB and recurrences not amenable to locoregional therapy:* Anthracyclines and platinum compounds as single agents or in combinations have some activity, but experience is limited to small case series.[c, i] Taxane-based therapy also is reasonable, given efficacy in other gynecologic malignancies.[j] Considering the rarity of cases, care providers should consider clinical trials

[a]Hoskins WJ, Perez CA, Young RC eds. Principles and Practice of Gynecologic Oncology, 2nd ed. Philadelphia: Lippincott-Raven, 1997
[b]Kurman RJ et al. Tumors of the Cervix, Vagina, and Vulva. Atlas of Tumor Pathology, 3rd series, #4. AFIP, Washington, DC, 1992
[c]Carosi RJ, Bornalaski JJ, Hoffman MS. Diagnosis and management of vulvar and vaginal intraepithelial neoplasia. Gynecologic Oncology for the Generalist 2001;28(4)
[d]Davis KP et al. Gynecol Oncol 1991;42:131–136
[e]Dancuart F et al. Int J Radiat Oncol Biol Phys 1988;14:745–749
[f]Kucera H, Vavra N. Gynecol Oncol 1991; 40:12-6
[g]Evans LS et al. Int J Radiat Oncol Biol Phys 1988; 15:901–6
[h]PW. Curr Treat Opt Oncol 2002;3:125–130
[i]Piver MS et al. Am J Obstet Gynecol 1978;131:311–313 Grisbgy
[j]Curtin JP et al. JCO 2001;19:1275–1278

REGIMEN

DOXORUBICIN (SINGLE AGENT)

Piver MS et al. Am J Obstet Gynecol 1978;31:311–313

Doxorubicin 60–90 mg/m^2 single dose intravenously per push on day 1 every 4 weeks (total dosage/cycle = 60–90 mg/m^2)

Emetogenic potential: Moderately high (Emetogenicity score 4). See Chapter 39 for antiemetic regimens

Patient Population Studied

Cervical or vaginal malignancies; 7 of 100 patients with advanced vaginal squamous cell carcinoma

Efficacy (N = 7 with Vaginal Cancer)

Complete response	1 patient
Partial response	1 patient*

*Treated with combination doxorubicin, cyclophosphamide, and fluorouracil

Toxicity

Myelosuppression	Dose-limiting toxicity. Leukopenia more common than thrombocytopenia or anemia. Nadir usually on days 10–14, with recovery by day 21 after treatment
Nausea and vomiting	Moderate severity on the day of treatment; delayed symptoms (>24 hours after treatment) uncommon
Mucositis and diarrhea	Common, but not dose limiting
Cardiotoxicity (acute)	Incidence not related to dosage. Presents within 3 days after treatment as arrhythmias, conduction abnormalities, ECG changes, pericarditis, and/or myocarditis; usually transient and asymptomatic
Cardiotoxicity (chronic)	Dosage-dependent dilated cardiomyopathy associated with congestive failure. Risk increases with cumulative doses >550 mg/m^2)
Strong vesicant	Avoid extravasation
Skin	Hand-foot syndrome, with skin rash swelling, erythema, pain, and desquamation. Onset at 5–6 weeks after starting treatment Hyperpigmentation of nails, rarely skin rash, urticaria. Potential for radiation recall
Alopecia	Common, but generally reversible within 3 months after discontinuing doxorubicin
Infusion reactions	Signs and symptoms include flushing, dyspnea, facial swelling, headache, back pain, chest and/or throat tightness, and hypotension. May occur with a first treatment. Symptoms resolve within several hours to a day after discontinuing doxorubicin
Urine discoloration	Red-orange discoloration usually within 1–2 days after drug administration

Chu E, DeVita VT Jr, eds. Physicians' Cancer Chemotherapy Drug Manual 2003. Sudbury, MA: Jones and Bartlett, pp. 135–139

Treatment Modifications

Adverse Event	Dose Modification
WBC <3000/mm^3 and platelet counts <100,000/mm^3	Delay start of next cycle until WBC >3000/mm^3 and platelet counts >100,000/mm^3
>2-week delay in start of cycle	Reduce doxorubicin dose by 15 mg/m^2
Doxorubicin total cumulative life-time dosage ≥400–450 mg/m^2	Obtain frequent MUGA scans to monitor cardiac function

Therapy Monitoring

1. *Before each treatment with doxorubicin (every 4 weeks):* H&P, CBC with differential, serum electrolytes, LFTs, BUN, and serum creatinine
2. *After patients receive a total cumulative lifetime doxorubicin dose of 400 to 450 mg/m^2:* Check radionuclide left ventricular ejection fraction periodically (every 2 cycles)

Piver MS et al. Am J Obstet Gynecol 1978;131:311–313

REGIMEN

CISPLATIN (SINGLE AGENT)

Thigpen JT et al. Gynecol Oncol 1986;23:101–104

Hydration before cisplatin: ≥1000 mL 0.9% NaCl injection (0.9% NS) with 20 mEq KCl/L, infused over a minimum of 3–4 hours. Monitor and replace electrolytes/magnesium as needed

Cisplatin 50 mg/m^2 single dose intravenously in 50–250 mL 0.9% NS at a rate of 1 mg/minute on day 1 every 3 weeks (total dosage/cycle = 50 mg/m^2)

Hydration after cisplatin: ≥1000 mL 0.9% NaCl injection (0.9% NS) with 20 mEq KCl/L, infused over a minimum of 3–4 hours. Encourage oral hydration

Emetogenic potential: High (Emetogenicity score = 5). See Chapter 39

Patient Population Studied

A study of 22 patients with advanced or recurrent vaginal cancers

Efficacy (N = 22)

One complete response out of 22 evaluable patients with vaginal cancer (most were heavily pretreated)

Toxicity (N = 22)

Hematologic

	% G1	% G2
Leukopenia[a]	9	13.6
Thrombocytopenia[b]	9	—

Nonhematologic

	Mild	Moderate	Severe
Nephrotoxicity[c]	27	—	—
Nausea/vomiting[d]	9	45	4.5
Fatigue	9	4.5	4.5

[a]Lowest WBC nadir = 2000 leukocytes/mm^3
[b]Lowest platelet nadir = 126,000 platelets/mm^3
[c]Dose-limiting toxicity in 35–40%
[d]Most common adverse effect

Toxicities Reported in Other Studies

Neurotoxicity	Usually peripheral sensory neuropathy with bilateral paresthesias and anesthesia in a "stocking and glove" distribution. Risk increases with high individual doses and cumulatively. Motor and autonomic neuropathies may also occur. Neurotoxic effects may be irreversible
Ototoxicity	High-frequency hearing loss and tinnitus
Hypersensitivity	Facial edema, wheezing, bronchospasm, and hypotension within minutes of drug exposure
Hepatic	Transient increases in LFTs
Gustatory	Dygeusia (metallic taste) and loss of appetite

Chu E, DeVita VT Jr, eds. Physicians' Cancer Chemotherapy Drug Manual 2003. Sudbury, MA: Jones and Bartlett, pp. 85–90
Thigpen JT et al. Gynecol Oncol 1986;23:101–104

Treatment Modifications

Adverse Event	Dose Modification
Serum creatinine ≥1.7 mg/dL (150 μmol/L)	Hold treatment until creatinine returns to pretreatment level, then reduce cisplatin dosage in subsequent cycles by 50%
G3/4 Ototoxicity	Hold treatment until ≤G2, then reduce cisplatin dosage in subsequent cycles by 50%
G3/4 Neurotoxicity	Hold treatment until ≤G2, then reduce cisplatin dosage in subsequent cycles by 50%

Therapy Monitoring

Before each treatment with cisplatin (every 4 weeks): H&P, attention to history and objective findings of neurotoxicity, CBC with differential, LFTs, serum electrolytes, and creatinine

REGIMEN

PACLITAXEL (SINGLE AGENT)

Curtin JP et al. JCO 2001;19:1275–1278

Premedications:
Dexamethasone 20 mg per dose orally or intravenously per push for 2 doses 14 hours and 7 hours before starting paclitaxel
Diphenhydramine 50 mg intravenously per push, 30 minutes before starting paclitaxel
Ranitidine 50 mg intravenously in 25–100 mL of 0.9% NaCl injection (0.9% NS) or 5% dextrose injection (D5W) over 30–60 minutes, 30 minutes before starting paclitaxel
Paclitaxel 170 mg/m^2 by continuous intravenous infusion diluted in 0.9% NS or D5W to a concentration of 0.3–1.2 mg/mL over 24 hours on day 1 every 3 weeks (total dosage/cycle = 170 mg/m^2
Note: Patients who previously received radiation treatment to the pelvis should be treated initially with a paclitaxel dosage of 135 mg/m^2. This may be increased according to the guidelines under dose modification

Emetogenic potential: Low (Emetogenicity score = 2). See Chapter 39 for antiemetic regimens

Patient Population Studied

A study of 42 patients with advanced nonsquamous cell cervical cancer who had either no benefit from or progressive disease on standard chemotherapy

Efficacy

Complete response	9.5%
Partial response	21.5%
Median duration of response	4.8 months

Toxicity (N = 42)

	No. of Patients				
	G0	G1	G2	G3	G4
Hematologic					
Leukopenia	5	3	11	16	7
Neutropenia	7	1	3	5	26
Thrombocytopenia	35	5	1	1	0
Anemia	21	7	10	4	0
Nonhematologic					
Nausea/vomiting	28	7	7	0	0
Gastrointestinal	31	5	5	0	1
Alopecia	16	7	19	0	0
Neurotoxicity	28	4	9	1	0
Edema	41	0	0	1	0

*The table identifies only toxicities in which at least one patient experienced a G3 or G4 toxicity

Other Toxicities

Febrile neutropenia	8 patients
Alopecia	26 patients
Mucositis	2 patients
Myalgias and arthralgias	Infrequent
Bradycardia grade 2	Incidence not specified

Treatment Modifications

Paclitaxel dosage levels:
110 mg/m^2 (minimum dosage)
135 mg/m^2
170 mg/m^2
200 mg/m^2 (maximum dosage)

Adverse Event	Dose Modification*
ANC <1500/mm^3	Hold treatment until ANC ≥1500/mm^3
Platelet count <100,000/mm^3	Hold treatment until platelets ≥100,000/mm^3
G1 Hematologic toxicity	Increase paclitaxel dosage by 1 level
G2/3 Hematologic toxicity	Administer same paclitaxel dosage
G4 Hematologic toxicity	Decrease paclitaxel dosage by 1 level
G2 Nonobstructive renal toxicity	Decrease paclitaxel dosage by 1 level
G3 hepatic toxicity	
G3 mucositis	
G4 GOG nonhematologic toxicity	

*Based on adverse events during previous cycles

Therapy Monitoring

Before each treatment: H&P, attention to history and objective findings of neurotoxicity, CBC with differential, LFTs, electrolytes, and creatinine

REGIMEN

CISPLATIN + FLUOROURACIL + RADIATION THERAPY

Roberts WS et al. Gynecol Oncol 1991;43:233–236

Cisplatin 50 mg/m^2 single dose intravenously in 100–1000 mL 0.9% NaCl injection (0.9% NS), over 6 hours on day 1 every 4 weeks for 2 cycles (total dosage/4-week cycle = 50 mg/m^2), *followed by:*
Fluorouracil 1000 mg/m^2 per day as a continuous intravenous infusion in 250–2000 mL 0.9% NS or 5% dextrose injection (D5W) over 24 hours on days 1–4 every 4 weeks for 2 cycles (total dosage/4-week cycle = 4000 mg/m^2)
Radiation therapy concurrent with chemotherapy:
External-beam radiation with 20-MeV linear accelerator, 180-cGy/day fractions to a total of 4000–5000 cGy to the whole pelvis ± periaortic radiation to a dose of 3600–4500 cGy

±

Additional external pelvic irradiation to limited fields to a total dose of 6480 cGy

±

Additional brachytherapy starting 2–3 weeks after external-beam radiation

Regimen for Delayed Diarrhea[1, 2]***:***
Loperamide 2 mg, administer orally every 2 h during waking hours (4 mg orally every 4 hours during hours of sleep). Continue for at least 12 h after diarrhea resolves
If diarrhea persists >48 h despite loperamide: Stop loperamide and hospitalize patient for IV hydration
For Persistent Diarrhea:
Octreotide 100–150 micrograms, administer subcutaneously 3-times-daily. Maximum total daily dose = 1500 micrograms
Antibiotic Therapy:
Ciprofloxacin 500 mg, administer orally twice daily, if absolute neutrophil count <500/mm^3 (even in the absence of fever or diarrhea), or patient is febrile in association with diarrhea. Antibiotics should also be administered if patient is hospitalized with prolonged diarrhea, and should be continued until diarrhea resolves[1]

[1]Rothenberg ML, et al. J Clin Oncol 2001; 19:3801–7
[2]Wadler S, et al. J Clin Oncol 1998; 16:3169–78

Emetogenic potential:
Day 1: High (Emetogenicity score ≥6)
Days 2–4: Low (Emetogenicity score ≥2). Potential for delayed symptoms after day 1. See Chapter 39 for antiemetic regimens

Patient Population Studied

A study of 67 patients with advanced carcinomas of the lower female genital tract, among whom 7 had vaginal cancers

Efficacy*

Complete clinical response (all histologies)	85%
Partial response (all histologies)	9%
Stable disease (all histologies)	3%

*Not stated for the subset of patients with vaginal cancer. However, 3 of 7 patients with vaginal cancer had no recurrence and no failure of treatment for a median follow-up of 13 months

Toxicity

Acute	
Neutropenia and thrombocytopenia	1 patient[a]
Radiation enteritis	5 patients[b]
Nausea, vomiting, and diarrhea	Very common
Renal, hepatic, or neurologic	Not significant
Delayed	
Rectovaginal fistula	3 patients[c]
Radiation proctitis	1 patient[c]
Small bowel fistula	2 patients[c]
Soft tissue necrosis	2 patients[c]
Hemorrhagic cystitis	1 patient

[a]Resulted in 8- to 14-day treatment delay
[b]Resulted in 8- to >14-day treatment delay
[c]Required surgery

Treatment Modifications

Adverse Event	Dose Modification
Serum creatinine ≥1.7 mg/dL (150 μmol/L)	Hold cisplatin until serum creatinine returns to pretreatment level, then reduce dosage by 50% in subsequent cycles
WBC ≤3000/mm^3 or platelet ≤100,000/mm^3	Delay cisplatin and fluorouracil until WBC ≥3000/mm^3 and platelet count ≥100,000/mm^3
>2-week delay in start of cycle	Reduce cisplatin and fluorouracil dosages by 50% each
G3/4 Hematologic toxicity	Hold radiation therapy until hematologic toxicity is ≤2
G ≥ RT-related toxicity	Hold RT, and resume RT when toxicity is G ≤ 2

Roberts WS et al. Gynecol Oncol 1991;43:233–236
Whitney CW et al. JCO 1999;17:1339–1348. Used a similar regimen for patients with cervical cancer; 91% completed both chemotherapy courses and had similar completion rates for radiation therapy

Therapy Monitoring

Weekly: CBC with differential, LFTs, electrolytes, and creatinine

SECTION II. Supportive Care, Drug Preparation, Complications, and Screening

39. Chemotherapy-Induced Nausea and Vomiting: Prophylaxis and Treatment

Thomas E. Hughes, PharmD, BCOP

Pathophysiology of Chemotherapy-Induced Nausea and Vomiting (CINV)

Neurotransmitters and the receptor targets

- Serotonin and the serotonin type 3 (5-HT_3) receptor
- Dopamine and the dopamine type 2 receptor
- Substance P and the neurokinin-1 or NK_1 receptor
- Histamine, acetylcholine, opiates, and their respective receptors

Two Phases of CINV

Acute phase

- Occurs in first 24 hours and is mediated by release of serotonin from enterochromaffin cells within GI tract
- Actual time of onset varies depending on the chemotherapeutic agent

Delayed phase

- Substance P and the NK_1 may be more important than serotonin in delayed CINV[6]
- Delayed CINV was initially described with cisplatin
- Although the onset of delayed emesis was initially defined at 24 hours postchemotherapy, more recent evidence suggests that referable symptoms may occur as early as 16 hours after cisplatin
- The incidence of delayed vomiting after cisplatin is greatest during the 24-hour period from 48 to 72 hours after treatment and progressively declines[5,6]
- Delayed CINV has also been described with a number of other chemotherapeutic agents, including carboplatin, cyclophosphamide, and the anthracyclines[6]

Anticipatory Nausea and Vomiting

- Occurs with poor emetic control with prior administration of chemotherapy
- Prevention is best approach
- Pharmacologic interventions are usually not successful, but behavioral methods with systematic desensitization is effective and has been used with some success[5]

Antiemetic Principles

- 5-HT_3-receptor antagonists are equally effective at equivalent doses. In general, they can be used interchangeably based on convenience, availability, and cost
- The lowest established proven dose of each 5-HT_3-receptor antagonist should be used
- Single-dose prophylactic regimens of 5-HT_3-receptor antagonists and corticosteroids for acute phase CINV prophylaxis are effective and preferred
- At biologically equivalent doses, oral antiemetic regimens are equivalent to intravenous antiemetic regimens
- All patients receiving chemotherapy should have antiemetics available on a PRN basis for breakthrough nausea and vomiting. The rescue agent should be selected to compliment and not duplicate the prophylactic regimen (ie, use a different pharmacologic class)
- For acute CINV prophylaxis, a regimen that includes a 5-HT_3-receptor antagonist and a corticosteroid is preferred for moderate to high emetic potential chemotherapy (emetic incidence of 30–90%)
- A corticosteroid alone is the recommended prophylactic regimen for low or intermediate emetic potential chemotherapy (emetic incidence of 10–30%)

Table 39–1. Antiemetic Pharmacologic Classes and Class Side Effects

Pharmacologic Class	Generic Name (Trade Name) [US FDA-approved]	Side-Effect Profile[12,16–21]
5-HT_3-receptor antagonists	Dolasetron (Anzemet®) Granisetron (Kytril®) Ondansetron (Zofran®) Palonesetron (Aloxi®)	Headache [C] Constipation [I] Lightheadedness or dizziness [I] Diarrhea [I] Transient elevations in liver enzymes [I] *ECG interval changes:* Prolongation of PR, QTc, and JT and widening of QRS (especially dolasetron) [R]
Corticosteroids	Dexamethasone (Decadron®) Methylprednisolone (Solu-Medrol®)	Hyperglycemia Mood changes Increased appetite Diarrhea Perineal irritation with rapid IV administration of dexamethasone Fluid retention
NK_1-receptor antagonists	Aprepitant (Emend®)	In randomized trials, side effects similar with or without aprepitant
Dopaminergic antagonists: Phenothiazines	Chlorpromazine (Thorazine®) Perphenazine (Trilafon®) Prochlorperazine (Compazine®) Promethazine (Phenergan®) Thiethylperazine (Torecan®)	Extrapyramidal side effects[a] Sedation Anticholinergic effects Hypotension with rapid IV administration Hypersensitivity Hepatotoxicity Cholestatic jaundice Leukopenia and agranulocytosis Hormonal dysfunction Neuroleptic malignant syndrome[b] Cardiovascular effects[c]
Dopaminergic antagonists: Butyrophenones	Droperidol (Inapsine®) Haloperidol (Haldol®)	Extrapyramidal side effects[a] Sedation Agitation Dizziness Chills Hallucinations Hypotension or hypertension Prolongation of ECG intervals (QT prolongation) Arrhythmias (eg, torsades de pointes)
Substituted benzamides	Metoclopramide (Reglan®) Trimethobenzamide (Tigan®)	Sedation Diarrhea Extrapyramidal side effects[a] Neuroleptic malignant syndrome[b] Hypotension Arrhythmias
Benzodiazepines	Lorazepam (Ativan®) Alprazolam (Xanax®)	Sedation Lethargy Weakness Impaired coordination

Table 39–1. *(continued)*

Pharmacologic Class	Generic Name (Trade Name) [US FDA-approved]	Side-Effect Profile[12,16–21]
Cannabinoids	Dronabinol (Marinol®)	Mood changes Memory loss Euphoria Dysphoria Hallucinations Sedation Paranoid ideation Ataxia Motor incoordination Blurred vision Hunger Cardiovascular effects[d] Syncope
Anticholinergics	Scopolamine (Transderm-Scop®)	Dry mouth Somnolence Sedation Constipation

C, common; I, infrequent; R, rare. For other agents, order of frequency is less clear

[a]Extrapyramidal side effects: Akathisia, tardive dyskinesia, parkinsonism, oculogyric crisis, torticollis

[b]Neuroleptic malignant syndrome: Hyperthermia, severe extrapyramidal dysfunction (eg, severe hypertonicity of skeletal muscles), altered mental status and/or level of consciousness, and autonomic instability

[c]Phenothiazine cardiovascular effects include hypotension, syncope, hypertension, bradycardia, and various ECG changes (nonspecific, reversible Q- and T-wave abnormalities). Cases of sudden death have also been reported, presumably secondary to verntricular arrhythmias

[d]The cardiovascular adverse effects of dronabinol are inconsistent but the following have been reported during therapy: hypotension, hypertension, syncope, tachycardia, palpitations, vasodilation, and facial flush

Table 39–2. Pharmacokinetic Parameters of 5-HT$_3$-Receptor Antagonists[16–20]

Parameter	Ondansetron (0.15 mg/kg IV)	Granisetron (40 mcg/kg IV)	Dolasetron[a] (1.8 mg/kg IV)	Palonosetron (10 mcg/kg IV)
Half-life (hour)	4.0[b]	8.95[b]	7.5[b]	40[c]
Protein binding	70–76%	65%	69–77%	62%
Oral bioavailability	56%	60%	75%	NR
Metabolism CYP isoenzymes	Hepatic 3A4 (major), 2D6, 1A2	Hepatic 3A4	Hepatic 2D6 (major), 3A4 (minor)	Hepatic 2D6 (major), 3A4, 1A2
Urinary excretion (parent compound)	5%	12%	67%	40%
Decreased clearance in elderly Dosage adjustment in elderly	Yes No	Yes No	No No	No No
Decreased clearance in hepatic dysfunction Dosage adjustment in hepatic dysfunction	Yes Yes (severe)	Yes No	No (IV); yes (PO) No	No No
Decreased clearance in renal dysfunction Dosage adjustment in renal dysfunction	Yes No	No No	Yes No	Yes No

[a]Dolasetron is rapidly converted to the active metabolite hydrodolasetron. All reported parameters refer to hydrodolasetron

[b]Data from cancer patients

[c]Data from studies in healthy volunteers

Table 39–3. Classification of Emetic Risk[5,9,15]

Method of Risk Classification

Identify the agent of highest emetic risk and determine the antiemetic regimen based on this agent

or

For combination chemotherapy regimens, use the following algorithm:

1. Identify the most emetogenic agent in the combination
2. Assess the relative contribution of other agents to the emetogenicity of the combination as follows:
   - Level 1 agents do not contribute to the emetogenicity of a given regimen
   - Adding one or more level 2 agents increases the emetogenicity of the combination by 1 level above that of the most emetogenic agent in the combination
   - Adding level 3 or 4 agents increases emetogenicity of the combination by 1 level per agent

Emetic Potential	Chemotherapy Drug	
High [level 5]/frequency of emesis >90%	Carmustine (>250 mg/m²) Cisplatin (≥50 mg/m²) Cyclophosphamide (>1500 mg/m²) Dacarbazine	Lomustine (>60 mg/m²) Mechlorethamine Streptozotocin
Moderately high [level 4]/ frequency of emesis 60–90%	Busulfan (>4 mg/day) Carboplatin Carmustine (≤250 mg/m²) Cisplatin (<50 mg/m²) Cyclophosphamide (750–1500 mg/m²) Cytarabine (>1 g/m²) Dactinomycin (>1.5 mg/m²)	Doxorubicin (>60 mg/m²) Epirubicin (>90 mg/m²) Melphalan (IV) Methotrexate (>1 g/m²) Mitoxantrone (>15 mg/m²) Procarbazine
Moderate [level 3]/frequency of emesis 30–60%	Aldesleukin (IL-2) Altretamine Arsenic trioxide Cyclophosphamide (<750 mg/m²) Dactinomycin (≤1.5 mg/m²) Daunorubicin Doxorubicin (20–60 mg/m²) Epirubicin (≤90 mg/m²) Idarubicin	Ifosfamide Irinotecan Lomustine (<60 mg/m²) Methotrexate (250–1000 mg/m²) Mitoxantrone (≤15 mg/m²) Oxaliplatin Pentostatin Plicamycin
Low [level 2]/frequency of emesis 10–30%	Asparaginase Capecitabine Cytarabine (<1 g/m²) Daunorubicin (liposomal) Docetaxel Doxorubicn (<20 mg/m²) Doxorubicin (liposomal) Etoposide Fluorouracil (<1000 mg/m²)	Gemcitabine Methotrexate (50–250 mg/m²) Mitomycin Paclitaxel Temozolamide Teniposide Thiotepa Topotecan
Nonemetogenic [level 1]/ frequency of emesis <10%	Bleomycin Busulfan (oral, <4 mg/kg) Chlorambucil Cladribine Fludarabine Hydroxyurea	Interferon alfa Melphalan (oral) Mercaptopurine Methotrexate (<50 mg/m²) Thioguanine Vinca alkaloids

Hesketh PJ et al. JCO 1997;15(1):103–109

Table 39–4. Antiemetic Regimens for Prophylaxis of CINV (Adults)[a]

Acute Nausea Vomiting (First 24 hours)	Delayed Nausea/Vomiting (Days 2–5)[b]	Comments
Emetic Potential: High [Level 5]/Frequency of Emesis >90%		
Cisplatin regimens 5-HT_3 antagonist + corticosteroid + aprepitant (all as single dose 30–60 minutes before chemotherapy) *Noncisplatin regimens* 5-HT_3 antagonist + corticosteroid ± aprepitant (all as single dose 30–60 minutes before chemotherapy)	*Cisplatin regimens* 1. Aprepitant + corticosteroid 2. One of the noncisplatin regimens *Noncisplatin regimens* 1. Aprepitant + corticosteroid (if aprepitant used on day 1) 2. Corticosteroid (single agent) 3. Metoclopramide + corticosteroid 4. 5-HT_3 antagonist + corticosteroid	1. Aprepitant is an inhibitor and/or inducer of a number of cytochrome p450 isoenzymes (e.g. CYP3A4, CYP2C9, CYP2D6). The patient's chemotherapy and concomitant drug therapy regimen should be screened for potential drug interactions. The addition of aprepitant to a combination antiemetic regimen adds significant expense and so its use should be reserved to those patients most likely to benefit. 2. Corticosteroids should NOT be used with regimens containing aldeslekin (IL-2)
Emetic Potential: Moderately High [Level 4]/Frequency of Emesis 60–90%		
5-HT_3 antagonist + corticosteroid ± aprepitant (all as single dose 30–60 minutes before chemotherapy)	1. Aprepitant + corticosteroid (if aprepitant used on day 1) 2. Corticosteroid (single agent) 3. Metoclopramide + corticosteroid 4. 5-HT_3 antagonist + corticosteroid 5. #1–#4 without corticosteroid	See level 5 comments
Emetic Potential: Moderate [Level 3]/Frequency of Emesis 30–60%		
5-HT_3 antagonist + corticosteroid	1. Corticosteroid (single agent) 2. Metoclopramide + corticosteroid 3. 5-HT_3 antagonist + corticosteroid	1. See level 5 comments 2. Aprepitant can be considered for risk level 3 regimens, particularly in refractory patients
Emetic Potential: Low [Level 2]/Frequency of Emesis 10–30%		
1. Corticosteroid (single dose 30 minutes before chemotherapy) 2. Dopaminergic antagonist (single dose 30 minutes before chemotherapy) *Note:* Antiemetic premedication often not necessary	Not necessary	Dopaminergic antagonists include: prochlorperazine, chlorpromazine, haloperidol, thiethylperazine, metoclopramide, perphenazine, and promethazine.
Emetic Potential: Nonemetogenic [Level 1]/Frequency of Emesis <10%		
Antiemetic premedication usually not necessary	Not necessary	See level 5 comments

[a]See Table 39–3 for emetic risk classification of chemotherapy agents and regimens. See Table 39–5 for dosing recommendations for antiemetic agents
[b]Agents associated with **delayed CINV** include cisplatin, carboplatin, cyclophosphamide, anthracyclines (eg, doxorubicin, epirubicin) and combinations including these agents

Table 39–5. Dosing Recommendations for CINV Prophylaxis (Adults) for Moderate to Highly Emetic Chemotherapy (Levels 3–5)[5,7–12,19]

Agent	Acute CINV Prophylaxis (Day 1) (Single dose given 30 minutes before chemotherapy)[a]		Delayed CINV Prophylaxis (Days 2–5)[b]	Tablet/Capsule Size for Oral Administration
	Oral (PO)	Intravenous (IV)		
5-HT_3 Receptor Antagonists				
Dolasetron (Anzemet)	100–200 mg PO	100 mg or 1.8 mg/kg IV	100–200 mg PO daily × 2–4 days	50 mg, 100 mg
Granisetron (Kytril)	2 mg PO	10 mcg/kg IV	1 mg PO twice daily × 2–4 days	1 mg
Ondansetron (Zofran)	24 mg PO	8 mg or 0.15 mg/kg IV	8 mg PO twice daily × 2–4 days	4 mg, 8 mg, 24 mg
Palonosetron (Aloxi)	NA	0.25 mg IV	NA	
Because of its extended half-life, palonosetron should be given only on day 1. Repeat doses within a 7-day interval are not recommended. Efficacy in prevention of delayed CINV has been demonstrated after the day 1 dose in moderately emetogenic chemotherapy				
Corticosteroids				
Dexamethasone (Decadron)	8–20 mg PO	8–20 mg IV	4–8 mg PO twice daily × 2–4 days	Variety
Methylprednisolone (Solu-Medrol)	NA	40–125 mg IV	NA	NA
When combined with aprepitant, IV doses of dexamethasone should be reduced by 25% and PO doses of dexamethasone reduced by 50%.				
NK_1-Receptor Antagonists				
Aprepitant (Emend)	125 mg PO	NA	80 mg PO daily × 2 days	80 mg, 125 mg
Aprepitant has only been evaluated in single-day chemotherapy regimens and is therefore recommended to be given for 2 days following chemotherapy (days 2 and 3). If used in a multiple-day chemotherapy regimen, longer durations may be indicated, although durations >5 days have not been studied				
Substituted Benzamide				
Metoclopramide (Reglan)	NA	*Prechemotherapy:* 2–3 mg/kg IV, then every 2–4 hours	20–40 mg (or 0.5 mg/kg) PO 4 times daily × 2–4 days	5 mg, 10 mg
Metoclopramide is not a first-line agent for acute CINV prophylaxis and should be reserved for refractory patients. Multiple-dose regimens are required, and concomitant use of diphenhydramine or benztropine are usually required to prevent extrapyramidal side effects				

NA, not applicable

[a]For chemotherapy /biologic regimens in which emetogenic agents are given either multiple times within the same day or by continuous IV infusions, alternative multiple-dose antiemetic regimens may be indicated

[b]Delayed CINV has been associated with cisplatin, carboplatin, cyclophosphamide, and anthracyclines (eg, doxorubicin, epirubicin)

Table 39–6. Antiemetics for Treatment of Chemotherapy-Induced Nausea and Vomiting (Adults)

Agents	Dosage Form [Tablet/Capsule/Suppository Sizes]	Dosages, Routes, and Schedules
Dopaminergic Antagonists: Phenothiazines		
Chlorpromazine (Thorazine®, others)	Tablets [25 mg, 50 mg]	25–50 mg PO q4–6h
	Injection	25–50 mg IVPB/IM q4–6h1
Perphenazine (Trilafon®)	Tablets [2 mg, 4 mg]	2–4 mg PO q8h
Prochlorperazine (Compazine®, others)	Tablets [5 mg, 10 mg, 25 mg]	5–20 mg PO q4–6h
	Suppositories [2.5 mg, 10 mg, 25 mg]	25 mg PR q4–6h
	Injection	5–20 mg IVPB/IM q4–6h[a]
Promethazine (Phenergan®)	Tablets [25 mg, 50 mg]	12.5–25 mg PO q4–6h
	Suppositories [12.5 mg, 25 mg, 50 mg]	12.5–25 mg PR q4–6h
	Injection	12.5–25 mg IV q4–6h[b]

[a]Rapid intravenous administration may induce hypotension. Administer by slow intravenous infusion (eg, 30 minutes)
[b]Promethazine injection is an irritant. Use caution with intravenous administration, particularly during administration into a peripheral vein. Dilution with IVPB administration may be considered to reduce irritation

Agents	Dosage Form [Tablet/Capsule/Suppository Sizes]	Dosages, Routes, and Schedules
Dopaminergic Antagonists: Butyrophenones		
Haloperidol (Haldol®, others)	Tablets [variety]	1–4 mg PO q6h
	Injection	1–4 mg IVPB/IM q6h
Substituted Benzamide		
Metoclopramide (Reglan®, others)	Tablets [5 mg, 10 mg]	20–40 mg (0.5 mg/kg) PO q6h
	Injection	20–40 mg (0.5 mg/kg) IV q6h[c]

[c]Higher doses of metoclopramide have been used for prophylaxis of CINV for highly emetic chemotherapy

Agents	Dosage Form [Tablet/Capsule/Suppository Sizes]	Dosages, Routes, and Schedules
Corticosteroids		
Dexamethasone	Tablets/oral solution [variety]	4–10 mg PO q6–12h
	Injection	4–10 mg IV q6–12h
Methylprednisolone	Injection	20–125 mg IV/IM q6h
Benzodiazepines[d]		
Alprazolam (Xanax®)	Tablets [0.25 mg, 0.5 mg, 1 mg, 2 mg]	0.125–0.5 mg PO q8h
Lorazepam (Ativan®)	Tablets [0.5 mg, 1 mg, 2 mg]	0.5–1 mg PO q6–12h
	Injection	0.5–1 mg IV q6–12h

[d]Benzodiazepines lack intrinsic antiemetic effects and should not be used as single agents against emetogenic chemotherapy

Agents	Dosage Form [Tablet/Capsule/Suppository Sizes]	Dosages, Routes, and Schedules
Cannabinoids		
Dronabinol (Marinol®)	Capsules [2.5 mg, 5 mg, 10 mg]	2.5–10 mg PO q6h

IM, intramuscularly; IVPB, intravenously by piggyback; PO, orally; PR by rectum

References

1. Gralla RJ. New agents, new treatment, and antiemetic therapy. Semin Oncol 2002;29:119–124
2. Griffin AM et al. On the receiving end. V: Patient perceptions of the side effects of cancer chemotherapy in 1993. Ann Oncol 1996;7:189–195
3. Poli-Bigelli S et al. Addition of the neurokinin 1 receptor antagonist aprepitant to standard antiemetic therapy improves control of chemotherapy-induced nausea and vomiting. Cancer 2003;97:3090-8
4. Hesketh PJ et al. The oral neurokinin-1 antagonist aprepitant for the prevention of chemotherapy-induced nausea and vomiting: a multinational, randomized, double-blind, placebo-controlled trial in patients receiving high-dose cisplatin–the aprepitant protocol 052 study group. JCO 2003;21:4112–4119
5. Anon. ASHP therapeutic guidelines on the pharmacologic management of nausea and vomiting in adult and pediatric patients receiving chemotherapy or radiation therapy or undergoing surgery. Am J Health-Syst Pharm 1999;56(15):729–764
6. Kris MG et al. Delayed emesis following anticancer chemotherapy. Support Care Cancer 1998;6:228–232
7. Gralla RJ et al. Recommendations for the use of antiemetics: evidence-based, clinical practice guidelines. JCO 1999;17:2971–2994
8. Anon. NCCN Antiemesis Practice Guidelines. Oncology 1997;11(11A): 57–89
9. Ettinger DS et al. Antiemesis. National Comprehensive Cancer Network (NCCN) Clinical Practice Guidelines in Oncology, version 2.2003; www.nccn.org
10. Anon. Prevention of chemotherapy- and radiotherapy-induced emesis: results of the Perugia Consensus Conference. Ann Oncol 1998;9:811–819
11. Koeller JM et al. Antiemetic guidelines: creating a more practical treatment approach. Support Care Cancer 2002;10:519–522
12. Emend (Aprepitant) [package insert]. Whitehouse Station, NJ: Merck & Co., Inc, March 2003
13. Eisenberg P et al. Improved prevention of moderately emetogenic chemotherapy-induced nausea and vomiting with palonosetron, a pharmacologically novel 5-HT_3 receptor antagonist. Cancer 2003;98:2473–2482
14. Gralla R et al. Palonosetron improves prevention of chemotherapy-induced nausea and vomiting following moderately emetogenic chemotherapy: results of a double-blind randomized phase III trial comparing single doses of palonosetron with ondansetron. Ann Oncol 2003;14:1570–1577
15. Hesketh PJ et al. Proposal for classifying the acute emetogenicity of cancer chemotherapy. JCO 1997;15:103–109
16. Zofran (Ondansetron) [package insert]. Research Triangle Park, NC: GlaxoSmithKline, April 2002
17. Kytril (Granisetron) [package insert]. Nutley, NJ: Roche Laboratories, Inc, August 2002
18. Anzemet (Dolasetron) [package insert]. Kansas City, MO: Aventis Pharmaceuticals. October 2003
19. Aloxi (Palonosetron) [package insert]. Bloomington, MN: MGI Pharma, Inc, July 2003
20. DiVall MV, Cersosimo RJ. Palonosetron, a novel 5-HT_3 receptor antagonist for chemotherapy-associated nausea and vomiting. Formulary 2003;38:414–430
21. Graves Davidson T. Causes and prevention of chemotherapy-induced emesis. Philadelphia: Medical Education Systems, Inc, 1996;34–35

40. Drug Preparation and Administration

David R. Kohler, PharmD

The following tables describe appropriate handling and storage, and drug product preparation and administration procedures for antineoplastics and other selected medications (so-called chemoprotectants and rescue agents) that are approved by the US Food and Drug Administration (FDA) for commercial use. The tables describe drug use under a variety of commonly encountered conditions, but do not identify all applications or conditions of product stability and compatibility. Clinicians are referred to product labeling for more complete information about individual products and to up-to-date focused reference sources for information about drug compatibility and stability. Likewise, the tables are not an exhaustive list of all marketed products and should not be construed as an endorsement of any manufacturer or as discriminating against products that were not specifically identified.

The information contained in this chapter is derived from contemporary product labeling and, in some cases, from published studies and personal communications with pharmaceutical manufacturers

Key to Abbreviations

0.45% NaCl	0.45% Sodium Chloride Injection, USP
0.9% NS	0.9% Sodium Chloride Injection, USP
3% NaCl	3% Sodium Chloride Injection [hypertonic]
AUC	Area under the concentration versus time curve
B0.9% NS	Bacteriostatic (antimicrobially preserved) 0.9% Sodium Chloride Injection
BWFI	Bacteriostatic Water for Injection, USP
CSF	Cerebrospinal fluid
D10W	10% Dextrose Injection, USP
D2.5W	2.5% Dextrose Injection, USP
D5W	5% Dextrose Injection, USP
D5W/0.2% NaCl	5% Dextrose and 0.20% Sodium Chloride Injection, USP
D5W/0.33% NaCl	5% Dextrose and 0.33% Sodium Chloride Injection, USP
D5W/0.45% NaCl	5% Dextrose and 0.45% Sodium chloride Injection, USP
D5W/0.9% NS	5% Dextrose and 0.9% Sodium chloride Injection, USP
D5W/LR	5% Dextrose Injection in Lactated Ringer's Injection, USP
D5W/RI	5% Dextrose Injection in Ringer's Injection, USP
DEHP	di-2-ethylhexyl phthalate (a plasticizing ingredient commonly used in flexible PVC containers)
LRI	Lactated Ringer's Injection, USP
PICC	Peripherally inserted central catheter
PK	Pharmacokinetic
PVC	Polyvinyl chloride
Q.S.	*Quantum suficiat or quantum satis* [Latin]: "As much as is sufficient"
RI	Ringer's Injection, USP
SICC	Subclavian-inserted central catheter
SWFI	Sterile Water for Injection, USP
VAD	Vascular access device (eg, catheter, port, other cannula)

ALDESLEUKIN

PROLEUKIN® Aldesleukin for injection product label, September 2000. Chiron Therapeutics, Emeryville, CA

Trissel LA. Handbook on Injectable Drugs, 13th ed. Bethesda: American Society of Health-System Pharmacists, Inc, 2005

Product Identification, Preparation, Storage, and Stability

- PROLEUKIN® is packaged in single-use vials containing 22 million International units, which is equivalent to 1.3 mg of aldesleukin protein. NDC 53905-991-01
- Store intact vials and reconstituted and diluted aldesleukin under refrigeration at 2°–8°C (35.6°–46.4°F). Protect from light. Do not freeze aldesleukin
- *Reconstitute* each vial with 1.2 mL SWFI to produce a clear, colorless to slightly yellow solution with a concentration = 18 million International units aldesleukin (1.1 mg of protein)/mL
- During reconstitution, direct the stream of SWFI at the side wall of a vial rather than directly into the drug powder and gently swirl vials to avoid excessive foaming
- *Do not shake* vials to dissolve aldesleukin
- For intravenous administration, dilute aldesleukin only with D5W to a final concentration between 0.5 and 1.1 million International units/mL (30–70 mcg/mL; see chart below). Drug delivery may be adversely affected by aldesleukin concentrations <30 mcg/mL or >70 mcg/mL

Aldesleukin (million International units)	Diluent Volume (D5W)
5–11	10 mL
7.5–16.5	15 mL
12.5–27.5	25 mL
25–55	50 mL
50–110	100 mL

- If it is necessary to administer aldesleukin in a concentration <30 mcg/mL, the drug should be diluted in D5W that contains Albumin Human, USP in a concentration of 0.1% (1 mg/mL)
- Either glass bottles or PVC bags are acceptable containers for aldesleukin, but plastic containers provide for more consistent drug delivery than glass containers
- Reconstituted and diluted aldesleukin solutions are stable for up to 48 hours at 2°–25°C (35.6°–77°F), but the PROLEUKIN® product does not contain a preservative. Store reconstituted and diluted solutions under refrigeration

Selected incompatibility:

- *Do not combine* aldesleukin with other drugs in the same container
- *Do not reconstitute or dilute* aldesleukin with 0.9% NS or antimicrobially preserved diluents, which may increase protein aggregation

Recommendations for Drug Administration and Ancillary Care

General:

- Bring the solution to room temperature before administration
- Administer aldesleukin by intravenous infusion over 15 minutes
- *Do not filter* aldesleukin
- Complete administration within 48 hours after reconstitution

ALEMTUZUMAB

CamPath® (alemtuzumab) product label, November 2004. Manufactured by ILEX Pharmaceuticals, L.P., San Antonio, TX. Distributed by BERLEX®, Montville, NJ

Product Identification, Preparation, Storage, and Stability

- CamPath® is packaged in glass single-use vials containing 30 mg alemtuzumab/mL. NDC 50419-357-03 (3 vials/carton). NDC 50419-357-01 (single vial)
- Store intact vials under refrigeration at 2°–8°C (35.6°–46.4°F) and protect them from direct sunlight
- *Do not freeze* alemtuzumab. Discard any vials that have been frozen
- *Do not shake* the vials before use
  - Withdraw from a vial into a syringe an amount of alemtuzumab needed to prepare a patient's dose
  - Inject the amount of drug needed to prepare a patient's dose into (Q.S.) 100 mL 0.9% NS or D5W in a plastic parenteral product container
  - Gently invert the bag to mix the solution
- Diluted alemtuzumab solutions may be stored at room temperature (15°–30°C; 59°–86°F) or refrigerated
- The CamPath® product contains no antimicrobial preservatives. Use the product within 8 hours after dilution

Selected incompatibility:

- None has been observed between alemtuzumab and PVC bags, PVC- or polyethylene-lined PVC administration sets, or low-protein binding filters
- No data are available concerning the compatibility of alemtuzumab with other drugs. Do not add or simultaneously infuse other drugs through the same intravenous line with alemtuzumab

Recommendations for Drug Administration and Ancillary Care

General:

- Administer alemtuzumab only by intravenous infusion over ≥2 hours
- Do not administer alemtuzumab by intravenous push or bolus injection

Recommended dose escalation:

- Alemtuzumab administration can result in serious infusion reactions. Gradual escalation to the recommended maintenance dose/schedule is required when initiating therapy and after treatment interruptions ≥7 days. In most cases, escalation to a 30 mg dose can be accomplished in 3–7 days as follows:
  (1) Initiate treatment with alemtuzumab 3 mg intravenously over 2 hours
  (2) After a 3 mg DAILY dose is tolerated (eg, infusion-related toxicities are grade ≤ 2), escalate DAILY dose to 10 mg/day and continue until tolerated
  (3) After a 10 mg *daily* dose is tolerated, escalate to a maintenance dose and schedule of alemtuzumab 30 mg/dose on 3 nonconsecutive days for 3 doses per week (eg, Monday, Wednesday, and Friday) for up to 12 weeks

Concomitant medications:

- Give premedication 30 minutes before the first alemtuzumab dose, before dose escalations, and as clinically indicated, with:
  (1) Diphenhydramine 50 mg orally or intravenously
  (2) Acetaminophen 650 mg orally
- Treat severe infusion-related events with:
  (1) Hydrocortisone 200 mg intravenously
- Give antimicrobial primary prophylaxis during treatment and continue for at least 2 months after the last alemtuzumab administration or until CD4+ lymphocyte counts are ≥200/mm^3
  (1) Cotrimoxazole (trimethoprim 160 mg + sulfamethoxazole 800 mg) orally, twice daily, 3 days/week
  (2) Famciclovir (or equivalent) 250 mg orally twice daily

AMIFOSTINE

Ethyol® AMIFOSTINE for injection product label, March 2003. MedImmune Oncology, Inc, Gaithersburg, MD

Product Identification, Preparation, Storage, and Stability

- Ethyol® is packaged in 10-mL single-use vials containing 500 mg of anhydrous amifostine as a sterile lyophilized powder. NDC 58178-017-01
- Reconstitute amifostine with 9.7 mL 0.9% NS to produce a solution with concentration = 500 mg amifostine/10 mL
- When reconstituted as recommended, amifostine is chemically stable for up to 5 hours at approximately 25°C (77°F) or up to 24 hours at 2°–8°C (35.6°–46.4°F)
- Amifostine may be further diluted with 0.9% NS to concentrations ranging from 5–40 mg/mL

Selected incompatibility:

- After further dilution in PVC bags with 0.9% NS to concentrations ranging from 5–40 mg/mL amifostine is chemically stable for up to 5 hours when stored at room temperature or for up to 24 hours when stored under refrigeration
- Admixture with solutions other than 0.9% NS with or without other additives is not recommended

Recommendations for Drug Administration and Ancillary Care

General:

- Administer intravenously (see indication-specific recommendations below)
- Provide adequate hydration before amifostine infusion
- Monitor a patient's blood pressure frequently during and immediately after the infusion, and thereafter as clinically indicated
- Keep patients in a supine position during the infusion. Interrupt amifostine infusion if systolic blood pressure (SBP) decreases significantly from baseline as follows:

Baseline SBP (mm Hg)	Decrease in SBP That Warrants Interrupting Amifostine Infusion
<100	20 mm Hg
100–119	25 mm Hg
120–139	30 mm Hg
140–179	40 mm Hg
≥180	50 mm Hg

- If BP returns to normal within 5 minutes and the patient is asymptomatic, resume administration to complete the planned dose
- If the planned dose cannot be administered, decrease the amifostine dosage during subsequent chemotherapy cycles from 910 mg/m^2 to 740 mg/m^2

To reduce cumulative renal toxicity with chemotherapy:

- Administer amifostine 910 mg/m^2 once daily by intravenous infusion over 15 minutes, 30 minutes before chemotherapy
- A 15-minute infusion is better tolerated than longer infusions

To decrease moderate-to-severe xerostomia from head and neck radiation:

- Administer amifostine 200 mg/m^2 once daily by intravenous infusion over 3 minutes, 15–30 minutes before standard-fraction radiation therapy (ie, 1.8–2 Gy/fraction)

ARSENIC TRIOXIDE

TRISENOX® (arsenic trioxide) injection product label, November 2005. Manufactured for Cephalon Inc, Frazer, PA

Product Identification, Preparation, Storage, and Stability

- TRISENOX® is a clear, colorless, preservative-free solution packaged in single-use glass ampules containing 10 mg of arsenic trioxide (1 mg/mL). NDC 60553-111-10 (package of 10 ampules)
- Store intact ampules at 25°C (77°F). Temperature excursions are permitted to 15°–30°C (59°–86°F)
- Dilute arsenic trioxide in 100–250 mL 0.9% NS or D5W before clinical use. Unused drug should be discarded in a manner appropriate for hazardous drugs
- Diluted arsenic trioxide solutions are chemically and physically stable for 24 hours when stored at room temperature and for up to 48 hours under refrigeration

Selected incompatibility:

- Arsenic trioxide should not be mixed with other drugs

Recommendations for Drug Administration and Ancillary Care

General:

- Administer arsenic trioxide by intravenous infusion over 1–2 hours. The duration of administration may be extended to 4 hours for patients who experience acute vasomotor reactions
- QT interval prolongation, premature ventricular contractions, complete AV block, ventricular tachycardia, and torsade de pointes have been observed during clinical use
- 12-lead EKG and serum electrolytes (potassium, calcium, magnesium) and creatinine should be evaluated before initiating therapy with arsenic trioxide. Preexisting electrolyte abnormalities should be corrected and, if possible, drugs that are known to prolong the QT interval should be discontinued
- QTc intervals >500 msec, should be corrected and the QTc reassessed with serial EKGs before beginning arsenic trioxide administration
- Cardiac QT/QTc prolongation should be expected within 1–5 weeks after beginning treatment
- The risk of torsade de pointes is related to the extent of QT prolongation, concomitant administration of QT prolonging drugs, a history of torsade de pointes, preexisting QT interval prolongation, congestive heart failure, administration of potassium-wasting diuretics, and other conditions that result in hypokalemia or hypomagnesemia
- During arsenic trioxide treatment, maintain serum potassium concentrations >4 mmol/L (>4 mEq/L) and magnesium concentrations >0.74 mmol/L (>1.8 mg/dL)
- Patients who reach an absolute QT interval >500 msec should be reassessed and immediate action should be taken to correct concomitant risk factors. The risk-to-benefit of continuing or suspending arsenic trioxide therapy should be reevaluated
- Patients who develop syncope, or rapid or irregular heartbeat should be hospitalized for monitoring, and serum electrolytes assessment. Discontinue arsenic trioxide until the QTc interval regresses to <460 msec, electrolyte abnormalities are corrected, and the syncope and irregular heartbeat cease

ASPARAGINASE

ELSPAR® (ASPARAGINASE) product label, August 2002. Merck & Co, Inc, West Point, PA

Product Identification, Preparation, Storage, and Stability

ELSPAR® is packaged in 10-mL vial containing asparaginase 10,000 International units as a sterile, white lyophilized plug or powder for intravenous or intramuscular injection after reconstitution. NDC 0006-4612-00

- The product's specific activity is at least 225 International units/mg of protein
- Store intact vials under refrigeration at 2°–8°C (35.6°–46.4°F)
- After reconstitution, ELSPAR® is a clear, colorless solution
- Unused, reconstituted asparaginase should be stored at 2°–8°C and discarded after 8 hours or sooner if it becomes cloudy
- Administer asparaginase by either intravenous or intramuscular routes

For intravenous use:

- Reconstitute vials containing asparaginase 10,000 International units with 5 mL SWFI or 0.9% NS. Ordinary shaking during reconstitution does not inactivate the enzyme, but may cause foaming
- Further dilute asparaginase with 0.9% NS or D5W
- Administer asparaginase within 8 hours and only if the solution remains clear
  - (1) Occasionally, a small number of gelatinous fiber-like particles may develop on standing
  - (2) Filtration through a 5-micrometer filter during administration removes the particles with no resultant loss in potency
  - (3) SOME LOSS OF POTENCY has been observed with the use of a 0.2-micrometer filter

For intramuscular use:

- Add 2 mL 0.9% NS to a vial containing asparaginase 10,000 International units asparaginase
- Administer asparaginase within 8 hours and only if the solution remains clear

Recommendations for Drug Administration and Ancillary Care

Intradermal skin test:

- Asparaginase administration is associated with allergic reactions. An intradermal skin test may be performed before initial administration and when asparaginase is given after an interval ≥1 week has elapsed between doses
- Observe a skin test site for at least 1 hour for a wheal or erythema; either sign indicates a positive reaction

Note: A *negative* skin test reaction does not preclude the possibility of an allergic reaction to asparaginase treatment; that is, be wary of false-negative results

Prepare a skin test solution as follows:

1. Reconstitute asparaginase 10,000 International units with 5 mL 0.9% NS
2. From this solution (2000 International units/mL), withdraw 0.1 mL and inject it into a vial containing 9.9 mL 0.9% NS, yielding a skin test solution of approximately 20 International units/mL
3. Inject intradermally 0.1 mL of the skin test solution (about 2 International units)

Note: In patients who demonstrate hypersensitivity by skin testing, and in any patient who previously completed a course of asparaginase, retreatment should be instituted only after successful desensitization

Desensitization should be performed before administering a first dose of asparaginase in positive reactors, and before retreating any patient for whom therapy is deemed necessary

Desensitization:

Clarkson B et al. Cancer 1970;25:279–305
Tallal L et al. Cancer 1970;25:306–320

- Rapid intravenous desensitization may be attempted with progressively increasing amounts of asparaginase if adequate precautions are taken to treat an acute allergic reaction should it occur
- The following schedule begins with a total of 1 International Unit, intravenously, and provided no reaction has occurred, doubles the dose every 10 minutes, until the accumulated total amount given equals the planned dose for that day

Injection Number	Asparaginase Dose (International Units)	Accumulated Total Dose
1	1	1
2	2	3
3	4	7
4	8	15
5	16	31
6	32	63
7	64	127
8	128	255
9	256	511
10	512	1023
11	1024	2047
12	2048	4095
13	4096	8191
14	8192	16,383
15	16,384	32,767
16	32,768	65,535
17	65,536	131,071
18	131,072	262,143

Example: a patient weighing 20 kg who is to receive 4000 International Units would receive desensitization injections 1 through 12

Intravenous administration:

- Infuse over at least 30 minutes through the side arm of a running infusion of 0.9% NS or D5W

Intramuscular administration:

- Limit the volume at a single injection site to ≤2 mL

AZACITIDINE

Vidaza™ (azacitidine for injectable suspension) product label, August 31, 2004. Manufactured by Ben Venue Laboratories, Inc, Bedford, OH. Manufactured for Pharmion Corporation, Boulder, CO

Product Identification, Preparation, Storage, and Stability

Vidaza™ is packaged in single-use vials containing azacitidine 100 mg as a lyophilized powder. NDC 67211-102-01

- Store intact vials at 25°C (77°F); temperature excursions are permitted to 15°–30°C (59°–86°F)
- Reconstitute the lyophilized powder with 4 mL SWFI by slowly injecting the diluent into a vial
- Invert the vial 2–3 times, and gently rotate it until a uniform cloudy suspension is formed. The resulting suspension contains 25 mg azacitidine/mL

Preparation for immediate administration:

1. Divide doses >4 mL equally into 2 syringes
2. Store reconstituted azacitidine suspension for up to 1 hour at 25°C, but the product must be administered within 1 hour after reconstitution

Preparation for delayed administration:

1. The reconstituted product may be kept in the vial or drawn into a syringe
2. Immediately place the product under refrigeration (2°–8°C; 35.6°–46.4°F) where it may be maintained for up to 8 hours

Recommendations for Drug Administration and Ancillary Care

For subcutaneous administration only:

For azacitidine suspension that is not administered immediately after preparation:

1. After removal from refrigeration, allow the suspension to equilibrate to room temperature for up to 30 minutes before administration
2. Re-suspend the product before administration to provide a homogeneous suspension by inverting the product container (vial or syringe) 2–3 times and by gently rolling syringes between the palms for 30 seconds immediately before administration
3. Doses >4 mL should be divided equally into 2 syringes and injected into 2 separate sites. Rotate sites for each injection (thigh, abdomen, or upper arm). New injections should be given at least 1 inch from an old site and never into areas were the site is tender, bruised, red, or hard

BACILLUS CALMETTE-GUÉRIN (BCG)

TheraCys® BCG, LIVE (INTRAVESICAL) product label, October 1999. Manufactured by Aventis Pasteur Limited, Toronto, Ontario, Canada. Manufactured for Aventis Pasteur, Inc, Swiftwater, PA

BCG LIVE (for intravesical use) TICE® BCG product label, July 2002. Manufactured by Organon Teknika Corporation, Durham, NC. Manufactured for Organon, Inc, West Orange, NJ

PACIS® BCG, Live (For Intravesical Use) product label (FDA approval) 9. March, 2000. Manufactured by BioChem Pharma, Inc, Sainte-Foy, Quebec, Canada. Distributed by UroCor, Inc, Oklahoma City, OK

Product Identification, Preparation, Storage, and Stability

- Store BCG and any diluent for reconstitution at 2°–8°C and protected from light

Product-Specific Preparation Instructions

TheraCys® BCG, live:

- The product is packaged in vials containing 81 mg freeze-dried BCG, accompanied by a vial of diluent. NDC 49281-880-01
- Each vial contains $10.5 \pm 8.7 \times 10^8$ colony forming units (CFU) BCG
  (1) Do *not* remove the stopper from the vial
  (2) Add 3 mL of the provided diluent to 1 vial of TheraCys® BCG. Use only the provided diluent to ensure appropriate dispersion
  (3) Shake the vial to produce a homogeneous suspension
  (4) With a syringe, aspirate the suspension from the vial and add it to a syringe containing 50 mL preservative-free 0.9% NS
  (5) Do *not* use TheraCys® BCG that exhibits flocculation or clumping after reconstitution

BCG LIVE (for intravesical use) TICE® BCG:

- The product is packaged in vials containing a lyophilized (freeze-dried) powder. NDC 0052-0602-02
- Each vial contains $1–8 \times 10^8$ CFU, equivalent to 50 mg (wet weight)
  (1) To prepare TICE® BCG suspension, add 1 mL preservative-free 0.9% NS to 1 vial at 4°–25°C (39.2°–77°F)
  (2) *Do not shake* vials after reconstitution. Aggressive agitation may cause mycobacterial clumping. Swirl the vial to produce a homogeneous suspension
  (3) Withdraw the suspension from a vial with a syringe. *Do not filter* TICE® BCG

PACIS® BCG, Live:

- The product is packaged in vials containing a freeze-dried powder
- Each vial contains $2.4–12 \times 10^6$ CFU, equivalent to 120 mg (semisolid dry weight) per ampule
  (1) Draw up into a small syringe 1 mL preservative-free 0.9% NS at 4°–25°C (39°–77°F), and inject it into 1 ampule of PACIS® BCG. Leave the drug and diluent in contact for about 1 minute. Mix the suspension by withdrawing it into the syringe and expelling it gently back into the ampule 2–3 times. Avoid producing foaming
  (2) Do not expose the reconstituted product to sunlight. Exposure to artificial light should be minimized

TICE® BCG and PACIS® BCG, live:

[Instructions common to both products]

1. Inject 1 mL of the suspension into either a 50-mL-capacity plastic parenteral container or a catheter-tipped syringe that contains 49 mL 0.9% NS. Gently rotate or repeatedly invert the container to disperse the drug
2. Use BCG suspension immediately after preparation. Discard any unused portion within 2 hours after preparation
3. All equipment, supplies, and receptacles in contact with BCG should be handled as having been contaminated with a biohazardous material. To prevent cross-contamination, parenteral drugs should not be prepared in an area where BCG was prepared
4. Reconstituted TheraCys® BCG and TICE® BCG are stable for 2 hours at 2°–8°C if protected from exposure to direct sunlight

Recommendations for Drug Administration and Ancillary Care

TheraCys® BCG Induction:

A single dose of 81 mg is instilled *intravesically* into the bladder once weekly for 6 consecutive weeks

TheraCys® BCG Maintenance:

A single dose of 81 mg is instilled *intravesically* into the bladder 3, 6, 12, 18, and 24 months after the initial dose

TICE® BCG:

Allow 7–14 days to elapse after bladder biopsy before TICE® BCG is administered. A standard treatment schedule consists of 50 mg instilled *intravesically* into the bladder once weekly for 6 consecutive weeks. This schedule may be repeated once if tumor remission has not been achieved and if the clinical circumstances warrant. Thereafter, intravesical TICE® BCG administration should continue at approximately monthly intervals for at least 6–12 months

PACIS® BCG:

A single dose of 120 mg is instilled into the bladder once weekly for 6 consecutive weeks. Patients may be retreated on the same dose and schedule if clinically indicated

General:

- Patients should not drink fluids for 4 hours before treatment and should empty their bladder before BCG administration
- Determine a patient's tuberculin reactivity by PPD skin testing before treatment
  - BCG treatment may cause sensitivity to subsequent tuberculin testing
- BCG is instilled into the bladder by gravity flow using a catheter and should be retained in the bladder for 2 hours and then voided
- *Do not force* BCG flow during instillation
- BCG suspension must remain in the bladder for a maximum of 2 hours. During the first hour, a patient should lie for 15 minutes each in the prone and supine positions and also on each side to maximize bladder surface exposure
- Patients who are not able to retain the suspension for 2 hours should be allowed to void sooner
- Patients who receive BCG treatment should be instructed to void from a seated position to avoid aerosolizing biohazardous material
  - Urine voided within 6 hours after treatment should be treated as infectious waste
- Patients should be instructed to drink enough liquid after treatment to maintain adequate hydration

Caution:

1. Reconstitute BCG using aseptic technique
2. BCG meningitis has been attributed to nosocomial contamination of intrathecal methotrexate
3. Parenteral drugs should not be prepared in the same area where BCG has been reconstituted to avoid cross-contamination
4. All equipment, supplies, and receptacles in contact with TICE® BCG should be considered biohazardous
5. Persons with an immunologic deficiency should not handle BCG
6. There are no data to support the interchangeability of BCG LIVE products

Contraindications:

- Compromised immunity, whether congenital or acquired (comorbid diseases or iatrogenic)
- Urinary tract biopsy, transurethral resection, or traumatic catheterization, or gross hematuria within 7 days before treatment
- Urinary tract infection, acute febrile illness, or active tuberculosis
- Demonstrated hypersensitivity to BCG
- Antibiotic treatments
  - Postpone BCG administration; antimicrobials may interfere with BCG effectiveness
- Small bladder capacity has been associated with increased risk of severe local reactions

Monitoring:

- Compromised immunity, whether congenital or acquired (comorbid diseases or iatrogenic)
- Monitor for signs and symptoms of toxicity after each intravesical treatment
- The following suggest systemic BCG infection and may require anti-tuberculosis therapy:
  1. Febrile episodes with flu-like symptoms lasting >72 hours
  2. Fever ≥39.4°C (≥103°F)
  3. Systemic manifestations that increase in intensity after repeated instillations
  4. Persistent liver function test abnormalities
  5. Local symptoms (prostatitis, epididymitis, orchitis) lasting >2–3 days

BEVACIZUMAB

AVASTIN™ (bevacizumab) product label, December 2004. Genentech, Inc, South San Francisco, CA. Genentech, Inc, Data on file, April 13, 2004

Product Identification, Preparation, Storage, and Stability

- Avastin™ is packaged in single-use clear glass vials containing either 100 mg or 400 mg bevacizumab solution in a uniform concentration of 25 mg/mL. NDC 50242-060-01 (100 mg/4 mL). NDC 50242-061-01 (400 mg/16 mL)
- Store intact vials under refrigeration at 2°–8°C (35.6°–46.4°F), and protect them from light. *Do not freeze* Avastin™
- *Do not shake* intact vials or diluted solutions
- Withdraw from a vial an amount of bevacizumab sufficient to prepare a patient's dose and add it to a volume of 0.9% NS sufficient to produce a total volume of (Q.S.) 100 mL in a PVC, polyolefin, or glass container. Gently invert the container to mix diluted bevacizumab solution. Discard unused bevacizumab that remains in a vial
- *Do not mix* bevacizumab with dextrose solutions
- After dilution, bevacizumab solutions may be stored at 2°–8°C for up to 8 hours
- After dilution in 0.9% NS, bevacizumab was stable for up to 24 hours under the following conditions:

Bevacizumab Concentrations (mg/mL)	Storage Temperatures	Container Composition
0.9 2.25 3 6.6 7.5 16.5	30°C (86°F)	PVC, polyolefin, glass
1 12.5 25 (undiluted drug)	2°–8°C 30°C	Polyolefin

Selected incompatibility:

- Do not mix bevacizumab with dextrose solutions

Recommendations for Drug Administration and Ancillary Care

General:

- *Do not administer* bevacizumab by intravenous push or bolus injection
- Administer bevacizumab by intravenous infusion after chemotherapy. The INITIAL DOSE is given over 90 minutes. If the first infusion is well tolerated, the administration duration may be decreased to 60 minutes during a second infusion. If a 60-minute infusion was well tolerated, subsequent treatments may be administered over 30 minutes
- *Do not administer,* mix, or flush bevacizumab with dextrose solutions

BLEOMYCIN SULFATE

Bleomycin for Injection, USP product label, September 2001. Manufactured by Ben Venue Laboratories, Inc, Bedford, OH. Manufactured for Bedford Laboratories™, Bedford, OH
BLENOXANE® (bleomycin sulfate for injection) product label, April 1999. Manufactured by Nippon Kayaku Co, Ltd, Tokyo, Japan. Distributed by Mead Johnson Oncology Products, A Bristol-Myers Squibb Company, Princeton, NJ

Trissel LA. Handbook on Injectable Drugs, 13th ed. Bethesda: American Society of Health-System Pharmacists, Inc, 2005

Product Identification, Preparation, Storage, and Stability

- Bleomycin sulfate is generically available from numerous manufacturers, usually as a powder for reconstitution for injection
- Store intact vials under refrigeration at 2°–8°C (35.6°–46.4°F)
- Reconstitute with 0.9% NS, SWFI, or BWFI as follows:

	Diluent Volumes			
Bleomycin Content/Vial	**0.9% NS for Intravenous or Intrapleural Administration**		**0.9% NS, SWFI, or BWFI for Subcutaneous or Intramuscular Administration**	
15 units	5 mL	Bleomycin concentration = 3 units/mL	1 mL	Bleomycin concentration = 15 units/mL
30 units	10 mL		2 mL	

- For *intrapleural administration,* further dilute bleomycin 60 units in 50–100 mL 0.9% NS
- *Do not reconstitute or dilute* bleomycin with dextrose-containing solutions. Bleomycins A_2 and B_2 potency decreases after reconstitution in D5W , which does not occur in 0.9% NS
- After reconstitution in 0.9% NS, bleomycin is stable for 24 hours at room temperature
- Bleomycin is compatible with glass, PVC, and high-density polyethylene containers and with polyethylene, PVC, and polybutadiene administration sets

Recommendations for Drug Administration and Ancillary Care

General:

- Bleomycin is given by slow intravenous injection over 10 minutes; by intravenous infusion; and by the intramuscular, intrapleural, and subcutaneous routes
- Bleomycin has been successfully filtered during intravenous administration with filter membranes composed of cellulose ester, cellulose nitrate/cellulose acetate ester, or tetrafluoroethylene polymer (Teflon® [DuPont]), without a significant loss of drug potency

For intrapleural administration:

- Administer bleomycin through a thoracostomy tube after excess pleural fluid drainage and confirmation of complete lung expansion. The thoracostomy tube is clamped after bleomycin instillation. The patient is moved from the supine to the left and right lateral positions several times during the next 4 hours. The clamp is then removed, and thoracostomy tube suction is reestablished

BORTEZOMIB

VELCADE® (bortezomib) for injection product label, March 2005. Millennium Pharmaceuticals, Inc, Cambridge, MA

Product Identification, Preparation, Storage, and Stability

- VELCADE® is packaged in single-use vials containing bortezomib 3.5 mg as a white to off-white cake or powder. NDC 63020-049-01
- Store unopened vials at controlled room temperature 25°C (77°F); temperature excursions are permitted from 15°–30°C (59°–86°F). Retain the product in its original packaging carton to protect it from light
- Reconstitute bortezomib powder with 3.5 mL 0.9% NS to produce a solution with concentration = 1 mg bortezomib/mL
- The reconstituted product should be a clear and colorless solution. It should be administered within 8 hours after preparation
- Before administration, reconstituted bortezomib solution may be stored in its original vial or a syringe at 25°C (excursions are permitted from 15°–30°C)
- The product may be stored for up to 3 hours in a syringe, but total storage time for the reconstituted solution must be <8 hours if it is exposed to normal indoor lighting

Recommendations for Drug Administration and Ancillary Care

General:

- For administration by intravenous push over 3–5 seconds
- The reconstituted product is suitable for direct injection

BUSULFAN

IV Busulfex® (busulfan) Injection product label, September 2003. Distributed by ESP Pharma, Inc, Edison, NJ

Trissel LA. Handbook on Injectable Drugs, 13th ed. Bethesda: American Society of Health-System Pharmacists, Inc, 2005

Product Identification, Preparation, Storage, and Stability

- Busulfex® is supplied as a sterile solution in 10-mL single-use clear glass ampules containing busulfan 60 mg/10 mL (6 mg/mL). NDC 67286-0053-8 (8 ampules per pack; package includes 8 syringe filters with filter pore size = 5 micrometers)
- Unopened Busulfex® ampules are stable until the date indicated on the package when stored under refrigeration between 2°and 8°C (35.6°–46.4°F)
- Preparation:
  - (1) Calculate the volume of busulfan needed to prepare a patient's dose. Add to the calculated volume 0.16 mL, which will remain in a syringe filter during fluid transfer
  - (2) Withdraw from an ampule into a syringe an amount of busulfan needed to prepare a patient's dose
  - (3) Filter the drug by injecting it into a diluent fluid through a 5-micrometer syringe filter (packaged with the commercial product)
    - (a) DO NOT use syringe filters other than the type included in the product package
    - (b) DO NOT use polycarbonate syringes or polycarbonate filter needles with Busulfex®
  - (4) Dilute busulfan with either 0.9% NS or D5W
    - (a) The diluent volume should be 10 times the volume of busulfan, so that the final product concentration is ≥0.5 mg busulfan/mL
    - (b) Always inject busulfan solution into the diluent, not the reverse
  - (5) Mix the product thoroughly by inverting the product container several times
- After dilution in 0.9% NS or D5W, Busulfex® is stable at room temperature (25°C; 77°F) for up to 8 hours, but the infusion must be completed within that time
- After dilution in 0.9% NS, busulfan is stable at refrigerated temperatures for up to 12 hours, but the infusion must be completed within that time

Selected incompatibility:

- *Do not mix* Busulfex® with another solution unless compatibility is known

Recommendations for Drug Administration and Ancillary Care

General:

- Administer busulfan by intravenous infusion via a central VAD over 2 hours. Rapid infusion is not recommended
- Before and after busulfan administration, flush the VAD with approximately 5 mL 0.9% NS or D5W. *Do not mix* Busulfex® with another solution unless compatibility is known
- All patients should be premedicated with phenytoin. Busulfan crosses the blood brain barrier and induces seizures. Although phenytoin decreases busulfan AUC_{plasma} by 15%, other anticonvulsants may increase busulfan AUC_{plasma}, and increase the risk of veno-occlusive disease or seizures

Busulfan Dosage as a Component of the "BuCy" Conditioning Regimen Before Hematopoietic Stem Cell Transplantation:

- The usual adult dosage is based on the lesser of either ideal or actual body weight, and is 0.8 mg/kg per dose, every 6 hours for a total of 16 doses (total daily dosage = 3.2 mg/kg for 4 consecutive days, or total dosage/4-day course = 12.8 mg/kg)
- Busulfan dosage is adjusted in obese patients based on Adjusted Ideal Body Weight (**AIBW**) as follows:

  Ideal Body Weight (IBW) Calculations:

  - IBW for men (kg) = 50 + 0.91 × ([height in cm]−152)
  - IBW for women (kg) = 45 + 0.91 × ([height in cm]−152)
  - **AIBW** (kg) = IBW + 0.25 × ([actual weight]−IBW)

CARBOPLATIN

PARAPLATIN® (carboplatin for injection) product label, June 2001. Bristol-Myers Squibb Oncology, Bristol-Myers Squibb Company, Princeton, NJ
PARAPLATIN® (carboplatin aqueous solution) Injection product label, January 2004. Bristol-Myers Squibb Oncology, Bristol-Myers Squibb Company, Princeton, NJ

Product Identification, Preparation, Storage, and Stability

- PARAPLATIN® (lyophilized powder formulation) is packaged in single-dose vials containing carboplatin 50 mg (NDC 0015-3213-30), 150 mg (NDC 0015-3214-30), or 450 mg (NDC 0015-3215-30)
- PARAPLATIN® INJECTION is an aqueous solution (10 mg carboplatin/mL) packaged in multidose vials containing carboplatin 50 mg/5 mL (NDC 0015-3210-30), 150 mg/15 mL (NDC 0015-3211-30), 450 mg/45 mL (NDC 0015-3212-30), or 600 mg/60 mL (NDC 0015-3216-3
- Store unopened vials of both formulations at 25°C (77°F). Temperature excursions to 15°–30°C (59°–86°F) are permitted. Protect unopened vials from light

Product-Specific Instructions

- PARAPLATIN® (carboplatin for injection) Lyophilized Powder: Immediately before use, reconstitute each vial with either SWFI, D5W , or 0.9% NS as follows:

Carboplatin Content per Vial	Diluent Volume	Concentration After Dilution
50 mg	5 mL	10 mg carboplatin/mL
150 mg	15 mL	
450 mg	45 mL	

- PARAPLATIN® (carboplatin aqueous solution) INJECTION is an aqueous solution containing 10 mg carboplatin/mL.
- Carboplatin may be further diluted to concentrations as low as 0.5 mg/mL with either D5W or 0.9% NS. After dilution, carboplatin may be stored at room temperature (25°C; 77°F) for up to 8 hours before use

Selected incompatibility:

- Avoid admixture with solutions with pH >6.5 (eg, solutions containing fluorouracil or sodium bicarbonate)
- Avoid admixture with mesna
- *Do not prepare or administer* carboplatin with needles or intravenous sets that contain aluminum parts that may come into contact with the drug

Recommendations for Drug Administration and Ancillary Care

General:

- Administer carboplatin by intravenous infusion over at least 15 minutes. Pre- or post-treatment hydration and forced diuresis are not required
- Aluminum reacts with carboplatin causing precipitation and loss of drug potency. *Do not prepare or administer* carboplatin with needles or intravenous sets that contain aluminum parts that may come into contact with the drug
- Prescriptions and medication orders should identify the drug by its complete generic name, CARBOPLATIN

CARMUSTINE

BiCNU® carmustine for injection product label, October 2003. Manufactured by Ben Venue Laboratories, Inc, Bedford, OH. Distributed by Bristol-Myers Squibb Oncology, Bristol-Myers Squibb Company, Princeton, NJ

Arbus MH. Am J Hosp Pharm 1988;45:531
Colvin M et al. Am J Hosp Pharm 1980;37:677–678
Fredriksson K et al. Acta Pharm Suec 1986;23:115–124

Product Identification, Preparation, Storage, and Stability

- The BiCNU® product includes 2 vials: one contains carmustine 100 mg and the other vial contains 3 mL sterile Dehydrated Alcohol Injection, USP for use as an initial diluent. NDC 0015-3012-38 (available only in packages containing 10 vials)
- Unopened vials are stable for 2 years if stored under refrigeration at 2°–8°C (35.6°–46.4°F), but for only 7 days when stored at room temperature (<25°C; <77°F). The lyophilized formulation does not contain a preservative and is intended for a single use
  - (1) Dissolve carmustine with 3 mL of the supplied sterile diluent (Dehydrated Alcohol Injection, USP)
  - (2) After the drug product has been completely dissolved, aseptically add 27 mL SWFI
    - (a) The resulting solution is clear, colorless to yellowish, and contains 3.3 mg carmustine/mL in 10% ethanol
    - (b) After reconstitution as recommended, carmustine is stable for 8 hours at room temperature (25°C) if it is protected from light exposure
  - (3) For administration to patients, carmustine should be further diluted with D5W and STORED ONLY in GLASS OR POLYETHYLENE-LINED parenteral product containers
    - (a) Carmustine adsorption to PVC, ethylene vinyl acetate (EVA), and polyurethane containers results in substantial drug loss

Stability as a Function of Carmustine Concentration and Storage Temperature

Favier M et al. Am J Health Syst Pharm 2001; 58:238–241
Hadji-Minaglou-Gonzalvez M-F et al. Clin Ther 1992;14:821–824

Diluent Solution	Carmustine Concentration	Storage Temperature	Duration of Stability
D5W	0.5–1 mg/mL	25°C	4 hours
	0.1–1 mg/mL	4°C (39.2°F)	24 hours

Important:

- Carmustine has a low melting point, 30.5°–32°C (86.9°–89.6°F). At these or greater temperatures, carmustine will liquefy and appear as an oily film on the walls of its original container vial. This is a sign of decomposition and affected vials should be discarded
- If adequate refrigeration during shipping is uncertain, inspect the vial containing carmustine (the larger of the two packaged vials) by holding it to bright light for inspection. Carmustine should appear as a very small amount of dry flakes or dry congealed mass. If this is evident, the product is suitable for use and should be refrigerated immediately
- Initial solubilization with ethanol produces a carmustine solution that can be very irritating to vascular endothelium during intravenous administration. Consequently, several investigators have evaluated alternative preparation schemes to decrease or eliminate ethanol from carmustine for intravenous administration. Although these methods are not advocated by the product manufacturer, and may present some logistical challenges with respect to material resources, two methods for producing an ethanol-free solution for intravenous administration are described at right

Alternative Preparation Schemes

Method 1:

1. To a vial containing 100 mg carmustine, add 30 mL preservative-free D5W
2. Heat the vial to 60°C (140°F) in a water bath for 5 minutes, and during heating, vigorously shake the vial 3 times
3. The preparation scheme produces a solution with a carmustine concentration of 3.3 mg/mL and a stability half-life of 46 hours
   - The investigators demonstrated an 8% loss in concentration after product filtration
   - Although carmustine must be diluted before it is administered to patients, the investigators did not describe secondary dilution

Levin VA, Levin EM. Sel Cancer Ther 1989;5:33–35

Method 2:

1. To a vial containing 100 mg carmustine, add 25 mL preservative-free D5W warmed to 37°C (98.6°F)
2. Shake the vial by hand or in a water bath warmed to 37°C for approximately 5 minutes
3. The preparation scheme produces a solution with a carmustine concentration of ~4 mg/mL and a mean stability half-life of 6.8 hours
   - When prepared with ethanol according to the manufacturer's instruction, carmustine must be diluted before it is administered to patients. Tepe et al. did not describe secondary dilution

Tepe P et al. J Neurooncol 1991;10:121–127

Selected incompatibility:

- Avoid admixture with solutions of pH >6 (eg, solutions containing sodium bicarbonate)
- Photodegradation occurs after exposure to strong light sources (>500 Lux; >46 foot-candles)

Recommendations for Drug Administration and Ancillary Care

General:

- Administer by intravenous infusion over 1–2 hours
- Carmustine is irritating to vascular endothelium largely because of the ethanol used to initially dissolve the drug. Administration over <1 hours may produce intense pain and burning at the site of injection
- *Use only* polyethylene or polyethylene-lined administration sets.
  - A substantial amount of carmustine may be lost from solution due to adsorption to the surfaces of ethylene vinyl acetate, PVC, and polyurethane product containers and administration sets
- Do *not* mix carmustine with solutions containing sodium bicarbonate
- Carmustine should not be given more frequently than every 6 weeks
- Myelosuppression associated with carmustine is cumulative; dosage adjustment must be considered on the basis of nadir blood counts from prior treatment
- Pulmonary toxicity from carmustine appears to be dose-related. Patients who receive cumulative carmustine dosages >1400 mg/m^2 are at significant risk. Delayed pulmonary toxicity can occur years after treatment and can result in death

CETUXIMAB

ERBITUX™ (Cetuximab) product label, August 2005. Manufactured by ImClone Systems Incorporated, Branchburg, NJ. Distributed and marketed by Bristol-Myers Squibb Company, Princeton, NJ

Product Identification, Preparation, Storage, and Stability

- Erbitux™ is supplied in single-use, 50-mL vials containing cetuximab 100 mg as a sterile, preservative-free, clear and colorless injectable liquid at a concentration of 2 mg/mL. NDC 66733-948-23
- The product may contain a small amount of easily visible, white, amorphous particulates
- *Do not shake or dilute* cetuximab
- Store vials under refrigeration at 2°–8°C (35.6°–46.4°F)
- Do *not* freeze the product. Increased particulate formation may occur at temperatures ≤0°C

Cetuximab stored in infusion containers is chemically and physically stable for up to 12 hours at 2°–8°C and up to 8 hours at controlled room temperature (20°–25°C; 68°–77°F). Discard unused cetuximab within 8 hours or 12 hours after preparation for products maintained at controlled room temperature or 2°–8°C, respectively

Recommendations for Drug Administration and Ancillary Care

General:

- Administer cetuximab by intravenous infusion with an infusion pump or syringe pump
- *Do not administer* by intravenous push or bolus injection

Infusion pump method:

1. Withdraw the contents from a vial of cetuximab using a sterile syringe attached to an appropriate needle, vented spike, or another appropriate transfer device
2. Inject a measured volume of cetuximab into a sterile evacuated container (glass containers; bags made of polyolefin, ethylene vinyl acetate, DEHP-plasticized or other PVC bags)
3. Using a new needle for each vial, repeat the procedure until the volume needed to complete a patient's dose has been injected into the container

Syringe pump method:

1. Withdraw from a vial a measured volume of cetuximab using a sterile syringe attached to an appropriate needle (a vented spike may be used)
2. Place the syringe into a syringe pump driver and set the rate

For both administration methods:

1. Administer cetuximab through a low protein binding 0.22-micrometer in-line filter (placed as proximal to the patient as practical)
2. Cetuximab should be piggybacked into a primary infusion line
3. Attach an administration set, and prime it with cetuximab before starting drug administration
4. The MAXIMUM INFUSION RATE should be ≤5 mL/min
5. Use 0.9% NS to flush the line at the end of infusion

Patient Monitoring:

1. A 1-hour observation period is recommended after completing cetuximab administration. Longer observation periods may be required in patients who experience infusion reactions
2. Patients should be periodically monitored for hypomagnesemia, hypocalcemia, and hypokalemia, during and following cetuximab administration. Monitoring should continue for approximately 8 weeks after the last dose administered; i.e., a period of time commensurate with the half-life and persistence of cetuximab
3. The onset of electrolyte abnormalities has been reported to occur from days to months after cetuximab administration. Electrolyte repletion may be necessary in some patients and, in severe cases, intravenous replacement may be required. The time to resolution of electrolyte abnormalities is not known

CISPLATIN

PLATINOL®-AQ (cisplatin injection) product label, November 2002. Bristol-Myers Squibb Oncology, Bristol-Myers Squibb Company, Princeton, NJ

Heung YW, et al. Am J Hosp Pharm 1987;44:124–130

Product Identification, Preparation, Storage, and Stability

- Cisplatin is generically available from several manufacturers as an aqueous solution for injection
- PLATINOL®-AQ is a sterile solution in multiple-dose vials containing 1 mg cisplatin/mL. The product does not contain an antimicrobial preservative. NDC 0015-3220-22 (50 mg/vial). NDC 0015-3221-22 (100 mg/vial)
- Store intact vials at 15°–25°C (59°–77°F). Do not refrigerate. Protect unopened containers from light
- Dilute PLATINOL®-AQ in a convenient volume of fluid. The diluting fluid MUST CONTAIN a chloride concentration ≥0.225% sodium chloride (≥38.5 mEq/L); eg, 0.45% NaCl, 0.9% NS, 3% NaCl, and saline and dextrose solutions with a chloride concentration >0.225%
- Mannitol is compatible and may be added to cisplatin solutions
- Protect cisplatin solutions that are not used within 6 hours after preparation from exposure to light
- Cisplatin that remains in an amber vial after initial entry is stable for 28 days if protected from light or for 7 days under fluorescent room light

Selected incompatibility:

- *Aluminum* reacts with cisplatin causing precipitation and loss of drug potency. *Do not prepare or administer* cisplatin with needles or intravenous sets that contain aluminum parts that may come into contact with the drug
- Dilution in solutions with less chloride content than the concentration found in 0.225% NaCl (<38.5 mEq/L)
- Cisplatin is incompatible in admixtures with mesna

Caution: Cisplatin dosages rarely exceed 100 mg/m² per cycle. Avoid inadvertent cisplatin (Platinol®) overdose due to confusion with carboplatin (Paraplatin®) or prescribing practices that fail to differentiate daily doses or dosages from total dose or dosage per cycle, respectively

– Prescriptions and medication orders should identify the drug by its complete generic name, CISPLATIN

– Product labeling advises pharmacists to contact health care providers who prescribe cisplatin dosages >100 mg/m² per cycle for dose confirmation

Recommendations for Drug Administration and Ancillary Care

General:

- Hydration is recommended with 1000–2000 mL of fluid by intravenous infusion starting 2–12 hours before cisplatin administration, which may be continued during and after administration is completed. Maintain oral or parenteral hydration and urine output for at least 24 hours after cisplatin administration is completed
- Administer cisplatin by intravenous infusion. Infusion duration generally is within a range of 15–120 minutes, but in some regimens, may be prolonged (8–24 hours)

CLADRIBINE

Cladribine injection product label, January 2000. Manufactured by Ben Venue Laboratories, Inc, Bedford, OH. Manufactured for Bedford Laboratories™, Bedford, OH

Product Identification, Preparation, Storage, and Stability

- Cladribine injection is packaged in a single-use, clear flint glass, 20-mL vial containing cladribine 10 mg (1 mg/mL) as a sterile, preservative-free, isotonic solution. NDC 55390-124-01
- Store intact vials under refrigeration 2°–8°C (35.6°–46.4°F) and protected from light
- Cladribine *must be diluted* before administration
- Dilute in 500 mL 0.9% NS an amount of cladribine needed to provide treatment for a single day. Dilution with D5W is not recommended
- A 7-day infusion solution should only be prepared with B0.9% NS (preserved with 0.9% benzyl alcohol) as follows:
  (1) Add to a plastic container an amount of cladribine needed for a 7-day supply of medication
  (2) Add to the same plastic container a calculated amount of B0.9% NS sufficient to produce a total volume of (Q.S.) 100 mL
  (3) Both cladribine and the diluent solution should be transferred into a parenteral product container through a sterile, disposable, hydrophilic syringe filter with pore size ≤0.22 micrometers to minimize the risk of microbial contamination
- Cladribine admixtures in 0.9% NS in PVC containers are chemically and physically stable for at least 24 hours at room temperature under normal room fluorescent light
- Solutions prepared with B0.9% NS for individuals weighing >85 kg may have reduced preservative effectiveness due to displacement of the benzyl alcohol-containing diluent by the volume of drug
- Admixtures prepared with antimicrobially preserved diluent have demonstrated acceptable chemical and physical stability for at least 7 days in a SIMS Deltec MEDICATION CASSETTE™ Reservoir
- Cladribine may precipitate when exposed to low temperatures, but can be resolubilized by warming at ambient room temperature and vigorous shaking
- Freezing does not adversely affect the solution. If freezing occurs, thaw at room temperature, but DO NOT thaw cladribine by radiant thermal or microwave heating
- After thawing, vials are stable until the expiration date on the product label if stored under refrigeration
- DO NOT refreeze cladribine

Recommendations for Drug Administration and Ancillary Care

General:

- Administer only by intravenous infusion
- After dilution, cladribine should be administered promptly or stored in the refrigerator (2°–8°C; 35.6°–46.4°F) for not more than 8 hours before starting administration
- Cladribine should not be mixed with other intravenous drugs or additives or infused simultaneously via a common intravenous line

CLOFARABINE

CLOLAR™ FOR INTRAVENOUS INFUSION (clofarabine) product label, October 2005. Manufactured by AAI Development Services, Charleston, SC. Manufactured for Genzyme Corporation, San Antonio, TX. Distributed by Genzyme Corporation, Cambridge, MA

Product Identification, Preparation, Storage, and Stability

- CLOLAR™ is packaged in flint glass, single-use, 20-mL vials containing clofarabine 20 mg (1 mg/mL) as a clear, practically colorless, preservative-free solution. NDC 58468-0100-2 (4 vials/box)
- Store intact vials at 25°C (77°F). Temperature excursions are permitted to 15°–30°C (59°–86°F)
- Undiluted clofarabine solution must be filtered. Use a sterile filter with a pore size equal to 0.2 micrometers either when aspirating the drug into a syringe *or* when expelling drug from the syringe into a diluent solution
- Dilute clofarabine with a convenient volume of 0.9% NS or D5W before administering it to patients
- Diluted solutions may be stored at room temperature for up to 24 hours after preparation

Recommendations for Drug Administration and Ancillary Care

General:

- Administer diluted clofarabine solutions by intravenous infusion over 2 hours
- Continuous intravenous hydration is recommended throughout a 5-day treatment course with clofarabine to reduce the effects of tumor lysis and other adverse events
- Glucocorticoid prophylaxis (eg, hydrocortisone 100 mg/m^2 per day for 3 days [days 1–3]) may prevent signs or symptoms of systemic inflammatory response (SIR) or capillary leak syndromes (e.g., hypotension)
- Early signs of SIR or capillary leak syndromes are indications to immediately discontinue clofarabine administration and provide appropriate supportive measures
- Close monitoring of renal and hepatic function during a 5-day treatment course with clofarabine are advised. Clofarabine should be immediately discontinued if substantive increases in creatinine or bilirubin are observed during treatment
- Clofarabine treatment may resume, possibly at a lower dose, after a patient's condition has stabilized and organ function has returned to baseline
- Although clofarabine has not been studied in patients with renal or hepatic impairment, 49–60% of a dose was renally eliminated as unchanged drug within 24 hours after administration to pediatric patients. Drugs that adversely affect kidney and liver function and those that produce or exacerbate hypotension should be avoided during the days on which clofarabine is administered
- If hyperuricemia is anticipated (indicative of tumor lysis), patients should receive allopurinol prophylactically
- Clofarabine compatibility with other drugs is not yet known

CYCLOPHOSPHAMIDE

CYTOXAN® (cyclophosphamide for injection) product label, USP November 2003. Manufactured by Baxter Healthcare Corporation, Deerfield, IL. Distributed by Bristol-Myers Squibb Oncology, Bristol-Myers Squibb Company, Princeton, NJ

Product Identification, Preparation, Storage, and Stability

- Cyclophosphamide is generically available from numerous manufacturers, packaged in vials as a powder for reconstitution for injection
- CYTOXAN®, the product marketed by Bristol-Myers Squibb as a powder for reconstitution for injection was reformulated in 2004 and no longer contains mannitol NDC 0015-0502-41 (500 mg/vial), NDC 0015-0505-41 (1000 mg/vial), NDC 0015-0506-41 (2000 mg/vial)
- Neither the former nor the current CYTOXAN® formulations contain an antimicrobial preservative
- Reconstitute CYTOXAN® with 0.9% NS[a] or SWFI[b], as follows:

Cyclophosphamide Content per Vial	Diluent Volume	Cyclophosphamide Concentration After Reconstitution
500 mg	25 mL	20 mg/mL
1000 mg	50 mL	
2000 mg	100 mL	

[a]After reconstitution with 0.9% NS, cyclophosphamide is suitable for direct intravenous injection
[b]After reconstitution with SWFI, the product is hypotonic, but may be administered by infusion after further dilution with one of the following solutions: D5W , 0.45% NaCl, 0.9% NS, D5W/RI, D5W/0.9% NS, LRI, Sodium Lactate Injection (1/6 molar sodium lactate), USP

- After reconstituting (nonlyophilized) CYTOXAN® with SWFI, the resulting solution is hypotonic. Reconstitution with SWFI and 0.9% NS to a concentration of 20 mg/mL yields solutions with the following osmolarities:

Cyclophosphamide and Diluent	Osmolarity
100 mg cyclophosphamide in 5 mL SWFI	74 mOsm/L
100 mg cyclophosphamide in 5 mL 0.9% NS	374 mOsm/L

- After reconstitution to a concentration of 20 mg/mL, cyclophosphamide is chemically and physically stable for 24 hours at room temperature or for 6 days under refrigeration (2°–8°C; 35.6°–46.4°F)

Recommendations for Drug Administration and Ancillary Care

General:

- After reconstitution with 0.9% NS, cyclophosphamide solutions may be given by intravenous push, intravenous infusion, intramuscularly, intraperitoneally, or intrapleurally
- Solutions prepared by reconstituting CYTOXAN® with SWFI are *hypotonic* and *are not recommended* for direct administration, but may be administered by infusion if diluted with any of the following: D5W, 0.45% NaCl, 0.9% NS, D5W/RI, D5W/0.9% NS, LRI, Sodium Lactate Injection, USP

CYTARABINE

Cytarabine for injection for intravenous, intrathecal or subcutaneous use only product label, August 2000. Manufactured by Ben Venue Laboratories, Inc, Bedford, OH. Manufactured for Bedford Laboratories™, Bedford, OH

Product Identification, Preparation, Storage, and Stability

- Cytarabine is generically available from several manufacturers. Products are formulated either as lyophilized powder or solution in single- or multiple-dose containers for intravenous, intramuscular, intrathecal, or subcutaneous injection
- *Do not use* bacteriostatically preserved drug and diluent products for intrathecal use and for preparing cytarabine for high-dose treatments ($\geq$1000 mg/m^2)
- Refer to product packaging and labeling for correct handling conditions; however, for the product identified above, store intact vials at 25°C (77°F). Temperature excursions are permitted to 15°–30°C (59°–86°F)
- Reconstitute cytarabine as follows (diluent selection depends on route of administration; see below):

Cytarabine Content per Vial	Diluent Volume	Reconstituted Cytarabine Concentration
100 mg	5 mL	20 mg/mL
500 mg	10 mL	50 mg/mL
1000 mg	10 mL	100 mg/mL
2000 mg	20 mL	100 mg/mL

- Promptly use cytarabine solutions that are reconstituted without a preservative
- Solutions reconstituted with BWFI may be stored at controlled room temperature, 15°–30°C, for up to 48 hours
- Discard solutions in which a slight haze develops

For intravenous or subcutaneous use:

- Reconstitute cytarabine with 0.9% NS, SWFI, or BWFI preserved with benzyl alcohol
- The reconstituted product may be further diluted to a convenient volume in 0.9% NS or D5W

For intrathecal use:

- Reconstitute cytarabine with PRESERVATIVE-FREE 0.9% NS to produce a solution with concentration $\leq$20 mg/mL. Typical administration volumes range from 5–10 mL, and should correspond with the volume of cerebrospinal fluid removed
- Admixtures with hydrocortisone sodium succinate for intrathecal administration (with or without methotrexate) should be prepared just before use and administered as soon as possible (within minutes) after preparation due to the instability of the hydrocortisone component

Caution: **Do not use an antimicrobially preserved diluent to prepare cytarabine for intrathecal use**

Recommendations for Drug Administration and Ancillary Care

General:

- Administer by intravenous, intrathecal, or subcutaneous routes only
- If cytarabine is given intramuscularly, administration sites should be rotated
- Use products prepared for intrathecal administration immediately after they are prepared
- Although the amount of drug administered is a modulating factor, patients generally can tolerate higher total doses given intravenously by rapid injection than by slow infusion due to cytarabine's rapid inactivation and the relatively brief cellular exposure to cytotoxic concentrations that occur after rapid injection

CYTARABINE LIPOSOME INJECTION

DEPOCYT® (cytarabine liposome injection) for intrathecal use only product label, October 2003. Manufactured by SkyePharma Inc, San Diego, CA. Distributed by ENZON Pharmaceuticals, Inc, Bridgewater, NJ

Product Identification, Preparation, Storage, and Stability

- DEPOCYT® is packaged in glass single-use vials containing a sterile, white to off-white suspension of cytarabine encapsulated into multivesicular lipid-based particles. NDC 57665-331-01
- DEPOCYT® does not contain a preservative and should be stored under refrigeration at 2°–8°C (36°–46°F)
- Protect DEPOCYT® from freezing and avoid aggressive agitation
- The DEPOCYT® product is intended for direct administration without further dilution
- Administer DEPOCYT® immediately after entering a vial. If treatment is delayed, do not use DEPOCYT® more than 4 hours after withdrawing the product from a vial. Unused portions should be discarded

Selected incompatibility:

- *Do not mix* DEPOCYT® with other medications

Recommendations for Drug Administration and Ancillary Care

General:

- Patients should receive either orally or intravenously dexamethasone 4 mg twice daily for 5 days, beginning on the day of DEPOCYT® injection
- Inject DEPOCYT® slowly, over a period of 1–5 minutes directly into the cerebrospinal fluid via an intraventricular reservoir or by direct injection into the lumbar sac
- *Do not use* in-line filters when administering DEPOCYT®
- After administration by lumbar puncture, a patient should be instructed to lie flat for 1 hour

DACARBAZINE

Dacarbazine for Injection, USP product label, May 2001. Manufactured by Ben Venue Laboratories, Inc, Bedford, OH. Manufactured for Bedford Laboratories™, Bedford, OH
Dacarbazine for Injection, USP product label, April 2002. American Pharmaceutical Partners, Inc, Schaumburg, IL

Trissel LA. Handbook on Injectable Drugs, 13th ed. Bethesda: American Society of Health-System Pharmacists, Inc, 2005

Product Identification, Preparation, Storage, and Stability

- Dacarbazine is generically available from several manufacturers. In general, dacarbazine is packaged in single-use amber glass vials containing either 100 mg or 200 mg dacarbazine
- Store intact vials under refrigeration at 2°–8°C (35.6°–46.4°F)
- Reconstitute dacarbazine with SWFI as follows:

Dacarbazine Content per Vial	Diluent (SWFI) Volume	Dacarbazine Concentration After Reconstitution
100 mg	9.9 mL	10 mg/mL
200 mg	19.7 mL	

- After reconstitution and before use, dacarbazine solution may be stored at 4°C for up to 72 hours or at normal room temperature and lighting conditions for up to 8 hours
- Dacarbazine is suitable for intravenous injection after reconstitution or may be further diluted in up to 250 mL of D5W or 0.9% NS and given by intravenous infusion
- After dilution in D5W or 0.9% NS, the resulting product may be stored at 4°C for up to 24 hours or at normal room conditions for up to 8 hours

Recommendations for Drug Administration and Ancillary Care

General:

- Administer dacarbazine by intravenous injection over 1 minute or by intravenous infusion over 15–30 minutes
- Dacarbazine is degraded by exposure to light. Cover parenteral containers with opaque material to protect dacarbazine solutions from light

DACTINOMYCIN

COSMEGEN® FOR INJECTION (DACTINOMYCIN FOR INJECTION) (Actinomycin D) product label, June 2005. Merck & Co, Inc, Whitehouse Station, NJ

Product Identification, Preparation, Storage, and Stability

- COSMEGEN® is supplied in vials containing dactinomycin 0.5 mg as a lyophilized powder. NDC 0006-3298-22
- Store intact vials at 25°C (77°F). Temperature excursions to 15°–30°C (59°–86°F) are permitted. Protect vials from light and humidity
- Reconstitute by adding 1.1 mL SWFI (without preservative) to a vial containing dactinomycin 0.5 mg to produce a solution that contains approximately 0.5 mg (500 mcg) dactinomycin/mL
- Reconstituted dactinomycin is chemically stable, but does not contain an antimicrobial preservative. Diluents preserved with benzyl alcohol or parabens will cause drug precipitation
- *Do not filter* dactinomycin during preparation. Filtration through cellulose ester filters may remove dactinomycin from the solution being filtered
- Use a "two-needle technique" to prepare dactinomycin if it is to be directly injected directly into a vein through a hypodermic needle. The "two-needle technique" prevents soft tissue exposure to dactinomycin that may remain on the external surface of a needle used during percutaneous injection

Two-needle technique:

1. Use 1 sterile needle to reconstitute and withdraw from a vial the calculated dose
2. Aspirate all the measured drug from the needle and needle hub into the syringe, and replace the first needle with a second needle
3. With a second sterile needle on the syringe, express air from the syringe and inject dactinomycin directly into the selected vein

Dactinomycin may be added to the tubing or side-arm of a rapidly flowing intravenous infusion of D5W or 0.9% NS or prepared as an admixture in the same solutions

Recommendations for Drug Administration and Ancillary Care

General:

- For administration by intravenous push or intravenous infusion only
- Please review the two-needle technique for direct intravenous push (see above). The procedure prevents soft tissue exposure to dactinomycin that may remain on the external surface of a needle used during percutaneous injection
- DO NOT FILTER dactinomycin during administration. Filtration through cellulose ester membrane filters may partially remove dactinomycin from the solution being filtered

Caution: Dactinomycin is a vesicant and may cause severe local soft tissue necrosis if extravasated

DAUNORUBICIN HCl

CERUBIDINE (Daunorubicin HCl) FOR INJECTION product label, December 1999. Manufactured by Ben Venue Laboratories, Inc, Bedford, OH. Manufactured for Bedford Laboratories, Bedford, OH

DAUNORUBICIN HYDROCHLORIDE INJECTION product label, July 1999. Manufactured by Ben Venue Laboratories, Inc, Bedford, OH. Manufactured for Bedford Laboratories™, Bedford, OH

Product Identification, Preparation, Storage, and Stability

- Daunorubicin injection (solution) and daunorubicin HCl for injection (lyophilized powder) are generically available from several manufacturers. Products are formulated either as powder or solution and packaged in glass single-use vials
- Store vials containing unreconstituted daunorubicin at controlled room temperature, 15°–30°C (59°–86°F). Protect daunorubicin from exposure to light
- Reconstitute powdered daunorubicin HCl with SWFI to produce a solution as follows:

Daunorubicin Content per Vial	Diluent (SWFI) Volume	Daunorubicin Concentration After Reconstitution
20 mg	4 mL	5 mg/mL
50 mg	10 mL	

- Reconstituted solutions are stable for 24 hours at room temperature and 48 hours under refrigeration (2°–8°C; 35.6°–46.4°F)
- The calculated dose is withdrawn into a syringe containing 0.9% NS 10–15 mL for injection

Selected incompatibility:

- Product labeling recommends NOT MIXING daunorubicin with heparin or other drugs

Recommendations for Drug Administration and Ancillary Care

General:

- Inject daunorubicin into the tubing or side-arm of a rapidly flowing intravenous infusion of D5W or 0.9% NS

Caution: Daunorubicin is a vesicant and can produce severe local soft tissue necrosis if extravasation occurs. *Never inject daunorubicin by the intramuscular, subcutaneous, or intrathecal routes*

DAUNORUBICIN, LIPOSOME INJECTION

DaunoXome® (daunorubicin citrate liposome injection) product label, July 2002. Gilead Sciences, Inc, San Dimas, CA

Product Identification, Preparation, Storage, and Stability

- DaunoXome® is a translucent, red liposomal dispersion of daunorubicin citrate equivalent to 50 mg daunorubicin base in 25 mL (2 mg/mL) packaged in single-use vials (NDC 61958-0301-1)
- Store DaunoXome® under refrigeration at 2°–8°C (35.6°–46.4°F). Do not freeze DaunoXome®. Protect it from exposure to light
- Withdraw the calculated volume of DaunoXome® needed for a patient's dose from a vial into a syringe, and transfer it into a sterile parenteral product container containing an equivalent volume of D5W (1:1 dilution) to produce a concentration after dilution = 1 mg daunorubicin/mL
- The product does not contain a preservative or bacteriostatic agent. Partially used vials should be discarded as hazardous waste
- If diluted DaunoXome® is not used immediately, it should be refrigerated at 2°–8°C (35.6°–46.4°F) for a maximum of 6 hours

Caution: The only fluid with which DaunoXome® may be admixed is D5W

Selected incompatibility:

- *Do not mix* DaunoXome® with any solution other than D5W

Recommendations for Drug Administration and Ancillary Care

General:

- Administer DaunoXome® intravenously over 60 minutes immediately after dilution
- *Do not filter* DaunoXome® during administration
- *Do not mix* DaunoXome® with other drugs

DECITABINE

Dacogen™ (decitabine) for Injection product label, May 2006. MGI Pharma, Inc., Bloomington, MN

Product Identification, Preparation, Storage, and Stability

- Decitabine is a white to almost white, sterile, lyophilized powder packaged in clear, colorless, single-use, 20-mL glass vials containing 50 mg decitabine, 68 mg monobasic potassium phosphate (potassium dihydrogen phosphate) and 11.6 mg sodium hydroxide (NDC 58063-600-50)
- Store intact vials at 25°C (77°F); excursions permitted to 15°–30°C

Caution: BEFORE BEGINNING reconstitution, evaluate whether decitabine administration will begin within 15 minutes after the lyophilized product is reconstituted. Decitabine hydrolyzes spontaneously after reconstitution. If drug administration will begin within 15 minutes after reconstitution began, there is no need to used pre-chilled diluents, but preparation should not commence until just before the drug is needed. If drug administration will begin >15 minutes to within 7 hours after reconstitution, use pre-chilled (2°–8°C; 35.6°–46.4°F) solutions to reconstitute and dilute decitabine

- Reconstitution with 10 mL SWFI produces a solution with concentration of 5 mg decitabine/mL at pH 6.7–7.3
- After powdered decitabine is completely dissolved, immediately withdraw the calculated volume of decitabine needed for a patient's dose from a vial into a syringe, and transfer it into a sterile plastic or glass parenteral product container containing a volume of 0.9%NS, D5W , or LRI sufficient to produce a concentration between 0.1–1.0 mg/mL
- If decitabine cannot be used within 15 minutes after diluent was introduced into a vial, the product should be promptly removed to refrigeration and may be stored for up to 7 hours after reconstitution. Reconstituted and diluted products that have not been used within the time limits identified above and trace contaminated materials should be discarded as hazardous waste
- If a decitabine-containing solution was prepared and refrigerated as described (above) and used within 7 h after reconstitution, administration should be completed within 3 hours after the product was transferred from refrigeration to room temperature conditions

Recommendations for Drug Administration and Ancillary Care

General:

- If decitabine is not prepared with chilled solutions and promptly refrigerated after preparation, administration MUST BEGIN within 15 minutes after reconstitution
- If decitabine was prepared with chilled solutions and stored under refrigeration promptly after preparation, administration MAY BEGIN up to 7 hours after reconstitution
- Drug administration should begin promptly after transfer from refrigerated to room temperature conditions

DENILEUKIN DIFTITOX

ONTAK® (denileukin diftitox) product label, February 2006. Manufactured by Seragen, Incorporated, San Diego, CA. Distributed by Ligand Pharmaceuticals Incorporated, San Diego, CA

Product Identification, Preparation, Storage, and Stability

- ONTAK® is packaged in single-use vials containing a sterile, frozen solution of recombinant denileukin diftitox 150 mcg/mL, (300 mcg/vial) (6 vials/package NDC 64365-503-01)
- Store ONTAK® at ≤ −10°C (≤14°F)
  - (1) Allow ONTAK® to equilibrate with room temperature (up to 25°C [77°F]) before preparing a dose. Thaw vials either [1] under refrigeration at 2°–8°C (35.6°–46.4°F) for not more than 24 hours, or [2] at room temperature for 1–2 hours
    - (a) *Do not heat* ONTAK® to thaw the product
    - (b) *Do not refreeze* ONTAK® after thawing
    - (c) ONTAK® solution in a vial may be mixed by gentle swirling. DO NOT VIGOROUSLY SHAKE ONTAK® solution
    - (d) After thawing, a haze may be visible. The haze should clear when the solution is at room temperature. *Do not use* the solution unless it is clear, colorless, and without visible particulate matter
  - (2) Prepare and contain diluted denileukin diftitox in plastic syringes or soft plastic parenteral product containers. *Do not use glass containers* because an unpredictable portion of the drug may be lost due to adsorption to glass surfaces
  - (3) Withdraw from 1 or more vials with a syringe the amount of denileukin diftitox needed to prepare a patient's dose and inject it into an empty plastic parenteral product container (bag or syringe)
    - (a) Denileukin diftitox *concentration must be* ≥15 mcg/mL during all preparation steps
  - (4) Add to the product container NOT MORE THAN 9 mL preservative-free 0.9% NS for each 1 mL denileukin diftitox ® in the container
- *Do not* mix denileukin diftitox with other drugs
- Partially used vials should be discarded immediately

Selected incompatibility:

- Product labeling recommends NOT MIXING denileukin diftitox with other drugs

Recommendations for Drug Administration and Ancillary Care

General:

- Administer denileukin diftitox by intravenous infusion over at least 15 minutes. There is no clinical experience with prolonged infusion times (>80 minutes)
- *Do not administer* denileukin diftitox as a bolus injection
- If infusion-related adverse events occur, Ontak® administration should be discontinued, or the delivery rate should be decreased depending on the severity of the reaction
- *Do not mix* denileukin diftitox with other drugs
- *Do not filter* denileukin diftitox during administration

DEXRAZOXANE

Zinecard® dexrazoxane for injection product label, October 2004. Distributed by Pharmacia & Upjohn Company, a division of Pfizer Inc., New York, NY

Product Identification, Preparation, Storage, and Stability

- Zinecard® is available in single-dose vials in two product strengths containing lyophilized dexrazoxane 250 mg (NDC 0013-8715-62) or dexrazoxane 500 mg (NDC 0013-8725-89). Both product packages contain a vial of 0.167 mol (1/6 M) Sodium Lactate Injection, USP for reconstitution
- Store dexrazoxane at 25°C (77°F). Temperature excursions are permitted to 15°–30°C (59°–86°F)
- Reconstitution with 0.167 mol (ie, 1/6 mol) Sodium Lactate Injection, USP produces a solution with concentration of dexrazoxane 10 mg/mL:

Dexrazoxane Content per Vial	Diluent Volume (0.167 M Sodium Lactate)
250 mg	25 mL
500 mg	50 mL

- Dexrazoxane is stable for 6 hours after the time of reconstitution when stored at controlled room temperature, 15°–30°C or under refrigeration, 2°–8°C (35.6°–46.4°F).
- The reconstituted solution may be diluted in a parenteral product container with either 0.9% NS or D5W to a concentration between 1.3 and 5 mg/mL
- Diluted dexrazoxane is stable for 6 hours when stored at controlled room temperature or under refrigeration
- Dexrazoxane degrades rapidly at pH > 7.0
- Discard any portion of unused dexrazoxane

Selected incompatibility:

- Product labeling recommends *not* mixing dexrazoxane with other drugs

Recommendations for Drug Administration and Ancillary Care

General:

- Administer dexrazoxane by slow intravenous push or a rapid intravenous infusion over a period of <30 minutes due to the relationship between dexrazoxane and doxorubicin administration
- **Complete doxorubicin administration within 30 minutes after dexrazoxane administration began**
- The recommended dosage ratio of dexrazoxane to doxorubicin is 10:1 (eg, 500 mg dexrazoxane/m^2:50 mg doxorubicin/m^2)

DOCETAXEL

TAXOTERE® (docetaxel) for injection concentrate product label, February 2005. Aventis Pharmaceuticals, Inc, Bridgewater, NJ

Product Identification, Preparation, Storage, and Stability

- TAXOTERE® is a concentrated solution in polysorbate 80. Product packaging includes a second vial that contains 13% [w/w] ethanol in SWFI, which is used as a diluent during product preparation. NDC 0075-8001-20 (20 mg docetaxel/0.5 mL), NDC 0075-8001-80 (80 mg docetaxel/2 mL)
- Store intact vials between 2° and 25°C (36°–77°F). Retain vials in the original packaging to protect them from bright light. Freezing does not adversely affect the undiluted product
- *Avoid* bringing docetaxel into contact with containers, syringes, tubing, and other materials used during drug preparation and administration that are made of plasticized PVC. Commercial Taxotere® Injection Concentrate has been shown to leach DEHP plasticizer from PVC containers and administration sets. *Store docetaxel solutions only* in bottles (glass, polypropylene) or plastic bags (polypropylene, polyolefin)
- Taxotere® injection concentrate requires 2 dilutions before administration. Both the Taxotere® injection concentrate and the diluent vials contain overfill to compensate for liquid that is lost during preparation. Overfill ensures that the initially diluted solution contains 10 mg docetaxel/mL after dilution with the entire contents of the diluent vial

Prepare an initial dilution:

1. Taxotere® vials should be stored between 2° and 25°C (36°–77°F). If Taxotere® and diluent vials are stored under refrigeration, allow to stand at room temperature approximately 5 minutes before proceeding
2. Aseptically withdraw the entire contents of an appropriate diluent vial (approximately 1.8 mL for Taxotere® 20 mg and approximately 7.1 mL for Taxotere® 80 mg) into a syringe by partially inverting the vial, and transfer it to the appropriate vial of Taxotere® Concentrate to produce an initially diluted solution containing 10 mg docetaxel/mL
3. Mix the initially diluted solution by repeated inversions for at least 45 seconds. Do not shake the vials. The initially diluted solution may be used immediately or stored under refrigeration or at room temperature for a maximum of 8 hours
4. The initially diluted Taxotere® solution should be clear; however, there may be some foam on top of the solution. Allow the vials to stand for a few minutes to allow any foam to dissipate. It is not necessary to wait for all foam to dissipate prior to continuing preparation

Prepare a final dilution for infusion:

1. Aseptically withdraw the required amount of initially diluted Taxotere® solution (10 mg/mL) with a calibrated syringe and inject into an infusion bag or bottle containing a volume of either 0.9% NS or D5W sufficient to produce a final docetaxel concentration within the range 0.3–0.74 mg/mL
   - *Do not exceed* docetaxel product concentrations of 0.74 mg/mL
2. Thoroughly mix the infusion by manually inverting the product container and by rotation
   - When prepared as described and stored between 2° and 25°C, docetaxel solutions are stable for 4 hours

Recommendations for Drug Administration and Ancillary Care

General:

- Visually inspect the infusion product for particulate matter or discoloration prior to administration. All docetaxel-containing solutions that are not clear or appear to contain a precipitate should be discarded
- Administer docetaxel by intravenous infusion over 1 hour under ambient room temperature and lighting conditions
- Administer fully prepared docetaxel within 4 hours after preparation (including the time needed to complete drug administration)
- *Do not use* PVC containers and administration sets to administer docetaxel. *Administer docetaxel only* through polyethylene-lined administration sets

Ancillary medication:

- FDA-approved product labeling recommends that all patients who are treated with docetaxel should receive a steroid such as dexamethasone 8 mg orally twice daily for 3 days (6 doses), starting 1 day before docetaxel to decrease the severity of fluid retention and hypersensitivity reactions that are associated with docetaxel

DOXORUBICIN HCI

ADRIAMYCIN® (doxorubicin HCI) for Injection, USP, and ADRIAMYCIN® (doxorubicin HCI) Injection, USP, product label, December 2002. Manufactured by Ben Venue Laboratories, Inc, Bedford, OH. Manufactured for Bedford Laboratories™, Bedford, OH

Product Identification, Preparation, Storage, and Stability

- ADRIAMYCIN® for Injection, USP, is a sterile red-orange lyophilized powder packaged in single-dose vials as follows:

Content Doxorubicin HCl	No. Vials/Package Unit	NDC No.
10 mg/vial	Carton of 10 vials	55390-231-10
20 mg/vial	Carton of 10 vials	55390-232-10
50 mg/vial	Individually boxed	55390-233-01

- Store unreconstituted vials at controlled room temperature, 15°–30°C (59°–86°F) and protect them from light. Retain vials in the packaging carton until they are used. Discard any unused portion
- Reconstitute the lyophilized powder with 0.9% NS as follows to produce a final concentration of 2 mg doxorubicin HCl/mL:

Doxorubicin HCl Content per Vial	Diluent Volume
10 mg	5 mL
20 mg	10 mL
50 mg	25 mL

- After adding the diluent, vials should be shaken and the contents allowed to dissolve
- After initially entering a sealed vial, doxorubicin solution is stable for 7 days at room temperature and under normal room light (100 foot-candles) and for 15 days at 2°–8°C (35.6°–46.4°F). Protect doxorubicin from exposure to sunlight. Promptly discard partially used vials of the Adriamycin® for injection product

- ADRIAMYCIN® Injection, USP, is a red-orange solution (2 mg doxorubicin HCl/mL) packaged in single-dose vials as follows:

Content Doxorubicin HCl	No. Vials/Package Unit	NDC No.
10 mg in 5 mL	Carton of 10 vials	55390-235-10
20 mg in 10 mL	Carton of 10 vials	55390-236-10
50 mg in 25 mL	Individually boxed	55390-237-01

- Store under refrigeration at 2°–8°C (36°–46°F) and protect from light. Retain vials in the packaging carton until they are used. Discard any unused portion

- ADRIAMYCIN® Injection, USP, is a red-orange solution (2 mg doxorubicin HCl/mL) packaged in sterile, multiple-dose individually boxed vials containing 200 mg/100 mL. NDC 55390-238-01
- Store under refrigeration at 2°–8°C (36°–46°F) and protect from light. Retain vials in the packaging carton until they are used. Discard unused solution that remains after the labeled storage time

Selected incompatibility:

- Antimicrobially preserved diluents are not recommended
- *Do not mix* doxorubicin with heparin or fluorouracil. The admixtures are incompatible and will precipitate

Recommendations for Drug Administration and Ancillary Care

General:

- Administer doxorubicin by slow intravenous injection into the tubing of a freely running intravenous infusion of 0.9% NS or D5W. The tubing should be attached to a needle or cannula inserted preferably into a large vein. If possible, avoid veins over joints and in extremities with compromised venous or lymphatic drainage
- The rate of administration is dependent on vein size and the dosage, but a dose should be administered over not less than 3–5 minutes
- Erythematous streaking along a vein as well as facial flushing may indicate an administration rate that is too rapid. Burning or stinging sensations may be indicative of perivenous infiltration and the infusion should be immediately terminated and restarted in another vein. Extravasation also may occur painlessly

Caution: Doxorubicin is a powerful vesicant and can produce severe local soft tissue necrosis if extravasation occurs. Doxorubicin *must not be given* by the intramuscular, subcutaneous, or intrathecal routes

DOXORUBICIN HCl LIPOSOME INJECTION

DOXIL® (doxorubicin HCl liposome injection) product label, November 2004. Manufactured by Ben Venue Laboratories, Inc, Bedford, OH. Distributed by Tibotec Therapeutics, Inc, Division of Ortho Biotech Products L.P., Raritan, NJ

Product Identification, Preparation, Storage, and Stability

- Doxil® contains doxorubicin HCl encapsulated in liposomes; it is not clear and it is not a solution
- The product is packaged in 10- or 30-mL glass, single-use vials containing either 20 mg doxorubicin HCl/10 mL (NDC 17314-9600-1) or 50 mg doxorubicin HCl/25 mL (NDC 17314-9600-2), respectively, as a translucent, red, liposomal dispersion
- Doxil® does not contain an antimicrobial preservative. Store unopened vials of Doxil® at 2°–8°C (35.6°–46.4°F)
- Avoid freezing. Prolonged freezing may adversely affect liposomal drug products; however, freezing for periods <1 month do not appear to adversely affect Doxil®
- Dilute Doxil® with D5W before administration as follows:

Note: Do not dilute Doxil® with any diluent other than D5W

Dose to Administer	Volume of D5W for Dilution
≤90 mg	250 mL
>90 mg	500 mL

- Diluted Doxil® may be stored under refrigeration at 2°–8°C, but should be administered within 24 hours
- *Do not filter* Doxil® before or after dilution

Selected incompatibility:

- Do not mix Doxil® with other drugs
- Do not mix Doxil® with a solution containing a bacteriostatic agent, such as benzyl alcohol

Recommendations for Drug Administration and Ancillary Care

General:

- Administer Doxil® by intravenous infusion over 30 minutes
- *Do not filter* Doxil® during administration
- *Caution:* Doxil® is a vesicant and may produce severe local soft tissue necrosis if extravasation occurs
- Extravasation may occur during intravenous administration with or without an accompanying stinging or burning sensation, and in spite of easy blood aspiration (good blood return) from the vascular access device through which Doxil® is administered
- If signs or symptoms of extravasation occur during Doxil® administration, the infusion should be immediately terminated and may be restarted in another vein. Doxil® must not be given by the intramuscular or subcutaneous routes

EPIRUBICIN HCl

ELLENCE® epirubicin hydrochloride injection product label, March 2, 2005. Manufactured by Pharmacia (Perth) Pty Limited, Bentley WA 6102 Australia. Manufactured for Pharmacia & Upjohn Company, A subsidiary of Pharmacia Corporation, Kalamazoo, MI

Product Identification, Preparation, Storage, and Stability

- ELLENCE® is packaged in polypropylene single-use vials as a sterile, preservative-free, ready-to-use solution in two product strengths: 50 mg epirubicin/25 mL (NDC 0009-5091-01) or 200 mg epirubicin/100 mL (NDC 0009-5093-01)
- Store epirubicin under refrigeration between 2° and 8°C (36°–46°F)
- *Do not freeze* epirubicin
- Protect epirubicin from light
- Ellence® solution is suitable for direct intravenous administration
- Use Ellence® solution within 24 hours after first vial penetration
- Discard partially used vials after dose preparation

Selected incompatibility:

- *Do not mix* epirubicin with other drugs in the same container
- Epirubicin is most stable at pH 4–5, and hydrolyzes spontaneously at alkaline pH

Recommendations for Drug Administration and Ancillary Care

General:

- Administer epirubicin by slow intravenous injection into the tubing of a freely running intravenous infusion of 0.9% NS or D5W over 3–20 minutes, depending on the dosage to be given and vein size
- Do *not* inject epirubicin directly into a vein due to the risk of extravasation, which may occur even in the presence of adequate blood return. Venous sclerosis may result from injection into small vessels or repeated injections into the same vein
- Avoid administration into veins over joints or in extremities with compromised venous or lymphatic drainage.
- *Caution*: Epirubicin is a vesicant and can produce severe local soft tissue necrosis if extravasation occurs. Epirubicin *must not be given* by the intramuscular, subcutaneous, or intrathecal routes
- Erythematous streaking along the vein as well as facial flushing may indicate too rapid an administration rate. Burning or stinging sensations may be indicative of perivenous infiltration and the infusion should be immediately terminated and restarted in another vein. Perivenous infiltration may occur painlessly

ETOPOSIDE

VePesid® (etoposide) for injection and capsules product label, September 1998. Bristol Laboratories Oncology Products, A Bristol-Myers Squibb Co. Princeton, NJ
ETOPOSIDE INJECTION product label, June 2003. Manufactured by Ben Venue Laboratories, Inc, Bedford, OH. Manufactured for Bedford Laboratories™ Bedford, OH
Toposar™ etoposide injection, product label, December 1998. Manufactured by SP Pharmaceuticals LLC, Albuquerque, NM. Manufactured for Pharmacia & Upjohn Company, Kalamazoo, MI
Information from Bristol-Myers Oncology Division. "VePesid® stability above 0.4 mg/mL", April 26, 1993

Product Identification, Preparation, Storage, and Stability

- Etoposide is generically available from several manufacturers. In general, formulations for parenteral use are packaged in single-use glass vials containing a viscous solution of etoposide 20 mg/mL that may also contain benzyl alcohol, polysorbate 80, and polyethylene glycol
- Store intact vials and diluted solutions at controlled room temperature of 15°–30°C (59°–86°F)
- Etoposide is marketed as a solution that MUST BE DILUTED before administration with either D5W or 0.9% NS to a concentration between 0.2 and 0.4 mg/mL in either glass or plastic containers
- Product stability is affected by the concentration of etoposide and the temperature at which the diluted product is maintained. Solutions with concentrations >0.1 mg/mL are supersaturated and potentially may precipitate. The time to precipitation at concentrations >0.4 mg/mL is unpredictable and may occur earlier than the times indicated in the following table, particularly if the product is stored at cool temperatures or agitated, as during delivery with a peristaltic pump

Etoposide Concentration	Duration of Stability
0.1 mg/mL	96 hours
0.2 mg/mL	96 hours
0.4 mg/mL	24–48 hours
0.6 mg/mL	8 hours
1 mg/mL	2 hours

Note: Plastic devices made of acrylic or ABS (acrylonitrile, butadiene, and styrene polymer) may crack and leak when used with undiluted etoposide injection

Recommendations for Drug Administration and Ancillary Care

General:

- *Do not administer* etoposide by rapid intravenous injection. Administer etoposide by intravenous infusion over at least 30–60 minutes to prevent hypotension. Longer infusion durations may be used when clinically appropriate for the volume of fluid that must be administered

ETOPOSIDE PHOSPHATE

ETOPOPHOS® (etoposide phosphate) for injection product label, February 2004. Bristol-Myers Squibb Co., Princeton, NJ

Product Identification, Preparation, Storage, and Stability

- Etoposide phosphate is packaged in single-dose vials containing etoposide phosphate equivalent to 100 mg etoposide (NDC 0015-3404-20)
- Store intact vials under refrigeration (2°–8°C; 35.6°–46.4°F) in the original package to protect the product from light
- Reconstitute etoposide phosphate with 5 mL or 10 mL of SWFI, D5W, 0.9% NS, BWFI with benzyl alcohol, or B0.9% NS with benzyl alcohol as follows:

		Concentration	
Etoposide Phosphate Content per Vial	Diluent Volume	Etoposide Phosphate	Etoposide
100 mg	5 mL	22.7 mg/mL	20 mg/mL
	10 mL	11.4 mg/mL	10 mg/mL

- When reconstituted as directed, solutions may be stored in glass or plastic containers under refrigeration for up to 7 days
- Solutions that were reconstituted with SWFI, D5W, or 0.9% NS may be stored in glass or plastic containers at controlled room temperature (20°–25°C; 68°–77°F) for up to 24 hours
- Solutions that were reconstituted with antimicrobially preserved diluents may be stored in glass or plastic containers at controlled room temperature for up to 48 hours
- After reconstitution, etoposide phosphate is suitable for direct administration to human subjects, or it may be further diluted to concentrations as low as 0.1 mg etoposide/mL with either D5W or 0.9% NS
- After dilution, etoposide phosphate solutions may be stored under refrigeration or at controlled room temperature for up to 24 hours

Recommendations for Drug Administration and Ancillary Care

General:

- Administer etoposide phosphate by intravenous infusion over 5 minutes to 3.5 hours

FLOXURIDINE (FUDR)

Floxuridine for Injection product label, February 2000. Manufactured by Ben Venue Laboratories, Inc, Bedford, OH. Manufactured for Bedford Laboratories™, Bedford, OH

Trissel LA. Handbook on Injectable Drugs, 13th ed. Bethesda: American Society of Health-System Pharmacists, Inc, 2005

Product Identification, Preparation, Storage, and Stability

- Floxuridine is packaged in 5-mL vials containing 500 mg floxuridine as a lyophilized powder. NDC 55390-135-01
- Store intact vials at 15°–30°C (59°–86°F)
- Reconstitute floxuridine with SWFI 5 mL to yield a solution containing approximately 100 mg floxuridine/mL
- Reconstituted floxuridine may be stored under refrigeration 2°–8°C (36°–46°F) for up to 2 weeks
- Floxuridine may be further diluted with D5W or 0.9% NS to a volume appropriate for the apparatus used to administer the drug
- Floxuridine was stable after dilution with either D5W or 0.9% NS to 0.5 mg/mL and storage in PVC or glass containers at 20°C or 37°C for 7 days

Selected incompatibility:

- Floxuridine is optimally stable at pH = 4–7. Avoid admixture with highly acidic or alkaline solutions

Recommendations for Drug Administration and Ancillary Care

General:

- Floxuridine has received FDA approval only for administration by continuous intra-arterial infusion

FLUDARABINE

Fludara® (fludarabine phosphate) for injection product label, October 2003. Manufactured by Ben Venue Laboratories, Inc, Bedford, OH. Manufactured for Berlex, Montville, NJ

Product Identification, Preparation, Storage, and Stability

Fludara® is packaged in single-use 6-mL clear glass vials containing 50 mg of lyophilized fludarabine phosphate. NDC 50419-511-06

- Store intact vials under refrigeration between 2° and 8°C (35.6°–46.4°F)
- Reconstitute fludarabine by aseptically adding to a vial 2 mL SWFI to produce a solution containing fludarabine phosphate 25 mg/mL
- Although reconstituted fludarabine is chemically stable for up to 16 days when stored at room temperature under ambient lighting, the Fludara® product does not contain an antimicrobial preservative and should be used within 8 hours after reconstitution
- Fludarabine may be further diluted in 100–125 mL D5W or 0.9% NS in glass or plastic containers

Recommendations for Drug Administration and Ancillary Care

General:

- Administer fludarabine by intravenous infusion over approximately 30 minutes

FLUOROURACIL

ADRUCIL® (fluorouracil injection, USP) product label, July 2003. SICOR Pharmaceuticals, Inc, Irvine, CA

Trissel LA. Handbook on Injectable Drugs, 13th ed. Bethesda: American Society of Health-System Pharmacists, Inc, 2005

Product Identification, Preparation, Storage, and Stability

- Fluorouracil is generically available from several manufacturers. In general, the products designed for parenteral use are formulated as an injectable solution containing 50 mg fluorouracil/mL
- Store at room temperature 15°–30°C (59°–86°F)
- Fluorouracil is subject to photodegradation and should be protected from light. Store the product in its original packaging until time of use
- Fluorouracil is characteristically colorless to faint yellow. Dark yellow indicates degradation and may result from prolonged storage in excessive heat or exposure to light. Discolored solutions should be discarded
- Fluorouracil may be given undiluted or diluted in dextrose or sodium chloride solutions, or solutions in which dextrose and sodium chloride are combined

Selected incompatibility:

- Prepare, store, and administer fluorouracil with plastic containers and administration sets. Fluorouracil adsorbs to glass surfaces more extensively than plastic surfaces (polyvinyl chloride, polyethylene, polypropylene)
- Fluorouracil and leucovorin calcium should not be combined in the same product container
- Fluorouracil should not be combined in the same product container with doxorubicin or simultaneously administered through the same administration set or VAD lumen

Recommendations for Drug Administration and Ancillary Care

General:

- Fluorouracil may be given by direct intravenous push over ≤2 minutes or as an intravenous infusion for durations of minutes to days
- Fluorouracil also has been given by prolonged infusion intra-arterially and by regional venous perfusion (eg, via the portal vein)
- Fluorouracil solutions may be given via peripheral or central vascular access; however, the undiluted solution has an osmolality of 650 mOsm/kg, a pH of approximately 9.2 (range 8.6–9.4) and can be irritating to small veins

GEMCITABINE HCI

GEMZAR® (GEMCITABINE HCI) FOR INJECTION product label, April 26, 2005. Eli Lilly and Company. Indianapolis, IN

Trissel LA. Handbook on Injectable Drugs, 13th ed. Bethesda: American Society of Health-System Pharmacists, Inc, 2005

Product Identification, Preparation, Storage, and Stability

- GEMZAR® is packaged in 10-mL or 50-mL single-use vials containing gemcitabine HCl 200 mg or 1000 mg, respectively, as a white, lyophilized powder. NDC 0002-7501-01 (200 mg/vial); NDC 0002-7502-01 (1000 mg/vial)
- Store intact vials at controlled room temperature (20°–25°C; 68°–77°F)
- Reconstitute gemcitabine as follows:

Gemcitabine Content per Vial	Volume of 0.9% NS Diluent per Vial	Gemcitabine Concentration After Reconstitution
200 mg	5 mL	38 mg/mL*
1000 mg	25 mL	

Note: The amount of gemcitabine powder within a vial causes the volume of the reconstituted product to be greater then the volume of diluent added during reconstitution.

Gemcitabine has limited solubility in aqueous media. Reconstitution to concentrations >40 mg/mL may prevent complete solubilization

- Shake the vial to dissolve gemcitabine
- Completely withdrawing a vial's contents will provide 200 mg/5.26 mL or 1000 mg/26.3 mL of gemcitabine, respectively
- DO NOT REFRIGERATE reconstituted gemcitabine solution to prevent crystallization. Gemzar® solutions are stable for at least 24 hours at controlled room temperature
- Reconstituted gemcitabine is suitable for direct administration or may be further diluted with 0.9% NS to concentrations as low as 0.1 mg/mL
- Gemcitabine is compatible with either glass or PVC containers and PVC administration sets

Recommendations for Drug Administration and Ancillary Care

General:

- Administer gemcitabine by intravenous infusion over 30 minutes

Fixed Dose-Rate Administration:

- Gemcitabine also may be administered intravenously at a fixed dose-rate (FDR) of 10 mg/m² per min

Notes: Experimental data have demonstrated that small increases in intracellular concentrations of gemcitabine's active triphosphate metabolite profoundly affect its intracellular area under the curve, and that a fixed gemcitabine administration rate of 10 mg/m² per min maximize the rate at which the metabolite accumulates in peripheral blood mononuclear cells

This observation is the basis for recent clinical trials with FDR gemcitabine administration which attempt to correlate increases in intracellular gemcitabine triphosphate concentrations with improved objective responses to treatment and survival

Tempero M et al. J Clin Oncol 2003;21:3402–3408. Comment in: J Clin Oncol 2003;21:3383–3384

GEMTUZUMAB OZOGAMICIN

Mylotarg® (gemtuzumab ozogamicin for injection) product label, August 2005. Wyeth Pharmaceuticals, Inc, Philadelphia, PA

Product Identification, Preparation, Storage, and Stability

- Mylotarg® is packaged in single-use amber glass vials containing 5 mg gemtuzumab ozogamicin as a lyophilized powder. NDC 0008-4510-01
- Store intact vials under refrigeration at 2°–8°C (35.6°–46.4°F)
- *Gemtuzumab is light-sensitive*: Protect from direct and indirect sunlight and unshielded fluorescent light during product preparation and administration. All preparation should take place in a biologic safety cabinet with shielded fluorescent light
- Reconstitute the contents of each vial with SWFI 5 mL to produce a solution with concentration = 1 mg/mL. Gently swirl each vial to aid dissolution. Inspect vial contents to ensure complete drug dissolution
- *Do not refrigerate* the reconstituted solution (1 mg/mL)
- Further dilute the reconstituted drug by injecting reconstituted gemtuzumab solution into 0.9% NS 100 mL in either a PVC or ethylene/polypropylene copolymer (non-PVC) container covered by material that will block ultraviolet (UV) light
- Gemtuzumab ozogamicin should be diluted only with 0.9% NS. DO NOT MIX gemtuzumab with other drugs
- Gemtuzumab protein in solution normally scatters light; consequently, the solution in the vial, a transfer syringe, or a parenteral container may appear hazy
- Maximum product storage times from the time of reconstitution until administration is completed are as follows:

Storage Temperature	Time After Reconstitution	Time After Dilution	Time For Administration	Total Duration
2°–8°C	≤8 hours	Immediate use	2-hour infusion	10 hours
Room temperature	≤2 hours	≤16 hours	2-hour infusion	20 hours

Recommendations for Drug Administration and Ancillary Care

General:

- Before gemtuzumab ozogamicin administration, give acetaminophen and diphenhydramine as primary prophylaxis to decrease the incidence of a postinfusion adverse symptom complex
- Do *not* administer gemtuzumab by intravenous push or bolus injection
- After diluting gemtuzumab ozogamicin with 0.9% NS, the resulting solution should be administered by intravenous infusion over 2 hours via peripheral or central venous access devices
- Protect the parenteral container from light during drug administration. It is not necessary to protect the administration set tubing
- Administer gemtuzumab through an in-line, low protein-binding filter with the following characteristics:

Filter Membrane Pore Sizes	Membrane Composition
0.22 micrometers	Polyether sulfone
1.2 micrometers	
1.2 micrometers	Acrylic copolymer hydrophilic filter
0.8 micrometers	Cellulose mixed ester (acetate and nitrate)
0.2 micrometers	Cellulose acetate membrane

- *Do not administer* other drugs through the same infusion line with gemtuzumab ozogamicin

IDARUBICIN HCl

Idamycin PFS® idarubicin hydrochloride injection product label, May 2003. Manufactured by Pharmacia Italia S.p.A. Milan, Italy (glass vials) and Pharmacia (Perth) Pty Limited, Bentley, WA 6102, Australia (polypropylene vials) . Manufactured for Pharmacia & Upjohn Company, Kalamazoo, MI
Idamycin® (idarubicin hydrochloride for injection, USP) product label, August 2000. Manufactured by Pharmacia & Upjohn S.p.A. Milan, Italy. Manufactured for Pharmacia & Upjohn Company, Kalamazoo, MI

Trissel LA. Handbook on Injectable Drugs, 13th ed. Bethesda: American Society of Health-System Pharmacists, Inc, 2005
Trissel LA, Martinez JF. Am J Hosp Pharm 1993;50:1134,1137

Product Identification, Preparation, Storage, and Stability

Idamycin PFS® idarubicin hydrochloride injection:

- The product is available as a sterile, red-orange, isotonic parenteral preservative-free solution of idarubicin HCl with a concentration of 1 mg/mL

Idamycin PFS®	Single-Dose Glass Vials	Single-Dose Cytosafe™ Vials
5 mg/5 mL	NDC 0013-2200-01	NDC 0013-2576-91
10 mg/10 mL	NDC 0013-2201-01	NDC 0013-2586-91
20 mg/20 mL	NDC 0013-2202-01	NDC 0013-2596-91

Note: Store Idamycin PFS® solution under refrigeration 2°–8°C (35.6°–46.4°F) and protected from light

Idamycin® (idarubicin hydrochloride [powder for reconstitution] for injection):

- The product is packaged in single-dose vials containing 20 mg idarubicin HCl. NDC 0013-2526-86
- Store the lyophilized powder formulation at room temperature and protected from light
- Reconstitute Idamycin® lyophilized powder formulation with 20 mL SWFI to produce a solution with a concentration of 1 mg/mL

Instructions Common to Both Products

- Idarubicin HCl 1 mg/mL is suitable for direct administration to patients. It also may be diluted to a concentration of 1–10 mg/100 mL in 0.9% NS or D5W , or to a concentration of 10 mg/100 mL in LRI
- *Note:* Idarubicin HCl solutions in 0.9% NS exhibit a low level of haziness that is visible under high-intensity light and measurable with a turbidimeter. The haziness increases to maximum with increasing drug dilution from a concentration of 1 mg/mL to 0.05 mg/mL. The haze is not indicative of drug instability or incompatibility

Selected incompatibility:

- Idarubicin is subject to photodegradation. Diluted products that are not administered within a few hours after preparation should be protected from light exposure
- Idarubicin is physically incompatible with heparin

Recommendations for Drug Administration and Ancillary Care

General:

- Administer idarubicin by slow push over 10–15 minutes into the tubing of a freely running intravenous infusion of 0.9% NS or D5W
- *Caution*: Idarubicin is a vesicant and may produce severe local soft tissue necrosis if extravasation occurs. Idarubicin *must not be given* by the intramuscular, subcutaneous, or intrathecal routes

IFOSFAMIDE

IFEX® (ifosfamide for injection) product label, November 2002. Manufactured by Baxter Healthcare Corporation, Deerfield, IL. Distributed by Bristol-Myers Squibb Oncology, Bristol-Myers Squibb Company, Princeton, NJ

Product Identification, Preparation, Storage, and Stability

- IFEX® is packaged in combination packages with the uroprotective agent MESNEX® (mesna) Injection or as single-dose vials as follows:
  - Five single-dose vials containing ifosfamide 1000 mg/vial + 3 multidose vials containing mesna 1000 mg/vial (NDC 0015-3556-26)
  - Ten single-dose vials containing ifosfamide 1000 mg/vial + 10multidose vials containing mesna 1000 mg/vial (NDC 0015-3554-27)
- Two single-dose vials containing ifosfamide 3000 mg/vial + 6 multidose vials containing mesna 1000 mg/vial (NDC 0015-3564-15)
- Single-dose vials containing ifosfamide 1000 mg/vial (NDC 0015-0556-05)
- Single-dose vials containing ifosfamide 3000 mg/vial (NDC 0015-0557-41)
- Store intact vials at controlled room temperature 20°–25°C (68°–77°F). Protect ifosfamide from temperatures >30°C (>86°F)
- Reconstitute ifosfamide with either SWFI or BWFI as follows:

  [Shake the vials to dissolve the drug]

Ifosfamide Content per Vial	Diluent Volume	Ifosfamide Concentration After Reconstitution
1000 mg	20 mL	50 mg/mL
3000 mg	60 mL	

- Ifosfamide solutions may be further diluted to produce concentrations between 0.6 and 20 mg/mL in any of the following fluids: D5W , 0.9% NS, LRI, D2.5W, 0.45% NaCl, or D5W/0.9% NS
- Ifosfamide is physically and chemically stable in a variety of parenteral fluid containers, including those made of glass, ethylene and propylene copolymers, PVC plasticized with phthalates, and other polyolefin materials
- Ifosfamide solutions should be refrigerated and used within 24 hours after preparation

Recommendations for Drug Administration and Ancillary Care

General:

- On the days of ifosfamide administration, give intravenous or oral fluid hydration consisting of at least 2000 mL/day greater than a patient's routine daily fluid consumption. Aggressive hydration has been shown to decrease the urothelial toxicity associated with ifosfamide
- Administer ifosfamide by intravenous infusion over a minimum of 30 minutes
- Give mesna concomitantly with ifosfamide to protect the urinary tract from exposure to reactive ifosfamide metabolites that are highly concentrated in urine
- Mesna may be added to the same container as ifosfamide without compromising the stability of either product

INTERFERON ALFA-2b

INTRON® A interferon alfa-2b, recombinant for injection product label, March 2004. Schering Corporation, Kenilworth, NJ

Product Identification, Preparation, Storage, and Stability

- INTRON® A is available in several formulations and package formats; however, the powder for injection is packaged in vials containing 10 million International units (NDC 0085-0571-02), 18 million International units (NDC 0085-1110-01), or 50 million International units (NDC 0085-0539-01) recombinant interferon alfa-2b
- The product packaging also contains a second vial of SWFI for use in reconstituting the powder
- Recombinant interferon alfa-2b also is formulated as a solution for injection, which is *not* recommended for intravenous infusion
- Store recombinant interferon alfa-2b powder for injection between 2° and 8°C (35.6°–46.4°F) both before and after reconstitution
- Prepare a solution for intravenous infusion immediately before use by reconstituting the powder formulation of interferon alfa-2b with the BWFI diluent provided
- Add an amount of interferon appropriate for a patient's dose to a bag containing 0.9% NS to produce a solution with an interferon concentration ≥10 million International units/100 mL
- Each of the 3 powdered interferon alfa-2b products identified contain 1 mg albumin, which prevents drug adsorption to containers and administration set surfaces during preparation and administration

Recommendations for Drug Administration and Ancillary Care

General:

- Administer interferon alfa-2b by intravenous infusion over 20 minutes

IRINOTECAN HCl

Camptosar® irinotecan hydrochloride injection product label, July 2005. Distributed by Pharmacia & Upjohn Co., Division of Pfizer Inc, New York, NY

Product Identification, Preparation, Storage, and Stability

- Camptosar® is packaged in single-dose amber glass vials containing an aqueous solution of irinotecan hydrochloride 40 mg/2 mL (NDC 0009-7529-02) or 100 mg/5 mL (NDC 0009-7529-01)
- The products are packaged in a plastic blister that is designed to prevent leaking if a product vial is broken. Dispose of broken product vials by incineration without opening the blister packaging
- Store intact vials at controlled room temperature (15°–30°C; 59°–86°F), and protect the product from light until it is used
- Camptosar® is physically and chemically stable for up to 24 hours at room temperature (approximately 25°C) under ambient fluorescent lighting
- Irinotecan *must be diluted* before infusion with D5W (preferred) or 0.9% NS to a concentration within the range of 0.12–2.8 mg/mL
- After dilution, irinotecan is physically and chemically stable for up to 24 hours at room temperature (approximately 25°C) under ambient fluorescent lighting
- After dilution in D5W , solutions that are stored at approximately 2°–8°C and protected from light are physically and chemically stable for 48 hours
- *Do not refrigerate* admixtures prepared with 0.9% NS to prevent the formation of visible particulates
- Because of possible microbial contamination during dilution, use irinotecan admixtures prepared with D5W within 24 hours if they were refrigerated after preparation. Admixtures prepared with D5W or 0.9% NS should be used within 6 hours if they were kept at room temperature (15°–30°C)

Selected incompatibility:

- Irinotecan is maximally stable at pH ≤6. *Avoid* admixture with neutral or alkaline solutions

Recommendations for Drug Administration and Ancillary Care

General:

- Administer irinotecan by intravenous infusion over 90 minutes
- Atropine may be administered prophylactically or therapeutically to patients who experience cholinergic symptoms in association with irinotecan
- Irinotecan is metabolically activated to SN-38, which is metabolized by the polymorphically expressed uridine diphosphate glucuronosyltransferase enzyme, UGT1A1. Approximately 10% of the North American population express homozygously the UGT1A1*28 allele and, consequently, are at greater risk for neutropenia from irinotecan than persons who express the wild phenotype, UGT1A1
- Initial irinotecan dosage should be decreased for persons who homozygously express UGT1A1*28

LEUCOVORIN CALCIUM

LEUCOVORIN CALCIUM FOR INJECTION product label, December 2003. Mayne Pharma (USA) Inc, Paramus, NJ
LEUCOVORIN CALCIUM INJECTION USP, LEUCOVORIN CALCIUM FOR INJECTION product label, September 2000. Manufactured by Ben Venue Laboratories, Inc, Bedford, OH. Manufactured for Bedford Laboratories™, Bedford, OH

Product Identification, Preparation, Storage, and Stability

Leucovorin calcium for injection:

- Leucovorin calcium for injection is generically available in a variety of product strengths
- Leucovorin calcium for injection is a sterile, lyophilized powder indicated for intramuscular or intravenous administration. In general, the lyophilized powdered products do not contain an antimicrobial preservative
- Reconstitute with BWFI (preserved with benzyl alcohol) or SWFI as follows:

Amount of Leucovorin Calcium per Vial	Volume of Diluent per Vial	Concentration After Reconstitution
50 mg	5 mL	10 mg/mL
100 mg	10 mL	
200 mg	20 mL	
350 mg	17.5 mL	20 mg/mL
500 mg	50 mL	10 mg/mL

- After reconstitution with BWFI, the resulting solution must be used within 7 days. If reconstituted with SWFI, use the product immediately and discard any unused portion
- FDA-approved product labeling recommends reconstituting leucovorin with SWFI for dosages >10 mg/m^2 (for adult patients) because of the amount of benzyl alcohol in BWFI. Avoid administering benzyl alcohol-containing products to adolescent and younger patients

Leucovorin calcium injection:

- Leucovorin calcium injection is generically available in a variety of product strengths as a sterile, preservative-free solution indicated for intramuscular or intravenous administration in single-use vials
- Store intact vials under refrigeration at 2°–8°C (35.6°–46.4°F)
- Protect from light. Discard partially used vials. Retain the product in its packaging carton until it is used.
- Each milliliter contains leucovorin calcium equivalent to 10 mg leucovorin

Leucovorin calcium for injection and jeucovorin calcium injection:

- Leucovorin calcium may be further diluted with D5W , 0.9% NS, D5W/0.9% NS, D10W , RI, or LRI for clinical use

Selected incompatibility:

- *Do not mix* leucovorin with fluorouracil. Admixture results in particulate formation

Recommendations for Drug Administration and Ancillary Care

General:

- For intravenous or intramuscular administration
- *Do not inject* leucovorin intravenously more rapidly than 160 mg per minute due to the rate at which calcium will be injected
- One milligram of leucovorin calcium contains:

Calcium	0.004 mEq
Calcium	0.002 mmol
Leucovorin	0.002 mmol

MESNA

Mesnex® (mesna) Injection, Mesnex® (mesna) Tablets product label, May 2002. Manufactured by Baxter Healthcare Corporation, Deerfield, IL (Mesnex® Injection). Distributed by Bristol-Myers Squibb Oncology, Bristol-Myers Squibb Company, Princeton, NJ

Product Identification, Preparation, Storage, and Stability

- Mesnex® (mesna) is packaged in multidose vials containing mesna 1000 mg/10 mL (single vial, NDC 0015-3563-02; package of 10 vials, NDC 0015-3563-03)
- For intravenous administration, dilute mesna within the concentration range of 1–20 mg mesna/mL in any of the following fluids: D5W, D5W/0.2% NaCl, D5W/0.33% NaCl, D5W/0.45% NaCl, 0.9% NS, or LRI.
- Diluted solutions are chemically and physically stable for 24 hours at 25°C (77°F)

Selected incompatibility (compatibility):

- Mesna is compatible and may be mixed in the same container with ifosfamide and cyclophosphamide
- Mesna is *not compatible* and should not be mixed in a container or in administration set tubing with cisplatin or carboplatin

Recommendations for Drug Administration and Ancillary Care

General:

- Mesna may be administered by intravenous injection, intermittent intravenous infusion, or continuous intravenous infusion
- If mesna tablets are not available for use, the parenteral product also may be given orally, diluted just before use in a small volume (60–120 mL; 2–4 oz) of a very cold (preferably) carbonated beverage to mask the drug's unpleasant flavor
- Avoid exposing mesna injection to the air. Mesna spontaneously oxidizes to dimesna on exposure to oxygen
- FDA-approved product labeling describes intermittent administration of mesna with ifosfamide as follows:

Intravenous administration:

- Mesna in a dosage equal to 20% of the ifosfamide dosage is given at the same time as ifosfamide, and then at 4 hours and 8 hours after each ifosfamide dose; that is, the total daily mesna dose is approximately 60% of the daily ifosfamide dose

Intravenous and oral administration:

- Mesna in a dosage equal to 20% of the ifosfamide dosage is given intravenously at the same time as ifosfamide, and then mesna tablets are given orally in a dose equal to 40% of the ifosfamide dose at 2 hours and 6 hours after each ifosfamide dose; that is, the total daily mesna dose approximately equals the daily ifosfamide dose

METHOTREXATE

Methotrexate injection product label, August 2000. Manufactured by Ben Venue Laboratories, Inc, Bedford, OH. Manufactured for Bedford Laboratories™, Bedford, OH

Product Identification, Preparation, Storage, and Stability

- Methotrexate is generically available in a variety of product strengths in liquid and lyophilized formulations
- Store methotrexate products at controlled room temperature of 15°–30°C (59°–86°F)
- In general, reconstitute lyophilized products to a concentration not greater than 25 mg methotrexate/mL
- Protect methotrexate products from light. Methotrexate is susceptible to photodegradation, the extent of which correlates inversely with methotrexate concentration and is exacerbated by admixture with sodium bicarbonate
- After reconstitution, lyophilized formulations and methotrexate injection (product in solution) are suitable for direct intravenous injection
- Methotrexate also may be further diluted for clinical use. A therapeutic indication often determines the volume in which a dose is prepared and administered; that is, whether dilution is necessary, or clinically or logistically appropriate. Compatible diluents include 0.9% NS, D5W , and combinations of saline and dextrose

For intrathecal injection and high-dose regimens:

- Use only preservative-free methotrexate and diluent solutions

For intrathecal injection:

- Use preservative-free 0.9% NS to dilute methotrexate for intrathecal injection to a concentration within the range of 1–2.5 mg/mL
- Admixtures with hydrocortisone sodium succinate for intrathecal administration (with or without cytarabine) should be prepared just before use and administered as soon as possible (within minutes) after preparation due to the instability of the hydrocortisone component

Recommendations for Drug Administration and Ancillary Care

General:

- Methotrexate may be given parenterally by intravenous push, short intravenous infusions over <1 hour, or continuous intravenous infusions for periods up to 24–36 hours, and by the intramuscular, intra-arterial, and intrathecal routes

For intravenous use:

- The duration of methotrexate administration varies among treatment protocols and published reports, and in the case of moderate and high-dose regimens ($\geq$100 mg/m^2), often correlates with schemes for concomitant hydration, urinary alkalinization, serum level monitoring and expectations for the rate at which methotrexate will be eliminated, and leucovorin rescue

For intrathecal injection:

- Use only products that *do not contain antimicrobial preservatives* (eg, alcohols, parabens)
- Administration should be completed as soon as possible after product preparation
- When possible, inject methotrexate in a volume equivalent to the volume of cerebrospinal fluid removed

MITOMYCIN

MUTAMYCIN® (Mitomycin for Injection, USP) product label, January 2000. Bristol-Myers Squibb Oncology, Bristol-Myers Squibb Company, Princeton, NJ
MITOMYCIN FOR INJECTION, USP product label, June 2000. Manufactured by Ben Venue Laboratories, Inc, Bedford, OH. Manufactured for Bedford Laboratories™, Bedford, OH
MITOMYCIN FOR INJECTION, USP product label, August 2000. Manufactured for SuperGen, Inc, San Ramon, CA

Product Identification, Preparation, Storage, and Stability

- Mitomycin is available generically from several manufacturers as a lyophilized powder in vials containing 5 mg, 20 mg, or 40 mg of the active drug
- Store intact vials at 15°–30°C (59°–86°F). Avoid temperatures >40°C (>104°F)
- Reconstitute mitomycin as follows:

Amount of Mitomycin per Vial	Volume of SWFI Diluent	Mitomycin Concentration After Reconstitution
5 mg	10 mL	0.5 mg/mL
20 mg	40 mL	
40 mg	80 mL	

- After adding the diluent, shake the vials to dissolve mitomycin. If the product does not dissolve immediately, allow it to stand at room temperature until a solution is obtained
- After reconstitution with SWFI, the product is stable for 14 days under refrigeration or 7 days at room temperature
- Mitomycin stability is not adversely affected by exposure to fluorescent lighting
- Reconstituted mitomycin (0.5 mg/mL) is suitable for intravenous administration, but the product may be further diluted to a concentration of 20–40 mcg/mL (0.02–0.04 mg/mL) in the following fluids at room temperature:

Vehicle/Diluent Solution	Duration of Stability
D5W	3 hours
0.9% NS	12 hours
0.167 M Sodium Lactate Injection, USP	24 hours

Recommendations for Drug Administration and Ancillary Care

General:

- Mitomycin may be injected directly into any suitable vein, but preferably is injected into the side-arm of a freely flowing intravenous infusion
- Mitomycin diluted in 20–50 mL SWFI or 0.9% NS has also been given intravesically into the urinary bladder as a treatment for transitional cell carcinoma

Caution: Mitomycin is a powerful vesicant and may produce severe local soft tissue necrosis if extravasation occurs

MITOXANTRONE HCl

NOVANTRONE® mitoxantrone for injection concentrate product label, March 2005. Manufactured for Serono Inc, Rockland, MA. Marketed by (OSI)™ oncology, OSI Pharmaceuticals, Inc, Melville, NY (for oncological indications)

Product Identification, Preparation, Storage, and Stability

- NOVANTRONE® is packaged in vials for multidose use containing mitoxantrone HCl (equivalent to 2 mg mitoxantrone free base/mL) as a sterile aqueous solution. NDC 44087-1520-1 (20 mg/10 mL); NDC 44087-1525-1 (25 mg/12.5 mL); NDC 44087-1530-1 (30 mg/15 mL)
- Store NOVANTRONE® intact vials between 15° and 25°C (59°–77°F)
- Partially used vials may be stored for up to 7 days at 15°–25°C or for 14 days under refrigeration (2°–8°C; 35.6°–46.4°F). DO NOT FREEZE mitoxantrone.
- *Mitoxantrone must be diluted* before administration to at least 50 mL (after dilution) in D5W or 0.9% NS

Selected incompatibility:

- Admixture with heparin may result in precipitation

Recommendations for Drug Administration and Ancillary Care

General:

- Mitoxantrone is usually given as a short, intravenous infusion over 5–30 minutes into the side-arm of a freely flowing intravenous solution, but it may be given by continuous intravenous infusion over 24 hours
- *Do not administer* a dose of mitoxantrone over <3 minutes

Caution: Mitoxantrone is a vesicant and may produce severe local soft tissue necrosis if extravasation occurs

NELARABINE

ARRANON® (nelarabine) Injection product label, October 2005. GlaxoSmithKline, Research Triangle Park, NC

Product Identification, Preparation, Storage, and Stability

- Arranon® is packaged in Type I clear glass vials with a gray butyl rubber (latex-free) stopper and a red, snap-off, aluminum seal. Vials contain nelarabine 250 mg (5 mg/mL) and sodium chloride (4.5 mg/mL) and SWFI in a total volume of 50 mL. Product vials are packaged in cartons containing one NDC 0007-4401-01 or six vials NDC 0007-4401-06
- Store Arranon® at 25°C (77°F). Temperature excursions to 15°–30°C (59°–86°F) are permitted.

Preparation for Administration:

- DO NOT DILUTE Arranon® prior to administration. Transfer a volume of nelarabine appropriate for a patient's dose into a PVC or glass container
- Transfer an amount appropriate for a patient's dose to a PVC or glass container

- Undiluted nelarabine is stable in PVC and glass containers for up to 8 hours at temperatures up to 30°C

Recommendations for Drug Administration and Ancillary Care

General:

- Administer by intravenous infusion over 2 hours to adult patients and over 1 hour in pediatric patients

OXALIPLATIN

ELOXATIN™ (oxaliplatin for injection) product label, April 2005. Manufactured by Ben Venue Laboratories, Bedford, OH. Manufactured for Sanofi-Synthelabo Inc, Distributed by Sanofi-Synthelabo Inc, New York, NY

Product Identification, Preparation, Storage, and Stability

- ELOXATIN™ (oxaliplatin) is packaged in single-use clear glass vials with gray elastomeric stoppers and flip-off seals containing 50 mg or 100 mg of oxaliplatin as a sterile, preservative-free aqueous solution with a concentration of 5 mg oxaliplatin/mL. NDC 0024-0590-10 (50-mg vial); NDC 0024-0591-20 (100-mg vial)
- Store intact vials under normal lighting conditions at 25°C (77°F). Temperature excursions are permitted to 15°–30°C (59°–86°F). Protect oxaliplatin from exposure to light in the original packaging carton
- After reconstitution in the original vial, store oxaliplatin for up to 24 hours under refrigeration at 2°–8°C (35.6°–46.4°F)
- Dilute oxaliplatin in 250–500 mL D5W before clinical use
- After dilution with D5W 250–500 mL, the product shelf life is 6 hours at room temperature (20°–25°C [68°–77°F]) or up to 24 hours under refrigeration
- Protection from light exposure is not required after dilution

Selected incompatibility:

- *Do not mix* oxaliplatin with alkaline media (eg, fluorouracil) in a container or through the same line during simultaneous administration
- Aluminum has been reported to degrade platinum compounds. Needles and intravenous administration sets containing aluminum parts that may contact oxaliplatin should not be used to prepare or administer the drug

Recommendations for Drug Administration and Ancillary Care

General:

- Oxaliplatin is usually given by intravenous infusion over 2 hours
- Increasing the infusion time for from 2 hours to 6 hours decreases maximum oxaliplatin concentrations by an estimated 32% and may mitigate acute toxicities
- Administration sets and vascular access device used to administer oxaliplatin should be flushed with D5W before using it to administer other medications
- Prescriptions and medication orders should identify the drug by its complete generic name, OXALIPLATIN

PACLITAXEL

TAXOL® (paclitaxel) injection product label, March 2003. Bristol-Myers Squibb Oncology, Bristol-Myers Squibb Company, Princeton, NJ
ONXOL™ (paclitaxel) injection product label, September 2001. Manufactured by FH Faulding & Co. Ltd, Mulgrave Victoria, Australia 3170. Manufactured for IVAX Research, Inc, Miami, FL. Distributed by IVAX Pharmaceuticals, Inc, Miami, FL

Chin A et al. Ann Pharmacother 1994;28:35–36
Trissel LA. Handbook on Injectable Drugs, 13th ed. Bethesda: American Society of Health-System Pharmacists, Inc, 2005

Product Identification, Preparation, Storage, and Stability

- Paclitaxel is generically available in a variety of product strengths
- Commercial products are packaged in multidose glass vials containing a viscous concentrated solution of paclitaxel 6 mg/mL formulated in a solvent system of dehydrated alcohol, 49.7% (v/v) and either polyoxyethylated castor oil (Cremophor® EL, 527 mg/mL) or polyoxyl 35 castor oil (527 mg/mL)
- Store unopened vials at 20°–25°C (68°–77°F) in the original package
- *Avoid bringing paclitaxel into contact* with containers, syringes, tubing, and other materials made of PVC during drug preparation and administration. Paclitaxel-containing solutions characteristically leach DEHP and other phthalate plasticizers from flexible PVC containers and infusion sets. Paclitaxel solutions should be stored in polypropylene or polyolefin containers and administered through polyethylene- or polyolefin-lined administration sets
- Neither freezing nor refrigeration adversely affects product stability. After refrigeration, components in the formulation may precipitate, but will redissolve with little or no agitation after reaching room temperature without adversely affecting product quality. Discard the product if the solution remains cloudy after warming to room temperature and gentle agitation, or if an insoluble precipitate is noted
- For clinical use, *concentrated paclitaxel must be diluted* in a polyolefin container to a concentration between 0.3 and 1.2 mg/mL in 0.9% NS, D5W, D5W/0.9% NS, or D5W/LRI. After dilution, paclitaxel solutions are physically and chemically stable for up to 48 hours at ambient temperature (20°–23°C; 68°–73.4°F) and fluorescent lighting
- Paclitaxel should be inspected visually for particulate matter and discoloration before administration whenever solution and container permit. After preparation, paclitaxel solutions may show haziness, which is attributed to the formulation vehicle
- *Administer paclitaxel through an in-line filter* that has a membrane with a pore size of 0.22 micrometers. Filtration does not cause significant losses in potency
- Do not use chemotherapy dispensing pins and similar admixture devices with spikes with paclitaxel, because they can cause a vial's stopper to collapse and compromise the sterility of its contents

Recommendations for Drug Administration and Ancillary Care

General:

- Administer paclitaxel by intravenous infusion over periods from 1 to ≥24 hours (commonly, 3 hours)
- Use non-PVC containers, administration sets, and filters to administer paclitaxel. *Avoid vented* administration sets
- All patients should receive primary prophylaxis against hypersensitivity reactions, particularly with paclitaxel infusion duration ≤3 hours. Prophylaxis may consist of:
  1. Dexamethasone 20 mg orally or intravenously for 2 doses, at approximately 12 hours and 6 hours before paclitaxel, *plus*
  2. Diphenhydramine (or an equivalent H_1 antihistamine) 50 mg intravenously 30–60 minutes before paclitaxel, *and*
  3. Ranitidine 50 mg or cimetidine 300 mg (or an equivalent H_2 antihistamine) intravenously, 30–60 minutes before paclitaxel administration
- After dilution within the recommended concentration range (0.3–1.2 mg/mL), paclitaxel may unpredictably precipitate in a product container or administration set tubing. The mechanism underlying spontaneous precipitation and predisposing conditions are not well defined. Consequently, care providers should remain vigilant for drug precipitation throughout the duration of paclitaxel administration

PACLITAXEL PROTEIN-BOUND PARTICLES FOR INJECTABLE SUSPENSION

ABRAXANE™ for injectable suspension (paclitaxel protein-bound particles for injectable suspension; albumin-bound) product label, January 2005. ABRAXIS™ ONCOLOGY A Division of American Pharmaceutical Partners, Inc, Schaumburg, IL

Product Identification, Preparation, Storage, and Stability

- ABRAXANE™ is available in single-use vials containing paclitaxel 100 mg and approximately 900 mg Albumin Human as a sterile lyophilized powder. NDC 68817-134-50. The product does not contain Cremophor® or other solvents
- Store unopened vials at 20°–25°C (68°–77°F), in the original package
- The following reconstitution procedure yields a suspension for intravenous injection containing 5 mg paclitaxel/mL:
  1. Slowly inject 20 mL 0.9% NS against the inside wall of a product vial over a minimum of 1 minute. To prevent foaming, *do not inject* the diluent directly into the lyophilized drug
  2. After all diluent has been added to a vial, allow each vial to sit for a minimum of 5 minutes to ensure that the lyophilized drug is properly wetted, *then*
  3. Gently swirl and invert the vial slowly for at least 2 minutes until the drug is homogenously dispersed. Avoid aggressively agitating the vial contents to prevent foaming
  4. If foaming or clumping occurs, allow the solution to stand undisturbed for at least 15 minutes until foam subsides
- Reconstituted ABRAXANE™ (5 mg paclitaxel/mL) should be milky and homogenous without visible particulates. If particulates or drug settling are observed, gently invert affected product vials to completely re-suspend the product before it is administered to a patient
- The reconstituted product may be stored under refrigeration for a maximum of 8 hours. Although freezing and refrigeration do not adversely affect product stability, reconstituted ABRAXANE™ suspension should be stored in its original carton and protected from bright light
- Discard the reconstituted suspension if precipitates are observed. After preparing ABRAXANE™ as recommended and transfer to a parenteral product container, the drug product is stable at ambient temperature (approximately 25°C) and lighting conditions for up to 8 hours
- Inject an amount of reconstituted ABRAXANE™ appropriate for a patient's dose into an empty, sterile, PVC container. DEHP-free solution containers and administration sets are not necessary to prepare or administer ABRAXANE™ but may be used. *Do not filter* ABRAXANE™ during preparation
- Suspended particles may settle if the product is not used soon after reconstitution. Ensure complete re-suspension by mildly agitating ABRAXANE™ before it is used
- Discard any unused reconstituted ABRAXANE™ after preparing a patient's dose

Recommendations for Drug Administration and Ancillary Care

General:

- Premedication to prevent hypersensitivity reactions is not required before administering ABRAXANE™
- Administer ABRAXANE™ suspension by intravenous infusion over 30 minutes to reduce the likelihood of infusion-related reactions
- It is not necessary to prepare or administer ABRAXANE™ with DEHP-free containers and administration, but they may be used
- *Do not filter* ABRAXANE™ during administration
- If ABRAXANE™ administration does not commence within 30 minutes after product preparation, the product container should be gently inverted (several repetitions) to re-suspend the drug particles before administering the drug

PEMETREXED

ALIMTA® pemetrexed for injection product label, August 9, 2004. Manufactured by Lilly France S.A.S. F-67640 Fegersheim, France. Manufactured for Eli Lilly and Company, Indianapolis, IN

Product Identification, Preparation, Storage, and Stability

- ALIMTA® is packaged in sterile single-use vials containing pemetrexed 500 mg. NDC 0002-7623-01
- Intact ALIMTA® vials should be stored at 25°C (77°F). Temperature excursions to 15°–30°C (59°–86°F) are permitted
- Reconstitute vials containing 500 mg pemetrexed with 20 mL of preservative-free 0.9% NS to produce a solution containing 25 mg pemetrexed/mL. Gently swirl each vial until the powder is completely dissolved
- The resulting solution is not suitable for direct administration to patients. *Further dilution is required to a total volume of* 100 mL (Q.S.) with preservative-free 0.9% NS.
- Pemetrexed is chemically and physically stable for up to 24 hours after reconstitution, when stored between 2° and 8°C (35.6°–46.4°F), or at 25°C. Temperature excursions to 15°–30°C are permitted

Selected incompatibility:

- Pemetrexed is physically incompatible with diluents containing calcium, including lactated Ringer's injection, and Ringer's injection

Recommendations for Drug Administration and Ancillary Care

General:

- Administer pemetrexed by intravenous infusion over 10 minutes

Supportive Ancillary Care:

- To reduce treatment-related hematologic and gastrointestinal toxicities, patients treated with pemetrexed should take folic acid 400–1000 mcg orally daily. At least five daily doses of folic acid must be taken during the 7-day period before the first dose of pemetrexed. Folic acid supplementation should continue throughout treatment and for 21 days after the last dose of pemetrexed
- Give one intramuscular injection of vitamin B_{12} (cyanocobalamin) 1000 mcg during the week before the first dose of pemetrexed and every 3 cycles thereafter. Repeated vitamin B_{12} injections may be given the same day as pemetrexed
- Primary prophylaxis with dexamethasone (or an equivalent glucocorticoid) reduces the incidence and severity of cutaneous reactions in patients treated with pemetrexed. In clinical trials, dexamethasone 4 mg orally was given twice daily the day before, the day of, and the day after pemetrexed administration

PENTOSTATIN

Nipent® (pentostatin for injection) product label, April 1998. Manufactured by Parkedale Pharmaceuticals Inc, Rochester, MI. Manufactured for SUPERGEN, Inc, San Ramon, CA

Product Identification, Preparation, Storage, and Stability

- Nipent® is packaged in single-dose vials containing pentostatin 10 mg as a white to off-white, sterile, lyophilized powder. NDC 62701-800-01
- Store intact vials of Nipent® under refrigeration at 2°–8°C (35.6°–46.4°F).
- Reconstitute the lyophilized product in single-use vials with 5 mL SWFI to produce a solution with a concentration of 2 mg pentostatin/mL
- After reconstitution, pentostatin solution is suitable for direct intravenous injection, or it may be diluted in 25–50 mL D5W or 0.9% NS
- When diluted with D5W or 0.9% NS to concentrations in the range of 0.18–0.33 mg/mL, pentostatin does not interact with PVC infusion containers or administration sets
- When reconstituted and diluted as directed pentostatin is stable for at least 48 hours, but the product should be used within 8 hours because it does not contain an antimicrobial preservative

Recommendations for Drug Administration and Ancillary Care

General:

- Administer pentostatin intravenously by rapid injection over 5 minutes, or by infusion over 20–30 minutes
- Give intravenous hydration with D5W/0.9% NS or D5W/0.45% NS, 500–1000 mL before pentostatin administration plus 500 mL D5W after pentostatin is given

RITUXIMAB

RITUXAN® (Rituximab) product label, December 2004. Manufactured by Genentech, Inc, South San Francisco, CA. Jointly marketed by Biogen IDEC Inc, San Diego, CA and Genentech, Inc

Product Identification, Preparation, Storage, and Stability

- Rituxan® is packaged in single-use vials containing 100 mg/10 mL (NDC 50242-051-21) or 500 mg/50 mL (NDC 50242-053-06) of sterile, preservative-free rituximab at a uniform concentration of 10 mg/mL
- Store intact vials under refrigeration at 2°–8°C (35.6°–46.4°F). Protect rituximab vials from direct sunlight
- Withdraw from a vial an amount of rituximab appropriate for a patient's dose and dilute it in either D5W or 0.9% NS to a concentration within the range of 1–4 mg/mL
- Gently invert the bag to mix the solution
- After dilution to a concentration within the range of 1–4 mg/mL, rituximab solutions may be stored under refrigeration for up to 24 hours after preparation, and may then be removed from refrigeration to room temperature conditions and used within 48 hours after preparation
- Discard any partially used vials
- No incompatibilities between rituximab and PVC or polyethylene bags have been observed

Recommendations for Drug Administration and Ancillary Care

General:

Premedication:

- Primary prophylaxis with acetaminophen 650–1000 mg and diphenhydramine 50–100 mg orally 30 minutes to 1 hour before rituximab administration to mitigate infusion reactions

Standard dosage:

- Rituximab 375 mg/m^2 intravenously in 0.9% NS or D5W, diluted to a concentration within the range of 1–4 mg/mL, once weekly for 4 weeks (total dosage/4-week course = 1500 mg/m^2)

Infusion rate:

- Initially at 50 mg/hour. If hypersensitivity or infusion reactions do not occur during the first 30 minutes, increase the rate by 50 mg/hour every 30 minutes, to a maximum rate of 400 mg/hour
- Subsequently, if previous administration was well tolerated, start at 100 mg/hour, and increase by 100 mg/hour every 30 minutes, to a maximum rate of 400 mg/hour

STREPTOZOCIN

Zanosar® (streptozocin sterile powder) product label, May 2003. SICOR Pharmaceuticals, Inc, Irvine, CA

Trissel LA. Handbook on Injectable Drugs, 13th ed. Bethesda: American Society of Health-System Pharmacists, Inc, 2005

Product Identification, Preparation, Storage, and Stability

- Zanosar® is packaged in vials containing streptozocin 1000 mg as a pale yellow freeze-dried powder. NDC 0703-4636-01
- Store intact vials containing freeze-dried streptozocin 1000 mg under refrigeration at 2°–8°C (35.6°–46.4°F) in the original packaging
- Reconstitute the product with 9.5 mL of either D5W or 0.9% NS to produce a solution with a concentration of 10 mg streptozocin/mL
- Reconstituted streptozocin (10 mg/mL) is stable at room temperature (15°–30°C; 59°–86°F) for 48 hours or for 96 hours under refrigeration
- The reconstituted product may be further diluted to a volume convenient for clinical use in either D5W or 0.9% NS. After dilution to 2 mg/mL in D5W or 0.9% NS, streptozocin is stable for 48 hours at room temperature and 96 hours under refrigeration
- The commercial product does not contain an antimicrobial preservative and the manufacturer recommends storage for not greater than 12 hours after reconstitution

Recommendations for Drug Administration and Ancillary Care

General:

- Administer streptozocin either by rapid intravenous injection (push) or by intravenous infusion over a period within the range of 15 minutes to 6 hours
- The commercial product does not contain an antimicrobial preservative and the manufacturer recommends storage for not greater than 12 hours after reconstitution

TENIPOSIDE

VUMON® (teniposide injection) product label, August 2004. Bristol-Myers Squibb Company; Princeton, NJ

Product Identification, Preparation, Storage, and Stability

- Vumon® is available in clear, colorless, glass ampules containing a nonaqueous solution of teniposide 50 mg/5 mL. Each milliliter of the product contains teniposide 10 mg, 30 mg benzyl alcohol, 60 mg *N,N*-dimethylacetamide, 500 mg purified Cremophor® EL (polyoxyethylated castor oil), and 42.7% (v/v) dehydrated alcohol. Single ampules, NDC 0015-3075-19; carton of 10 ampules, NDC 0015-3075-97
- Store intact ampules under refrigeration at 2°–8°C (35.6°–46.4°F) in the original packaging. Freezing does not adversely affect the product
- *Do not permit plastic* equipment or devices to remain in contact with undiluted teniposide. Prolonged exposure may cause syringes and other plastic solution transfer devices to soften or crack, which may increase the risk of drug leakage. The effect has not been reported with teniposide solutions after dilution
- Teniposide solutions may leach phthalate plasticizers from PVC containers and administration set tubing. The extent of leaching correlates directly with the concentration of drug and the duration of exposure
- *Use only non-DEHP* containers and administration sets (glass or polyolefin containers; polyolefin-lined sets) to prepare and administer teniposide. Stability and use times are identical in glass and plastic containers
- Dilute teniposide with either D5W or 0.9% NS to produce final teniposide concentrations = 0.1 mg/mL, 0.2 mg/mL, 0.4 mg/mL, or 1 mg/mL
- Teniposide stability at room temperature after dilution in D5W or 0.9% NS:

Teniposide Concentration	Duration of Stability
0.1 mg/mL	24 hours
0.2 mg/mL	
0.4 mg/mL	
1 mg/mL	4 hours

- Do not refrigerate teniposide solutions after dilution
- Although solutions are chemically stable under the conditions indicated, precipitation still may occur, especially if a diluted solution is subjected to more agitation than is needed to prepare a homogeneous admixture
  - Spontaneous precipitation has been reported during 24-hour infusions in which teniposide was diluted to concentrations of 0.1–0.2 mg/mL
- To prevent precipitation, *minimize the storage time* before administering diluted teniposide

Selected incompatibility:

- Do not permit diluted teniposide to come into contact with other drugs and fluids
- Admixture with heparin can cause teniposide precipitation

Recommendations for Drug Administration and Ancillary Care

General:

- Administer teniposide by intravenous infusion over at least 30–60 minutes as soon as possible after preparation to avoid precipitation
- In general, administration sets designed for infusing intravenous fat emulsion or paclitaxel, and low-DEHP-containing nitroglycerin sets, are suitable for use with teniposide
- Hypotension has been reported after rapid intravenous administration
- *Thoroughly flush* administration sets and VADs with D5W or 0.9% NS before and after teniposide administration. *Do not permit* diluted teniposide to come into contact with other drugs and fluids

THIOTEPA

Thiotepa for injection product label, April 2001. Manufactured by Ben Venue Laboratories, Inc, Bedford, OH. Manufactured for Bedford Laboratories™, Bedford, OH

Grossman SA et al. JCO 1993;11:561–569
Gutin PH, et al. Cancer 1976; 38:1471–1475
Murray KM et al. Am J Health Syst Pharm 1997;54:2588–2591
Strong JM et al. Cancer Res 1986;46(12 pt 1):6101–6104

Product Identification, Preparation, Storage, and Stability

- Thiotepa is packaged in single-use vials containing 15 mg of nonpyrogenic, sterile lyophilized powder (NDC 55390-030-10)
- Store intact single-use vials under refrigeration at 2°–8°C (35.6°–46.4°F) and protect the product from exposure to light
- Reconstitute thiotepa with 1.5 mL SWFI to produce a drug concentration of approximately 10.4 mg/mL
- The actual withdrawable quantities and concentration achieved are as follows:

Labeled content per vial	15 mg
Actual content per vial	15.6 mg
Approximate withdrawable volume per vial	1.4 mL
Approximate withdrawable amount (mass) per vial	14.7 mg

- After reconstitution with SWFI, store thiotepa under refrigeration at 2°–8°C for up to 8 hours
- Reconstituted solutions should be clear. Solutions that are opaque or precipitate should not be used
- The reconstituted solution (concentrations ≥3 mg/mL) is hypotonic and should be further diluted with 0.9% NS, D5W , D5W/0.9% NS, RI, or LRI before clinical use
- Dilution with 0.9% NS to concentrations <1.8 mg/mL are nearly isotonic; *but*
  –Thiotepa solutions that have been diluted with 0.9% NS to a concentration <1 mg/mL should be *used immediately* after preparation due to the formation of drug adducts with chloride

Recommendations for Drug Administration and Ancillary Care

General:

- Thiotepa is usually given by rapid intravenous administration, but has also been given by intravesical, intracavitary, intrathecal, intramuscular, and intratumoral routes
- To eliminate haze, filter solutions through a 0.22-micrometer filter before or during administration (hydrophilic polyethersulfone or cellulose ester filter membranes [Aerodisc®, Pall Corp.; MILLEX®-GS, Millipore Corp.]). Filtering does not alter potency

Intravenous administration:

- Thiotepa 0.3–0.4 mg/kg body weight may be given by rapid intravenous injection over 5 minutes

Intracavitary administration:

- The tubing that is used to drain fluid from the cavity often is used to instill thiotepa

Intravesical administration:

- Fluids are withheld for 8–12 hours before treatment. Thiotepa 60 mg in 30–60 mL 0.9% NS is instilled into the bladder by a catheter. For maximum effect, the solution should be retained for 2 hours. If it is not possible to retain 60 mL for 2 hours, the dose may be given in a volume of 30 mL. A patient is repositioned every 15 minutes for maximum area contact

Intrathecal administration:

- Thiotepa 2–10 mg/m^2 per dose, or a fixed amount of 10 mg/dose by either intralumbar or intraventricular routes, diluted with 0.9% NS to a concentration of 1–5 mg/mL
- There is no PK advantage for intrathecal versus intravenous administration. Thiotepa clearance from the CSF is approximately 9 times greater than CSF bulk outflow

TOPOTECAN HCl

HYCAMTIN® (topotecan hydrochloride) for injection product label, July 2003. GlaxoSmithKline, Research Triangle Park, NC

Craig SB et al. J Pharm Biomed Anal 1997;16:199–205
Krämer I, Thiesen J. J Oncol Pharm Practice 1999;5:75–82

Product Identification, Preparation, Storage, and Stability

- HYCAMTIN® is packaged in single-dose vials containing topotecan hydrochlorideequivalent to 4 mg topotecan (free base) as a sterile, buffered, light yellow to yellow-green lyophilized powder. Single vial, NDC 0007-4201-01; package of 5 vials, NDC 0007-4201-05
- Store intact vials in the original cartons to protect them from light at controlled room temperature between 20°–25°C (68°–77°F)
- Reconstitute lyophilized topotecan HCl with 4 mL SWFI to produce a solution with concentration = 1 mg/mL
- After reconstitution with SWFI, topotecan HCl 1 mg/mL, stored for 28 days at 4°C or 25°C and protected from light was found to be physically and chemically stable by HPLC analysis without color change or visible precipitation
- After reconstitution with BWFI (preserved with benzyl alcohol) to a concentration of 1 mg/mL and further diluted in a PVC container, topotecan HCl stability was as follows:

Diluting/Vehicle Solution	Diluted Concentration	Storage Conditions	% Loss of Topotecan
0.9%NS	10 mcg/mL	Room temperature × 4 days	<3%
	500 mcg/mL		
D5W	10 mcg/mL		
	500 mcg/mL		
BWFI	10 mcg/mL	Room temperature × 21 days	<4%

- Dilute an amount of drug appropriate for a patient's dose in 50–250 mL of either 0.9% NS or D5W
- After dilution with 0.9% NS or D5W and storage at room temperatures, topotecan is stable for at least 24 hours
- Topotecan is susceptible to photodegradation during storage:
  –*Protect stored solutions* from light exposure
  –Protection from light is not necessary during topotecan administration

Selected incompatibility:

- Topotecan is formulated with tartaric acid to maintain a pH between 2.5 and 3.5. Topotecan solubility and stability decrease with increasing pH; its lactone ring spontaneously hydrolyzes at pH >4

Recommendations for Drug Administration and Ancillary Care

General:

- Administer topotecan by intravenous infusion over 30 minutes

TRASTUZUMAB

HERCEPTIN® (Trastuzumab) product label February 2005. Genentech, Inc, South San Francisco, CA

Product Identification, Preparation, Storage, and Stability

- Herceptin® is packaged in vials that contain 440 mg of trastuzumab as a sterile, preservative-free, lyophilized powder under vacuum (NDC 50242-134-68). The package includes a second vial that contains 20 mL BWFI preserved with 1.1% benzyl alcohol. Store intact vials under refrigeration at 2°–8°C (35.6°–46.4°F)
- The diluent provided with the Herceptin® product is formulated to maintain product stability and sterility for up to 28 days. Other diluents have not been shown to contain effective preservatives and should not be used
- Reconstitute trastuzumab with the supplied BWFI to produce a multidose solution containing 21 mg trastuzumab/mL
  1. Slowly inject 20 mL of the provided diluent directly into the lyophilized drug
  2. Gently swirl vials to aid reconstitution. *Do not shake* trastuzumab during reconstitution to avoid excessive foaming, which may make dissolution difficult and compromise the amount of solution that can be withdrawn from a vial

     [Trastuzumab may be sensitive to shear-induced stresses that can be produced during agitation or rapid expulsion from a syringe]
  3. Slight foaming is not unusual during reconstitution. After adding the diluent, allow vials to stand undisturbed for approximately 5 minutes
  4. After reconstitution, dilute an amount of trastuzumab appropriate for a patient's dose in 250 mL 0.9% NS. *Do not use dextrose* solutions to dilute trastuzumab
  5. Gently invert the container to mix the solution

     [Trastuzumab is compatible with PVC and polyethylene containers]
- For patients with known hypersensitivity to benzyl alcohol, trastuzumab may be reconstituted with SWFI, then diluted in 250 mL 0.9% NS and used immediately. All partially used vials reconstituted in this manner must be discarded after a single use
- Trastuzumab solutions diluted in 0.9% NS in PVC or polyethylene bags may be stored at 2°–25°C (35.6°–77°F) for up to 24 hours before use, but the diluted solution will not inhibit microbial growth. Therefore, store reconstituted and diluted trastuzumab solutions under refrigeration

Selected incompatibility:

- *Do not mix or dilute* trastuzumab with other drugs

Recommendations for Drug Administration and Ancillary Care

General:

- Administer a 4-mg/kg trastuzumab loading dose by intravenous infusion over 90 minutes
- *Do not administer* trastuzumab by rapid injection techniques (push or bolus)
- Observe patients for fever and chills and other infusion-associated symptoms
- If administration is well tolerated, subsequent *weekly* maintenance doses of trastuzumab 2 mg/kg may be administered over 30 minutes
- Trastuzumab may be administered in an outpatient setting
- *Do not mix* or dilute trastuzumab with other drugs

VINBLASTINE SULFATE

VINBLASTINE SULFATE FOR INJECTION, USP product label, December 1998. Manufactured by Ben Venue Laboratories, Inc, Bedford, OH. Manufactured for Bedford Laboratories™, Bedford, OH
VINBLASTINE SULFATE INJECTION product label, March 2003. American Pharmaceutical Partners, Inc, Schaumberg, IL

Product Identification, Preparation, Storage, and Stability

- Vinblastine is generically available in a variety of product strengths in liquid and lyophilized formulations
- Store vials under refrigeration at 2°–8°C (35.6°–46.4°F) to assure product stability

Vinblastine Sulfate for Injection, USP:

- Vials contain vinblastine sulfate as a lyophilized powder, without excipients
- Protect the lyophilized powder and vinblastine solutions from light
- Reconstitute vials containing 10 mg vinblastine sulfate with 10 mL of B0.9% NS (preserved with benzyl alcohol) or 0.9% NS to produce a solution with a concentration of 1 mg/mL
- After reconstitution with 10 mL B0.9% NS (preserved with benzyl alcohol), vinblastine sulfate solution may be kept under refrigeration for 30 days without significant loss of potency
- *Discard* partially used vials containing vinblastine sulfate reconstituted with 0.9% NS (without an antimicrobial preservative)

Vinblastine sulfate injection:

- Multiple-use vials contain a sterile solution of vinblastine sulfate, 1 mg/mL (10 mg/10-mL; 25 mg/25 mL) that is preserved with benzyl alcohol 0.9% (v/v)
- *Discard* partially used vials not more than 28 days after initial use

Vinblastine sulfate for injection and vinblastine sulfate injection:

- For continuous intravenous infusion, vinblastine sulfate solutions may be further diluted in D5W, 0.9% NS, or LRI
- Vinblastine in powdered form and in solution should be protected from light during storage
- Vinblastine may be further diluted with a volume of 0.9% NS, D5W, or LRI that is convenient for administration

Recommendations for Drug Administration and Ancillary Care

General:

- Vinblastine is *for intravenous use only*
- Vinblastine sulfate (1 mg/mL) is suitable for direct intravenous injection, or it may be injected into the tubing of a running intravenous solution. In either case, injection may be completed in about 1 minute
- Administration through a nylon filter may cause drug loss due to absorption to the filter. Vinblastine concentration was not affected by filtration through filter membranes made of cellulose acetate, cellulose nitrate, cellulose ester, Teflon®, or polysulfone
- FDA-approved labeling recommends rinsing the syringe and needle by aspirating blood into the syringe after completing drug injection before the needle is withdrawn. The procedure is intended to minimize the possibility of extravasation after administration by venipuncture
- Vinblastine doses should not be further diluted after reconstitution or given intravenously for prolonged periods (≥15 minutes), unless administration technique is based on continuous infusion through central VADs, subcutaneously implanted 'ports,' or peripherally inserted central VADs (eg, PICC, SICC)
- *Do not inject* vinblastine by intravenous injection into a lower extremity, or an extremity in which the circulation is impaired or potentially impaired to decrease a potential for treatment-related thrombosis
- *Caution*: Vinblastine is a vesicant and may produce severe local soft tissue necrosis if extravasation occurs

Warnings: When vinblastine is dispensed in something other than its original container (eg, a syringe), the product should be labeled: "WARNING—FOR INTRAVENOUS USE ONLY. FATAL IF GIVEN INTRATHECALLY." Any material used to package or overwrap a syringe or another container for vinblastine should be labeled, "WARNING—DO NOT REMOVE COVERING UNTIL MOMENT OF INJECTION. FOR INTRAVENOUS USE ONLY. FATAL IF GIVEN INTRATHECALLY."

VINCRISTINE SULFATE

VINCRISTINE Sulfate Injection, USP preservative-free solution product label, September 2002. Faulding Pharmaceutical Co, A Mayne group Company, Paramus, NJ

Product Identification, Preparation, Storage, and Stability

- Vincristine Sulfate Injection, USP is a sterile, preservative–free solution that is suitable for clinical use without further dilution. In general, products are packaged in single-use vials containing either 1 mg or 2 mg of vincristine sulfate, both in a concentration of 1 mg/mL
- Store vincristine sulfate under refrigeration at 2°–8°C (35.6°–46.4°F)
- Vincristine should not be added to solutions with a pH outside the range of 3.5–5.5
- Vincristine may be diluted with a volume of 0.9% NS or D5W that is convenient for administration

Selected incompatibility:

- When used in combination with **asparaginase**, vincristine should be given 12–24 hours *before* asparaginase to minimize toxicity. If asparaginase is administered before vincristine, it may decrease vincristine's hepatic clearance

Recommendations for Drug Administration and Ancillary Care

General:

- Vincristine is *for intravenous use only*
- Vincristine may be injected either directly into a vein or into the tubing of a running intravenous solution. Injection should be completed within 1 minute
- Vincristine sulfate injection should not be given to patients while they are receiving radiation therapy through fields that include the liver
- Vincristine doses should not be further diluted after reconstitution or given intravenously for prolonged periods (≥15 minutes) unless administration technique is based on continuous infusion through central VADs, subcutaneously implanted "ports," or peripherally inserted central VADs (eg, PICC, SICC)
- *Do not inject* vincristine into a lower extremity, or an extremity in which the circulation is impaired or potentially impaired to decrease a potential for treatment-related thrombosis
- *Do not filter* vincristine solutions:

  –Administration through cellulose acetate, cellulose nitrate, cellulose ester, nylon, or Teflon® filters has demonstrated variable drug loss due to absorption. In general, the extent of drug loss due to filtration is inversely proportional to the concentration of vincristine in solution
- *Caution*: Vincristine is a vesicant and may produce severe local soft tissue necrosis if extravasation occurs

Warnings: When vincristine is dispensed in something other than its original container (eg, a syringe), the product should be labeled: "WARNING—FOR INTRAVENOUS USE ONLY. FATAL IF GIVEN INTRATHECALLY." Any material used to package or overwrap a syringe or another container for vincristine should be labeled, "WARNING—DO NOT REMOVE COVERING UNTIL MOMENT OF INJECTION. FOR INTRAVENOUS USE ONLY. FATAL IF GIVEN INTRATHECALLY."

VINORELBINE TARTRATE

NAVELBINE® (vinorelbine tartrate) injection product label, April 2003. Manufactured by Pierre Fabre Médicament Production, Idron, France. Manufactured for GlaxoSmithKline, Research Triangle Park, NC
Vinorelbine tartrate injection product label, October 2003. Manufactured by Ben Venue Laboratories, Inc, Bedford, OH. Manufactured for Bedford Laboratories™, Bedford, OH

Product Identification, Preparation, Storage, and Stability

- Vinorelbine tartrate is generically available. In general, commercial products are packaged in single-use glass vials containing vinorelbine tartrate as a clear, colorless to pale yellow solution equivalent to 10 mg vinorelbine/1 mL or 50 mg vinorelbine/5-mL
- Store vinorelbine under refrigeration at 2°–8°C (35.6°–46.4°F), and protect it from light
- Intact vials are stable at temperatures up to 25°C (77°F) for up to 72 hours, but *do not freeze* vinorelbine
- Vinorelbine *must be diluted* before administration

Syringe container:

- Dilute vinorelbine in a syringe to a concentration between 1.5 and 3 mg/mL with either D5W or 0.9% NS

Bag or bottle container:

- Dilute vinorelbine in a parenteral container to a concentration between 0.5 and 2 mg/mL with one of the following solutions: D5W , 0.9% NS, 0.45% NaCl, D5W/0.45% NaCl, RI, LRI

Syringe, bag, or bottle container:

- Diluted vinorelbine may be used for up to 24 hours under normal room light when stored in polypropylene syringes or PVC bags at 5°–30°C (41°–86°F)

Recommendations for Drug Administration and Ancillary Care

General:

- Administer vinorelbine by slow intravenous injection over 6–10 minutes into the side port of a free-flowing intravenous solution closest to the fluid container followed by flushing with at least 75–125 mL of D5W , 0.9% NS, 0.45% NaCl, D5W/0.45% NaCl, RI, LRI
- *Caution*: Vinorelbine is a vesicant and may produce severe local soft tissue necrosis if extravasation occurs

41. Chemotherapy Dose Modifications

Michael Menefee, MD, Pamela McDevitt, Pharm D, and Tito Fojo MD, PhD

Anticancer Therapeutics Requiring Dose Modification for Patients with Hepatic Dysfunction

Aldesleukin (interleukin-2)	Fluorouracil	Procarbazine
Altretamine		Sorafenib
		Sunitinib
		Tegafur
Amsacrine	Flutamide	Teniposide
	Gemcitabine	
	Gemtuzumab	
	Hydroxyurea	
Anastrozole	Idarubicin	Thioguanine
Asparaginase	Ifosfamide	
Bicalutamide	Imatinib	Thiotepa
Bortezomib		
Capecitabine		
Carmustine		
Clofarabine		
Cyclophosphamide	Irinotecan	Tretinoin (all-*trans*-retinoic acid)
Cytarabine	Isotretinoin (13-*cis*-retinoic acid)	Trimetrexate
Dacarbazine	Mercaptopurine	
Dactinomycin	Methotrexate	Vinblastine
Daunorubicin		
Daunorubicin Citrate Liposomal		
Dexrazoxane		
Docetaxel	Mitotane	Vincristine
Doxorubicin	Mitoxantrone	Vinorelbine
	Nelarabine	
Doxorubicin liposome injection	Nilutamide	
Epirubicin		
Erlotinib		
Etoposide	Paclitaxel	
	Pemetrexed	

Anticancer Therapeutics Requiring Dose Modification for Patients with Renal Dysfunction

		Lenalidomide
Aldesleukin	Cyclophosphamide	Lomustine
Aminoglutethimide		
Amsacrine		
Arsenic trioxide	Cytarabine	Melphalan
Asparginase	Dacarbazine	Mercaptopurine
Azacitidine		
Bleomycin	Daunorubicin	Methotrexate
Bortezomib	Daunorubicin Citrate Liposome	Mitomycin
	Dexrazoxane	Nelarabine
	Epirubicin	
Capecitabine	Etoposide	Pemetrexed
Carboplatin	Fludarabine	Pentostatin
	Gemcitabine	
Carmustine	Hydroxyurea	Procarbazine
Cisplatin	Idarubicin	Raltitrexed
Clofarabine	Ifosfamide	Sorafenib
	Interferon alfa 2-B	Sunitinib
		Streptozocin
		Teniposide
		Thiotepa
		Topotecan
		Tretinoin
		Trimetrexate

Guidelines for Chemotherapy Dosage Adjustments

	Hepatic Dysfunction			Renal Dysfunction	
Drug	**Bilirubin (mg/dL)**	**AST/SGOT (units/L)**	**% Dose Administered**	**Creatinine Clearance (mL/min) or Serum Creatinine (mg/dL)**	**% Dose Administered**
Aldesleukin	Omit if signs of hepatic failure (ascites, encephalopathy, jaundice) are observed. *Do not* restart sooner than 7 weeks after recovery from severe hepatic dysfunction[1]			Hold or discontinue if serum creatinine >4.5 mg/dL or serum creatinine >4.0 mg/dL in the presence of fluid overload[1]	
Alemtuzumab	No dosage adjustment recommended			No dosage adjustment recommended	
Altretamine	No dosage adjustment recommended			No dosage adjustment recommended	
Amifostine	No dosage adjustment recommended			NA	
Aminoglutethimide	No dosage adjustment recommended			No dosage adjustment recommended[2]	
Amsacrine	>2		75%[3]	Scr 1.5	75%[3]
Anastrozole	No formal recommendation, but reduction may be necessary with hepatic dysfunction			No dosage adjustment recommended[4]	
Arsenic trioxide	No dosage adjustment recommended			No formal recommendation, but dosage reduction may be necessary[5]	
Azacitidine	No dosage adjustment recommended			Increased BUN/Scr	50%[6]
Asparaginase	No dosage adjustment recommended[7]			NA[7]	
Bevacizumab	No dosage adjustment recommended			No dosage adjustment recommended	
Bicalutamide	No formal recommendation, but reduction may be necessary if bilirubin >3 mg/dL[8]			No dosage adjustment recommended	
Bleomycin	No dosage adjustment recommended			10–60	75%
				<10	50%[9]
Bortezomib	NA[10]			NA[10]	
Buserelin	No dosage adjustment recommended			No dosage adjustment recommended	
Busulfan	No dosage adjustment recommended			No dose reduction necessary	
Capecitabine	No dosage adjustment recommended[11]			30–50	75%
				<30	Hold[11]
Carboplatin	No dosage adjustment recommended			If CrCl < 60 AUC dose is modified according to creatinine clearance CrCl[12,13]	
Carmustine	No dosage adjustment recommended[14]			<60	Hold[15]
Cetuximab	No dosage adjustment recommended			No dosage adjustment recommended	
Chlorambucil	No dosage adjustment recommended			No dosage adjustment recommended	
Cisplatin	No dosage adjustment recommended			30–45	50%
				<30	Hold[16]

	Hepatic Dysfunction			Renal Dysfunction	
Drug	Bilirubin (mg/dL)	AST/SGOT (units/L)	% Dose Administered	Creatinine Clearance (mL/min) or Serum Creatinine (mg/dL)	% Dose Administered
Cladribine	No dosage adjustment recommended			No dosage adjustment recommended	
Clofarabine	NA[17]			NA[17]	
Cyclophosphamide	3–5		75%	10–50	75%
		>180	75%	<10	50%[18]
	>5		Hold[19]		
Cytarabine	No formal recommendation, but reduction may be necessary with hepatic dysfunction			No formal recommendation, but dosage reduction may be necessary[20]	
Cytarabine liposome	No dosage adjustment recommended			No dosage adjustment recommended	
Dacarbazine	No dosage adjustment recommended[21]			No formal recommendation, but dosage reduction may be necessary[22]	
Dactinomycin	>3		50%[23]	NA	
Daunorubicin	1.5–3		75%	Scr >3	50%[24]
	3–5		50%		
	>5		Hold		
Daunorubicin liposome	1.2–3		75%	>3	50%[25]
	>3		50%		
Denileukin diftitox	No dose reduction necessary			No dosage adjustment recommended	
Dexrazoxane	Because a doxorubicin dose reduction is recommended in the presence of hyperbilirubinemia, the dexrazoxane dosage should be proportionately reduced (maintaining the 10:1 ratio) in patients with hepatic impairment[26]			The recommended dosage ratio of dexrazoxane:doxorubicin is 10:1 (eg, 500 mg/m² dexrazoxane:50 mg/m² doxorubicin). In patients with CrCl <40 mL/min the recommended dosage ratio of dexrazoxane:doxorubicin is 5:1 (eg, 250 mg/m² dexrazoxane:50 mg/m² doxorubicin)[26, 27]	
Docetaxel	>ULN	>1.5 ULN	Hold[28]	No dosage adjustment recommended	
	Hold if alkaline phosphatase >2.5 × upper limit of normal (ULN)				
Doxorubicin	1.5–3		50%	No dosage adjustment recommended	
	3.1–5		25%[29]		
	>5		Hold[30]		
Doxorubicin liposome	1.5–3		50%	No dosage adjustment recommended	
	3.1–5		25%[31]		
	>5		Hold[32]		

Epirubicin	1.2–3		50%	Limited data precludes specific recommendations, but lower doses should be considered in patients with serum creatinine >5 mg/dL[33]	
	>3		25%		
		2–4 × ULN	50%		
		>4 × ULN	25%[33]		
Erlotinib	Erlotinib is eliminated by hepatic metabolism and biliary excretion. Use caution when administering to patients with hepatic impairment[34]			Dose reduction likely unnecessary because <9% of a single dose is excreted in the urine[34]	
Estramustine	No dosage adjustment recommended			No dosage adjustment recommended	
Etoposide	1.5–3		50%	15–50	75%
	>3		Hold	<15	consider 50%[35]
		60–180	50%		
		>180	Hold[36]		
Etoposide phosphate	1.5–3		50%	15–50	75%
	>3		Hold	<15	consider 50%[37]
		60–180	50%		
		>180	Hold[38]		
Floxuridine	No dosage adjustment recommended			No dosage adjustment recommended	
Fludarabine	No dosage adjustment recommended			30–70/1.73 m^2	80% in U.S. 50% in U.K.[39] (different product formulations)
Fluorouracil	>5		Hold[40]	No dosage adjustment recommended	
	Avoid fluorouracil in patients with dihydropyrimidine deficiency (DPD). Evaluate for DPD any patient who develops unexpectedly severe toxicity after fluorouracil treatment[41]				
Flutamide	No formal recommendation, but reduction may be necessary if bilirubin >3.0 mg/dL[42]			No dosage adjustment recommended	
Gefitinib	No dosage adjustment is required in patients with moderate to severe hepatic impairment due to liver metastases			No dosage adjustment recommended	
Gemcitabine	NA[43]			No dosage adjustment recommended[43]	
Gemtuzumab ozogamicin	Use extra caution when administering in patients with hepatic impairment[44]			No dosage adjustment recommended	
Goserelin	No dosage adjustment recommended			No dosage adjustment recommended	
Hydroxyurea	NA[45]			<10	consider reducing[45]

Drug	Hepatic Dysfunction			Renal Dysfunction	
	Bilirubin (mg/dL)	AST/SGOT (units/L)	% Dose Administered	Creatinine Clearance (mL/min) or Serum Creatinine (mg/dL)	% Dose Administered
Idarubicin	1.5–3		75%	No formal recommendation, but dose reduction may be necessary[46]	
	3–5		50%		
	>5		Hold		
		60–180	75%		
		>180	50%[47]		
Ifosfamide	NA[48]			No dosage adjustment recommended[49]	
Imatinib	>3		Hold	No dosage adjustment recommended	
		>5 × ULN	Hold		
	Once bilirubin <1.5 or AST (SGOT) <2.5 × ULN, reduce dose from 400 mg to 300 mg or from 600 mg to 400 mg[50]				
Interferon alfa	No dosage adjustment recommended			No dosage adjustment recommended[51]	
Irinotecan	No formal recommendation, but dosage reduction may be necessary[52]			No dosage adjustment recommended	
Isotretinoin	No formal recommendation, but dosage reduction may be necessary[53]			No dosage adjustment recommended	
Lenalinomide	No dosage adjustment recommended			NA[54]	
Leucovorin	No dosage adjustment recommended			No dosage adjustment recommended	
Leuprolide	No dosage adjustment recommended			No dosage adjustment recommended	
Lomustine	No dosage adjustment recommended			<60	Hold[55]
Mechlorethamine	No dosage adjustment recommended			No dosage adjustment recommended	
Megestrol acetate	No dosage adjustment recommended			No dosage adjustment recommended	
Melphalan	No dosage adjustment recommended			No dose reduction is necessary. However, use with caution in the presence of renal dysfunction[56, 57]	
Mercaptopurine	In general, no dosage reduction is necessary, but consider decreasing mercaptopurine dosage by 10% for patients who lack thiopurine methyltransferase, an enzyme responsible for mercaptopurine catabolism[58]			No formal recommendation but can adjust for renal dysfunction by either increasing interval or decreasing dose[58]	
Mesna	No dosage adjustment recommended			No dosage adjustment recommended	
Methotrexate	3.1–5		75%	10–50	50%
	>5		Hold	<10	Hold[59]
		>180	75%[60]		
Mitomycin	No dosage adjustment recommended			Scr >1.7	Hold[61]

Drug	Hepatic impairment	Hepatic dose	Renal impairment	Renal dose
Mitotane	No formal recommendation for dose reduction. Monitor serum levels[62]		No formal recommendation for dose reduction. Monitor serum levels	
Mitoxantrone	>3	75%[63]	No dosage adjustment recommended	
Nelarabine	Risk of adverse reaction with bilirubin >3mg/dL[64]		No dosage adjustment for CrCl >50 mL/min; Insufficient data if <50 mL/min[64]	
Nilutamide	No formal recommendation, but reduction may be necessary if bilirubin >3 mg/dL[65]		No dosage adjustment recommended	
Oxaliplatin	No dosage adjustment recommended		Safety and efficacy in combination with FU/LV in renal impairment has not been evaluated therefore caution is advised with preexisting renal dysfunction[66] data support the recommendation that dose reductions of single-agent oxaliplatin are not necessary if CrCl >20 mL/min[67]	
Paclitaxel Note: Dosage recommendations are for the first course of therapy; further dose reduction in subsequent courses should be based on individual tolerance or published protocols. Data are not available for dose adjustments for regimens other than 135 mg/m² over 24 hours or 175 mg/m² over 3 hours	24-hour infusion			
	≤1.5 mg/dL AND <2 × ULN	135 mg/m²	No dosage adjustment recommended	
	≤1.5 mg/dL AND 2-<10 × ULN	100 mg/m²		
	1.6–7.5 mg/dL AND <10 × ULN	50 mg/m²		
	>7.5 mg/dL OR ≥10 × ULN	Not recommended		
	3-hour infusion			
	≤1.25 × ULN AND <10 × ULN	175 mg/m²		
	1.26–2.0 × ULN AND <10 × ULN	135 mg/m²		
	2.01–5.0 × ULN AND <10 × ULN	90 mg/m²		
	>5.0 × ULN OR ≥10 × ULN	Not recommended[68]		
Paclitaxel protein-bound particles	No dosage adjustment recommended		No dosage adjustment recommended	
Pegaspargase	No dosage adjustment recommended		No dosage adjustment recommended	
Pemetrexed	Data unavailable with bilirubin >1.5 × ULN or transaminases >3 × ULN; patients with transaminases 3–5 × ULN were included in trials if they had hepatic metastases. Patients with grade 3/4 non-hematologic toxicity (except grade 3 transaminase elevation) should receive 75% of previous dose. Discontinue after 2 dose reduction[69]		CrCl < 45mL/min	Hold[69]
Pentostatin	No dosage adjustment recommended		No formal recommendation for dosage reduction but may be necessary if CrCl 30–60 mL/min[70]	
Procarbazine	No formal recommendation, but dosage reduction may be necessary[71]		<30	Hold[72]
Raltitrexed	NA		25–65	50%
			<25	Hold[73]

	Hepatic Dysfunction			Renal Dysfunction	
Drug	**Bilirubin (mg/dL)**	**AST/SGOT (units/L)**	**% Dose Administered**	**Creatinine Clearance (mL/min) or Serum Creatinine (mg/dL)**	**% Dose Administered**
Rituximab	No dosage adjustment recommended			No dosage adjustment recommended	
Sorafenib	No dose adjustment necessary for Child-Pugh A and B hepatic impairment. Patients with Child-Pugh C hepatic impairment not studied[74]			No studies in patients with CrCI < 30 mL/min[74]	
Streptozotocin	No dosage adjustment recommended			NA[76]	
Sunitinib	No clinical studies in patients with impaired hepatic function (eg, ALT or AST >2.5 × ULN or, if due to underlying disease, >5 × ULN)[75]			No clinical studies in patients with SCr >2 × ULN.[75]	
Tamoxifen	No dosage adjustment recommended			No dosage adjustment recommended	
Tegafur	NA[77]			No dosage adjustment recommended	
Temozolomide	No dosage adjustment recommended			No dosage adjustment recommended	
Teniposide	No formal recommendation, but dosage reduction may be necessary[78]			No formal recommendation, but dosage reduction may be necessary with sufficient renal impairment[78]	
Thalidomide	No dosage adjustment recommended			No dosage adjustment recommended	
Thioguanine	>5.0		Hold[79]	No dosage adjustment recommended	
Thiotepa	No formal recommendation, but dosage reduction may be necessary[80]			No formal recommendation, but dosage reduction may be necessary[80]	
Topotecan	No dosage adjustment recommended[81]			20–39	0.75 mg/m²
				<10	NA
Trastuzumab	No dosage adjustment recommended			No dosage adjustment recommended	
Tretinoin	3.1–5		≤25 mg/m²	≤60	≤25 mg/m²[82]
	>5		Hold		
		>180	≤25 mg/m²[82]		
Trimetrexate	No formal recommendation, but dose reduction may be necessary[83]			No dosage adjustment recommended	
Vinblastine	1.5–3		50%	No dosage adjustment recommended	
	>3		Hold		
		60–180	50%		
		>180	Hold[84]		
Vincristine	1.5–3		50%	No dosage adjustment recommended	
	>3		Hold		
		60–180	50%		
		>180	Hold[85]		
Vinorelbine	2–3		50%	No dosage adjustment recommended	
	3.1–5		25%[86]		
	>5		Hold[87]		

Note: Clinicians are strongly recommended to review the dose modifications of agents; either used alone or in combination with other agents, from appropriate and applicable peer-reviewed publications for additional clinical guidance

References

1. Proleukin® Aldesleukin for Injection, USP, product label, September 2000. Chiron Therapeutics, Emeryville, CA
2. Santen RJ & Misbin RI. Pharmacotherapy 1981;1;95–120
3. Grove WR, et al. Clin Pharm 1982;1:320
4. Arimidex® (anastrozole) product label, December 1995. Zeneca Pharmaceuticals-US, Wilmington DE
5. Trisenox® (arsenic trioxide) injection product label, June 2003. Manufactured for Cell Therapeutics, Inc., Seattle, WA
6. Vidaza™ (azacitadine for injectable suspension) product label, August 31, 2004. Manufactured by Ben Venue Laboratories, Inc., Bedford, OH. Manufactured for Pharmion Corporation, Boulder, CO
7. Elspar® (Asparaginase) product label, August 2002. Merck & Co., Inc., West Point, PA
8. Casodex® (bicalutamide) product label, May 2005. Zeneca Pharmaceuticals-US, Wilmington DE
9. Skeel RT: Handbook of Cancer Chemotherapy, 3rd Little, Brown and Co, Boston, MA, 1991
10. Velcade® (bortezomib) for Injection product label, March 2005. Millennium Pharmaceuticals, Inc., Cambridge, MA
11. Xeloda® (capecitabine) product label, 2001. Roche Pharmaceuticals, Nutley, NJ, USA
12. Chu E, DeVita VT, eds. Cancer Chemotherapy Drug Manual. Sudbury NA: Jones and Bartlett Publishers, 2006:379–386
13. Paraplatin® (carboplatin) product label, 1999. Bristol-Myers Squibb, Princeton, NJ
14. Lessner HE & Vogler WR. Cancer Chemother Rep 1974;58:407–411
15. Chu E, DeVita VT, eds. Cancer Chemotherapy Drug Manual. Sudbury NA: Jones and Bartlett Publishers, 2006:379–386
16. Kintzel PE, et al Cancer Treat Reviews 1995;21:33–64
17. Clolar™ (clofarabine) product label, 2005. Manufactured for Genzyme Corporation, San Antonio, TX
18. Bennett WM, et al: Drug Prescribing in Renal Failure, American College of Physicians, Philadelphia, PA, 1987
19. Chu E, DeVita VT, eds. Cancer Chemotherapy Drug Manual. Sudbury NA: Jones and Bartlett Publishers, 2006:379–386
20. Cytosar-U® (cytarabine) product label, 1999. Upjohn Company, Kalamazoo, MI
21. Ignoffo RJ. Applied Therapeutics The Clinical Use of Drugs, 4th. Applied Therapeutics, Vancouver, WA, 1998
22. DTIC-Dome PI® (dacarbazine) product label, 1998. Bayer Corporation, West Haven, CT
23. Chu E, DeVita VT, eds. Cancer Chemotherapy Drug Manual. Sudbury NA: Jones and Bartlett Publishers, 2006:379–386
24. Chu E, DeVita VT, eds. Cancer Chemotherapy Drug Manual. Sudbury NA: Jones and Bartlett Publishers, 2006:379–386
25. DaunoXome® (daunorubicin citrate liposome injection) product label, 1999. Gilead Sciences, Inc., San Dimas, CA
26. Chu E, DeVita VT, eds. Cancer Chemotherapy Drug Manual. Sudbury NA: Jones and Bartlett Publishers, 2006:379–386
27. Zinecard® (dexrazoxane) product label, 2005. Pharmacia & Upjohn Company, New York, NY
28. Taxotere® (docetaxel) product label, 2003. Aventis Pharmaceuticals, Bridgewater, NJ
29. Adriamycin RDF®/PFS® (doxorubicin), product label, 2000. Pharmacia & Upjohn, Inc. Kalamazoo, MI
30. Chu E, DeVita VT, eds. Cancer Chemotherapy Drug Manual. Sudbury NA: Jones and Bartlett Publishers, 2006:379–386
31. Doxil® (doxorubicin hydrochloride liposome injection) product label, 1997. SEQUUS Pharmaceuticals, Inc., Menlo Park, CA
32. Chu E, DeVita VT, eds. Cancer Chemotherapy Drug Manual. Sudbury NA: Jones and Bartlett Publishers, 2006:379–386
33. Ellence® (epirubicin hydrochloride) product label, 2003. Pharmacia & Upjohn, Kalamazoo, MI
34. Tarceva® (erlotinib) product label, 2005. Genentech, Inc, South San Francisco, CA
35. Vepesid® (etoposide) product label, 2000. Bristol Laboratories, Princeton, NJ
36. Perry MC. Semin Oncol 1982;9:65–74.
37. Vepesid® (etoposide) product label, 2000. Bristol Laboratories, Princeton, NJ
38. Vepesid® (etoposide) product label, 2000. Bristol Laboratories, Princeton, NJ
39. Fludara® (fludarabine phophosphate) SPC (UK) product label, 2003. Berlex Laboratories, Quebec, Canada.; Fludara® (fludarabine) product label, October 2003. Berlex, Montville, NJ
40. Chu E, DeVita VT, eds. Cancer Chemotherapy Drug Manual. Sudbury NA: Jones and Bartlett Publishers, 2006:379–386
41. Harris BE, et al. *Cancer,* 1991:68:499–501
42. Chu E, DeVita VT, eds. Cancer Chemotherapy Drug Manual. Sudbury NA: Jones and Bartlett Publishers, 2006:379–386
43. Gemzar® (gemcitabine HCI) product label, 1999. Eli Lilly & Co, Indianapolis, IN
44. Mylotarg™ (gemtuzumab ozogamicin) product label, 2001. Wyeth Laboratories, Philadelphia, PA
45. Hydrea® (hydroxyurea) product label, October 2005. Bristol-Myers Squibb Co., Princeton, NJ
46. Idamycin® (idarubicin) product label, 1997. Adria Laboratories, Columbus, OH
47. Chu E, DeVita VT, eds. Cancer Chemotherapy Drug Manual. Sudbury NA: Jones and Bartlett Publishers, 2006:379–386
48. Ifex® (ifosfamide) product label, 1999. Bristol-Myers Oncology Division, Princeton, NJ
49. Norpoth K, et al. Klin Wchenschr 1975;53:1075–76.
50. Gleevec™ (imatinib capsules) product label, 2002. Novartis Pharmaceuticals Corp, East Hanover, NJ
51. Interferon alfa-2B drug evaluation, 1974–2006 Thomson Micromedex® Healthcare Series Vol 127
52. Camptosar® (irinotecan hydrdochloride injection) product label, March 2005. Distributed by Pharmacia & Upjohn Co., Division of Pfizer Inc., New York, NY
53. Isotretinon drug evaluation, 1974–2006 Thomson Micromedex® Healthcare Series Vol 127
54. Revlimid® (lenalidomide) product label, 2005. Celgene Corporation, Summit, NJ
55. Chu E, DeVita VT, eds. Cancer Chemotherapy Drug Manual. Sudbury NA: Jones and Bartlett Publishers, 2006:379–386
56. Alkeran® (melphalan) product label, November 2004. GlaxoSmithKline, Research Triangle Park, NC
57. Knoben JE & Anderson PO (Eds): Handbook of Clinical Drug Data, 6th. Drug Intelligence Publications, Inc. Hamilton, IL, 1988
58. Chu E, DeVita VT, eds. Cancer Chemotherapy Drug Manual. Sudbury NA: Jones and Bartlett Publishers, 2006:379–386
59. Bennett WM, et al: Drug Prescribing in Renal Failure, American College of Physicians, Philadelphia, PA, 1987
60. Chu E, DeVita VT, eds. Cancer Chemotherapy Drug Manual. Sudbury NA: Jones and Bartlett Publishers, 2006:379–386
61. Mutamycin® (Mitomycin for Injection, USP) product label, January 2000. Bristol-Myers Squibb Oncology, Bristol-Myers Squibb Company, Princeton, NJ
62. Lysodren® (mitotane tablets, USP) product label, 1998. Bristol-Myers Squibb Co., Princeton, NJ
63. Chu E, DeVita VT, eds. Cancer Chemotherapy Drug Manual. Sudbury NA: Jones and Bartlett Publishers, 2006:379–386
64. Arranon® (nelarabine) product label, October 2005. GlaxoSmithKline, Research Triangle Park, NC
65. Chu E, DeVita VT, eds. Cancer Chemotherapy Drug Manual. Sudbury NA: Jones and Bartlett Publishers, 2006:379–386
66. Eloxatin®, (oxaliplatin for injection) product label, April 2005. Manufactured by Ben Venue Laboratories, Bedford OH. Manufactured for Sanofi-Synthelabo Inc., New York, NY
67. Takimoto CH, et al. J Clin Oncol 2003;21:2664–2672
68. Taxol® (paclitaxel) Injection product label, March 2003. Bristol-Myers Squibb Oncology, Bristol-Myers Squibb Company, Princeton, NJ
69. Alimta® (pemtrexed for injection) product label, August 9, 2004. Manufactured by Lilly France S.A.S. F-67640 Fegersheim, France. Manufactured for Eli Lilly and Company, Indianapolis, IN
70. Nipent® (pentostatin for injection) product label, April 1998. Manufactured by Parkedale Phrmaceuticals Inc., Rochester, MI. Manufactured for SUPERGEN, Inc., San Ramon, CA
71. Matulane® (procarbazine hydrochloride), 2002. Sigma-Tau Pharmaceuticals, Inc., Gaithersburg, MD
72. Chu E, DeVita VT, eds. Cancer Chemotherapy Drug Manual. Sudbury NA: Jones and Bartlett Publishers, 2006:379–386
73. Judson I, et al. Br J Cancer 1998; 78(9):1188–1193
74. Nexavar® (sorafenib) product label, December 2005. Bayer Pharmaceuticals Corporation, West Haven, CT
75. Sutent® (sunitinib malate) product label, January 2006. Pfizer Labs, New York, NY
76. Chu E, DeVita VT, eds. Cancer Chemotherapy Drug Manual. Sudbury NA: Jones and Bartlett Publishers, 2006:379–386
77. Bedikian AY, et al. Am J Clin Oncol 1983:6:181–186
78. Vumon® (teniposide injection) product label, October 1998. Bristol Laboratories Oncology products, a Bristol-Myers Squibb Company; Princeton, NJ
79. Chu E, DeVita VT, eds. Cancer Chemotherapy Drug Manual. Sudbury NA: Jones and Bartlett Publishers, 2006:379–386
80. Thiotepa for Injection USP, product label, April 2001. Manufactured by Ben Venue Laboratories, Inc., Bedford, OH. Manufactured for Bedford Laboratories™, Bedford OH
81. Hycamtin® (topotecan hydrochloride) For Injection product label, July 2003. GlaxoSmithKline, Research Triangle Park, NC
82. Chu E, DeVita VT, eds. Cancer Chemotherapy Drug Manual. Sudbury NA: Jones and Bartlett Publishers, 2006:379–386
83. Neutrexin® (trimetrexate glucuronate for injection), 2000. MedImmune Oncology Inc., Gaithersburg, MD
84. Chu E, DeVita VT, eds. Cancer Chemotherapy Drug Manual. Sudbury NA: Jones and Bartlett Publishers, 2006:379–386
85. Chu E, DeVita VT, eds. Cancer Chemotherapy Drug Manual. Sudbury NA: Jones and Bartlett Publishers, 2006:379–386
86. Navelbine® (vinorelbine tartrate) Injection product label, April 2003. Manufactured by Pierre Fabre Medicament Production, Idron, France. Manufactured for GlaxoSmithKline, Research Triangle Park, NC
87. Chu E, DeVita VT, eds. Cancer Chemotherapy Drug Manual. Sudbury NA: Jones and Bartlett Publishers, 2006:379–386

42. Antineoplastic Drugs: Preventing and Managing Extravasation

David R. Kohler, PharmD

Irritants

Irritants may produce any of the following reactions: erythema along a vein or phlebitis, with sensations of tenderness, warmth, or burning, and pain. As a consequence of extravasation, local swelling, erythema, induration with sensations of itching, aching, tightness, or pain may occur but not tissue necrosis. Drugs are intrinsically more or less irritating owing to differences in physical and chemical properties and the excipient products with which they are formulated. The manifestations and severity of reactions after extravasation with irritant drugs often correlate with the concentration of drug, the amount and volume extravasated, and the duration of exposure. Symptoms are typically of short duration and, except for local hyperpigmentation, there are no lasting sequelae

Vesicants

Vesicants cause severe tissue injury, usually resulting in necrosis; consequently, vesicant extravasation is a medical emergency. Vesicant extravasation injuries may be subtle with a delayed onset of morbidity, or they may be immediately apparent with a rapid onset of symptoms. The severity of lesions, the time over which they develop, and the likelihood of spontaneous healing without intervention also vary among vesicant drugs. DNA-binding agents (eg, anthracyclines, anthracenediones, mitomycin) tend to produce more severe and indolent lesions than non–DNA-binding drugs (eg, vinca alkaloids, taxanes). Over a period of days to weeks, erythema, swelling, induration, and pain may increase and progress to brawny discoloration, blistering, or dry desquamation. Lesions may ulcerate and form eschars. Ulcers are characteristically painful with erythematous borders and necrotic bases. Evidence for spontaneous re-epithelialization is typically absent. Lesions caused by DNA-binding agents may continue to expand laterally and deepen for weeks to months after an extravasation event, involving adjacent structures by cytolytic release of active drug from necrotic tissue

What to Avoid in Placement of Vascular Access Devices (VADs)

Peripheral VADs	Central VADs and Implanted Ports
• Fragile, small, or low-flow vessels such as the dorsal aspect of the wrist • Areas of hematoma, edema, impaired lymphatic drainage, phlebitis, inflammation, induration or obvious infection, and sites of previous irradiation • Veins in extremities with decreased sensation, paresthesias, or neurologic weakness. Impaired tactile sensation may prevent a patient from feeling and promptly reporting discomfort associated with extravasation • Using veins that have been accessed within the previous 24 hours • Sites distal to previous venipuncture sites or previous sites of extravasation • Vessels of the hand, wrist, and antecubital fossa for administering irritants or vesicants • A site that does not allow for continuous visual inspection	• Port placement in suboptimal locations, such as the groin or axillae • Areas where needle stability is compromised (eg, the side on which a patient prefers to sleep)

Assessing VADs

New Peripheral VADs	Preexisting Peripheral VADs	Central VADs and Implanted Ports
• Obtain peripheral vascular access in a large vessel in the upper extremities. Peripheral venous access in a lower extremity is *not* recommended	• Assess preexisting peripheral VADs for patency by verifying a brisk blood return and ease of flushing. Flush solutions should flow freely to gravity • Assess site for swelling, erythema, pain, drainage • Assess for signs or symptoms of venous obstruction	Assess central VADs and ports for patency by verifying a brisk blood return and ease of flushing

Note: A new peripheral VAD placed just before drug administration is strongly recommended for administering vesicant drugs

General Principles for Irritant and Vesicant Drug Administration

1. Verify VAD patency by checking for a brisk blood return both before and after drug administration
2. Advise patients to immediately report pain, burning, stinging, or other discomfort they experience during and after parenteral drug administration

Note: Complaints of discomfort often occur during drug administration or promptly afterward, but may be delayed by ≥48 hours after completing drug administration. The onset of clinically apparent morbidity may be delayed by weeks after an extravasation incident

3. After drug administration is completed, flush the administration set with a compatible solution to ensure complete drug delivery

IV Push

Peripheral VADs	Central VADs and Implanted Ports
• Administer intravenously a freely flowing compatible solution before beginning chemotherapy administration • Introduce chemotherapy into an administration set at a Y-site or injection port most proximal to the patient • Check for a blood return before starting chemotherapy administration, check during drug administration after every 1–2 mL of drug administered, and check after drug administration is completed. *Do not* check for VAD patency with a chemotherapy drug • Flush the VAD and vein with the freely flowing compatible solution every 2–3 minutes when injecting large volumes, flush between different drugs, and flush after completing drug administration • Advise patients to immediately report pain, burning, stinging, or other discomfort they experience during and after parenteral drug administration *Note:* Complaints of discomfort often occur during drug administration or promptly afterward, but may be delayed by ≥48 hours after completing drug administration. The onset of clinically apparent morbidity may be delayed by weeks after an extravasation incident • Observe the vascular access site continuously during drug administration	

IV Piggyback (Secondary Infusions)

Peripheral VADs		Central VADs and Implanted Ports
• Administer a cytotoxic agent as a secondary infusion piggy-backed to the primary line at a Y-site or injection port between the flush solution container and the infusion device (pump) used to control the rate of administration. If more than 1 injection port is available, use the port most proximal to the pump • Secure the administration set tubing using tape or a secure locking device		• Secure the administration set tubing using tape or a secure locking device • Administer as a secondary infusion piggybacked to the primary line at a Y-site or injection port • Every hour, observe the vascular access site for erythema or edema, and evaluate all fluid pathway connections • Advise ambulatory outpatients to monitor their VAD exit site or their port entry site for erythema or edema, and advise them whom to contact if complications arise
Irritant	**Vesicant**	
• Check for a brisk blood return before administering chemotherapy and after drug administration is completed • Observe the IV site every 15 minutes for erythema or edema until drug delivery is completed • An infusion pump should be used to administer irritant drugs in large volumes through peripheral veins via continuous (prolonged) infusion	• *Do not use* an infusion pump to administer vesicant drugs • Check for a brisk blood return before administering chemotherapy, check every 5 minutes during administration, and check after drug administration is completed • Observe the vascular access site continuously for erythema or edema • *Do not administer* large volumes of vesicant drugs into peripheral veins unless using a peripherally inserted central catheter	

Continuous or Prolonged (Primary Infusions)

Peripheral VADs	Central VADs and Implanted Ports
• *Not* recommended	• An infusion device is required • Every 1–4 hours, observe the vascular access site for erythema or edema, and monitor the connections • Advise ambulatory outpatients to monitor their VAD exit site or their port entry site for erythema or edema and whom to contact if complications arise

Extravasation is suspected if:

- A patient complains of pain, stinging, burning, or other discomfort at an injection site or in an area that is referable to the distal end of a catheter or implanted port
- There is erythema or blanching in the epidermis overlying an injection site, and swelling or induration around the site
- A blood return cannot be obtained from the VAD
- Parenteral fluids used to "carry" or flush the drug no longer flow freely

  Note: Extravasation from a tunneled VAD may produce discomfort and edema along the subcutaneous track or erythema where the VAD exits the skin. Patients with tunneled VADs or implanted ports may complain of tingling, burning, aching, or other types of pain over the chest wall, the infraclavicular area, neck, or shoulder (sites referable to the location of the port body) ± fever

Dermal reactions that must be distinguished from extravasation include:

- *Flare reactions:* A local allergic reaction that occurs without pain, usually characterized by red blotches along the vein through which a drug was administered. Flare reactions typically subside within 30 minutes with or without treatment
- *Urticarial reactions*: Associated with pruritus along the vein through which a drug was administered
- *Other nonextravasation reactions*: Aching along the vein through which a drug was administered, supra- or perivascular hyperpigmentation, and wheals

If drug extravasation occurs or is suspected:

- *Stop* drug administration
- Remove the syringe used to administer push doses or disconnect the administration set at the point closest to the VAD, *but do not* dislodge or remove the VAD or a needle used to access implanted ports from its current location
- With a fresh syringe, attempt to aspirate from the VAD (or a needle left in an implanted port) any drug it contains and any accessible drug that can be retrieved from the extravasation site
- Implement appropriate pharmacologic and nondrug interventions as directed by a medically responsible care provider or as indicated by local policy, procedure, or standards of practice

  Note: If appropriate and practical, seek consultation with care providers experienced in managing extravasation of antineoplastic drugs. Nurses and pharmacists who are certified or experienced in oncology practice may be excellent resources for information about appropriate management
- As appropriate for the situation: remove peripheral VADs (this does not include PICC, SICC, or midline catheters), or remove the needle from an implanted port before applying topical interventions
- Apply a dressing if indicated, but protect the site from unnecessary compression
- Record in a patient's medical record details about the event and any interventions used in management

  Note: Documentation should identify the date and time of extravasation, the dimensions of the injured site (perpendicular length and width at their greatest dimensions), relevant patient complaints, drugs extravasated, an estimate of the amount of extravasated drugs, all interventions used in management, instructions given to the patient, and a record of subsequent evaluations and consultations. When recording measurements, identify what was measured (eg, swelling, erythema, induration, ulceration), and the time it was measured with respect to when extravasation occurred

VAD, vascular access device. In the present document, the term includes short, peripherally inserted catheters [SICCs]; long-line peripherally inserted central catheters [PICCs]); and subcutaneously tunneled central catheters [CCs])

The preceding recommendations are adapted from the following resources:

The National Institutes of Health Clinical Center Nursing and Patient Care Services Department's Standard of Practice: Care of the Patient Receiving Intravenous Cytotoxic or Biologic Agents

Camp-Sorrell D. Developing extravasation protocols and monitoring outcomes. J Intraven Nurs 1998;21:232–239

Schrijvers DL. Extravasation: A dreaded complication of chemotherapy. Ann Oncol 2003;14 (suppl 3):iii26–30

Schulmeister L, Camp-Sorrell D. Chemotherapy extravasation from implanted ports. Oncol Nurs Forum 2000;27:531–538

Susser WS et al. Mucocutaneous reactions to chemotherapy. J Am Acad Dermatol 1999;40:367–398

Table 42–1. Drug-Specific Extravasation Management Guidelines

Risk Category	Antidote Intervention and Preparation	Local Care	Comments
Actinomycin D	See guidelines for Dactinomycin		
Adriamycin®	See guidelines for Doxorubicin		
Alimta®	See guidelines for Pemetrexed		
BCNU	See guidelines for Carmustine		
Camptosar®	See guidelines for Irinotecan HCl		
Carboplatin (PARAPLATIN®; Bristol-Myers Squibb Oncology, Bristol-Myers Squibb Company, Princeton, NJ)			
Unknown[a]	No known antidotes	• No specific local therapy is indicated	
Carmustine (BiCNU®; distributed by Bristol-Myers Squibb Oncology, Bristol-Myers Squibb Company, Princeton, NJ)[1]			
Irritant	No known antidotes	• Aspirate back through the VAD to remove any accessible extravasated drug • No specific local therapy is indicated	• Patients may complain of irritation and stinging pain during administration—a result of ethanol used to reconstitute carmustine • Carmustine should be diluted in at least 250 mL fluid • Topical sodium bicarbonate solution inactivates carmustine spilled or splashed on the skin, but *must not* be injected locally in the event of carmustine extravasation
Cisplatin (PLATINOL®-AQ; Bristol-Myers Squibb Oncology, Bristol-Myers Squibb Company, Princeton, NJ)[2–5]			
Irritant	See Comments	• No local therapy is indicated after extravasation with small volumes of dilute cisplatin solutions (see Comments) • Extravasation with large volumes or highly concentrated cisplatin solutions may be treated as an extravasation with mechlorethamine (see Comments)	• Extravasation injury has been reported after extravasation of concentrated cisplatin solutions (>0.4 mg/mL) • Although sodium thiosulfate has been recommended to chemically neutralize cisplatin, the conditions under which cisplatin extravasation will produce severe morbidity and tissue necrosis remain undefined (with respect to a threshold concentration or volume); therefore, the most appropriate use of sodium thiosulfate is not known
Cosmegen®	See guidelines for Dactinomycin		
Dacarbazine (also called DTIC; available generically)[6, 7]			
Irritant	No known antidotes	• Aspirate back through the VAD to remove any accessible extravasated drug • No local therapy is indicated • Protect exposed tissues from light following extravasation • Avoid applying pressure to the extravasation site	• Increased skin toxicity was produced in some animal models when dacarbazine was administered intradermally followed by light exposure
Dactinomycin (COSMEGEN®; Merck & Co, Whitehouse Station, NJ)			
Vesicant	No known antidotes	• Treat as for doxorubicin extravasation	• Topical cooling has been inconsistently effective in animal studies
Daunorubicin HCl (CERUBIDINE™; Bedford Laboratories, Bedford, OH; also called daunomycin; available generically)			
Vesicant	No known antidotes	Treat as for doxorubicin extravasation	
Daunorubicin citrate liposome injection (DaunoXome®; Gilead Sciences, Inc, San Dimas, CA)[8–10]			
Irritant	No known antidotes	• Aspirate back through the VAD to remove any accessible extravasated drug • Apply cold to the involved area with circulating ice water, an ice pack, or other cold pack for 15–60 minutes every 2 hours for at least 48 hours after extravasation[b] • Elevate the involved extremity • Avoid applying pressure to the extravasation site	

Risk Category	Antidote Intervention and Preparation	Local Care	Comments
DaunoXome®	See guidelines for Daunorubicin citrate liposomal		
Docetaxel (TAXOTERE®; Aventis Pharmaceuticals, Inc, Bridgewater, NJ)[11, 12]			
Irritant	No known antidotes	• Treat as for paclitaxel extravasation	• It is not yet clear whether application of either cold or heat provides benefit in managing docetaxel extravasation. In one case report, erythema and hyperpigmentation may have been exacerbated by application of warmth[13] • Extravasation often presents acutely with swelling and tenderness of the involved site. Blistering and onset or exacerbation of pain may be delayed by several days. Erythema and edema may increase markedly during the first week. Skin desquamation characteristically occurs within 2–3 weeks • Involved site dysesthesias or loss of sensation occurs commonly. Locally altered tactile sensation may persist for months after an extravasation event[14]
Doxil®	See guidelines for Doxorubicin, liposomal		
Doxorubicin HCl (ADRIAMYCIN®; Bedford Laboratories™, Bedford, OH)[15–18]			
Vesicant	No known antidotes	• Aspirate back through the VAD to remove any accessible extravasated drug • Apply cold to the involved area with circulating ice water, an ice pack, or other cold pack for 15–60 minutes at least 4 times daily for 24–48 hours after extravasation[b] • Elevate the involved extremity • Avoid applying pressure to the extravasation site	• Seek surgical consultation, especially if a patient reports pain at the extravasation site within 10 days after the event. Surgical debridement or excision may be required to remove nonviable tissues, release trapped drug, and prevent more extensive prolonged tissue injury • Early surgical intervention should be reserved for patients with local uncontrolled pain, repeated infections, or limb restriction attributed to extravasation injury[19] • Case reports suggest that dexrazoxane may mitigate local morbidity after extravasation with doxorubicin and other anthracycline drugs[c] • Anecdotes and at least one prospective study suggest DMSO may mitigate local morbidity after extravasation with doxorubicin[d]
Doxorubicin HCl liposome injection (DOXIL®; Tibotec Therapeutics, Inc, division of Ortho Biotech Products LP, Raritan, NJ)[20, 21]			
Vesicant	No known antidotes	• Treat as for doxorubicin extravasation	• The severity of tissue injury may be related to the volume and duration for which the extravasated drug remains in contact with the affected site[21]
Ellence®	See guidelines for Epirubicin		
Eloxatin®	See guidelines for Oxaliplatin		
Epirubicin HCl (ELLENCE®; Pharmacia & Upjohn Company, a subsidiary of Pharmacia Corporation, Kalamazoo, MI)[22]			
Vesicant	No known antidotes	• Treat as for doxorubicin extravasation	• Case reports suggest that dexrazoxane may mitigate local morbidity following extravasation with anthracycline drugs[c] • Anecdotes and at least one prospective study suggest DMSO may mitigate local morbidity following extravasation with epirubicin[d]
Etoposide (VePesid®; Bristol Laboratories Oncology Products, A Bristol-Myers Squibb Co. Princeton, NJ. Toposar™; Pharmacia & Upjohn Company, Kalamazoo, MI)[23]			
Irritant (see Comments)		• Treat as for vinblastine extravasation	• Skin ulceration is unlikely when etoposide injection is diluted to concentrations used clinically
Fluorouracil (ADRUCIL®; SICOR Pharmaceuticals, Inc, Irvine, CA)			

(*continued*)

Table 42–1. Drug-Specific Extravasation Management Guidelines (*continued*)

Risk Category	Antidote Intervention and Preparation	Local Care	Comments
Irritant		• No specific local therapy is indicated	
Gemcitabine HCl (GEMZAR®; Eli Lilly and Company, Indianapolis, IN)			
Unknown[a] (see Comments)	No known antidotes	• No specific local therapy	• Based on clinical trial data, gemcitabine is not a vesicant (personal communication with Eli Lilly and Company, November 7, 2005)
Gemzar®	See guidelines for Gemcitabine HCl		
Hycamtin®	See guidelines for Topotecan HCl		
Idarubicin HCl (Idamycin®; Pharmacia & Upjohn Company, Kalamazoo, MI)[24]			
Vesicant	No known antidotes	• Treat as for doxorubicin extravasation	
Irinotecan HCl (Camptosar®; Pharmacia & Upjohn Company, division of Pfizer, New York, NY)			
Unknown[a]	No known antidotes	• Aspirate back through the VAD to remove any accessible extravasated drug • Apply cold to the involved area with circulating ice water, an ice pack, or other cold pack for 15–60 minutes at least 4 times daily for 24–48 hours after extravasation[b] • Elevate the involved extremity • Avoid applying pressure to the site	• The recommendations for Local Care are based on the manufacturer's product label (Camptosar®, dated July 21, 2005), which specifies in the event of extravasation: "[intradermally] flushing the site with sterile water and application of ice. . . ." Health care providers should note that the value of subcutaneous and intradermal flushing with saline and other solutions and subsequently aspirating the flush solutions in an effort to dilute and remove an extravasated drug is controversial
Mechlorethamine HCl (also called HN_2 TRITURATION OF MUSTARGEN®; Merck & Co, Whitehouse Station, NJ)[25–28]			
Vesicant	Isotonic sodium thiosulfate 0.167 mol/L (1/6 M $Na_2S_2O_3$) solution	• Aspirate back through the VAD to remove any accessible extravasated drug • Inject 1/6 M $Na_2S_2O_3$ solution through the IV access device: 2–5 mL for each milligram of mechlorethamine that was extravasated • Remove the IV access device • With a 25-G needle, inject subcutaneously, 1/6 M $Na_2S_2O_3$ solution circumferentially, into the tissue surrounding the site • Avoid applying pressure to the site	• *Rapid* intervention is essential in treating nitrogen mustard extravasation • $Na_2S_2O_3$ solution chemically neutralizes mechlorethamine • The intervention is clinically accepted, but reports confirming benefit are scant. ***Preparation of a 1/6 M*** $Na_2S_2O_3$ *solution:* Starting with 10% $Na_2Ss_2O_3$ solution (1 g/10 mL). In a syringe, mix 4 mL $Na_2S_2O_3$ with 6 mL water for injection Starting with 25% $Na_2S_2O_3$ solution (2.5 g/10 mL). In a syringe, mix 1.6 mL $Na_2S_2O_3$ with 8.4 mL water for injection
Mithramycin	See guidelines for Plicamycin		
Mitomycin (mitomycin-C, MUTAMYCIN®; Bristol-Myers Squibb Oncology, Bristol-Myers Squibb Company, Princeton, NJ. Available generically)[29–33]			
Vesicant	No known antidotes	• Treat as for doxorubicin extravasation	• Extravasation is typically accompanied by pain and swelling, but initially may be painless • Mitomycin is associated with ulceration at areas of recent vascular damage, including venipuncture sites that are distant from the site of extravasation • Dermal injury after mitomycin extravasation may be delayed from 1 to 29 weeks after administration • Mitomycin extravasation injury may occur, may be exacerbated, or may recur after the affected area is exposed to sunlight[29] • Anecdotes and at least one prospective study suggest that DMSO may mitigate local morbidity after extravasation with mitomycin[d]

Risk Category	Antidote Intervention and Preparation	Local Care	Comments
Mitoxantrone HCl (NOVANTRONE®; marketed by (OSI)™ Oncology, OSI Pharmaceuticals, Inc, Melville, NY)[5, 34]			
Vesicant	No known antidotes	• Treat as for doxorubicin extravasation	• Causes blue discoloration in soft tissues where infiltration has occurred • Inconsistently produces tissue necrosis after extravasation • When ulceration occurs, lesions may spontaneously resolve with conservative treatment
Navelbine®	See guidelines for Vinorelbine		
Nitrogen mustard	See guidelines for Mechlorethamine		
Novantrone®	See guidelines for Mitoxantrone		
Oncovin®	See guidelines for Vincristine		
Oxaliplatin (ELOXATIN™; Sanofi-Synthelabo Inc, New York, NY)[35–37]			
Irritant	No known antidotes	• Aspirate back through the VAD to remove any accessible extravasated drug • Avoid applying pressure to the extravasation site • Orally administered nonsteroidal analgesics may be useful in managing pain and inflammation	• Inflammatory reactions were reported after oxaliplatin extravasation (approximate amount extravasated: 40–104 mg)[36] • Clinical appearance within 2–3 days after extravasation is described as resembling erysipelas, with swelling, pain, induration, erythema, local heat, impaired movement when joints are involved • Although there is concern that cold compresses may trigger the cold temperature-induced neuropathy associated with oxaliplatin,[37] both cold and warm compresses have been used to manage oxaliplatin extravasation without any report of deleterious effects from either intervention[36, 38] • Induration, inflammation, and paresthesias may persist for weeks after an extravasation event[37]
Paclitaxel (TAXOL®; Bristol-Myers Squibb Oncology, Bristol-Myers Squibb Company, Princeton, NJ. ONXOL™; IVAX Pharmaceuticals, Inc, Miami, FL. Available generically)[39–42]			
Vesicant	No known antidotes	• Aspirate back through the VAD to remove any accessible extravasated drug • Apply cold to the involved area with circulating ice water, an ice pack, or other cold compresses for 15–20 minutes at least 4 times daily for 24–48 hours after extravasation[b] • Avoid applying pressure to the site	• It is not yet clear whether application of either cold or heat provides benefit in managing paclitaxel extravasation. In one case report, blisters, erythema, and hyperpigmentation may have been exacerbated by application of warmth[13] • Skin overlying the extravasation site may become inflamed (mimicking a first-degree thermal burn) and desquamate • In two cases, subcutaneous perilesional infiltration with hyaluronidase after paclitaxel extravasation may have delayed healing[43] • Gross and microscopic examination of biopsied and excised tissues from paclitaxel extravasation injuries reveals tissue necrosis[42, 44] but, in general, administration and extravasation management follow procedures developed for irritant (nonvesicant) hazardous drugs • Involved site dysesthesias or sensory loss are common sequelae; motor weakness also has been reported
Paraplatin®	See guidelines for Carboplatin		

(continued)

Table 42–1. Drug-Specific Extravasation Management Guidelines (*continued*)

Risk Category	Antidote Intervention and Preparation	Local Care	Comments
Pemetrexed (ALIMTA®; Eli Lilly and Company, Indianapolis, IN)			
Unknown[a] (see Comments)	No known antidotes	• No specific recommendations for local therapy	• Based on clinical trial data, pemetrexed is not a vesicant (personal communication with Eli Lilly and Company, November 7, 2005)
Platinol®	See guidelines for Cisplatin		
Plicamycin (No longer marketed in the United States)			
Irritant	No known antidotes	• Aspirate back through the VAD to remove any accessible extravasated drug • No specific local therapy is indicated • Avoid applying pressure to the site	
Taxol®	See guidelines for Paclitaxel		
Taxotere®	See guidelines for Docetaxel		
Teniposide (VUMON®; Bristol Laboratories Oncology products, a Bristol-Myers Squibb Company, Princeton, NJ)			
Irritant		• Treat as for vinblastine extravasation	
Topotecan HCl (HYCAMTIN®; GlaxoSmithKline, Research Triangle Park, NC)			
Nonirritant	No known antidotes	• Aspirate back through the VAD to remove any accessible extravasated drug • Apply cold to the involved area with cold circulating ice water, an ice pack, or other compresses for 15–20 minutes four times daily for 24 hours after extravasation[b] • Avoid applying pressure to the site	• In two cases, extravasation was accompanied by pain and swelling, which resolved within 24 hours after topical cooling. There were no sequelae in either case, and no recurrence of morbidity in one of the two patients who received additional topotecan on the day after the extravasation event[45] • "Inadvertent extravasation … has been associated only with mild local reactions such as erythema and bruising" (Hycamtin® product labeling, July 2003)
Velban®	See guidelines for Vinblastine		
Vinblastine sulfate (available generically)[46–49]			
Vesicant	No known antidotes	• Aspirate back through the VAD to remove any accessible extravasated drug • Consider dispersing the drug by administering hyaluronidase injection 150–300 units diluted in 1–6 mL 0.9% NaCl injection into the VAD through which the extravasated drug was administered, by subcutaneous injection with a fine-gauge needle circumferentially around the involved site, or by both techniques *Note:* Hyaluronidase is marketed in the United States in several formulations: solutions containing 150 units or 200 units/mL, and a lyophilized powder for reconstitution for injection • Apply warm packs for 15–20 minutes at least 4 times daily for 24–48 hours after extravasation[b] • Avoid applying pressure to the site	• Warmth increases local blood flow, enhancing drug absorption and removal from the site • Hyaluronidase may aid dispersing the extravasated drug • Do not apply topical steroid products. Topical steroids have exacerbated extravasation injury in animal models

Risk Category	Antidote Intervention and Preparation	Local Care	Comments
Vincristine sulfate (available generically)[49, 50]			
Vesicant	No known antidotes	Treat as for vinblastine extravasation	
Vindesine sulfate (no longer marketed in the United States)[51, 52]			
Vesicant	No known antidotes	Treat as for vinblastine extravasation	
Vinorelbine tartrate (available generically)[49, 53, 54]			
Vesicant	No known antidotes	Treat as for vinblastine extravasation	
VM-26	See guidelines for Teniposide		
VP-16, VP-16-213	See guidelines for Etoposide		

[a]When it is not known whether a drug is an irritant or a vesicant, take the most conservative approach to intervention; that is, follow the recommendations for managing doxorubicin extravasation

[b]Optimal temperatures and the frequency and duration for applying warm and cold compresses over areas of extravasation injury are not known. Caregivers should instruct patients to apply heat or cold intermittently, when appropriate, for as long as possible during each application, but not for durations that may compromise a patient's quality of life

The following interventions cannot yet be recommended; nevertheless, they are noteworthy

[c]**Dexrazoxane**

Anecdotal reports suggest that dexrazoxane may mitigate tissue injury after extravasation of doxorubicin or epirubicin:

Dexrazoxane 1000 mg/m^2 per day intravenously, diluted in a volume of 0.9% NaCl injection (0.9% NS) or 5% Dextrose Injection (D5W) sufficient to produce a concentration of 1.3–5 mg/mL over 10–30 minutes for 2 consecutive days, *followed by:*

Dexrazoxane 500 mg/m^2 intravenously, diluted in a volume of 0.9% NaCl or D5W sufficient to produce a concentration of 1.3–5 mg/mL over 10–30 minutes on the third day after extravasation[55–57] (total dexrazoxane dosage = 2500 mg/m^2)

Note: Dexrazoxane administration began approximately 2 hours after extravasation with epirubicin

[d]**Dimethyl sulfoxide (DMSO)**

Anecdotes and at least one prospective study suggest that dimethyl sulfoxide may mitigate local morbidity after extravasation of anthracyclines, mitomycin, and other drugs. (*Note:* The following regimens are not ranked by preference or effectiveness)

Regimen 1: Dimethyl sulfoxide 50% (w/w) 1–2 mL applied topically over the involved site once, followed by cold compresses applied topically for 15–20 minutes every hour for 12–24 hours[33]

Regimen 2: Dimethyl sulfoxide 99% 4 drops/10 cm^2 of involved skin surface area, applied topically over an area twofold greater than the affected area (including the involved site) every 8 hours for 1 week. The solution is left to dry in air without an occlusive dressing, and DMSO administration is followed by local cooling with a cold pack applied topically to the involved site for 60 minutes every 8 hours for the first 3 days after the extravasation event[58]

Regimen 3: Dimethyl sulfoxide 99% applied topically over an area twofold greater than the affected area (including the involved site) every 6 hours for 14 days. The solution is left to dry in air without an occlusive dressing[59]

Regimen 4: Dimethyl sulfoxide 99% or 50% 15 mL or **dimethyl sulfoxide 75%** volume not specified, applied topically over the involved site every 4–6 hours for 3 days after the extravasation event with topical cooling[60]

Note: The US Food and Drug Administration has approved dimethyl sulfoxide 50% (w/w) for administration to human subjects only for the symptomatic relief of patients with interstitial cystitis. Dimethyl sulfoxide 99.0% is commercially marketed for cryopreservation, and the compound is also available in various concentrations and purity grades for veterinary and laboratory use and as an industrial solvent. Health care providers are discouraged from using DMSO that is not intended for use in human subjects, because the product may facilitate systemic absorption of chemical impurities and contaminants after topical use

Adverse Reactions From Dimethyl Sulfoxide

DMSO 50%	DMSO 99%	Reference
Unpleasant taste, halitosis, and body odor (often described as garlic-like)		58–60
Blistering if the application site is not permitted to dry before a dressing is applied		59
Tingling, stinging, or burning sensation Histamine release with itching, erythema, rash, and urticaria DMSO is hydroscopic. Application to moist or wet skin produces an exothermic reaction (heat)		
	Local tingling or burning	58, 59, 61, 62
	Severe pain	63, 64
	Burning, swelling, erythema	64

General References

Boyle DM, Engelking C. Vesicant extravasation: myths and realities. Oncol Nurs Forum 1995;22:57–67

Dorr RT. Antidotes to vesicant chemotherapy extravasations. Blood Rev 1990;4:41–60

Drug-Specific References

1. Colvin M, Hartner J, Summerfield M. Stability of carmustine in the presence of sodium bicarbonate. Am J Hosp Pharm 1980;37:677–678
2. Lewis KP, Medina WD. Cellulitis and fibrosis due to *cis*-diamminedichloroplatinum(II) (Platinol) infiltration. Cancer Treat Rep 1980;64:1162–1163
3. Howell SB, Taetle R. Effect of sodium thiosulfate on *cis*-dichlorodiammineplatinum(II) toxicity and antitumor activity in L1210 leukemia. Cancer Treat Rep 1980;64:611–616
4. Leyden M, Sullivan J. Full-thickness skin necrosis due to inadvertent interstitial infusion of cisplatin [letter]. Cancer Treat Rep 1983;67:199
5. Dorr RT, Alberts DS, Soble M. Lack of experimental vesicant activity for the anticancer agents cisplatin, melphalan, and mitoxantrone. Cancer Chemother Pharmacol 1986;16:91–94
6. Buesa JM, Gracia M, Valle M et al. Phase I trial of intermittent high-dose dacarbazine. Cancer Treat Rep 1984;68:499–504
7. Dorr RT, Alberts DS, Einspahr J et al. Experimental dacarbazine antitumor activity and skin toxicity in relation to light exposure and pharmacologic antidotes. Cancer Treat Rep 1987;71:267–272
8. Cabriales S, Bresnahan J, Testa D et al. Extravasation of liposomal daunorubicin in patients with AIDS-associated Kaposi's sarcoma: a report of four cases [see comments]. Oncol Nurs Forum 1998;25:67–70. Comment in: Oncol Nurs Forum 1998;25:653–654
9. Keenan A. Reader seeks clarification on the role of glucocorticoids and sodium bicarbonate [comment]. Oncol Nurs Forum 1998;25:653–654. Comment on: Oncol Nurs Forum 1998;25:67–70
10. Cabriales S. Reader seeks clarification of the role of glucocorticoids and sodium bicarbonate. The author responds [comment, letter]. Oncol Nurs Forum 1998;25:654. Comment on: Oncol Nurs Forum 1998;25:653–654
11. Raley J, Geisler JP, Buekers TE, Sorosky JI. Docetaxel extravasation causing significant delayed tissue injury. Gynecol Oncol 2000;78:259–260
12. Ascherman JA, Knowles SL, Attkiss K. Docetaxel (Taxotere) extravasation: a report of five cases with treatment recommendations. Ann Plast Surg 2000;45:438–441
13. Goodman M, Stewart I, Lydon J et al. Use caution when managing paclitaxel and taxotere infiltrations. Oncol Nurs Forum 1996;23:541–542
14. Ho C-H, Yang C-H, Chu C-Y. Vesicant-type reaction due to docetaxel extravasation [letter]. Acta Derm Venereol 2003;83:467–468
15. Rudolph R, Stein RS, Pattillo RA. Skin ulcers due to Adriamycin. Cancer 1976;38:1087–1094
16. Larson DL. Treatment of tissue extravasation by antitumor agents. Cancer 1982;49:1796–1799
17. Linder RM, Upton J, Osteen R. Management of extensive doxorubicin hydrochloride extravasation injuries. J Hand Surg 1983;8:32–38
18. Loth TS, Eversmann WW Jr. Treatment methods for extravasations of chemotherapeutic agents: a comparative study. J Hand Surg [Am] 1986;11:388–396
19. Langstein HN, Duman H, Seelig D et al. Retrospective study of the management of chemotherapeutic extravasation injury. Ann Plast Surg 2002;49:369–374
20. Madhavan S, Northfelt DW. Lack of vesicant injury following extravasation of liposomal doxorubicin [letter]. J Natl Cancer Inst 1995;87:1556–1557
21. Lokich J. Doxil extravasation injury: a case report [letter]. Ann Oncol 1999;10:735–736
22. Wilson J, Carder P, Gooi J, Nishikawa H. Recall phenomenon following epirubicin. Clin Oncol 1999;11:424–425
23. Dorr RT, Alberts DS. Skin ulceration potential without therapeutic anticancer activity for epipodophyllotoxin commercial diluents. Invest New Drugs 1983;1:151–159
24. Lu K, Savaraj N, Kavanagh J et al. Clinical pharmacology of 4-demethoxydaunorubicin (DMDR). Cancer Chemother Pharmacol 1986;17:143–148
25. Hatiboglu I, Mihich E, Moore GE, Nichol CA. Use of sodium thiosulfate as a neutralizing agent during regional administration of nitrogen mustard: an experimental study. Ann Surg 1962;156:994–1001
26. Fasth A, Sörbo B. Protective effect of thiosulfate and metabolic thiosulfate precursors against toxicity of nitrogen mustard (HN_2). Biochem Pharmacol 1973;22:1337–1351
27. Owen OE, Dellatorre DL, Van Scott EJ, Cohen MR. Accidental intramuscular injection of mechlorethamine. Cancer 1980;45:2225–2226
28. Dorr RT, Soble M, Alberts DS. Efficacy of sodium thiosulfate as a local antidote to mechlorethamine skin toxicity in the mouse. Cancer Chemother Pharmacol 1988;22:299–302
29. Fuller B, Lind M, Bonomi P. Mitomycin C extravasation exacerbated by sunlight [letter]. Ann Intern Med 1981;94(4 pt 1):542
30. Johnston-Early A, Cohen MH. Mitomycin C-induced skin ulceration remote from infusion site [letter]. Cancer Treat Rep 1981;65:529
31. Khanna AK, Khanna A, Asthana AK, Misra MK. Mitomycin C extravasation ulcers. J Surg Oncol 1985;28:108–110
32. Aizawa H, Tagami H. Delayed tissue necrosis due to mitomycin C. Acta Derm Venereol 1987;67:364–366
33. Patel JS, Krusa M. Distant and delayed mitomycin C extravasation. Pharmacotherapy 1999;19:1002–1005
34. Peters FTM, Beijnen JH, ten Bokkel Huinink WW. Mitoxantrone extravasation injury [letter]. Cancer Treat Rep 1987;71:992–993
35. Baur M, Kienzer H-R, Rath T, Dittrich C. Extravasation of Oxaliplatin (Eloxatin®)—Clinical Course. Onkologie 2000;23:468–471
36. Kretzschmar A, Pink D, Thuss-Patience P, Dörken B, Reichert P, Eckert R. Extravasations of oxaliplatin [letter]. JCO 2003;21:4068–4069
37. Foo KF, Michael M, Toner G, Zalcberg J. A case report of oxaliplatin extravasation [letter]. Ann Oncol 2003;14:961–962
38. Kennedy JG, Donahue JP, Hoang B, Boland PJ. Vesicant characteristics of oxaliplatin following antecubital extravasation. Clin Oncol 2003;15:237–239
39. Lubejko BG, Sartorius SE. Nursing considerations in paclitaxel (Taxol) administration. Semin Oncol 1993;20:26–30
40. Ajani JA, Dodd LG, Daugherty K et al. Taxol-induced soft-tissue injury secondary to extravasation: characterization by histopathology and clinical course [see comments]. J Natl Cancer Inst 1994;86:51–53. Comment in: Oncol Nurs Forum 1994;21:973
41. Rogers BB. An author responds [letter; comment]. Oncol Nurs Forum 1994;21:973. Comment on: J Natl Cancer Inst 1994;86:51–53
42. Herrington JD, Figueroa JA. Severe necrosis due to paclitaxel extravasation. Pharmacotherapy 1997;17:163–165
43. du Bois A, Fehr MK, Bochtler H, Koechli OR. Clinical course and management of paclitaxel administration. Oncol Rep 1996;3:973–974
44. Bicher A, Levenback C, Burke TW et al. Infusion site soft-tissue injury after paclitaxel administration. Cancer 1995;76:116–120
45. Oostweegel LMM, van Warmerdam LJC, Schot M et al. Extravasation of topotecan, a report of two cases. J Oncol Pharm Practice 1997;3:115–116
46. Britton RC, Habif DV. Clinical uses of hyaluronidase: a current review. Surgery 1953;33:917–940
47. Laurie SW, Wilson KL, Kernahan DA et al. Intravenous extravasation injuries: the effectiveness of hyaluronidase in their treatment. Ann Plast Surg 1984;13:191–194
48. Dorr RT, Alberts DS. Vinca alkaloid skin toxicity: antidote and drug disposition studies in the mouse. J Natl Cancer Inst 1985;74:113–120
49. Bertelli G, Dini D, Forno GB et al. Hyaluronidase as an antidote to extravasation of Vinca alkaloids: clinical results. J Cancer Res Clin Oncol 1994;120:505–506
50. Bellone JD. Treatment of vincristine extravasation [letter]. JAMA 1981;245:343
51. Dorr RT, Jones SE. Inapparent infiltrations associated with vindesine administration. Med Pediatr Oncol 1979;6:285–288
52. Mateu J, Llop C. Delayed treatment of vindesine extravasation [letter]. Ann Pharmacother 1994;28:967–968
53. Bertelli G, Garrone O, Bighin C, Dini D. Correspondence re: Cicchetti S, Jemec B, Gault DT: Two case reports of vinorelbine extravasation: management and review of the literature. Tumori 86: 289–292, 2000. Tumori 2001;87:112–113
54. Moreno de Vega MJ, Dauden E, Abajo P et al. Skin necrosis from extravasation of vinorelbine. J Eur Acad Dermatol Venereol 2002;16:488–490
55. Langer SW, Sehested M, Jensen PB et al. Dexrazoxane in anthracycline extravasation [letter]. JCO 2000;18:3064
56. Langer SW, Sehested M, Jensen PB. Treatment of anthracycline extravasation with dexrazoxane. Clin Cancer Res 2000;6:3680–3686
57. Jensen JN, Lock-Andersen J, Langer SW, Mejer J. Dexrazoxane—a promising antidote in the treatment of accidental extravasation of anthracyclines. Scand J Plast Reconstr Surg Hand Surg 2003;37:174–175
58. Bertelli G, Gozza A, Forno GB et al. Topical dimethylsulfoxide for the prevention of soft tissue injury after extravasation of vesicant cytotoxic drugs: a prospective clinical study. JCO 1995;13:2851–2855
59. Olver IN, Aisner J, Hament A et al. A prospective study of topical dimethyl sulfoxide for treating anthracycline extravasation. JCO 1988;6:1732–1735
60. Lawrence HJ, Walsh D, Zapotowski KA et al. Topical dimethylsulfoxide may prevent tissue damage from anthracycline extravasation. Cancer Chemother Pharmacol 1989;23:316–318
61. St. Germain B, Houlihan N, D'Amato S. Dimethyl sulfoxide therapy in the treatment of vesicant extravasation. Two case presentations. J Intraven Nurs 1994;17:261–266
62. Alberts DS, Dorr RT. Case report: topical DMSO for mitomycin-C-induced skin ulceration. Oncol Nurs Forum 1991;18:693–695
63. Llinares ME, Bermúdez M, Fuster JL et al. Toxicity to topical dimethyl sulfoxide in a pediatric patient with anthracycline extravasation. Pediatr Hematol Oncol 2005;22:49–52
64. Creus N, Mateu J, Massó J et al. Toxicity to topical dimethyl sulfoxide (DMSO) when used as an extravasation antidote. Pharm World Sci 2002;24:175–176

43. Indications for Growth Factors in the Hematology-Oncology Setting

Pamela W. McDevitt, PharmD, BCOP, and James N. Frame, MD, FACP

Neutropenia

Epidemiology

The incidence of grade 4 neutropenia in chemotherapy regimens ranges from 1.2% to 98%.[1] The incidence of febrile neutropenia is 25–40% in chemotherapy-naive patients.[1]

Regimen	% Grade 3/4 Neutropenia
Carboplatin/Taxol[2]	63
Cisplatin/VP16[3]	85
Topotecan[4]	88
Vinorelbine[5]	53
Adriamycin/Cytoxan (AC)[6] (doxorubicin/cyclophosphamide)	7
5-Fluoruracil/epirubicin Cytoxan (FEC)[7]	25
Cisplatin/5-fluorouracil[8]	9
Irinotecan/5-fluorouracil/leucovorin (IFL)[9]	54
5-Fluorouracil/irinotecan/leucovorin (FOLFIR)[10]	46
5-Fluorouracil/oxaliplatin/leucovorin (FOLFOX4)[11]	44
Cytoxan/Adriamycin/vincristine/prednisone (CHOP/CNOP)[12]	91
Adriamycin/bleomycin/vinblastine/dacarbazine (ABVD)[13]	21
Melphalan/prednisone (MP)[14]	37
Fludarabine[15]	56
Gemcitabine/cisplatin (GC)[16]	71

NCI Common Toxicity Criteria

Grade	ANC/AGC
0	Normal
1	≥1500–<2000/mm^3
2	≥1000–<1500/mm^3
3	≥500–<1000/mm^3
4	<500/mm^3

WHO Toxicity Criteria

Grade	ANC/AGC
0	>2000
1	1500–1900/mm^3
2	1000–1400/mm^3
3	500–900/mm^3
4	<500/mm^3

Preparations

1. Filgrastim (G-CSF)
2. Pegfilgrastim (pegylated G-CSF)
3. Sargramostim (GM-CSF)

REGIMEN

FILGRASTIM G-CSF (NEUPOGEN®)

Cancer patients receiving myelosuppressive chemotherapy:
Filgrastim 5 μg /kg/day, round to nearest vial size, either 300 μg or 480 μg,[1] subcutaneously daily after chemotherapy continuing until ANC reaches 10,000/mm^3 or clinically sufficient neutrophil count is achieved after nadir
[The FDA-approved dose is subcutaneous or intravenous administration for up to 2 weeks after expected chemotherapy-induced ANC nadir[18]]
Note: It is recommended not to use filgrastim in the period 24 hours before or 24 hours after chemotherapy

Cancer patients receiving bone marrow transplant (BMT):
Filgrastim 10 mcg/kg/day by intravenous infusion over 4 or 24 hours or as a continuous 24-hour subcutaneous infusion
Note: Administered at least 24 hours after cytotoxic CT and at least 24 hours after bone marrow infusion

Dose adjustment:
1. When ANC > 1000/mm^3 for 3 consecutive days, reduce dose to 5 μg/kg/day
2. If ANC > 1000/mm^3 for 3 more consecutive days, discontinue G-CSF
3. If ANC < 1000/mm^3, resume at 5 μg/kg/day
4. If ANC decreases to <1000/mm^3 at any time during the 5 μg/kg/day administration, increase dose to 10 μg/kg/day and follow dose adjustment guidelines

Notes on dosing:
1. Doses recommended are for adult patients
2. Obese patients should be dosed on actual body weight, even morbidly obese patients
3. Do not reduce doses in elderly

Peripheral blood progenitor cells (PBPCs) collection:
Filgrastim 10 μg/kg/day subcutaneously or 5–8 μg/kg subcutaneously twice daily
Note: The optimal timing and duration of growth factor stimulation have not been determined[19,20]

Filgrastim G-CSF (Neupogen®) is available in the United States in single-dose vials or prefilled syringes containing 300 or 480 μg per syringe or vial

Efficacy

1. In a phase III placebo-controlled trial of small cell lung cancer patients, filgrastim reduced the incidence of febrile neutropenia after chemotherapy by 37% (77% versus 40%)[25]
2. Increase in ANC seen ~24 hours after administration; 50% decrease in circulating neutrophils occurs within 1–2 days after discontinuation and returns to pretreatment levels within 4–7 days

Indications (Cancer Patients)

1. Myelosuppressive chemotherapy
2. Acute myeloid leukemia (AML) receiving induction or consolidation chemotherapy
3. BMT
4. Peripheral blood progenitor cell (PBPC) collection
5. Severe chronic neutropenia

Toxicity

>10% of Patients

Fever	Alopecia
Nausea/vomiting	Diarrhea
Mucositis	↑ LDH (19%)
Medullary bone pain (24–26%)	
Splenomegaly (more common when treatment >14 days; usually subclinical)	

Bone pain is reported more frequently in patients treated at higher doses (20–100 μg/kg/day) administered intravenously compared with lower subcutaneous doses. Bone pain is generally controlled with non-narcotic analgesics but may infrequently require narcotic analgesics

1–10% of Patients

Chest pain	Fluid retention
Headache	Skin rash
↑ Uric acid (8%)	Anorexia
Stomatitis	Constipation
Leukocytosis	Pain at injection site
Weakness	Dyspnea
Cough	Sore throat
↑ Alkaline phosphatase (9%)	

<1% of Patients (Important or Life-Threatening)

Pericarditis	Thrombophlebitis
ARDS, hypoxia	Splenic rupture
Sickle cell crisis	
Transient supraventricular arrhythmia	
Cutaneous vasculitis with high ANC (1/7000)	
Allergic reactions (including urticaria, rash or anaphylaxis)	

Therapy Monitoring

1. *During G-CSF therapy after cytotoxic chemotherapy:* CBC with differential twice weekly
2. *After BMT:* CBC at least 3 times per week
3. *During initiation of therapy for severe chronic neutropenia:* CBC twice weekly for the first 4 weeks and for 2 weeks following dose adjustment, then monthly while stable
4. *PBPC collection:* ANC after 4 days of G-CSF, and consider dose modifications if WBC > 100,000/mm^3

Notes

1. The manufacturer does not recommend concurrent use with myelosuppressive chemotherapy or radiation therapy
2. Patients must be instructed to report abdominal or shoulder tip pain, prompting evaluation for splenomegaly or splenic rupture, especially healthy donors receiving filgrastim for mobilization of PBPC
3. Patients must be instructed to report respiratory distress, prompting evaluation for acute respiratory distress syndrome (ARDS)
4. Use with caution in patients with sickle cell disease; sickle cell crises have been reported following therapy
5. Safety has not been established in patients with chronic myeloid leukemia (CML) or myelodysplastic syndromes (MDS), in those receiving chemotherapy associated with delayed-myelosuppression, or those receiving mitomycin C or myelosuppressive doses of antimetabolites such as 5-fluorouracil
6. In all clinical studies of the use of G-CSF for PBPC collection, G-CSF was administered after re-infusion of the collected cells
7. G-CSF is contraindicated in patients with a hypersensitivity to *Escherichia coli*–derived proteins, filgrastim, or any component of the formulation[18]
8. NCCN Guidelines (V. 2. 2005) recommend routine use of G-CSF support for patients at high risk (defined > 20%) of development of febrile neutropenia receiving treatment with curative intent, adjuvant therapy, or treatment expected to prolong survival or to improve QOL

REGIMEN

PEGFILGRASTIM (NEULASTA®)

Cancer patients receiving myelosuppressive chemotherapy

Pegfilgrastim (Neulasta®) 6 mg subcutaneously once per chemotherapy cycle. Administer at least 24 hours after cytotoxic chemotherapy and at least 14 days before the next administration of cytotoxic chemotherapy[21,22]

Dosing:

Dose recommended is for adult patients ≥45 kg

Pegfilgrastim (Neulasta®) is available in the United States in single-dose prefilled syringes containing 6 mg per syringe

Efficacy

1. In a phase III trial of breast cancer patients, the efficacy of pegylated G-CSF was similar to that of filgrastim, based on duration of severe neutropenia (1.8 days versus 1.6 days) and incidence of febrile neutropenia (13% versus 20%)[21]
2. Pegylated G-CSF is primarily cleared by neutrophil receptor binding; thereafter, pegylated G-CSF concentrations decline rapidly at the onset of neutrophil recovery

Toxicity

15%–72% of Patients

Neutropenic fever	Fever
Nausea/vomiting	Alopecia
Mucositis	Diarrhea
Medullary bone pain (24–26%)*	↑ LDH (19%)
Constipation	Fever
Anorexia	Skeletal pain
Taste perversion	Headache
Dyspepsia	Myalgia
Insomnia	Abdominal pain
Generalized weakness	Peripheral edema
Arthralgia	Granulocytopenia
Dizziness	Fatigue
Stomatitis	

*Bone pain is generally controlled with non-narcotic analgesics but may infrequently require narcotic analgesics

<10% of Patients

Leukocytosis (WBC > 100,000/mm³) <1%
Hypoxia (1 case in clinical trials)
↑ Alkaline phosphatase (9%)
↑ Uric acid (8%)
<1% of Patients (Important or Life Threatening)
Splenic rupture
Sickle cell crisis
Allergic reactions including urticaria, rash or anaphylaxis

Indications (Cancer Patients)

To reduce incidence of febrile neutropenia after myelosuppressive chemotherapy

Therapy Monitoring

Recommended only with regard to patient's hematologic status and ability to tolerate myelosuppressive chemotherapy

Notes

1. The manufacturer does not recommend concurrent use of pegfilgrastim with myelosuppressive chemotherapy or radiation therapy
2. Patients must be instructed to report abdominal or shoulder tip pain, prompting evaluation for splenomegaly or splenic rupture
3. Patients must be instructed to report respiratory distress, prompting evaluation for ARDS
4. Use with caution in patients with sickle cell disease; sickle cell crises have been reported following therapy
5. Safety has not been established in patients with CML or MDS, in those receiving chemotherapy associated with delayed myelosuppression, or in patients receiving mitomycin C or myelosuppressive doses of antimetabolites such as 5-fluorouracil
6. Pegylated G-CSF is contraindicated in patients with known hypersensitivity to *E. coli*-derived proteins, pegfilgrastim, filgrastim, or any other component of the formulation[22]

REGIMEN

SARGRAMOSTIM, GM-CSF (LEUKINE®)

Following chemotherapy in AML (adults)[23]*:*
Sargramostim 250 μg/m²/day intravenously over 4 hours until ANC >1500/mm³ for 3 consecutive days or a maximum of 42 days is reached

Notes:
1. Start therapy on day 11 of cycle or 4 days after completion of induction chemotherapy if the bone marrow on day 10 is hypoblastic with <5% blasts
2. This regimen may be repeated if a second cycle of induction chemotherapy is needed
3. Discontinue immediately if leukemia re-grows

Mobilization of peripheral blood progenitor cells (PBPCs)[24]*:*
Sargramostim 250 μg/m²/day intravenously over 24 hours or subcutaneously once daily throughout the entire course of PBPC collection

Following transplantation of autologous PBPCs: **Sargramostim** 250 μg/m²/day intravenously over 24 hours or subcutaneously once daily beginning immediately after the infusion of PBPCs and continuing until an ANC >1500 cells/mm³ for 3 consecutive days is attained

Myeloid reconstitution after autologous or allogeneic BMT:
Sargramostim 250 μg/m²/day as a 2-hour intravenous infusion beginning 2–4 hours after the marrow infusion and ≥24 hours after the last dose of chemotherapy or radiation therapy. Patients should not receive sargramostim until the post-marrow infusion ANC is <500 cells/mm³. Continue therapy until ANC >1500 cell/mm³ for 3 consecutive days

Notes:
1. If severe adverse reaction occurs, reduce dose by 50% or temporarily discontinue the dose until the reaction abates
2. If blast cells appear or progression of the underlying disease occurs, discontinue treatment immediately
3. Interrupt or reduce the dose by half if ANC is >20,000 cells/mm³

BMT failure or engraftment delay:
Sargramostim 250 μg/m²/day intravenously as a 2-hour infusion for 14 days

Notes:
1. After 7 days off therapy if engraftment has not occurred, repeat **sargramostim** 250 μg/m²/day intravenously as a 2-hour infusion for 14 days
2. After another 7 days off therapy if engraftment still has not occurred, administer **sargramostim** 500 μg/m²/day as a 2-hour infusion for 14 days. If there is still no improvement, it is unlikely that further dose escalation will be beneficial

Dosing:
1. If a severe adverse reaction occurs, temporarily reduce the dose by 50% or temporarily discontinue the dose until reaction abates
2. Doses recommended are for adult patients
3. Obese patients should be dosed on actual body weight, even in morbidly obese patients
4. Do not reduce doses in elderly

Sargramostim (Leukine®) is available in the United States in vials containing 250 μg (powder) or 500 μg/mL (solution) per vial

Efficacy

1. After AML induction chemotherapy, GM-CSF significantly shortened the duration of neutropenia (ANC < 500/mm³ by 4 days, ANC < 1000/mm³ by 7 days) and decreased incidence of grade IV/V infection (10% versus 36%) and death from infection (6% versus 15%)[23]
2. PBPC collections from patients treated with GM-CSF were significantly higher (11.41×10^4 CFU-GM/kg versus 0.96×10^4/kg) [24]

Indications (Cancer Patients)

1. Following induction chemotherapy in AML
2. Mobilization of PBPCs for collection and myeloid reconstitution after autologous PBPC transplantation
3. Myeloid reconstitution after autologous or allogeneic BMT
4. BMT failure or engraftment delays

Toxicity

>10% of Patients

Hypotension*	Tachycardia*
Flushing*	Syncope*
Peripheral edema (11%)	Dyspnea (28%)
Mucositis	Stomatitis
Diarrhea (52–89%)	Rash
Alopecia	Polydypsia
Headache (26%)	Myalgia (18%)
Arthralgia (21%)	Bone pain
↑ Serum creatinine (14%)	
Local reactions at injection site (~50%)	

*First-dose effects

1–10% of Patients

Chest pain	Headache
Nausea	Vomiting
Leukcocytosis	Thrombocytopenia
Weakness	Pleural effusion (1%)
Capillary leak syndrome	
Supraventricular arrhythmias	
Pericardial effusion (4%)	

<1% of Patients (Important or Life-Threatening)

Pericarditis	Anaphylaxis
Thrombophlebitis	Thrombosis
Other arrhythmias	

Therapy Monitoring

CBC with differential twice weekly during therapy. Interrupt therapy or reduce dose by half for excessive leukocytosis as defined by manufacturer: ANC >20,000 cells/mm^3 or WBC >50,000 cells/mm^3

Notes[24]

1. Use with caution in patients with:
   - Preexisting cardiac problems
   - Hypoxia
   - Fluid retention
   - Pulmonary infiltrates of CHF
   - Renal or hepatic impairment
   - Rapid increase in peripheral blood counts
2. Do not use in patients with >10% leukemic myeloid blasts in the bone marrow or peripheral blood
3. Discontinue GM-CSF immediately if blast cells appear after bone marrow infusion
4. Contraindications:
   - Patients with known hypersensitivity to GM-CSF, yeast-derived products, or any component of the formulation
   - Simultaneous administration with cytotoxic chemotherapy or radiation therapy
   - Administration 24 hours preceding or following chemotherapy or radiation therapy[24]

References

1. Ozer H et al. JCO 2000;18(20):3558–3585
2. Schiller JH et al. NEJM 2002;346:92–98
3. Pujol JL et al. J Natl Cancer Inst. 2001;93:300–308
4. von Pawel J et al. JCO 1999;17:658–667
5. LeChevalier T et al. JCO 1994;12:360–367
6. Fisher B et al. JCO 1997;15:1858–1869
7. French Adjuvant Study Group. JCO 2001;19:602–611
8. Forastiere AA et al. JCO 1992;10:1245–1251
9. Saltz LB et al. NEJM 2000;343:905–914
10. Douillard JY et al. Lancet 2000;355:1041–1047
11. Sanofi-Synthelabo Inc. Eloxatin package insert. New York: 2002 Aug
12. Bjorkholm M et al. Blood 1999;94:599a
13. Cannellos GP et al. NEJM 1992;327:1478–1484
14. Oken MM et al. Cancer 1997;79:1561–1567
15. Keating MJ et al. Blood 1989;74:19–25
16. vonder Maase H et al. JCO 2000;17:3068–3077
17. Perry MC, ed. The Chemotherapy Source Book, 3rd ed. Philadelphia: Lippincott Williams & Wilkins; 2001:907
18. Amgen, Inc. Neupogen package insert. Thousand Oaks, CA: 2002 May
19. Weaver CH et al. JCO 2000;18:43–53
20. Nademanee A et al. JCO 1994;12:2176–2186
21. Green MD et al. Ann Oncol 2003;14: 29–35
22. Amgen, Inc. Neulasta package insert. Thousand Oaks, CA: 2002 Jan
23. Rowe JM et al. Blood 1995;86(2):1773–1778
24. Berlex Laboratories, Inc. Leukine package insert. Richmond, CA: 2002 June
25. Crawford J et al. NEJM 1991;325:164–170

Chemotherapy-Induced Anemia

Epidemiology

Incidence rates of 50–60% for chemotherapy-induced anemia have been reported in retrospective reviews of patients with nonmyeloid malignancies who were receiving myelosuppressive chemotherapy and who have required RBC transfusion during therapy[1]

Cancer	% Anemia Cases[2]
Breast cancer	22
Lung cancer	17
Non-Hodgkin lymphoma	15
Ovarian cancer	9
Multiple myeloma	8
Colorectal cancer	6

NCI Common Toxicity Criteria

Grade	Hemoglobin
0	Normal
1	10.0 g/dL–<Lower limit of normal
2	8.0–<10.0 g/dL
3	6.5–8.0 g/dL
4	<6.5 g/dL

WHO Toxicity Criteria

Grade	Hemoglobin
0	Normal
1	10.0–Lower limit of normal
2	8.0–9.9 g/dL
3	6.5–7.9 g/dL
4	<6.5 g/dL

Preparations

1. Epoetin alfa
2. Darbepoetin (Aranesp)

Treatment Overview

1. Baseline and periodic monitoring of iron, total iron-bind capacity, transferring saturation, and ferritin levels is recommended
2. Iron supplementation (usual oral dosing of 325 mg 2–3 times/day) should be instituted as necessary to provide for increased requirements during therapy
3. Blood pressure in patients treated with epoietin (EPO) therapy should be carefully monitored, particularly in patients with a history of hypertension or cardiovascular disease
4. Increases in dosage should not be made more frequently than once a month
5. The possibility that epoetin alfa can act as a growth factor for any tumor type, particularly myeloid malignancies, cannot be excluded[4–6]
6. Monitor CBC with differential and serum chemistries according to treatment routine
7. Pure red blood cell aplasia (PRCA) has been reported in a limited number of patients. If patient shows evidence of PRCA, contact Amgen/Ortho Biotech Products, L.P. (US Amgen Medical Information 1-800-772-6436)
8. There have been rare reports of potentially serious allergic reactions
9. Intravenous iron optimizes EPO response as manifested by a greater percentage of patients with hemoglobin response (68% versus 36%), a significantly greater mean hemoglobin response ($P <.02$), and increases in overall quality of life including energy and activity level[12]
10. Contraindications to EPO therapy are uncontrolled hypertension and known hypersensitivity to mammalian cell-derived products and albumin (human)[4,5]
11. Increased incidence of thrombotic events reported in patients treated with erythropoietic agents

REGIMEN

EPOETIN ALFA (PROCRIT)

In adult cancer patients on chemotherapy, initiate therapy when Hgb ≤ 10 g/dL, or <12 g/dL if symptomatic, with a goal of maintaining a target Hgb not to exceed 12 g/dL[4–6,8]

Cancer patients receiving myelosuppressive chemotherapy:
Epoetin alfa 40,000 units subcutaneously once weekly*

Notes:

1. Escalate dose to 60,000 units subcutaneously once weekly[6,9] if the patient has not had a reduction in transfusion requirements or if the Hgb rise is <1 g/dL
2. Hold dose if Hgb > 13 g/dL; resume at 25% dose reduction when Hgb ≤ 12 g/dL[4,6]

Alternative dosing schedule:
Epoetin alfa 150 units/kg as a subcutaneous injection 3 times per week

Notes:

1. Escalate dose to 300 units/kg subcutaneously 3 times per week after a minimum of 4 weeks if the patient has not had a reduction in transfusion requirements or if the Hgb rise is not satisfactory
2. If there has been no response at a dose of 300 units/kg subcutaneously 3 times per week after an additional 4–8 weeks, discontinue therapy[4,6]
3. Hold dose if Hgb > 13 g/dL; resume at 25% dose reduction when Hgb ≤ 12 g/dL[4,6]

*This schedule is more convenient and more practical

Anemia of chronic kidney disease (CKD) in adults:
Epoetin alfa 50–100 units/kg subcutaneously or intravenously 3 times/week
Reduce dose by 25% when Hgb:

- Approaches 12 g/dL
- Increases >1 g/dL in any 2-week period

Increase dose by 25% when Hgb:

- Does not ↑ by 2 g/dL after 8 weeks of therapy
- Is below suggested target range (10–12 g/dL)

Maximum epoetin alfa dose: 300 units/kg 3 times per week

Epoetin alfa (Procrit) is available in the United States in vials containing 2000, 3000, 4000, 10,000, and 40,000 units/vial

Efficacy

1. Clinical studies have demonstrated a reduction in RBC transfusion requirements (25% versus 40%) in chemotherapy patients receiving epoetin alfa, as well as significant differences in quality of life scales including energy level and ability to do daily activities[13]
2. In CKD studies, 95% of patients had a clinically significant rise in Hgb and virtually all patients were transfusion-independent by 2 months

Indications

1. Anemia from chemotherapy in patients with nonmyeloid malignancies
2. Anemia of CKD[4,5]
3. Other nononcologic indications include zidovudine-related anemia in HIV patients and reduction of allogeneic blood transfusion in surgery patients
4. In addition to the FDA-approved indications, ASCO/ASH 2002 guidelines recognizes EPO use in low-risk myelodysplasia patients with a low (<200 mU/L) endogenous erythropoietin level.[6] Use in patients with multiple myeloma, NHL, or CLL should be considered only if chemotherapy and/or corticosteroids treatment fail to produce a rise in Hgb[6]

Toxicity

>10% of Patients

Hypertension	Headache
Fatigue	Fever

1–10% of Patients

Arthralgia	Nausea
Chest pain	Polycythemia
Clotted access	Seizures
Diarrhea	Vomiting
Dizziness	Weakness
Edema	

<1% of Patients (Important or life-threatening)

CVA/TIA
Myocardial infarction

Therapy Monitoring

1. *Until maintenance dose is established:* Monitor Hgb twice weekly
2. *After any dose adjustment:* Monitor Hgb twice weekly for 2–6 weeks
3. *After maintenance dose is established:* Monitor Hgb at regular intervals (≈2–4 times/month)

REGIMEN

DARBEPOETIN (ARANESP)

In adult cancer patients on chemotherapy, initiate therapy when Hgb ≤ 10 g/dL, or <12 g/dL if symptomatic with a goal of maintaining a target Hgb not to exceed 12 g/dL[4–6,8]

Cancer patients receiving myelosuppressive chemotherapy:
Darbepoetin 2.25 μg/kg subcutaneously every week with dose adjusted to achieve target Hgb, *or*
Darbepoetin 200 μg subcutaneously every 2 weeks[10]
Notes:
1. If Hgb rises <1 g/dL after 6 weeks of therapy, increase dose to 4.5 μg/kg/week
2. If Hgb increases >1 g/dL in a 2-week period or Hgb exceeds 11 g/dL, reduce dose by 40%
3. If Hgb >13 g/dL hold dose until Hgb ≤ 12g/dL, then reinitiate at 40% dose reduction[5]

For anemia of chronic kidney disease in adult:
Darbepoetin Initial dosage 0.45 mcg/kg subcutaneously or intravenously weekly

Conversion from Epoetin alfa to Darbepoetin[5]

Epoetin alfa (units/wk)	Darbepoetin (μg/wk)
<1500	6.25
1500–2499	6.25
<2500	6.25
2500–4999	12.5
5000–10,999	25
11,000–17,999	40
18,000–33,999	60
34,000–89,999	100
>90,000	200

Darbepoetin (Aranesp) is available in the United States in vials or prefilled syringes containing 25, 40, 60, 100, 150, 200, 300, and 500 μg per vial or syringe

Therapy Monitoring

1. *Until maintenance dose established or after any dose adjustment:* Monitor weekly Hgb for 4 weeks
2. *After Hgb stabilized:* Monitor Hgb at regular intervals (≃2–4 times monthly)

Indications

1. Anemia from chemotherapy in patients with nonmyeloid malignancies
2. Anemia of CKD[4,5]

Efficacy

Darbepoetin significantly reduced RBC transfusion requirements (27% versus 52%); treated patients required fewer units of blood (0.67 versus 1.92) and had better improvement in FACT-Fatigue scores (56% versus 44%) than patients receiving placebo for chemotherapy-associated anemia[14]

Toxicity

>10% of Patients

Hypertension	Headache
Fatigue	Fever

1–10% of Patients

Chest pain	Edema
Nausea	Vomiting
Diarrhea	Polycythemia
Clotted access	Arthralgia
Dizziness	Seizures
Weakness	

<1% of Patients (Important or Life-Threatening)

CVA/TIA
Myocardial infarction

References

1. Groopman JE, Itri LM. J Natl Cancer Inst 1999;91(19):1616–1634
2. Tchekmedyian NS. Oncology 2002;16(suppl 9): 17–24
3. Perry MC, ed. The Chemotherapy Source Book, 3rd ed. Philadelphia: Lippincott Williams & Wilkins, 2001:906
4. Ortho Biotech Products, L.P. Procrit package insert. Raritan (NJ): 2004 Jun
5. Amgen, Inc. Aranesp package insert. Thousand Oaks, CA: 2006 Mar
6. Rizzo JD et al. JCO 2002;20(19):4083–4107
7. MacDougall IC et. al. J Am Soc Nephrol 1999;10:2392–2395
8. Crawford J et al. Cancer 2002;95:888–895
9. Gabrilove JL et. al. JCO 2001;19:2875–2882
10. Jumbe N et. al. Oncology 2002;16(10 suppl 1): 45–55
11. Data on file. Ortho Biologics, Inc
12. Auerbach M et al. JCO 2004;22(7):1301–1307
13. Littlewood TJ et al JCO 2001;19(11):2865–2874
14. Vansteenkiste J et al J Natl Cancer Inst 2002;94(16):1211–1220

Chemotherapy-Induced Thrombocytopenia

Epidemiology

Among patients receiving dose-intensive myelosuppressive chemotherapy for solid tumors or lymphoma, 20–25% have developed clinically significant platelet counts with nadirs $<50,000/mm^3$; 10–15% of these patients experienced nadir counts of $20,000/mm^3$ or less[1]

NCI Common Toxicity Criteria

Grade	Platelet Count
0	Normal
1	$75,000/mm^3$– <Lower limits of normal
2	$\geq 50,000$–$<75,000/mm^3$
3	$\geq 10,000$–$<50,000/mm^3$
4	$<10,000/mm^3$

WHO Toxicity Criteria

Grade	Platelet Count
0	Normal
1	75,000–normal
2	$50,000$–$74,900/mm^3$
3	$25,000$–$49,900/mm^3$
4	$<25,000/mm^3$

Preparations

Oprelvekin

REGIMEN

rhIL-11 (OPRELVEKIN, NEUMEGA®)

Cancer patients receiving myelosuppressive chemotherapy:

rhIL-11 50 μg/kg/day subcutaneously daily, beginning 6–24 hours after completion of chemotherapy until platelet count is ≥ 50,000/mm³ or for a maximum of 21 days

Notes:

1. Do not round dose
2. Administer rhIL-11 for a maximum of 21 days for up to 6 cycles
3. Discontinue rhIL-11 at least 2 days before next chemotherapy
4. Administer subcutaneously in the abdomen, thigh, hip, or upper arm
5. In renal impairment (creatinine clearance <30 mL/min), reduce dose to 25 μg/kg/day[3]
6. Recommended dose in obese adults does not differ from the standard recommended adult dose of 50 μg/kg/day, which is based on actual body weight. The maximum patient weight treated with rhIL-11 in clinical trials was 147 kg[4]

rhIL-11 is available in the United States in single-dose vials containing 5 mg rhIL-11 per vial

Efficacy

1. In a randomized placebo-controlled trial of 93 patients with various nonmyeloid malignancies who had recovered from an episode of severe chemotherapy-induced thrombocytopenia (platelets ≤20,000/mm³), the number of patients who required platelet transfusions was significantly lower for patients receiving rhIL-11 (50 μg/kg/day) than for the placebo group (70% versus 96%, $P < .05$)[5]
2. At present, rhIL-11 therapy should be reserved for patients experiencing therapy-limiting thrombocytopenia; not recommended for routine use[3]
3. Platelet increase is seen within 5–9 days

Therapy Monitoring

1. *Platelet counts:* Monitor during the time of the expected nadir and until adequate recovery has occurred. Discontinue oprelvekin when post-nadir platelet counts are ≥50,000/mm³[3]
2. *Fluid and electrolytes:* Monitor especially in patients receiving chronic diuretic therapy

Notes

1. Not indicated after myeloablative chemotherapy. Effectiveness not demonstrated in phase II study
2. *Severe or fatal adverse reaction reported postmarketing in BMT setting:* Fluid retention or overload (facial edema, pulmonary edema), capillary leak syndrome, pleural and pericardial effusion, papilledema and renal failure
3. Safety and efficacy has also not been established in the following settings:
   - Agents that cause delayed myelosuppression such as nitrosoureas or mitomycin-C
   - Regimens of > 5 days' duration
   - Chronic administration
4. Use with caution in patients who have a history of atrial arrhythmia or CHF or whose clinical condition can be exacerbated by fluid retention
5. Patients with a history of stroke or TIA may be at increased risk for these events[3]
6. rhIL-11 is contraindicated in patients with a history of hypersensitivity to oprelvekin or any component of the formulation

References

1. Dutcher JP et al. Cancer 1984;53:557–562
2. Perry MC, ed. The Chemotherapy Source Book, 3rd ed. Philadelphia: Lippincott Williams & Wilkins, 2001:907
3. Genetics Institute. Oprelvekin package insert. Cambridge, MA: June 2004
4. Personal correspondence, Genetics Institute. Cambridge, MA: Oct 2003
5. Tepler I et al. Blood 1996;87:3607–3614

Indications

Prevention of severe thrombocytopenia (≤20,000/mm³) and the reduction of the need for platelet transfusion in adult patients who are at high risk for thrombocytopenia after myelosuppressive chemotherapy for nonmyeloid malignancies[3]

Toxicity[b]

Boxed warning: Allergic or hypersensitivity reactions, including anaphylaxis, have been reported in the postmarketing setting

>10% of Patients

Anemia[a]	Edema[b] (59%)
Neutropenic fever (48%)	Dyspnea[b] (48%)
Headache (41%)	Rhinitis (42%)
Nausea/vomiting (77%)	Dizziness (38%)
Fever (36%)	Mucositis (43%)
Diarrhea (43%)	Insomnia (33%)
Increased cough (29%)	Pharyngitis (25%)
Rash (25%)	Tachycardia[b] (20%)
Vasodilatation (19%)	Conjunctival injection[b] (19%)
Palpitations[b] (14%)	Atrial fibrillation/flutter[b] (12%)
Oral moniliasis[b] (14%)	Pleural effusion[b] (10%)
Syncope (13%)	Asthenia[b] (14%)

[a]Probably a dilutional phenomena; appears within 3–5 days of initiation of therapy and resolves in about 1 week after cessation of rhIL-11

[b]Occurred in significantly more rhIL-11-treated patients than placebo-treated patients

1–10% of Patients

Papilledema (2%)
Antibody development (1%)
Stroke (unknown rate)

Note: In clinical studies, most adverse events resolved within days of rhIL-11 discontinuation

Sudden death (2 patients): Relation to rhIL-11 uncertain

44. Indications for Bisphosphonates in the Hematology-Oncology Setting

Reem A. Shalabi, PharmD, BCOP, David R. Kohler, PharmD, and James N. Frame, MD

Primary Indications in Cancer Patients

1. To protect bone from new metastatic lesions
2. To treat hypercalcemia of malignancy
3. To prevent treatment-related bone demineralization, osteolysis, and pathologic fractures
4. To treat osteolytic lesions, decrease the incidence of pathologic fractures, prevent skeletal deformities, and prevent and decrease the severity of pain

Intravenous versus Oral Bisphosponates

Intravenous

1. Much more effective than oral agents at reversing hypercalcemia and relieving bone pain, particularly in patients with breast cancer and multiple myeloma
2. Can overcome disadvantages associated with oral agents, including poor absorption from the GI tract (<3% oral bioavailability); have a lower incidence of adverse GI events
3. Require clinic/hospital administration

Oral

1. Convenient
2. Absorption can be impaired by food and beverages other than water
3. Associated with greater incidence of upper GI toxicity than with intravenous administration, including dysphagia; esophagitis; and esophageal, gastric, or duodenal erosion; ulceration; and perforation

Body JJ et al. JCO 1998;16:3890–3899
Riccardi A et al. Tumori 2003;89:223–236

Hypocalcemic Effects

Bisphosphonate	Median Time to Normocalcemia	Duration of Normocalcemia	% Achieving Normocalcemia
Zoledronic acid[a]	4 days	32 days	87
Pamidronate[b,c]	4 days	28 days	70–100
Clodronate[c]	3 days	14 days	80
Alendronate[d]	4 days	15 days	74

[a]Major P et al. JCO 2001;19:558–567
[b]Body JJ, Dumon JC. Ann Oncol 1994;5:359–363
[c]Purohit OP et al. Br J Cancer 1995;72:1289–1293
[d]Nussbaum SR et al. JCO 1993;11:1618–23

Adapted from Riccardi A et al. Tumori 2003;89:223–236; and Body J-J. Semin Oncol 2001;28(4 suppl 11):49–53

References

1. Ibrahim A et al. Clin Cancer Res 2003;9:2394–2399
2. Zometa® (zoledronic acid) Injection product label, November 2004. Novartis Pharmaceuticals Corporation; East Hanover, NJ

REGIMENS

Key to abbreviations and symbols: 0.9% NS = 0.9% NaCl injection; 0.45% NS = 0.45% NaCl injection; D5W = 5% dextrose injection; ASCO, American Society of Clinical Oncology; AUC, area under the plasma concentration versus time curve; SCr, serum creatinine; CrCl, creatinine clearance

ZOLEDRONIC ACID [ZOMETA®]

Oncology-Related Indication(s)	Usual Dosages	Dose Adjustments Baseline CrCl ≤60 mL/min*
Multiple myeloma with lytic bone lesions on plain radiographs Metastatic breast cancer with abnormal bone radiographs ± pain	**Zoledronic acid** 4 mg[a] intravenously in 100 mL 0.9% NS or D5W over at least 15 minutes every3–4 weeks [a]Recommended for patients with CrCl > 60 mL/min	Baseline CrCl: 50–60 mL/min → Recommended Dose: 3.5 mg Baseline CrCl: 40–49 mL/min → Recommended Dose: 3.3 mg Baseline CrCl: 30–39 mL/min → Recommended Dose: 3 mg *Doses are calculated to produce an AUC (0.6 mg·hour/L) similar to that achieved in patients with CrCl 2= 75 mL/min
Bone metastases from solid tumors[1,2]	Supplementation for myeloma and bone metastases from solid tumors: **Calcium** 500 mg/day orally, *plus* **Vitamin D** 400 International units/day orally	Baseline SCr: Within normal limits; SCr Increase: ≥0.5 mg/dL Baseline SCr: Abnormal; SCr Increase: ≥1 mg/dL Action (both): Withhold zoledronic acid until SCr decreases to within 10% of baseline, then resume with the same dose given previously
Hypercalcemia of malignancy: Serum Ca^{2+} ≥ 12 mg/dL (≥3 mmol/L)[1]	**Zoledronic acid** 4 mg intravenously in 100 mL 0.9% NS or D5W over at least 15 minutes every 3–4 weeks	1. Initiate treatment only after (1) adequate hydration with 0.9% NS, (2) adequate urine output, and (3) with doses appropriate for a patient's creatinine clearance (see Dose Adjustments above) 2. Encourage ambulatory patients to maintain hydration orally 3. If hypercalcemia persists or recurs, there should be ≥7 days between consecutive treatments *Note:* Patients with SCr ≥ 4.5 mg/dL (≥400 μmol/L) have been excluded from trials of hypercalcemia of malignancy

Toxicity

>10%	Fever (30–40%), nausea/vomiting (29%), constipation (26.7%), hypomagnesemia (10.5%), hypotension (10.5%)
1–10%	Bone/back pain (10%), flulike syndrome, injection site reaction, dyspepsia, hypocalcemia, hypophosphatemia, hypermagnesemia, increased serum creatinine
<1%	Rash, pruritus, increased liver transaminases, chest pain, ocular inflammation, uveitis, iritis, scleritis, episcleritis, conjunctivitis

References

1. Ibrahim A et al. Clin Cancer Res 2003;9:2394–2399
2. Zometa® (zoledronic acid) Injection product label, November 2004. Novartis Pharmaceuticals Corporation; East Hanover, NJ

PAMIDRONATE DISODIUM [AREDIA®]

Oncology-Related Indication(s)	Usual Dosages	Adjustments for Serum Creatinine		
Multiple myeloma with osteolytic bone lesions on plain radiographs[1,2]	**Pamidronate** 90 mg intravenously in 250–500 mL 0.9% NS, 0.45% NS, or D5W, over 1–4 hours, every 3–4 weeks	In patients with Bence-Jones proteinuria and dehydration, ensure adequate hydration with 0.9% NS before administering pamidronate		
Metastatic breast cancer with abnormal bone radiographs ± pain[1,2]		**Baseline**	**Re-treatment**	**Action**
		Normal SCr	SCr increased ≥0.5 mg/dL (≥44 μmol/L)	Hold until SCr is within 10% of baseline[b]
		Abnormal SCr	SCr increased ≥1.0 mg/dL (≥88 μmol/L)	Hold until SCr is within 10% of baseline[b]
Steroid-induced osteoporosis[a3,4]	**Pamidronate** 60 mg intravenously in 250 mL 0.9% NS, 0.45% NS, or D5W over 2 hours every 12 weeks for 48 weeks, *or* **Pamidronate** 150 mg orally, daily for 12–24 months[c]	Pamidronate is available outside the United States in a tablet formulation containing 150 mg of the active drug		

Toxicity

>10%	Nausea/vomiting (27%), injection site reaction (18%), abdominal pain/GI complaints (15%), hypertension (15%), constipation (12.6%), and fever
1–10%	Anemia (6%), tachycardia (6%), hypothyroidism (6%), hypomagnesemia (4.9%), leukopenia (4%), hypophosphatemia (1.9%), hypotension (1.9%), rash (1%), flulike syndrome, bone/back pain, anorexia, hypocalcemia, and fluid overload
<1%	Allergic reaction (dyspnea, angioedema, anaphylaxis), hypokalemia, transient proteinuria, ocular inflammation, uveitis, iritis, scleritis, episcleritis, jaw osteonecrosis

[a]Not an FDA-approved indication
[b]When resuming treatment after a hiatus for renal impairment, administer pamidronate over at least 2 hours at doses not >90 mg and not more frequently than every 4 weeks after renal function returns to baseline
[c]An oral formulation is not available for commercial use in the United States

References

1. ASCO Practice Guidelines. JCO 2000;18:1378–1391
2. Aredia® product label, October 2003. Novartis Pharmaceutical Corporation; East Hanover, NJ
3. Smith MR et al. NEJM 2001;345:948–955
4. Reid IR et al. Lancet 1988;331:143–146

CLODRONATE DISODIUM [BONEFOS™, OSTAC®][a]

<table>
<tr><th>Oncology-Related Indication(s)</th><th>Usual Dosages</th><th>Dose Modification for Renal Impairment</th></tr>
<tr><td>Treatment of hypercalcemia of malignancy[b1]: serum Ca^{2+} ≥12 mg/dL (≥3 mmol/L)[1]</td><td>Clodronate 300 mg/day intravenously in 500 mL 0.9% NS or D5W over 2 hours for up to 5 days,
or
Clodronate 1500 mg single dose intravenously in 500 mL 0.9% NS or D5W over 4 hours</td><td>Treatment with intravenous clodronate may continue for >5 days but should be limited to not exceed 10 days for a single hypercalcemic episode
<table><tr><th>CrCl (mL/min)</th><th>Dose Reduction</th></tr><tr><td>50–80</td><td>25%</td></tr><tr><td>12–50</td><td>25–50%</td></tr><tr><td><12</td><td>50%</td></tr></table></td></tr>
<tr><td>Maintenance treatment after effective IV treatment for hypercalcemia[b2–5]</td><td>Clodronate 1600-mg/day (range: 400–3200 mg) orally, indefinitely
Note: Data from published studies are for 3 months. Treatment likely will continue for longer durations with clodronate or another agent</td><td rowspan="3">Clodronate disodium is available outside the Unites States in:
400-mg capsules
520-mg tablets (higher bioavailability)
800-mg tablets
The oral bioavailability of one 520-mg tablet approximately equals two 400-mg capsules or one 800-mg tablet

Clodronate should be taken with water 1 hour before or 2 hours after eating, drinking, or taking other medications</td></tr>
<tr><td>Multiple myeloma (regression of bone lesions)[b5–7]</td><td>Clodronate 1600–3200 mg/day orally,
or
Clodronate 1040–2080 mg/day orally</td></tr>
<tr><td>Metastatic bone disease[b5,7–13]</td><td>Clodronate 300 mg/day intravenously in 250–500 mL D5W or 0.9% NS over 2–3 hours, for 8–14 consecutive days, followed by:
Clodronate 1040–2080 mg/day orally, indefinitely, or
Clodronate 1600 mg 2 times daily or 1600 mg/day (as a single 1600 mg dose, 800 mg twice daily, or 400 mg 4 times daily) orally, indefinitely
Note: Studies have examined treatment durations of 4–11 weeks. Treatment likely will continue for longer durations with clodronate or another agent</td></tr>
</table>

Toxicity

>10%	Dysgeusia (50%)
1–10%	Bone/back pain, nausea/vomiting, constipation, diarrhea, dyspepsia, abdominal pain, flatulence, abdominal distention, dysphagia, transient proteinuria (IV form)
<1%	Hyperparathyroidism (0.6%), increased serum creatinine, gastritis, gastric ulceration, increase in liver transaminases, ocular inflammation, uveitis, respiratory impairment in aspirin sensitive patients, hypersensitivity (respiratory symptoms), rash, hypocalcemia, hypomagnesemia

[a]Clodronate is not available for commercial use in the United States
[b]Not an FDA-approved indication

References

1. Bonefos™ (disodium clodronate) European SPC. Revised 10 April, 2002
2. Percival RC et al. Br J Cancer 1985;51:665–669
3. Rastad J et al. Acta Med Scand 1987;221:489–494
4. Ziegler R, Scharla SH. Recent Results Cancer Res 1989;116:46–53
5. Clodronic acid. In: Sweetman SC, ed. Martindale, the Complete Drug Reference, 33rd ed. London: Pharmaceutical Press, 2002:751–52
6. Coleman RE. Am J Clin Oncol 2002;25(6 suppl 1):S32–8
7. Diel IJ et al. NEJM 1998;339:357–363
8. Adami S et al. J Urol 1985;134:1152–1154
9. Heidenreich A et al. J Urol 2001;165:136–140
10. Rizzoli R et al. Bone 1996;18:531–537
11. Kanis JA et al. Bone 1996;19:663–667
12. Body J-J et al. JCO 1998;16:3890–3899
13. McCloskey EV et al. Br J Haematol 1998;100:317–325

ALENDRONATE SODIUM [FOSAMAX®]

Oncology-Related Indication(s)	Usual Dosages	Dose Adjustments	
For the prevention[a] and treatment of steroid-induced osteoporosis in men and women receiving a daily dose equivalent to ≥7.5 mg prednisone[1]	**Alendronate** 5 mg orally daily	**Elderly patients**	**No adjustments**
		CrCl ≥ 35 mL/min	No adjustments
Postmenopausal women not receiving estrogen[1]	**Alendronate** 10 mg orally daily	CrCl < 35 mL/min	Do not administer drug
		Alendronate is available as 5-mg and 10-mg tablets	
Hypercalcemia of malignancy[a,b2]: serum Ca^{2+} ≥12 mg/dL (≥3 mmol/L)[1]	**Alendronate** 5, 10, or 15 mg intravenously[b] over 2 hours	Not recommended if CrCl < 35 mL/min	

Toxicity

>10%	Fever (intravenous formulation)
1–10%	Constipation (3.1%), diarrhea (3.1%) headache (2.6%), gastritis/gastric ulceration (1.5%), nausea/vomiting, abdominal pain, flatulence, abdominal distention, dysphagia, hypocalcemia, hypophosphatemia
<1%	Increases in liver transaminases (intravenous formulation), iritis, scleritis, episcleritis

[a]Not an FDA-approved indication
[b]A parenteral formulation is not available for commercial use in the United States

References

1. Fosamax® tablets and oral solution product label, September 2003. Merck & Co., Inc., Whitehouse Station, NJ
2. Nussbaum SR et al. JCO 1993;11:1618–1623

RISEDRONATE SODIUM [ACTONEL®]

Oncology-Related Indication(s)	Usual Dosage	Dosage Adjustments
For the prevention and treatment of steroid-induced osteoporosis in men and women receiving a daily dose equivalent to ≥7.5 mg prednisone	**Risedronate** 5 mg orally daily	**Elderly patients**: **No adjustments** CrCl ≥ 30 mL/min: No adjustments CrCl < 30 mL/min: Do not administer drug Risedronate is available as 5-mg tablets

Toxicity

>10%	Arthralgia (32.8%), bone/back pain (26.1%), headache (18%), nausea/vomiting (10.9%), abdominal pain (11.6%), diarrhea (10.6%)
1–10%	Flulike syndrome (9.8%), rash (7.7%), chest pain (5%), asthenia (4.9%), hypercholesterolemia (4.8%), flatulence (4.6%), gastritis/gastric ulceration (4.1%), conjunctivitis (3.1%), pruritus (3%), abdominal distention, dysphagia
<1%	Iritis, scleritis, episcleritis

Actonel® product label, March 2003. Proctor and Gamble Pharmaceuticals, Cincinnati, OH

Therapy Monitoring[a,b]

Tests	Zoledronic acid[1,2]	Pamidronate[1,3]	Clodronate[1,4,5]	Alendronate[1,6]	Risedronate[1,7]
SCr before single-dose	+	Renal Impairment[c]	—	+	+
SCr before repeated treatments	+		+	+	+
Serum albumin and BUN	Unexplained albuminuria or azotemia | d,e |		—	—	—
CBC with differential	—	+	—	—	—
Calcium	+	—	—	+	+
Phosphorus	+	—	—	—	—
Magnesium	+	—	—	—	—
Hemoglobin and hematocrit	+	—	+	—	—

+, complete the test before drug administration; —, no need to test

[a]Evaluation is recommended before initial and each repeated administration of parenteral bisphosphonates, and at the time of routine repeated visits for patients receiving oral agents (eg, monthly to quarter annually)

[b]Product labeling for some products warns about a potential for fetal harm if pregnant females receive bisphosphonate treatment during gestation

[c]When resuming treatment after a hiatus for renal impairment, administer pamidronate over at least 2 hours, at doses not greater than 90 mg, and at administration frequencies not more often than every 4 weeks after renal function returns to baseline

[d]In patients with multiple myeloma, discontinue bisphosphonate treatment until renal problems resolve in patients with:

- Unexplained albuminuria >500 mg/24 hours, *or*
- Azotemia (an increase in serum Cr ≥0.5 mg/dL (44 μmol/L), or an absolute Cr value >1.4 mg/dL (126 μmol/L), among patients with normal baseline creatinine[1]

Reassess every 3–4 weeks with a 24-hour urine collection for total protein and urine protein electrophoresis

[e]In patients with multiple myeloma for whom pamidronate treatment was withheld for renal dysfunction, reinstitute pamidronate only after renal function returns to baseline, with infusion durations >2 hours and at doses/schedules ≤90 mg every 4 weeks[1]

References

1. Berenson JR. JCO 2002;20:3719–3736
2. Zometa® (zoledronic acid) Injection product label, November 2004. Novartis Pharmaceuticals Corporation; East Hanover, NJ
3. Aredia® product label, October 2003. Novartis Pharmaceutical Corporation; East Hanover, NJ
4. Ostac® (clodronate disodium) tablets and injection product label, 4 June 1998. Boehringer Mannheim Standard; Hoffmann-La Roche Ltd/Ltee, Mississauga, Ontario, Canada
5. Bonefos™ (disodium clodronate) European SPC. Revised, 10 April 2002.
6. Fosamax® (alendronate sodium) capsules & oral solution product label, September 2003. Merck & Co. Inc, Whitehouse Station, NJ
7. Actonel® (risedronate sodium) product label, March 2003. Proctor and Gamble Pharmaceuticals, Cincinnati, OH

Note

Bisphosphonates have been implicated in causing necrotic mandibular and maxillary lesions in patients with malignant diseases (pamidronate and zoledronic acid) or with osteoporosis who had no history of malignancy (alendronate and risedronate). The typical presentation was a non-healing extraction socket or exposed jawbone. Surgical debridement was not completely effective in eradicating necrotic bone and hyperbaric oxygen treatments were not consistently effective in limiting its progression. Viable bone may remain exposed after debridement, and necrosis has progressed in spite of ceasing bisphosphonates treatment. Most patients required surgical removal of the involved bone. Lesion pathogenesis was most consistent with a process that is clinically and radiographically similar to osteoradionecrosis. Most patients developed jaw disease that was not detected by their medical care providers. In each case, the diagnosis was established only after a dental examination. Health care providers are urged to include a complete dental evaluation for all patients with appropriate preventive dentistry before initiating bisphosphonate treatment

Ruggiero SL et al. J Oral Maxillofac Surg 2004;62:527–534

45. Transfusion Therapy

Ashok Nambiar, MD, and Susan Leitman, MD

PRODUCT

WHOLE BLOOD[1,2]

Preparation/Composition

1. Donor blood 450–500 mL containing red blood cells (RBCs), plasma, clotting factors, and anticoagulant
2. Platelets and granulocytes are not functional

Indications

RBC replacement in acute blood loss with pronounced hypovolemia

Administration

Whole blood is given over a maximum of 4 hours through a 170-micron filter or a leukocyte reduction filter

Notes

1. Whole blood is not routinely available and is rarely required in hematology-oncology patients. It is not a source of viable white blood cells (WBCs) or platelets
2. *Shelf life:* 21 days in CPD (citrate-phosphate-dextrose); 35 days in CPDA-1 (citrate-phosphate-dextrose-adenine) preservative

PRODUCT

RED BLOOD CELLS[1–4]

Preparation/Composition

1. RBCs obtained by apheresis collection or prepared from whole blood by centrifugation
2. RBCs collected in CPDA-1 anticoagulant have a hematocrit of 65–80% and a storage volume of 250–300 mL
3. RBC collections from which plasma has been removed and 100 mL of adenine-containing RBC nutrient solution (eg, AS-1) has been added, have a hematocrit of 55–60% and a volume of 300–350 mL

Indications

1. Improve oxygen carrying capacity in anemic patients
2. In most stable, asymptomatic patients, transfusion is initiated if hemoglobin ≤7 g/dL
3. Patients with cardiopulmonary or cerebrovascular disease may be transfused at higher hemoglobin levels[5]

Administration

1. RBCs are administered over a maximum period of 4 hours through a 170-μm leukocyte reduction filter
2. Do not add medications to blood products. 0.9% NaCl injection is the only compatible intravenous solution that may be added to RBCs, if needed to decrease hematocrit

Notes

1. Patients with allergic and febrile nonhemolytic transfusion reactions benefit from premedication with benadryl 25 to 50 mg orally or intravenously and acetaminophen, 650 to 1000 mg orally respectively
2. *Shelf life:* 35 days in CPDA-1; 42 days if stored in additive solutions like AS-1

PRODUCT

WASHED RED BLOOD CELLS[1,2]

Preparation/Composition

Washing RBCs with 1 L saline removes more than 98% of plasma proteins. RBCs are then resuspended in saline at an approximate hematocrit of 75%

Indications

1. Patients with a history of severe or recurrent allergic reactions
2. For patients with paroxysmal nocturnal hemoglobinuria, routine washing of group-specific RBCs is not required
3. Washed RBCs are used in neonates to decrease potassium load in patients with cardiac or renal disease

Administration

Washed RBCs must be transfused within 24 hours

Notes

1. RBCs washed with larger volumes of saline or units collected from IgA-deficient donors are required for patients with severe IgA deficiency
2. *Shelf life:* Washed RBCs have a shelf life of only 24 hours

PRODUCT

LEUKOCYTE-REDUCED RED BLOOD CELLS[1,2]

Preparation/Composition

Contains $<5 \times 10^6$ WBCs per unit. Leukocyte reduction filters remove $> 99.9\%$ of the contaminating leukocytes

Indications

1. In a patient with recurrent febrile non-hemolytic transfusion reactions (FNHTR)
2. To decrease the likelihood of HLA alloimmunization and immune-mediated platelet destruction
3. To decrease the risk of transmission of cytomegalovirus (CMV) infection in high-risk CMV-seronegative patients

Administration

The product is transfused over a maximum period of 4 hours through a 170-μm filter ok?

Notes

1. Pre-storage leukoreduction is preferred over bedside filtration
2. The use of bedside leukoreduction filters has been associated with "hypotensive" reactions and facial flushing
3. *Shelf life:* Depends on the preservative; 35 days for CPDA-1; 42 days for additive solutions such as AS-1

PRODUCT

FROZEN-DEGLYCEROLIZED RED BLOOD CELLS[1,2]

Preparation/Composition

Goal: Remove glycerol in which RBCs are suspended

1. Deglycerolization is achieved by first thawing RBCs and then washing them with saline solutions of decreasing osmolarity to remove the glycerol
2. The final product has few leukocytes and <0.1% of the original plasma

Indications

RBCs are frozen with glycerol as the cryoprotectant to maintain integrity after thawing. Indications for use include:

1. Storing autologous collections
2. Storing units with rare blood types

Administration

Deglycerolized RBCs must be transfused within 24 hours

Notes

1. RBCs washed with larger volumes of saline or units collected from IgA-deficient donors are required for patients with severe IgA deficiency
2. *Shelf life:* Washed RBCs have a shelf life of only 24 hours

PRODUCT

PLATELETS[1,2]

Preparation/Composition

1. *Single-donor apheresis platelets:* Collected from single donors by apheresis. Contain $\geq 3 \times 10^{11}$ platelets in 250–300 mL plasma
2. *Random-donor platelets (RDPs):* Platelet concentrates prepared from units of whole blood. RDPs contain $\geq 5.5 \times 10^{10}$ platelets suspended in 45–60 mL of plasma

Administration

1. When administering RDPs, an adult dose is obtained by pooling 5–6 units of RDP into a single pack
2. Use a standard 170-μm filter or a leukocyte reduction filter, and infuse within 4 hours

Notes

1. Platelets are not routinely recommended for correction of thrombocytopenia in patients with ITP or TTP in the absence of a risk for severe bleeding
2. Washed, irradiated, and leukoreduced platelets have indications similar to those described under RBCs
3. *Platelet increments and HLA-matched platelets*[7]

   Of chronically transfused patients, 20–30% will develop alloimmunization to HLA antigens and will not experience an increment in their platelet count when platelets from randomly selected donors are administered. Platelet count should be obtained 15–60 minutes after transfusion, and the corrected count increments (CCIs; see equation) should be calculated. CCIs should be obtained for two consecutive transfusions. With no clinical explanation such as splenomegaly, fever, or ongoing bleeding to explain the poor increment in the platelet count, patients with poor CCIs are usually found to have an immune-mediated cause for the poor increments. In these patients, platelet cross-matching is carried out to select compatible products. Alternatively, HLA and platelet antibody screening tests are done. If the HLA antibody screen is positive, patients are supported with HLA-matched platelet products. Rarely, the antibodies may be directed against platelet-specific antigens, in which case phenotype-matched platelet donors are recruited. IVIG may offer a short-term benefit, but it does not produced sustained responses; its routine use in alloimmunized patients is not recommended

$$\text{CCI} = \frac{(\text{Post-transfusion platelet count/mm}^3 - \text{pretransfusion platelet count/mm}^3) \times \text{body surface area (m}^2)}{\text{Number of platelets transfused (multiples of }10^{11})}$$

Note: In above formula can instead divide by number of units transfused. A CCI of <5000 to 7500/mm^3 suggests platelet refractoriness

4. *Shelf life:* 5 days. Pooled platelets must be transfused within 4 hours

Indications[6]

1. Actively bleeding patients with thrombocytopenia
2. Actively bleeding patients with congenital or acquired platelet function disorders, regardless of platelet counts
3. Prophylactic treatment when:
   - Platelet counts are <10,000/mm^3 in stable afebrile patients with hematologic disease without underlying coagulopathy
   - Platelet counts are <20,000/mm^3 in patients with active mucosal bleeding or fever
   - Platelet counts are <50,000/mm^3 in patients requiring line placement or minor surgery
   - Platelet counts are <75,000/mm^3 in patients undergoing major surgical procedures
   - Platelet counts are <100,000/mm^3 in patients requiring ophthalmic surgery, or surgical procedures involving the upper airway, brain, or spinal cord

PRODUCT

FRESH FROZEN PLASMA (FFP)[1,2]

Preparation/Composition

Fresh frozen plasma (FFP) (200–250 mL) is

- Obtained by apheresis, *or*
- Prepared by centrifugation of whole blood and frozen within 8 hours of collection

Indications

1. Replacement of coagulation factors in patients with coagulopathy of liver disease, massive transfusion, warfarin overdose, and DIC. The INR should be >1.6 or the PT/PTT must be elevated at least >1.5 times the normal
2. Therapeutic plasma exchange in patients with TTP. Cryo-poor plasma is FFP from which the cryoprecipitate fraction has been removed through cold precipitation. This may be used as the plasma exchange replacement fluid in patients with refractory/relapsing TTP
3. Patients with rare disorders such as isolated factor (V, X, XI) deficiencies or C-1 esterase inhibitor deficiency

Administration

When replacing coagulation factors, a dose of 10–15 mL/kg is recommended, with periodic monitoring of coagulation tests to determine efficacy and appropriate dosing intervals

Notes

1. Vitamin K therapy should be used to correct minimally altered PT/PTT values in patients with liver disease who are not actively bleeding. Similarly, FFP is unnecessary for patients with warfarin overdose in the absence of active bleeding or risk for bleeding from an emergent procedure. Patients with INR <5 are initially managed with cessation of therapy for 48 hours with watchful return of coagulation tests to baseline levels
2. IgA-deficient FFP is indicated for patients with IgA-deficiency
3. *Shelf life:* One year when stored frozen at −18°C or lower; 24 hours when thawed and kept at 1–6°C

PRODUCT

CRYOPRECIPITATE[1,2]

Preparation/Composition

1. Cryoprecipitate is the cold-insoluble precipitate formed when FFP is thawed at 1–6°C
2. Cryoprecipitate contains >150 mg fibrinogen, >80 units factor VIII, as well as 40–70% of the VWF and 20–30% of the factor XIII present in the initial unit of FFP

Indications

1. Fibrinogen replacement during dilutional coagulopathy
2. The hypofibrinogenemia/dysfibrinogenemias of liver disease, DIC, and L-asparaginase therapy
3. Factor XIII deficiency

Administration

Each unit (bag) of cryoprecipitate increases fibrinogen level by 5–10 mg/dL. Eight to ten bags are pooled and infused as a single dose in a 70-kg adult

Notes

1. Cryoprecipitate is no longer used to treat patients with hemophilia A or VWD
2. *Shelf life:* 1 year when kept frozen at −18°C or lower; 6 hours after thawing when kept at 1–6°C; 4 hours after pooling

PRODUCT

GRANULOCYTE TRANSFUSIONS[1,2]

Preparation/Composition

1. Granulocytes collected by leukapheresis from donors stimulated either with steroids or G-CSF plus steroids
2. Product contains $\geq 1 \times 10^{10}$ granulocytes suspended in 200–300 mL plasma

Indications

1. Severely neutropenic patients (ANC $<500/\text{mm}^3$) with bacterial sepsis without improvement despite 48–72 hours of optimum antibiotic therap, provided there is a reasonable expectation of bone marrow recovery
2. Possible role in severely neutropenic patients with serious fungal infection not responding to antifungal therapy
3. Patients with granulocyte function disorders such as chronic granulomatous disease and leukocyte adhesion deficiency with refractory bacterial or fungal infections may also benefit from granulocyte transfusions

Administration

1. Transfusions are given daily until clinical improvement or neutrophil recovery occurs
2. Given the large number of RBCs in the product, the donor should be RBC crossmatch–compatible with the recipient
3. Granulocyte products are routinely irradiated
4. The product is stored at room temperature (outdated in 24 hours) and is preferably infused soon after its collection
5. One hour after transfusion, differential counts must be obtained to document neutrophil increments (usually $0.5–1 \times 10^3/\text{mm}^3$)
6. Do not use leukocyte reduction filters; use standard 170-μm filters

Notes

1. HLA-matched granulocyte donors should be used for HLA-alloimmunized patients
2. CMV-seronegative donors should be selected for CMV-seronegative recipients
3. Severe febrile and pulmonary reactions, especially in HLA alloimmunized patients, may occur. Amphotericin administration should be at least 2–4 hours separated from the granulocyte infusion.
4. *Shelf life:* 24 hours

PRODUCT

IRRADIATED CELLULAR BLOOD PRODUCTS[1,2]

Preparation/Composition

RBCs, platelets, and granulocytes are irradiated with 25 Gy of gamma radiation

Indications

1. All patients that are at risk for transfusion-associated graft-versus-host disease (TA-GVHD) must receive irradiated cellular products. These include patients with:
   - Hematologic malignancy receiving fludarabine-based chemotherapy or intensive chemoradiotherapy or undergoing peripheral blood stem cell and bone marrow transplantations
   - Hodgkin and non-Hodgkin lymphoma
   - Certain solid tumors (neuroblastoma and sarcoma)
   - Congenital severe immunodeficiency
2. Receiving HLA-matched platelets or directed donations from blood relatives
3. Blood products for infants < 4 months are routinely irradiated

Administration

The guidelines for administering irradiated products are similar to those described for the individual products that have not been irradiated

Notes

1. Plasma products such as FFP and cryoprecipitate are not required to be irradiated
2. Leukoreduction does not prevent TA-GVHD and should not be substituted for irradiation
3. *Shelf life:* RBCs must be used within 28 days after they are irradiated or before their original outdate, whichever is earlier. The shelf life of platelets and granulocytes is not affected by irradiation

PRODUCT

RH IMMUNE GLOBULIN (RHIG)[1,2]

Preparation/Composition

High titer IgG, anti-D immunoglobulin derived from pooled human plasma

Indications

Prophylaxis against alloimmunization to Rh(D) antigen in Rh(D)-negative individuals, especially children and women of child bearing age who have been exposed to Rh(D)-positive RBCs via RBC, platelet, or granulocyte transfusions

Administration

1. Rh(D)-negative mothers receive a standard 300 μg dose (IM/IV) of RHIG at 28 weeks antepartum. Another dose, given within 72 hours after delivery of an Rh(D)-positive infant, protects against up to 15 mL of Rh(D)-positive RBCs
2. An IV preparation (WinRho, 300 μg) should be used in thrombocytopenic patients exposed to Rh(D)-positive products

Notes

1. RHIG is also given after miscarriage, termination of pregnancy, amniocentesis, chorionic villous biopsy, or other obstetric manipulations/trauma. The optimum RHIG dosages vary with indication/gestation
2. IV RHIG (50–75 μg/kg) is FDA-approved for use in Rh(D)-positive non-splenectomized patients with ITP. A 1–2 g/dL drop in hemoglobin may occur after therapy; patients should be monitored for hemolysis

PRODUCT

CMV-NEGATIVE CELLULAR BLOOD PRODUCTS[1,2]

Preparation/Composition

1. RBCs, platelets, and granulocytes are collected from CMV-seronegative donors
2. Only 30–50% of donors are CMV-seronegative; hence, this product is frequently in short supply
3. Leukoreduced products are provided when CMV-seronegative products are unavailable

Indications

1. CMV-seronegative patients undergoing myelosuppressive chemotherapy and/or radiation therapy
2. CMV-seronegative, bone marrow/PBSC transplantation candidates, when the donor is CMV-seronegative. For T-cell–depleted transplants, CMV-negative products may be indicated even if the donor is CMV-seropositive
3. CMV-seronegative patients with immunodeficiency disorders
4. CMV-seronegative patients receiving solid organ transplants from CMV-seronegative donors
5. CMV-negative products are recommended for pregnant women and routinely provided for all intrauterine transfusions and transfusions in very low birth weight infants
6. CMV-negative products are not indicated for CMV-seronegative, immunocompetent patients
7. CMV-negative products are not indicated for immunosuppressed patients, if they are CMV-seropositive

Administration

CMV-seronegative products are infused following the same guidelines described earlier for RBCs, platelets, and granulocytes

Notes

1. CMV is a cell-associated virus; hence, plasma products such as FFP and cryoprecipitate are not tested for CMV
2. Blood products that have been leukoreduced with third-generation filters are considered to be equivalent to CMV-negative products; several centers routinely use leukoreduced products in lieu of CMV-negative components
3. *Shelf life:* Not affected by the CMV status of the blood product

TRANSFUSION COMPLICATIONS[8]

ACUTE HEMOLYTIC TRANSFUSION REACTION (AHTR)

General

1. The estimated risk per unit transfused is 1 in 25,000
2. Infusion of ABO-incompatible blood is the leading cause of AHTR. Phlebotomy errors and blood administration errors account for the majority of cases
3. *Immune-mediated AHTR can* result in intravascular or extravascular hemolysis

   Donor RBCs may be lysed by naturally occurring anti-A/anti-B alloantibodies, drug-induced antibodies, or RBC autoantibodies in the recipient plasma

   Recipient RBCs may undergo destruction if incompatible antibodies are present in plasma-containing products such as FFP and platelets, or even in plasma-derived products such as IVIG
4. *Non–immune-mediated* hemolysis may mimic AHTR:

   Donor RBCs may be lysed by the addition of medications/hypotonic solutions to the blood bag, malfunctioning blood warmers, and damage in the extracorporeal circuit

   Recipient RBCs may be lysed by the administration of large amounts of hypotonic replacement fluids
5. Hemolytic transfusion reactions must be distinguished from episodes of hemolysis in patients with G6PD deficiency, hereditary spherocytosis, sickle cell disease, or paroxysmal nocturnal hemoglobinuria

Pathophysiology

1. Antigen–antibody complexes are formed on the surface of RBCs, complement is activated, and RBCs are lysed
2. The C3a and C5a anaphylatoxins, free hemoglobin, TNF-α, IL-1, IL-6, and IL-8 that are liberated mediate the hypotension, bronchospasm, renal ischemia, and activation of the coagulation cascade seen in AHTR

Clinical picture

1. Clinical presentation is more severe in immune-mediated compared with non–immune-mediated hemolysis. In general, the clinical course of intravascular hemolysis is more severe than extravascular hemolysis
2. Severity depends on the volume and rate of infusion of incompatible RBCs and on the nature of the antigen and titers of antibody involved
3. Signs and symptoms include fever, rigors, severe anxiety, vomiting, pain in the chest, abdomen, flank or infusion site, dyspnea, hypotension, hemoglobinuria, and diffuse bleeding

Management

Clinical

1. Stop the transfusion. Replace the infusion set and keep intravenous line open with normal saline
2. Assess cardiopulmonary status and provide support as necessary
3. Notify the blood bank, check the patient's identity with identifiers on the issued blood unit, and return the remaining blood product along with attached labels and infusion set
4. Draw fresh blood samples and send to the blood bank. Send additional samples for CBC, plasma hemoglobin, bilirubin, LDH, haptoglobin, electrolytes, BUN, and creatinine. A delayed urine sample is preferred for hemoglobin testing
5. Achieve brisk diuresis using furosemide 20–40 mg intravenously or dosed as needed to achieve a urine output >100 mL/hour
6. Provide maintenance IV fluid infusion at 3000 mL/m^2/day, paying attention to fluid balance and alkalinization of urine. Deteriorating renal function may require dialysis
7. Monitor for ongoing hemolysis and DIC
8. RBC exchange may be considered if there is severe ongoing hemolysis

Blood bank

1. Clerical check is carried out to verify that all labels on the blood unit match the recipient
2. The post-transfusion plasma sample is visually inspected for hemoglobinemia
3. A direct antiglobulin test (direct Coombs' test) is done on the post-transfusion sample. If positive, the eluate is examined to identify the coating antibody. However, the direct antiglobulin test may be negative if all incompatible RBCs have been hemolyzed
4. Additional testing may include reconfirmation of the ABO and Rh type of the patient (using both pre- and post-transfusion specimens) and of the donor unit. The antibody screen and cross-match may also be repeated to confirm donor–patient compatibility
5. Nonimmune hemolysis must be excluded when the work-up is negative for antibody-mediated RBC destruction

TRANSFUSION COMPLICATIONS

DELAYED HEMOLYTIC TRANSFUSION REACTION (DHTR)

General

1. A newly formed alloantibody or an anamnestic increase in the titer of a previously undetectable antibody results in the destruction of transfused RBCs 3–14 days after a serologically compatible RBC transfusion
2. Patients have typically been previously alloimmunized through transfusion or pregnancy

Pathophysiology

1. Antibodies are commonly directed against the Rh/Kell antigens and rarely fix complement
2. RBC destruction occurs extravascularly with minimal cytokine release

Clinical picture

1. Patients may be asymptomatic or may present with fever, jaundice, or malaise. Decreased hematocrit, reticulocytosis, hyperbilirubinemia, or elevated LDH may be seen on testing
2. In patients with sickle cell disease, DHTR may mimic a painful crisis or present with severe hemolysis
3. Intravascular hemolysis, renal dysfunction, and progression to DIC are rare with DHTR

Management

Clinical

1. Future RBC transfusions must be negative for the antigen against which the patient has made an antibody, even if the antibody is undetectable at the time of transfusion
2. Patients with sickle cell disease who have made RBC antibodies should receive RBC transfusions that are at least partially phenotype-matched

Blood bank

1. A DAT is performed on the post-transfusion sample and any coating antibody identified. The antibody screen is also repeated on this sample

TRANSFUSION COMPLICATIONS

FEBRILE NONHEMOLYTIC TRANSFUSION REACTION (FNHTR)

General

1. FNHTRs are fairly common (0.5%/unit transfused), with higher rates seen in frequently transfused patients and multiparous women
2. Other causes of fever, including bacterial contamination and AHTR must be ruled out

Pathophysiology

1. Antibodies in patient's plasma directed against HLA/platelet/granulocyte antigens form antigen–antibody complexes on the surface of transfused platelets and granulocytes. Less commonly, such antibodies in the donor plasma can complex with corresponding antigens present on recipient cells. Complement activation, with release of complement components and inflammatory cytokines, follows
2. During the storage process, leukocytes can elaborate IL-1, IL-6, IL-8, and TNF-α, which are known to mediate FNHTR. Pre-storage leukoreduction decreases the concentration of inflammatory mediators in the product

Clinical picture

1. Rise in temperature of $\geq 1°C$ or more, typically with shaking chills, occurring during or up to 4 hours after a transfusion
2. In addition to fever, the patient may have chills, rigors, headache, and severe anxiety
3. The severity of the reaction is dose-related. With continued infusion, high fever and debilitating symptoms may develop

Management

Clinical

1. Stop the transfusion, keep the line open with normal saline, perform all clerical checks, and return the remaining product to the blood bank
2. The fever is usually self-limited and responds to antipyretics
3. Control of rigors may require meperedine 25–50 mg intravenously per push
4. Complete the full work-up of AHTR if a hemolytic reaction cannot be ruled out
5. Obtain blood cultures if bacterial contamination is being considered in the differential diagnosis
6. Individuals with FNHTR benefit from premedication with oral acetaminophen 650–1000 mg

Blood bank

1. The returned product should be sent to microbiology laboratory for Gram's stain and culture whenever there is a suspicion of bacterial contamination
2. Other components made from this donation are immediately quarantined
3. Patients with two or more febrile reactions should receive leukoreduced products

TRANSFUSION COMPLICATIONS

ALLERGIC TRANSFUSION REACTION

General

1. Similar to FNHTR, allergic transfusion reaction is fairly common, especially in chronically transfused patients
2. Severe IgA deficiency should be ruled out in patients with anaphylactic reactions
3. Rare cases of anaphylaxis mediated by antibodies to haptoglobin or complement component C4 have been reported in patients with deficiencies of these proteins

Pathophysiology

1. Hypersensitivity to allergens (eg, plasma proteins) or drugs in donor plasma

Clinical picture

1. Symptoms range from mild uncomplicated urticaria to fatal anaphylaxis
2. Mild allergic reactions are very common, limited to localized rash, pruritus, and flushing and do not require detailed work-up
3. Infrequently, patients present with severe bronchospasm, tongue and laryngeal swelling, hypotension, vomiting, diarrhea, and shock

Management

Clinical: For uncomplicated allergic reactions

1. Stop transfusion. Administer diphenhydramine 50 mg intravenously per push or another H_1-blocking antihistamine. If symptoms improve, restart the transfusion
2. If symptoms reappear and progress on restarting the transfusion, stop the transfusion and do not restart
3. For future transfusions, premedicate the patient with diphenhydramine 50 mg intravenously per push or orally or with another H_1-blocking antihistamine, 30–45 minutes before the transfusion
4. For patients with recurrent reactions, consider adding hydrocortisone 50–100 mg, administered intravenously prior to the start of the transfusion
5. For patients with severe reactions to platelets, use volume-reduced or washed platelets; for reactions to RBCs, use saline washed products

Clinical: For anaphylactoid and anaphylactic reactions

1. Stop transfusion; maintain IV access and initiate resuscitation with fluids, vasopressors, bronchodilators, and respiratory support as needed
2. Investigate recipient for severe IgA deficiency
3. If the allergen has not been identified, cellular components for future transfusions must be extensively washed. Adequate preparation of the patient with H_1-blockers and steroids is recommended
4. For patients with severe IgA deficiency, all cellular products must be extensively washed and plasma must be obtained from IgA-deficient donors (see next section)

TRANSFUSION COMPLICATIONS

ALLERGIC TRANSFUSION REACTION: PATIENTS WITH IgA DEFICIENCY[9] [TRANSFUSION STRATEGY FOR PATIENTS WITH IgA DEFICIENCY]

General

1. IgA deficiency (IgAD) affects approximately 1 in 600 people
2. IgA deficiency must be excluded when anaphylactic reactions develop to blood products
3. Newer enzyme immunoassays have replaced passive hemagglutination and passive hemagglutination inhibition assays, used for the detection of anti-IgA antibodies and very low levels of IgA, respectively
4. All patients with IgA deficiency do not have anti-IgA antibodies
6. Individuals lacking anti-IgA antibodies with no history of previous transfusion reactions can be safely transfused with regular blood components
7. Patients with severe IgA deficiency and anti-IgA antibodies are at risk for developing an anaphylactic reaction when receiving blood products containing even small amounts of IgA immunoglobulin

Pathophysiology

1. IgA exists as two subclasses, IgA1 and IgA2; the IgA2 subclass is associated with two allotypic determinants, α2m [1] and α2m [2]
2. Anti-IgA antibodies may be class-specific (anti-IgA), subclass-specific (anti-IgA1 or IgA2) or allotype-specific [anti-IgA2 m (1) or IgA2m (2)]

Clinical picture

1. Patients may present with severe bronchospasm, tongue and laryngeal swelling, hypotension, vomiting, diarrhea, and shock

Management

Clinical: For anaphylactoid and anaphylactic reactions:

1. Stop transfusion; maintain IV access and initiate resuscitation with fluids, vasopressors, bronchodilators, and respiratory support as needed
2. For patients with severe IgA deficiency, all cellular products must be extensively washed, and plasma must be obtained from IgA-deficient donors

Blood bank: Guide to selecting components for patients at risk for IgA-anaphylaxis

RBCs

1. RBC units washed with 1–2 L of sterile normal saline have a 99% reduction in their plasma protein content. For IgA-sensitized individuals, it is recommended that RBCs be washed with higher volumes of saline (2–3 L) for satisfactory removal of IgA
2. Frozen deglycerolized RBCs are essentially free of IgA and are probably as safe as RBCs collected from IgA-deficient donors
3. Freezing of autologous units should be considered for IgA-sensitized individuals who have recurrent reactions with washed RBCs

Platelets

- Platelets can be rendered IgA-deficient by washing them free of the plasma IgA. All hospital blood banks may not provide this service

Fresh frozen plasma and cryoprecipitate

- Plasma-derived components such as FFP and cryoprecipitate should be collected only from IgA-deficient donors

Immunoglobulins and plasma derivatives

- IgA-deficient products, chosen after scrutiny of the manufacturer's product insert and confirmed to contain < 0.05 mg/dL of IgA, can be safely transfused in IgA-sensitized patients

TRANSFUSION COMPLICATIONS

POST-TRANSFUSION PURPURA (PTP)

General

1. PTP is a rare complication, presenting as sudden onset of severe thrombocytopenia 7–10 days after transfusion in a previously transfused or pregnant patient
2. About 200 cases have been reported worldwide

Pathophysiology

1. In > 90% of cases, platelet destruction is mediated by an alloantibody directed against the human platelet specific antigen, HPA-1a
2. Rapid destruction of the autologous HPA-1a–negative platelets by a poorly defined "innocent bystander" mechanism contributes to the thrombocytopenia

Clinical picture

1. Severe unexplained thrombocytopenia developing 7–10 days after transfusion of a blood product should raise the suspicion of PTP
2. Patients may be asymptomatic or may present with purpura, ecchymoses, mucosal bleeding, or life-threatening hemorrhage

Management

Clinical

1. The thrombocytopenia is usually self-limiting and spontaneously resolves in 2–3 weeks
2. Routine platelet transfusions do not improve platelet counts, may in fact be detrimental, and should be avoided if there is time to begin specific treatment
3. For patients with life-threatening hemorrhage, high-dose IVIG is preferred over therapeutic plasma exchange as the first line of therapy, and it leads to the recovery of platelet counts in 3–4 days

Blood bank

1. Platelet antibody studies may show the presence of anti–HPA-1a platelet antibody. Rarely, other specificities have been described
2. Platelet genotyping studies are done to confirm antibody specificities
3. Patients with anti–HPA-1a antibody should receive HPA-1a–negative platelets
3. Leukoreduced platelets from random donors may be successful once IVIG therapy has been initiated
4. RBC requirements are best met by providing washed products

TRANSFUSION COMPLICATIONS

TRANSFUSION-ASSOCIATED CIRCULATORY OVERLOAD

General

1. Circulatory overload occurs in up to 1% of transfusions in elderly patients

Pathophysiology

1. A rapid increase in the intravascular volume in patients with severe chronic anemia or in those with compromised cardiorespiratory or renal function can precipitate acute pulmonary edema

Clinical picture

1. Signs and symptoms are those of congestive heart failure

Management

Clinical

1. The transfusion should be stopped
2. Provide supplemental oxygen, begin IV diuresis, and reassess fluid balance
3. Further transfusions may require more diuresis and slower infusion rates (1 mL/kg/hour)
4. The differential diagnosis includes transfusion-related acute lung injury (TRALI)

Blood bank

1. Blood components may be divided into smaller aliquots
2. Platelet volume can be reduced

TRANSFUSION COMPLICATIONS

TRANSFUSION-ASSOCIATED GRAFT-VERSUS-HOST-DISEASE (TA-GVHD)

General

1. The provision of gamma-irradiated cellular blood components for all patient groups at risk for TA-GVHD effectively prevents this frequently fatal complication of transfusion

Pathophysiology

1. Similar to GVHD seen in the hematopoietic transplant setting, the immunocompetent lymphocytes in the donor unit proliferate in a susceptible (immunodeficient or immunosuppressed) host and launch a destructive immune response against host tissues expressing foreign HLA antigens
2. In rare instances, a directed donation from a family member (donor with a homozygous haplotype) has caused TA-GVHD in an immunocompetent host (recipient heterozygous for the donor haplotype)

Clinical picture

1. Symptoms and signs appear 10–14 days after transfusion
2. Marrow hypoplasia is a distinguishing hallmark of TA-GVHD
3. The fulminant cutaneous, gastrointestinal, and hepatic manifestations of acute GVHD are also seen with TA-GVHD
4. More than 90% of patients have a fatal outcome

Management

Clinical

1. Unlike transplant-associated GVHD, TA-GVHD responds poorly to interventions
2. Responses have been reported to combination therapies involving ATG, cyclosporine, methylprednisolone, anti-CD3 monoclonal antibodies, nafamostat mesylate, and G-CSF
3. Prevention of TA-GVHD is achieved by identifying all groups at risk and by the meticulous attention to irradiation of all cellular components transfused to these patients

Blood bank

1. The blood bank should be notified about all patients at risk for TA-GVHD even before any blood products are ordered
2. All HLA-matched products are irradiated
3. All cellular components from blood relatives are irradiated
4. Microchimerism studies may aid in the diagnosis of TA-GVHD

TRANSFUSION COMPLICATIONS

TRANSFUSION RELATED ACUTE LUNG INJURY (TRALI)[8,10]

General

Estimated incidence: 1 in 5000 transfusions of plasma-containing components

Pathophysiology

1. TRALI results from the transfusion of any plasma containing blood component (RBCs, platelets, FFP, cryoprecipitate, or granulocytes) or plasma-derivative (IVIG)
2. Antibodies (HLA class I/II, antineutrophil) in donor plasma react with patient's WBCs or antibodies in the recipient plasma form complexes with donor leukocytes
3. Antigen–antibody complex formation and complement activation lead to aggregation, margination and sequestration of neutrophils in the pulmonary microvasculature
4. Tissue-disruptive enzymes and free radicals released from neutrophils damage the vascular endothelium, and fluid extravasates into the interstitium and alveolar spaces
5. Alternatively, a lipid-priming agent in stored blood, acting in concert with a "priming" lung injury that preceded the transfusion, has been proposed in the two-hit hypothesis for the development of TRALI

Clinical picture

1. Signs and symptoms occur within 1–6 hours of the transfusion
2. Fever and mild-to-moderate hypotension are frequently seen. Less frequently, hypertension is present
3. Respiratory distress can rapidly progress to severe hypoxemia and respiratory failure
4. *Chest x-rays:* Bilateral extensive white-out pattern or more patchy changes
5. The pulmonary edema is noncardiogenic in origin. Central venous and pulmonary capillary wedge pressures are normal
6. A transient drop in the WBC count has also been described

Management

Clinical

1. Achieve optimum oxygenation with rapid and intensive respiratory support
2. Exclude AHTR, anaphylaxis, bacterial contamination, and fluid overload
3. Most patients improve clinically and radiologically in 72–96 hours
4. Blood products may continue to be used cautiously. Leukoreduction of all cellular components might be beneficial where TRALI is mediated by anti-HLA/antineutrophil antibody in the patient

Blood bank

1. Other blood components prepared from this donor are quarantined, and the blood donor center is notified
2. Donor and patient are worked up for anti-HLA and antineutrophil antibodies. The patient is typed for HLA class I and II, and neutrophil antigens, to confirm the specificity of the antibody
3. Antibody-positive donors implicated in fatal TRALI are permanently deferred

TRANSFUSION COMPLICATIONS

BACTERIAL CONTAMINATION

General

1. Until recently, an important cause of transfusion-related mortality
2. Mandatory bacterial testing of platelets in the United States, beginning March 2004, has significantly reduced this risk
3. *Risk of bacterial contamination of platelet unit:* Approximately 1 in 5000 based on 2004–2005 data
4. RBC units have a much lower risk of bacterial contamination

Pathophysiology

1. Bacteria enter donor unit during collection process/component preparation
2. Components (eg, platelets) stored at room temperature are commonly associated with gram-positive organisms such as *Staphylococcus*
3. Components (eg, RBCs) stored at 4°C are associated with gram-negative organisms, such as *Enterobacter, Yersinia, Pseudomonas,* and *Serratia*

Clinical picture

1. High fever, chills, rigors, dyspnea, hypotension, and shock may develop rapidly
2. Milder presentations, particularly in a previously febrile patient, may go unrecognized

Management

Clinical

1. Stop the transfusion and resuscitate aggressively
2. Send the remaining product for bacterial culture; send patient samples for blood cultures
3. Commence broad-spectrum antibiotics to cover both gram-positive and gram-negative organisms; modify therapy based on culture results

Blood bank

1. The implicated product should be sent immediately for gram stain and culture
2. All other components (RBC/FFP/cryo) made from this donation should be quarantined
3. Depending on the identity of the organism, donor follow-up may be indicated. A review of all donor collection and processing procedures may also be appropriate in certain instances

TRANSFUSION COMPLICATIONS

INFECTIOUS RISKS OF TRANSFUSION[11]

Viruses

1. All blood donations in the United States are tested for human immune deficiency virus (HIV-1/2), human T-cell lymphotropic virus (HTLV-I/II), hepatitis B virus (HBV), hepatitis C virus (HCV), and West Nile virus (WNV) infections
2. Routine testing for hepatitis A virus and parvovirus B19 is not done
3. On rare occasions, donors with window-phase infections can transmit disease
4. Currently, the estimated risks of viral transmission from a blood unit are:
    - HIV: 1 in 2.14 million
    - HTLV: 1 in 3 million
    - HBV: 1 in 488,800
    - HCV: 1 in 1.94 million

Parasites

1. Post-transfusion malaria, babesiosis, and Chagas' disease have been reported in the United States
2. Routine screening of donor blood for these agents is not carried out

Prions

1. A screening test for variant Creutzfeldt-Jakob disease (vCJD) is not currently available
2. Donor exclusion criteria are based on a history of travel and residence in Europe
3. Two possible cases of transfusion-transmitted vCJD have been reported from United Kingdom[12]

References

1. Brecher M, ed. Technical Manual, 14th ed. Bethesda: American Association of Blood Banks, 2002
2. Simon T, Dzik W , Snyder E et al, eds. Rossi's Principles of Transfusion Medicine. Philadelphia: Lippincott Williams & Wilkins, 2002:69–88
3. Goodnough LT et al. Transfusion medicine. First of two parts-blood transfusion. NEJM 1999;340(6):438–447
4. Goodnough LT et al. Transfusion medicine. Second of two parts-blood conservation. NEJM 1999; 340(7):525–533
5. Hébert PC et al. A multicenter, randomized, controlled clinical trial of transfusion requirements in critical care. NEJM 1999;340:409
6. Schiffer CA et al. American Society of Clinical Oncology. Platelet transfusion for patients with cancer: clinical practice guidelines of the American Society of Clinical Oncology. JCO 2001;19(5):1519–1538
7. Sacher RA et al. Management of patients refractory to platelet transfusion. Arch Pathol Lab Med 2003;127:409–414
8. Popovsky MA, ed. Transfusion Reactions, 2nd ed. Bethesda: American Association of Blood Banks, 2001
9. Gilstad CW. Anaphylactic transfusion reactions. Curr Opin Hematol 2003;10(6):419–423
10. Kleinman S et al. Toward an understanding of transfusion-related acute lung injury: statement of a consensus panel. Transfusion 2004;44(12):1774–1789
11. Dodd RY et al. Current prevalence and incidence of infectious disease markers and estimated window-period risk in the American Red Cross blood donor population. Transfusion 2002;42:975
12. Llewelyn CA et al. Possible transmission of variant Creutzfeldt-Jakob disease by blood transfusion. The Lancet 2004;363:417

46. Oncologic Emergencies

Michael M. Boyiadzis, MD, MHSc, and Tito Fojo, MD, PhD

Spinal Cord Compression (SCC)[1-13]

Etiology

Lifetime incidence of SCC in cancer patients:	1–6%
Median overall survival of patients with SCC:	3–16 months
SCC as the initial manifestation of cancer:	20–30% of all cases of SCC
SCC as the initial manifestation of cancer:	Lung cancer Cancer of unknown primary Non-Hodgkin lymphoma Myeloma
SCC distribution along spine: Thoracic spine Lumbar spine Cervical spine	 60–80% 15–30% 4–13%

Sites of Involvement	% SCC	Histology (% of All Cases)
Extradural metastases*	90–95	Prostate cancer (15–20) Breast cancer (15–20) Lung cancer (15–20) Non-Hodgkin lymphoma (5–10) Multiple myeloma (5–10) Renal cancer (5–10) Other (10–15)
Intradural masses	5–10	Meningioma Nerve sheath tumors Large leptomeningeal metastases
Transforaminal progression of paravertebral tumor	Uncommon	Lymphomas Neuroblastomas
Primary hematogenous seeding to epidural space	Rare	

*The most common mechanisms are:
- Direct extension into the epidural space of a hematogenous metastasis to a vertebral body
- Pathologic fracture of a vertebral body infiltrated by a metastatic deposit, resulting in cord injury by a bone fragment or spinal instability

- Differential diagnosis of SCC:
  1. Epidural abscess
  2. Subdural abscess
  3. Hematoma
  4. Herniated disk
  5. Leptomeningeal disease
  6. Hypertropic arthritic changes
  7. Radiation myelopathy
  8. Myelopathy secondary to intrathecal chemotherapy

Evaluation/Work-Up

Symptoms

Back pain	95%
Weakness	60–85%
Sensory deficits	40–90%
Autonomic dysfunction	50%
Ataxia	5%

- Spinal cord compression has been associated with most cancers. Consequently, any cancer patient with new back pain or a change in character of preexisting back pain should receive appropriate evaluation
- Suspected spinal cord compression requires immediate imaging studies and consultation with a radiation oncologist and a neurosurgeon
- Because multiple spinal epidural metastasis are found in one-third of patients, imaging of the entire spinal cord or at least the thoracic and lumbar spine in addition to the symptomatic region is recommended

Imaging Studies

Gadolinium-enhanced MRI	• The standard for diagnosis of spinal cord compression • Sensitivity: 93%; specificity: 97%; overall diagnostic accuracy: 95%
CT scan	• Useful for assessing the degree of bone destruction and whether bone or tumor is causing the spinal cord compression
Myelography	• Myelography and postmyelogram CT is used for patients in whom MRI is contraindicated, such as patients with pacemakers, mechanical valves, and other metal implants • Myelography is contraindicated in the presence of brain masses, thrombocytopenia, and coagulopathy and carries a small risk of worsening the neurologic deficit because of pressure shifts in the event of complete spinal subarachnoid block

Treatment Strategies

1. Supportive care

a. Pain control with opioids as Clinically indicated. See Chapter 52, Cancer Pain: Assessment and Management

b. Corticosteroids to lessen pain, reduce vasogenic cord edema, and avoid radiation-induced spinal edema

Dexamethasone 96 mg as an intravenous bolus *followed by*
Dexamethasone 96 mg in 4 divided doses orally daily for 3 days. Taper in 10 days

Note: This regimen was used in a randomized controlled trial that compared high-dose dexamethasone with no therapy in 57 patients with metastatic SCC treated with RT alone. Eighty-one percent of the participants were ambulatory after treatment in the intervention arm compared with 63% in the control group. Significant side effects were reported in 11% of those who received high-dose dexamethasone

Sorensen PS et al. Eur J Cancer 1994;30:22–27

or

Dexamethasone 10 mg as an intravenous bolus *followed 6 hours later by*
Dexamethasone 4 mg orally every 6 hours. Taper to zero within 2 weeks
Note: Used because of increased incidence in side effects observed with higher doses

Heimdal K et al. J Neuro-Oncol 1992;12:141–144
Vecht CJ et al. Neurology 1989;39:1255–1257

Dexamethasone is marketed in the United States in numerous generic formulations for oral administration, including immediate-release tablets containing 0.25, 0.5, 0.75, 1, 2, 4, and 6 mg, and in elixirs (which contain alcohol) and solutions for oral administration

Treatment Strategies (continued)

2. Radiation therapy

a. Preferred treatment for most patients with metastatic SCC: 30 Gy in 10 fractions over 2 weeks

b. Important variables: (1) Early diagnosis
(2) Favorable histology

Radiosensitive tumors	Lymphoma Myeloma Seminoma Ewing's sarcoma
Moderately radiosensitive tumors	Breast cancer Prostate cancer
Relative radioresistant tumors	Melanoma Lung cancer Colon cancer

Note: In a prospective analysis of 209 patients treated with radiation and steroids:

- Of those who were ambulatory, nonambulatory, or paraplegic before treatment, 98%, 60%, and 11%, respectively, were able to ambulate
- Early diagnosis was the most important response predictor of success so that a majority of patients able to walk and with good bladder function maintained these capacities
- When diagnosis was late, tumors with favorable histologies (ie, myeloma, breast, and prostate carcinomas) responded best to radiation therapy
- Duration of response was also influenced by histology. A favorable histology was associated with higher median response duration: myeloma, breast, and prostate carcinomas, 16, 12, and 10 months, respectively
- Median survival time was 6 months, with a 28% probability of survival at 1 year. There was a correlation between patient survival and duration of response, with systemic relapse of disease generally being the cause of death

Maranzano E et al. Int J Radiat Oncol Biol Phys 1995;32:959–967

- Transient myelopathy can develop 2–6 months after radiation therapy secondary to transient demyelination of the posterior columns
- The symptoms of transient myelopathy often resolve spontaneously within a year in most cases
- Chronic progressive myelitis is a late delayed complication of radiation

3. Surgery ± Radiation

Surgery should be considered in patients with:

- Spinal instability
- Paraplegia at diagnosis
- Retropulsion of bones within the vertebral canal
- Radioresistant tumors
- Deterioration during radiation therapy
- Prior radiation therapy in the same areas
- No tissue diagnosis

Note: The first phase III randomized trial evaluating the efficacy of direct decompressive surgery in patients with metastatic SCC compared the standard 30 Gy in 3-Gy daily fractions without a break with decompressive and stabilization surgery within 24 hours of diagnosis followed by the same radiation therapy started within 2 weeks. The trial was terminated early at interim analysis when early-stopping rules were met regarding the primary end points of ambulatory rate and time ambulatory after treatment. Regarding the primary end point of ambulation, the combined treatment had a median ambulation time of 126 days compared with 35 days for radiation alone ($P = .006$). Furthermore, baseline ambulatory and nonambulatory patients who had surgery and radiation had half the likelihood of being nonambulatory compared with those who had radiation only. Among nonambulatory patients, the combined-treatment patients had a significantly higher chance of regaining the ability to walk after therapy (56% versus 19%; $P = .03$). Although the study included only 101 patients, the results of this study challenge the accepted status quo of radiation alone in the management of metastatic SCC

Patchell R et al Proc Am Soc Clin Oncol 2003;22:1

4. Chemotherapy ± Radiation

Chemotherapy can be used in combination with radiation therapy for treatment of SCC or alone in patients who are not surgery or radiation candidates for chemosensitive tumors, including neuroblastoma, Ewing's sarcoma, osteogenic sarcoma, germ cell tumors, and lymphomas

Superior Vena Cava (SVC) Syndrome (SVCS)[14–22]

Etiology

Obstruction of the SVC due to all causes affects approximately 15,000 people per year in the United States

Causes of SVC Syndrome

Malignant	**85–95% of all cases**
Bronchogenic carcinoma[a]	80%
Non-Hodgkin lymphoma[b]	15%
Metastatic cancers[c]	5–10%
Nonmalignant[d]	**10–15%**

[a]Small cell lung cancer accounts for up to 60% of all cases of SVC obstruction

[b]Diffuse large cell and lymphoblastic lymphomas are the most common subtypes associated with SVC syndrome. Despite a common presentation with mediastinal lymphadenopathy, Hodgkins' disease rarely causes SVC syndrome

[c]*Most common primary tumor sites:* Breast cancer >> germ cell malignancies and gastrointestinal cancers

[d]Causes include granulomatous infections, goiter, aortic aneurysms, fibrosing mediastinitis, tension pneumothorax, and SVC thrombosis. Many cases of SVC thrombosis are caused by indwelling central venous devices

Evaluation/Work-Up

Symptoms

Dyspnea	60%	Dysphagia	9%
Facial swelling	50%	Dizziness	<5%
Cough	20%	Headache	<5%
Arm swelling	18%	Lethargy	<5%
Chest pain	15%	Syncopal attacks	<5%

- Appropriate management of SVC syndrome requires identification of the condition and its antecedent cause
- As many as 60% of patients with SVC syndrome secondary to cancer present without a known diagnosis of cancer
- The rapidity of onset of symptoms and signs from SVC obstruction is dependent on the rate at which complete obstruction of the SVC occurs in relation to the recruitment of venous collaterals. Patients with malignant disease develop symptoms of SVC syndrome within weeks to months because the rapidity of tumor growth does not allow adequate time to develop collateral flow

1. **Contrast-enhanced chest CT**
   - Is the preferred imaging modality once the diagnosis is suspected
   - Defines the level and extent of venous blockage
   - Maps collateral pathways of venous drainage
   - Often permits identification of the underlying cause of venous obstruction
2. **Bilateral upper extremity venography**
   - Can define the site and extent of SVC obstruction and visualize collateral pathways
   - Does not identify the cause of SVC obstruction unless thrombosis is the sole cause
3. **Biopsy**
   - To establish histologic diagnosis when indicated
   - Bronchoscopy, mediastinoscopy, or thoracotomy may be indicated when less invasive procedures do not provide a definitive diagnosis

Treatment Strategies

General Principles

- Treatment should be selected according to the histologic disorder and stage of the primary process
- Goals of treatment are to relieve symptoms and attempt the cure of the primary malignant process
- Deferring therapy until a full diagnostic work-up has been completed does not pose a hazard for most patients, provided the evaluation is efficient and the patient is clinically stable
- Treatment recommendations should be determined by a multidisciplinary team to include the radiation oncologist, medical oncologist, and a surgeon or pulmonologist, when appropriate
- Prognosis and life expectancy are related to the histologic type and stage of the underlying malignancy at presentation

1. Radiation therapy

a. Most often chosen as the initial modality of treatment

b. Provides quick relief of symptoms; often within 72 hours;

c. 70–90% of patients are free of symptoms by 2 weeks

d. Complications:

- Esophagitis
- Nausea and vomiting
- Skin irritation
- Possible worsening of symptoms secondary to edema

e. Recurrence of SVC syndrome is reported in 10–19% of patients treated with RT. Causes include:

- Tumor recurrence
- Radiation fibrosis
- Thrombosis

f. The optimal total dose fraction has not been established, and dosage must be individualized to the patient and the underlying malignancy

2. Chemotherapy

a. An acceptable alternative in patients with chemosensitive malignancies. Choice of therapy is guided by evaluation

Note: Radiation Therapy versus Chemotherapy

- Systematic review of two randomized and 44 nonrandomized studies were performed to determine the effectiveness of different treatment modalities for SVC obstruction in patients with carcinoma of the bronchus
- *Small cell lung cancer:* Chemotherapy and/or radiation therapy relieved SVC obstruction in 77%; 17% of those treated had a recurrence of SVC obstruction
- *Non–small cell lung cancer:* Chemotherapy and/or radiation therapy relieved SVC obstruction in 60%; 16% of those treated had a recurrence of SVC obstruction
- *Conclusions*: It is reasonable to choose between radiation therapy and chemotherapy treatment on the basis of stage and performance status. Effectiveness was not clearly related to any particular radiation therapy fractionation schedule or chemotherapy regimen

Rowell NP, Gleeson FV. JCO 2002;14:338–351

3. Endovascular therapies: expandable wire stents

a. Successfully used to open and maintain the patency of SVC obstruction resulting from malignant causes

b. Complete resolution of SVC syndrome occurs in 68–100% of patients treated with a metallic stent

c. Prompt resolution achieved regardless of stent type

- Several investigators report immediate relief of disabling headaches caused by SVC syndrome
- Facial cyanosis and facial edema usually resolve within 1–2 days
- Truncal and upper extremity edema usually resolve within 2–3 days but may take up to 1 week

d. Recurrence rates range from 4–45%; secondary to:

- Tumor in-growth through the interstices of the stent
- Tumor growth around the ends of the stent, leading to thrombosis

e. Recurrence can be treated with anticoagulation, angioplasty of the stented area, or repeat stenting

f. Thrombolysis is often an integral part of the endovascular management of SVCS because thrombosis is frequently a critical component of the obstruction and lysis necessary to allow the passage of the wire. Using these techniques, technical success can be achieved in 90–100% of cases

g. Indications:

- Patients with reduced life expectancy
- SVC obstruction recurring after first-line therapy
- Patients with symptoms that are acute and so severe that immediate treatment is needed

Treatment Strategies (*continued*)

h. Contraindications:

- Thrombus or complete SVC obstruction are not contraindications for stent placement

i. Complication (rates) of endovascular therapy:

- Stent misplacement (10%)
- Stent migration (5%)
- Stent occlusion (10%)
- Cardiac arrthymias (rare)

j. There is no consensus regarding anticoagulation (warfarin/aspirin) after stent placement

Notes:

- Use especially in patients with the presence of thrombus visualized on venography
- *Autopsy studies*: 30–50% of patients with SVC syndrome have evidence of thrombosis
- Suspect an obstructing thrombus if symptoms do not improve within the first week of radiation therapy or chemotherapy
- Many patients have large necrotic friable tumor masses, and the area of tumor is under increased pressure. For these patients, anticoagulant or fibrinolytic therapy poses a considerable risk of bleeding
- For treatment of catheter-related SVC see Chapter 49 on venous catheter-related thrombosis

Tumor Lysis Syndrome (TLS)[23–30]

Etiology

1. TLS describes the metabolic derangements that occur with tumor breakdown after the initiation of cytotoxic therapy and is characterized by:
   - Hyperkalemia
   - Hyperphosphatemia with secondary hypocalcemia
   - Hyperuricemia
2. TLS may also occur spontaneously before cytotoxic therapy, is less common, and is usually associated with normal phosphorus levels
3. TLS can lead to acute renal failure and can be life threatening
4. Risk factors for TLS
   a. Bulky disease
      - Bulky adenopathy
      - Hepatosplenomegaly
      - High leukocyte count
      - Elevated pretreatment LDH (LDH >500 units/L)
      - Elevated pretreatment uric acid
      - Chemosensitive tumors

   b. Compromised renal function
      - Biochemical abnormalities
      - Decreased urine output
      - Use of potentially nephrotoxic drugs

Degree of Risk	Tumor Type	Supporting Data
Highest	• Burkitt's lymphoma • Lymphoblastic lymphoma • T-cell acute lymphoblastic leukemia • Other acute leukemias	Frequent cases
Moderate	• Low-grade lymphoma treated with chemotherapy, radiation therapy, or steroids • Multiple myeloma • Breast carcinoma treated with chemotherapy or hormonal therapy • Small cell carcinoma • Germ cell	Recognized complication, but few occurrences
Lowest	• Low-grade lymphoma treated with interferon • Merkel's cell carcinoma • Medulloblastoma •Adenocarcinoma of the gastrointestinal tract	Case reports only

Evaluation/Work-Up

- It is essential to maintain a high index of suspicion to identify patients at risk for developing TLS
- Patients at high risk should received preventive measures and be treated in a proactive fashion. See Treatment Strategies section

Treatment Strategies

1. **Hydration and diuresis—mainstay of therapy**
   a. **Hydration with 3000 mL/m^2** perday unless a patient presents with signs of acute renal dysfunction and oliguria
   b. **Furosemide (Lasix)** 20–40 mg intravenously per push to maintain urine output of >> 100 mL/m^{2}per hour if there is no evidence of acute obstructive uropathy or hypovolemia

2. **Correction of hyperkalemia**
   - Can develop within 12–24 hours of initiation of chemotherapy
   - Emergent treatment indicated if cardiac toxicity or muscular paralysis is present or if the hyperkalemia is severe (serum potassium >6.5–7 mEq/L) even with no electrocardiographic changes

   a. Calcium infusions
      - **Calcium gluconate** 10%, 5–30 mL intravenously, *or*
      - **Calcium chloride** 5%, 5–30 mL intravenously

        –Indicated when it is potentially dangerous to wait the 30–60 minutes for insulin and glucose or sodium bicarbonate to act
        –May be repeated after 5 minutes if ECG does not improve
        –Protective effect of calcium begins within minutes, but is *relatively short-lived (<60 minutes)*

   b. Glucose and insulin
      - **50% glucose** 25 g (1 ampule) intravenously, *plus*
      - **Regular insulin** 5–10 units intravenously per push

        –Effective therapy usually leads to a 0.5–1.5 mEq/L decrease in the plasma potassium concentration, an effect that begins in 15 minutes, peaks at 60 minutes, and *lasts for 4–6 hours*

   c. Sodium bicarbonate
      - **Sodium bicarbonate** ($NaHCO_3$) 44–88 mEq (1–2 ampules) intravenously

        –Onset of action in 15–30 minutes with a *duration of action of 1–2 hours*

   d. Nebulizer therapy
      - **Nebulized albuterol** 10–20 mg in 4 mL normal saline by inhalation over 10–15 minutes

   e. Potassium-binding resins
      - **Sodium polystyrene sulfonate** 15–50 g orally; may be *repeated every 6 hours* until serum potassium is within normal limits

   f. Dialysis
      - Definitive therapy for patients with severe hyperkalemia
      - May be indicated if pharmacologic measures are ineffective or in patients with renal failure and other metabolic derangements

   Sodium polystyrene sulfonate is generically available in the United States in several formulations for oral administration, including a liquid suspension containing 16 g/15 mL and a finely ground powder containing approximately 15 g per 4 level teaspoonfuls. The finely ground powder is mixed in an aqueous vehicle or a syrupy solution (eg, sorbitol) before administration

3. **Correction of hyperphosphatemia (and hypocalcemia)**
   - Hyperphosphatemia develops within 24–48 hours after initiation of chemotherapy
   - Hyperphosphatemia may result in tissue precipitation of calcium phosphate leading to hypocalcemia, intrarenal calcifications, nephrocalcinosis, and acute obstructive uropathy
   - Treatment of hyperphosphatemia usually corrects any related hypocalcemia; thus, calcium administration should be given only to patients with symptoms related to hypocalcemia

   a. Oral phosphate binders
      - **Aluminium hydroxide** 15–30 mL orally every 6 hours

   b. Hemodialysis
      - The most effective therapeutic strategy
      - Consider if hyperphosphatemia is severe, especially in the setting of renal failure and symptomatic hypocalcemia
      - The clearance of phosphorus is better with hemodialysis than with continuous venovenous hemofiltration or continuous peritoneal dialysis

Treatment Strategies (*continued*)

4. **Correction of hyperuricemia**
   - Hyperuricemia develops within 24–48 hours after initiation of chemotherapy when the excretory capacity of the renal tubules is exceeded
   - In the presence of an acid pH, uric acid crystals form in the renal tubule, leading to intraluminal renal tubular obstruction and acute renal obstructive uropathy and renal dysfunction

   a. Xanthine oxidase inhibitor
   - **Allopurinol** 100 mg/m^2 orally every 8 hours (maximum 800 mg/day), *or*
   - **Allopurinol** 10 mg/kg/day orally in 3 doses, one every 8 hours (maximum 800 mg/day), *or*
   - **Allopurinol** 200–400 mg/m^2 per day intravenously in 1–3 divided doses (maximum 600 mg/day)

   Note: Patients with no evidence of laboratory or clinical tumor lysis syndrome and low risk for developing TLS are candidates for allopurinol
   - Dose adjustment for creatinine clearance:

Creatinine Clearance	Oral Allopurinol Dose
10–20 mL/min	200 mg/day
3–10 mL/min	100 mg/day
<3 mL/min	100 mg every 36–48 hours

   - The incidence of allergic reactions is increased in patients receiving amoxicillin, ampicillin, or thiazide diuretics
   - Allopurinol inhibits the metabolism of **azathioprine and mercaptopurine;** thus, a **dose reduction** by 65–75% of these purine analogs is recommended with concomitant use of allopurinol
   - Side effects include rash (1.5%), nausea (1.3%), vomiting (1.2%), and renal insufficiency (1.2%)

   Allopurinol is available in the United States generically as immediate-release tablets for oral administration containing 100 mg or 300 mg allopurinol

   b. Recombinant urate oxidase
   - **Rasburicase/Elitek®** (recombinant urate oxidase) 0.15–0.2 mg/kg daily intravenously for up to 5 days. Chemotherapy should be initiated 4 to 24 hours after the first dose

   Notes:
   - Rasburicase administration for <5 days may be sufficient and less expensive
   - Rasburicase does not require adjustment with a decrease in the creatinine clearance
   - Side effects include skin rash, nausea and vomiting, and rarely a hypersensitivity reaction including anaphylaxis. Antibodies against rasburicase or its epitopes occur in about 10% of patients
   - Potential candidates for the treatment and prophylaxis of TLS with rasburicase include patients with either TLS or clinical manifestations of TLS and those at high risk for TLS
   - Rasburicase is contraindicated in patients with G6PD deficiency and/or methemoglobinemia
   - *Rasburicase has not been approved by the FDA for use in adults*

5. **Alkalinization of the urine**

   a. **Sodium bicarbonate** 100 mEq/day administer intravenously to alkalinize the urine

   Note: Urinary alkalization increases the solubility and excretion of uric acid and helps avoid crystallization of uric acid. However, *alkalinization is not uniformly recommended and in the majority of cases should be avoided because:*

   (1) It favors precipitation of calcium–phosphate complexes in renal tubules, a concern in patients with concomitant hyperphosphatemia
   (2) The metabolic alkalemia that may result from the administration of bicarbonate can worsen the neurologic manifestations of hypocalcemia
   (3) At alkaline urine with a pH >6.5, the solubility of **xanthine** and **hypoxanthine** significantly decreases, leading to the development of urinary xanthine crystals during and after allopurinol therapy

Syndrome of Inappropriate Secretion of Antidiuretic Hormone (SIADH)[31–35]

Etiology

1. Among cancer patients, 1–2% of develop SIADH
2. The hyponatremia is initially mediated by ADH-induced water retention. The ensuing volume expansion activates secondary natriuretic mechanisms, resulting in sodium and water loss and the restoration of near euvolemia. The combination of water retention due to inappropriate ADH secretion and secondary solute loss (sodium and potassium) accounts for the fall of the plasma sodium concentration. Thus, patients with SIADH have normal volume status, hyponatremia with hypo-osmolality, elevated renal excretion of sodium (>20 mEq/L), and urine osmolality greater than plasma osmolality

Causes of SIADH

Tumors	• *Small-cell lung cancer (SCLC)* is most commonly associated with SIADH; occurs in 10% of SCLC patients • Other tumors
Pulmonary conditions	• Pneumonia • Tuberculosis • Pulmonary abscess • Acute respiratory failure • Positive-pressure ventilation
Central nervous system disease	• Stroke • Acute psychosis • Inflammatory & demyelinating disorders • Trauma • Mass lesions • Seizures • Infection • Hemorrhage
Drugs	• *Cytotoxic drugs:* Cyclophosphamide, ifosfamide, vinca alkaloids • *Other drugs*: Phenothiazines, tricyclic antidepressants, chlorpropamide, clofibrate, oxytocin, desmopressin phenothiazides, opiate derivatives, serotonin reuptake inhibitors
Miscellaneous	• Severe pain • Postoperative state

Evaluation/Work-Up

1. Careful history with attention to excluding other possible causes
   - Diuretic administration
   - Preexisting renal disease
   - Adrenal insufficiency
   - Hypothyroidism
2. Review of recent chemotherapy agents and ancillary medications looking for a causative agent (see above)
3. Search for pulmonary or CNS disease if clinically indicated
4. Serum sodium as part of serum electrolytes including BUN and creatinine
5. Urine sodium, urine osmolality, plasma osmolality
6. Thyroid function tests
7. AM serum cortisol; ACTH if clinically indicated

Treatment Strategies

General Principles

- Correction of the hyponatremia is guided by the severity of the clinical presentation and the pace with which the hyponatremia developed. If it developed slowly, correct over several days
- The rate of correction should not exceed 8–10 mmol/L on any day of treatment. The initial rate of correction can be 1–2 mmol/L per hour for several hours in patients with severe symptoms of hyponatremia
- Indications for stopping the rapid correction are the cessation of life-threatening manifestations or a serum sodium of 125–130 mmol/L (or lower if the baseline serum sodium concentration is <100 mmol/L

1. **Water restriction**
   a. **The mainstay in asymptomatic hyponatremia 500–1000 mL/24 hours**
   - The associated negative water balance raises the plasma sodium concentration toward normal. It can also lead to volume depletion due to unmasking of the sodium deficit
2. **Salt (sodium) administration**
   - Severe, symptomatic or resistant hyponatremia often requires the administration of salt. Although both sodium and water are retained in hypovolemia, sodium handling is intact in patients with SIADH. Thus, when isotonic saline is administered, the sodium is excreted in the urine, whereas some of the water may be retained, leading to possible worsening of hyponatremia. Consequently, to elevate the plasma sodium in patients with SIADH, 3% hypertonic saline may need to be administered

Formula used to estimate the effect of 1 liter of any infusate on serum Na^+:

$$\text{Change in serum } Na^+ \text{ (mmol/L)} = \frac{\text{Infusate } Na^+ \text{ concentration} - \text{serum } Na^+ \text{ concentration}}{\text{Total body water} + 1}$$

Infusate	Infusate Na^+ in mmol/L
5% NaCl in water	855
3% NaCl in water	513
0.9% NaCl in water	154
Ringer's lactate solution	130
0.45% NaCl in water*	34
5% Dextrose in water*	0

*Should never be used in management of hyponatremia

Estimated total body water (in liters)*	
Patient	Fraction of body weight
Non-elderly men	0.6
Non-elderly women	0.5
Elderly men	0.5
Elderly women	0.45

*Calculated as a percentage of body weight

Example: Clinical case to calculate amount of Na^+ needed in a patient with SIADH (NEJM 2000;342:1581–1589)
A 58-year-old man with SCLC presented with confusion and lethargy and was diagnosed with SIADH. He weighs 60 kg, is euvolemic, and has a serum sodium concentration of 108 mmol per liter, serum osmolality 220 mOsm per kilogram of water, and urine osmolality 600 mOsm per kilogram of water. Treatment plan includes water restriction and the administration of 3% NaCl. According to the above formula, the administration of 1 liter of 3% NaCl is estimated to increase the serum concentration by 10.9 mmol per liter

$$\text{Change in serum } Na^+ \text{ (mmol/L)} = \frac{\text{Infusate } Na^+ \text{ concentration } [513] - \text{serum } Na^+ \text{ concentration } [108]}{\text{Total body water}[36]^* + 1} = 10.9 \text{ mmol/L}$$

*Patient's total body water is 36 liters: 0.60 × 60 (wt in kg) for this non-elderly man

Note: The initial goal in this case is to increase the serum sodium concentration by 5 mmol/L over the first 12 hours. One liter of 3% NaCl will increase the serum sodium concentration by 10.9 mmol/L. To increase it by 5 mmol/L, only 0.46 liter is required [5/10.9 = 0.46]. Therefore, 0.46 liter over the first 12 hours or 38 mL per hour is required. Twelve hours after starting the 3% NaCl infusion, the patient's clinical condition improved, and his serum sodium increased to 114 mmol/L. The hypertonic infusion was stopped, but fluid restriction continued

3. **Salt plus loop diuretics**
   - The effect of hypertonic saline can be enhanced if given with a loop diuretic. This lowers the urine osmolality and increases water excretion by impairing the renal responsiveness to ADH
   a. **Furosemide (Lasix)** 20–40 mg intravenously per push

Treatment Strategies (continued)

4. **Demeclocycline**
   - Use to induce nephrogenic diabetes insipidus if the above measures do not improve the hyponatremia
   a. **Demeclocycline** 600–1200 mg orally each day
      Note:
      - Monitoring of renal function is required because demeclocycline has nephrotoxic effects
      - *Side effects:* Nausea, vomiting, diarrhea, glossitis, dysphagia, hepatotoxicity, nephrotoxicity
      - *Contraindications*: Hypersensitivity to tetracyclines

      Demeclocycline is available in the United States generically as immediate-release tablets for oral administration, containing 150 mg or 300 mg demeclocycline HCl

Hypercalcemia Associated with Cancer[36–40]

Etiology

1. Hypercalcemia is the most common metabolic complication of malignancy occurring in 10% of cancer patients
2. Hypercalcemia of malignancy is a grave complication with median survival rates between 6 and 10 weeks

Most Common Types of Hypercalcemia Associated with Cancer

Type	Frequency	Bone metastasis	Causative factors	Typical Tumor
Humoral	80%	Absent—minimal	PTHrP*	SCC of lung SCC of esophagus SCC of cervix SCC of head and neck Renal cell carcinoma Breast cancer Ovarian cancer
Local osteolytic	20%	Common—extensive	Cytokines Chemokines PTHrP	Breast cancer Multiple myeloma Lymphoma

PTH, parathyroid hormone; PTHrP, PTH-related protein; SCC, squamous cell cancer
*Circulating PTHrP levels are increased in virtually all patients with humoral hypercalcemia of malignancy and up to two-thirds of patients with bone metastases

Evaluation/Work-Up

The tumors in a patient with hypercalcemia associated with malignant disease are generally large and readily apparent. However, a further evaluation should consider not only mechanisms potentially related to the cancer but also causes of calcium elevation that are unrelated to the cancer

1. Serum calcium as part of serum electrolyte, mineral and hepatic panel to include serum albumin
2. Ionized calcium [see Note below]
3. Levels of intact PTH should be measured routinely
4. PTHrP only in selected cases

(Although most patients with typical humoral hypercalcemia of malignancy have increased levels of circulating PTHrP, the diagnosis is usually obvious on clinical grounds. Therefore, PTHrP should be measured only in the occasional cases in which the diagnosis of humoral hypercalcemia of malignancy cannot be made on clinical grounds or when the cause of hypercalcemia is obscure)

Note: Approximately 55% of the total serum calcium is bound to serum proteins and is biologically inert. About 45% is in the ionized form and metabolically active. In general, the plasma calcium concentration falls by 0.8 mg/dL (0.2 mmol/L) for every 1.0 g/dL fall in the plasma albumin concentration. Because of the high prevalence of low protein levels in cancer patients, direct measurement of ionized serum calcium is preferred because it avoids the variability of the serum protein concentration. If an ionized calcium level is not available, the measured serum calcium can be adjusted for variations in serum albumin by the formula:

$$\text{Corrected calcium (mg/dL)} = \text{Measured total calcium} + 0.8 \times [4.5 - \text{albumin (g/dL)}]$$

Treatment Strategies

- Several agents commonly used before the introduction of bisphosphonates are now used infrequently, usually when bisphosphonates are ineffective or contraindicated

1. Hydration
   - Extracellular volume deficits exist in all patients with symptomatic hypercalcemia of malignancy. Therefore, the first intervention should be intravenous hydration with isotonic saline
   - The volume replacement depends on the baseline level of dehydration, renal function, cardiovascular status, degree of mental impairment, and severity of hypercalcemia

   a. **Hydration** with 1–2 liters of 0.9% normal saline (0.9% NS) intravenously over 2–4 hours

   Note: This will result at most in a decrease in serum calcium levels of 0.5 mmol/L (1–2 mg/dL)

2. Diuretics

   a. **Furosemide (Lasix)** 20–40 mg intravenously per push

   Notes:
   - The use of diuretics should be avoided until the volume deficit has been fully corrected. Loop diuretics (such as furosemide) cause calciuresis and may be effective in acutely decreasing calcium levels after volume repletion.
   - Thiazide diuretics decrease renal calcium excretion and should be avoided

3. **Bisphosphonates (first-line therapy)** [See Chapter 44 for more information on bisphosphonates]
   - Bisphosphonates should be initiated as soon as hypercalcemia is diagnosed
   - Initiate treatment only after (1) adequate hydration with 0.9% NS; (2) adequate urine output; and (3) determining the dose appropriate for a patient's creatinine clearance
   - Encourage ambulatory patients to maintain hydration orally
   - If hypercalcemia persists or recurs, there should be ≥ 7 days between consecutive treatments

Hypocalcemic Effects of Bisphosphonates

Adapted from Riccardi A et al and Body J-J[41]

Bisphosphonate	Median Time to Normocalcemia	Duration of Normocalcemia	% Achieving Normocalcemia
Pamidronate[42,43]	4 days	28 days	70–100%
Zoledronate acid[44]	4 days	32 days	87%
Clodronate[42]	3 days	14 days	80%
Alendronate[45]	4 days	15 days	74%

a. **Pamidronate** 90 mg intravenously in 250–500 mL 0.9% NS, 0.45% NS, or D5W over 1–4 hours every 3–4 weeks, *or*

Dose Modifications for Renal Impairment for Doses Other Than the First Dose

Baseline	Retreatment	Action
Normal SCr	SCr increased ≥0.5 mg/dL (45 micromol/L)	Hold until SCr within 10% of baseline
Abnormal SCr	SCr increased ≥1.0 mg/dL (90 micromol/L) above baseline	Hold until SCr within 10% of baseline

b. **Zoledronate** 4–8 mg intravenously in 100 mL 0.9% NS or D5W over at least 15 minutes every 3–4 weeks

Dose Adjustments for Patients with Baseline CrCl ≤60 mL/min* for Doses Other Than the First Dose

Baseline CrCl	Recommended Dose
50–60 mL/min	3.5 mg
40–49 mL/min.	3.3 mg
30–39 mL/min	3 mg

*Doses are calculated to produce an AUC (0.6 mg/hour/L) similar to that achieved in patients with CrCl = 75 mL/min

c. **Clodronate** 300 mg/day intravenously in 500 mL 0.9% NS or D5W over 2 hours for up to 5 days (treatment with intravenous clodronate may continue for >5 days but should be limited to not more than 10 days for a single hypercalcemic episode), *or*
Clodronate 1500 mg single dose intravenously in 500 mL 0.9% NS or D5W over 4 hours

Dose Modifications for Renal Impairment for Doses Other Than the First Dose

CrCl (mL/min)	Dose Reduction
50–80	25%
12–50	25–50%
<12	50%

d. **Alendronate** 5, 10, or 15 mg intravenously over 2 hours
(A parenteral formulation is not available for commercial use in the United States)

Dose Modifications for Renal Impairment for Doses Other Than the First Dose

Elderly patients	No adjustments
CrCl ≥35 mL/min	No adjustments
CrCl <35 mL/min	Do not administer drug

4. **Gallium nitrate (second-line therapy)**
   a. **Gallium nitrate** 100–200 mg/m^2/day intravenously continuously over a 24-hour period for 5 days

   Notes:
   - Results in a gradual reduction of serum calcium over the 5-day infusion. If the serum calcium levels are lowered into normal levels in <5 days of infusion, treatment may be discontinued
   - The 5-day schedule of administration is more cumbersome than the 1-day administration of the biphosphonates, often limiting its use to the acute setting
   - *Contraindications*: Renal impairment (serum creatinine >2.5 mg/dL or 220 μmol/L)
   - *Adverse effects*: Renal failure, hypophosphatemia, hypocalcemia, respiratory alkalosis, vomiting, hypotension, tachycardia, nausea, vomiting, diarrhea, acute optic neuritis

5. **Plicamycin (second-line therapy)**
   Plicamycin is a highly toxic antibiotic with antineoplastic and hypocalcemic activity that acts by blocking RNA synthesis in osteoclasts.
   Plicamycin is not available is the United States
   a. **Plicamycin** 25 μg/kg intravenously over 4–6 hours
   (Further courses may be given at intervals of 1 week or more if required. Plicamycin lowers serum calcium levels within 12 hours with a maximum effect at about 48 hours)

   Notes:
   - Although widely used in the past, side effects, including thrombocytopenia, myelosuppression, hepatotoxicity, nephrotoxicity, coagulopathy nausea, vomiting, as well as the availability of other agents, currently limits its use
   - *Contraindications*: Bone marrow suppression, thrombocytopenia, coagulation disorder, bleeding

6. **Calcitonin (second-line therapy)**
   a. **Calcitonin** 4–8 units/kg intramuscularly or by subcutaneous injection every 12 hours

   Note:
   - Calcitonin can bring about a rapid decline of serum calcium within 2–6 hours of administration. The need for frequent administration and the occurrence of tachyphylaxis within a few days of instituting therapy limits its usefulness in the acute setting, where it should be used in combination with longer-acting agents
   - *Adverse effects*: Flushing, nausea, vomiting, local inflammatory reaction at the site of injection

7. **Corticosteroids (second-line therapy)**
   - May be useful in patients with steroid-sensitive cancers such as lymphomas and multiple myeloma by decreasing the 1,25-dihydroxycholecalciferol levels

   a. **Prednisone** 60 mg orally daily for 7–10 days (or equivalent steroid dose)

   Note: Steroids have a slow onset of action (7 days) and a short duration of action (3–4 days)

8. **Phosphorus**
   a. **Neutral phosphate salts** 500–1500 mg/day of elemental phosphorus orally in 2–4 divided doses

   Note: Hypophosphatemia develops in most patients with hypercalcemia associated with cancer and the presence of hypophosphatemia increases the difficulty of treating hypercalcemia. Phosphorous should be replaced orally or administered through a nasogastric tube

Anaphylaxis[46–50]

Etiology

- Anaphylaxis is an acute hypersensitivity reaction that is often an unpredictable and potentially catastrophic complication of cancer treatment. It can occur at any time during the administration of therapy
- Almost all the antineoplastic drugs and many biological agents including monoclonal antibodies, have been reported to cause hypersensitivity reactions
- Certain classes of chemotherapeutic agents commonly associated with hypersensitivity reactions include the **taxanes, platinum compounds, asparaginase,** and **epipodophyllotoxins**
- Despite prophylactic measures with steroids or antihistamines to reduce the incidence of hypersensitivity reactions, hypersensitivity reactions still occur. Severe reactions may require immediate medical management with the drugs listed below

Evaluation

1. Focused physical examination
2. Establishment of a stable airway
3. Establishment of intravenous access
4. Administration of epinephrine

Note: Parenteral epinephrine is the cornerstone of management

Treatment Strategies

Drug	Dose	Route	Frequency
Epinephrine 1:1000	0.3–0.5 mL	IM, SC[a]	Immediately, then every 5–15 minutes
Epinephrine 1:10,000	0.5–1.0 mL	IV[b]	Immediately, then every 5–10 minutes
	3–5 mL	ET[c]	Immediately
Diphenyhydramine[d]	25–50 mg	IV, PO or IM	Immediately, then every 4–6 hours as needed
Cimetidine *or* Ranitidine	300 mg	IV	Every 8–12 hours as needed
	50 mg	IV	Every 8–12 hours as needed
Hydrocortisone[e]	100 mg	IV	Every 6 hours as needed
Albuterol[f]	2.5–5 mg	Via nebulizer	Every 20 minutes up to 3 doses
Glucagon[g]	1–2 mg	IV	Immediately, then every 5–15 minutes

ET, via endotracheal tube; IM, intramuscularly; IV, intravenously; PO, orally; SC, subcutaneous

[a]Intramuscular administration is preferred over subcutaneous, because intramuscular epinephrine is better absorbed

[b]Patients with severe airway edema, severe hypotension, or severe bronchospasm should receive IV epinephrine 0.5–1 mL of a 1:10,000 dilution at intervals of 5–10 minutes with cardiac monitoring

[c]If IV access cannot be obtained, administer 3–5 mL of a 1:10,000 epinephrine dilution via the endotracheal tube

[d]Antihistamines should be given to all patients with anaphylaxis and continued until symptoms resolve completely

[e]Corticosteroids are administered to prevent recurrent or protracted anaphylaxis. Use hydrocortisone or equivalent dose of another steroid

[f]Persistent respiratory distress or wheezing requires the use of nebulized β-adrenergic agents (albuterol)

[g]Patients on β-blockers may be resistant to treatment with epinephrine and can develop refractory hypotension and bradycardia. Glucagon has inotropic and chronotropic effects that are not mediated through β-receptors and should be administered in this subsets of patients

References

1. Gabriel K et al Semin Neurol 2004;24:375–383
2. Schiff D. Neurol Clin 2003;21:67–86, viii
3. Prasad D et al Lancet Oncol 2005;6:15–24
4. Schiff D et al.. Neurology 1997;49:452–456
5. Bilsky MH et al. Oncologist 1999;4:459–469
6. Yalamanchili M et al. Curr Treat Options Oncol 2003;4:509–516
7. Loblaw DA et al JCO 2005;23:2028–2037
8. Loblaw DA et al JCO 1998;16:1613–1624
9. Sze WM , Clin Oncol (R Coll Radiol) 2003;15:345–352
10. Hardy JR et al. Clin Oncol (R Coll Radiol) 2002;14:132–134
11. Maranzano E et al JCO 2005;23:3358–3365
12. Kwok Y et al. JCO 2005;23:3308–3310
13. Greenberg HS et al. Ann Neurol 1980;8:361–366
14. Wudel LJ Jr et al. Curr Treat Options Oncol 2001;2:77–91
15. Markman M, Cleve Clin J Med 1999;66:59–61
16. Ostler PJ et al. Clin Oncol (R Coll Radiol) 1997;9:83–89
17. Armstrong BA et al. Int J Radiat Oncol Biol Phys 1987;13:531–539
18. Spiro SG et al. Thorax 1983;38:501–505
19. Pignon JP et al. N Engl J Med 1992;327:1618–1624
20. Hochrein J et al. Am J Med 1998;104:78–84
21. Yim CD et al. Radiol Clin North Am 2000;38:409–424
22. Schindler N et al. Surg Clin North Am 1999;79:683–694, xi
23. Cairo MS et al. Br J Haematol 2004;127:3–11
24. Arrambide K et al. Semin Nephrol 1993;13:273–280
25. Cairo MS et al. Clin Lymphoma 2002;3 Suppl 1:S26–31
26. Baeksgaard L et al. Cancer Chemother Pharmacol 2003;51:187–192
27. Nicolin G et al. Eur J Cancer 2002;38:1365–1377; discussion 1378–1369
28. Davidson MB et al. Am J Med 2004;116:546–554
29. Locatelli F et al. Contrib Nephrol 2005;147:61–68
30. Yarpuzlu AA. Clin Chim Acta 2003;333:13–18
31. Adrogue HJ et al. Int J Biochem Cell Biol 2003;35:1495–1499
33. Silverman P et al. Semin Oncol 1989;16:504–515
34. Flombaum CD et al. Semin Oncol 2000;27:322–334
35. Goh KP et al. Am Fam Physician 2004;69:2387–2394
36. Stewart AF et al. N Engl J Med 2005;352:373–379
37. Davidson TG, Am J Health Syst Pharm 2001;58 Suppl 3:S8–15
38. Mundy GR et al. Hypercalcemia of malignancy. Am J Med 1997;103:134–145
39. Ralston SH et al. Calcif Tissue Int 2004;74:1–11
40. Ratcliffe WA et al. Lancet 1992;339:164–167
41. Riccardi A et al. Tumori 2003;89:223–236; and Body JJ. Semin Oncol 2001;28(4 suppl 11):49–53
42. Purohit OP. Br J Cancer 1995;72:1289–1293
43. Body JJ. Ann Oncol 1994;5:359–363
44. Major P. JCO 2001;19:558–567
45. Nussbaum SR et al. JCO 1993;11:1618–1623
46. Zanotti KM et al. Drug Saf 2001;24:767–779
47. Shepherd GM. Clin Rev Allergy Immunol 2003;24:253–262
48. Ellis AK et al. Cmaj 2003;169:307–311
49. Tang AW. Am Fam Physician 2003;68:1325–1332
50. Simons FE et al. J Allergy Clin Immunol 2001;108:871—873

47. Fever and Neutropenia

Juan Gea-Banacloche, MD, and Thomas J. Walsh, MD

Definitions According to the Current Recommendations of the Infectious Diseases Society of America

Fever: Single oral temperature of 38.3°C (101°F) or a temperature of 38.0°C (100.4°F) for ≥1 hour
Neutropenia: A neutrophil count of <500 cells/mm^3 or a count of <1000 cells/mm^3 predicted to decrease to <500 cells/mm^3

Hughes WT et al. Clin Infect Dis 2002;34:730–751

Etiology

Fever and neutropenia

- 10–20%: Microbiologically documented infection (most commonly bacteremia)
- 20–30%: Clinically documented infection (eg, cellulitis, pneumonia, typhlitis)
- 50–70%: No clinically or microbiologically documented infection

Infectious causes

1. Bacteria make up the most commonly documented cause of fever and neutropenia
2. Gram-positive bacteria predominate in recent series; however, the incidence of gram-negative bacteria is increasing
3. Gram-negative bacteremia may be associated with faster clinical decompensation and death compared with gram-positive bacteremia. Hence, empirical treatment is targeted to cover gram-negative pathogens, particularly *Pseudomonas aeruginosa*
4. *Candida* and *Aspergillus* species are the most common causes of invasive fungal infections in neutropenic patients. They are uncommon early or during short episodes of neutropenia, but they become more comon with longer duration of neutropenia

Factors contributing to immune compromise of an individual patient

1. Corticosteroids, fludarabine, and alemtuzumab (Campath-1H) produce severe defect in cellular immunity
2. Myeloma and CLL are accompanied by defects in humoral immunity
3. Patients without a spleen are at risk of overwhelming sepsis caused by encapsulated bacteria, mainly *Streptococcus pneumoniae*
4. Obstruction (biliary, ureteral, bronchial) facilitates local infection (cholangitis, pyelonephritis, postobstructive pneumonia)
5. Intravascular devices, drainage tubes, or stents may become colonized and lead to local infection, bacteremia, or fungemia

Treatment Overview

1. Expeditious evaluation is mandatory, with special attention to skin, mouth, perianal region, and lungs
2. Cultures of blood*, urine, and sputum should be obtained in all patients
3. In patients with diarrhea, stool culture with a test to rule out *Clostridium difficile* (culture or toxin assay) should be obtained
4. In patients with signs or symptoms of upper respiratory tract infection, a nasopharyngeal wash to screen for viruses (respiratory syncytial virus, influenza A and B, adenovirus and parainfluenza 1, 2, 3) should be obtained
5. CBC with differential count, chemistry panel, and chest radiograph should be obtained as baseline
6. Antimicrobial treatment should be instituted without delay (for dosage, route of administration, dose adjustment for renal and hepatic impairment on specific agents, see Appendix I)

***Standard practice of blood cultures:**

- Adequate volume of blood drawn is critical for successful isolation of microorganisms
- Aerobic and anaerobic blood culture bottle should be obtained with 10 mL of blood collected in each bottle (adult)
- Minimum of 2 sets of cultures (2 aerobic and 2 anaerobic blood culture bottles) should be obtained
- In case of a line with multiple lumens, each lumen should be sampled
- Peripheral cultures are not necessary unless single-lumen catheter

Antibiotic Therapy

A flow diagram with suggested antibiotic therapy for inpatients with fever and neutropenia is presented in Figure 47–1. We recommend a systematic approach in which specific questions are answered in order:

1. Is the patient clinically stable?

In a *clinically stable patient* who does not need vancomycin (uncomplicated fever and neutropenia), intravenous monotherapy with an anti–pseudomonal β-lactam (cephalosporin or carbapenem)* is recommended. Combination therapy with a β-lactam + aminoglycoside has been associated with more toxicity and no better outcome and is not recommended in uncomplicated fever and neutropenia

- **Ceftazidime** 2000 mg intravenously every 8 hours
- **Cefepime** 2000 mg intravenously every 8 hours
- **Imipenem-cilastatin** 500 mg intravenously every 6 hours
- **Meropenem** 1000 mg intravenously every 8 hours

*It is critically important for clinicians to be familiar with the pattern of resistance to the various β-lactam antibiotics in their institutions. In vitro susceptibility may vary widely among different institutions and make some of these alternatives unacceptable

Furno P et al. Lancet Infect Dis 2002;2:231–242
Paul M et al. Br Med J 2003;326:1111–1115

2. Is the addition of vancomycin required?

Indications for use of vancomycin:

1. Severe sepsis or septic shock
2. Clinically apparent catheter-related infection
3. Known colonization with methicillin-resistant *Staphylococcus aureus* (MRSA) or penicillin-resistant *Streptococcus pneumoniae*
4. Severe mucositis (risk of infection with *viridans* group *Streptococcus*)

- **Vancomycin** 1000 mg intravenously every 12 hours

3. Is sepsis or septic shock present?

In the presence of severe sepsis or septic shock, broad-spectrum coverage for gram-negative bacilli and viridans group streptococci should be instituted. Many authorities recommend dual therapy (β-lactam + aminoglycoside or β-lactam + fluoroquinolone) to maximize the antimicrobial spectrum. Vancomycin is typically added in this situation. Common regimens include:

β-Lactam + **aminoglycoside** + vancomycin *or* β-lactam + **fluoroquinolone** + vancomycin

β-Lactam:	**Ceftazidime** 2000 mg intravenously every 8 hours, *or* **Cefepime** 2000 mg intravenously every 8 hours, *or* **Meropenem** 1000 mg intravenously every 8 hours, *or* **Imipenem** 500 mg intravenously every 6 hours
Aminoglicoside:	**Gentamicin** 4–7 mg/kg intravenously every day, *or* **Tobramycin** 4–7 mg/kg intravenously every day, *or* **Amikacin** 15 mg/kg intravenously every day
Fluoroquinolone:	**Ciprofloxacin** 400 mg intravenously every 8 hours, *or* **Levofloxacin** 750 mg intravenously every day, *or* **Moxifloxacin** 400 mg intravenously every day
Vancomycin:	**Vancomycin** 1000 mg intravenously every 12 hours

Hughes WT et al. Clin Infect Dis 2002;34:730–751

4. Is oral therapy acceptable?

If a patient has a MASCC (Multinational Association for Supportive Care in Cancer) Index ≥21, (Klastersky J et al.), oral antibiotics may be used. This scoring system has good sensitivity and specificity to identify patients at low risk for complications. A recommended regimen is:

- **Ciprofloxacin** 750 mg + **amoxicillin/clavulanic acid** 875 mg/125 mg orally twice a day (Freifeld A et al.)

[Start oral treatment in the inpatient setting. After 24 hours of observation, selected patients with support from a personal caregiver (friend, relative, or professional), reliable telecommunications, readily available transportation, and close access to emergency medical care may be discharged]

Freifeld A et al. NEJM 1999;341:305–311
Klastersky J et al. JCO 2000;18:3038–3051

(*continued*)

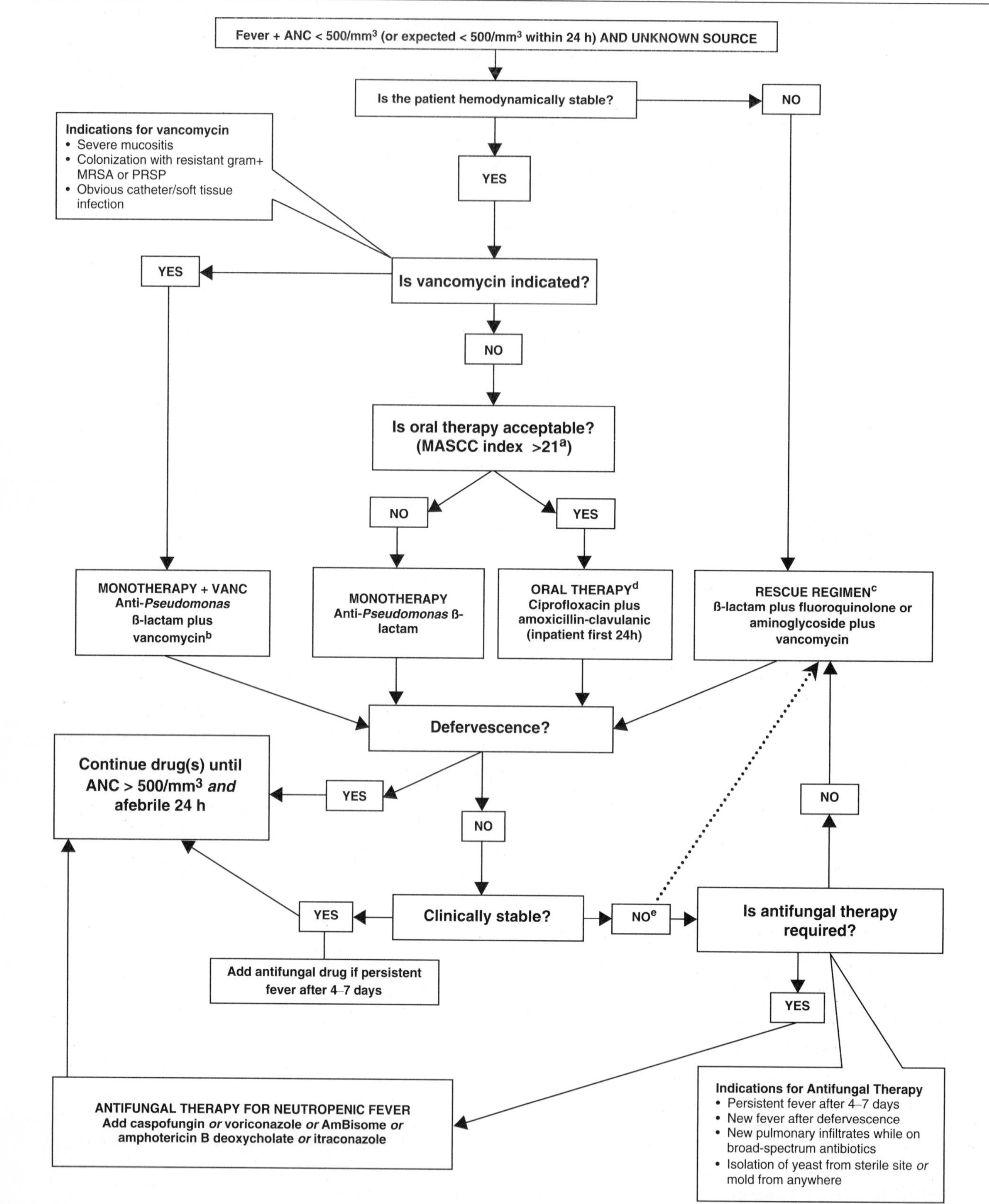

Figure 47–1. [a]MASCC Index (Multinational Association of Supportive Care in Cancer. Burden of illness: no or mild symptoms, +5; moderate symptoms, +3; no hypotension, +5; no chronic obstructive pulmonary disease, +4; solid tumor or no previous fungal infection, +4; no dehydration, +3; outpatient status, +3; age <60 years, +2. A MASCC Index ≥21 has been associated with a relatively low risk of severe complications.

[b]Vancomycin should be discontinued after 48 hours if there is no bacteriologic documentation of a pathogen requiring its use, except in soft tissue or tunnel infections.

[c]This "rescue" antibacterial regimen varies among institutions depending on the local patterns of antibiotic resistance. β-lactum + fluoroquinolone/aminogylcoside + vancomycin is typical, but it may be broader depending on the prevalence of multiresistant pathogens.

[d]We recommend initiating oral therapy in the hospital (see text for a detailed discussion).

[e]Dashed line used to indicate that a change in antibacterial agents may not be needed

MRSA, methicillin (oxacillin)-resistant *Staphylococcus aureus*; PRSP, penicillin-resistant *Streptococcus pneumoniae*.

Antibiotic Therapy (*continued*)

5. Does the patient have a fever, and is the patient clinically stable?

a. If the fever resolves, then antibiotics are continued until ANC $\geq$500/mm^3

b. For a **clinically or microbiologically documented** bacterial infection, antibiotics should be continued for the standard amount of time typically used to treat such infection or until resolution of neutropenia, whichever is longer

c. For uncomplicated fever and neutropenia **of uncertain origin**, antibiotics should be continued until the fever has resolved and the ANC is >500/mm^3 for 24 hours. If there was no documented fungal infection, antifungal agents can also be discontinued at this time

d. If fever persists and the patient remains neutropenic but with no other clinical changes, continue the initial regimen, performing daily meticulous physical exam and cultures, and add an antifungal agent after 4 days of fever. In many of these cases, the fever abates with neutrophil recovery and no infection is documented. The common practice of empirically adding vancomycin in this setting has been shown to be ineffective in a randomized placebo-controlled clinical trial and should be discouraged

e. If fever persists and the patient's condition deteriorates, change the antibacterial agents and evaluate exhaustively for an invasive fungal infection. In some cases, an change in antibacterial agents *may not be needed* (indicated by the dashed line in the figure). The introduction of antifungal agents has been made easier by the availability of less toxic drugs

Cometta A et al. Clin Infect Dis 2003;37:382–389

Antibiotic Choices in Special Clinical Circumstances

Penicillin-allergic patient:
- **Aztreonam** 2000 mg intravenously every 6 hours , *plus*
- **Vancomycin** 1000 mg intravenously every 12 hours

Abdominal pain (consider neutropenic enterocolitis):
- **Imipenem-cilastatin** 500 mg intravenously every 6 hours, *or*
- **Meropenem** 1000 mg intravenously every 8 hours, *or*
- **Ceftazidime** 2000 mg intravenously every 8 hours, *plus*
  Metronidazole 500 mg intravenously every 6 hours[a], *or*
- **Cefepime** 2000 mg intravenously every 8 hours, *plus*
  Metronidazole 500 mg intravenously every 6 hours[a]

[a]The addition of metronidazole may be the preferred approach until *Clostridium difficile* is ruled out

Pulmonary infiltrates in the setting of neutropenia + fever[b]:
- **Imipenem-cilastatin or meropenem or ceftazidime or cefepime**[c] intravenously, *plus*
  Levofloxacin 750 mg intravenously every 24 hours, *or*
- **Imipenem-cilastatin, meropenem, ceftazidime, or cefepime**[c] intravenously, *plus*
  Moxifloxacin 400 mg intravenously every 24 hours, *or*
- **Imipenem-cilastatin, meropenem, ceftazidime, or cefepime**[c] intravenously, *plus*
  Gatifloxacin 400 mg intravenously every 24 hours

[b]Early CT and bronchoalveolar lavage is recommended, because the array of potential pathogens in these patients makes empirical management of pneumonia particularly risky. The inclusion of a fluoroquinolone in this situation aims to provide adequate coverage for the common causes of community-acquired pneumonia

[c]dose as for abdominal pain above

Maschmeyer G et al. Ann Hematol 2003;82(suppl 2):S118–126

Empirical Antifungal Therapy (see table that follows)

See table that follows

Initial anti-infective therapy is aimed at bacterial infection. Invasive fungal infections are uncommon early in the course of neutropenia, but their risk increases with the duration and degree of neutropenia. *Candida* infections tend to appear earlier than mold infections. These infections may be difficult to diagnose and are associated with high mortality. Over the years, empirical addition of antifungal therapy in neutropenic fever has become standard practice. Empirical addition of antifungal agents should not replace a thorough search for invasive fungal infection. This should usually include a CT of the chest and serum galactomannan antigen. The choice of empirical antifungal therapy should be based on the clinical picture, prior use of antifungal drugs, toxicity of the agent, and its spectrum of action

Indications:

- Persistent fever after 4–7 days of antibacterial antibiotics
- New fever after defervescence
- New pulmonary infiltrates while on broad-spectrum antibiotics
- Isolation of yeast from sterile site *or* mold from anywhere

European Organization for Research on Therapy of Cancer International Antimicrobial Therapy Cooperative Group. Am J Med 1989;86(6 Pt 1):668–672
Klastersky J [Editorial]. NEJM 2004;351:1445–1447
Pizzo PA et al. Am J Med 1982;72:101–111

<table>
<tr><th>Drug Name</th><th>Administration</th><th>Spectrum of Activity</th><th colspan="2">Toxicity</th><th>References</th></tr>
<tr><td>Amphotericin B desoxycholate</td><td>0.6–1 mg/kg per day intravenously over 2–6 hours</td><td>Amphotericin B (as desoxycholate or in a lipid formulation) has activity against most yeasts, Aspergillus, and Zygomycetes. It is not active against Scedosporium, Fusarium, and dematiaceous molds</td><td colspan="2">Most toxic. High incidence of renal insufficiency. One liter of 0.9% NS before or around the infusion may prevent nephrotoxicity</td><td>Pizzo PA et al. AM J Med 1982;72:101–111
Am J Med 1989; 86:668–672</td></tr>
<tr><td colspan="6">Acetaminophen 650 mg PO ± diphenhydramine 12.5–50 mg PO/IV may be given before amphotericin. Additional doses of acetaminophen and diphenhydramine may be given PRN or on a preset schedule. Alternatively, one can observe a patient's response to an initial dose and give premedication only if amphotericin was not tolerated
Meperidine 25 mg/dose may be given intravenously for rigors (oral administration not effective). An additional two doses of meperidine may be administered at 10-minute intervals (total: 3 doses) if rigors persist. Decreasing rate of administration may mitigate infusion-related effects</td></tr>
<tr><td>Liposomal amphotericin B (Ambisome®)</td><td>3–7.5 mg/kg per day intravenously over 120 minutes [duration of administration may be reduced to 60 minuets if infusion over 120 minutes is tolerated]</td><td>Activity against most yeasts, Aspergillus, and Zygomycetes. It is not active against Scedosporium, Fusarium, and dematiaceous molds</td><td colspan="2">Less toxic than amphotericin B desoxycholate, but not more effective</td><td>Walsh TJ et al. NEJM 1999; 340:764–771</td></tr>
<tr><td>Voriconazole</td><td>Initial dose: 6 mg/kg intravenously every 12 hours for 24 hours (2 doses), followed by Maintenance dose: 4 mg/kg intravenously every 12 hours</td><td>No significant activity against Zygomycetes (Mucor, Rhizopus, etc). May be preferable to lipid formulations of amphotericin B against Fusarium and Scedosporium</td><td rowspan="3">Interacts with multiple drugs metabolized by cytochrome P450 so that the dose of other drugs may need to be adjusted. Liver enzyme abnormalities have been described with all the azoles, and hepatic failure has been reported. Monitor LFTs weekly to biweekly, then monthly</td><td>No need for adjustment in renal insufficiency</td><td>Walsh TJ et al. NEJM 2002; 346:225–234</td></tr>
<tr><td>Itraconazole</td><td>Initial dose: 200 mg intravenously every 12 hours for 48 hours (4 doses), followed by Maintenance dose: 200 mg intravenously daily</td><td>Active against yeast, Aspergillus, and some dematiaceous molds</td><td>The carrier used in the intravenous formulation is nephrotoxic</td><td>Boogaerts M et al. Ann Intern Med 2001;135: 412–422</td></tr>
<tr><td>Fluconazole</td><td>400 mg intravenously or orally once or twice daily</td><td>Inactive against molds. Empirical administration for persistent fever and neutropenia should be considered only when risk of aspergillosis is very low</td><td>Adjust dose in renal insufficiency: 50% doses for creatinine clearance <50 mL/min</td><td>Winston DJ et al. Am J Med 2000; 108:282–289</td></tr>
<tr><td>Caspofungin</td><td>Loading dose: 70 mg intravenously on the first day of treatment, followed by Maintenance dose: 50 mg intravenously daily</td><td>Active only against Candida and Aspergillus</td><td colspan="2">Caspofungin has been shown to be equivalent to liposomal amphotericin B in the management of uncomplicated fever and neutropenia, but its efficacy compared with other agents in the treatment of established fungal infections in neutropenic patients is unknown</td><td>Walsh TJ et al. NEJM 2004; 351:1391-402</td></tr>
</table>

Management of Specific Clinical Syndromes During Neutropenia

Diagnostic Considerations	Management
Skin/Soft Tissue Infections	
1. Prompt biopsy with histologic staining and culture for bacteria, mycobacteria, viruses, and fungi 2. A vesicle should be unroofed and a scraping of the base examined by direct fluorescence assay to make the diagnosis of varicella zoster virus. The scrapings should also be sent for herpes simplex virus culture **Pathogens:** • Gram-negative bacilli (eg, *P. aeruginosa*, *Aeromonas* spp, *Plesiomonas shigelloides*) • *Streptococcus pyogenes* • *Staphylococcus aureus* • Varicella zoster virus (VZV) • Herpes simplex virus (HSV) • *Candida* spp • *Zygomycetes* (eg, *Rhizopus*, *Mucor*)	• For ecthyma gangrenosum include coverage of *Pseudomonas:* **Ceftazidime** 2000 mg intravenously every 8 hours, *or* **Cefepime** 2000 mg intravenously every 8 hours, *or* **Ciprofloxacin** 400 mg intravenously every 8 hours • Treat *S. pyogenes* infections aggressively with: **Penicillin** G 4 million units intravenously every 4 hours, *plus* **Clindamycin** 900 mg intravenously every 8 hours, *plus* surgical debridement • In case of streptococcal shock syndrome, IVIG may be helpful: **IVIG** 1000 mg/kg of body weight on day 1, *followed by* **IVIG** 500 mg/kg on days 2 and 3 • Treat perianal cellulitis with broad-spectrum coverage including anaerobes: **Imipenem** 500–1000 mg intravenously every 6 hours, *or* **Meropenem** 1000 mg intravenously every 8 hours • *VZV:* **Acyclovir** 10 mg/kg intravenously every 8 hours • *HSV:* **Acyclovir** 5 mg/kg intravenously every 8 hours
Sinusitis	
1. Evaluate with CT scan and examination by otolaryngologist 2. Take tissue biopsy if there is suspicion of fungal infection or there is no response to antibiotic therapy after 72 hours **Pathogens:** • *P. aeruginosa* • *S. aureus* • Fungi: *Aspergillus* spp, *Zygomycetes* (eg, *Mucor*, *Rhizopus*), dematiaceous molds	• Broad-spectrum coverage including *Pseudomonas* and *S. aureus* **Imipenem** 500–1000 mg IV every 6 hours, *or* **Meropenem** 1000 mg intravenously every 8 hours, *or* **Cefepime** 2000 mg intravenously every 8 hours • Consider fungal coverage: **Amphotericin B sodium desoxycholate** 1 mg/kg intravenously every day, *or* An **amphotericin B lipid formulation** 5 mg/kg intravenously every day
Pulmonary Infections	
1. CT scan and bronchoalveolar lavage should be performed early 2. Pneumonia during neutropenia is often caused by gram-negative bacilli and *S. aureus*, but can also be caused by community-acquired pneumonia pathogens 3. Neutropenic patients are at risk for invasive fungal infections, particularly aspergillosis **Pathogens:** • Gram-negative bacilli • *S. aureus* • *Streptococcus pneumoniae* • *Haemophilus influenzae* • *Legionella* spp • *Chlamydiophyla pneumoniae* • Invasive fungal infections: *Aspergillus*, *Zygomycetes*, *Fusarium*	• Cefepime, imipenem, and meropenem have better activity than ceftazidime against *S. pneumoniae* **Cefepime** 2000 mg intravenously every 8 hours, *or* **Imipenem** 500–1000 mg intravenously every 6 hours, *or* **Meropenem** 1000 mg intravenously every 8 hours • Adding coverage for atypical pathogens is recommended: **Levofloxacin** 750 mg intravenously every day, *or* **Moxifloxacin** 400 mg intravenously every day, *or* **Azithromycin** 500 mg intravenously every day • If pneumonia develops while the patient is on antibiotics, antifungal coverage should be added: **Amphotericin B desoxycholate** 1 mg/kg intravenously every day, *or* **Amphotericin B lipid formulation** 5 mg/kg intravenously every day, *or* **Voriconazole** 6 mg/kg intravenously every 12 hours × 2 loading doses, followed by 4 mg/kg intravenously every 12 hours *or* **Caspofungin 70 mg** intravenously loading dose, followed by 50 mg every day

(continued)

Diagnostic Considerations	Management
Gastrointestinal Tract Infections	
1. Lesions associated with mucositis or esophagitis can become superinfected **Pathogens:** • *Candida* (oral mucositis and esophagitis) • HSV (oral mucositis and esophagitis) • CMV (esophagitis)	• Mucositis or esophagitis: **Acyclovir** 5 mg/kg intravenously every 8 hours, *and* **Fluconazole** 400 mg intravenously every day
2. Diarrhea is most commonly caused by *Clostridium difficile* (send toxin assay) but can also be caused by other organisms **Pathogens:** • *Salmonella* spp • *Shigella* spp • *Aeromonas* spp • *Escherichia coli* • Viruses: Rotavirus, adenovirus, astrovirus, calicivirus • Parasites: *Giardia, Cryptosporidium*	• For diarrhea caused by *C. difficile*: **Metronidazole** 500 mg intravenously or orally every 6–8 hours for 10–14 days **Vancomycin** 125–250 mg orally every 6 hours if refractory to metronidazole [For *C. difficile*, no follow-up testing is recommended, because treatment of carriers is not recommended]
3. Enterocolitis in neutropenic patients (typhlitis) is most commonly caused by a mix of bowel organisms, including *Clostridium* species and *Pseudomonas* **Pathogens:** • Enteric gram-negative bacilli • *Clostridium* species • *P. aeruginosa*	• For enterocolitis in neutropenic patients, use broad-spectrum coverage including *Pseudomonas* coverage: **Imipenem** 500–1000 mg intravenously every 6 hours, *or* **Meropenem** 1000 mg intravenously every 8 hours, *or* **Ceftazidime** 2000 mg intravenously every 8 hours, *plus* **Metronidazole** 500 mg intravenously every 6 hours ± **Vancomycin** 1000 mg intravenously every 12 hours
Urinary Tract Infections	
1. Treat bacteriuria in febrile neutropenic patients 2. Consider whether candiduria may represent disseminated candidiasis **Pathogens:** • Enteric gram-negative bacilli: *E. coli, Klebsiella* spp • *P. aeruginosa* (prior antibiotics, instrumentation, stents) • *Enterococcus* spp (including VRE) • *Candida spp*	• Remove Foley catheter to clear colonization • In a neutropenic patient, treat bacteriuria/ candiduria regardless of symptoms –Candiduria may be treated with **fluconazole** 400 mg intravenously or orally every day –Treat bacteriuria according to susceptibility testing
CNS Infections	
1. Bacteria cause most cases of meningitis (*S. pneumoniae, Listeria monocytogenes, Neisseria meningitidis*, other gram-negative bacilli) 2. In patients with cell-mediated immunodeficiency, also consider *Listeria* or *Cryptococcus neoformans* 3. Encephalitis is most commonly caused by HSV, but consider other viruses 4. Brain abscesses during neutropenia are almost always caused by fungi **Pathogens:** • *S. pneumoniae* • *L. monocytogenes* • *N. meningitidis* • *Candida* spp, *Aspergillus* spp (brain abscess during neutropenia) • Cryptococcus (meningitis in T-cell immunodeficiency) • Herpes simplex 1	Bacterial meningitis during neutropenia: **Ceftazidime** 2000 mg intravenously every 8 hours, *plus* **Vancomycin** 1000 mg intravenously every 12 hours, *plus* **Ampicillin** 2000 mg intravenously every 4 hours Cryptococcal meningitis: **Amphotericin B desoxycholate** 1 mg/kg intravenously every day, *or* An **amphotericin B lipid formulation** 6 mg/kg intravenously every day, *with* **Flucytosine** 25 mg/kg per dose orally every 6 hours (adjust dosage for renal insufficiency) Encephalitis: **Acyclovir** 10 mg/kg intravenously every 8 hours until HSV encephalitis has been ruled out

Viral Infections During Neutropenia

Diagnostic Considerations	Management
Herpes Simplex Virus	
1. HSV may reactivate during neutropenia and worsen chemotherapy or radiation therapy-induced mucositis 2. Suspicious oral and genital lesions should be cultured for HSV 3. Pending culture results, empirical treatment of suspicious lesions should be initiated 4. Reactivation during one cycle of chemotherapy does not imply that HSV recurrence will follow each cycle, and prophylactic treatment is not necessary. If reactivation occurs after several cycles of chemotherapy, attempt prevention with valacyclovir 500 mg per dose orally twice daily 5. When to use intravenous versus oral therapy? Oral agents may be as effective as intravenous acyclovir; the decision is based on the presence of nausea, vomiting, or clinical situations that make absorption questionable	**Acyclovir** 5 mg/kg per dose intravenously every 8 hours, *or* **Valacyclovir** 500 mg per dose orally twice daily, *or* **Famciclovir** 250 mg per dose orally twice daily
Varicella Zoster	
1. VZV reactivation is related more to defects in cell-mediated immunity than to neutropenia 2. A maculopapular and vesicular rash in a dermatomal distribution suggests VZV infection, although HSV may have a similar presentation 3. A vesicle should be unroofed and a scraping of the base examined by direct fluorescence assay to establish a diagnosis 4. The main risk of VZV in immunocompromised patients is visceral dissemination. If infection is documented, respiratory precautions should be instituted and treatment started with high-dose intravenous acyclovir	**Acyclovir** 10 mg/kg per dose intravenously every 8 hours, *or* **Acyclovir** 500 mg/m^2 per dose intravenously every 8 hours
Cytomegalovirus	
1. CMV is an uncommon pathogen during neutropenia, but it can occur in the setting of coexisting severe defects of cell-mediated immunity 2. Determination of pp65 antigenemia cannot be used during neutropenia because the test requires an ANC >1000/mm^3 to quantify the number CMV-infected white blood cells 3. CMV disease (rather than CMV reactivation determined by PCR or pp65 antigenemia) is unusual except in HIV (retinitis, colitis) and after allogeneic stem cell transplantation (pneumonitis, enterocolitis) 4. Diagnosis of CMV colitis requires rectosigmoidoscopy or colonoscopy with biopsy. The tissue sample should be processed both for viral culture and immunohistochemistry, since there are cases diagnosed by one modality and not the other. A common differential diagnosis involves acute graft-versus-host disease, *C. difficile* colitis, and neutropenic enterocolitis (typhlitis). Tissue examination is mandatory because more than one process may be present 5. The diagnosis of CMV pneumonitis requires the appropriate host (typically an allogeneic stem cell transplant recipient), a consistent clinical presentation, and the presence of CMV in the respiratory secretions (Ljungman P et al. Clin Infect Dis 2002;34:1094–1097) 6. For CMV pneumonitis, the treatment of choice is ganciclovir	CMV pneumonitis: **Ganciclovir** 5 mg/kg intravenously every 12 hours for 21 days (adjust dose for renal insufficiency), *plus* **IVIG** 500 mg/kg intravenously every 48 hours for 3 weeks, *or* **Foscarnet** 90 mg/kg intravenously every 12 hours [As a single agent Foscarnet may be substituted for ganciclovir to avoid the potential bone marrow toxicity of ganciclovir]

Antibacterial, Antifungal and Antiviral Agents

Dose/Dosage and Administration Route and Schedule	Adjustments for Renal Impairment (Clcr = Creatinine Clearance)	Adjustments for Hepatic Impairment

Antibacterials

Amikacin

Multiple-Daily Administration (MDA):
Loading Dose: Amikacin 8 mg/kg, administer intravenously over 30–60 minutes × 1 dose, followed by
Maintenance Doses: Amikacin 7.5 mg/kg/dose, administer intravenously over 30–60 minutes every 12 hours[a]

or

Once-Daily Administration (ODA):
Amikacin 15 mg/kg/dose, administer intravenously over 30–60 minutes every 24 hours[a]

	MDA	ODA
Peak	15–30 μg/mL	56-54 μg/mL
Trough	5–10 μg/mL	<1 μg/mL
Toxic Trough	>10μg/mL	>35 μg/mL

SI: μmol/L = 1.71 × mg/L

Adjustments for Renal Impairment: In patients with renal impairment, dosage and/or administration intervals should be adjusted based on amikacin serum levels

Adjustments for Hepatic Impairment: In patients with cirrhosis and ascites, amikacin dosage should be based on whole body weight rather than lean weight to reflect an increase in drug distribution volume

Ampicillin + Sulbacta (2 mg:1 mg) [Unasyn®]

Unasyn® 3000 mg (contains ampicillin 2000 mg + sulbactam 1000 mg), administer intravenously by push over 10–15 minutes every 6 hours

or

Unasyn® 3000 mg (contains ampicillin 2000 mg + sulbactam 1000 mg), administer intravenously by infusion over 15–30 minutes every 6 hours

Adjustments for Renal Impairment:

Clcr (mL/min)	Dose & Schedule
≥30	3000 mg q 6–8 h
15–29	3000 mg q 12 h
5–14	3000 mg q 24 h

Adjustments for Hepatic Impairment: No treatment modifications are indicated

Cefazolin

Cefazolin 2000 mg, administer intravenously by push over 3–5 minutes every 6–8 hours

or

Cefazolin 2000 mg, administer intravenously by infusion over 15–30 minutes every 6–8 hours

Adjustments for Renal Impairment:

Clcr (mL/min)	Dose & Schedule
≥55	2000 mg q 6–8 h
35–54	2000 mg q 8 h
11–34	1000 mg q 12 h
≤10	1000 mg q 24 h

Adjustments for Hepatic Impairment: No treatment modifications are indicated

(*continued*)

Antibacterial, Antifungal and Antiviral Agents (*continued*)

Dose/Dosage and Administration Route and Schedule	Adjustments for Renal Impairment (Clcr = Creatinine Clearance)	Adjustments for Hepatic Impairment

Cefepime

Dose/Dosage and Administration Route and Schedule: Cefepime 2000 mg, administer intravenously over 30 minutes every 8–12 hours

Adjustments for Renal Impairment:

Clcr (mL/min)	Dose & Schedule	
>60	2000 mg q 12h	2000 mg q 8h
30–60	2000 mg q 24h	2000 mg q 12h
11– 29	1000 mg q 24h	2000 mg q 24h
<10	500 mg q 24h	1000 mg q 24h

Adjustments for Hepatic Impairment: No treatment modifications are indicated

Ceftazidime

Dose/Dosage and Administration Route and Schedule: Ceftazidime 2000 mg, administer intravenously by push over 3–5 minutes every 8–12 hours

or

Ceftazidime 2000 mg, administer intravenously by infusion over 15–30 minutes every 8–12 hours

Adjustments for Renal Impairment:

Clcr (mL/min)	Dose & Schedule
≥51	2000 mg q 8–12h
31–50	1000 mg q 12h
16–30	1000 mg q 24h
6–15	500 mg q 24h
<5	500 mg q 48h

Adjustments for Hepatic Impairment: No treatment modifications are indicated

Ciprofloxacin

Dose/Dosage and Administration Route and Schedule: Ciprofloxacin 400 mg, administer intravenously over 60 min every 12 hours (every 8h in fever and neutropenia)

or

Ciprofloxacin 750 mg, administer orally every 12 hours

[In the USA, Ciprofloxacin is available in various formulations for oral administration, including: immediate-release tablets (100-, 250-, 500-, 750-mg strengths), extended-release tablets (500- & 1000-mg strengths), powder for preparing a liquid suspension, and a liquid product containing microencapsulated ciprofloxacin]

Adjustments for Renal Impairment:

	Dose & Schedule by Administration Route	
Clcr (mL/min)	Intravenous	Oral
>50	400 mg q 12h	750 mg q 12h
>30		—
30–50	—	250–500 mg q 12h
5–29	200–400 mg q 18–24h	250–500 mg q 18h
On dialysis	—	250–500 mg q 24h after dialysis

Adjustments for Hepatic Impairment: No treatment modifications are indicated, but monitor closely for adverse events

(*continued*)

Antibacterial, Antifungal and Antiviral Agents (*continued*)

<table>
<tr><th>Dose/Dosage and Administration Route and Schedule</th><th>Adjustments for Renal Impairment (Clcr = Creatinine Clearance)</th><th>Adjustments for Hepatic Impairment</th></tr>
<tr><th colspan="3">Clarithromycin</th></tr>
<tr><td>Clarithromycin 500 mg, administer orally every 12 hours

In the USA, Clarithromycin is available in several formulations for oral administration, including: immediate-release tablets (250 or 500-mg/tablet), an extended-release 500-mg tablet, and granulated products for preparing liquid suspensions (125-mg/5 mL or 250-mg/5 mL). BiaxinAE FilmtabAE (clarithromycin tablets, USP), BiaxinÆ XL FilmtabÆ (clarithromycin extended-release tablets), BiaxinÆ Granules (clarithromycin for oral suspension, USP) product label, December 2003. Abbott Laboratories, North Chicago, IL</td><td><table><tr><th>Clcr (mL/min)</th><th>Dose & Schedule</th></tr><tr><td>60</td><td>500 mg q 12h</td></tr><tr><td>30-60</td><td>250 mg q 12h</td></tr><tr><td><30</td><td>125 m g q 12h</td></tr></table></td><td>No treatment modifications are indicated</td></tr>
<tr><th colspan="3">Erythromycin Lactobionate</th></tr>
<tr><td>Erythromycin Lactobionate 1000 mg administer intravenously over 20–60 minutes every 6 hours</td><td><table><tr><th>Clcr (mL/min)</th><th>Dose & Schedule</th></tr><tr><td>≥10</td><td>1000 mg q 6h</td></tr><tr><td><10</td><td>500–750 mg q 6h, BUT NOT >2000 mg/d</td></tr></table></td><td>No treatment modifications are indicated, but monitor closely for adverse events</td></tr>
<tr><th colspan="3">Gentamicin</th></tr>
<tr><td>Multiple-Daily Administration (MDA):
Loading Dose: Gentamicin 2 mg/kg × 1 dose administer intravenously over 30–60 minutes, followed by
Maintenance Doses: Gentamicin 1.7 mg/kg/dose, administer intravenously over 30–60 minutes every 8 hours[a]
or
Once-Daily Administration (ODA):
Gentamicin 4–7 mg/kg/dose, administer intravenously over 30–60 minutes every 24 hours[a]
<table><tr><th></th><th>MDA</th><th>ODA</th></tr><tr><td>Peak</td><td>4–10 μg/mL</td><td>16–24 μg/mL</td></tr><tr><td>Trough</td><td>1–2 μg/mL</td><td><1 μg/mL</td></tr><tr><td>Toxic Trough</td><td>≥2 μg/mL</td><td>≥2 μg/mL</td></tr></table>SI: μmol/L = 2.09 × mg/L</td><td>In patients with renal impairment, dosage and/or administration intervals should be adjusted based on gentamicin serum levels.</td><td>No treatment modifications are indicated</td></tr>
</table>

(*continued*)

Antibacterial, Antifungal and Antiviral Agents (*continued*)

Dose/Dosage and Administration Route and Schedule	Adjustments for Renal Impairment (Clcr = Creatinine Clearance)	Adjustments for Hepatic Impairment

Imipenem-Cilastatin

Dose/Dosage and Administration Route and Schedule: Imipenem-cilastatin 500 mg administer intravenously over 20–60 minutes every 6 hours

[Maximum total daily dosage should not exceed 50 mg/kg/day]

Adjustments for Renal Impairment:

Body Weight	Clcr (mL/min/1.73 m²) 6–20	21–40	41–70	≥71
≥70 kg		250 mg q 6h	500 mg q 8h	500 mg q 6h
60 kg	250 mg q 12h	250 mg q 8h	250 mg q 6h	500 mg q 8h
50 kg		250 mg q 12h	250 mg q 8h	
40 kg				250 mg q 6h
30 kg	125 mg q 12h	125 mg q 8h	125 mg q 6h	250 mg q 8h

- Patients with Clcr ≤5 mL/min/1.73 m² should not receive imipenem-cilastatin unless hemodialysis is instituted within 48 hours
- There is inadequate information to recommend imipenem-cilastatin use for patients undergoing peritoneal dialysis.
- For hemodialyzed patients with Clcr ≤5 mL/min/1.73 m², use the weight-appropriate dosage recommendations for patients with Clcr = 6–20 mL/min/1.73 m². (see Table) Administer the imipenem-cilastatin after hemodialysis and at 12 hour intervals after the end of hemodialysis

Adjustments for Hepatic Impairment: No treatment modifications are indicated

Levofloxacin

Dose/Dosage and Administration Route and Schedule: Levofloxacin 500–750 mg, administer intravenously over at least 60 minutes (500-mg dose) to 90 minutes (750-mg dose), once daily

or

Levofloxacin 500–750 mg, administer orally once daily

In the USA, Levofloxacin is available in three formulations for oral administration, including: immediate-release tablets (250, 500, and 750 mg/tablet) and an oral solution (25 mg/mL). Levaquin® (levofloxacin) Tablets, Levaquin® (levofloxacin) Oral Solution product label, October 2004. Ortho-McNeil Pharmaceutical, Inc., Raritan, NJ

Adjustments for Renal Impairment:

Clcr (mL/min)	Initial Dose	Subsequent Doses
Acute bacterial exacerbation of chronic bronchitis, community-acquired pneumonia, acute maxillary sinusitis, uncomplicated SSSI, chronic bacterial prostatitis		
50–80 mL/min	No dose adjustment is required	
20–49 mL/min	500 mg	250 mg q 24h
10–19 mL/min	500 mg	250 mg q 48h
Hemodialysis	500 mg	250 mg q 48h
CAPD	500 mg	250 mg q 48h
Complicated SSSI, nosocomial pneumonia, community-acquired pneumonia		
50–80 mL/min	No dose adjustment is required	
20–49 mL/min	750 mg	750 mg q 48h
10–19 mL/min	750 mg	500 mg q 48h
Hemodialysis	750 mg	500 mg q 48h
CAPD	750 mg	500 mg q 48h
Complicated UTI, acute pyelonephritis		
≥20 mL/min	No dosage adjustment required	
10–19 mL/min	250 mg	250 mg q 48 h
Uncomplicated UTI		
No dosage adjustment required		

SSSI, skin and skin structure infections; CAPD, chronic ambulatory peritoneal dialysis

Adjustments for Hepatic Impairment: No modification is necessary

(*continued*)

<table>
<tr><th colspan="3">Antibacterial, Antifungal and Antiviral Agents (continued)</th></tr>
<tr><th>Dose/Dosage and Administration Route and Schedule</th><th>Adjustments for Renal Impairment (Clcr = Creatinine Clearance)</th><th>Adjustments for Hepatic Impairment</th></tr>
<tr><th colspan="3">Linezolid</th></tr>
<tr><td>Linezolid 600 mg, administer intravenously over 30–120 minutes every 12 hours
or
Linezolid 600 mg, administer orally every 12 hours
In the USA, Linezolid is available in several formulations for oral administration, including: immediate-release film-coated tablets (400 or 600 mg linezolid/tablet) and powdered linezolid for preparing a liquid suspension (100 mg/5 mL). Zyvox® Linezolid Injection. Linezolid Tablets, Linezolid for Oral Suspension product label, September 2004. Pharmacia & Upjohn Division of Pfizer Inc, NY, NY</td><td>No treatment modifications are indicated, but monitor closely for adverse events</td><td>No modification is necessary for patients with mild-to-moderate hepatic insufficiency (Child-Pugh classes A & B). Linezolid use has not been studied in patients with more severe hepatic insufficiency</td></tr>
<tr><th colspan="3">Meropenem</th></tr>
<tr><td>Meropenem 1000 mg, administer intravenously by push over 3–5 minutes every 8 hours
or
Meropenem 1000 mg, administer intravenously by infusion over 15–30 minutes every 8 hours</td><td><table><tr><th>Clcr (mL/min)</th><th>Dose & Schedule</th></tr><tr><td>>51</td><td>1000 mg q 8h</td></tr><tr><td>26–50</td><td>1000 mg q 12h</td></tr><tr><td>10–25</td><td>500 mg q 12h</td></tr><tr><td><10</td><td>500 mg q 24h</td></tr></table></td><td>No modification is necessary</td></tr>
<tr><th colspan="3">Metronidazole</th></tr>
<tr><td>Metronidazole 500 mg, administer intravenously over 60 minutes every 6 hours
or
Metronidazole 500 mg, administer orally every 6 hours
or
Metronidazole 2000 mg/day, administer by continuous intravenous infusion over 24 hours
In the USA, Metronidazole is available generically in various formulations for oral administration, including: immediate-release tablets (250 & 500 mg), capsules (375 mg), and extended-release tablets (750 mg)</td><td><table><tr><th>Clcr (mL/min)</th><th>Dose & Schedule</th></tr><tr><td><10 mL/min</td><td>250 mg q 6h</td></tr></table></td><td>Metronidazole metabolism decreases in severe hepatic disease; however, correlates between hepatic dysfunction and altered metronidazole metabolism have not been identified, and guidelines for modifying metronidazole use have not been established</td></tr>
<tr><th colspan="3">Nafcillin</th></tr>
<tr><td>Nafcillin 2000 mg, administer intravenously by push over 5–10 minutes every 4 hours
or
Nafcillin 2000 mg, administer intravenously by infusion over 30–60 minutes every 4 hours</td><td>No modification is necessary</td><td>Dosage reduction may be required in patients with concomitant renal and hepatic dysfunction. When possible, serum levels should be monitored and doses adjusted accordingly</td></tr>
</table>

(*continued*)

Antibacterial, Antifungal and Antiviral Agents (*continued*)

<table>
<tr><th>Dose/Dosage and Administration Route and Schedule</th><th>Adjustments for Renal Impairment (Clcr = Creatinine Clearance)</th><th>Adjustments for Hepatic Impairment</th></tr>
<tr><td colspan="3">Ofloxacin</td></tr>
<tr><td>Ofloxacin 400 mg, administer intravenously over 30 minutes (200-mg dose) or 60 minutes (400-mg dose) every 12 hours
or
Ofloxacin 400 mg, administer orally every 12 hours
In the USA, Ofloxacin is available in generic formulations for oral administration as immediate-release tablets containing 200, 300, or 400 mg/tablet</td><td>Clcr (mL/min) | Dose & Schedule
20–50 | 400 mg q 24h
<20 | 200 mg q 24h</td><td>In patients with severe liver function disorders (e.g., cirrhosis ± ascites), do not exceed a maximum daily dose of 400 mg</td></tr>
<tr><td colspan="3">Piperacillin</td></tr>
<tr><td>Piperacillin 3000 mg, administer intravenously by push over 3–5 minutes, every 4–6 h
or
Piperacillin 3000 mg, administer intravenously by infusion over 20–30 minutes every 4–6 h</td><td>Clcr (mL/min) | Uncomplicated UTI | Complicated UTI | Serious Systemic Infection
>40 | No modifications are necessary
20–40 | 3000 mg q 8h | 3000 mg q 8h | 4000 mg q 8h
<20 | 3000 mg q 12h | 3000 mg q 12h | 4000 mg q 12h</td><td>For patients on hemodialysis, administer 2000 mg every 8 hours. Hemodialysis removes 30–50% of piperacillin in 4 hours. Give an additional dose of 1000 mg piperacillin after each dialysis period</td></tr>
<tr><td colspan="3">Tobramycin</td></tr>
<tr><td>Multiple-Daily Administration (MDA):
Loading Dose: Tobramycin 2 mg/kg ×1 dose over 30–60 minutes, followed by
Maintenance Doses: Tobramycin 1.7 mg/kg/dose, administer intravenously over 30–60 minutes every 8 hours[a]
or
Once-Daily Administration (ODA):
Tobramycin 4–7 mg/kg/dose, administer intravenously over 30–60 minutes every 24 hours[a]

 | MDA | ODA
Peak | 4–10 μg/mL | 16–24 μg/mL
Trough | 1–2 μg/mL | <1 μg/mL
Toxic Trough | > 2 μg/mL | >2 μg/mL

SI: μmol/L = 2.09 × mg/L</td><td>In patients with renal impairment, dosage and/or administration intervals should be adjusted based on tobramycin serum levels</td><td>No treatment modifications are indicated</td></tr>
</table>

(*continued*)

<table>
<tr><th colspan="3">Antibacterial, Antifungal and Antiviral Agents (continued)</th></tr>
<tr><th>Dose/Dosage and Administration Route and Schedule</th><th>Adjustments for Renal Impairment (Clcr = Creatinine Clearance)</th><th>Adjustments for Hepatic Impairment</th></tr>
<tr><th colspan="3">Vancomycin</th></tr>
<tr>
<td>Vancomycin 1000 mg, administer intravenously over 1–2 hours every 12 hours
or
Vancomycin 2000 mg/day, administer by continuous intravenous infusion over 24 hours
<table>
<tr><th></th><th>Every 12 hours administration</th></tr>
<tr><td>Peak</td><td>5–15 mg/mL</td></tr>
<tr><td>Trough</td><td>20– 40 μg/mL</td></tr>
<tr><td>Toxic Peak</td><td>>80 mg/mL</td></tr>
<tr><td>Toxic Trough</td><td>>15 μg /mL</td></tr>
</table>
SI: μmol/L = 0.69 × mg/L</td>
<td>In patients with renal impairment, dosage and/or administration intervals should be adjusted based on vancomycin serum levels
Manufacturer recommendations for daily dosing based on renal function:
<table>
<tr><th>Clcr (mL/min)</th><th>Daily Vancomycin Dose (mg/24 h)</th></tr>
<tr><td>100</td><td>1545</td></tr>
<tr><td>90</td><td>1390</td></tr>
<tr><td>80</td><td>1235</td></tr>
<tr><td>70</td><td>1080</td></tr>
<tr><td>60</td><td>925</td></tr>
<tr><td>50</td><td>770</td></tr>
<tr><td>40</td><td>620</td></tr>
<tr><td>30</td><td>465</td></tr>
<tr><td>20</td><td>310</td></tr>
<tr><td>10</td><td>155</td></tr>
</table>
• For functionally anephric patients, give an initial dosage of 15 mg/kg of body weight
• The dosage required to maintain stable concentrations is 1.9 mg/kg per 24 hours
• In patients with severe renal impairment, it may be convenient to give a maintenance dose every few days</td>
<td>No treatment modifications are indicated</td>
</tr>
<tr><th colspan="3">Antifungals</th></tr>
<tr><th colspan="3">Amphotericin B Sodium Desoxycholate and Amphotericin Liposomal [Ambisome® (Amphotericin B) Liposome for Injection]</th></tr>
<tr>
<td>Amphotericin B Sodium Desoxycholate 0.3–1.5 mg/kg per day, administer intravenously over 2–6 hours
or
Amphotericin Liposomal [AmBisome® (amphotericin B) liposome for injection] 3–7.5 mg/kg per day, administer intravenously over 2 hours (initially) to 60 minutes (in patients who have previously tolerated administration)</td>
<td>Amphotericin B is nephrotoxic, but the severity of renal impairment and modifications in either amphotericin dosage or administration schedule have not been established</td>
<td>No treatment modifications are indicated</td>
</tr>
<tr><th colspan="3">Caspofungin</th></tr>
<tr>
<td>Loading dose: Caspofungin 70 mg, administer intravenously over 60 min on day 1, followed by
Maintenance dose: Caspofungin 50–70 mg/day, administer intravenously over 60 min</td>
<td>No treatment modifications are indicated</td>
<td>Child Pugh Score 5–6:
No adjustment
Child Pugh Score 7–9:
Loading Dose: 70 mg
Maintenance Dose: 35 mg
Child Pugh Score > 9:
No recommendation (insufficient experience, increased potential for toxicity)</td>
</tr>
</table>

(*continued*)

Antibacterial, Antifungal and Antiviral Agents (*continued*)

Dose/Dosage and Administration Route and Schedule	Adjustments for Renal Impairment (Clcr = Creatinine Clearance)	Adjustments for Hepatic Impairment
Fluconazole		
Prophylaxis against Candidal Infection in persons undergoing HSCT and others who may experience prolonged neutropenia (ANC <500/mm³) as a consequence of treatment: Fluconazole 400 mg daily, administer orally **Vaginal Candidiasis:** Fluconazole 150 mg administer orally for 1 dose **Oropharyngeal Candidiasis:** Fluconazole 200 mg orally or IV on the first day, then 100 mg once daily; treatment should be continued for at least 2 weeks to decrease the likelihood of relapse **Esophageal Candidiasis:** Fluconazole 200 mg orally or IV on the first day, then 100 mg once daily (MAX daily dose 400 mg); treatment should last for at least 3 weeks and for at least 2 weeks following resolution of symptoms **Systemic Candidiasis:** Fluconazole up to 400 mg orally or IV once daily for 4–6 weeks **Candidal UTI or Peritonitis:** Fluconazole 50–200 mg orally or IV per day **Cryptococcal Meningitis — Treatment:** Fluconazole 400 mg orally or IV on the first day, then 200 mg once daily (MAX dosage 400 mg once daily); treat for 10–12 weeks after the cerebrospinal fluid becomes culture negative **Cryptococcal Meningitis—Suppression:** Fluconazole 200 mg daily, administer orally In the USA, Fluconazole is available in various formulations for oral administration, including: immediate-release tablets (50-, 100-, 150-, 200-mg strengths) and powdered fluconazole for preparing liquid suspensions	Single-dose therapy for vaginal candidiasis not adjusted for impaired renal function In patients with impaired renal function who are to receive multiple doses, give an initial loading dose of fluconazole 50–400 mg, then maintenance doses (according to indication) are based on creatinine clearance as follows: Clcr (mL/min): Percent of Recommended Dose >50: 100% ≤50: (Without dialysis) 50% With regular dialysis: 100% after each dialysis	No treatment modifications are indicated, but fluconazole has been associated with rare cases of serious hepatic toxicity, including fatalities primarily in patients with serious underlying medical conditions Discontinue fluconazole in patients who develop signs and symptoms consistent with liver disease or elevations in hepatic function tests
Itraconazole		
Loading dose: Itraconazole 200 mg/dose, administer intravenously over 1 hour every 12 hours for 4 doses, followed by **Maintenance dose:** Itraconazole 200 mg/day, administer intravenously over 1 hour Itraconazole 50–400 mg/day generally produces steady-state serum concentrations of itraconazole + hydroxyitraconazole (combined) of 0.3–7 μg/mL. Therapeutic range is usually considered >0.5–1 μg/mL	No treatment modifications are indicated Injectable formulations containing hydroxypropyl-β-cyclodextrin (e.g., SPORANOX®, Janssen Pharmaceutica Products, L.P., Titusville, NJ) should not be used in patients with Clcr <30 mL/min due to decreased clearance of vehicle used	No treatment modifications are indicated, but monitor closely for adverse events. Itraconazole elimination half-life was prolonged in cirrhotic patients in a clinical trial with orally administered itraconazole capsules

(*continued*)

<table>
<tr><th colspan="3">Antibacterial, Antifungal and Antiviral Agents (continued)</th></tr>
<tr><th>Dose/Dosage and Administration Route and Schedule</th><th>Adjustments for Renal Impairment (Clcr = Creatinine Clearance)</th><th>Adjustments for Hepatic Impairment</th></tr>
<tr><th colspan="3">Voriconazole</th></tr>
<tr>
<td>Loading dose:
Voriconazole 6 mg/kg per dose, administer intravenously over 1–2 hours every 12 hours for 2 doses, followed by
Maintenance dose:
Voriconazole 4 mg/kg per dose, administer intravenously over 1–2 hours every 12 hours
or
Oral maintenance dose for patients with body weight = 40 kg: Voriconazole 200 mg administer orally every 12 hours
Oral maintenance dose for patients with body weight <40 kg: Voriconazole 100 mg administer orally every 12 hours
In the USA, Voriconazole is available in three formulations for oral administration, including: including: immediate-release tablets (50 and 200-mg/tablet) and a powdered product for preparing liquid suspensions (40-mg/mL). VFENDAE Tablets (voriconazole) VFENDAE (voriconazole) for Oral Suspension product label, December 2004. Roerig Division of Pfizer Inc, NY, NY</td>
<td>No treatment modifications are indicated for patients with mild-moderate renal impairment

Patients with Clcr <50 mL/min should not receive parenteral voriconazole formulated with sulfobutyl ether β-cyclodextrin sodium (e.g., VFEND® IV, Roerig Division of Pfizer, Inc., NY, NY)</td>
<td>Decrease the maintenance dose of voriconazole in patients with mild to moderate hepatic cirrhosis</td>
</tr>
<tr><th colspan="3">Antivirals</th></tr>
<tr><th colspan="3">Acyclovir</th></tr>
<tr>
<td>Cutaneous & Mucosal HSV1 & HSV2 Infections in Immune Compromised Patients (Ages ≥12 years):
Acyclovir 5 mg/kg per dose, administer intravenously over 1 hour every 8 hours for 7 days
Herpes Genitalis—Severe Initial Episodes (Ages ≥12 years):
Acyclovir 5 mg/kg per dose, administer intravenously over 1 hour every 8 hours for 5 days or Acyclovir 200 mg/dose, administer orally every 4 hours for 5 doses/day for 10 days
Herpes Genitalis—Chronic Suppression:
Acyclovir 400 mg/dose, administer orally twice daily for up to 12 months
HSV Encephalitis (Ages ≥12 years):
Acyclovir 10 mg/kg per dose, administer intravenously over 1 hour every 8 hours for 10 days
Herpes Zoster Infections in Immune Compromised Patients (Ages ≥12 years):
Acyclovir 10 mg/kg per dose, administer intravenously over 1 hour every 8 hours for 7 days or Acyclovir 800 mg/dose, administer orally every 4 hours for 5 doses/day for 7–10 days
Chicken Pox (all patients with body weight >40 kg):
Acyclovir 800 mg/dose, administer orally 4 times daily for 5 days
In the USA, Acyclovir is available generically in formulations for oral administration, including: immediate-release tablets (400 and 800-mg/tablet), immediate-release capsules (200-mg/capsule), and a powdered product for preparing a liquid suspension (200-mg/5 mL)</td>
<td>Treatment modifications for parenterally administered acyclovir formulations
<table>
<tr><th>Clcr (mL/min/1.73 m²)</th><th>Percent of Recommended Dose</th><th>Dosing Interval (h)</th></tr>
<tr><td>>50</td><td>100%</td><td>q 8h</td></tr>
<tr><td>25–50</td><td>100%</td><td>q 12h</td></tr>
<tr><td>10–25</td><td>100%</td><td>q 24h</td></tr>
<tr><td>0–10</td><td>50%</td><td>q 24h</td></tr>
</table>
Treatment modifications for orally administered acyclovir formulations
<table>
<tr><th>Normal Dose & Schedule</th><th>Clcr (mL/min/1.73 m²)</th><th>Modified Dose & Schedule</th></tr>
<tr><td rowspan="2">200 mg q 4h</td><td>>10</td><td>200 mg q 4h for 5 doses/day</td></tr>
<tr><td>0–10</td><td>200 mg q 12h</td></tr>
<tr><td rowspan="2">400 mg q 12h</td><td>>10</td><td>400 mg q 12h</td></tr>
<tr><td>0–10</td><td>200 mg q 12h</td></tr>
<tr><td rowspan="3">800 mg q 4h for</td><td>>25</td><td>800 mg q 4h 5 doses/day</td></tr>
<tr><td>10–25</td><td>800 mg q 8h</td></tr>
<tr><td>0–10</td><td>800 mg q 12h</td></tr>
</table>
</td>
<td>No treatment modifications are indicated</td>
</tr>
</table>

(*continued*)

<table>
<tr><th colspan="3">Antibacterial, Antifungal and Antiviral Agents (continued)</th></tr>
<tr><th>Dose/Dosage and Administration Route and Schedule</th><th>Adjustments for Renal Impairment (Clcr = Creatinine Clearance)</th><th>Adjustments for Hepatic Impairment</th></tr>
<tr><th colspan="3">Amantadine</th></tr>
<tr><td>Adults, ages < 65 years:
Amantadine 200 mg/day, administer orally as a single dose,
or
Amantadine 100 mg, administer orally, twice daily
Adults, ages ≥65 years:
Amantadine 100 mg/day, administer orally
In the USA, Amantadine is available generically in formulations for oral administration, including: immediate-release tablets (100-mg/tablet), immediate-release capsules (100-mg/capsule), and a syrup (50-mg/5 mL)</td><td><table><tr><th>Clcr (mL/min/1.73 m²)</th><th>Dose & Schedule</th></tr><tr><td>30–50</td><td>200 mg on the first day followed by 100 mg/d on subsequent days</td></tr><tr><td>15–29</td><td>200 mg on the first day followed by 100 mg on alternate days</td></tr><tr><td><15
Patients on hemodialysis</td><td>200 mg every 7 days</td></tr></table></td><td>No treatment modifications are indicated</td></tr>
<tr><th colspan="3">Foscarnet</th></tr>
<tr><td>HYDRATION:
Adnminister 750–1000 mL 0.9% Sodium Chloride Injection (0.9%NS) or 5% Dextrose Injection (D5W) before the first foscarnet infusion to establish diuresis. With subsequent treatment, give 750–1000 mL hydration during the foscarnet administration when administering 90–120 mg/kg and 500 mL during the foscarnet administration when administering 40–60 mg/kg. Hydration volume may be decreased as clinically indicated
CMV retinitis:
Induction:
Foscarnet 90 mg/kg, administer intravenously over 60–90 minutes every 12 hours for 2–3 weeks depending on clinical response
or
Foscarnet 60 mg/kg, administer intravenously over at least 60 minutes every 8 hours for 2–3 weeks depending on clinical response
Maintenance:
Foscarnet 90–120 mg/kg per day, administer intravenously over 120 minutes
Acyclovir-resistant HSV:
Foscarnet 40 mg/kg, administer intravenously over at least 60 minutes every 8–12 hours for 2–3 weeks or until healed</td><td>Dosages and schedules based on renal function for acyclovir resistant HSV and induction therapy of CMV retinitis*<table><tr><th></th><th colspan="2">Indication: HSV</th><th colspan="2">Indication: CMV</th></tr><tr><th rowspan="2">Clcr (mL/min/kg)</th><th colspan="4">Dosages (in mg/kg/dose) equivalent to:</th></tr><tr><th>80 mg/kg/d</th><th>120 mg/kg/d</th><th colspan="2">180 mg/kg/d</th></tr><tr><td>>1.4</td><td>40 mg/kg q 12h</td><td>40 mg/kg q 8h</td><td>60 mg/kg q 8h</td><td>90 mg/kg q 12h</td></tr><tr><td>>1–1.4</td><td>30 mg/kg q 12h</td><td>30 mg/kg q 8h</td><td>45 mg/kg q 8h</td><td>70 mg/kg q 12h</td></tr><tr><td>>0.8–1</td><td>40 mg/kg q 12h</td><td>35 mg/kg q 12h</td><td>50 mg/kg q 12h</td><td>50 mg/kg q 12h</td></tr><tr><td>>0.6–0.8</td><td>35 mg/kg q 24h</td><td>25 mg/kg q 12h</td><td>40 mg/kg q 12h</td><td>80 mg/kg q 24h</td></tr><tr><td>>0.5–0.6</td><td>25 mg/kg q 24h</td><td>40 mg/kg q 24h</td><td>60 mg/kg q 24h</td><td>60 mg/kg q 24h</td></tr><tr><td>≥0.4–0.5</td><td>20 mg/kg q 24h</td><td>35 mg/kg q 24h</td><td>50 mg/kg q 24h</td><td>50 mg/kg q 24h</td></tr><tr><td><0.4</td><td colspan="4">Not recommended</td></tr></table></td><td>No treatment modifications are indicated</td></tr>
</table>

(*continued*)

Antibacterial, Antifungal and Antiviral Agents (*continued*)

Dose/Dosage and Administration Route and Schedule	Adjustments for Renal Impairment (Clcr = Creatinine Clearance)	Adjustments for Hepatic Impairment
	Foscarnet	
	Dosages and schedules based on renal function for **maintenance therapy** of CMV retinitis*	

Clcr (mL/min/kg)	Indication: CMV — Dosages (mg/kg/dose) equivalent to: 90 mg/kg/d (Once daily)	120 mg/kg/d (Once daily)
>1.4	90 mg/kg q 24h	90 mg/kg q 24h
>1–1.4	90 mg/kg q 24h	90 mg/kg q 24h
>0.8–1	90 mg/kg q 24h	90 mg/kg q 24h
>0.6–0.8	80 mg/kg q 48h	80 mg/kg q 48h
>0.5–0.6	80 mg/kg q 48h	80 mg/kg q 48h
≥ 0.4–0.5	80 mg/kg q 48h	80 mg/kg q 48h
<0.4	Not recommended	

*If the creatinine clearance falls below ≤0.4 mL/min/kg, Foscarnet should be discontinued. Affected patients should receive hydration and be monitored daily until renal impairment resolves

Ganciclovir

CMV Retinitis:
Induction:
Ganciclovir 5 mg/kg per dose, administer intravenously over 1 hour every 12 hours for 14–21 days
Maintenance:
Ganciclovir 5 mg/kg per day, administer intravenously over 1 hour 7 days/week
or
Ganciclovir 6 mg/kg per day, 5 days/week

CMV Prevention in Transplant Recipients:
Induction:
Ganciclovir 5 mg/kg per dose, administer intravenously over 1 hour every 12 hours for 7–14 days
Maintenance:
Ganciclovir 5 mg/kg per day, administer intravenously over 1 hour 7 days/week
or
Ganciclovir 6 mg/kg per day, 5 days/week

Clcr (mL/min)	Induction Dose & Schedule	Maintenance Dose & Schedule
≥70	5 mg/kg q 12h	5 mg/kg q 24h
50–69	2.5 mg/kg q 12h	2.5 mg/kg q 24h
25–49	2.5 mg/kg q 24h	1.25 mg/kg q 24h
10–24	1.25 mg/kg q 24h	0.625 mg/kg q 24h
<10	1.25 mg/kg 3× per week after hemodialysis	0.625 mg/kg 3× per week after hemodialysis

Adjustments for Hepatic Impairment: No treatment modifications are indicated

[a] The amount of drug and interval between repeated doses should be adjusted based on measured drug concentrations in serum, plasma, or blood and individualized pharmacokinetic assessment
[b] The amount of drug given per dose should correlate with the severity of infection

Prepared by David Kohler, PharmD and Juan Gea-Banacloche, MD

48. Catheter-Related Bloodstream Infections: Management and Prevention

Naomi P. O'Grady, MD

Epidemiology and Microbiology

The organisms causing bloodstream infections have changed over the last 15 years

Most Common Organisms 1986 to 1989

Coagulase-negative staphylococci
Staphylococcus aureus

Most Common Organisms 1992 to 1999

Organism	Frequency	Antimicrobial Resistance
Coagulase-negative staphylococci	37 %	
Enterococci	13.5%	Dramatic rise in enterococcal isolates resistant to vancomycin—from 0.5% in 1989 to 25.9% in 1999[1]
S. aureus	12.6%	>50% of all *S. aureus* nosocomial isolates are oxacillin resistant[1]
Gram-negative bacilli	14%	Increasing prevalence of Enterobacteriaceae with extended-spectrum β-lactamases (ESBLs), particularly *Klebsiella pneumoniae*. Such organisms are resistant to many commonly used cephalosporins
Candida infections	8%	Growing resistance of *Candida albicans* to antifungals; 50% of *Candida* bloodstream infections are caused by non-*albicans* species including *C. glabrata* and *C. krusei,* which are more likely than *C. albicans* to demonstrate resistance to fluconazole and itraconazole. Resistance to voriconazole has not been reported thus far, although continued surveillance is needed

Definitions[2]

- **Catheter colonization:** Significant growth of a microorganism in a quantitative or semi quantitative culture of the catheter tip, subcutaneous catheter segment, or catheter hub
- **Exit-site infection:** Erythema, induration, and/or tenderness within 2 cm of the catheter exit site; may be associated with other signs and symptoms of infection, such as fever or pus emerging from the exit site with or without concomitant bloodstream infections
- **Tunnel infection:** Tenderness, erythema, and/or induration 12 cm from the catheter exit site along the subcutaneous tract of a tunneled catheter (eg, Hickman or Broviac) with or without concomitant bloodstream infections
- **Pocket infection:** Infected fluid in the subcutaneous pocket of a totally implanted intravascular device; often associated with tenderness, erythema, and/or induration over the pocket; spontaneous rupture and drainage, or necrosis of the overlying skin, with or without concomitant bloodstream infection, may also occur
- **Catheter-related bloodstream infection:** Bacteremia or fungemia in a patient who has an intravascular device and one positive result from culture of blood samples from the peripheral vein, clinical manifestations of infection (eg, fever, chills, and/or hypotension), and no apparent source for bloodstream infection (except for the catheter). One of the following should be present: a positive result of semiquantitative (>15 cfu per catheter segment) or quantitative ($>10^2$ cfu per catheter segment) catheter culture, whereby the same organism (species and antibiogram) is isolated from a catheter segment and a peripheral blood sample; simultaneous quantitative cultures of blood samples with a ratio of >5:1 (central venous catheter [CVC] versus peripheral catheter); differential time to positivity (ie, a positive result of culture from a CVC is obtained at least 2 hours earlier than a positive result from a culture from peripheral blood)

Diagnosis

1. Blood cultures

- Clinical findings for establishing the diagnosis of catheter-related infection are unreliable because of poor sensitivity and specificity
- When catheter infection is suspected, two sets of blood cultures should be sent with at least one drawn percutaneously[2]
- Paired quantitative or qualitative blood cultures with continuously monitored differential time to positivity are recommended when long-term catheters cannot be removed[3–5]

2. Catheter cultures

- Culture catheters only when catheter-related bloodstream infection is suspected[2]
- Quantitative or semiquantitative cultures are recommended[2]
- When culturing a catheter segment, either the tip or the subcutaneous segment should be submitted for culture[6]
- For suspected pulmonary artery catheter infection, the introducer tip should be cultured[2]

Management[2]

Nontunneled central venous catheters (CVCs) [see Figures 48–1 and 48–2]

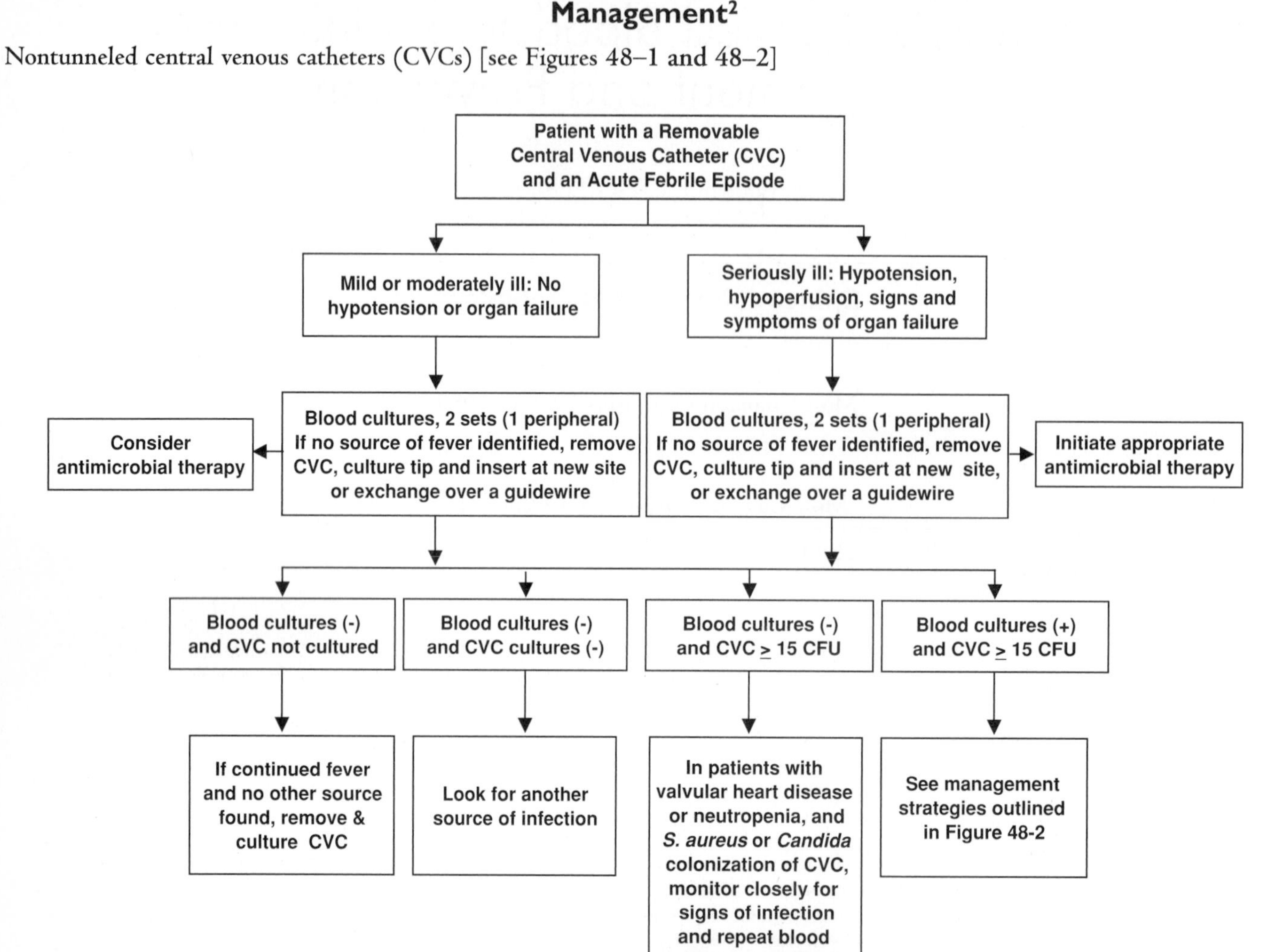

Figure 48–1. CFU, colony-forming unit; CVC, central venous catheter. (From Guidelines for the Management of Intravascular Catheter-Related Infections)

- CVCs in patients with fever and mild to moderate symptoms do not need to be routinely removed
- CVCs should be removed and cultured if the patient has a tunnel infection (erythema or purulence overlying the catheter exit site) or clinical signs of sepsis
- If blood culture results are positive or if the CVC is exchanged over the guidewire and has significant colonization according to results of quantitative or semiquantitative cultures, the catheter should be removed and placed into a new site
- In some patients without evidence of persistent bloodstream infection or if the infecting organism is a coagulase-negative staphylococci and if there is no suspicion of local or metastatic complications, the CVC may be retained
- A transesophageal echocardiogram (TEE) should be obtained to rule out vegetations (endocarditis) in patients with a catheter-related *S. aureus* bloodstream infection
- If a TEE is not available and the results of a transthoracic echocardiography are negative, the duration of therapy should be decided clinically
- After removal of a colonized catheter associated with bloodstream infection, if there is persistent bacteremia or fungemia or a lack of clinical improvement, aggressive evaluation for septic thrombosis, infective endocarditis, and other metastatic infections should commence
- Febrile patients with valvular heart disease or patients with neutropenia whose catheter tip culture reveals significant growth of *S. aureus* or *Candida* species on semiquantitative or quantitative culture with no bloodstream infection should be followed up closely for development of infection, and samples of blood for culture should be obtained accordingly
- After a catheter is removed from a patient with a catheter-related bloodstream infection, nontunneled catheters may be reinserted after appropriate systemic antimicrobial therapy is begun

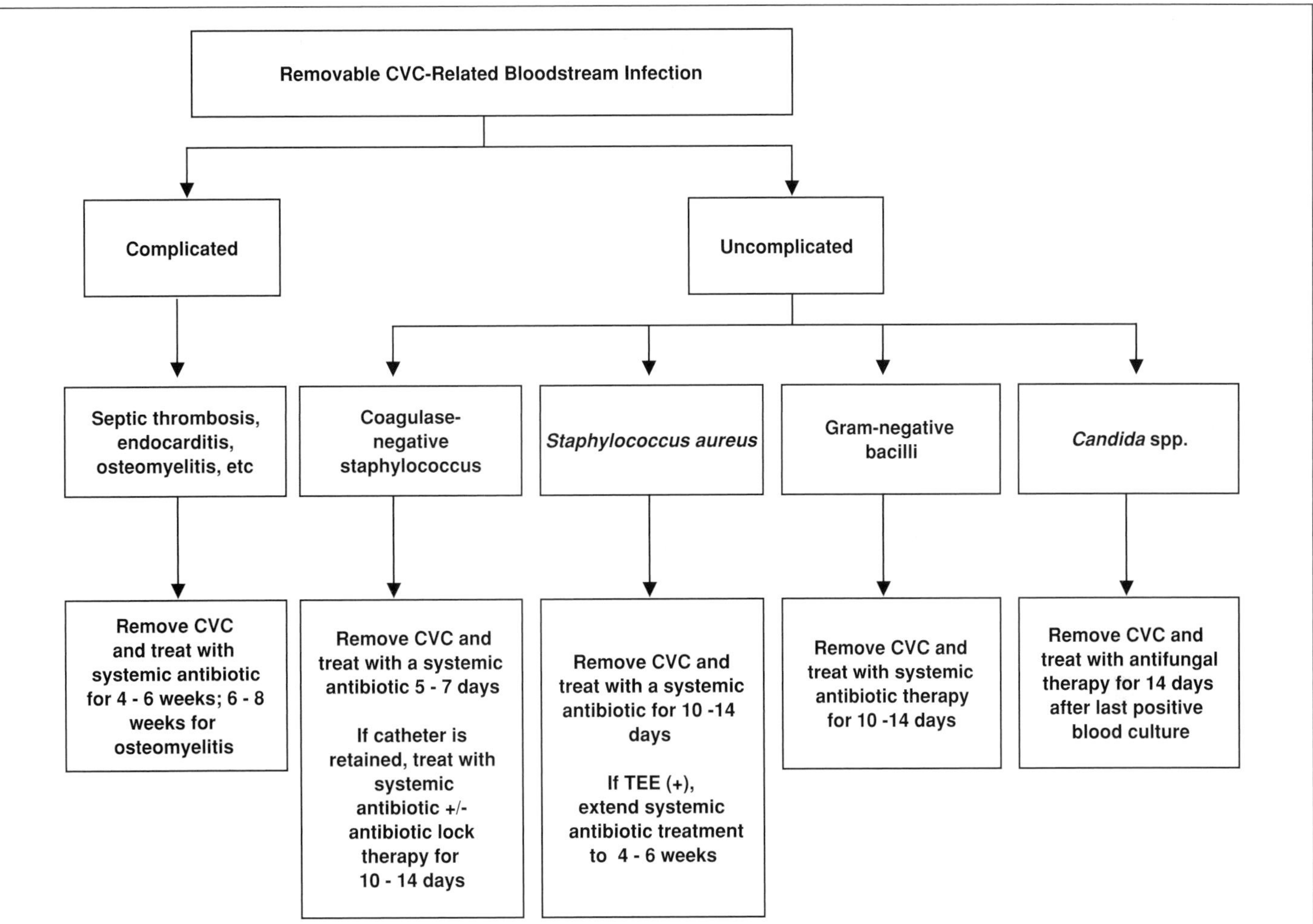

Figure 48–2. CVC, central venous catheter; TEE, transesophageal echocardiography. (From Guidelines for the Management of Intravascular Catheter-Related Infections)

Tunneled CVCs and intravascular devices (IDs) [see Figure 48–3]

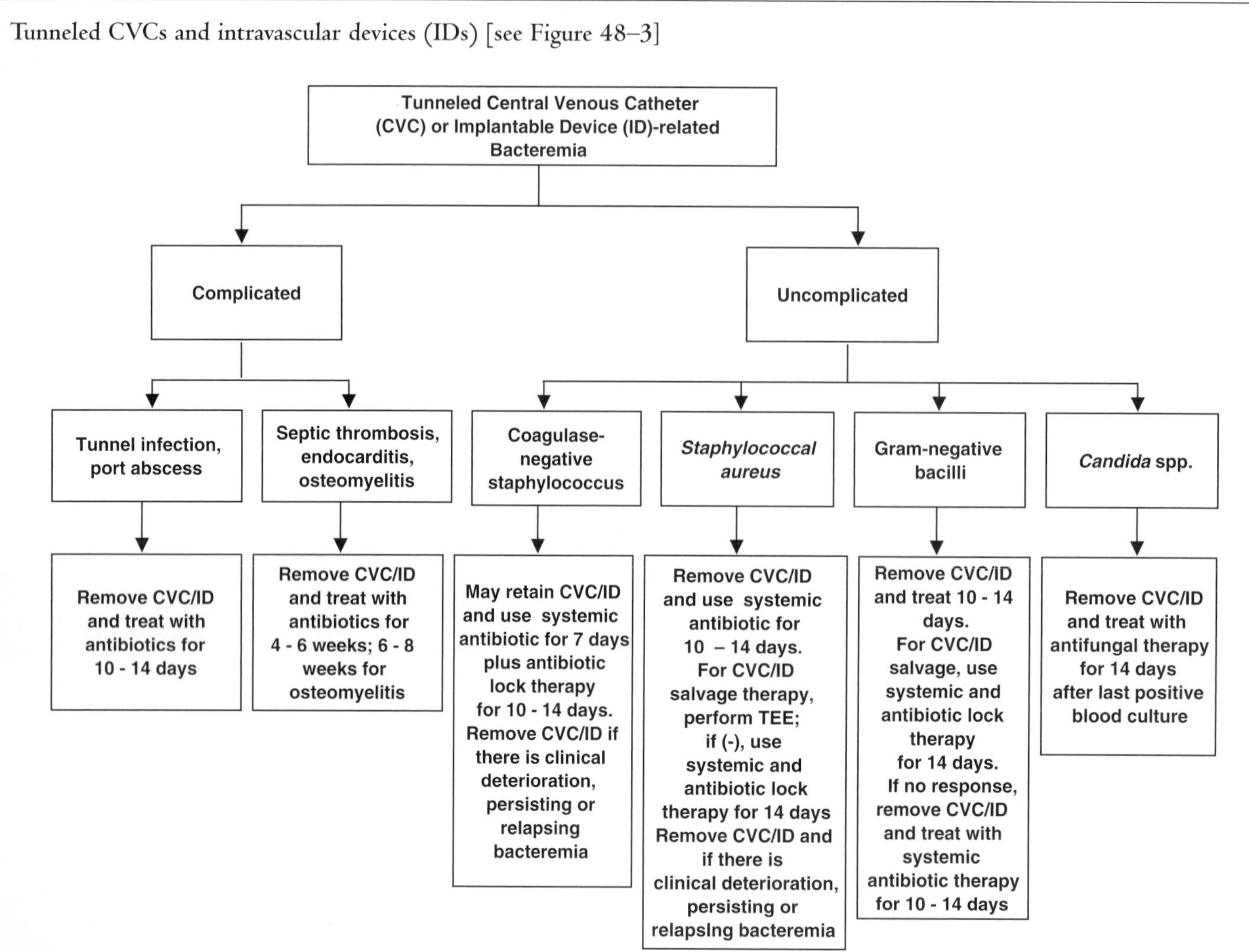

Figure 48–3. CVC, central venous catheter; TEE, transesophageal echocardiography. (From Guidelines for the Management of Intravascular Catheter-Related Infections)

- Clinical assessment is recommended to determine whether the CVC or the ID is the source of infection or bloodstream infection
- For complicated infections, the CVC or the ID should be removed
- For salvage of the CVC or the ID in patients with uncomplicated infections, antibiotic lock therapy should be used for 2 weeks with standard systemic therapy for treatment of catheter-related bacteremia due to *S. aureus*, coagulase-negative staphylococci, and gram-negative bacilli for suspected intraluminal infection in the absence of tunnel or pocket infection
- Tunneled catheter pocket infections or port abscess require removal of catheter and usually 7–10 days of appropriate antibiotic therapy
  Reinsertion of tunneled intravascular devices should be postponed until after appropriate systemic antimicrobial therapy is begun, based on susceptibilities of the bloodstream isolate and after repeat cultures of blood samples yield negative results

Prevention[7]

1. **Site of catheter insertion**
   - Subclavian site has lowest rate of infectious complications
   - Catheters inserted into an internal jugular vein have been associated with higher risk of infection than that of those inserted into a subclavian or femoral vein[8,9]
2. **Skin antisepsis**
   - **2% chlorhexidine gluconate** is superior to 10% povidone-iodine or 70% alcohol in preventing catheter colonization. Chlorhexidine should be used in adult and adolescent patients unless there is a contraindication to its use
3. **Catheter site dressing regimens**
   - Transparent, semipermeable polyurethane dressings are reliable, secure, and convenient
   - **Chlorhexidine-impregnated sponge dressings** can reduce the risk of bacteremia with CVCs in place >4 days. This small disk can be placed over the insertion site and left in place for up to 7 days
   - **Mupirocin ointment** applied at the insertion sites of CVCs prevents catheter-related bloodstream infections, but it has also been associated with mupirocin resistance and selection for fungal organisms. This ointment may adversely affect the integrity of polyurethane catheters and is therefore not recommended
   - Mupirocin ointment has been used intranasally to decrease nasal carriage of *S. aureus* and reduce the risk of catheter related bloodstream infections. However, this practice is not recommended because of the development of resistance
4. **Antimicrobial/antiseptic impregnated catheters**
   - Certain antimicrobial or antiseptic-impregnated or antiseptic-coated catheters have been shown to decrease the risk of catheter-related bloodstream infection[10]
   - Catheters coated with **chlorhexidine/silver sulfadiazine** on the external luminal surface only reduced the risk of bacteremia compared with standard noncoated catheters. [11,12] Selection of resistance to chlorhexidine/silver sulfadiazine is a concern; however, this has not yet been demonstrated. These catheters may be cost-effective in the ICU and in burn patients, neutropenic patients, and patients who have had catheters placed under emergency conditions
   - Catheters impregnated on the internal and external surfaces with **minocycline/rifampin** are associated with lower rates of bacteremia when compared with chlorhexidine/silver sulfadiazine–impregnated catheters. [13] No minocyline/rifampin–resistant organisms were reported, although this is a theoretical risk
   - A second-generation catheter is now available with a chlorhexidine coating on both the internal and external luminal surfaces
   - The decision to use chlorhexidine/silver sulfadiazine– or minocyline/rifampin–impregnated catheters should be based on the need to enhance prevention of catheter-related bloodstream infections in these patients and balanced against the concern for possible emergence of resistant pathogens and the cost of implementing this strategy
5. **Antibiotic lock prophylaxis**
   - Antibiotic lock prophylaxis can be useful in neutropenic patients with long-term catheters using a solution of heparin plus 25 mcg/mL of vancomycin
   - This practice can increase the risk of VRE. [14] Antibiotic lock prophylaxis is not recommended routinely, although in patients with difficult access who have had multiple episodes of bacteremia, it is not an unreasonable strategy
6. **Replacement of catheters**
   - There are no studies that show an advantage of routine catheter replacement at scheduled time intervals as a method to reduce catheter related bloodstream infections[15–17]
   - Replacement of temporary catheters over a guidewire in the setting of bacteremia is not an acceptable replacement strategy, because the source of infection is usually colonization of the skin tract from the insertion site to the vein[18,19]

References

1. Centers for Disease Control and Prevention. National Nosocomial Infections Surveillance (NNIS) System report, data summary from January 1990 to May 1999, issued June 1999. Am J Infect Control 1999;27:520–532
2. Mermel LA et al. Guidelines for the management of intravascular catheter-related infections. Clin Infect Dis 2001;32:1249–1272
3. Maki DG et al. NEJM 1977;296:1305–1309
4. DesJardin JA et al. Ann Intern Med 1999;131:641–647
5. Blot F et al. Lancet 1999;354:1071–1077
6. Sherertz RJ et al. J Clin Microbiol 1997;35:641–646
7. O'Grady NP et al. Guidelines for the prevention of intravascular catheter-related infections. MMWR Recomm Rep 2002;51:1–29
8. Merrer J et al. JAMA 2001;286:700–707
9. Mermel LA et al Am J Respir Crit Care Med 1994;149:1020–1036
10. Raad I et al et al. Ann Intern Med 1997;127:267–274
11. Mermel LA. Ann Intern Med 2000;132:391–402
12. Veenstra DL et al. JAMA 1999;281:261–267
13. Darouiche RO et al. NEJM 1999;340:1–8
14. Centers for Disease Control and Prevention. Recommendations for preventing the spread of vancomycin resistance. Recommendations of the Hospital Infection Control Practices Advisory Committee (HICPAC). MMWR Morb Mortal Wkly Rep 1995;44:1–13
15. Eyer S et al .Crit Care Med 1990;18:1073–1079
16. Uldall PR et al. Lancet 1981;1:1373
17. Cook D et al. Crit Care Med 1997;25:1417–1424
18. Mermel LA et al. Am J Med 1991;91:197S–205S
19. Cobb DK et al. NEJM 1992;327:1062–1068

49. Venous Catheter-Related Thrombosis

McDonald Horne, MD

Common Venous Access Devices

Design	Blood Draw	IV Fluid	Blood Product	Duration of Use	Routine Flush
Tunneled					
Open-ended (Hickam)	++++	++++	++++	Weeks to years	Daily
Valved (Groshong)	++++	++++	++++	Weeks to years	Weekly
Ports (open or valved end)	++++	++++	++++	Months to years	Monthly
Nontunneled					
Peripheral (PICC, open or valved)	+	++++	+	<3 months	Daily or weekly
Central	++++	++++	++++	<3 months	Daily

Reproduced, with permission, from: Horne MK, Mayo DJ, Freifeld AG. In: Beutler E, Lichtman MA, Coller BS, Kipps TJ, Seligsohn U, eds. Williams Hematology, 6th ed. New York: McGraw-Hill, 2001.

Contraindications for Placement of Venous Access Devices

1. Active infection
2. Neutropenia
3. Thrombocytopenia (<50,000/mm^3)
4. Coagulopathy

Optimal Catheter Placement

The catheter tip should be in the mid superior vena cava, just outside the right atrium. Opinions differ about the risks and benefits of placing the tip within the right atrium

Epidemiology of Venous Catheter-Related Thrombosis

Incidence	Central Venous Catheters (CVCs)	Peripherally Inserted Central Catheters (PICCs)
Symptomatic DVT	1–10%	1–4%
Asymptomatic DVT (documented by venography)	~30%	~20%
Catheter occlusion (without DVT)	~10%	

Chemaly RF et al. Clin Infect Dis 2002;34:1179–1183
Horne MK et al. Ann Surg Oncol 1995;2:174–178
Kuriakose P et al. J Vasc Interv Radiol 2002;13:179–184
Stephens LC et al. J Parent Enter Nutr 1995;19:75–79
Verso M et al. JCO 2003;21:3665–3675

Other Complications of Venous Access Devices

Arrhythmia	13%
Arterial puncture	2.8–3.8%
Malposition of reservoir	2%
Pneumothorax	1–1.8%
Wound dehiscence	1.5%
Hemorrhage	1.1–1.2%
Failure of insertion	1.2%

Kuter JD. Oncologist 2004;9:207–216

Complications of Upper Limb-DVT

1. *Pulmonary embolism (PE):* The incidence of clinical overt PE is estimated at 12%, with the incidence of PE in cancer patients being higher at 15–25%
2. Postphlebitic syndrome occurs in ~15%

Verso M et al. JCO 2003;21:3665–3675

Work-Up of Venous Catheter-Related Thrombosis

Differential diagnosis

1. Cellulitis
2. Fluid retention
3. Local vein compression by tumor

Imaging procedures

1. *Ultrasound:* Use for jugular, axillary, and subclavian veins (sensitivity and specificity 80%)
2. *Venography:* Use for more central veins including innominate and vena cava and when there is high clinical suspicion despite negative ultrasound

Baarslag H-J et al. Ann Intern Med 2002;136:865–872
Haire WD et al. J Vasc Surg 1991;13:391–397
Verso M et al. JCO 2003;21:3665–3675

Prevention of Venous Catheter-Related Thrombosis

1. Daily low-dose warfarin (1 mg) has been recommended in cancer patients with CVC, but this is controversial and not without risk. If it is used, the INR should be kept <1.5 and checked monthly or more frequently when a patient is unstable
2. Low molecular weight heparin (2500 units/day Fragmin) subcutaneously every day

Bern MM et al. Ann Intern Med 1990;112:423–428
Kuriakose P et al. J Vasc Interv Radiol 2002;13:179–184
Monreal M et al. Thromb Haemost 1996;75:251–253

Treatment of Venous Catheter-Related Thrombosis

1. There is no consensus on the optimal treatment of patients with CVC-related DVT
2. If the CVC is functioning and does not appear to be infected, there is no imperative to remove it

	Acute Care	Subacute Care
CVC-related DVT; restoring patency not imperative	1. Standard doses of unfractionated **heparin** for 5–7 days *Loading dose*: 80 units/kg *Maintenance dose:* 18 units/kg/hour 2. Leave CVC in place	1. **Warfarin** orally to maintain an INR of 2–3 for 4–6 weeks, *or* 2. **Enoxaparin** (LMWH) 1 mg/kg subcutaneously once per day for 4–6 weeks
CVC-related DVT; restoring patency imperative	1. **tPA** by direct injection into clot under fluoroscopic guidance, *or* 2. **Urokinase** by direct injection into clot under fluoroscopic guidance 3. Remove CVC 4. Standard doses of **unfractionated heparin** for 5–7 days *Loading dose:* 80 units/kg *Maintenance dose*: 18 units/kg/hour	1. **Warfarin** orally to maintain an INR of 2–3 for 4–6 weeks, *or* 2. **Enoxaparin** (LMWH) 1 mg/kg subcutaneously once per day for 4–6 weeks
Superior vena cava thrombosis	1. **tPA** by direct injection into clot under fluoroscopic guidance, or 2. **Urokinase** by direct injection into clot under fluoroscopic guidance 3. Standard doses of **unfractionated heparin** for 5–7 days *Loading dose:* 80 units/kg *Maintenance dose:* 18 units/kg/hour	1. **Warfarin** orally to maintain an INR of 2–3 for 4–6 weeks, *or* 2. **Enoxaparin** (LMWH) 1 mg/kg subcutaneously once per day for 4–6 weeks
Internal jugular vein thrombosis	1. Heat 2. Anti-inflammatory agents 3. *For severe or progressive symptoms:* Standard doses of unfractionated heparin for 5–7 days *Loading dose:* 80 units/kg *Maintenance dose*: 18 units/kg/hour	
Peripheral vein thrombophlebitis	1. Heat 2. Anti-inflammatory agents 3. Consider line removal	

Becker DM et al. Arch Intern Med 1991;151:1934–1943
Chang R et al. J Vasc Intervent Radiol 1996;7:845–851
Gould JR et al. Am J Med 1993;95:419–423
Mayo DJ et al. Clin J Oncol Nurs 1997;1:5–10

Management of Catheter Tip Occlusion with a Fibrin Sheath

Mechanism

Accumulation of a fibrin coating (sheath) at the tip of the catheter, forming a one-way valve that blocks withdrawal from the CVC but allows infusion

Differential diagnosis

1. Catheter migration out of the superior vena cava into a smaller vein, where it abuts the vein wall more easily
2. Perpendicular abutment of the catheter tip against the wall of the superior vena cava
3. Catheter compression by kinking or a suture
4. Catheter lumen occlusion with precipitated salts or lipid

Evaluation

1. Reposition the patient to relieve a reversible malposition of the catheter tip
2. Obtain chest x-ray to identify catheter tip location
3. Inject x-ray contrast material through the occluded lumen(s) to identify pericatheter backtracking indicative of a fibrin sheath and to rule out an extensive fibrin sheath that could lead to extravasation of infused fluids

Treatment

1. If an occlusive fibrin sheath is identified but there is no evidence that infused fluid will extravasate, the catheter can be used for infusion
2. To restore the ability to withdraw from the catheter: Instill 2 mg alteplase (Cathflo™ Activase, Genentech, Inc.) in 2 mL of diluent into the occluded lumen and allow it to dwell for 2 hours. If this does not restore the ability to withdraw, the alteplase treatment can be repeated once

Crain MR et al. Am J Roentgenol 1998;171:341–346
Mayo DJ et al. Oncol Nurs Forum 1995;22:675–680
Semba CP et al. J Vasc Interv Radiol 2002;13:1199–1205
Stephens LC et al. J Parent Enter Nutri 1995;19:75–79
Tschirhart JM et al. Am Surg 1988;54:326–328

50. Complications and Follow-Up After Hematopoietic Stem Cell Transplantation (HSCT)

Michael M. Boyiadzis, MD, MHSc, Juan Gea-Banacloche, MD, and Michael R. Bishop, MD

Infectious Complications[1–4]

Preengraftment Period (<30 days After HSCT)

Autologous and allogeneic transplant recipients are similar with respect to early infectious complications. The risk of infection during this period is related to neutropenia and mucositis resulting from the conditioning regimen

Bacterial	Principal causes of sepsis • Gram-negative bacilli (eg, *Pseudomonas* species, Enterobacteriaceae) • Gram-positive bacteria (eg, *viridans* group *Streptococcus*, coagulase-negative *Staphylococci*) Common sources include gastrointestinal tract and intravascular devices
Fungal	Fungal infections become more common with prolonged and profound neutropenia • *Candida* infections occur early and are often prevented with fluconazole (for dose and duration of prophylaxis, see Fluconazole under Prophylactic Agents) • *Aspergillus* infections occur later (generally after 10–14 days of neutropenia). There is no proven effective prophylaxis for *Aspergillus* infections (some experts recommend itraconazole, voriconazole, caspofungin, or micafungin)
Viral	Herpes simplex virus (HSV) reactivates commonly during this period and can worsen mucositis. Prophylaxis with acyclovir or valacyclovir reduces HSV reactivation (for dose and duration of prophylaxis, see Acyclovir/Valacyclovir under Prophylactic Agents)

Early Postengraftment Period (30–100 Days After HSCT)

The risk of infection is greater and different for allogeneic recipients than for autologous recipients during this period

Autologous HSCT

There is some degree of immunodeficiency, but opportunistic infections are the exception rather than the rule

Bacterial	Related to the intravascular device
Fungal	Uncommon Some centers continue prophylaxis against *Pneumocystis jiroveci* (formerly *Pneumocystis carinii*) for 6 months after transplant
Viral	Varicella-zoster virus (VZV) reactivation and community respiratory virus infections

Allogeneic HSCT

The infection risk during this period is related to severely impaired cell-mediated immunity, acute graft-versus-host disease (GVHD) and its treatment and cytomegalovirus (CMV) reactivation. The latter two increase the risk of viral and fungal infections

Factors That Increase Risks	Factors That Lower Risks
Haplo-identical stem cell transplantation	Transplants from an HLA-identical sibling
Matched-unrelated donor	
Cord blood	

(continued)

Early Postengraftment Period (30–100 Days After HSCT) (*continued*)

Bacterial	In the absence of acute GVHD and its treatment, the most common pathogens are related to the intravascular device, and include: • Gram-positive organisms (eg, coagulase-negative staphylococci) • Nonfermentative gram-negative bacilli (including *Pseudomonas, Acinetobacter,* and *Stenotrophomonas*) In the presence of acute GVHD and its treatment, the most common pathogens are: • Enteric gram-negative bacilli (eg, *E. coli, Klebsiella, Enterobacter, Citrobacter, Serratia*) and *Pseudomonas*
Fungal	Risk factors CMV disease and steroid use[5]: • *Aspergillus* is the most common mold, but reports of *Zygomycetes* infections are increasing (perhaps due to the common use of voriconazole) • Non-*albicans Candida* infections, which may be resistant to fluconazole, are increasing
Viral	• CMV reactivation occurs in up to 70% of recipients at risk –*At risk:* CMV+ recipient with a CMV+ or CMV− donor and CMV− recipients with a CMV+ donor • VZV and HSV can cause disease, although antiviral prophylaxis has made them less common • HHV6 commonly reactivates after allogeneic transplantation. In most cases, reactivation is asymptomatic. However, in some cases it has been associated with fever, rash, pneumonitis, and meningoencephalitis[6] • *Respiratory viruses:* Adenovirus, respiratory syncytial virus, and parainfluenza cause significant morbidity and mortality[7,8] • Co-infections (particularly *Aspergillus*) have been documented with parainfluenza and other respiratory viruses[9]

Late Postengraftment Period (>100 Days After HSCT)

The risk of infection is higher for allogeneic recipients than for autologous recipients

Allogeneic HSCT

Risk of sepsis from bacterial pathogens after an allogeneic transplantation persists particularly in patients with chronic GVHD, which induces a state of functional hyposplenism. The treatment of chronic GVHD consists of immunosuppressive agents that increase the risk of infection. There is also persistent humoral immunodeficiency

Bacterial	Encapsulated bacteria, particularly *Streptococcus pneumoniae* are significant pathogens[10]
Fungal	Fungal infections are uncommon except in the presence of active immunosuppression
Viral	• CMV reactivation is an ever-present risk, higher if the patient received ganciclovir prophylaxis or treatment[11] • Most patients have a VZV reactivation in the first few months after discontinuing acyclovir prophylaxis • Respiratory virus infections continue to be a problem for months. Influenza vaccination should be restarted 6 months after transplantation

Prophylactic Agents Commonly Used to Reduce the Rates of Infections and Virus Reactivation After HSCT[1]

FLUCONAZOLE

Indications:
• To prevent invasive disease with *Candida* species
• Administration of fluconazole should commence at the time of transplantation and continue for at least 75 days after HSCT

Therapy:
Fluconazole 400 mg orally or intravenously daily for at least 75 days after HSCT

Fluconazole is available in the United States in various formulations for oral administration, including immediate-release tablets (50-, 100-, 150-, 200-mg strengths) and powdered fluconazole for preparing liquid suspensions

(*continued*)

Prophylactic Agents Commonly Used to Reduce the Rates of Infections and Virus Reactivation After HSCT[1] *(continued)*

ACYCLOVIR

Indications:

- Acyclovir prophylaxis reduces **HSV** reactivation by 75%
- Acyclovir prophylaxis in adults can also be administered in HSV-negative patients
- Administration of acyclovir or valacyclovir should commence at the time of transplant
- Routine acyclovir prophylaxis for >30 days after HSCT is not recommended
- Valacyclovir for 6 months or after the patient is off immunosuppression, whichever takes longer

Therapy:

Acyclovir 200 mg orally every 8 hours, *or*
Acyclovir 250 mg/m^2 per dose intravenously every 12 hours, *or*
Valacyclovir 500 mg orally once daily

Acyclovir is available in the United States generically in formulations for oral administration, including: immediate-release tablets (400 and 800 mg/tablet), immediate-release capsules (200 mg/capsule), and a powdered product for preparing a liquid suspension (200 mg/5 mL)
Valacyclovir hydrochloride is available in the United States as tablets for oral administration containing either 500 or 1000 mg valacyclovir HCl (Valtrex® caplets. GlaxoSmithKline, Research Triangle Park, NC)

COTRIMOXAZOLE (TRIMETHOPRIM + SULFAMETHOXAZOLE IN A 1:5 RATIO)

Indications:

- Trimethoprim + sulfamethoxazole **(TMP + SMZ)** is the prophylactic agent of choice for PCP prophylaxis and confers some degree of protection against toxoplasmosis
- PCP prophylaxis is recommended from the time of engraftment until 6 months after HSCT and after 6 months if the patient has GVHD or is receiving immunosuppressive therapy

Therapy:

TMP + SMZ 160 mg/800 mg orally, daily, *or*
TMP + SMZ 80 mg/400 mg orally, daily, *or*
TMP + SMZ 160 mg/800 mg orally 3 days per week
Alternate:
Dapsone 50 mg orally twice daily, *or*
Dapsone 100 mg daily orally
Note: Rule out G6PD deficiency before starting dapsone
Aerosolized pentamidine 300 mg by inhalation every 3–4 weeks.

Dapsone is available generically in the United States in tablets for oral administration that contain 25 mg or 100 mg dapsone
Pentamidine isethionate is available generically in the United States as a sterile solution or lyophilized powder for intravenous administration, and a solution for aerosolization and administration by inhalation

VARICELLA-ZOSTER IMMUNOGLOBULIN

Indication: Prevention of VZV disease after exposure of HSCT recipients to a person with chickenpox or shingles (use if <24 months after HSCT or >24 months after HSCT if patient is receiving immunosuppressive therapy or has chronic GVHD)

Therapy:

Varicella-zoster immunoglobulin 625 units intramuscularly, preferably within 48 hours of exposure. It is not efficacious if given >96 hours after the exposure

IMMUNE GLOBULIN, INTRAVENOUS (IVIG)

Indication: IgG levels <500 mg/dL [monitor IgG levels monthly beginning before transplantation]

Therapy:

IVIG 400–500 mg/kg intravenously every 2–4 weeks; continue until IgG is >500 mg/dL for 3 consecutive months, then monitor level monthly

Cytomegalovirus Surveillance and Treatment During The Post-Transplantation Period[1]

Ganciclovir prophylaxis (the systematic administration of ganciclovir to all patients at risk for CMV reactivation) reduces the incidence of CMV disease to 2–4%, but does not improve outcome and is associated with late CMV reactivation. The preferred approach is "preemptive," based on monitoring CMV reactivation by measuring antigenemia or PCR and intervening with ganciclovir only when reactivation is detected before active disease occurs.

Indications for monitoring:
- HSCT recipients who are CMV IgG–positive or who received graft from a donor who is CMV IgG–positive

Monitoring:
- Weekly CMV antigenemia, *or*
- Weekly CMV PCR if CMV antigenemia is not feasible or patient has ANC <500 mm^3

Duration of monitoring:
- Continue beyond day + 100 if immune suppression continues (excluding immune suppression produced by cyclosporine or tacrolimus) or if there is a history of late CMV reactivation (after day + 75)[4]

Treatment indications:
- A patient with CMV+ antigenemia or two consecutive PCR assays positive for CMV

Note: The best evidence pertains to the use of CMV antigenemia (pp65 detection). CMV PCR is a newer assay, and the sensitivity and specificity tend to vary depending on the kind of PCR and primers used. The current CDC/ASBMT/IDSA guidelines suggest one positive antigenemia test or two consecutive CMV PCR tests as triggers for preemptive administration of ganciclovir or foscarnet

Therapy:
- **Ganciclovir** 5 mg/kg per dose intravenously every 12 hours for 7 days, *followed by*
- **Ganciclovir** 5 mg/kg per dose intravenously daily 5 days per week

Alternative:
- **Foscarnet** 60 mg/kg per dose intravenously every 12 hours for 7 days, *followed by*
- **Foscarnet** 60 mg/kg per dose intravenously daily 5 days per week

Alternative:
- **Valganciclovir** 900 mg orally every 12 hours, *followed by*
- **Valganciclovir** 900 mg orally daily 5 days per week

Note: Discontinue acyclovir when either ganciclovir or foscarnet is used

Duration of treatment:
Continue treatment until 2 consecutive weekly CMV antigenemia tests or PCR for CMV are negative

Noninfectious Complications After Allogeneic HSCT[12–15]

1. Acute graft-versus-host disease after allogeneic HSCT[16,17]
2. Chronic graft-versus-host disease after allogeneic HSCT

Note: Except for acute GVHD and chronic GVHD, autologous transplant recipients may develop post-transplantation complications similar to those of allogeneic transplant recipients. Monitoring recommendations for autologous transplant recipients are similar to those included in the chapter for allogeneic transplant recipients

ACUTE GRAFT-VERSUS-HOST DISEASE (ACUTE GVHD)

Epidemiology and Staging of Acute GVHD

Incidence

Source of Stem Cells	Incidence
HLA-identical sibling donor	20–50%
HLA-mismatched sibling	50–80%
HLA-identical unrelated donor	50–80%

Risk Factors

1. Unrelated HLA-identical donor
2. HLA-mismatch
3. Gender mismatch
4. Increasing donor or recipient age
5. Ineffective GVHD prophylaxis

Organs Involvement

Organ Involved	% of Patients
Skin	81
Gastrointestinal	54
Liver	50

Staging and Grading of Acute GVHD

Staging of Acute GVHD

Skin, liver, and gastrointestinal tract are staged independently and combined for an overall grade

Stage	Skin[a]	Liver	Gastrointestinal Tract[b]
Stage I	Rash on <25% of skin	Total bilirubin 2–3 mg/dL	Diarrhea >500 mL/day
Stage II	Rash on 25–50% of skin	Total bilirubin 3.1–6 mg/dL	Diarrhea >1000 mL/day
Stage III	Generalized erythroderma	Total bilirubin 6.1–15 mg/dL	Diarrhea >1500 mL/day
Stage IV	Bullae	Total bilirubin >15 mg/dL	Severe abdominal pain, bleeding ± ileus

[a]A maculopapular rash initially involving the face, ears, palms, soles, and upper trunk. If GVHD advances rash spreads to rest of body, generally sparing the scalp. Histologic examination is needed to establish diagnosis

[b]A pan-intestinal process that can present with nausea, vomiting, anorexia, diarrhea and or abdominal pain. The diagnosis of gastrointestinal GVHD must be made by mucosal biopsy

Grading for Acute GVHD

Grade	Skin	Liver		Gut
I	1–2	0		0
II	1–3	1	and/or	1
III	2–3	2–4	and/or	2–3
IV	2–4	2–4	and/or	2–4

Przepiorka D et al. Bone Marrow Transplant 1995;15:825–828
Rowlings P et al. Br J Hematol 1997;97:855–864

Prophylaxis and Treatment of Acute GVHD

Standard prophylaxis for acute GHVD:
Cyclosporine + methotrexate

Treatment options for acute GVHD:

1. *First-line therapy*: Corticosteroids
2. *Investigational therapies for patients with acute GVHD who do not respond to steroids:* Mycophenolate mofetil, tacrolimus, antithymocyte globulin, daclizumab, infliximab, pentostatin, visilizumab, denileukin diftitox, keratinocyte growth factor-2

REGIMEN FOR STANDARD PROPHYLAXIS

CYCLOSPORINE + METHOTREXATE

Arai S et al, Blood Review 2000;14:190–204
Jacobsohn DA. Expert Opin Investig Drugs 2002;11(9):1271–1280
Storb R et al. Blood 1989;73(6):1729–1734
Storb R et al. Blood 1992;80(2):560–561
Storb R et al. NEJM 1986;314(12):729–735

Cyclosporine 2–5 mg/kg per dose intravenously or orally twice daily (every 12 hours) starting 1–2 days before graft infusion and continuing for a total of 6 months

Notes:
1. Begin with intravenous administration and then continue with oral administration
2. A 12-hour schedule increases trough concentrations and decreases peak concentrations. However, cyclosporine may also be given once a day
3. Oral cyclosporine is incompletely absorbed. Changing from intravenous to oral administration (or the reverse) requires a conversion

Intravenous:Oral Dose (mg:mg)	
Cyclosporine (Sandimmune®)	Cyclosporine [modified] (Neoral®)
1:2–3	1:1–2

Methotrexate 15 mg/m² intravenously on day 1 after transplantation (total dose: 15 mg/m²),
followed by
Methotrexate 10 mg/m² per dose intravenously for 3 doses on days 3, 6, and 11 after transplantation (total for 3 doses: 30 mg/m²)

Cyclosporine is available in the United States in two encapsulated and solution formulations for oral administration: cyclosporine (Sandimmune®; Novartis) and cyclosporine [modified]. The modified and unmodified products are distinguished by marked differences in oral bioavailability and cannot be used interchangeably without carefully monitoring cyclosporine blood concentrations and dose adjustments based on individual response. Both formulations are marketed in two strengths, containing 25 mg or 100 mg cyclosporine. Cyclosporine and cyclosporine [modified] also are available in solution formulations for oral administration

Sandimmune® 25-mg and 100-mg capsules contain cyclosporine
Sandimmune® Oral Solution contains cyclosporine 100 mg/mL
NEORAL® 25-mg and 100-mg capsules contain cyclosporine [modified]
NEORAL® Oral Solution contains cyclosporine [modified] 100 mg/mL
GENGRAF® 25-mg and 100-mg capsules contain cyclosporine [modified]
GENGRAF® Oral Solution contains cyclosporine [modified] 100 mg/mL

Emetogenic potential: Low (Emetogenicity score 2–3). See chapter 39 for antiemetic regimens

Patient Population Studied

Several studies of many patients with hematologic malignancies who had undergone HLA-identical sibling HSCT

Efficacy

Storb R et al. NEJM 1986;314(12):729–735

In a seminal randomized trial comparing the effect of a methotraxate and cyclosporine combination with cyclosporine alone there was a significant reduction in the cumulative incidence of grades II–IV acute GVHD in patients who received the combination regimen (33%) compared with those receiving cyclosporine alone (54%) $P = .014$

Treatment Modifications

General guidance:
1. Cyclosporine dose modifications may be guided by pharmacokinetics when these are available. Often, however, therapeutic targets can be effectively achieved by making small incremental changes of 10–25%
2. If levels are high, or in the presence of toxicity, hold cyclosporine and resume a lower dose after:
   - Demonstrating a level within the targeted range
   - Adverse events are diminished or resolved

Adverse Event	Dose Modification
Baseline serum creatinine within normal limits and serum creatinine increases to 1.5–2 mg/dL (132–176 μmol/L)	Reduce cyclosporine dose by 50%
Baseline serum creatinine within normal limits and serum creatinine increases to >2 mg/dL (>176 μmol/L)	Hold cyclosporine and check daily creatinine and cyclosporine levels. Restart cyclosporine when creatinine is <2 mg/dL (<176 μmol/L) at 50% of the initial dose
Hypertension develops while on cyclosporine	Consider calcium channel blockers or β-blockers as first line therapy
Voriconazole therapy in a patient with therapeutic cyclosporine levels	Reduce cyclosporine dose by ≃ 50%

Adverse Event	Methotrexate dose modification
Bilirubin 2.1–3.0 mg/dL (35.9–51.3 μmol/L)	Reduce dose by 25%
Bilirubin 3.1–4.0 mg/dL (53–68.4 μmol/L)	Reduce dose by 50%
Bilirubin >4.1 mg/dL (>70.1 μmol/L)	Hold Methotrexate
Serum creatinine 1.6–2.0 mg/dL (141–176 μmol/L)	Reduce dose by 25%
Serum creatinine 2.1–2.5 mg/dL (185–220 μmol/L)	Reduce dose by 50%
Serum creatinine >2.5 mg/dL (>220 μmol/L)	Hold Methotrexate
Severe mucositis	Hold Methotrexate

Toxicity

Cyclosporine

Common

Headache
Hirsutism, hypertrichosis
Nausea, vomiting, diarrhea
Tremor
Hypertension
Nephrotoxicity
Hyperlipidemia

Serious

Posterior encephalopathy (seizures, blindness)
Gum hyperplasia
Hepatotoxicity
Hypomagnesemia
Anaphylaxis with IV formulations (rare)
Hyperkalemia (rare)
Pancreatitis (rare)
Paresthesia (rare)

Methotrexate

Common

Alopecia, photosensitivity, rash
Anorexia, diarrhea
Nausea, vomiting
Stomatitis

Serious

Cirrhosis
Elevated liver function test
Hepatic fibrosis, atrophy, necrosis, and failure
Gastrointestinal bleeding
Mucositis, ulceration
Hyperuricemia
Nephropathy, renal failure
Interstitial pneumonitis (acute, chronic)
Methotrexate-induced lung disease
Myelosuppression

Therapy Monitoring

1. *Daily cyclosporine levels:*
   - At the start of therapy
   - When clinical toxicity is encountered
   - When potentially interacting agents are added or withdrawn
2. *Cyclosporine level 24–72 hours after change in:*
   - Dose
   - Schedule
   - Route of administration
   - Product formulation
3. *Weekly to every 2 weeks:* BUN and creatinine

Notes:

1. Cyclosporine assay methodologies vary among clinical laboratories
2. The therapeutic target concentrations also vary with:
   - Type of sample assayed (if specimen other than whole blood is analyzed)
   - Dosing interval
   - Temperature
   - Clinician preferences
3. Therapeutic monitoring strategies also vary and may include the following samples:
   - *Traditional*: predose, trough, or C0
   - *2-hour post-dose*: C2 or absorption profiling
4. Verify whether aberrant levels are correct, particularly when they occur unexpectedly. Factors that perturb cyclosporine levels include:
   - Noncompliance with an oral regimen
   - The introduction, modification, and discontinuation of drugs that potentially interfere with cyclosporine absorption (after oral administration), metabolism, and elimination
   - Incorrect sampling time
   - Blood drawn through a catheter lumen used to administer the drug intravenously
   - Drawing specimens while administering cyclosporine intravenously

Notes

1. Cyclosporine is extensively metabolized by the cytochrome P450 CYP3A subfamily enzymes; its metabolism and elimination can be markedly perturbed by drugs that induce or inhibit CYP3A enzymes
2. Cyclosporine is an inhibitor of P-glycoprotein
3. At some transplantation centers, tacrolimus has replaced cyclosporine because two phase III trials have shown a decrease in grades II–IV acute GVHD when comparing tacrolimus/methotrexate with cyclosporine/methotrexate. However, disease-free survival was not different. Patients received **methotrexate** 15 mg/m^2 on day 1 and 10 mg/m^2 on days 3, 6, and 11 after marrow transplantation. **Tacrolimus** was started on the day before transplantation at 0.03 mg/kg/day by continuous IV infusion. The route of administration was converted from IV to PO at the ratio of 1:4 in 2 divided doses per day when the patients were able to tolerate oral intake. Tacrolimus dose was reduced by 25% when the creatinine was elevated > twice the baseline and by 50% for patients with a creatinine >3 times baseline. Levels of tacrolimus were maintained between 10 and 30 ng/mL. The dose was tapered by 20% per month starting 2 months post-transplantation and discontinued at the end of 6 months

Tacrolimus side effects

Common: Constipation, diarrhea, nausea, vomiting, headache, insomnia, tremor
Serious: Hyperglycemia (frequent), hyperkalemia, hypomagnesemia, hypertension, myocardial hypertrophy, QT prolongation, torsades de pointes, nephrotoxicity

Nash RA et al. Blood 2000;96:2062–2068
Ratanatharathorn V et al. Blood 1998;92:2303–2314

Tacrolimus is generically available in the United States in a variety of formulations and product strengths, including capsules for oral administration containing the equivalent of 0.5 mg, 1 mg, and 5 mg of anhydrous tacrolimus (Prograf®; Fujisawa Healthcare, Inc, Deerfield, IL)

4. In a prospective randomized trial comparing a 3-drug regimen (cyclophosphamide [CSP], methotrexate [MTX], prednisone) with a 2-drug regimen (CSP, MTX), there was no significant impact on the incidence of acute GVHD or event-free or overall survival Chao NJ et al. Biol Blood Marrow Transplant 2000;6:254–261

REGIMEN FOR FIRST-LINE TREATMENT

CORTICOSTEROIDS

Martin PJ. Blood 1990;76:1464–1472
Vogelsang GB. Annu Rev Med 2003:29–52
Weisdorf D. Blood 1990;75:1024–1030

Grade I GVHD (limited skin disease):
Low-dose corticosteroids: Prednisone 1 mg/kg per day (or equivalent) orally, continuously, *or*
Topical corticosteroids: 0.1% triamcinolone applied to the body rash every 12 hours, and **1% hydrocortisone** applied to the face every 12 hours
Note: Taper gradually after GVHD is controlled

Grade II-IV GVHD (systemic or severe skin disease):
High dose corticosteroids: Methylprednisolone 62.5 mg/m^2 per dose intravenously twice a day for 4 to 7 days [If no response after 4 days, continue until response (7-day maximum trial)
If response occurs within 7 days, taper as follows:

- 50 mg/m^2 per dose intravenously twice a day for 2 days
- 37.5 mg/m^2 per dose intravenously twice a day for 2 days
- 25 mg/m^2 per dose intravenously twice a day for 2 days
- After this, steroids are reduced by 10% each week until a dose of 10 mg/day prednisone or its equivalent is reached. Subsequent reductions will be made at the clinician's discretion

Notes:

1. Convert methylprednisolone to oral **prednisone** (equivalent of intravenous dose) when clinically appropriate at the clinician's discretion
   Example: **Prednisone** 100 mg orally daily for 2 days after attaining a methylprednisolone dose of 25 mg/m^2
2. If GVHD worsens during taper, steroids should be increased to previous dose
3. **During steroid taper, maintain cyclosporine at therapeutic levels**
4. If no response is observed within 7 days of methylprednisolone treatment, increase methylprednisolone to 500 mg/m^2 per dose intravenously twice a day for 2 days. If there is no improvement, consider using second-line immunosuppressive therapy for acute GVHD
   Prednisone is marketed in the United States in numerous generic formulations for oral administration, including immediate-release tablets containing 1, 2.5, 5, 10, 20, and 50 mg, and in solutions and syrups

Emetogenic potential: Nonemetogenic to low (Emetogenicity score ≤2). See Chapter 39 for antiemetic regimens

Patient Population Studied

Multiple studies of patients who develop acute GVHD after allogeneic-HSCT

Efficacy

Less than 50% of patients who develop acute GVHD show durable improvement after initial steroid treatment

Toxicity

Common: Cataracts, Cushing's syndrome euphoria/depression, GI distress, peptic ulcer, mild elevations in liver function tests, hypertension, sodium and fluid retention, impaired wound healing, muscle weakness, skin atrophy
Serious: Osteoporosis, tuberculosis reactivation, adrenocortical insufficiency, glaucoma, hyperglycemia, increased intracranial pressure, seizures, CHF

Therapy Monitoring

Criteria to determine response to acute GVHD treatment
Complete response:
Complete resolution of all clinical signs and symptoms of acute GVHD
Partial response:
≥50% reduction in skin rash, stool volume or frequency, and/or total bilirubin
Maintenance of adequate performance status (Karnofsky score ≥70%)
No response:
<50% reduction in skin rash, stool volume or frequency, and/or total bilirubin
Failure to maintain adequate performance status (Karnofsky score ≤70%)
Progressive disease:
Further progression of signs and symptoms of acute GVHD, *and/or*
Decline in performance status after the initiation of therapy

Notes

1. If there is no improvement on corticosteroid therapy, consider using second-line therapy
2. No second-line therapy has proved to have better efficacy
3. *Investigational therapies for patients with acute GVHD who do not respond to steroids:* Mycophenolate mofetil, tacrolimus, antithymocyte globulin, daclizumab, infliximab, pentostatin, visilizumab, denileukin diftitox, keratinocyte growth factor, sirolimus

Jacobsohn DA. Expert Opin Invest Drugs 2002;11(9):1271–1280
Javier Bolanos-Meade et al. Curr Opin Hematol 2004;12:40–44

CHRONIC GRAFT-VERSUS-HOST DISEASE AFTER ALLOGENEIC HSCT[18–20]

Epidemiology and Staging of Chronic GVHD

The majority of patients with chronic GVHD had prior acute GVHD. Their disease may evolve directly from acute GVHD (progressive) or may be followed a period of resolution (quiescent) or develop with no history of acute GHVD (de novo)

Incidence

Source of Stem Cells	Incidence
HLA-identical sibling donor	40%
HLA-nonidentical related SCT	>50%
HLA-matched unrelated donor	70%

Risk Factors

1. Older age
2. Gender mismatch
3. Mismatched or unrelated donor
4. Peripheral blood stem cells
5. Donor lymphocyte infusion
6. T-cell–replete graft
7. History of acute GVHD

Organ Involvement

	% of Patients
Skin	65–80
Mouth	48–72
Liver	40–73
Eye	18–47
Gastrointestinal	16–26
Lung	10–15
Joints	2–12

Timing of Onset of Chronic GVHD

HCST Source	Median Time to Diagnosis
HLA-identical sibling donor	201 days
HLA-nonidentical related donor	159 days
Unrelated donor	133 days

Diagnosis and Staging of Chronic GVHD

The First NIH Consensus Development Project on Criteria for Clinical Trials in Chronic Graft Versus Host Disease in June 2005 developed new diagnostic criteria, clinically staging criteria, and standardized response criteria that are clinical meaningful

Diagnosis requirements of chronic GVHD:

- Patients may be classified as having limited disease if they have localized skin involvement with or without hepatic dysfunction
- Patients may be classified as having extensive disease if they have generalized skin involvement or limited skin involvement combined with eye involvement, mouth or liver dysfunction with abnormal histology of any other target organ. Although this classification system is highly reproducible, it has no proven prognostic value
- Multivariate analysis of patients with chronic GVHD found three variables that are risk factors for shortened survival: Extensive skin GVHD involving >50% of the body surface area, platelet count <100,000/μL and progressive onset

Akpek G et al. Blood 2001;97:1219–1226

- Distinction from acute GVHD
- Presence of at least one diagnostic clinical sign of chronic GVHD or an appropriate constellation of distinctive signs confirmed by biopsy or other relevant diagnostic tests
- Exclusion of other possible diagnoses

Notes:

- Scoring of organ manifestations requires careful assessment of signs, symptoms, laboratory values, and other study results
- A clinical scoring system (0–3) is recommended for scoring of individual organs, and global assessment of severity (none, mild, moderate, severe) derived by combining organ-specific scores
- Systemic therapy should be considered for patients who meet criteria for moderate to severe overall severity

Global scoring of chronic GVHD

Mild chronic GVHD: Presence of mild abnormalities not associated with clinically significant functional impairment (maximum of score 1 in all affected organs or sites) that involves one or two organs or sites (except lung involvement, see below)

Moderate chronic GVHD: Presence of moderate abnormalities associated with functional impairment in at least one organ or site (maximum of score 2 in any affected organ or site) or mild abnormalities involving three or more organs (maximum of score 1 in all affected organs or sites). A lung score of 1 is considered moderate chronic GVHD

Severe chronic GVHD: Abnormalities affecting any organ or site scored as 3 along with clinically significant functional impairment. A lung score of 2 or 3 is also considered severe chronic GVHD

Filipovich AH et al. Biology of Blood and Marrow Transplantation 2005;11:945–956

Signs and Symptoms of Chronic GVHD[a]

Organ or Site	Diagnostic (Sufficient to establish the diagnosis of chronic GVHD)	Distinctive (Seen in chronic but not acute GVHD, but insufficient alone to establish a diagnosis of chronic GVHD)
Skin	Poikiloderma Lichen-planus-like features Sclerotic features Morphea-like features Lichen sclerosus-like features	Depigmentation
Nails		Dystrophy Longitudinal ridging, splitting, or brittle features Onycholysis Pterygium unguis Nail loss (usually symmetric; affects most nails)
Scalp and body hair		New onset of scarring or nonscarring scalp alopecia (after recovery from chemoradiotherapy) Scaling, papulosquamous lesions
Mouth	Lichen-type features Hyperkeratotic plaques Restriction of mouth opening from sclerosis	Xerostomia Mucocele Mucosal atrophy Pseudomembranes[a] Ulcers[a]
Eyes		New-onset dry, gritty, or painful eyes[b] Cicatricial conjunctivitis Keratoconjunctivitis sicca[b] Confluent areas of punctate keratopathy
Genitalia	Lichen-type features Vaginal stricture or stenosis	Erosion[a] Fissures[a] Ulcers[a]
GI tract	Esophageal web Strictures or stenosis in the upper to mid third of the esophagus	
Lung	Bronchiolitis obliterans diagnosed with lung biopsy	Bronchiolitis obliterans diagnosed with PFTs and radiology[b]
Muscles, fascia, joints	Fasciitis Joint stiffness or contractures secondary to sclerosis	Myositis or polymyositis[b]

[a]In all patients, infection, drug effect, and other causes must be excluded. (NIH Consensus Development Project on Criteria for Clinical Trials in Chronic Graft Versus Host Disease)
[b]Diagnosis of chronic GVHD requires biopsy or radiology confirmation (or Schirmer's test for eyes)

Chronic GVHD: Treatment Options

First Line: Prednisone ± Cyclosporine A (CSA)
Investigational therapies for chronic GVHD that do not respond to prednisone + cyclosporine include: High-dose corticosteroids, mycophenolate mofetil, tacrolimus, thalidomide, extracorporeal photophoresis, psoralen and UVA, hydroxychloroquine

Chronic GVHD: Antimicrobial Prophylaxis

Infections are a common cause of death in chronic GVHD. Recommendations regarding prophylaxis are based on expert opinion rather than controlled trials.[2,3] A common practice is to start antimicrobial prophylaxis as soon as the diagnosis of chronic GVHD is made, or at least when active immunosuppression for the treatment of chronic GVHD is started

Antibacterial Prophylaxis

First Choice	Alternative
Penicillin V potassium 500 mg orally twice daily	*Penicillin allergy:* **Cotrimoxazole** (trimethoprim 80 mg + sulfamethoxazole 400 mg) orally daily *Penicillin and sulfonamide allergy:* **Clarithromycin** 500 mg orally daily

Penicillin V (phenoxymethyl penicillin) potassium is generically available in the United States in two formulations for oral administration, including immediate-release tablets containing either 250 or 500 mg penicillin V, and powdered products for preparing liquid suspensions containing either 125 mg or 250 mg penicillin V per 5 mL)
Clotrimazole is generically available in the United States in a variety of formulations and product strengths, including tablets and liquids
Clarithromycin is available in the United States in several formulations for oral administration, including immediate-release tablets (250 or 500 mg/tablet), an extended-release 500-mg tablet, and granulated products for preparing liquid suspensions (125 mg/5 mL or 250 mg/5 mL). Biaxin® Filmtab® (clarithromycin tablets), Biaxin® XL Filmtab® (clarithromycin extended-release tablets), Biaxin® Granules (clarithromycin for oral suspension) product label, December 2003. Abbott Laboratories, North Chicago, IL

Antiviral Prophylaxis

First Choice	Alternative
Acyclovir 200 mg orally every 12 hours *Note:* most experience is with Acyclovir	**Valacyclovir** 500 mg orally daily *Note:* Valacyclovir is more convenient and is an acceptable alternative

Valacyclovir hydrochloride is available in the United States as tablets for oral administration containing either 500 or 1000 mg valacyclovir HCl (Valtrex® caplets. GlaxoSmithKline, Research Triangle Park, NC)
Acyclovir is available in the United States generically in formulations for oral administration, including immediate-release tablets (400 and 800 mg/tablet), immediate-release capsules (200 mg/capsule), and a powdered product for preparing a liquid suspension (200 mg/5 mL)

Antifungal Prophylaxis

It is unknown whether administering antifungal prophylaxis during GVHD is efficacious in terms of decreasing the incidence of invasive fungal infections or improving outcome. Some experts, concerned with the risk of invasive aspergillosis in this setting, advocate the use of voriconazole, but this approach is off-label and must be considered experimental

Pneumocystis carinii Pneumonia (PCP)Prophylaxis

Prophylaxis for *Pneumocystis carinii* pneumonia should be administered to all patients undergoing treatment for chronic GVHD and for 6 months beyond the discontinuation of immunosuppressive medications

First Choice	Alternative
Cotrimoxazole DS (trimethoprim 160 mg + sulfamethoxazole 800 mg) per day orally 3 days/week	**Aerosolized pentamidine** 300 mg by inhalation every 4 weeks

Clotrimazole is generically available in the United States in a variety of formulations and product strengths, including tablets and liquids
Pentamidine isethionate is available in the United States generically as a sterile solution or lyophilized powder for intravenous administration and as a solution for aerosolization and administration by inhalation

Note: patients with chronic GHVD undergoing dental work or other invasive procedures should receive standard antibiotic prophylaxis

CHRONIC GVHD REGIMEN FOR FIRST-LINE TREATMENT

PREDNISONE AND CYCLOSPORINE A (CSA)

Sullivan KM. Blood 1988;72:555–561
Vogelsang GB, Blood 2001;97:1196–1201

Prednisone 1 mg/kg per day orally continuously, *and*
Cyclosporine 5 mg/kg per dose twice daily orally continuously (total dose: 10 mg/kg/day)
Notes:

1. If disease is stable or improving after 2 weeks, prednisone is tapered by 25% per week to a target dose of 1 mg/kg every other day
2. After successfully completing a steroid taper, cyclosporine dosage is reduced by 25% per week. Administer prednisone and cyclosporine on alternate days such that the patient takes cyclosporine on 1 day and alternates with prednisone the next day
3. *After 9 months:* If disease has completely resolved, wean patient from both medications with dose reductions every 2 weeks
4. *After 9 months:* If response is incomplete, continue therapy for an additional 3 months and then reevaluate patients. If a patient does not have a beneficial response after an additional 3 months or demonstrates progressive disease, salvage regimens are warranted

Prednisone is marketed in the United States in numerous generic formulations for oral administration, including immediate-release tablets containing 1, 2.5, 5, 10, 20, and 50 mg, and in solutions and syrups for oral administration
Cyclosporine is available in the United States in two different encapsulated and solution formulations for oral administration; that is, cyclosporine (Sandimmune®; Novartis) and cyclosporine [modified]. The modified and unmodified products are distinguished by marked differences in oral bioavailability and cannot be used interchangeably without carefully monitoring cyclosporine blood concentrations and dose adjustments based on individual response. Both formulations are marketed in two strengths, containing 25 mg or 100 mg cyclosporine. Cyclosporine and cyclosporine [modified] also are available in solution formulations for oral administration

Sandimmune® 25-mg and 100-mg capsules contain cyclosporine (Novartis Pharmaceuticals Corporation, East Hanover, NJ)
Sandimmune® Oral Solution contains cyclosporine 100 mg/mL (Novartis Pharmaceuticals Corporation)
NEORAL® 25-mg and 100-mg capsules contain cyclosporine [modified] (Novartis Pharmaceuticals Corporation) NEORAL® Oral Solution contains cyclosporine [modified] 100 mg/mL (Novartis Pharmaceuticals Corporation)
GENGRAF® 25-mg and 100-mg capsules contain cyclosporine [modified] (Abbott Laboratories, North Chicago, IL) GENGRAF® Oral Solution contains cyclosporine [modified] (Abbott Laboratories)

Emetogenic potential: Nonemetogenic to low (Emetogenicity score ≤2). See Chapter 39 for antiemetic regimens

Treatment Modifications

General guidance:

1. Cyclosporine dose modifications may be guided by pharmacokinetics when these are available. Often, however, therapeutic targets can be effectively achieved by making small incremental changes of 10–25%
2. If levels are high, or in the presence of toxicity, hold cyclosporine and resume a lower dose after:
   - Demonstrating a level within the targeted range
   - Adverse events are diminished or resolved

Adverse Event	Dose Modification
Baseline serum creatinine within normal limits and serum creatinine increases to 1.5–2 mg/dL (132–176 μmol/L)	Reduce cyclosporine dose by 50%
Baseline serum creatinine within normal limits and serum creatinine increases to >2 mg/dL (>176 μmol/L)	Withhold cyclosporine and check daily creatinine and cyclosporine levels. Restart cyclosporine when creatinine is <2 mg/dL (<176 μmol/L) at 50% of the initial cyclosporine dose
Hypertension develops while on cyclosporine	Consider calcium channel blockers or β-blockers as first line therapy
Voriconazole therapy in a patient with therapeutic cyclosporine levels	Reduce cyclosporine dose by ≃ 50%

Patient Population Studied

Patients with chronic GVHD

EFFICACY

Five-year survival rate is ~50%

Toxicity

Prednisone

Incidence and severity depend on dose administered and duration of administration

Common
Mood and behavioral abnormalities
GI distress
Hypertension, sodium and fluid retention
Impaired skin healing
Increased risk of infection
Osteoporosis
Skin atrophy

Serious
Adrenocortical insufficiency
Cataracts, glaucoma
Cushing's syndrome
Hyperglycemia
Tuberculosis reactivation

Cyclosporine A

Common
Headache
Hirsutism, hypertrichosis
Nausea, vomiting, diarrhea
Tremor
Hypertension
Nephrotoxicity
Hyperlipidemia

Serious
Anaphylaxis (with IV use; rare)
Posterior encephalopathy (seizures, blindness)
Gum hyperplasia
Hepatotoxicity
Hypomagnesemia
Hyperkalemia (rare)
Pancreatitis (rare)
Paresthesia (rare)

Therapy Monitoring

1. *Cyclosporine level:*
   - At the start of therapy
   - When clinical toxicity is encountered
   - When potentially interacting agents are added or withdrawn
2. *Cyclosporine level 24–72 hours after change in:*
   - Dose
   - Schedule
   - Route of administration
   - Product formulation
3. *Weekly to every 2 weeks:* BUN and creatinine

Notes:

1. Cyclosporine assay methodologies vary among clinical laboratories
2. The therapeutic target concentrations also vary with:
   - Type of sample assayed (if specimen other than whole blood is analyzed)
   - Temperature
3. Verify whether aberrant levels are correct, particularly when they occur unexpectedly. Factors that perturb cyclosporine levels include:
   - Noncompliance with an oral regimen
   - The introduction, modification, and discontinuation of drugs that potentially interfere with cyclosporine, metabolism, and elimination
   - Incorrect sampling time

Note

In a randomized trial, patients with newly diagnosed extensive GVHD and platelet count >100,000/μL were treated with cyclosporine alternating with prednisone every other day or alternate-day prednisone alone. Treatment with cyclosporine and prednisone reduced the risk for steroid-related toxicity, but there was no difference in overall mortality, recurrent malignancy, and discontinuation of all immunosuppressive therapy

Koc S et al. Blood 2002;100:48–51

OCULAR COMPLICATIONS

Cataracts

Incidence	• *Single-dose total-body irradiation (TBI):* > 85% of patients develop cataracts within 3–4 years • *Fractionated radiation:* 30% incidence at 3 years; 80% at 5–10 years
Risk factors	• Age >23 years • 0.04 Gy/minute radiation dose rate • >3 months steroid administration
Monitor	HSCT recipients should be evaluated by an ophthalmologist before transplantation, 3 months after transplantation, then yearly
Treatment	Surgery when indicated

Keratoconjunctivitis Sicca Syndrome [Reduced tear flow, keratoconjunctivitis sicca, sterile conjunctivitis, corneal epithelial defects, corneal ulceration]

Incidence	• *Patients with GVHD:* 40% • *Patients without GVHD:* 10%
Risk factors	• Chronic GVHD • Single-dose TBI • Age >20 years • Use of methotrexate for GVHD prophylaxis
Monitor	HSCT recipients should be evaluated by an ophthalmologist before transplantation, 3 months after transplantation, then yearly If a patient develops keratoconjunctivitis sicca syndrome, more frequent evaluations may be needed If a patient is asymptomatic beyond 3 months, perform ophthalmologic examination and Schirmer test yearly
Treatment	• Topical lubricants and topical immunosuppressants (corticosteroids and cyclosporine) *Note:* patients on topical corticosteroids should have eye pressures monitored monthly. Temporary punctal occlusion using punctal plugs can be performed to enhance the moisture on the surface of the eyes

Ischemic Retinopathy [Cotton-wool spots and optic disc edema]

Incidence	Occurs in 10% of patients after HSCT
Risk factors	• TBI • Cyclosporine therapy • Use of cyclophosphamide and busulfan
Monitor	HSCT recipients should be evaluated by an ophthalmologist before transplantation, 3 months after transplantation, then yearly
Treatment	• Cotton wool spots (CWS) are frequently seen as an incidental finding at 3 months post-transplantation and can resolve spontaneously. Asymptomatic patients need follow-up for 1 to 3 months until CWS resolve – Symptomatic CWS are rare and occur when they are located in the central of the macula causing scotomas (small field defects). Patients with extensive CWS may have had TBI and may have poorly controlled hypertension or diabetes mellitus. Consider tapering cyclosporine if a symptomatic patient has >0–15 CWS in the macular region – Extensive CWS may actually represent CMV retinitis, and consultation with an ophthalmologist is recommended • Optic disc edema can be more ominous, suggesting cyclosporine toxicity when other causes, such as CNS lesions, have been ruled out. Tapering cyclosporine is recommended, especially if the patient has other neurologic signs of cyclosporine toxicity

ENDOCRINE DYSFUNCTION

Subclinical Hypothyroidism [Elevated TSH with normal free T_4]	
Incidence	*During the first year after HSCT:* 7–16%. May resolve spontaneously
Risk factors	Radiation therapy
Monitor	TSH and free T_4 levels twice yearly for the first year, then yearly
Treatment	Consider levothyroxine treatment if TSH concentration remains high or is increasing
Overt Hypothyroidism [Elevated TSH with low free-T_4 levels]	
Incidence	• *After 10 Gy, single-dose TBI:* 90% • *After fractionated TBI:* 14–15% • Diagnosed a median 50 months post-HSCT
Risk factors	Radiation therapy
Monitor	TSH and free T_4 levels twice yearly for the first year, then yearly
Treatment	*Levothyroxine:* Thyroid hormone levels should be measured 4–6 weeks after commencement of replacement therapy, and dosage should be tailored thereafter to the individual patient and adjusted according to thyroid function evaluation every 6 months

GONADAL FAILURE AND FERTILITY

Male Patients	
Incidence	Most of the patients given TBI conditioning experience gonadal failure Only 17–20% of men recover gonadal function. Fathering a child is rare
Risk factors	• Radiation therapy • Use of chemotherapy (busulfan/cyclophosphamide)
Monitor	Measure testosterone levels in symptomatic patients
Treatment	• Testosterone levels after HSCT are usually normal because Leydig cells are less vulnerable to radiation and chemotherapy even when spermatogenesis is reduced or absent. Thus, most males do not require testosterone replacement • Sex hormone replacement therapy with testosterone derivatives is indicated in patients with uncompensated hypogonadism • Symptomatic patients should be referred to endocrinologist and/or urologist
Female Patients	
Incidence	• Most patients given TBI conditioning as part of HSCT undergo premature ovarian failure • After HSCT for malignant diseases, ovarian function recovers in 10–14% of females • Pregnancy after HSCT transplantation is rare, but can occur with the use of donor oocytes as part of assisted reproductive technology
Risk factors	• Radiation therapy • Cytotoxic chemotherapy (such as busulfan/cyclophosphamide) • Increasing age
Monitor	• If clinical symptoms of menopause occur, measure FSH level • To assess ovarian function, measure FSH and estradiol levels off hormone replacement • Annual gynecologic examination is recommended
Treatment	• Because iatrogenic premature ovarian failure occurs with radiation and chemotherapy, young women without contraindications to hormones (eg, breast cancer) may benefit from hormone replacement therapy (HRT) • HRT can be initiated soon after HSCT (within the first month post-transplantation) • For HSCT recipients ≤35 years, use monophasic oral contraceptive preparations • For HSCT recipients >36 years. use postmenopausal hormone replacement preparations with estrogens and progestins • HSCT recipients who have had a hysterectomy may use estrogen alone • HRT can be interrupted once every 2–3 years to evaluate for spontaneous recovery of ovarian function

SKELETAL COMPLICATIONS

Avascular Necrosis (AVN) of Bone	
Incidence	• *Overall incidence:* 4–10% • Hips are most commonly affected (80%), followed by knee (10%) and wrist and ankle (< 10%) • *Mean time from transplantation to AVN:* 18 months • Multiple joints are affected in most patients
Risk factors	• Steroid use • TBI >10 Gy or >12 Gy in fractionated doses
Monitor	Screening for avascular necrosis is not recommended In symptomatic patients, MRI of the affected areas
Treatment	Joint replacement of the affected joins
Osteopenia/Osteoporosis	
Incidence	• *Osteopenia*: 33% • *Osteoporosis*: 10%
Risk factors	• Steroids • Cyclosporine A • Tacrolimus therapy • Iatrogenic hypogonadism
Monitor	Dual photon densitometry at 1 year for adult women or any patient with prolonged corticosteroid or calcineurin inhibitor exposure. Subsequent densitometry testing determined by defects or to assess response to therapy
Treatment	• Sex hormone replacement in patients with gonadal failure if clinically indicated • Bisphosphonates (see Chapter 44 for more information on bisphosphonates) calcium and vitamin D

HEPATIC COMPLICATIONS

Veno-occlusive Disease (VOD) [Hepatomegaly, right upper quadrant pain, jaundice, and ascites usually beginning within 6 weeks of HSCT. Not all features may be present, and the severity of signs and symptoms can vary]	
Incidence	• *After high-dose chemotherapy and TBI:* 20–50% • After high-dose cyclophosphamide and busulfan without TBI
Risk factors	• Preexisting liver dysfunction • Intensive conditioning regimens • Graft from mismatched or unrelated donor • Therapy with acyclovir, amphotericin, vancomycin, methotraxate, busulfan • Prior radiation to the liver
Monitor	For patients suspected of having VOD, perform ultrasound and Doppler studies to determine whether there is attenuation or reversal of venous flow or portal vein thrombosis
Treatment	• Because >70% of patients recover spontaneously, therapy is mainly supportive • For severe VOD, no therapy has proved more efficacious. Two therapies that have been used for the treatment of VOD are human tissue-type plasminogen activator and defibrotide *Note:* Prophylactic administration of ursodeoxycholic acid is recommended in HSCT recipients (*dose*: 600 mg day orally; *duration*: from −1 to day +80 post-transplantation) to reduce hepatic complications Ursodiol (ursodeoxycholic acid) is available in the United States as immediate-release capsules for oral administration containing 300 mg of the active drug
Iron Overload	
Incidence	*Iron overload on the basis of an elevated serum ferritin:* 88% of long-term survivors of HSCT
Risk factors	Heavy red blood cell transfusion history
Monitor	• All HSCT recipients should be screened for iron overload • Measure serum ferritin levels every 6 months for 2 years, then yearly. Serum ferritin should be measured 1 year post transplant and if abnormal, confirmatory liver biopsy considered based upon the magnitude of elevation and clinical context. Subsequent monitoring is suggested for the evaluation of elevated LFTs with continued RBC transfusions or hepatitis C infection
Treatment	• Phlebotomy • Chelation therapy

PULMONARY COMPLICATIONS

Chronic Obstructive Pulmonary Disease

Incidence	20% of long term survivors after HSCT
Risk factors	• GVHD • TBI • Hypogammaglobulinemia • Methotraxate use for GVHD prophylaxis • Recurrent infections
Monitor	• HSCT candidates should have baseline pulmonary function tests (PFTs) • In asymptomatic HSCT recipients PFTs every 3 months during the first post-transplantation year, then yearly • Patients with chronic GVHD PFTs every 1–2 months
Treatment	Obstructive pulmonary disease generally does not respond to bronchodilator treatment, and only 30–40% of patients respond on immunosuppressive therapy given alone or in combination with cyclosporine

Obliterative Bronchiolitis

Incidence	• *After HSCT:* 2–14% • *Mortality rate:* 50%
Risk factors	• Chronic GVHD • Low immunoglobulin levels
Monitor	• HSCT candidates should have baseline pulmonary function tests (PFTs) • In asymptomatic HSCT recipients, PFTs every 3 months during the first post-transplantation year, then yearly • Patients with chronic GVHD, PFTs every 1–2 months
Treatment	• Characteristically, patients with obliterative bronchiolitis disease do not respond well to conventional therapy for chronic GVHD with glucocorticoids. Combination therapy with glucocorticoids and steroids is indicated. If pulmonary function continues to deteriorate, some investigators add azathioprine • Prompt treatment of infections is an important element of clinical management and may help to alter the clinical course of a disease whose pace can vary from slow progression to rapidly fatal respiratory failure • Lung transplantation may be an option for patients with advanced disease, although the transplanted lung may be also be a target for immune mediated damage

SECONDARY MALIGNANCIES[21–23]

Post-Transplantation Lymphoproliferative Disorder (PTLD)

Incidence	1% *Median time from HSCT*: 2.5 months. B-cell PTLD > T-cell PTLD > late-onset lymphoma
Risk factors	• Use of antithymocyte globulin (ATG) for prophylaxis or treatment of acute GVHD • TBI in the preoperative regimen • T-cell depletion of donor marrow • Unrelated donor or HLA-nonidentical–related donor • Primary immune deficiency disease • EBV-negative patients transplanted from EBV-positive donors • Grade III-IV acute GVHD
Treatment	1. Removal of immunosupression 2. Donor lymphocyte infusion 3. Rituximab

Solid Tumors

Incidence	• Patients receiving a allo-HSCT have a 2- to 3 fold increased risk of developing solid tumor compared with an age-, gender, and region adjusted population. • 2.2% at 10 years and 6.7% at 15 years after transplantation • *Median time from HSCT to the development of solid tumors:* 5–6 years • Most common histologies: –Malignant melanoma –Cancers of the buccal mucosa –Liver –Brain and other parts of the central nervous system –Thyroid –Bone –Connective tissue
Risk factors	In an analysis of 19,229 patients who received allogeneic HSCT (97.2%) and syngeneic HSCT (2.8%), the risk was higher for recipients who were younger at the time of transplantation than those who were older. Higher doses of radiation were associated with higher risk Chronic GVHD and male sex were strongly linked with an excess risk of squamous cell cancers of the buccal cavity and skin
Monitor	HSCT patients should be followed up indefinitely to detect early cancer following current cancer screening recommendations (see Chapter 54 for cancer screening recommendations)
Treatment	As clinically indicated for specific cancer and stage

Recommended Vaccinations For Adult HCST Recipients (Autologous and Allogeneic)

Vaccine or Toxoid	Amount	Route	Time (Months)		
Tetanus-diphtheria toxoid (Td)	0.5 mL	IM	12	14	24
Haemophilus influenzae type b conjugate vaccine	0.5 mL	IM	12	14	24
Inactivated poliovirus vaccine	0.5 mL	IM	12	14	24
23-Valent pneumococcal polysaccharide	0.5 mL	IM	12		24
Hepatitis B	1 mL	IM	12	14	24
Measles-mumps-rubella attenuated live vaccine	0.5 mL	SC			24
Influenza virus	0.5 mL	IM	Lifelong annual administration beginning before HSCT and resuming 6 months after HSCT		

- Recommendations of CDC, the Infectious Disease Society of America, and the America Society of Blood and Marrow Transplantation http://www.cdc.gov/mmwr/preview/mmwrhtml/rr4910a1.htm
- For the guidelines, HSCT recipients are presumed immunocompetent at ≥24 months after HSCT if they are not on immunosuppressive therapy and do not have GVHD

References

1. MMWR Recomm Rep 2000;49:1–125, CE121–127
2. Roy V et al. Leuk Lymphoma 1997;26:1–15
3. Hughes WT et al. Clin Infect Dis 2002;34:730–751
4. Wingard JR. Transpl Infect Dis 1999;1:3–20
5. Fukuda T et al. Blood 2003;102:827–833
6. Hentrich M et al. Br J Haematol 2005;128:66–72
7. Bowden RA. Am J Med 1997;102:27–30; discussion 42–43
8. Whimbey E et al. Am J Med 1997;102:10–18; discussion 25–26
9. Nichols WG et al. Blood 2001;98:573–578
10. Kulkarni S et al. Blood 2000;95:3683–3686
11. Boeckh M et al. Blood 2003;101:407–414
12. Socié G et al. Blood 2003;101:3373–3385
13. Wingard JR et al. Hematology (Am Soc Hematol Educ Program) 2002:422–444
14. Tabbara IA et al. Arch Intern Med 2002;162:1558–1566
15. Antin JH. NEJM 2002;347:36–42
16. Arai S et al. Blood Rev 2000;14:190-204
17. Vogelsang GB et al. Ann Rev Med 2003;54:29–52
18. Vogelsang GB. Blood 2001;97:1196–1201
19. Lee S et al. Biol Blood Marrow Transplant 2003;9:215–233
20. Bhushan V et al. JAMA 2003;2003:2599–2603
21. Adè s L et al. Blood Rev 2002;16:135–46
22. Socié G et al. N Engl J Med 1999;341:14–21
23. Curtis RE et al. NEJM 1997;336:897–904

51. Radiation Complications

Diana Stripp, MD, and Eli Glatstein, MD

Radiation therapy (RT) is a major cancer treatment potential, both in definitive and palliative treatment. The aim of RT is to achieve the maximum tumor killing with minimal normal tissue damage

Factors Affecting Side-Effect Profile

Clinical: The site and the radiation responsiveness of the primary tumor
The tolerance of the surrounding normal tissue to RT
The associated use of chemotherapy

Physical: Arrangement and energy of the radiation beams and the anatomic structures in their path

Biological: The tissue response to RT at the molecular level
The individual's sensitivity to radiation

Radiation Side Effects: Acute and Late Phases

Early or acute side effects

- Largely represent killing of rapidly proliferating cells, such as mucosa, skin, and bone marrow
- Occur during or shortly after RT
- Usually begin 2–3 weeks into RT, increase progressively, and reach a plateau in the 5th to 7th weeks. Recovery is often seen during the last week of RT
- A majority recover without long-term sequelae as a result of the repopulation of normal stem cells
- The use of concomitant chemotherapy may significantly prolong and worsen acute reactions

Late or chronic side effects

- Largely represent cell loss from apoptosis and organ or tissue atrophy. Inflammation is rarely seen unless infection becomes superimposed
- Occur months or years after RT
- Generally progress slowly
- Can result in permanent undesirable effects of RT without sacrificing the tumor control

Morbidity Scoring

Common Toxicity Criteria for Adverse Events version 3.0 (CTCAE v3.0)[1]

Tolerance Dose (TD)

- Refers to the normal tissue tolerance of each organ to radiation
- TD5/5 is the dose that results in a 5% rate of major complications within 5 years after treatment (presumes that RT is given with the conventional fraction size of 1.8–2 Gy/day). TD 50/5 is the dose that results in a 50% rate of major complications within 5 years after treatment.
- Attempts have been made to define the TD5/5 for each organ[2]
- The defined TD5/5 should be used only as a guideline and not as an absolute. In the current era of combining chemotherapy and radiation or using altered fractionation schedules, adjustments in the tolerance doses are necessary

Normal Tissue Tolerance to Therapeutic Irradiation

	TD 5/5 Volume*			TD 50/5 Volume*			
Organ	**1/3**	**2/3**	**3/3**	**1/3**	**2/3**	**3/3**	**Selected end point**
Kidney	5000	3000[a]	2300		4000[a]	2800	Clinical nephritis
Bladder		8000	6500		8500	8000	Symptomatic bladder contracture and volume loss
Bone							
Femoral head			5200			6500	Necrosis
TM joint	6500	6000	6000	7700	7200	7200	Marked limitation of joint function
Rib cage	5000			6500			Pathologic fracture
Skin			100 cm^2/5000			100 cm^2/6500	Telangiectasis
	10 cm^2/7000	30 cm^2/6000	100 cm^2/5500			100 cm^2/7000	Necrosis, ulceration
Brain	6000	5000	4500	7500	6500	6000	Necrosis, infarction
Brain stem	6000	5300	5000			6500	Necrosis, infarction
Optic nerve			5000			6500	Blindness
Chiasma			5000			6500	Blindness
Spinal cord	5 cm/5000	10 cm/5000	20 cm/4700	5 cm/7000	10 cm/7000		Myelitis, necrosis
Cauda equine			6000			7500	Clinically apparent nerve damage
Brachial plexus	6200	6100	6000	7700	7600	7500	Clinically apparent nerve damage
Eyes Lens			1000			1800	Cataract requiring intervention
Retina			4500			6500	Blindness
Ears Mid/external	3000	3000	3000[a]	4000	4000	4000[a]	Acute serous otitis
Mid/external	5500	5500	5500[a]	6500	6500	6500[a]	Chronic serous otitis
Parotid[a]		3200[a]	3200[a]		4600[a]	4600[a]	Xerostomia[b]
Larynx	7900[a]	7000[a]	7000[a]	9000[a]	8000[a]	8000[a]	Cartilage necrosis
		4500	4500[a]			8000[a]	Laryngeal edema
Lungs	4500	3000	1750	6500	4000	2450	Pneumonitis
Heart	6000	4500	4000	7000	5500	5000	Pericarditis
Esophagus	6000	5800	5500	7200	7000	6800	Clinical stricture/perforation
Stomach	6000	5500	5000	7000	6700	6500	Ulceration, perforation
Small intestine	5000		4000[a]	6000		5500	Obstruction, perforation/fistula
Colon	5500		4500	6500		5500	Obstruction, perforation/ulceration/fistula
Rectum			6000			8000	Severe proctitis/necrosis/fistula, stenosis
Liver	5000	3500	3000	5500	4500	4000	Liver failure

*Values shown are tolerance doses for 1/3, 2/3 and 3/3 partial volumes of all listed organs

[a] <50% of volume doesn't make a significant change

[b] TD100/5 is 5000

Emami B et al. Int J Radiat Oncol Biol Phys 1991;21(1):109–122

SKIN

Skin: Early (Acute) Side Effects

Presentation

1. Seen as early as 7–10 days after starting RT
2. Erythema → increased dryness → hyperpigmentation → loss of hair (epilation) → dry desquamation at 4–5 weeks
3. Moist (wet) desquamation is seen 5–7 days after dry desquamation with continuation of RT dose

Management

1. Erythema, dryness, hyperpigmentation, and epilation

   General:
   - Avoid topical products on the skin within the RT portal during the radiation delivery
   - Wash skin gently and pat it dry
   - Keep skin well moisturized[3] and encourage regular moisturization after RT with nonirritating, fragrance-free lotions such as **Eucerin®** Original Moisturizing Lotion or **Keri®** Original Moisture Therapy lotion
   - *Pruritus*: Add **hydrocortisone cream 1%** or **2.5%** to the moisturizer; apply topically to intact skin twice daily
2. Moist desquamation

   General:
   - Apply compresses with **0.9% NaCl** or **aluminum acetate solution** (Burow's or Modified Burow's Solution) 3 or 4 times daily to clean and remove dead skin
   - Use **nonionic moisturizers** such as **Aquaphor®** Healing Ointment or a **vitamin A and E ointment** to provide a barrier to infection and loss of body fluid
   - Use a nonadhesive dressing when necessary to prevent added irritation

   Antibiotics: Use a topical antibiotic cream if infection occurs
   - Apply **triple antibiotic ointment (polymyxin B sulfate + neomycin + bacitracin zinc)** twice daily to affected area, *or*
   - Apply **silver sulfadiazine** twice daily to affected area

   Analgesia: Use medication for pain control as needed. See Chapter 52.
   - **Oxycodone, hydromorphone,** or **morphine**

Skin: Late (Chronic) Side Effects

Presentation

1. Hyper- or hypopigmentation
2. Telangiectasia
3. Permanent alopecia
4. Chronic ulceration, cutaneous atrophy
5. Fibrosis
6. Edema
7. Increased risk of basal cell carcinoma and melanoma

Management

1. Hyper- or hypopigmentation/increased risk of basal cell carcinoma and melanoma
   - Permanent use of **skin moisturizers with SPF > 15** and **protection from the sun** are advised
2. Chronic ulceration not responding to conservative therapy
   - Usually requires surgical repair
   - **Hyperbaric oxygen** treatment can lead to re-epithelialization and eliminate the need for surgical intervention. Hyperbaric oxygen is considered after the failure of conservative management
   - **Pentoxifylline** 400 mg orally 2–3-times per day. May increase blood flow and promote healing[4]
3. Radiation-induced fibrosis: **Pentoxifylline and α-tocopherol** can significantly reduce fibrosis[4]
   - **Pentoxifylline** 400 mg orally 2–3-times per day
   - **α-Tocopherol** 1000 units/day

Pentoxifylline is available in the United States in generic products for oral administration formulated as controlled-release and extended-release tablets containing 400 mg/tablet

D-α-Tocopherol and **DL-α-tocopherol acetate** (vitamin E) are available in the United States in numerous formulations for oral administration, including immediate-release tablets containing 100, 200, 400, 500, and 800 units of tocopherol; immediate-release capsules containing 100, 200, 400, and 1000 units of tocopherol; and drops and solutions

SOFT TISSUES AND BONE

Soft tissues and bone: Early (Acute) Side Effects

Presentation:

Soft tissue edema can develop especially in treatment of the head and neck region

Management:

Soft tissue edema

- **A temporary tracheostomy** may be required when patient develops laryngeal edema (when the possibility of laryngeal edema is high, a prophylactic **tracheostomy** can be performed before starting RT)
- Short course of steroids:
  - –**Dexamethasone** orally 2–4 times per day. Begin with a dose of 4 mg per day, tapering over 14 days, with dose and duration of treatment depending on response

Dexamethasone is marketed in the United States in numerous generic formulations for oral administration, including immediate-release tablets containing 0.25, 0.5, 0.75, 1, 2, 4, and 6 mg, and in elixirs (which contain alcohol) and solutions for oral administration

Soft tissues and bone: Late (Chronic) Side Effects

Presentation

1. Soft tissue edema
   - Common late effect; more common with RT + neck dissection
   - Edema can occur in the neck, oral cavity, pharynx, or larynx
2. Soft tissue necrosis
   - Rare late complication. May present as unhealed wound, chronic ulceration
3. Soft tissue fibrosis of the neck
   - Common late effect, especially with RT + neck dissection
   - Woody fibrosis of cervical soft tissues with limited range of motion
4. Trismus
   - Caused by temporomandibular joint fibrosis and/or masticator fibrosis
5. Osteoradionecrosis of the mandible
   - Uncommon late effect of RT to head and neck. Risk increased by xerostomia and poor dental/oral hygiene

Management

1. Soft tissue edema
   - Elevation of head and neck while in bed
   - Short course of steroids:
     - –**Dexamethasone** orally 2–4 times per day. Begin with 4 mg per day, tapering over 14 days, with dose and duration of treatment depending on response
2. Soft tissue necrosis
   - Conservative management:
     - –Good oral hygiene
     - –**Pentoxifylline** 400 mg orally 2–3 times per day
     - –**α-Tocopherol** 1000 units per day
     - –**Antibiotics** for possible underlying infection that prevents healing. Choice depends on the sites of infection. Use anaerobic coverage for mucosal lesions; gram-positive coverage for skin ulcers. See Chapter 47
   - **Hyperbaric oxygen** and, if necessary, surgical intervention with planned hyperbaric oxygen in persistent cases is recommended after failure of conservative management
3. Soft tissue fibrosis of neck
   - Range-of-motion exercises of the neck and shoulder for prevention
4. Trismus
   - Preventive jaw stretching exercise
5. Osteoradionecrosis of the mandible
   - Xerostomia and poor dental and oral hygiene increase the risk of developing ORN. See Head and Neck: Salivary Gland and Taste Buds, for recommendations
   - Prevention:
     - –Full dental evaluation with correction of periodontal disease before starting RT is necessary
     - –*To maintain healthy teeth*: Daily **topical fluoride application using a fluoride tray: 1.1% (w/w) sodium fluoride toothpaste (PreviDent® 5000 Plus)** topically for 10–15 minutes twice daily during and after completion of RT

Dexamethasone is marketed in the United States in numerous generic formulations for oral administration, including immediate-release tablets containing 0.25, 0.5, 0.75, 1, 2, 4, and 6 mg, and in elixirs (which contain alcohol) and solutions for oral administration
Pentoxifylline is available in the United States, in generic products for oral administration that are formulated as controlled-release or extended-release products that contain 400 mg/tablet
D-α-Tocopherol acetate and DL-α-tocopherol acetate (vitamin E) are available in the United States in numerous formulations for oral administration: containing 100, 200, 400, 500, and 800 units of tocopherol; immediate-release capsules containing 100, 200, 400, and 1000 units of tocopherol; and drops and solutions

EARS

Ears: Early (Acute) Side Effects

Presentation

1. Otitis externa
2. Serous otitis media, or infectious otitis externa or media
   - Usually occurs after the 3rd to 4th week of RT and can persist after completion of RT treatment

Management

1. Otitis externa
   - **Hydrocortisone** otic drops; instill into the ear 3 times daily, *or*
   - **Hydrocortisone 1% + neomycin 5 mg + polymyxin B 10,000 units** otic drops. Instill solution into the ear 3 times daily, *or*
   - **Anesthetic otic drops;** instill into the ear 3 times daily for pain in the external ear canal
2. Serous otitis media or infectious otitis externa or media
   - Decongestants or antihistamines:
     –**Diphenhydramine** 25–50 mg orally 3 times per day
     –**Loratadine** 10 mg orally once per day, or another **nonsedating antihistamine**
   - If medical therapy is not effective:
     –Insert a myringotomy tube
   - If infection is suspected, oral antibiotics should be used:
     –**Amoxicillin** 500 mg orally every 8 hours for 10 days

Diphenhydramine HCl is available in the United States generically in numerous formulations for oral administration, including immediate-release tablets containing 25 mg or 50 mg diphenhydramine, chewable immediate-release tablets containing 12.5 mg diphenhydramine, immediate-release capsules containing 25 mg or 50 mg diphenhydramine, orally disintegrating strips containing 12.5 mg or 25 mg diphenhydramine, and liquids, solutions, elixirs (contain alcohol), and syrups in various concentrations
Three **nonsedating antihistamine products** are available for oral administration:
Loratadine is generically available as tablets containing 10 mg, or as orally disintegrating tablets containing 10 mg, rapidly disintegrating tablets containing 10 mg, and a syrup containing 1 mg/mL. Doses are administered once daily
Cetirizine HCl is available for oral administration as tablets containing 5 mg or 10 mg, chewable tablets containing 5 mg or 10 mg, and a syrup containing 5 mg/5 mL (ZYRTEC®)
Fexofenadine HCl is available for oral administration as tablets containing 30 mg, 60 mg, and 180 mg, and as capsules containing 60 mg (Allegra®). Administration schedule varies with patient age and renal function and the dose administered
Amoxicillin is available in the United States generically in various formulations for oral administration, including immediate-release tablets containing 500 mg or 875 mg/tablet; chewable tablets containing 125 mg, 200 mg, 250 mg, and 400 mg/tablet; immediate-release capsules containing 250 mg or 500 mg/capsule; tablets containing 200 mg or 400 mg for producing a liquid suspension; and powdered products for preparing liquid suspensions with concentrations equal to 50 mg/mL, 125 mg/5 mL, 200 mg/5 mL, 250 mg/5 mL, and 400 mg/5 mL

Ears: Late (Chronic) Side Effects

Presentation:

Permanent hearing loss
- Can occur in patients who receive a high dose to the auditory organs (>45–50 Gy)[5]

Management:

Permanent hearing loss
- Prevention is the best treatment. However, in a situation in which a high dose to the cochlea is unavoidable, a hearing aid may be needed

HEAD AND NECK: ORAL AND ORAL PHARYNGEAL MUCOSA

Oral and Oral Pharyngeal Mucosa: Early (Acute) Side Effects

Presentation

1. Mucositis
   - Starts at about 1–2 weeks
   - Oral discomfort → injected mucosa → patchy ulceration → confluent mucositis at about the 4th to 5th weeks
   - Plateau for about 1–2 weeks
   - Recovery starts close to the end of the treatment course
   - Complete mucosal healing usually occurs within 2–3 weeks after RT completion
   - Concomitant chemoradiation can be associated with a severe and long-lasting mucositis
2. Oral/mucosal candidiasis
3. Bacterial infection

Management

1. Mucositis

   General:
   - **Baking soda or saline (0.9% NaCl for irrigation) oral rinse:** Baking soda 1 tsp or table salt 1 tsp in 1 quart (~946 mL) of water. Gargle a minimum of 3 times per day
   - Use a water pik to remove sticky materials from the mucosa
   - **Sucralfate suspension** 1000 mg/10 mL orally 3–4 times daily, *or*
   - Other mucosal coating products (with emollient properties to soothe irritated tissues but without an anesthetic component). These rinses relieve the pain of oral lesions by adhering to injured tissue of the oral mucosa and protecting it from further injury while providing a moist wound environment necessary for healing:
     - –**Gelclair®** bioadherent oral gel (polyvinylpyrrolidone, sodium hyaluronate, and glycerrhetinic acid); mix Gelclair® with 1–3 tbsp (15–45 mL) tap water (or may be used undiluted); swish the product around the oral cavity or gargle with it for at least 1 minute. Use as needed. The product is usually expectorated, but is harmless if swallowed
     - –**Biotene® Mouthwash** (glucose oxidase, lactoperoxidase, and lysozyme); administer by swishing the product around the oral cavity or gargling with it for at least 30 seconds, then expectorate. Use as needed
     - –**RadiaCare™** Oral Wound Rinse; mix the powder with the specified amount of water. A usual dose is approximately 1 tbsp, which should be swished or gargled in the mouth for about 1 minute [safe if swallowed]. Repeat 4 times per day or as needed

   Analgesia:
   - Topical anesthetics
     - –**Viscous lidocaine 2%:simethicone liquid:with or without diphenhydramine liquid (12.5 mg/5 mL)** in 1:1:1 mixture, 15 mL every 4–6 hours as needed

     Note: This may be swallowed, but the lidocaine component can numb the hypopharynx, increasing the risk of aspiration
     - –**Topical morphine** rinse 15 mL of a 2% morphine solution every 3 hours 6 times per day

     Note: Topical morphine has been shown to be superior to other topical anesthetics in a small, randomized trial. It has better pain control with decreased duration of functional impairment[6]
   - Oral or parenteral opioids: Medication for pain control is used as needed
     - –**Oxycodone, hydromorphone, or morphine. See Chapter 52.**

     Note: Systemic opioids are mostly used to control pain associated with mucositis
2. Oral/mucosal candidiasis
   - Topical antifungal agents: Continue treatment for at least 48 hours after perioral symptoms resolve and cultures return to normal (see Chapter 47)
     - –**Nystatin suspension** 500,000–1,000,000 units (5–10 mL) orally 4 times per day
     - –**Nystatin troches** 1–2 troches (200,000–400,000 units); dissolve slowly in mouth 4–5 times daily

     Notes:

     (1) Patients with esophageal candidiasis require systemic antifungal treatment

     (2) Topical antifungal agents such as nystatin require contact with the affected area and results among patients may be inconsistent (see Chapter 47)
   - Oral antifungal agents:
     - –**Fluconazole** 200 mg orally on day 1, followed by **fluconazole** 100 mg per day orally for 13 days on days 2–14
3. Bacterial infection (see Chapter 47)
   - Antibiotics that provide good anaerobic coverage:
     - –**Amoxicillin with or without clavulonic acid** orally until symptoms resolve (typically 7–10 days amoxicillin + clavulonic acid [875/125] every 12 hours orally)
     - –**Metronidazole** 500 mg orally every 6 hours

Sucralfate is available in the United States generically as a suspension for oral administration containing 1000 mg sucralfate/10 mL
Lidocaine 2% viscous is available in the United States generically in various product sizes
Simethicone is generically available in the United States in several formulations for oral administration, including liquid drops containing 40 mg simethicone/0.6 mL
Diphenhydramine HCl is available in the United States generically in numerous liquid formulations for oral administration, including solutions, elixirs (contain alcohol), and syrups in various concentrations
Morphine sulfate is commercially available in the United States in various liquid formulations for oral administration, or it may be extemporaneously compounded from immediate-release tablets formulated for oral administration or from morphine sulfate powder
Nystatin is available in the United States generically in a variety of formulations for oral administration, including a suspension containing 100,000 units/mL and troches containing 200,000 units
Co-amoxiclav (amoxicillin + clavulonic acid) is available in the United States generically in various formulations for oral administration, including:

Description	Amoxicillin Content	Clavulonic Acid Content
Immediate-release tablets	250 mg	125 mg
	500 mg	125 mg
	875 mg	125 mg
Chewable tablets	125 mg	31.25 mg
	200 mg	28.5 mg
	250 mg	62.5 mg
	400 mg	57 mg
Extended-release tablets	1000 mg	62.5 mg

Metronidazole is available in the United States generically in various formulations for oral administration, including immediate-release tablets containing 250 mg or 500 mg, immediate-release capsules containing 375 mg, and extended-release tablets containing 750 mg

Oral & Oral Pharyngeal Mucosa: Late (Chronic) Side Effects

Presentation

1. Pallor, telangiectasis, thinning of the mucosa
2. Persistent ulceration of soft tissue
   - Can be very painful

Management

1. Pallor, telangiectasis, thinning of the mucosa
   - Maintain meticulous oral hygiene
2. Persistent ulceration of soft tissue
   - *Analgesia*: Adequate pain control, may need opioids
     –**Codeine, morphine, hydromorphone,** or **fentanyl. See Chapter 52**
   - Exposed bone needs prompt attention
     –**Hyperbaric oxygen** may promote soft tissue and bony healing. If bone remains exposed, surgical repair with or without planned hyperbaric oxygen is needed to prevent osteomyelitis

HEAD AND NECK: SALIVARY GLAND AND TASTE BUDS

Salivary Gland and Taste Buds: Early (Acute) Side Effects

Presentation

1. Acute sialadenitis
   - Tenderness and swelling of the salivary glands
   - May occur within hours after the first RT session and subside within a few days
2. Xerostomia
   - Progressive thickening of saliva with decrease in salivary output within the first 2–3 weeks
3. Loss of taste
   - Common side effect of head and neck RT
   - Return of taste, with/without some degree of permanent impairment → 4–6 months > completion of RT

Management

1. Acute sialadenitis and xerostomia

   General:
   - **Hydration** during RT is essential, especially in symptomatic patients
   - Baking soda rinse, glyceride, guaifenesin, carbonated drinks (sugar and alcohol-free), or papain, 3–4 times per day

     Note: All these have been tried with variable results
   - **Pilocarpine** 5–10 mg/dose orally 3–4 times/day up to a total daily dose of 30 mg

     Note: Compared with placebo, pilocarpine maintains significantly better salivary function in patients undergoing RT, although quality of life is not different[7]

   Prevention:
   - Radioprotector for the salivary gland during postoperative RT for head and neck cancer: **Amifostine** 200 mg/m^2 intravenously 15–30 minutes before daily RT

     Note: Recommended especially in the postoperative setting[8]

Salivary Gland and Taste Buds: Late (Chronic) Side Effects

Presentation:

Permanent xerostomia
- Occurs in patients who receive high doses of RT to both parotid glands

Management:

Permanent xerostomia
- Mixed results have been achieved with either:
  - –**Artificial saliva products** may be used as often as needed to moisten and lubricate the mouth and throat in xerostomia (products are available in spray and moistened swab forms), *or*
  - –**Glyceride** preparations, *or*
  - –**Pilocarpine** 5–10 mg/dose orally 3–4 times/day up to a total daily dose of 30 mg

Pilocarpine HCL is available in the United States in film-coated tablets for oral administration containing 5 mg or 7.5 mg. Salagen® Tablets; MGI Pharma, Inc, Bloomington, MN

HEAD AND NECK: PHARYNX AND ESOPHAGUS

Pharynx and Esophagus: Early (Acute) Side Effects

Presentation:

Pharyngitis/esophagitis

- Dysphagia and odynophagia occur in the 2nd or 3rd week of RT; resolve 2–3 weeks after completion of RT
- Characterized by somatic pain when swallowing
- Severe oropharyngitis → intermittent aspiration. Silent aspiration occurs in >60% of patients[9]

Management:

Pharyngitis/esophagitis

General:

- **Soft diet** to maintain nutritional intake
- **Biotene® Mouthwash** (glucose oxidase, lactoperoxidase, and lysozyme); swish the product around the oral cavity or gargle with it for at least 30 seconds, then expectorate. Use as needed
- **Gelclair®** bioadherent oral gel (polyvinylpyrrolidone, sodium hyaluronate, and glycerrhetinic acid); mix Gelclair® with 1–3 tbsp (15–45 mL) tap water (or may be used undiluted); swish the product around the oral cavity or gargle with it for at least 1 minute. The product is usually expectorated, but is harmless if swallowed
- **RadiaCare™** Oral Wound Rinse, mix the powder with the specified amount of water. A usual dose is approximately 1 tbsp, which should be swished or gargled in the mouth for about 1 minute (safe if swallowed). Repeat 4 times per day or as needed

Analgesia:

- Topical anesthetics
  - –**Viscous lidocaine 2%:simethicone liquid: with or without diphenhydramine liquid (12.5 mg/5 mL)** in 1:1:1 mixture, 15 mL every 4–6 hours as needed

    Note: This may be swallowed, but the lidocaine component can numb the hypopharynx, increasing the risk of aspiration
  - –**Topical morphine** rinse 15 mL of a 2% morphine solution every 3 hours 6 times daily

    Note: This has been shown to be superior to other topical anesthetics in a small, randomized trial. Better pain control with decreased duration of functional impairment[5]
- Oral or parenteral opioids: For pain control to maintain comfort
  - –**Morphine, oxycodone, hydromorphone, fentanyl. See Chapter 52**

    Note: Systemic opioids often used to control pain are associated with pharyngitis/esophagitis

Prevention in patients at high risk for severe mucositis, pharyngitis, and esophagitis:

- Placement of a **feeding tube** before starting RT is recommended

  Note: Most patients who receive chemotherapy and radiation concurrently become totally dependent on tube feeding for nutritional support. Most regain swallowing ability

Rehabilitation:

- Speech and swallowing therapy aid in recovery

Pharynx and Esophagus: Late (Chronic) Side Effects

Presentation

1. Soft tissue changes including pallor, telangiectasia, and fibrosis, which may lead to stricture formation
2. Persistent inability to swallow
3. Chronic aspiration

Management

1. Strictures
   - Surgical dilation
2. Persistent inability to swallow
   - Speech and swallowing therapy
   - Severe cases that persist despite speech and swallowing therapy may need permanent feeding tube
3. Chronic aspiration
   - Nothing by mouth with nutritional support via permanent feeding tube
   - Severe cases may need laryngectomy for airway protection

LUNGS

Lungs: Early (Acute) Side Effects

Presentation:

Dry, nonproductive cough
- Likely due to transient injury to the airway mucosa soon after completing RT

Management:

Dry, nonproductive cough
- Symptomatic treatment including **cough suppressants, bronchodilators,** or **humidification**

Lungs: Subacute Side Effects

Presentation:

Radiation pneumonitis (RP)
- Uncommon side effect, usually seen 1–3 months after RT
- Can be lethal if it involves sufficient lung volume
- *Acute symptoms of RP*: Dry cough, low-grade fever, congestion, dyspnea, pleuritic chest pain, and hemoptysis
- *Findings on imaging studies:* Changes corresponding to the RT portal
- Factors increasing risk
  - –Low performance status[11]
  - –History of cigarette smoking
  - –Comorbid illnesses
  - –Lung volume irradiated

Notes:

(1) Risk starts when >22% of total lung volume is exposed to 20 Gy.[11] RP is not seen if <22% of total lung volume is exposed to 20 Gy compared with an 8% frequency when 22–31% of lung is exposed to 20 Gy[10]

(2) RP is a clinical diagnosis of exclusion. Typical imaging findings in the absence of clinical symptoms does not warrant the diagnosis of RP

(3) No solid data to indicate that chemotherapy used in combination with thoracic radiation (as in lung or esophageal cancer) leads to increased RP. However, if one uses chemotherapy agents that have known toxicity to lung, such as bleomycin, mitomycin, or cyclophosphamide, then the risk increases dramatically

Management:

Radiation pneumonitis (RP)

Prevention:
- Limit the lung volume exposed to <22% of total lung volume and <20 Gy[10]

General:
- –*Superinfection*: Use antibiotics including penicillin based, cephalosporin, macrolides, or quinolones (see Chapter 47)
- –Supplemental **oxygen** as needed
- –*Corticosteroids*: **Prednisone** 30–60 mg/dose orally every day for 2–3 weeks followed by a gradual taper. Reduce daily dose by 5–10 mg/day each week or every other week, depending on patient's symptoms

  Note: Initiate corticosteroids only when symptoms are associated with hypoxemia. It is often very difficult to taper steroids in the setting of RP because of persistent symptoms. The rate of tapering should depend on the response of the patient

Prednisone is marketed in the United States in numerous generic formulations for oral administration, including immediate-release tablets containing 1, 2.5, 5, 10, 20, or 50 mg, and in solutions and syrups for oral administration

Lungs: Late (Chronic) Side Effects

Presentation:

Pulmonary fibrosis
- May occur 1–2 years after radiation
- May or may not be preceded by RP; usually develops silently in radiated area
- Most patients are asymptomatic when small volumes of the lung are affected
- If a sufficient or significant amount of lung is involved: → dyspnea → progressive cor pulmonale. This process is irreversible

  Note: Occurs nearly always in the radiated area. In general, consider the area of the lung that receives >20 Gy as functionless. Therefore, it is prudent for the radiation oncologist to select patients and to minimize the lung exposure to radiation

Management:

Pulmonary fibrosis
- Supportive care
  - –Supplemental oxygen
  - –Bronchodilators

(1) **Ipratropium bromide inhalation aerosol.** Start with 2 actuations (18 mcg/actuation) 4 times per day. Additional doses may be given as required to a maximum of 12 inhalations/24 hours, *or*

(2) **Ipratropium bromide inhalation solution 0.02%.** The usual dose is 500 mcg orally 3–4 times/day by nebulization every 6–8 hours

- Prevention

  Note: It has been reported that amifostine is effective in reducing acute severe esophagitis and pneumonitis in locally advanced non–small cell lung cancer treated with chemoradiation[12,13]. However, a recent RTOG report failed to confirm objective improvement in esophagitis, although patient self-assessment showed statistically significant improved swallowing function with amifostine[14]

Ipratropium bromide is marketed in the United States as a 0.02% solution for inhalation by nebulization and in metered-dose inhalers that deliver 18 mcg/actuation

HEART

Heart: Early (Acute) Side Effects

Presentation

1. Cardiac damage
   - Uncommon when (less than 30% of the heart receives 40 Gy
2. Acute pericarditis
   - Rare

Management:

Pericarditis

- Observation
- Nonsteroidal anti-inflammatory agents (NSAIDS)
  –**Aspirin, ibuprofen, naproxen,** or **indomethacin**
- Steroids
  –**Prednisone** 30–60 mg/dose orally daily for 2–3 weeks, followed by a gradual taper. Reduce daily dose by 5–10 mg/day each week or every other week, depending on patient's symptoms

Prednisone is marketed in the United States in numerous generic formulations for oral administration, including immediate-release tablets containing 1, 2.5, 5, 10, 20, and 50 mg, and in solutions and syrups for oral administration

Heart: Late (Chronic) Side Effects

Presentation

1. Pericarditis
   - May develop 6 months to years after RT
   - *Presentation*: Chest pain, dyspnea, fever, and abnormalities on ECG
   - Pericardial effusion with tamponade may develop
2. Cardiomyopathy or pancarditis
   - Uncommon but can occur if RT + cardiotoxic chemotherapy such as doxorubicin is administered
3. Other cardiac effects of uncertain etiology: Coronary artery disease, valvular defects, conduction abnormalities

Management

1. Pericarditis
   - Pericardiocentesis and pericardiotomy are necessary for impending tamponade; both visceral and parietal pericardium must be removed
2. Cardiomyopathy or pancarditis
   - Avoid cardiomyopathy by adjusting anthracycline dosages and meticulously designing radiation portals

GASTROINTESTINAL SYSTEM: ESOPHAGUS

Esophagus: Early (Acute) Side Effects

Presentation

1. Esophagitis: Sensation of food getting stuck while swallowing (contrast with somatic pain that occurs when swallowing with pharyngitis from head and neck RT)

2. Gastroesophageal reflux disease (GERD)
3. Colonization by *Candida* species

Management

1. Esophagitis

General:

- **Soft diet** to maintain nutritional intake
- *Sucralfate slurry*: 1000 mg/10 mL orally 3–4 times per day

Analgesia:

- Topical anesthetics:
  –**Viscous lidocaine 2%:simethicone liquid: with or without diphenhydramine liquid (12.5 mg/5 mL)** in 1:1:1 mixture, 15 mL every 4–6 hours as needed
  Note: This may be swallowed, but the lidocaine component can numb the hypopharynx, increasing the risk for aspiration
  –**Topical morphine** rinse 15 mL of a 2% morphine solution every 3 hours 6 times per day
  Note: This has been shown superior to other topical anesthetics in a small, randomized trial. Better pain control with decreased duration of functional impairment[5]
- Oral or parenteral opioids
  –For pain control to maintain comfort
  –**Morphine, oxycodone, hydromorphone, fentanyl, codeine. See Chapter 52**
  Note: Systemic opioids often used to control pain associated with pharyngitis/esophagitis

Prevention in patients at high risk for severe esophagitis:

- Placement of a **feeding tube** before starting RT is recommended
  Note: Most patients receiving concurrent chemoradiation become totally dependent on tube feeding for nutritional support. Most do regain swallowing ability

Rehabilitation:

- Speech and swallowing therapy aid in recovery

2. GERD
   - Antacids and proton pump inhibitors

Esophagus: Late (Chronic) Side Effects

Presentation

1. Persistent esophagitis
2. Stricture
3. Chronic ulceration
4. Fistula

Management

1. Persistent esophagitis
   - Symptomatic relief, supportive care, similar to management of acute esophagitis
2. Stricture
   - Esophageal dilation
3. Chronic ulceration
   - Surgical intervention may be needed

GASTROINTESTINAL SYSTEM: STOMACH

Stomach: Early (Acute) Side Effects

Presentation

1. Nausea and vomiting
   - Occurs frequently with gastric RT. Resolves after the completion of RT
2. Acute gastritis with ulceration
   - 2–3 weeks after the start of RT. Resolves after the completion of RT

Management

1. Nausea and vomiting

Antiemetics before RT:
- **Ondansetron** 4–8 mg orally 30–60 minutes before RT. *For intractable nausea:* 4–8 mg orally twice daily continually
- **Granisetron** 2 mg orally 30–60 minutes before RT. *For intractable nausea:* 1 mg twice daily continually if needed
- **Metoclopramide** 40 mg orally 30–60 minutes before RT. *For intractable nausea:* 20–40 mg 4 times daily continually
- **Prochlorperazine** 20 mg orally 30–60 minutes before RT. *For intractable nausea* 5–20 mg orally every 4–6 hours continually
- **Lorazepam** 1 mg orally 30–60 minutes before RT. *For intractable nausea:* 0.5–1 mg orally every 6–12 hours continually
- **Dronabinol** 10 mg orally 30–60 minutes before RT. *For intractable nausea:* 2.5–10 mg orally every 6 hours continually
- **Chlorpromazine** 50 mg orally 30–60 minutes before RT. *For intractable nausea:* 25–50 mg orally every 4–6 hours continually

2. Nausea and vomiting and acute gastritis with ulceration
   - Smaller daily fraction size of RT
   - 1.5 Gy may be required when irradiating an intact stomach

Ondansetron is available in the United States in several formulations for oral administration, including immediate-release tablets containing 4 mg or 8 mg ondansetron HCl dihydrate, orally disintegrating tablets containing 4 mg or 8 mg ondansetron base, and as an oral solution containing 5 mg ondansetron HCl dihydrate/5 mL (Zofran®)
Granisetron is manufactured in the United States in tablets for oral administration containing 1 mg granisetron and as an oral solution containing 2 mg granisetron/10 mL (KYTRIL®)
Metoclopramide HCl is available in the United States generically as immediate-release tablets for oral administration containing 5 mg or 10 mg metoclopramide HCl and as an oral solution containing 5 mg/mL
Prochlorperazine is available in the United States generically in several formulations, including immediate-release tablets for oral administration containing 5 mg, 10 mg, and 25 mg prochlorperazine maleate, an oral solution containing 5 mg prochlorperazine edisylate/5 mL, and suppositories for rectal insertion containing 2.5 mg, 5 mg, and 25 mg prochlorperazine
Lorazepam is available in the United States generically in immediate-release tablets for oral administration containing 0.5 mg, 1 mg, and 2 mg lorazepam and as a concentrated oral solution containing 2 mg lorazepam/mL
Dronabinol is available in the United States as a solution in sesame oil and in soft gelatin capsules for oral administration that contain 2.5 mg, 5 mg, and 10 mg dronabinol (Marinol®)
Chlorpromazine is available in the United States generically in several formulations, including immediate-release tablets for oral administration containing 10 mg, 25 mg, 50 mg, 100 mg, and 200 mg chlorpromazine HCl, a concentrated oral solution containing 100 mg chlorpromazine HCl/mL, and suppositories for rectal insertion containing 100 mg chlorpromazine base

Stomach: Late (Chronic) Side Effects

Presentation (a few months to years after the completion of RT)
1. Dyspepsia, chronic gastritis
2. Persistent ulceration
3. Gastric outlet obstruction
4. Perforation

Management
1. Dyspepsia, chronic gastritis
   - H_2-blockers:
     –**Ranitidine** 150 mg orally 2 times per day, or 300 mg orally at bedtime, *or*
     –**Famotidine** 40 mg orally at bedtime, or 20 mg orally 2 times per day, *or*
     –**Cimetidine** 300 mg orally 4 times per day, or 400 mg orally 2 times per day
   - Proton pump inhibitors:
     –**Rabeprazole** 20 mg orally daily, *or*
     –**Esomeprazole** 20 mg orally daily, *or*
     –**Lansoprazole** 15 mg orally daily, *or*
     –**Pantoprazole** 40 mg orally daily
     Note: The proton pump inhibitors' doses and schedules vary by indication. Dose adjustment and duration of administration must be tailored to individual patients
   - Sucralfate suspension 1000 mg in 15 mL orally 3–4 times per day
2. Persistent ulceration, gastric outlet obstruction, and perforation
   - Surgical intervention

Sucralfate is available in the United States generically as a suspension for oral administration containing 1000 mg sucralfate/10 mL
Rabeprazole is available in the United States in enteric-coated delayed-release tablets containing 20 mg (Aciphex®)
Esomeprazole magnesium is available in the United States in delayed-release capsules containing 20 mg or 40 mg as enteric-coated pellets (NEXIUM®)
Lansoprazole is available in the United States in several formulations, including: enteric-coated granules in delayed-release capsules containing 15 mg or 30 mg lansoprazole, delayed-release orally disintegrating tablets containing 15 mg or 30 mg lansoprazole as enteric-coated microgranules,

and in unit-dosed packets containing 15 mg or 30 mg lansoprazole as enteric-coated granules for preparing a delayed-release oral suspension (PREVACID®)
Pantoprazole is available in the United States in delayed-release tablets containing 20 mg or 40 mg (PROTONIX®)

GASTROINTESTINAL SYSTEM: SMALL AND LARGE INTESTINE

Small and Large Intestine: Early (Acute) Side Effects

Presentation

1. Fatigue, nausea, vomiting, early satiety, anorexia, and diarrhea
2. Enteritis
   - Crampy abdominal pain and watery diarrhea
3. Proctocolitis
   - Occurs 2–3 weeks after the start of pelvic RT
   - Frequent bowel movement with or without watery diarrhea; rectal urgency; and tenesmus
4. Proctitis

Management

1. Antidiarrhea medications
   - **Psyllium fiber** 1 tsp in 8 oz water orally 3–4 times per day
   - **Cholestyramine** 1 g orally 1–4 times per day as needed
   - **Loperamide** 4 mg orally at the first onset of loose stools, followed by **loperamide** 2 mg orally every 2 hours around the clock until the patient is free from diarrhea for 12 hours
   - **Diphenoxylate-atropine** 2 tablets orally after each bowel movement to a maximum of 8 tablets per day
   - **Octreotide acetate injection** 100–500 mcg per dose subcutaneously 2 or 3 times daily, doubling the dose at 3- to 4-day intervals until maximum control of symptoms is achieved

     Note: Octreotide has been shown to be more effective compared with conventional treatments mentioned above in the control of radiation induced diarrhea[15]
2. Enteritis and proctocolitis
   - Low-residue diet
3. Mild proctitis
   - **Anusol® Ointment** externally to the affected area up to 5 times daily
   - **Anusol® hemorrhoidal suppositories**, insert 1 suppository rectally 4 times daily
   - Hydrocortisone-containing preparations

     –**Anucort HC** 25 mg hydrocortisone acetate suppository rectally in the morning and at night as needed
     –**Anusol HC-I® Ointment** containing 1.12% hydrocortisone acetate equivalent to 1% hydrocortisone topically, as needed
     –**Hemorrhoidal HC** hydrocortisone-containing suppositories for rectal insertion as needed
     –**Protocort** 30 mg hydrocortisone acetate suppository rectally in the morning and at night as needed
4. Severe proctitis
   - **Mesalamine suppositories** 500 mg rectally twice daily
   - **Glucocorticoid retention enemas**

     –**Hydrocortisone retention enema** 100 mg in 60 mL of an aqueous suspension once daily
     –**Predsol retention enema** 20 mg/100 mL of prednisolone (as sodium phosphate) in an aqueous solution once daily
   - **Sucralfate** 2000 mg as a retention enema in 15–30 mL water for 10–20 minutes twice daily

     Note: This use of sucralfate is off-label because sucralfate is not marketed in the United States in a formulation intended for rectal administration. Therefore, one administers as an enema the oral suspension product (1000 mg sucralfate/10 mL)

Anhydrous cholestyramine resin is available in the United States generically in various powdered formulations for preparing a suspension or adding to foods
Loperamide is available in the United States generically as immediate-release capsules and tablets containing 2 mg loperamide and in liquid formulations containing loperamide 1 mg/mL or 5 mg/mL
Diphenoxylate-atropine is available in the United States generically for oral administration in immediate-release tablets that contain diphenoxylate HCL 2.5 mg plus atropine sulfate 0.025 mg, and as an oral liquid that contains diphenoxylate HCL 2.5 mg plus atropine sulfate 0.025 mg/5 mL
Octreotide acetate is available in the United States as an injectable solution. The short-acting product, Sandostatin®, is for administration by intravenous or subcutaneous injection and is marketed in the following concentrations: 0.05 mg/mL, 0.1 mg/mL, 0.2 mg/mL, 0.5 mg/mL, and 1 mg/mL
Octreotide acetate for injectable suspension (Sandostatin LAR®) is a long-acting formulation for intragluteal administration only and is marketed in the following concentrations: 10 mg/5 mL, 20 mg/5 mL, and 30 mg/5 mL

Anusol® Ointment contains the following active ingredients: mineral oil 46.6% (skin protectant), pramoxine HCl 1% (pain reliever), zinc oxide 12.5% (skin protectant). The product is indicated for the relief of anorectal pain, soreness, itching, and burning
Anusol® hemorrhoidal suppositories contain topical starch 51% as a skin protectant. It is indicated for the relief of rectal itching, burning, and discomfort
Anusol HC-1 Ointment in the United States contains 1.12% hydrocortisone acetate equivalent to 1% hydrocortisone. It is indicated for the relief of external anal itching
Anucort HC is available in the United States as suppositories containing 25 mg hydrocortisone acetate
Hemorrhoidal HC suppositories are available in the United States generically. In general, the products contain hydrocortisone 25 mg in a suppository base
Protocort is available in the United States as suppositories containing 30 mg hydrocortisone acetate
Hydrocortisone retention enemas are available in the United States containing 100 mg hydrocortisone acetate in 60 mL water as an aqueous suspension
Predsol retention enemas are available in the United States containing 20 mg/100 ml of prednisolone (as sodium phosphate) in an aqueous solution
Sucralfate is available in the United States as an oral suspension product containing 1000 mg sucralfate/10 mL

Small and Large Intestine: Late (Chronic) Side Effects

Presentation

1. Radiation injury to small bowel
   - Malabsorption of fat, diarrhea, persistent bleeding, ulceration, perforation, and fistulas
   - *Small bowel obstruction:* Uncommon; occurs 1–5 years after RT. Obstruction may be preceded by episodic, crampy, abdominal pain
2. Radiation injury to colon
   - Strictures, persistent painless bleeding, ulceration, tenesmus, obstipation, diarrhea and rectal urgency
3. Rectovaginal fistulas may occur because of the high local RT dose from a brachytherapy implant

Management

1. Malabsorption
   - Lactaid 1 capsule orally with dairy product
   - Pancreatic or lactase enzyme preparations:

     –**Pancrelipase** start with 400 units lipase/kg per meal orally and titrate to 2500 units lipase/kg per meal

     Note: In some patients, enteric-coated **pancrelipase** enzyme tablets may not dissociate as intended and may pass through the bowel intact. Administer pancrelipase with meals or snacks. Individualize dosage by giving the number of tablets or capsules that optimally minimize steatorrhea. Adjust doses slowly; monitor symptoms and response

     (1) Select products with a high lipase content to avoid steatorrhea

     (2) Do not crush or chew enteric-coated products or the enteric-coated contents of opened capsules

     (3) Capsules may be opened and shaken onto a small quantity of soft food that is not hot and does not require chewing

     (4) Pancrelipase should be swallowed immediately without chewing to prevent mucosal irritation

     (5) Ingested doses should be followed with a glass of juice or water to ensure complete ingestion

     (6) Avoid mixing pancrelipase with foods that have a pH >5.5, which can dissolve enteric coatings
2. Surgical intervention for persistent symptoms should be considered as last resort

LIVER

Liver: Early (Acute) Side Effects

Presentation:

A relatively silent period, because more extensive radiation injury is required before onset of clinically significant acute inflammation of the hepatic tissue. Usually, symptoms occur subacutely

Management:

Expectant

Liver: Subacute to Late (Chronic) Side Effects

Presentation

1. Radiation-induced liver disease (RILD)
   - The incidence of these severe toxicities is dose- and volume-related
   - Increased risk of liver damage in patients who receive >30 Gy to the whole liver

- Liver dose <30 Gy; the incidence is <1%
- Development of anicteric ascites 2–4 months after RT
- Veno-occlusive disease of the lobular central veins occurs
  –Vague to intense right upper quadrant discomfort
  –Ascites
  –Jaundice occurs later; alkaline phosphatase level >>bilirubin and other LFTs[16,17]
- *Computed tomography (CT) findings*: Low-density changes

2. Combined-modality–induced liver disease (CMILD) occurs with bone marrow preparative regimens
   - Occurs earlier, usually within 4–6 weeks after RT
   - Veno-occlusive disease of the lobular central veins:
     –Vague to intense right upper quadrant discomfort
     –Ascites
     –Jaundice occurs early; bilirubin >>alkaline phosphatase
   - There are no imaging findings in CMILD patients

Management
1. No specific therapy exists for treatment of RILD or CMILD
2. No proven benefit to anticoagulants or corticosteroids
3. Conservative management of ascites using diuretics, including spironolactone

GENITOURINARY SYSTEM: BLADDER

Urinary Bladder: Early (Acute) Side Effects

Presentation: Usually begin 2 weeks after starting RT
1. Cystitis with dysuria
2. Urinary frequency and urgency
3. Obstructive urinary symptoms

Management
1. Dysuria
   - Topical analgesics
     –**Phenazopyridine hydrochloride** 200 mg orally 3 times daily
   - NSAIDs:
     –**Ibuprofen** 200 mg orally 3–4 times daily as needed
     –**Naproxen** 220 mg orally 1–2 times daily as needed
2. Urinary frequency and urgency
   - Antispasmodics
     –**Oxybutynin chloride** 5 mg orally 2–3 times per day as needed
     –**Flavoxate hydrochloride** 100–200 mg orally 3–4 times daily as needed
     –**Hyoscyamine sulfate** 0.15–0.30 mg orally 3–4 times daily as needed
3. Obstructive urinary symptoms
   - **Terazosin** start 1 mg orally at bedtime; titrate as needed over 4–6 weeks to a maximum of 20 mg/day
   - **Doxazosin** start 1 mg orally once a day; titrate as needed over 4–6 weeks to a maximum of 8 mg/day
   - **Tamsulosin** start 0.4 mg orally once a day; increase to 0.8 mg each day after 1–2 weeks
   - **Finasteride** 5 mg orally once daily

Phenazopyridine HCl is available in the United States generically as immediate-release tablets for oral administration containing 100 mg, 150 mg, and 200 mg

Oxybutynin Cl is available in the United States generically in several formulations, including immediate-release tablets for oral administration that contains 5 mg oxybutynin, extended-release tablets that contain 5 mg, 10 mg, or 15 mg, a syrup containing 5 mg oxybutynin/5 mL, and in a transdermal (patch) system for application to the skin that delivers 3.9 mg oxybutynin/day (total content is 36 mg oxybutynin)

Flavoxate HCl is available in the United States generically in tablets for oral administration that contain 100 mg

Hyoscyamine sulfate is available in the United States generically in many solid and liquid formulations for oral administration, including immediate-release tablets that contain 0.125 mg or 0.15 mg, sublingual tablets that contain 0.125 mg, extended-release and sustained-release tablets that contain 0.375 mg, orally disintegrating tablets that contain 0.125 mg, extended-release and timed-release capsules that contain 0.375 mg, an oral solution (0.125 mg/mL), an elixir (0.125 mg/5 mL), and an oral spray solution (1 spray delivers 0.125 mg in 1 mL)

Terazosin HCl is available in the United States generically in a variety of solid formulations for oral administration, including tablets that contain 1 mg, 2 mg, 5 mg, and 10 mg terazosin base and capsules that contain 1 mg, 2 mg, 5 mg, and 10 mg terazosin base

Doxazosin mesylate is available in the United States generically in tablet formulations for oral administration that contain 1 mg, 2 mg, 4 mg, or 8 mg doxazosin base
Tamsulosin HCl is commercially available in the United States as immediate-release capsules for oral administration that contain 0.4 mg tamsulosin HCl (Flomax®)
Finasteride is commercially available in the United States as immediate-release tablets for oral administration that contain 1 mg finasteride/tablet (Propecia®) or 5 mg finasteride/tablet (Proscar®)

Urinary Bladder: Late (Chronic) Side Effects

Presentation

1. Persistent dysuria
1. Persistent frequency and urgency
2. Obstructive urinary symptoms
3. Hematuria or hemorrhage due to telangiectasis or ulceration
4. Decreased bladder capacity
5. Urethral stricture, especially in patients with history of transurethral resection of the prostate
6. Fistula
7. Sphincter insufficiency is less common. Injury to ureters is rarely seen

Management

1. Persistent dysuria, frequency, urgency, and obstructive symptoms:
   - Symptomatic relief is the goal
   - Use agents recommended for acute management, as above
2. Hematuria or hemorrhage:
   - May require endoscopy with cauterization
3. Severe decreased bladder capacity:
   - May require cystectomy

GENITOURINARY SYSTEM: KIDNEY

Kidneys: Early (Acute) Side Effects

Presentation:

Acute radiation nephropathy is rarely symptomatic. Symptoms are similar to those with nephropathy of other causes
Note: Renal damage is rarely reversible

Management

- Limit the volume of kidney irradiated
- TD 5/5 (5% incidence at 5 years) is 20 Gy if both kidneys are irradiated

Kidneys: Late (Chronic) Side Effects

Presentation

Note: The incidence of renal toxicity is dose- and volume-dependent. With increased volume irradiated and increased radiation dose, there is an increased risk of renal toxicity

(1) When both kidneys are irradiated to 20 Gy, the rate of renal failure is 5% at 5 years

(2) When both kidneys are irradiated to 28 Gy, the rate of renal failure is 50% at 5 years

Note: Renal damage is rarely reversible
Progression to chronic radiation nephropathy can occur ≈ 1–2 years after completion of RT. Associated symptoms include:

- Hyperreninemic hypertension
- Nephrotic syndrome

Management

1. Limit the volume of kidney irradiated. TD 5/5 (5% incidence at 5 years) is 20 Gy if both kidneys are irradiated
2. For end-stage renal disease, dialysis or transplantation is needed

GENITOURINARY SYSTEM: TESTIS AND ERECTILE FUNCTION

Testis and Erectile Function: Early (Acute) Side Effects

Presentation:

Azoospermia, oligospermia, and hormonal changes

- Can occur even in patients receiving low-dose testicular RT

  Note: Sperm count may recover; however, it may take up to months or years after RT

Management:

Azoospermia and oligospermia

- Sperm banking before starting RT is recommended in men with fertility concerns

Testis and Erectile Function: Late Side Effects

Presentation:

Erectile dysfunction

- Can occur with high RT dose to the prostate

Management:

Erectile dysfunction

- **Sildenafil citrate** 25–100 mg orally once daily 1 hour before sexual activity
- **Vardenafil HCL** 5–20 mg orally once daily 1 hour before sexual activity
- **Tadalafil** 5–20 mg orally once daily 1 hour before sexual activity
- Local therapy (consult a urologist):
  - –**Alprostadil** (prostaglandin E_1) for intracavernosal injection or suppository for intraurethral insertion
  - –Urethral implants

Sildenafil citrate is commercially available in the United States as immediate-release tablets for oral administration that contain 25 mg, 50 mg, and 100 mg sildenafil citrate (Viagra®)
Vardenafil HCl is commercially available in the United States as immediate-release tablets for oral administration that contain 2.5 mg, 5 mg, 10 mg, and 20 mg vardenafil HCl (LEVITRA®)
Tadalafil is commercially available in the United States as immediate-release tablets for oral administration that contain 5 mg, 10 mg, and 20 mg tadalafil (CIALIS®)

GENITOURINARY SYSTEM: VULVA

Vulva: Early (Acute) Side Effects

Presentation:

Vulvar reactions to radiation are essentially skin reactions but are more severe because of the location

Management:

Vulvar reactions

- Attention to personal hygiene
- Topical steroids for symptoms of pruritus
  - –**Hydrocortisone cream** 1–2.5%; apply locally twice daily
- Topical antibiotics may be necessary if signs of infection are present
  - –**Triple antibiotic ointment (polymyxin B sulfate + neomycin + bacitracin zinc)** apply twice daily to affected area
- Treatment break from RT may be warranted if confluent grade 4 (moist desquamation) reaction occurs

Vulva: Late (Chronic) Side Effects

Presentation

1. Pruritus
2. Pain
3. Telangiectasis
4. Pigmentation changes
5. Hair loss
6. Skin atrophy
7. Ulceration
8. Fibrosis with associated dyspareunia

Management

1. Atrophy of the skin
   - Topical estrogen or testosterone creams
     –**Estradiol gel 0.06%** (eg, EstroGel®) metered-dose pump 1.25 mg (1 metered application) topically to intact skin once daily
     Note: The recommended area of application is the arm, from shoulder to wrist
     –**Estrace®** cream topically once daily
2. Persistent ulceration
   - Surgical intervention
3. Fibrosis with narrowing of the introitus
   - Daily use of a dilator

GENITOURINARY SYSTEM: VAGINA

Vagina: Early (Acute) Side effects

Presentation

1. Vaginitis
2. Vaginal candidiasis

Management

1. Vaginitis
   - Vaginal douching with water or a 1:10 mixture of hydrogen peroxide and water 2–3 times daily
2. Vaginal candidiasis

Miconazole nitrate

- Intravaginal suppositories; insert 1 suppository intravaginally once daily at bedtime for 1 day (1200 mg/suppository), for 3 consecutive days (200 mg/suppository) or for 7 consecutive days (100 mg/suppository)
- Cream
  –*Intravaginal*: Insert 1 applicatorful intravaginally once daily at bedtime for 3–7 consecutive days
  –*Topical*: Apply to affected areas twice daily (morning and evening) for up to 7 consecutive days, or as needed

Clotrimazole

- *Intravaginal suppositories*: Insert 1 suppository intravaginally once daily at bedtime for 3 consecutive days (200 mg/suppository)
- Cream
  –*Intravaginal:* Insert 1 applicatorful intravaginally once daily at bedtime for 3–7 consecutive days
  –*Topical:* Apply to affected areas twice daily (morning and evening) for up to 7 consecutive days, or as needed

Nystatin

- *Vaginal tablets:* insert 1 tablet using an applicator, high in the vagina daily for 2 weeks (100,000 units/tablet)
- *Topical cream*: Apply to affected external areas 2–3 times daily until healing is complete
- *Topical powder:* Apply to affected external areas 2–3 times daily until healing is complete

Fluconazole 150 mg orally for one dose

Fluconazole is available in the United States in various formulations for oral administration, including immediate-release tablets containing 50 mg, 100 mg, 150 mg, and 200 mg, and powdered fluconazole for preparing liquid suspensions

Vagina: Late (Chronic) Side Effects

Presentation

1. Atrophy
2. Telangiectasia
3. Adhesion, dyspareunia, fibrosis
4. Ulceration, fistula formation

Management

1. Adhesion formation and fibrosis
   - Daily vaginal dilation to prevent adhesion formation and fibrosis
   - Topical estrogen creams to promote healing and prevent atrophy and dyspareunia
     –**Estradiol gel 0.06%** (eg, EstroGel®) metered-dose pump 1.25 mg (one metered application) topically to intact skin once daily
     Note: The recommended area of application is the arm, from shoulder to wrist
     –**Estrace®** cream topically once daily
3. Persistent ulcer or fistula
   - Surgical intervention may be necessary

GENITOURINARY SYSTEM: UTERINE CERVIX AND UTERUS

Uterine Cervix and Uterus: Early (Acute) Side Effects

Presentation:

Ulceration of the uterine cervix

- Unavoidable with RT for curative treatment of cervical cancer
- May present with persistent clear watery discharge

Management:

Ulceration of the uterine cervix

- Personal hygiene is essential to prevent superinfection
- Vaginal douching with water or a 1:10 mixture of hydrogen peroxide and water 2–3 times per day
- If ulceration persists, the patient may require surgical intervention

Uterine Cervix and Uterus: Late (Chronic) Side Effects

Presentation

1. Hematometra
   - Rare complication due to residual functioning endometrium and a stenotic cervical os
2. Cervical ulceration
   - Necrosis of the cervix (or uterus) can be seen with high-dose brachytherapy used in the treatment of the gynecologic cancers

Management

Hematometra

- Cervical os dilation and surgical debridement may be necessary

GENITOURINARY SYSTEM: OVARIES

Ovaries: Early (Acute) Side Effects

None

Ovaries: Late (Chronic) Side Effects

Presentation

1. Permanent menopause develops in premenopausal women who receive high-dose RT to the ovaries
2. Sexual dysfunction with dyspareunia frequently follows treatment for pelvic malignancies. The causes are both physical and psychological

Management

1. Permanent menopause
   - When fertility is an issue, one can surgically move ovaries out of the RT portal before starting RT
   - To reduce hot flashes
     –**Venlafaxine** 37.5 mg orally 2 times per day[18]
2. Sexual dysfunction with dyspareunia
   - Attention to personal hygiene
   - Hormone replacement therapy. Many commercial preparations are available. Consult a gynecologist
   - Lubrication and daily dilation of the vagina may aid in prevention of dyspareunia

Venlafaxine HCl is available in the United States in 2 formulations for oral administration, including immediate-release tablets that contain 25 mg, 37.5 mg, 50 mg, 75 mg, and 100 mg, and extended-release capsules that contain 37.5 mg, 75 mg, and 150 mg (Effexor® and Effexor XR®)

CENTRAL NERVOUS SYSTEM: BRAIN

Brain: Early (Acute) Side Effects

Presentation:

Increased intracranial pressure (ICP) due to RT-induced edema with the first few fractions of RT leads to:

- Nausea
- Vomiting
- Increased headache

- Changes in mental status (less commonly seen)
- Worsening of neurologic signs (less commonly seen)
- Seizures (less commonly seen)

Management:
Increased ICP

- **Dexamethasone** 10 mg orally or intravenously as a loading dose, followed by 4–6 mg 4 times a day. The dose can be tapered after symptoms have stabilized for 3–4 days

  Note: A fast tapering schedule with a reduction in dose of 50% every 3–4 days is recommended if patient has been on dexamethasone <1 week

Dexamethasone is marketed in numerous generic formulations for oral administration, including immediate-release tablets containing 0.25, 0.5, 0.75, 1, 2, 4, and 6 mg, and in elixirs (which contain alcohol) and solutions for oral administration

Brain: Subacute Side Effects

Presentation:
Somnolence syndrome

- Often noted ≈ 1–4 months after cranial RT
- Characterized by drowsiness, nausea, irritability, anorexia, apathy, and dizziness without focal neurologic abnormalities
- Resolves spontaneously within 2–5 weeks

  Note: Focal neurologic signs seen after RT may be related to intralesional or local reaction, such as edema, demyelination, or bleeding into the tumor

Management:
Somnolence syndrome may be alleviated by corticosteroids

- **Dexamethasone** 10 mg orally or intravenously as a loading dose followed by 4–6 mg 4 times a day. The dose can be tapered after symptoms have stabilized for 3–4 days

  Note: May need a slow taper depending on the patient's symptoms

Dexamethasone is marketed in the United States in numerous generic formulations for oral administration, including immediate-release tablets containing 0.25, 0.5, 0.75, 1, 2, 4, and 6 mg, and in elixirs (which contain alcohol) and solutions for oral administration

Brain: Late (Chronic) Side Effects

Presentation

1. Focal necrosis of the brain
   - Occurs 6 months to several years >RT
   - Occurs in 1–5% of patients who received ≥60 Gy to the brain
   - Associated with focal symptoms as well as symptoms associated with increased ICP
   - Abnormalities can be seen on CT scan or magnetic resonance imaging
   - A void of metabolic activity on PET (proton emission tomography) scan can confirm the clinical diagnosis
2. Leukoencephalopathy
   - Diffuse white matter injury
   - Characterized by lethargy, seizures, spasticity, paresis, ataxia, dementia, or even death
   - More severe form is seen in patients who receive combined chemotherapy and RT
   - Leukoencephalopathy has been reported to be as high as 45% when RT and intravenous or intrathecal methotrexate were given together, and <1% when RT is given alone[19]
3. Neuropsychological and intellectual deficits
   - Memory deficits and learning disabilities can be seen in children 6 months after RT
   - Global IQ decline can be observed 1–2 years after RT[20]
   - Risk factors for more severe deficits[21]:
     - –Young age when exposed to RT
     - –Higher RT doses
     - –Large volume of brain irradiated
4. In adults, memory loss, confusion, dementia, ataxia, and psychomotor retardation can also be seen
5. RT-induced glioma
   - Well documented in children's medical literature
   - 15-year cumulative risk estimated to be 2.7%[22]

Management

1. Focal necrosis
   - May be alleviated by corticosteroids

     –**Dexamethasone** 10 mg orally or intravenously as a loading dose, followed by 4–6 mg 4 times per day. The dose can be tapered after symptoms have stabilized for 3–4 days

     Note: May need a slow taper, depending on the patient's symptoms
   - Symptomatic treatment with anticonvulsant drugs
   - Surgical resection may be needed
2. Leukoencephalopathy
   - Supportive care

Dexamethasone is marketed in the United States in numerous generic formulations for oral administration, including immediate-release tablets containing 0.25, 0.5, 0.75, 1, 2, 4, and 6 mg, and in elixirs (which contain alcohol) and solutions for oral administration

CENTRAL NERVOUS SYSTEM: SPINAL CORD

Spinal Cord: Early (Acute) Side Effects

Presentation

Transient radiation effects on the spinal cord may be seen within 2–4 months after RT

- Incidence is as high as 15% after mantle RT for Hodgkin disease
- Presumed due to the transient demyelination within the RT portal[23]
- *L'Hermitte's sign:* Electric-like shock radiating down the spine to the extremities with flexion of the neck
- Spontaneous resolution expected within 6 months. No relationship to late injury reported

Management

- Symptoms may be alleviated by corticosteroids
  - –**Dexamethasone** 10 mg orally or intravenously as a loading dose followed by 4–6 mg 4 times per day. The dose can be tapered after symptoms have stabilized for 3–4 days

    Note: May need a slow taper, depending on the patient's symptoms. **Gabapentin** 100–600 mg orally 3 times per day

Dexamethasone is marketed in the United States in numerous generic formulations for oral administration, including immediate-release tablets containing 0.25, 0.5, 0.75, 1, 2, 4, and 6 mg, and in elixirs (which contain alcohol) and solutions for oral administration

Gabapentin is available in the United States as imprinted hard-shell capsules containing 100 mg, 300 mg, and 400 mg of gabapentin, elliptical film-coated tablets containing 600 mg and 800 mg of gabapentin, and as an oral solution containing 250 mg/5 mL of gabapentin

Spinal Cord: Late (Chronic) Side Effects

Presentation:

Chronic progressive radiation myelitis (CPRM)

- Rare but devastating late effect. Symptoms start 9–15 months after RT is completed
- Caused by intramedullary vascular damage that progresses to hemorrhagic necrosis or infarction and extensive demyelination with white matter necrosis
- Presents with progressive paresthesias, sensory changes, and weakness
- Risk factors for CPRM
  - –Large fraction size
  - –Length of the cord treated (higher risk with longer segment)
  - –Total dose (higher risk with higher total dose): A cord dose of 45 Gy in 1.8–2 Gy daily fractions has <0.2% chance of developing CPRM[24]
- The majority of patients die of secondary complications

Management:

CPRM

- High-dose corticosteroids
  - –**Dexamethasone** 10 mg orally or intravenously 4 times per day. The dose can be tapered slowly after symptoms have stabilized or improved for several days
- **Hyperbaric oxygen** may lead to remission

Dexamethasone is marketed in the United States in numerous generic formulations for oral administration, including immediate-release tablets containing 0.25, 0.5, 0.75, 1, 2, 4, and 6 mg, and in elixirs (which contain alcohol) and solutions for oral administration

ENDOCRINE SYSTEM

Endocrine System: Early (Acute) Side Effects

Presentation

1. Hyperthyroidism
   - Thyrotoxicosis has rarely been reported after mantle or cervical RT for Hodgkin disease
   - Subsequently evolves into hypothyroidism
2. Diffuse, symmetric thyroid enlargement representing Hashimoto's thyroiditis has been reported but is a rare reaction to RT

Management:

Hyperthyroidism

- Antithyroid agents maybe needed, such as methimazole or propylthiouracil. In addition, a β-blocker may also needed. Consult an endocrinologist for help in management

Endocrine System: Late (Chronic) Side Effects

Presentation

1. Hypothyroidism
   - Late RT effect, 1–2 years after RT
   - As high as 63% at 10 years after treatment of head and neck region and thorax[25]
   - Can also be seen in patients who receive moderate dose to the pituitary that leads to the decreased production of thyroid stimulating hormone
   - Risk factors:
     –*Dose:* Some studies have shown a relationship between dose and RT-induced hypothyroidism
     –*Age:* Young children tend to be more susceptible
     –*Chemotherapy*: Some studies have shown chemotherapy increases the risk of hypothyroidism when used in combination with moderate dose of RT
2. Thyroid cancer
   - A late effect of radiation exposure
   - Risk after RT is about 1.7% in adults[26]
   - Risk increased in children and young adults[27]

Management:

Hypothyroidism
- TSH and thyroxine (T_4) levels should be measured every 6 months after head and neck and upper thoracic RT
- If hypothyroidism develops, treat accordingly

References

1. Trotti A et al. Semin Radiat Oncol 2003;13(3):176–181
2. Emami B et al. Int J Radiat Oncol Biol Phys 1991;21(1):109–122
3. Momm F et al. Strahlenther Onkol 2003;179(10):708–712
4. Delanian S et al. 2003;21(13):2545–2550
5. Pan CC et al. Int J Radiat Oncol Biol Phys 2005;61(5):1393–1402
6. Cerchietti LC et al. Cancer 2002;95(10):2230–2236
7. Fisher J et al. Int J Radiat Oncol Biol Phys 2003;56(3):832–836
8. Brizel DM. JCO 2001;19(4):1233–1234
9. Eisbruch A et al. Int J Radiat Oncol Biol Phys 2002;53(1):23–28
10. Graham MV et al. Int J Radiat Oncol Biol Phys 1999;45(2):323–329
11. Robnett TJ et al. Int J Radiat Oncol Biol Phys 2000;48(1):89–94
12. Komaki R et al. Semin Radiat Oncol 2002;12(1 suppl 1):46–49
13. Antonadou D et al. Int J Radiat Oncol Biol Phys 2003;57(2):402–408
14. Movsas BJ. Clin Oncol 2005;23(10):2145–2154
15. Yavuz MN et al. Int J Radiat Oncol Biol Phys 2002;54(1):195–202
16. Piedbois P et al. Radiother Oncol 1990;18(suppl 1):125–127
17. Ganem G et al. Int J Radiat Oncol Biol Phys 1988;14(5):879–884
18. Loprinzi CL et al. Lancet 2000;356(9247):2059–2063
19. Griffin T. *In:* Gilbert H, Kagan A, eds. Radiation Damage of the Nervous System. New York: Raven Press, 1980:155–174
20. Palmer SL et al. JCO 2001;19(8):2302–2308
21. Mulhern RK et al. JCO 1998;16(5):1723–1728
22. Tsang RW et al. Cancer 1993;72(7):2227–2233
23. Jones A. Br J Radiol 1964;37:727–744
24. Marcus RB Jr, Million RR. Int J Radiat Oncol Biol Phys 1990;19(1):3–8
25. Pai HH et al. Int J Radiat Oncol Biol Phys 2001;49(4):1079–1092
26. Hancock SL, Cox RS, McDougall IR. NEJM 1991;325(9):599–605
27. Hanford JM, Quimby EH, Frantz VK. JAMA 1962;181:404–410

52. Cancer Pain: Assessment and Management

Ann Berger, MSN, MD

Definition of Pain

Pain is "an unpleasant sensory and emotional experience associated with actual or potential tissue damage" (IASP Subcommittee on Taxonomy, p. 250). What this tells us is that pain is far more than a physical phenomenon; it clearly has a sensory and emotional component. A very important definition of pain is: "Pain is whatever the experiencing person says it is, existing whenever he/she says it does" (McCaffery, p. 95). This is important in that it is critical to always believe the patient with cancer who says that he/she has pain

Pain terms: a list with definitions and notes on usage. Recommended by the IASP Subcommittee on Taxonomy. Pain 1979;6:249–252
McCaffery M. Nursing Practice theories related to cognition, bodily pain, and man-environment interactions. Los Angeles, UCLA Student Store, 1968

Prevalence

- Over 70% of patients with advanced cancer report having moderate to severe pain
- At time of diagnosis and during active treatment, 30–50% of patients have cancer pain
- In the advanced stages, 70–90% have pain (Levy)
- 40–50% of patients report their pain as being moderate or severe
- 25–30% of patients report very severe or excruciating pain
- In a large series of 2000 patients, one-third had one site of pain, one-third had two sites of pain, and one-third had three or more sites (Twycross)

Levy MH. NEJM 1996;335:1124–1132
Twycross R. In: Sykes N, Fallon MT, Patt RP, eds. Clinical Pain Management: Cancer Pain/Practical Applications & Procedures. London: Hodder & Stoughton Educational 2003:3–21

Table 52–1. Etiology of Cancer Pain

1. Pain secondary to tumor involvement

Invasion into cutaneous, deep tissues and bone, resulting in somatic pain:
- Bone pain
- Muscle and soft tissue pain
- Headache

Injury to sympathetically innervated organs, resulting in visceral pain:
- Hepatic distention syndrome
- Midline retroperitoneal syndrome
- Chronic intestinal obstruction
- Peritoneal carcinomatosis
- Malignant perineal pain
- Adrenal pain syndrome
- Ureteric obstruction

Aberrant somatosensory processes caused by injury to nervous system, resulting in neuropathic pain:
- Cranial neuralgias
- Radiculopathies
- Brachial plexopathy
- Lumbosacral plexopathy
- Peripheral mononeuropathies
- Spinal cord compression

2. Pain after diagnostic and therapeutic procedures
- Lumbar puncture
- Needle biopsy
- Bone marrow biopsy
- Paracentesis/thoracentesis

3. Treatment-related pain

Surgical removal of tumor or metastases:
- Postoperative pain
- Postmastectomy pain
- Post–radical neck dissection pain
- Post-thoracotomy pain
- Stump and phantom limb pain
- Lymphedema

Chemotherapy:
- Mucositis
- Peripheral neuropathy
- Arthralgia and myalgia due to paclitaxel
- Hand/foot syndrome (capecitabine)
- Flare of bone pain with hormonal therapy for breast and prostate cancer

Radiation therapy:
- Mucositis/esophagitis
- Enteritis and proctitis
- Myelitis
- Chronic myelopathy
- Plexopathy (brachial and lumbosacral)
- Osteoradionecrosis
- Skin "burns"

Other:
- Growth factor induced bone pain
- Postherpetic neuralgia
- Aldesleukin (IL-2)- and interferon-related myalgias

Portenoy RK, Conn M. Cancer pain syndromes. In: Bruera ED, Portenoy RK, eds. Cancer Pain: Assessment and Management. New York: Cambridge University Press, 2003:89–108
McGuire DB. Occurrence of cancer pain. J Natl Cancer Inst Monogr 2004;32:51–56

Table 52–2. Physical Pain Assessment

Where is it most painful now?
How long have you been in pain?
Has this changed from your initial complaint?
What is the temporal pattern of your pain? Is it continuous, or is it intermittent?
What are the characteristics of the pain: aching, cramping, burning, throbbing, numb, tingling, shooting?
What is its intensity: at present, at its lowest, and at its highest level. Scale: 0–10; or mild, moderate, severe
What is an acceptable or tolerable level of pain?
What factors aggravate the pain, such as moving, standing, or sitting?
What factors relieve pain, such as heat, cold, massage, or medications?
What treatments have you tried, what has been their effectiveness, and what side effects have you experienced? (Include over-the-counter medications and alternative and complementary therapies.)

Table 52–3. Types of Pain

Type	Description	Examples	Treatment
Somatic	Localized, aching, throbbing	Bone, joint pain Gnawing feeling	NSAIDs, opioids
Visceral	Pressure, tightening, aching	Pleural, hepatic disease Pulling, stretching	NSAIDs, opioids, steroids
Neuropathic	Severe, sharp, shooting, stabbing, burning, hot, numbing, tingling	Peripheral neuropathy Postherpetic neuralgia	Opioids, steroids, neuroleptics, tricyclic antidepressants, acupuncture
Myofascial	Tightness, pulling, spasm	Upper back, neck	NSAIDs, heat, stretching, TENS trigger point release

TENS, transcutaneous electrical nerve stimulation
**Suffering and pain issues:* Total pain is more than just physical pain. Total pain can involve a suffering component as well as a physical component. Suffering involves psychological and coping factors, social support and loss issues, fear of death, financial concerns, and spiritual concerns

Table 52–4. Assessment of Pain: Psychosocial Assessment

Initial Assessment	Reassessment
What are you most hoping for?	How do you feel things are going?
What are your goals, and how can we best achieve it?	What is the hardest part of your treatment?
What do you fear the most?	Are you having good days? Are you finding enjoyment in things?
Who do you turn to for support?	How is your family/spouse/significant other doing?
Why do you think this disease has occurred? What other losses have you endured during your life?	What helps you meet the challenges you endure?
Do you want others to be involved in decision making about your care?	Who would speak on your behalf if complications arise?

Reproduced, with permission, from Baker K, Berger A. Cancer Pain Assessment: Where Does It Hurt? In: Berger A, ed. Advances in Cancer Pain: A Bedside Approach. The Oncology Group, CMP Healthcare Media,© 2004.

Nature of Pain
Recreational Therapy
* Relaxation
* Stress Management
*Pet, Music, & Art Therapy
Core Team
* Comprehensive Assessment
* Coordinate Interventions
* Discharge Planning
Counseling
* Grief Counseling,
*Family Support, End of Life Issues
* Community Transition
Treatment Regimen
Co-morbidity/ Concomitant Disorder
Disease Process
Rehabilitation
* Functional Interventions
* Assistive Devices
* Energy Conservation
Physical Pain
Complementary
* Acupuncture / Acupressure
* Tai Chi
* Trigger Point Release
Total Pain Individuals' Quality of Life
Psychological Predisposition
Spirituality
Social work
* Socioeconomic Support
* Community Resources
*Coping Skills
Level of Function
Suffering
Roles & Relationships Isolation
Spiritual Ministry
* Pastoral Presence
* Prayer
* Meaning, Hope and Peace
Economic Burden
Grief
Emotional State
Pharmacy
*Pharmacological Counseling
*Equianalgesia
*Adjuvant Agents
Nutrition
* Satiety, Dysphagia
* Nausea
*Intake Modification, TPN /Tube Feedings

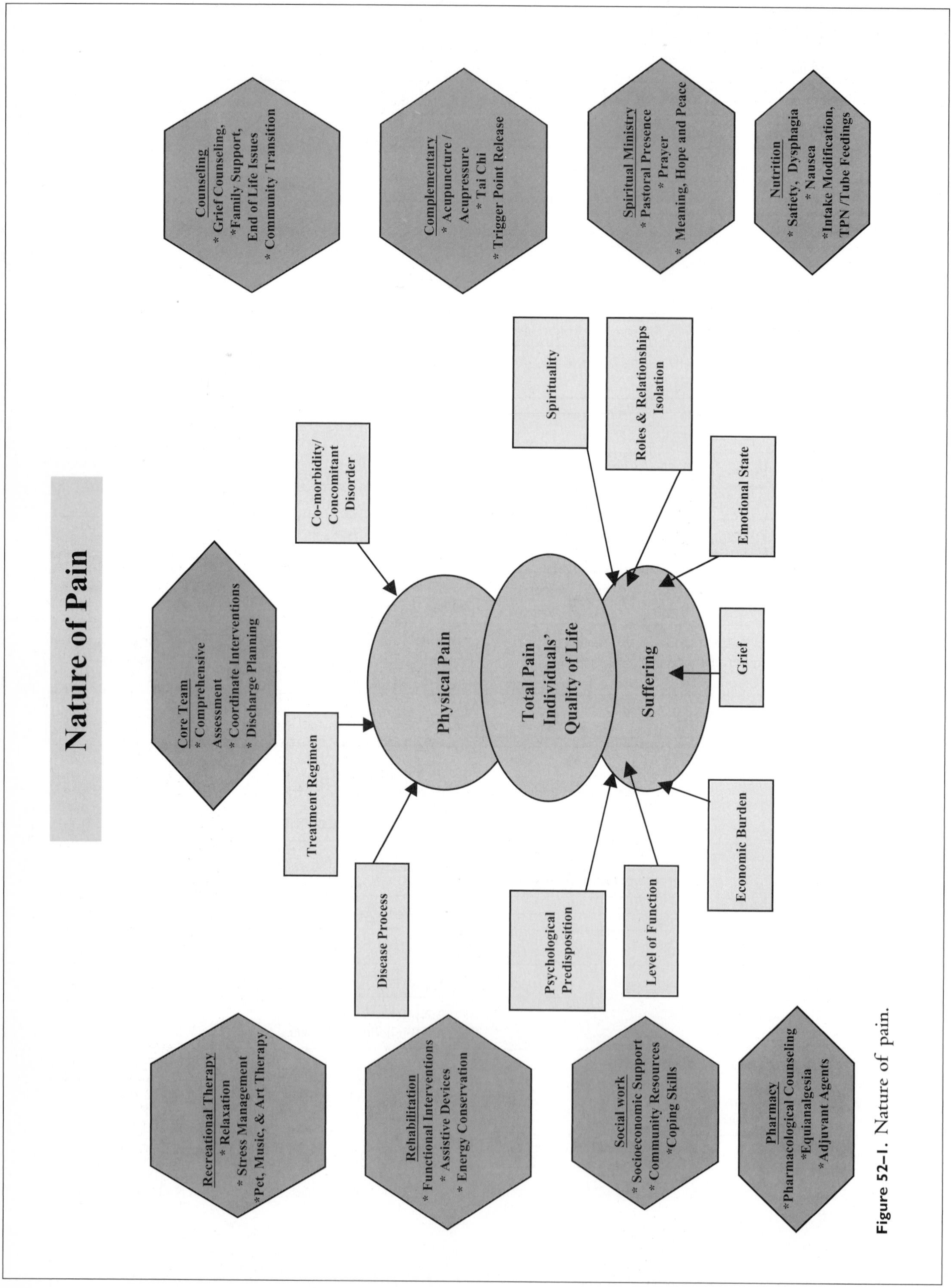

Figure 52–1. Nature of pain.

Table 52–5. Other Issues to Address in Pain Assessment

- Current mood state
- History of psychiatric disorders
- Social support
- Financial stress/insurance issues
- Access to health care/medications
- Current use of illicit drugs/alcohol
- Past history of substance abuse
- Coping skills
- Home environment (physical layout, who is living in the home)
- Primary language spoken, literacy
- Conflict within the family
- Loss/grief issues
- Fears
- Comorbidities
- Concurrent symptoms (fatigue, nausea, diarrhea/constipation, insomnia)
- Concurrent medications
- Cultural influences/preferences
- Functional status
- Patient goals
- Family concerns/issues

Table 52–6. Pain: The Spiritual History

- *Faith*: Is spirituality a part of your life?
- *Meaning*: What meaning do you place on having this cancer pain?
- What is your meaning of being?
- *Importance*: What significance does your belief have on your disease?
- *Community*: Do you have a supportive spiritual community?
- *Care*: How can we attend to these spiritual needs in your care?

Ambuel B. Taking a spiritual history #19. J Palliat Med 2003;6:932–933

Table 52–7. Important Terms with Opioid Use

- *Tolerance*: The need to escalate doses of opioids despite a lack of change in the pain being treated. This is a rare occurrence. Opioid doses usually require escalation because of worsening pain in the face of disease progression
- *Physical dependence*: After approximately 1 week on steady dosing of opioids, the body becomes physically dependent on the medication. If one were to abruptly stop the opioids, withdrawal symptoms would occur. Hence, all opioids should be tapered over time. Note that the experience of withdrawal can often be confused with addiction
- *Addiction*: A psychological and behavioral process that encompasses three types of aberrant phenomenon: loss of control over drug use, compulsive drug use, and continued use despite harm. There is a craving for the opioid, and extreme measures will be taken to gain access, that is, theft, prostitution, and so on. The risk involves those who take opioids for reasons other than pain. The risk of addiction is very low in individuals who take opioids for pain
- *Pseudoaddiction:* Occurs when pain is being undertreated. The individual monitors very closely the timing of the opioids and is frequently asking for opioids more frequently than ordered and/or for a higher dose. They are striving to get better pain control, not an inappropriate amount of opioids for other intentions

Table 52–8. Principles of Opioid Management

I. Dosing and dose titration
A. Consider prior exposure to opioids and dosing requirement
B. Dose according to pain intensity
C. Perform ongoing reassessment and titrate to therapeutic effect or toxicity
D. Titrate upward by 25–50%
E. Begin with as-needed (prn) dosing to determine opioid requirement
F. Should frequent prn dosing be required, pain is constant or severe, consider long-acting agent
G. Determine 24-hour opioid requirement and convert to long-acting agent
H. Provide short-acting agent for breakthrough dosing (5–15% of long-acting opioid dose)

II. Monitoring and treatment of side effects
A. Sedation

1. May develop tolerance 2–3 days after initiation of an opioid or dose adjustment
2. Assess use of other centrally acting agents
3. Check organ function
4. Adjust opioid dose by 30–50%
5. May consider use of a stimulant such as **methylphenidate** HCl 5–20 mg orally for 2 doses/day at 8 AM and 12 noon, or one dose after waking and a second dose approximately 4 hours later
6. Reassure staff and family that this might be secondary to sleep deprivation in the past

Methylphenidate HCl is available in the United States generically in a variety of products for oral administration, including prompt-release tablets containing 5 mg, 10 mg, and 20 mg

B. Respiratory depression
1. Monitor sedation in opioid-naive patients
2. Slow and safe titration

C. Nausea
1. Consider other causative factors
2. Assess bowel function
3. Review concurrent medications
4. Rotate opioids
5. If other opioids not an option:
   a. Medicate with an antiemetic to help central and peripheral mechanisms such as:
      • **Metoclopramide** 10–40 mg (or 0.5 mg/kg per dose) orally 4 times daily, *or*
   b. Medicate with an antiemetic to help vestibular (motion-related) nausea such as:
      • **Meclizine HCl** 6.25–25 mg orally 4 times per day, *or*
      • **Scopolamine** 1.5-mg patch applied to intact skin behind an ear every 72 hours
6. Consider use of acupressure bands

Metoclopramide HCl is available in the United States generically as prompt-release tablets for oral administration containing 5 mg and 10 mg metoclopramide HCl, and as an oral solution containing 5 mg/mL
Meclizine HCl is available generically in the United States in a variety of products for oral administration, including: prompt-release tablets containing 12.5 mg, 25 mg, or 50 mg; prompt-release capsules containing 25 mg; chewable tablets containing 25 mg
Scopolamine is available generically in the United States in a variety of formulations, including injectable solutions in various concentrations, and as a circular flat patch designed for continuous release of 1 mg scopolamine (base) over 72 hours after application to an area of intact skin behind an ear. Transderm Scop® product label, 2004. Novartis Consumer Health, Inc, Parsippany, NJ

Note: Although scopolamine is also available in products formulated for oral and parenteral administration, such products are less useful for continuous symptom management than the transdermal patch system because of a shorter duration of action and a greater incidence of anticholinergic adverse effects associated with transiently high systemic concentrations after intermittent use

D. Constipation
1. Tolerance does not develop
2. Prevent constipation with a daily bowel regimen which includes **Docusate** and **Senna**

(*continued*)

Table 52–8. Principles of Opioid Management (*continued*)

Docusate is generically available in the United States in numerous products for oral administration formulations as both the sodium and calcium salts, *including*:

Docusate Sodium (dioctyl sodium sulfosuccinate)		Docusate Calcium (dioctyl calcium sulfosuccinate)	
Formulation	**Strength**	**Formulation**	**Strength**
Prompt-release tablets	50 mg	Prompt-release capsules	240 mg
Prompt-release capsules	50 mg 100 mg 250 mg	Prompt-release soft-gelatin capsules	
Prompt-release soft-gelatin capsules	50 mg 100 mg 250 mg		
Syrups	20 mg/5 mL 50 mg/15 mL 60 mg/15 mL 100 mg/30 mL		
Liquid	150 mg/15 mL		

Docusate is also available in many combination products for oral administration
Senna (sennosides) is generically available in the United States in numerous single-entity products for oral administration, including: prompt-release tablets containing 6 mg, 8.6 mg, 15 mg, 17 mg, 25 mg; chewable tablets containing 10 mg; granules containing 20 mg/5 mL; syrup containing 8.8 mg/5 mL; liquid containing 8.8 mg/15 mL; concentrated liquid containing 33.3 mg/mL; and oral drops containing 8.8 mg/mL. Sennosides also are available in many combination products for oral administration

St. Germaine D, Berger A. Cancer pain management. In: Berger A, ed. Handbook of Supportive Oncology. Hackensack, NJ: Cambridge Medical Publications (in press)

Table 52–9. Opioid Equianalgesic Dosing

Drug	Oral Equivalent (mg)	IV Equivalent (mg)	Ratio
Morphine	30	10	3:1
Hydromorphone	7.5	1.5	5:1
Oxycodone	20–30		
Methadone	2.5–7.5	1–3.5	1:2.5

Morphine sulfate is commercially available in the United States in various liquid formulations for oral administration, or it may be extemporaneously compounded from prompt-release tablets formulated for oral administration or from morphine sulfate powder

Hydromorphone HCl is available in the United States generically in many solid and liquid formulations for oral administration, including prompt-release tablets containing 2 mg, 4 mg, and 8 mg hydromorphone; extended-release capsules containing 12 mg, 16 mg, 24 mg, and 32 mg; a solution containing 1 mg/mL in a variety of volumes per package; suppositories for rectal insertion containing 3 mg

Oxycodone HCl is available generically in the United States in many solid and liquid formulations for oral administration, including prompt-release tablets containing 5 mg; immediate-release tablets containing 15 mg and 30 mg; immediate-release capsules containing 5 mg; controlled-release tablets containing 10 mg, 20 mg, 40 mg, and 80 mg; a solution containing 5 mg/5 mL; a concentrated solution containing 20 mg/mL

Methadone HCl is available generically in the United States in a variety of formulations and product strengths for oral administration, including prompt-release tablets containing 5 mg and 10 mg; dispersible tablets containing 40 mg; solutions containing 5 mg methadone/5 mL and 10 mg methadone/5 mL; and a concentrated solution containing 10 mg methadone/mL

Morphine Equivalence

From	To	Oral:Oral Ratio	IV:IV Ratio
Morphine	Hydromorphone	4:1	7:1
Morphine	Oxycodone	1–1.5:1	
Morphine	Methadone	4–12:1	4–12:1

Morphine/Fentanyl Equivalence

Morphine 1 mg/hour intravenously	≈	Fentanyl 10 mcg/hour intravenously
Fentanyl 10 mcg/hour intravenously	≈	Fentanyl 10 mcg/hour transdermally
Transmucosal fentanyl (Actiq®) 200 mcg	≈	2 mg morphine intravenously

Oral Morphine Equivalent (mg/day)		Fentanyl Transdermal System (mcg/hour)
45–134	≈	25
135–224	≈	50
225–314	≈	75
314–404	≈	100
405–494	≈	125
495–584	≈	150

Fentanyl transdermal system (fentanyl patches) is available generically in the United States in several delivery rate strengths, including patches that deliver 12.5 mcg/hour, 25 mcg/hour, 50 mcg/hour, 75 mcg/hour, and 100 mcg/hour. Patch sizes vary directly with their labeled delivery rate and the amount of fentanyl they contain

Fentanyl citrate transmucosal system (fentanyl lozenge on a stick) is available in the United States in several product strengths, including 200, 400, 600, 800, 1200, and 1600 mcg as fentanyl base. Actiq® (oral transmucosal fentanyl citrate) product label, 2004. Cephalon, Inc, Salt Lake City, UT

Table 52–10. Principles of Adjuvant Medication Use

I. Choose Appropriate Analgesics
- A. Introduce adjuvant therapy when:
  - 1. Opioids/analgesics are ineffective or produce unacceptable side effects
  - 2. Mechanism of pain is identified
- B. Select adjuvant agent with lowest adverse-effect profile
- C. Consider drug–drug interactions
- D. Anticipate therapeutic response time
- E. Discuss goals of therapy with patient:
  - 1. Titration process
  - 2. Anticipated response time
- F. Begin at lowest recommended dose
- G. Titrate one agent at a time to effectiveness or dose-limiting toxicities:
  - 1. Titrate no sooner than every 72 hours
  - 2. Titration schedule is dependent on half-life of agent
- H. If partial response obtained with dose-limiting toxicities:
  - 1. Lower existing dose by 25%
  - 2. Add agent from a different drug class
- I. If partial response obtained at maximum dosing without toxicities: add agent from a different drug class

II. Reevaluate
- A. Determine response and side effects
- B. Decrease opioid dose as adjuvant agents reach effectiveness
- C. Consider combining adjuvant drugs with different mechanisms of action
- D. Introduce complementary modalities to optimize pain management

St. Germaine D, Berger A. Cancer pain management. In: Berger A, ed. Handbook of Supportive Oncology. Hackensack, NJ: Cambridge Medical Publications (in press)

Table 52–11. Neuropathic Pain Medications

Note on dosing: For some of the drugs, the maximum daily doses specified may produce systemic concentrations that are associated with pharmacologic toxicities, particularly in patients with impaired end-organ function. For these, information about toxic concentrations for the drug and relevant metabolites are provided as follows: TDM Toxic: [*analyte name*], concentrations at which drug-related toxicities typically occur (specimen in which the concentration is measured). TDM=Therapeutic Drug Monitoring

Drug	Analgesic Indication	Dosing (see note above)	Special Considerations	Side Effects
Anticonvulsants				
Carbamazepine	Trigeminal neuralgia Diabetic neuropathy	300 mg TID orally Max. 300 mg QID orally	Obtain CBC and LFTs before administration Monitor for agranulocytosis	Somnolence, dizziness, gait disturbance
Note: TDM Toxic: *carbamazepine* (blood) ≥15 mg/L (≥64 micromol/L) Carbamazepine is available in the United States generically in a variety of products for oral administration, including prompt-release tablets containing 200 mg carbamazepine; chewable tablets containing 100 mg carbamazepine; extended-release tablets containing 100 mg, 200 mg, and 400 mg carbamazepine; extended-release capsules containing 100 mg, 200 mg, and 300 mg carbamazepine; and liquid suspensions containing 100 mg carbamazepine/5 mL and 200 mg carbamazepine/5 mL				
Gabapentin	Postherpetic neuralgia Diabetic neuropathy Migraine headaches	300 mg TID orally Max. 1200 mg TID orally	Somnolence may require lower initial dosing Night-time dosing may facilitate sleep	Somnolence, diarrhea, mood swings, fatigue nausea, dizziness
Note: TDM Toxic: *gabapentin* (blood) ≥25 mcg/mL (≥25 mg/L) Gabapentin is available in the United States generically in a variety of products for oral administration, including prompt-release tablets containing 100 mg, 300 mg, 400 mg, 600 mg, and 800 mg of gabapentin; prompt-release capsules containing 100 mg, 300 mg, and 400 mg of gabapentin; and an oral solution containing 250 mg gabapentin/5 mL				
Lamotrigine	HIV neuropathy Trigeminal neuralgia Cold-induced allodynia	25–50 mg/day orally Max. 200 mg BID orally	Titrate slowly For pain refractory to phenytoin and carbamazepine Valproic acid reduces clearance	Rash, dizziness, ataxia, constipation, nausea, diplopia, somnolence
Note: TDM Toxic: not established. Be wary of *lamotrigine* (blood) >20 mcg/mL (>20 mg/L) Lamotrigine is available in the United States in two formulations for oral administration, including prompt-release tablets containing 25 mg, 100 mg, 150 mg, and 200 mg/tablet and as chewable tablets containing tablets containing 2 mg, 5 mg, and 25 mg/tablet. Lamictal® Tablets and Lamictal® Chewable Dispersible Tablets product label, August 2005. GlaxoSmithKline				
Oxcarbazepine	Trigeminal neuralgia	300–600 mg/day orally Max. 2400 mg/day orally	Similar to carbamazepine with less severe side effects	Skin sensitivity, hyponatremia
Oxcarbazepine is available in the United States in two formulations for oral administration, including prompt-release film-coated tablets containing 150 mg, 300 mg, and 600 mg/tablet; and a liquid suspension containing 300 mg oxcarbazepine/5 mL. Trileptal® Tablets and Oral Suspension product label, March 2005. Novartis Pharmaceuticals Corporation, East Hanover, NJ				
Phenytoin	Trigeminal neuralgia Diabetic neuropathy	300 mg/day orally 1000 mg initial loading dose orally or intravenously	Weak to moderate analgesic effect Obtain CBC and LFTs before administration	Gingival hyperplasia, hirsutism
Note: TDM Toxic: *total phenytoin* (blood) >20 mg/L (>79 micromol/L); TDM Toxic: *free phenytoin* (blood) ≥2.5 mg/L (≥9.9 micromol/L)				

<table>
<tr><td colspan="5">Phenytoin is available in the United States generically in a variety of formulations and strengths for oral administration, including prompt-release capsules containing 100 mg phenytoin sodium (equivalent to 92 mg phenytoin); extended-release capsules containing 30 mg or 100 mg phenytoin sodium (equivalent to 27.6 mg and 92 mg phenytoin, respectively); extended-release capsules containing 200 mg or 300 mg phenytoin sodium (equivalent to 184 mg and 276 mg phenytoin, respectively); chewable tablets containing 50 mg phenytoin; and a liquid suspension containing 125 mg phenytoin/5 mL and ≤6% alcohol</td></tr>
<tr><td>Topiramate</td><td>Post-thoracotomy
Reflex sympathetic dystrophy
Headaches,
Intercostal neuralgia</td><td>25–50 mg/day orally
Max. 200 mg BID orally</td><td>Prolonged use may cause renal calculi
Absorption slowed by food</td><td>Anorexia, weight loss</td></tr>
<tr><td colspan="5">Topiramate is available in the United States generically in two formulations for oral administration, including prompt-release tablets containing 25 mg, 50 mg, 100 mg, and 200 mg; and prompt-release (sprinkle) capsules containing topiramate 15 mg or 25 mg. Topamax® Tablets and Sprinkle Capsules product label, June 2005. Ortho-McNeil Neurologics, Inc</td></tr>
<tr><td>Valproic acid</td><td>Migraine headaches
Cluster headaches
Tension headaches</td><td>250 mg/day orally
Max. 600 mg TID orally</td><td>Multiple drug interactions</td><td>CNS depression, hepatic, hematologic toxicity</td></tr>
<tr><td colspan="5">Note: TDM Toxic: total valproic acid (blood) >120 mg/L (>832 micromol/L); TDM Toxic: free valproic acid (blood) >15 mg/L (>104 micromol/L)</td></tr>
<tr><td colspan="5">Valproic acid and derivatives are available in the United States generically in various formulations and strengths for oral administration, including prompt-release capsules containing 250 mg valproic acid; delayed-release, enteric-coated tablets containing 125 mg, 250 mg, and 500 mg as divalproex sodium; extended-release tablets containing 250 mg or 500 mg as divalproex sodium; sprinkle capsules containing 125 mg as divalproex sodium; and a liquid syrup containing 250 mg sodium valproate/5 mL</td></tr>
<tr><td colspan="5">Tricyclic Antidepressants</td></tr>
<tr><td>Amitriptyline
(Elavil®, and many generic products)</td><td>Neuropathic pain
Musculoskeletal pain</td><td>10–25 mg orally at bedtime
Max. 150 mg orally at bedtime</td><td>Take 10 hours before planned waking to decrease side effects</td><td>Dry mouth, sedation, cardiac arrhythmias, urinary retention</td></tr>
<tr><td colspan="5">Note: TDM Toxic: amitriptyline (blood) ≥ 500 mcg/L (≥ 1805 nmol/L);</td></tr>
<tr><td colspan="5">Amitriptyline is available in the United States generically, formulated for oral administration as prompt-release tablets containing 10 mg, 25 mg, 50 mg, 75 mg, 100 mg, and 150 mg amitriptyline HCl/tablet</td></tr>
<tr><td>Desipramine
(Norpramin®, and many generic products)</td><td>Neuropathic pain
Musculoskeletal pain</td><td>10–25 mg orally at bedtime
Max. 50–100 mg orally at bedtime</td><td>Less sedative and anticholinergic effects than amitriptyline</td><td>Dry mouth, sedation, cardiac arrhythmias, urinary retention</td></tr>
<tr><td colspan="5">Note: TDM Toxic: desipramine (blood) ≥500 mcg/L (≥1880 nmol/L)</td></tr>
</table>

Table 52–11. Neuropathic Pain Medications (*continued*)

Drug	Analgesic Indication	Dosing (see note above)	Special Considerations	Side Effects
Desipramine is available in the United States generically, formulated for oral administration as prompt-release tablets containing 10 mg, 25 mg, 50 mg, 75 mg, 100 mg, and 150 mg desipramine HCl/tablet				
Nortriptyline (Pamelor®, and many generic products)	Neuropathic pain Musculoskeletal pain	10–25 mg orally at bedtime Max. 100–150 mg orally at bedtime		Dry mouth, sedation, cardiac arrhythmias, urinary retention
Note: TDM Toxic: *nortriptyline* (blood) ≥500 mcg/L (≥1900 nmol/L)				
Nortriptyline is available in the United States generically in several formulations for oral administration, including prompt-release tablets containing 10 mg, 25 mg, 50 mg, and 75 mg nortriptyline HCl/tablet; and as a solution containing 10 mg nortriptyline base/5 mL				
Neuroleptic Agents				
Olanzapine	Opioid-induced cognitive impairment	2.5–5 mg/day orally Max 20 mg/day orally	Safer neuroleptic, with reduced extrapyramidal effects, drug interactions, and neutropenia	Agitation, headache, insomnia, somnolence
Olanzapine is available in the United States in two formulations for oral administration, including prompt-release tablets containing 2.5 mg, 5 mg, 7.5 mg, 10 mg, 15 mg, and 20 mg olanzapine and orally disintegrating tablets containing 5 mg, 10 mg, 15 mg, and 20 mg olanzapine. ZYPREXA® Olanzapine Tablets, ZYPREXA® ZYDIS® Olanzapine Orally Disintegrating Tablets, ZYPREXA® IntraMuscular Olanzapine for Injection product label, May 26, 2005. Eli Lilly and Company				
NMDA (N-methyl-d-aspartate) Receptor Antagonists (a glutamate receptor)				
Ketamine	Refractory neuropathic pain	0.1–1.5 mg/kg per hour, intravenously Use as continuous infusion in hospice setting; or intermittently for less severe pain	Poorly absorbed orally Do not use with increased ICP, hypertension, or psychosis Ketamine is hepatically metabolized. Pharmacodynamic effects may be prolonged in patients with impaired liver function	Confusion, hallucinations
Ketamine hydrochloride is available generically in the United States in several concentrations for parenteral administration, including 200 mg/vial (10 mg/mL, 20 mL/vial), 500 mg/vial (50 mg/mL, 10 mL/vial and 100 mg/mL, 5 mL/vial)				
Methadone	Somatic pain Neuropathic pain	2.5 mg QD or BID orally or intravenously	May reduce opioid tolerance	
Methadone hydrochloride is available generically in the United States in a variety of formulations and product strengths for oral administration, including prompt-release tablets containing 5 mg or 10 mg of methadone HCl; dispersible tablets containing 40 mg methadone HCl; solutions containing 5 mg/5 mL or 10 mg/5 mL; and a concentrated solution containing 10 mg methadone HCl/mL				

Dextromethorphan polistirex oral suspension, extended-release equivalent to 30 mg dextromethorphan HBr/5 mL (Delsym®)	Polyneuropathy	15 mg BID orally Maximum dose can vary and is determined empirically	Slow-release dextromethorphan Product contains 0.26% alcohol	Pharmacokinetic interaction between dextromethorphan and serotonin reuptake inhibitors or MAO inhibitors may result in serotonin syndrome
Dextromethorphan polystirex is available in the United States as an extended-release suspension that contains the equivalent of 30 mg dextromethorphan hydrobromide /5 mL and 0.26% alcohol (Delsym® ER Suspension; Celltech Pharmaceutical Co, Rochester, NY)				
Antiarrhythmics				
Mexiletine	Refractory neuropathic pain	50 mg TID orally Max. 10 mg/kg per day orally	May worsen preexisting cardiac arrhythmias. Do not use in second- and third-degree AV blocks. Monitor ECG at high doses	Nausea, anxiety, dizziness
Note: TDM Toxic: *mexiletine* (blood) >2 mcg/mL (>11.2 micromol/L)				
Mexiletine hydrochloride is available in the United States as prompt-release capsules for oral administration containing 150 mg, 200 mg, and 250 mg. Mexitil® product label, May 30, 2003. Boehringer Ingelheim Pharmaceuticals, Inc				
Lidocaine	Refractory neuropathic pain	Administer intravenously	Do not use with compromised cardiac contractility or conduction Avoid use of tricyclic antidepressants	
Note: TDM Toxic: *lidocaine* (blood) ≥6 mcg/mL (≥25.6 micromol/L)				
Local/Cutaneous Anesthetics				
Eutectic mixture of lidocaine 2.5% and prilocaine 2.5% (EMLA®)	Peripheral neuropathy allodynia	Apply topically to intact skin QID and cover with an occlusive dressing (eg, Opsite™ film dressing; Smith & Nephew Inc, Memphis, TN)		
A eutectic mixture of lidocaine and prilocaine is available in the United States as EMLA® Cream (lidocaine 2.5% and prilocaine 2.5%) product label, May 2005. AstraZeneca LP				
Lidocaine patch 5% (Lidoderm®)	Postherpetic neuralgia	Apply topically to intact skin for up to 12 hours every 24 hours		
Lidocaine HCl is available in the United States in Lidoderm®, a 10- × 14-cm patch for topical application to intact skin. Lidoderm® (lidocaine patch 5%) product label, September 2004. Endo Pharmaceuticals, Inc				

Table 52–11. Neuropathic Pain Medications (*continued*)

Drug	Analgesic Indication	Dosing (see note above)	Special Considerations	Side Effects
Topical Agents				
Capsaicin	Peripheral neuropathy Arthropathy Mucositis	Apply topically to intact skin QID		
Capsaicin is available in the United States in a variety of formulations and product strengths for topical application, including lotions 0.025% and 0.075%; creams 0.025% (with and without other active ingredients), 0.025% and 0.075% in an emollient base; and gel 0.025 and 0.05%				
Polyvinylpyrrolidone, sodium hyaluronate, and glycerrhetinic acid bioadherent oral gel (Gelclair®)	Mucositis	Dilute the contents of one Gelclair® packet with 1–3 tablespoons (15–45 mL) tap water (or may be used undiluted); "swish" the product around the oral cavity or gargle with it for at least 1 minute, QID. The product is usually expectorated, but is harmless if swallowed		
Gelclair® is available in the United States packaged in boxes of 21 single-dose packets containing 15 mL of concentrated bioadherent oral gel. Gelclair® product label, August 2003. (OSI)™ oncology, OSI Pharmaceuticals, Inc				
Corticosteroids				
Dexamethasone	Oncologic emergency (spinal cord or nerve compression) Refractory neuropathic pain Increased ICP Organ distention Bone metastasis	80–100 mg intravenously × 1, then 10–12 mg intravenously QID; or 1 mg–4 mg orally QID	Improves pain, nausea, appetite, and malaise Longer duration of action (36–72 hours) No mineralocorticoid effects (edema) Taper dosing to discontinue	Myopathy, delirium, depression
Dexamethasone is available in the United States in numerous formulations and product strengths for oral administration, including prompt-release tablets containing 0.25 mg, 0.5 mg, 0.75 mg, 1 mg, 2 mg, 4 mg, and 6 mg, and in elixirs (which contain alcohol) and solutions				
Prednisone		5–10 mg BID orally	Use to reduce myopathy Taper dose to discontinue Improves pain, nausea, and appetite	Hypotension, dry mouth, somnolence
Prednisone is available in the United States in numerous formulations and product strengths for oral administration, including prompt-release tablets containing 1, 2.5, 5, 10, 20, and 50 mg prednisone, and in solutions and syrups				

α_2-Adrenergic Agonists				
Clonidine	Diabetic neuropathy Cancer-related neuropathy Chronic headache	0.1 mg/day orally max. 2 mg/day orally; *or* Apply and replace topical patches to intact hairless skin every 7 days	Beneficial in less opioid-responsive patients May reduce opioid requirement	Hypotension, dry mouth, somnolence

Clonidine hydrochloride is available generically in the United States in a variety of products, including prompt-release tablets for oral administration containing 0.1 mg, 0.2 mg, and 0.3 mg; as a topical transdermal system (patch) for topical application that delivers 0.1 mg, 0.2 mg, or 0.3 mg per 24 hours continuously for 7 days (Catapres-TTS® Transdermal Therapeutic System product label, August 2004. Boehringer Ingelheim Pharmaceuticals, Inc); and a parenteral formulation for epidural use (Duraclon®, Xanodyne Pharmaceuticals Inc)

BID, twice per day; ICP, intracranial pressure; QD, once per day; QID, four times per day; TID, three times per day

Reproduced, with permission, from Pereira D, St. Germaine D. Pharmacologic Adjuvant Therapy for Cancer Pain. In: Berger A, ed. Advances in Cancer Pain: A Bedside Approach. The Oncology Group, CMP Healthcare Media,© 2004.

Table 52-12. Nonsteroidal Anti-Inflammatory Agents

Agent	Typical Starting Dose	Maximum Daily Dose	Comments
Aspirin	650 mg orally every 4 hours	4000 mg	Irreversibly inhibits platelet aggregation
Aspirin is available in the United States generically in various products for oral administration, including chewable tablets containing 81 mg; prompt-release tablets or caplets containing 165 mg, 325 mg, and 500 mg aspirin in formulations that are uncoated, film-coated, enteric-coated, or buffered; delayed-, extended-, or slow-release tablets or caplets containing 81 mg, 650 mg, and 800 mg. Aspirin is also available generically as suppositories for rectal insertion that contain 120 mg, 200 mg, 300 mg, and 600 mg/suppository			
Celecoxib (**Celebrex**®)	100–200 mg orally every 12 hours	400 mg	Contraindicated in patients who are allergic to sulfonamides
Celecoxib is available in the United States as capsules for oral administration containing 100 mg, 200 mg, and 400 mg. Celebrex® product label, July 2005. G.D. Searle LLC, Division of Pfizer Inc, New York, NY			
Choline magnesium trisalycylate (**Trilisate**®, and others)	500–1000 mg orally every 12 hours	3000 mg	Inexpensive Does not interfere with platelet aggregation Less gastric upset than aspirin and other salicylates
Choline magnesium trisalicylate is available in the United States generically in several formulations for oral administration, including prompt-release film-coated tablets containing 500 mg, 750 mg, and 1000 mg salicylate, and as a liquid containing 500 mg salicylate/5 mL			
Diclofenac (**Voltaren**®)	50–75 mg orally every 8–12 hours orally	225 mg	Available in sustained release form
Diclofenac is available in the United States generically in numerous formulations for oral administration, including prompt-release tablets containing 50 mg diclofenac potassium; in delayed-release enteric-coated tablets containing 25 mg, 50 mg, and 75 mg; and extended-release tablets containing 100 mg diclofenac sodium			
Diflunisal (**Dolobid**®, and others)	250–500 mg orally every 8–12 hours	1500 mg	Causes less gastric irritation compared with aspirin Increases acetaminophen level 50% when both drugs are administered concomitantly
Diflunisal is available in the United States generically in formulations for oral administration, including prompt-release tablets containing 250 mg or 500 mg			
Etodolac (**Lodine**®, and others)	200 mg orally every 6 hours to 400 mg orally every 8 hours	400 mg	Causes less gastric irritation especially in the elderly Antacids reduce peak concentration by 20%
Etodolac is available in the United States generically in numerous formulations for oral administration, including prompt-release film-coated tablets containing 400 mg and 500 mg; extended-release film-coated tablets containing 400 mg, 500 mg, and 600 mg; and capsules containing 200 mg and 300 mg			
Fenoprofen (**Nalfon**®, and others)	300–600 mg orally every 6 hours	3200 mg	Associated with higher incidence of renal toxicity compared with other NSAIDs
Fenoprofen is available in the United States generically in formulations for oral administration, including prompt-release capsules containing 200 mg and 300 mg, and tablets containing 600 mg			
Flurbiprofen (**Ansaid**®, and others)	50–100 mg orally every 6–8 hours	300 mg/day	May cause CNS stimulation
Flurbiprofen is available in the United States generically in formulations for oral administration, including prompt-release film-coated tablets containing 50 mg and 100 mg			

Ibuprofen (Motrin®, and others)	200–800 mg orally every 6–8 hours	3200 mg	Associated with less gastric toxicity compared with other NSAIDs
Ibuprofen is available in the United States generically in many solid and liquid formulations for oral administration, including prompt-release tablets that contain 100 mg, 200 mg, 400 mg, 600 mg, and 800 mg ibuprofen; prompt-release gelcaps, caplets, capsules, and captabs that contain 200 mg ibuprofen; chewable tablets that contain 50 mg and 100 mg ibuprofen; liquid suspensions that contain 100 mg ibuprofen/2.5 mL and 100 mg ibuprofen/5 mL; and liquid drops that contain 40 mg ibuprofen/mL			
Indomethacin (**Indocin®**, and others)	25–50 mg orally every 6–8 hours, *or* 25–50 mg rectally every 6–8 hours	200 mg	Associated with greater incidence and severity of toxicities than other NSAIDs
Indomethacin is available in the United States generically in a variety of products formulated for oral administration, including prompt-release capsules containing 25 mg or 50 mg; sustained-release capsules containing 75 mg; and a liquid suspension containing 25 mg indomethacin/5 mL. Indomethacin is also available generically as suppositories for rectal insertion that contain 50 mg/suppository			
Ketoprofen (**Orudis®**, and others)	50–75 mg orally every 6–8 hours	300 mg	Associated with higher incidence of dyspepsia compared with other NSAIDs
Ketoprofen is available in the United States generically in several formulations for oral administration, including prompt-release capsules containing 50 mg or 75 mg; and sustained-release capsules containing 100 mg, 150 mg, and 200 mg			
Ketorolac (**Toradol®**, and others)	15–30 mg intramuscularly (IM) every 6 hours 15–30 mg intravenously (IV) every 6 hours 10 mg orally every 4–6 hours	120 mg IM 120 mg IV 40 mg orally	Used only for pain (minor antipyretic properties) *An NSAID available in injectable form [indomethacin sodium trihydrate is also available in injectable form]* Not to be used for more than 5 days because of potential toxicity
Ketorolac is available in the United States generically in prompt-release tablets for oral administration containing 10 mg, and in formulations for injection with concentrations of 15 mg/mL and 30 mg/mL			
Meclofenamate sodium	50–100 mg orally every 6 hours	400 mg	Rarely used owing to gastric and neurologic toxicities Associated with high incidence of diarrhea
Meclofenamate sodium is available in the United States generically as capsules for oral administration containing the equivalent of either 50 mg or 100 mg meclofenamic acid			
Meloxicam (**Mobic®**)	7.5–15 mg orally daily	15 mg	Preferential COX-2 activity Less selective than other COX-2 inhibitors
Meloxicam is available in the United States as prompt-release tablets for oral administration containing 7.5 mg or 15 mg and as a liquid suspension containing 7.5 mg meloxicam/5 mL. Mobic® product label, August 10, 2005. Boehringer Ingelheim Pharmaceuticals, Inc			
Nabumetone (**Relafen®**, and others)	1000–2000 mg orally daily, *or* 500–750 mg orally 2 times per day	2000 mg	Associated with higher incidence of diarrhea than other NSAIDs
Nabumetone is available in the United States generically as prompt-release tablets for oral administration containing 500 mg or 750 mg			

Table 52–12. Nonsteroidal Anti-Inflammatory Agents (*continued*)

Agent	Typical Starting Dose	Maximum Daily Dose	Comments
Naproxen (**Naprosyn®**, and others)	250 every 8–500 mg every 12 hours, orally	1250 mg	May increase effects of phenytoin, warfarin, and sulfonylureas
Naproxen is available generically in the United States in a variety of products for oral administration, including prompt-release tablets containing 220 mg, 275 mg, and 550 mg naproxen sodium; prompt-release tablets containing 250 mg, 375 mg, and 500 mg naproxen; delayed-release tablets containing 375 mg and 500 mg naproxen; controlled-release tablets containing 375 mg and 500 mg naproxen sodium; and liquid suspensions containing 125 mg naproxen /5 mL			
Oxaprozin (**Daypro®**, and others)	600–1200 mg orally daily	1800 mg	
Oxaprozin is available in the United States from several sources as prompt-release tablets or caplets for oral administration containing 600 mg of oxaprozin and as prompt-release tablets for oral administration containing 678 mg oxaprozin potassium equivalent to 600 mg of oxaprozin			
Piroxicam (**Feldene®**, and others)	10–20 mg orally daily	20 mg	Optimum efficacy may not occur for 1–2 weeks Associated with high incidence of dyspepsia Increases the effect of phenytoin, warfarin, and sulfonylureas
Piroxicam is available in the United States generically as prompt-release capsules for oral administration containing 10 mg or 20 mg of piroxicam			
Sulindac (**Clinoril®**, and others)	150–200 mg orally every 12 hours	400 mg	Associated with less renal toxicity than other NSAIDs
Sulindac is available in the United States generically as prompt-release tablets containing 150 mg or 200 mg			

Data from Mosby's Drug Consult. St. Louis, CV Mosby, 2004.

Table 52–13. Visceral Pain Syndromes

Agent	Dosing	Comments
Bladder Spasm		
Opium tincture	Starting dose: 3 drops orally every 6 hours Titrate to therapeutic response or side effects	Shares the toxicities associated with opiate agonists; used commonly to inhibit gastric motility, but can provide analgesia for bladder spasms
Opium tincture, deodorized is available in the United States in liquid formulations for oral administration that contains 10 mg anhydrous morphine equivalents/mL and 19% ethanol		
Belladonna and opium rectal suppository	30–60 mg per rectum 1–2 times/day Maximum of 4 doses per day	Analgesic and antispasmodic agent Decreased effect with phenothiazines; increased effect with central nervous system depressants, tricyclic antidepressants
Belladonna and opium rectal suppositories are manufactured in the United States in at least two product formulations, including suppositories for rectal insertion containing powdered belladonna extract 16.2 mg and powdered opium 30 mg, or powdered belladonna extract 16.2 mg and powdered opium 60 mg. The product is marketed as a schedule II (CII) controlled substance. Paddock Laboratories, Inc, Minneapolis, MN		
Oxybutynin chloride (**Ditropan®**, and many generic products)	Starting dose: 5 mg orally 2–3 times per day Maximum dose of 5 mg 4 times per day	Antimuscarinic agent Use cautiously in individuals also receiving belladonna; may result in excessive anticholinergic activity
Oxybutynin Cl is available in the United States generically in several formulations, including prompt-release tablets for oral administration that contain 5 mg oxybutynin, extended-release tablets that contain 5 mg, 10 mg, or 15 mg, a syrup containing 5 mg oxybutynin/5 mL, and in a transdermal (patch) system for application to the skin that delivers 3.9 mg oxybutynin/day (total content is 36 mg oxybutynin)		
Phenazopyridine hydrochloride (**Pyridium®**, and many generic products)	100–200 mg orally 3 times per day	Produces topical analgesia on urinary tract mucosa Decreases urinary pain, burning, urgency, and frequency
Phenazopyridine HCl is available in the United States generically as prompt-release tablets for oral administration containing 100 mg, and 200 mg		
Bowel Obstruction		
Octreotide acetate (**Sandostatin®**)	50–300 mg per dose intravenously or subcutaneously for 2–4 doses per day	Very costly Useful in bowel obstruction for its antisecretory properties
Octreotide acetate is available in the United States as an injectable solution. The short-acting product, Sandostatin®, is for administration by intravenous or subcutaneous injection and is marketed in the following concentrations: 0.05 mg/mL, 0.1 mg/mL, 0.2 mg/mL, 0.5 mg/mL, and 1 mg/mL. Octreotide acetate for injectable suspension (Sandostatin LAR®) is a long-acting formulation for *intragluteal administration only* and is marketed in the following concentrations: 10 mg/5 mL, 20 mg/5 mL, and 30 mg/5 mL (Novartis Pharmaceuticals Corporation, East Hanover, NJ)		
Transdermal scopolamine	One patch delivers 1 mg scopolamine over 3 days Apply 1 patch to the hairless (intact) skin behind the ear every 3 days	Peak levels achieved within 24 hours Reduces motility and intraluminal secretions
Scopolamine is available in the United States generically in a variety of formulations, including injectable solutions in various concentrations, and as a circular, flat patch designed for continuous release of 1 mg scopolamine (base) over 72 hours after application to an area of intact skin on the head behind an ear. Transderm Scop® product label, 2004. Novartis Consumer Health, Inc, Parsippany, NJ		

Table 52–13. Visceral Pain Syndromes (*continued*)

Agent	Dosing	Comments
Hyoscyamine sulfate (**Levsin®**, and other generic products)	*Prompt-release products* 0.125 mg orally or sublingually 2 times per day Maximum dose: 0.25 mg, 3 times per day *Extended- and sustained-release products* 0.375–0.75 mg orally every 12 hours	Individual must be well hydrated to receive maximum dose
L-Hyoscyamine sulfate is available in the United States generically in many solid and liquid formulations for oral administration, including prompt-release tablets that contain 0.125 mg or 0.15 mg, sublingual tablets that contain 0.125 mg, extended-release and sustained-release tablets that contain 0.375 mg, orally disintegrating tablets that contain 0.125 mg, extended-release and timed-release capsules that contain 0.375 mg, an oral solution (0.125 mg/mL), an elixir (0.125 mg/5 mL), and an oral spray solution (1 spray delivers 0.125 mg in 1 mL)		
Glycopyrrolate (Robinul®, and other generic products)	1–2 mg orally 2–3 times per day	Anticholinergic and antispasmodic
Glycopyrrolate is available in the United States generically formulated in prompt-release tablets for oral administration containing 1 mg or 2 mg		
Corticosteroids	Variable dosing	Useful for analgesia and inflammation

Data from Mosby's Drug Consult. St. Louis: CV Mosby, 2004

53. Hospice Care and End-of-Life Issues

Charles F. Von Gunten, MD, and David Weismann, MD

Hospice Care

The number one complaint about hospice care from patients and families is that no one had told them about it sooner. Referral for hospice care is appropriate when the most important goal is comfort rather than making the cancer better. If patients improve or resume anticancer therapy, they can be discharged (graduate) and resume services later without penalty

Eligibility: Prognosis of <6 months if the patient's disease *runs its usual course.* Individual patients can continue to be eligible if they live >6 months as long as the physician believes death is *more likely than not* within 6 months. The patient does not need a DNR (do not resuscitate) order. There is no limit to the number of days a patient can receive hospice care. There is no penalty for the physician being wrong

Prognosis: Oncologists overestimate prognosis when compared with actual survival. Referral for hospice care is associated with an *increase* in survival compared with that of controls

General Indicators of Poor Prognosis	Specific Indicators of Poor Prognosis
Performance status: *Karnovsky 10 or 20 (ECOG/Zubrod 4):* <1 month *Karnovsky 30 or 40:* 1–2 month *Karnovsky 50 (or ECOG/Zubrod 3):* 2–3 months	*Hypercalemia:* 6 weeks *Multiple brain metastases:* 3–6 months *Anorexia:* <2 months *Delirium/confusion:* <1 month *Dyspnea* <1 month
Nutritional status *Serum albumin <2.5 mg/dL:* <6 months	**Specific cancers** *Stage IV NSCLC:* 6–12 months *Unresectable pancreas:* 4–7 months *Stage IV esophagus:* 3–6 months *Stage IV gastric:* 7 months

Discussing Hospice Care

One of the biggest barriers to timely referral for hospice care is physician discomfort with the discussion.
Clinical pearl: Discuss hospice care after determining broad goals of care (eg, comfort, to be as independent and comfortable as possible)

Steps	Suggested Phrases
1. Establish the setting: privacy, time	"I'd like to talk with you about our overall goals for your care"
2. What does the patient understand? Get the patient talking	"What do you understand about your current health situation?" *or* "What have the doctors told you about your cancer?"
3. What does the patient expect? Correct misperceptions	"What do you expect in the future?" *or* "What goals do you have for the time you have left—what is important to you?"
4. Discuss Hospice Care	"You've told me you want to be as independent and comfortable as possible. Hospice care is the best way I know to help you achieve those goals." **Never say, "There's nothing more we can do"**
5. Respond to emotions	Be quiet. The most profound initial response a physician can make is silence, providing a reassuring touch, and offering facial tissues. The most common mistake is to talk too much
6. Establish a plan	"I'll ask the hospice to come by to give information, then you and I can discuss it"

Discussing DNR Orders

Discuss DNR orders after discussions of overall goals of care following a stepwise approach

Steps	Suggested Phrases
1. Establish the setting: privacy, time	"I'd like to talk with you about our overall goals for your care"
2. What does the patient understand? Get the patient talking	"What do you understand about your current health situation?" *or* "What have the doctors told you about your cancer?"
3. What does the patient expect? Correct misperceptions. An informed decision about DNR status is only possible if the patient has a clear understanding of his or her illness and prognosis	"What do you expect in the future?" *or* What goals do you have for the time you have left—what is important to you? Do you ever think about dying? How do you want it to be?
4. Discuss DNR order *Clinical pearl:* Start general and become specific later in the conversation	**Never say, "Do you want us to do everything?"** "You have said you want to be comfortable when you die and you hope you'll just slip away in your sleep. Therefore, I recommend that I write a DNR order, which means that we won't try artificial or heroic means to keep you alive when that time comes"
5. Respond to emotions	Be quiet. The most profound initial response a physician can make is silence, providing a reassuring touch, and offering facial tissues. The most common mistake is to talk too much
6. Establish a plan. A DNR order does not address any aspect of care other than preventing the use of CPR	"We will continue maximal medical therapy"

When the Patient will not be DNR

The seemingly unreasonable persistent request for CPR typically stems from one of several themes

Steps	Suggested Phrases
1. Inaccurate information about CPR. For patients with advanced cancer, who undergo CPR in the hospital, the survival to discharge is zero	"What do you know about CPR?"
2. Hopes, fears, and guilt. Some need an explicit recommendation or permission to stop all efforts to prolong life, that death is coming and that they no longer have to continue "fighting"	"What do you expect to happen? What do you think would be done differently, after the resuscitation, that wasn't being done before?"
3. Distrust of the medical care system	"What you said makes me wonder if you may not trust the doctors and nurses to do what is best for you—will you tell me about your concerns?"

If patients are not ready for a DNR order, don't let it distract you from other important end-of-life care needs; emphasize the goals that you are trying to achieve; save a repeat discussion for a future time. Good care, relationship building, and time will help resolve most conflicts

Managing persistent requests for CPR

Decide whether you believe that CPR represents a futile medical treatment; that is, CPR cannot be expected to either restore cardiopulmonary function or to achieve the expressed goals of the patient. Physicians are not legally or ethically obligated to participate in a futile medical treatment. Some facilities have a policy that a physician may enter a DNR order in the chart against patient wishes. Your options at this time include:

- Transfer care to another physician chosen by the patient/family
- Plan to perform CPR at the time of death, **but don't end the discussion.** Tell the patient that you need guidance if he or she survives because it is very likely the patient will be on life support in the ICU and may not be capable of making decisions. Ask the patient (or the family) to help you determine guidelines for deciding whether to continue life-support measures. If not already done, clarify whether the patient has a legal surrogate decision-maker

Normal Dying

Weakness/fatigue	Give permission to patient, family, and other caregivers to accept weakness/fatigue. This does not represent loss of will; the patient is dying
Decreasing appetite/food intake, wasting	Loss of appetite and weight loss are normal at the end of life. Parenteral or enteral feeding neither improves symptom control nor lengthens life: The patient is dying of cancer—it is the cancer that is making the patient thin
Decreasing fluid intake, dehydration	Blood pressure or weak pulse is normal. Peripheral edema or ascites means excess body water and salt. Low oncotic pressure means parenteral fluids cause peripheral or pulmonary edema, worsened breathlessness, cough, and orotracheobronchial secretions
Decreasing blood perfusion, renal failure	Tachycardia, hypotension, peripheral cooling, peripheral and central cyanosis, and mottling of the skin (livedo reticularis) are normal. Venous blood may pool along dependent skin surfaces. Urine output falls as perfusion of the kidney diminishes. Oliguria or anuria is normal. Parenteral fluids do not reverse this circulatory shutdown: The body is shutting down
Neurologic dysfunction: Two patterns	Brain failure—the "usual road" with decreased level of consciousness that leads to coma and death. The "difficult road" that a few patients follow presents as an agitated delirium due to CNS excitation, with or without myoclonic jerks, which leads to coma and death
Pain	There is no evidence that there is a crescendo of pain near death. Terminal delirium frequently misdiagnosed as pain
Changes in respiration	Diminished tidal volume. Periods of apnea and/or Cheyne-Stokes pattern respirations are normal. Accessory respiratory muscle use may become prominent
Loss of ability to swallow	Gurgling, crackling, or rattling sounds with each breath may be heard. Some have called this the "death rattle." For unprepared families and professional caregivers, it may sound like the patient is choking
Loss of ability to close eyes	Wasting leads to loss of the retro-orbital fat pad, and the orbit falls posteriorly within the orbital socket. Eyelids are of insufficient length
Loss of sphincter control	Urinary and fecal incontinence are common. A marked increase in need for direct caregiving is required to keep patient clean

End-of-Life Issues

Medications at the End of Life

Limit medications to those needed to manage symptoms such as pain, breathlessness, excess secretions, terminal delirium, and seizures and their prevention. Choose the least invasive route of administration: Buccal mucosa or oral routes first, subcutaneous or intravenous routes only if necessary, and intramuscular route almost never

Symptom	Medication	Dosage
Terminal delirium	Lorazepam	1–2 mg orally or sublingually every 1 hour until settled
	Midazolam	1–2 mg subcutaneously or by intravenous push every 15 minutes until settled
	Haloperidol	1–5 mg orally or subcutaneously every hour until settled
	Chlorpromazine	10–25 mg orally, per rectum, or intravenously every 2–6 hours
Seizures	Any benzodiazepine	Lorazepam 2–5 mg orally, sublingually, subcutaneously, or intravenously every hour, *or* Midazolam 2–4 mg subcutaneously or by intravenous push every 15 minutes
	Fosphenytoin	Administer subcutaneously 4–6 mg/kg/day or a dose that substitutes the oral phenytoin sodium daily dose
	Phenobarbital	60–120 mg by intravenous push, intramuscularly or per rectum every 20 minutes until settled
Rattle	Scopolamine	0.2–0.4 mg subcutaneously every 4 hours, *or* Apply 1–3 transdermal patches every 72 hours, *or* 0.1–1.0 mg/hour by continuous intravenous or subcutaneous infusion

(*continued*)

Symptom	Medication	Dosage
	Glycopyrrolate	0.2 mg subcutaneously every 4–6 hours, *or* 0.4–1.2 mg/day by continuous intravenous or subcutaneous infusion
Bowel obstruction	Octreotide	50 mcg subcutaneously every 8 hours, *or* 10 mcg/hour by continuous infusion and titrate
Breathlessness	Morphine	*Opioid naive:* 5–10 mg orally every hour, *or* 1–2 mg subcutaneously every 20 minutes, *or* 1–2 mg intravenously every 15 minutes *Opioid tolerant:* Increase pain dose by 50%

Care at the Time of Death

Answer questions and review the signs and potential events that can be expected. For many families and caregivers, knowing ahead of time decreases anxiety. Most people do not know much about death

Signs of death discussed with family:
The heart stops beating; breathing stops; pupils become fixed; body color becomes pale and waxen as blood settles; body temperature drops; muscles and sphincters relax, urine and stool may be released; eyes may remain open; the jaw can fall open; the trickling of fluids internally may be heard

After expected death occurs:
Go to the bedside to comfort family members who are distressed and appreciate that the doctor shows that he or she cared. This need not take more than 5–10 minutes

Participate with nursing to create a visually peaceful and accessible environment. A few moments spent alone in the room positioning the patient's body, disconnecting any lines and machinery, removing catheters, and cleaning up any mess allow the family closer access to the patient's body. If eyes remain open, eyelids can be manually held closed for a few minutes and usually remain closed once they dry. If they remain open, a small amount of surgical tape or a short Steri-strip will hold them closed for longer without pulling on eyelashes when they are removed. If the jaw falls open as muscles relax, a rolled-up towel placed under the chin of a head elevated on pillows usually holds the jaw closed until muscles stiffen some 4–6 hours later

The doctor may need to tell the "bad news" of a patient death to someone who didn't have previous warning. Follow the guidelines for communicating bad news. Avoid breaking unexpected news by telephone, because communicating in person provides much greater opportunity for assessment and support. Tell them what to expect before they see the body (eg, changes in body color, temperature, and the scene they will see)

Writing a Condolence Note

A note or letter from the doctor after the death has been widely reported to be helpful to the bereaved. Such a note has two goals: to offer tribute to the deceased as someone who was important and to be a source of comfort to the survivors. It should be hand-written and sent promptly, generally within 2 weeks after the death. Use any standard stationery

Steps	Suggested Phrases
Acknowledge the loss and name the deceased	"The hospice called to let me know that your mother, Mary Smith, died on Thursday"
Express your sympathy	"I was so sad to hear the news"
Note special qualities of the deceased	"I will miss her sense of humor"
Recall a memory about the deceased	"I particularly remember when she had all of us in the office laughing at one of her jokes about the examination gown"
Name personal strengths of the bereaved	"I was impressed by the devotion you and your family showed your mother during her illness. I remember when she commented on it herself"
Offer help, but be specific. Don't say, "If there is anything I can do, please call"	"I'd be happy to answer any questions you or your family might have about her illness and her care. Just make an appointment with the office—no charge"
End with a word or phrase of sympathy	"I'll never forget your mother or the care you gave her"

Telephone Notification

There will be situations in which the people who need to know about the death are not present. In some cases, you may choose to tell someone by phone that the patient's condition has "changed," and wait for them to come to the bedside to tell the news. Factors to consider in weighing this include family member advice, whether death was expected, the anticipated emotional reaction, if the person is alone, if the person is able to understand, distance, availability of transportation, and time of day. There are times when notification of death by telephone is unavoidable. If this is anticipated, prepare for it. Determine who should be called and in what fashion. Some families prefer not to be awakened at night if there is an expected death

Steps	Suggested Phrases
1. Get the setting right	Ask to speak to the person closest to the patient
2. Ask what the person understands	"What have the doctors told you about M's condition?"
3. Provide a "warning shot"	"I'm afraid I have some bad news"
4. Tell the news	"I'm sorry to have to give you this news, but M just died"
5. Respond to emotions	Active listening is the best initial approach. I can hear how sad you are
6. Conclude with a plan	If the family chooses to come to see the body, arrange to meet them personally

References

Buckman R. How to Break Bad News: A Guide for Health Care Professionals. Baltimore: Johns Hopkins University Press, 1992

Centers for Medicare & Medicaid Services. Hospice Manual Chapter II-Coverage of Services.[Online] Available http://cms.hhs.gov/manuals/21_hospice/hs200.asp. October 11, 2002

Council Report: Medical futility in end-of-life care. JAMA 1999;281:937–941

Diem SJ, Lantos JD, Tulsky JA. Cardiopulmonary resuscitation on television. Miracles and misinformation. NEJM 1996;334(24):1578–1582

Emanuel LL, von Gunten CF, Ferris FD, eds. The EPEC Curriculum. 1999. The EPEC Project www.epec.net

Fast Facts and Concepts. www.eperc.mcw.edu. Last accessed February 10, 2004

Warm E. Improving EOL care–internal medicine curriculum project. J Pall Med 1999;2:339–340

54. Cancer Screening

Jennifer Eng-Wong, MD, Kathleen Calzone, RN, MSN, APNG, and Sheila A. Prindiville, MD

American Cancer Society Recommendations for the Early Detection of Cancer in Average-Risk, Asymptomatic People[1]

Cancer Site	Population	Test or Procedure	Frequency
Breast	Women >20 years	Breast self-examination	Monthly, starting at age 20
		Clinical breast examination	Every 3 years from ages 20–39 Annually, starting at age 40[a]
		Mammography	Annually, starting at age 40
Colorectal	Men and women, >50 years	Fecal occult blood test (FOBT)[b] *or*	Annually, starting at age 50
		Flexible sigmoidoscopy *or*	Every 5 years, starting at age 50
		Fecal occult blood test (FOBT) *and* flexible sigmoidoscopy[c] *or*	Annual FOBT and flexible sigmoidoscopy every 5 years, starting at age 50
		Double-contrast barium enema (DCBE) *or*	Every 5 years, starting at age 50
		Colonoscopy	Every 10 years, starting at age 50
Prostate	Men >50 years	Digital rectal examination (DRE) *and* prostate-specific antigen test (PSA)	The PSA test and the DRE should be offered annually, starting at age 50, for men who have a life expectancy of at least 10 years[d]
Cervix	Women	Pap test	Cervical cancer screening should begin ~3 years after a woman begins having vaginal intercourse, but no later than 21 years of age. Screening should be done every year with conventional Pap tests or every 2 years using liquid-based Pap tests. Women ≥30 years who have had 3 normal consecutive test results may get screened every 2–3 years. Women ≥70 years who have had ≥3 normal Pap tests and no abnormal Pap tests in the last 10 years and women who have had a total hysterectomy may choose to stop cervical cancer screening
Cancer-related check-up	Men and women >20 years		During a periodic health exam, the cancer-related check-up should include examination for cancers of thyroid, testicles, ovaries, lymph nodes, oral cavity, and skin, as well as health counseling about tobacco, sun exposure, diet and nutrition, risk factors, sexual practices, and environmental and occupational exposures

[a]Beginning at age 40, annual clinical breast examination should be performed before mammography

[b]FOBT as sometimes done in the physician's office, with the single stool sample on fingertip during a DRE is not an adequate substitute for the recommended at-home procedure of collecting 2 samples from 3 consecutive specimens. Toilet bowl FOBT tests also are not recommended. Compared with guaiac-based tests for the detection of occult blood, immunochemical tests are more patient-friendly and are likely to be equal or better in sensitivity and specificity. There is no justification for repeating FOBT in response to an initial positive finding

[c]Flexible sigmoidoscopy together with FOBT is preferred compared with FOBT or flexible sigmoidoscopy alone

[d]Information should be provided to men about the benefits and limitations of testing so that an informed decision about testing can be made with the clinician's assistance

Routine screening for lung cancer and ovarian cancer in high-risk individuals is currently under study. No routine screening method is currently recommended

Modified ACS Guidelines for Screening and Surveillance for Individuals at Increased Risk for Colon Cancer[1]

Risk Category	When to Begin	Recommendation	Comment
Single small (<1 cm) adenoma	3–6 years after the initial polypectomy	Colonoscopy	If exam is normal, the patient can thereafter be screened according to average-risk guidelines
Large (≥1cm) adenoma, multiple adenomas or adenomas with high-grade dysplasia or villous change	Within 3 years of the initial polypectomy	Colonoscopy	If normal, repeat exam in 3 years. If normal, then the patient can thereafter be screened according to average risk guidelines
Personal history of curative intent resection of colorectal cancer	Within 1 year of cancer resection	Colonoscopy	If normal, repeat exam in 3 years. If normal then, repeat examination every 5 years
Either colorectal cancer or adenomatous polyps in any first-degree relative before age 60 or in 2 or more first-degree relatives at any age (if not a hereditary syndrome)	Age 40, or 10 years before the youngest case in the immediate family	Colonoscopy Genetic counseling	Every 5–10 years
Family history of familial adenomatous polyposis (FAP)	Puberty	Early surveillance with endoscopy Genetic counseling	These patients are best referred to a center with experience in the management of FAP
Family history of hereditary nonpolyposis colon cancer (HNPCC)[2]	Age 21	Colonoscopy Genetic counseling	If the genetic test is positive or if the patient has not had genetic testing, screen every 1–2 years until age 40, then annually. These patients are best referred to a center with experience in the management of HNPCC
Inflammatory bowel disease, chronic ulcerative colitis, Crohn's disease	Significant cancer risk after onset of pancolitis, or 12–15 years after onset of left sided colitis	Colonoscopy with biopsies for dysplasia	Every 1–2 years. These patients are best referred to a center with experience in the surveillance and management of inflammatory bowel disease

Reproduced, with permission, from Smith RA, et al. American Cancer Society guidelines for the early detection of cancer. *CA: Cancer J Clin* 2002;52:8–22.

Modified NCCN Guidelines for Screening and Treating Women at Increased Risk for Breast Cancer[3,a]

Risk Category	BSE Encouraged	Clinical Breast Exam	Mammogram	Risk Reduction Strategy
Prior thoracic radiation therapy	Yes	Every 6–12 months	Obtain 8–10 years after radiation or at age 40, whichever is first	
Gail Model risk: >1.7% over next 5 years and ≥35 years[b]	Yes	Every 6–12 months	Yes	Consider: Tamoxifen 20 mg orally daily for 5 years
LCIS/atypical hyperplasia	Yes	Annual	Yes	
Strong family history or genetic predisposition[4]	Yes	Every 6–12 months	Start at age 25 or 5–10 years before index case in family	Consider: • Breast MR • Genetic testing • Prophylactic oophorectomy • Prophylactic mastectomy • Tamoxifen 20 mg orally daily for 5 years • Ovarian cancer screening with transvaginal ultrasound and CA-125

[a]See Chapter 55, Selected Criteria for Referring a Patient to a Genetics Professional for definition
[b]Determine Gail Model risk at: http://bcra.nci.nih.gov/brc/

References

1. Smith RA et al. American Cancer Society guidelines for the early detection of cancer. CA Cancer J Clin 2002;52:8–22
2. Burke W et al. Recommendations for follow-up care of individuals with an inherited predisposition to cancer. I. Hereditary nonpolyposis colon cancer. Cancer Genetics Studies Consortium. JAMA 1997;277:915–919
3. NCCN Practice Guidelines in Oncology, V.1.2005
4. Burke W et al. Recommendations for follow-up care of individuals with an inherited predisposition to cancer. II. *BRCA1* and *BRCA2*. Cancer Genetics Studies Consortium. JAMA 1997;277:997–1003

55. Genetics of Common Inherited Cancer Syndromes

Kathleen Calzone, RN, MSN, APNG, Jennifer Eng-Wong, MD, and Sheila A. Prindiville MD

Table 55–1. Indications for Genetic Testing for Cancer Susceptibility (American Society of Clinical Oncology (ASCO), 2003[1])

1. Personal and/or family history suggestive of a known cancer susceptibility syndrome
2. The genetic test can be adequately interpreted
3. Genetic test results will aid in diagnosis and/or influence medical or surgical management

Testing should be performed only in the context of both pre- and post-test genetic counseling including risks, benefits and limitations of testing, early detection, and risk reduction options[1,2]

Table 55–2. Selected Hereditary Cancer Syndromes

Syndrome	Gene	Mode of Inheritance	Clinical Manifestations
Breast/ovarian cancer syndrome[3–6]	*BRCA1*	Autosomal dominant	Cancers of the breast, ovary, fallopian tube, and possibly prostate, gastric, colon, and pancreas as well as other sites
	BRCA2	Autosomal dominant	Cancers of the breast, ovary, fallopian tube, prostate, pancreas, melanoma, and possibly gastric as well as other sites
Cowden's syndrome[7–9]	*PTEN*	Autosomal dominant	Multiple mucocutaneous lesions, vitiligo, angiomas, benign proliferative disease of multiple organ systems, breast cancer, thyroid cancer, colon cancer, macrocephaly
Familial adenomatous polyposis[9–11]	*APC*	Autosomal dominant	Multiple (>100) colon and/or rectal adenomatous polyps, polyps in the upper gastrointestinal tract, osteomas, epidermoid cysts, desmoid tumors, congenital hypertrophy of retinal pigment, dental abnormalities and cancers of the thyroid, small bowel, hepatoblastoma, and brain tumors
Fanconi anemia[9,12,13]	*FANCA* *FANCB* *FANCC* *FANCD2* *FANCE* *FANCF* *FANCG* *FANCL* *BRCA2/FANC D1*	Autosomal recessive	Leukemia, squamous cell carcinomas—head/neck, esophagus, cervix, vulva, anus, hepatoma, hepatic adenoma, myelodysplastic syndrome
Gorlin syndrome [basal cell nevus syndrome][9,14]	*PTCH*	Autosomal dominant	Basal cell carcinoma, medulloblastoma, ovarian cancer, fibrosarcoma, odontogenic keratocyst, palmar/plantar pits, macrocephaly
Hereditary nonpolyposis colorectal cancer[9,15–17]	*MLH1* *MSH2* *MSH6* *MSH3* *PMS1* *PMS2*	Autosomal dominant	Cancers of the colon, rectum, stomach, small intestine, liver and biliary tract, brain, endometrium and ovary; and transitional cell carcinoma of the ureters and renal pelvis

(continued)

Syndrome	Gene	Mode of Inheritance	Clinical Manifestations
Li-Fraumeni syndrome[9,18]	*p53*	Autosomal dominant	Breast cancer, sarcoma, brain tumors, leukemia, adrenocortical carcinoma
Melanoma[9,19,20]	*p16* *CDK4*	Autosomal dominant	Melanoma, astrocytoma, pancreatic cancer
Muir-Torre syndrome[9,21,22]	*MSH2* *MLH1*	Autosomal dominant	GI and GU cancers, sebaceous gland carcinomas, keratoacanthomas, breast cancer, benign breast tumors
Multiple endocrine neoplasm type I[9,23]	*MEN1*	Autosomal dominant	Pancreatic islet cell tumors, parathyroid disease, adrenal cortical tumors, carcinoids, lipomas
Multiple endocrine neoplasm type II[9,24]	*RET*	Autosomal dominant	Medullary thyroid cancer, pheochromocytoma, parathyroid disease
Neurofibromatosis[9,25,26]	*NF1*	Autosomal dominant	Neurofibromas, optic gliomas, café-au-lait macules, axillary or inguinal freckles, iris hamartomas, sphenoid wing dysplasia or congenital bowing/thinning of long bones
	NF2	Autosomal dominant	Neurofibromas, gliomas, vestibular schwannoma, schwannomas of other cranial and peripheral nerves, meningioma, ependymonas, astrocytomas
Prostate cancer[9,27–33]	*BRCA1* *BRCA2* *RNASEL* *ELAC2/HPC2* *MSR1* *Several other loci under study*	Varied: Autosomal dominant, X-linked	Prostate cancer; other cancers not fully defined
Retinoblastoma[9,34]	*RB1*	Autosomal dominant	Retinoblastoma, soft tissue and osteosarcoma, lipomas
von Hippel-Lindau disease[9,35]	*VHL*	Autosomal dominant	Renal cell cancer, hemangioblastoma of brain, spinal cord, and retina, renal cysts, pheochromocytomas, endolymphatic sac tumors
Wilms' tumor[9,36]	*WT1*	Autosomal dominant	Wilms' tumor, aniridia, embryologic tumors
Xeroderma pigmentosum[9,37]	*RAD2*	Autosomal recessive	Basal and squamous cell skin cancer, melanoma, brain, lung, and gastric cancers, leukemia, conjunctival papillomas, actinic keratosis, lid epithiomas, keratoacanthomas, angiomas, fibromas

Table 55–3. Selected Criteria for Referring a Patient to a Genetics Professional[6,38]

1. General indications:
   a. Family member with documented deleterious mutation in a cancer susceptibility gene
   b. Cancer in two or more close relatives (on same side of family)
   c. Early age at cancer diagnosis
   d. Multiple primary tumors
   e. Bilateral cancer in paired organs
   f. Multiple rare cancers in biologically related relatives
   g. Constellation of tumors consistent with known hereditary syndrome (eg, medullary thyroid cancer and pheochromocytoma)
   h. Evidence of autosomal dominant transmission

2. Breast and/or ovarian genetic syndrome assessment if patient has one or more of the following:
   a. Age ≤40 years at diagnosis of breast cancer
   b. Bilateral breast cancer and/or breast and ovarian cancer in the same individual or close relatives on the same side (maternal or paternal) of the family
   c. Clustering of breast cancer with male breast cancer, thyroid cancer, sarcoma, adrenocortical carcinoma, endometrial cancer, brain tumors, dermatologic manifestations, or leukemia/lymphoma in the same family
   d. Member of a family with a known mutation in a breast cancer susceptibility gene
   e. Populations at risk, such as women of Ashkenazi Jewish descent with breast cancer at before the age of 50 or ovarian cancer at any age

3. Li-Fraumeni syndrome criteria:
   a. Member of a kindred with a known positive TP53 mutation
   b. Individual diagnosed with a sarcoma under 45 years of age and with a first-degree relative diagnosed under 45 years of age with any cancer and an additional first- or second-degree relative in the same lineage with any cancer diagnosed under age 45 years of age or a sarcoma at any age

4. Li-Fraumeni–like syndrome criteria: Individual with:
   a. Any childhood tumor
   b. Any sarcoma, brain tumor, or adrenocortical carcinoma diagnosed under age 45, *and*
   c. A first- or second-degree relative with typical Li-Fraumeni syndrome at any age and another first- or second-degree relative with any cancer diagnosed <60 years

5. Colorectal cancer (FAP/HNPCC) syndrome criteria:
   a. Early age at onset of colorectal cancer (<age 50), *or*
   b. Clustering of same or related cancer in close relative
      (1) Colorectal
      (2) Endometrial
      (3) Ovarian
      (4) Duodenal/small bowel
      (5) Stomach
      (6) Ureteral/renal pelvis
      (7) Sebaceous adenomas or sebaceous carcinoma, *or*
   c. Multiple colorectal carcinomas or >10 adenomas in same individual, *or*
   d. Family with known hereditary syndrome associated with cancer with or without mutation (eg, polyposis)
   e. Cancer in an individual and/or family with congenital anomalies or birth defects

Table 55–4. Management Guidelines for Selected Inherited Cancer Syndrome

Cancer Risk Management Options for Selected Cancers Associated with Hereditary Breast/Ovarian Cancer Syndrome[38–40]			
Cancer	Test or Procedure	Frequency	Considerations
FEMALE			
Breast	Mammography	Every 12 months starting at age 25 or 5 years before earliest breast cancer case in family, whichever is earlier	Consider offering participation in ongoing high risk screening studies using MRI or other modalities.
	Prophylactic mastectomy	Consider once childbearing/breastfeeding is complete	
	Clinical breast exam	Every 6 months starting at age 25	
	Breast self-exam	Every month starting at age 20	
	Chemoprevention: Tamoxifen	Consider on a case-by-case basis	Only limited data available on the efficacy of tamoxifen in mutation carriers with conflicting efficacy data in *BRCA1* mutation carriers. Tamoxifen is relatively contraindicated in women with a history of thromboembolic disease
Ovarian	Transvaginal ultrasound with color-flow Doppler	Every 6 or 12 months starting at age 25	
	CA-125	Every 6 or 12 months starting at age 25	
	Prophylactic oophorectomy	Recommended when childbearing complete	
	Chemoprevention: Oral contraceptive	Consider on a case-by-case basis	Not routinely recommended for ovarian cancer risk reduction unless needed for another indication. Could be considered while awaiting prophylactic oophorectomy but may be associated with a small increased breast cancer risk
MALE			
Prostate	Digital rectal exam	Every year starting at age 40	
	PSA	Every year starting at age 40	
Breast	Mammography	Consider on a case-by-case basis.	Not routinely recommended but could be considered if technically feasible
	Clinical breast exam	Consider every year starting at age 25	There are no data to support this but it is a low-risk intervention

American Cancer Society Guidelines should be followed for cancer screening other than that outlined above
Refer to Chapter 54 for more information

Table 55–4. Management Guidelines for Selected Inherited Cancer Syndrome (*continued*)

Cancer Risk Management Options for Hereditary Nonpolyposis Colorectal Cancer (HNPCC)[38,41]

Cancer	Test or Procedure	Frequency	Considerations
		FEMALE	
Colon	Colonoscopy	Every 1–2 years starting at age 20–25 or 10 years before the earliest age of diagnosis in the family, whichever is earlier, then every year after age 40	
	Total colectomy with ileorectal anastomosis	Consider on a case-by-case basis	Not routine. Consider only if: (1) not a candidate for routine screening or (2) diagnosis of adenoma or adenocarcinoma
	Total proctocolectomy	Consider on a case-by-case basis if rectal cancer is present	
Ovarian	Transvaginal ultrasound with color-flow Doppler	Every year starting at age 25–35	
	CA-125	Every year starting at age 25–35	
	Prophylactic oophorectomy	Consider when childbearing complete	
	Chemoprevention Oral contraceptive	Consider on a case-by-case basis	Not routine. Recommend only if another indication is needed. Considered while awaiting prophylactic oophorectomy
Endometrial	Transvaginal ultrasound with color-flow Doppler	Every year starting at age 25–35	
	Endometrial aspirate	Every year starting at age 25–35	
	Prophylactic hysterectomy	Consider when childbearing complete	
Stomach	Upper endoscopy	Consider on a case-by-case basis	Benefit from screening with upper endoscopy unclear because of absence of precursor lesions
Urinary tract	Urine cytology	Consider on a case-by-case basis	No proven benefit to screening urine cytology, but consider because of minimal risks and low cost
		MALE	
Colon	Colonoscopy	Every 1–2 years starting at age 20–25 or 10 years before the earliest age of diagnosis in the family, whichever is earlier. Every year after age 40	
	Prophylactic total abdominal colectomy with ileorectal anastomosis	Considered on a case-by-case basis	Not routinely considered for risk reduction unless: (1) not a candidate for routine screening; (2) diagnosis of an adenoma or adenocarcinoma
Stomach and duodenal	Upper endoscopy	Considered on a case-by-case basis	Benefit from screening with upper endoscopy unclear because of absence of precursor lesions
Urinary tract	Urine cytology	Consider on a case-by-case basis	No data that urine cytology leads to early diagnosis, but consider because of minimal risks and lower cost

Table 55–5. Key Elements of Informed Consent for Genetic Testing for Cancer Susceptibility[1,2]

Topic	Content	
Purpose of test	*No history of cancer:* 1. Potential clarification of personal cancer risk 2. Risk for other family members *History of cancer:* 1. Establishing the basis for existing cancer 2. Identifying risk for other cancers 3. Risk for other family members	
Practical aspects of test	1. Type of analysis being performed 2. Cost 3. Insurance coverage 4. Biosample required (blood, buccal swab, etc) 5. Timeframe for results to be available 6. Plan for result disclosure	
Possible test outcomes	Specificity and sensitivity of test *Known deleterious mutation in family:* 1. Negative/informative 2. Positive for deleterious mutation in family *No known mutation in family:* 1. Negative/uninformative 2. Variant of uncertain significance 3. Positive for deleterious mutation 4. Cancer risks associated with gene if deleterious mutation identified	
Psychosocial implications	*Psychological:* 1. Relief 2. Anxiety 3. Vulnerability 4. Anger 5. Depression 6. Guilt 7. Regret over prior decisions	*Social:* 1. Family implications 2. Patterns of transmission 3. Family dissemination plan for results 4. Testing other family members 5. Insurance risks (health, life, disability and long-term care insurance) 6. Employment discrimination 7. Military discrimination
Options for medical follow-up	*Benefits, limitations, and recommendations:* 1. Surveillance options 2. Prophylactic surgery options 3. Chemoprevention options 4. Risk avoidance options 5. Participation in clinical research	
Privacy and confidentiality	1. Where test report will be stored 2. Who has access to test report 3. Process and considerations in disclosing to third parties	
Tissue storage and reuse	*Laboratories policy:* 1. Additional testing of identifiable samples 2. Length of storage of sample	
Alternatives to testing	*Options:* 1. Decline testing 2. Empiric risk calculations 3. Delay of testing 4. Delay in receiving results once tested 5. Research participation	

Table 55-6. Resources

Organization	Contact Information	Resource
American Society of Clinical Oncology	http://www.asco.org	Cancer Genetics and Cancer Predisposition Genetic Testing, first edition, an ASCO Curriculum including binders and CD-Rom slide set ONCOSEP: Genetics Tool for self-education and assessment in genetic testing, risk assessment, and specific areas of genetic disease. Policy statement on genetic testing for cancer susceptibility
Centers for Disease Control and Prevention (CDC)	http://www.cdc.gov/genomics	Genomics and Disease Prevention at CDC online information resource and listserve
Gene clinics	http://www.geneclinics.org	Genetics web-based information resource on genetic syndromes, genetic testing, and clinical resources
OMI™ Online Mendelian Inheritance in Man	http://www3.ncbi.nlm.nih.gov/omim	An online catalogue of information on human genes and genetic disorders
Physician's Database Query (PDQ®)	http://www.cancer.gov/cancerinfo/pdq/genetics	An NCI database that contains the latest information about genetics

References

1. ASCO, American Society of Clinical Oncology policy statement update. Genetic testing for cancer susceptibility. JCO 2003;21:2397–2406
2. Geller G et al. Genetic testing for susceptibility to adult-onset cancer. The process and content of informed consent [see comments]. JAMA 1997;277(18):1467–1474
3. Breast Cancer Linkage Consortium. Cancer risks in BRCA2 mutation carriers. J Natl Cancer Inst 1999;91(15):1310–1316
4. Thompson D et al. The Breast Cancer Linkage Consortium, Cancer incidence in BRCA1 mutation carriers. J Natl Cancer Inst 2002;94:1358–1365
5. Ford D et al. Genetic heterogeneity and penetrance analysis of the BRCA1 and BRCA2 genes in breast cancer families. The Breast Cancer Linkage Consortium. Am J Hum Genet 1998;62(3):676–689
6. Lindor NM et al. The concise handbook of family cancer syndromes. J Natl Cancer Inst 1998;90:1039–1071
7. Marsh DJ et al. Mutation spectrum and genotype-phenotype analyses in Cowden disease and Bannayan-Zonana syndrome, two hamartoma syndromes with germline PTEN mutation. 1998;7:507–515
8. Liaw D et al. Germline mutations of the PTEN gene in Cowden disease, an inherited breast and thyroid cancer syndrome. 1997;16:64–67
9. Lindor NM et al. The concise handbook of family cancer syndromes. Mayo Familial Cancer Program. J Natl Cancer Inst 1998;90(14):1039–1071
10. Bisgaard ML et al. Familial adenomatous polyposis (FAP): frequency, penetrance, and mutation rate. Hum Mutat 1994;3:121–125
11. Giardiello FM et al. Phenotypic variability of familial adenomatous polyposis in 11 unrelated families with identical APC gene mutation. Gastroenterology 1994;106:1542–1547
12. Rosenberg PS et al. Cancer incidence in persons with Fanconi anemia. Blood 2003;101:822–826
13. Joenje H et al. The emerging genetic and molecular basis of Fanconi anemia. Nat Rev Genet 2001;2:446–459
14. Shanley S et al. Nevoid basal cell carcinoma syndrome: review of 118 affected individuals. Am J Med Genet 1994;50:282–290
15. Aarnio M et al. Cancer risk in mutation carriers of DNA-mismatch-repair genes. Int J Cancer 1999;81:214–218.
16. Vasen HFA et al. Cancer risk in families with hereditary nonpolyposis colorectal cancer diagnosed by mutation analysis. Gastroenterology 1996;110:1020–1027
17. Griffioen G et al. Extracolonic manifestations of familial adenomatous polyposis: Desmoid tumours, and upper gastrointestinal adenomas and carcinomas. Scand J Gastroenterol Suppl 1998;225:85–91
18. Kleihues P et al. Tumors associated with p53 germline mutations: a synopsis of 91 families. Am J Pathol 1997;150:1–13
19. Greene MH. The genetics of hereditary melanoma and nevi. Cancer 1999;86(suppl):2464–2477
20. Rulyak SJ et al. Characterization of the neoplastic phenotype in the familial atypical multiple-mole melanoma-pancreatic carcinoma syndrome. Cancer 2003;98:798–804
21. Schwartz RA et al. The Muir-Torre syndrome: a 25-year retrospect. J Am Acad Dermatol 1995;33:90–104
22. Bapat B et al. The genetic basis of Muir-Torre syndrome includes the hMLH1 locus. Am J Hum Genet 1996;59:736–739
23. Giraud S et al. Germ-line mutation analysis in patients with multiple endocrine neoplasia type 1 and related disorders. Am J Hum Genet 1998;63:455–4467
24. Mulligan LM et al. Genotype-phenotype correlation in multiple endocrine neoplasia type 2: report of the International RET Mutation Consortium. J Intern Med 1995;238:343–346.
25. Friedman JM et al. Type 1 neurofibromatosis: a descriptive analysis of the disorder in 1,728 patients. Am J Med Genet 1997;70:138–143.
26. Evans DG et al. Genotype/phenotype correlations in type 2 neurofibromatosis (NF2): evidence for more severe disease associated with truncating mutations. J Med Genet 1998;35:450–455
27. Ostrander EA et al. Genetics of prostate cancer: too many loci, too few genes. Am J Hum Genet 2000;67(6):1367–1375
28. Easton DF and T.B.C.L. Consortium, Cancer Risks in BRCA2 Mutation carriers. J Natl Cancer Inst 1999;91(15):1310–1316
29. Edwards SM et al. Cancer Research UK/British Prostate Group UK Familial Prostate Cancer Study Collaborators. British Association of Urological Surgeons Section of Oncology. Two percent of men with early-onset prostate cancer harbor germline mutations in the BRCA2 gene. Am J Hum Genet 2003;72(1):1–12
30. Brose MS et al. Cancer risk estimates for BRCA1 mutation carriers identified in a risk evaluation program. J Natl Cancer Inst 2003;94(18):1365–1372
31. Rebbeck TR et al. Association of HPC2/ELAC2 genotypes and prostate cancer. Am J Hum Genet 2000;67(4):1014–1019
32. Xu J et al. Common sequence variants of the macrophage scavenger receptor 1 gene are associated with prostate cancer risk. Am J Hum Genet 2003;72(1):208–212
33. Carpten J et al. Germline mutations in the ribonuclease L gene in families showing linkage with HPC1. Nat Genet 2002;30(2):181–184
34. Li FP et al. Hereditary retinoblastoma, lipoma, and second primary cancers. J Natl Cancer Inst 1997;89:83–84
35. Chen F et al. Germline mutations in the von Hippel-Lindau disease tumor suppressor gene: correlation with phenotype. Hum Mutat 1995;5:66–72
36. Auber F et al. Surgical management and genotype/phenotype correlations in WT1 gene-related diseases (Drash, Frasier syndromes). J Pediatr Surg 2003;38:124–129.
37. Kraemer KH et al. Xeroderma pigmentosum: cutaneous, ocular, and neurologic abnormalities in 830 published cases. Arch Dermatol 1987;123:241–250
38. NCCN. NCCN Practice Guidelines in Oncology, 2003
39. Burke W et al. Recommendations for follow-up care of individuals with an inherited predisposition to cancer. II. BRCA1 and BRCA2. Cancer Genetics Studies Consortium [see comments]. JAMA 1997;277(12):997–1003
40. Liede A et al. Cancer risks for male carriers of germline mutations in BRCA1 or BRCA2: a review of the literature. JCO 2004;22:735–742
41. Burke W et al. Cancer Genetics Studies Consortium. Recommendations for follow-up care of individuals with an inherited predisposition to cancer: I. Hereditary non-polyposis colon cancer. JAMA 1997;277:915–919

SECTION III. Selected Hematologic Diseases

56. von Willebrand Disease

Michael M. Boyiadzis, MD, MHSc, and Margaret E. Rick, MD

Epidemiology

von Willebrand disease (VWD) is a congenital bleeding disorder resulting from a quantitative or qualitative deficiency of von Willebrand factor (VWF), a plasma glycoprotein with essential platelet-dependent function in primary hemostasis and a carrier for factor VIII in the circulation. Acquired von Willebrand syndrome presents as a similar bleeding disorder

Prevalence

Inherited:	1% in United States using laboratory screening (most common inherited bleeding disorder); estimated 1.0% of patients with VWD are symptomatic
Acquired:	0.04–0.13%
Male/female ratio:	**1:1**

Budde U et al. Rev Clin Exp Hematol 2001;5.4:355–568
Kumar S et al. Mayo Clin Proc 2002;77:181–187
Sadler JE et al. Thromb Haemost 2000;84:160–174

Classification of Inherited VWD

Type 1 (classic): 70–80%
Quantitative deficiency of VWF
Inheritance: Autosomal dominant

Type 2 (variant): 15–30%
Qualitative defect of VWF
Inheritance: Autosomal dominant or autosomal recessive

- *Type 2A:* 10–20% of VWD.

Inheritance: Autosomal dominant or recessive

Decreased platelet-dependent VWF function, with lack of high molecular weight VWF multimers

- *Type 2B:* 5–10% of VWD.

Inheritance: Autosomal dominant

Increased VWF affinity for platelet receptor (leading to decreased plasma levels of VWF) with lack of high molecular weight VWF multimers. Patients may have thrombocytopenia from clearance of small platelet aggregates formed by the binding of the VWF

- *Type 2M*: Uncommon type 2 VWD.

Inheritance: Autosomal dominant

Decreased platelet-dependent VWF function with normal high molecular weight VWF multimers

- *Type 2N:* Uncommon type 2 VWD.

Inheritance: Autosomal recessive

Decreased affinity for factor VIII. Lack of protection of factor VIII by VWF leads to rapid clearance and low levels of factor VIII

Type 3: Rare ($1–5/10^6$)
Complete deficiency of VWF
Inheritance: Autosomal recessive

Meyer D et al. Thromb Haemost 1997;78:451–456
Sadler JE et al. Thromb Haemost 2000;84:160–174

Work-Up

1. Activated partial thromboplastin time (aPTT); not a sensitive measure for VWD
2. Plasma VWF antigen (**VWF:Ag**)
3. Plasma VWF activity (ristocetin cofactor activity [**VWF:RCo**] and collagen binding activity [ELISA; limited availability])
4. Factor VIII activity (**FVIII:C**)
5. Bleeding time (**BT**) or automated platelet function analyzer testing (eg, PFA-100™); not sensitive measures for VWD

The tests below (6 and 7) should be performed to determine the VWD subtype after the diagnosis is established. Also, tests 6 and 7 may be performed if there is high index of suspicion for VWD, even if some of the above tests (tests 1–5) are normal

6. **VWF multimers** (gel electrophoresis for size distribution of plasma multimers)
7. Ristocetin-induced platelet aggregation (**RIPA**; test used to determine if the patient's VWF has an abnormally high affinity for the its platelet receptor)

Type	VWF:Ag	VWF:RCo	RIPA	Plasma Multimer Distribution	FVIII:C	BT
1	↓	↓	N/↓	N	↓/N	↑/N
2A	↓/N	↓↓/↓	↓	↓ HMW	N/↓	↑/N
2B	↓/N	↓↓/↓	↑↑	↓ HMW	N/↓	↑/N
2M	↓/N	↓↓/↓	↓	N	N/↓	↑/N
2N	N	N	N	N	↓↓	N
3	↓↓↓	↓↓↓	↓↓↓	Not detectable	↓↓↓	↑↑

N, normal; HMW: high molecular weight multimers

Favaloro EJ. Blood Rev 1999;13:185–204
Rick ME. Clin Lab Med 1994;14:781–793

Treatment Options

Unlike patients with hemophilia in whom treatment may be administered regularly to prevent bleeding, patients with VWD generally have less clinical bleeding and usually receive treatment only in anticipation of an invasive procedure and during the recovery period or for trauma. An exception may be patients with rare type 3 VWD who might receive replacement therapy regularly for some time, depending on an activity in which bleeding might be anticipated

1. DDAVP™ (desmopressin; 1-deamino-8-D-arginine vasopressin). Perform therapeutic trial before use
2. Replacement therapy: Virally inactivated concentrates containing factor VIII/VWF
3. Antifibrinolytic agents
4. Topical agents
5. Platelet concentrates (rarely used)

Management of Different Types of Inherited VWD

Type	Treatments of Choice		Alternative and Adjuvant Therapies
1	Desmopressin	Factor VIII/VWF concentrates	Antifibrinolytic agents
2A	Desmopressin	Factor VIII/VWF concentrates	Antifibrinolytic agents
2B	Desmopressin[a]	Factor VIII/VWF concentrates	Antifibrinolytic agents
2M	Desmopressin	Factor VIII/VWF concentrates	Antifibrinolytic agents
2N	Desmopressin[b]	Factor VIII/VWF concentrates	Antifibrinolytic agents
3	—	Factor VIII/VWF concentrates	Antifibrinolytic agents and platelet concentrates

[a]Desmopressin may decrease the platelet count and aggravate bleeding in type 2B patients
[b]Increase in factor VIII levels will be shorter in duration than expected

Federici AB et al. Curr Opin Pediatr 2002;14:23–33

REGIMEN

DDAVP® (DESMOPRESSIN ACETATE) (1-DEAMINO-8-D-ARGININE VASOPRESSIN) STIMATE® (INTRANASAL PREPARATION)

Mannucci PM. Blood 2001;97:1915–1919
Mannucci PM. NEJM 2004;351:683–694
Pasi KJ et al. Haemophilia 2004;10:218–231

Intravenous administration is preferred for treatment of acute bleeding episodes

Intravenous preparation:
Test dose

1. Measure VWF and factor VIII levels before the infusion
2. **Desmopressin acetate** 0.2–0.3 μg/kg (not to exceed 20 μg) intravenously in 50 mL 0.9% NaCl injection (0.9% NS) over 20–30 minutes
3. Measure VWF and factor VIII levels 1–2 and 4 hours after administration. Expect a 2- to 5-fold increase in VWF and factor VIII levels at 30–60 minutes, falling over 6–12 hours

Therapeutic dose
Desmopressin acetate 0.2–0.3 μg/kg (not to exceed 20 μg) intravenously in 50 mL 0.9% NS over 30 minutes; may be repeated every 12–24 hours for 2–4 doses

Intranasal preparation:
Test dose

1. Measure VWF and factor VIII levels before administration
2. *Patient weight <50 kg:* **Desmopressin acetate** 1 spray (150 μg) intranasally in 1 nostril
   Patient weight ≥50 kg: **Desmopressin acetate** 2 sprays (300 μg) intranasally, 1 spray in each nostril
3. Measure VWF and factor VIII levels 1–2 and 4 hours after administration. Expect a 1.5- to 3-fold increase at 1 hour after administration in VWF and factor VIII levels, falling over 6–12 hours

Therapeutic dose
Patient weight <50 kg: **Desmopressin acetate** 1 spray (150 μg) intranasally in 1 nostril
Patient weight ≥50 kg: **Desmopressin acetate** 2 sprays (300 μg) intranasally, 1 spray in each nostril. Repeat every 12–24 hours for 2–4 doses

Notes

1. Since the response to desmopressin acetate is generally consistent, a test dose at the time of diagnosis should be performed to establish the individual pattern of response and to predict clinical efficacy
2. Once the therapeutic trial is known to be successful, desmopressin acetate can be used without further therapeutic trials
3. When repeated doses are administered, tachyphylaxis may develop. Patients may be followed up clinically for response, and/or ristocetin cofactor levels may be measured after 3–4 doses or after 3–4 days of administration to assess response
4. For patients with type 2B VWD, platelet counts are usually obtained at each time point in the trial to check whether the platelet count drops to a level that might contribute to bleeding (<30,000 to 50,000/mm^3, depending on the procedure)
5. Adults should be warned to limit fluid intake to 1 liter in the 24 hours after desmopressin acetate
6. Desmopressin acetate should be avoided in patients with known atherosclerosis or unstable coronary artery disease
7. Although not absolutely contraindicated, desmopressin acetate is not usually administered to children younger than 2 years of age
8. The intranasal concentration of desmopressin acetate used in patients with VWD is higher than the dose used for non-VWD patients (diabetes insipidus patients)
9. The advantage of using desmopressin is its availability and the avoidance of plasma concentrates

Patient Population Studied

Patients with VWD type 1 or 2 with spontaneous bleeding or before an invasive procedure. In type 2B, thrombocytopenia may worsen, and desmopressin acetate has no therapeutic role in patients with in type 3 VWD

Efficacy

Type	Response
1	Usually effective; most effective in mild or moderate disease
2A	Often effective
2B	May be effective, but in some patients may cause transient thrombocytopenia and worsening of bleeding. Perform trial including platelet counts before use
2M	Limited experience; use if trial indicates response
2N	May be effective, but the duration of factor VIII increase will be shortened owing to a decreased survival of the factor VIII
3	Ineffective

Toxicity

1. Vasodilatation causing flushing: Common
2. Headache (often controlled by decreasing the rate of infusion): Common
3. Tachycardia: Common
4. Hypotension: Common
5. Hypertension: Uncommon
6. Volume overload: Uncommon
7. Hyponatremia: rare if excessive fluid intake is avoided and more than 4 doses are not administered

Tachyphylaxis with serious hyponatremia and seizures can occur with repeated doses. If desmopressin acetate is to be administered for more than 4 doses:

1. Limit doses to once daily
2. Restrict water intake
3. Monitor daily serum sodium levels, and measure VWF levels for evidence of tachyphylaxis (or follow response clinically)

REGIMEN

VIRALLY INACTIVATED FVIII/VWF CONCENTRATE (HUMATE P®)

Battle J et al. Hemophilia 2002;8:301–307
Mannucci PM. Blood 2001;97:1915–1919
Pasi KJ et al. Haemophilia 2004;10:218–231

Replacement therapy is given intravenously over 5–15 minutes within 10–30 minutes of the planned procedure by a slow intravenous infusion at a rate not greater than 4 mL/minute

Humate P® is approved for use in VWD and is labeled with ristocetin cofactor units. Use ristocetin cofactor units to calculate dose

Efficacy

A retrospective survey reported 97 patients with various types of VWD who were treated with Humate P® for 73 surgical interventions, 344 bleeding events, and 93 other events including invasive procedures
The efficacy was rated excellent to good in 99% of surgical operations, 97% of bleeding events, and 86% of the remaining events

Dobrkovska A et al. Haemophilia 1998;4(suppl 3):33–39

Toxicity (N = 97)

Adverse Event	Mild	Moderate
Chills	1	—
Phlebitis	1	—
Vasodilation	—	1
Paresthesia	1	—
Urticaria	—	1
Rash	—	1
Pruritus	—	1

Dobrkovska A et al. Haemophilia 1998;4(suppl 3):33–39

Replacement Therapy

[Monitor patients clinically, and give replacement according the clinical setting and judgment of the physician]

Clinical Situation	Dose of VWF	No. of Infusions	VWF Target Plasma Level*
Major surgery	40–60 units/kg	Every 12 hours initially; then once daily until wound healing is complete	50–100 units/dL; maintain levels for 3–10 days
Minor surgery	30–50 units/kg	Once daily (may require only 1–3 days)	>30 units/dL
Dental extraction	20–30 units/kg	Usually one dose prior to procedure	>30 units/dL for ≥12 hours
Spontaneous minor bleeding	20–30 units/kg	One dose is usually sufficient Monitor clinically	>30 units/dL

*Factor levels can be predicted based on pharmacokinetic data; 40–50 units/kg (VWF: RCO) will increase plasma VWF levels to 80–100% depending on the baseline levels and hematocrit

Patient Population Studied

Patients with type 3 VWD and patients who do not respond to DDAVP or in whom DDAVP is contraindicated

Monitoring Therapy

1. *Surgical procedures:* Measure plasma levels of factor VIII activity and/or VWF activity every 12 hours the day of surgery, then every 24 hours or as dictated by clinical circumstances
2. It is not usually necessary to monitor replacement therapy in patients with spontaneous minor bleeding
3. *Every physician encounter:* Careful clinical follow-up because bleeding may not correlate well with factor levels; careful clinical monitoring is needed

Notes

1. Fresh frozen plasma contains both factor VIII and VWF, but the large amounts that are needed to attain hemostatic concentrations may cause volume overload. In addition, plasma is not generally inactivated for infectious agents, and it is not recommended
2. Eight to 12 bags of cryoprecipitate (each bag contains 80–100 units of factor VIII, 5–10 × higher concentration than fresh frozen plasma) can normalize factor VIII and VWF levels and stop or prevent bleeding. However, methods for inactivating infectious agents are not routinely applicable to this plasma fraction. Thus, cryoprecipitate is not recommended. Use only for very serious bleeding when virally inactivated concentrates are not available

REGIMEN

ANTIFIBRINOLYTIC AGENTS
EPSILON-AMINO CAPROIC ACID (EACA), AMICAR®, TRANEXAMIC ACID

Mannucci PM. NEJM 2004;351:683–694
Mannucci PM. NEJM 1998;339:245–253

Epsilon aminocaproic acid (Amicar®) 50–60 mg/kg orally or intravenously every 4–6 hours (maximum dose of 24 g/day) or

Tranexamic acid 20–25 mg/kg orally or intravenously every 8–12 hours

Epsilon-aminocaproic acid (Amicar®) is available in the United States as 500 and 1000-mg tablets or as a 25% syrup for oral use containing 250 mg/mL of aminocaproic acid, and as an injectable product containing 250 mg/mL aminocaproic acid

Tranexamic acid is not marketed in the United States as tablets, only as an intravenous preparation

Toxicity

The side effects of tranexamic acid and amino caproic acid are dose dependent

1. Nausea: Common
2. Vomiting: Common
3. Abdominal pain: Occasional
4. Headache: Occasional
5. Thrombotic complications: Rare

Monitoring Therapy

No laboratory monitoring is usually necessary; assess response to antifibrinolytic agents clinically

Indications

1. Less severe forms of mucosal bleeding, menorrhagia, epistaxis, dental procedures.
2. Adjuncts to desmopressin acetate or replacement therapy with virally inactivated factor VIII/VWF concentrate

Efficacy

1. May be sufficient in managing the less severe forms of mucosal bleeding
2. More often, these are prescribed as adjuncts to replacement therapy with desmopressin and plasma concentrates during both minor and major surgery
3. Contraindicated in patients bleeding from the upper urinary tract because of risk that clots will be retained in the ureter and bladder

Mannucci PM. NEJM 1998;339:245–253

Notes

1. These synthetic agents inhibit the activation of plasminogen to plasmin and at high doses, inhibit plasmin
2. They should be used intermittently for bleeding episodes, since long-term use may lead to thrombosis; the duration of use for episodes of bleeding in VWD patients is usually 3–5 days
3. They are contraindicated in patients with bleeding from the upper urinary tract because clots that do not lyse may cause ureteral obstruction
4. Antifibrinolytic agents should not be used when there is evidence of an active intravascular clotting process

REGIMEN

TOPICAL AGENTS

Mannucci PM. NEJM 1998;339:245–253
Mannucci PM. Blood 2001;97:1915–1919

Topical therapies can be placed locally on accessible bleeding sites, such as oral or nasal bleeding; they may be used until the bleeding is controlled

1. Gelfoam; gelfoam soaked with topical thrombin
2. Micronized collagen strips (Avitene)
3. Topical fabric soaked with topical thrombin

REGIMEN

PLATELET CONCENTRATES

Mannucci PM. NEJM 2004;351:683–694

Platelet concentrates are used infrequently in VWD patients. When hemorrhage is not controlled despite adequate factor VIII and VWF levels, platelet concentrates (given together with factor VIII/VWF concentrates) at doses of 4×10^{11} to 5×10^{11} may help control bleeding. Transfused normal platelets are thought to be hemostatically effective because they contain VWF and transport and localize VWF from the rapidly flowing blood into sites of vascular injury

Platelets from human leukocyte antigen–compatible donors should be used if repeated or frequent use is likely

Special Therapeutic Settings

During Pregnancy and Delivery

General:

1. Patients with VWD have a higher rate of postpartum hemorrhage: 16–29% in the first 24 hours and 22–29% after 24 hours compared with 3–5% in the general population
2. In patients with VWD type 1 or 2, the levels of VWF and factor VIII rise 2–3 fold above baseline during the second and third trimesters of pregnancy, but fall rapidly after delivery
3. In patients with type 2 VWD, although the levels of VWF and factor VIII increase, a complete normalization of hemostasis may not occur because part of the increased VWF is qualitatively abnormal and may not correct VWF activity. In type 2B VWD, thrombocytopenia may develop or worsen
4. The risk of bleeding is higher with patients with type 3 VWD because there is no physiologic increase in the FVIII:C and VWF levels
5. Patients should be monitored for VWF and factor VIII levels once during the second and third trimesters of pregnancy and within 10 days of the expected delivery date. They should be monitored clinically for at least 2–4 weeks after delivery when the risk of bleeding is higher
6. Risk of bleeding at delivery is minimal when the factor VIII level is higher than 50 units/dL, and the risk of bleeding at delivery is higher if the factor VIII level is <20 units/dL
7. Cesarean section should be reserved for the usual obstetrical indications. VWF and factor VIII activity should be >50 units/dL for cesarean section or epidural anesthesia; replacement therapy should also be given if an episiotomy is required
8. Desmopressin is generally not used during pregnancy because of the theoretical possibility that it may cause uterine contractions

VWD Type 1 or 2:

VWD type 1 or 2 at the time of delivery with factor VIII level of <20 units/dL:

- In patient previously shown to respond to desmopressin acetate by a therapeutic trial, administer desmopressin acetate intravenously *after* onset of labor with 2–3 doses thereafter at 8- to 12-hour intervals
- In patient who has excessive bleeding despite desmopressin acetate or has not responded to desmopressin acetate by a therapeutic trial, use virally inactivated factor VIII/VWF concentrate as indicated for replacement therapy

VWD type 1 or 2 after delivery with factor VIII level of <20 units/dL:

- In patient previously shown to respond to desmopressin acetate by a therapeutic trial, administer desmopressin acetate at 12-hour intervals for 2–3 doses
- In patient who has excessive bleeding despite desmopressin acetate or has not been previously shown to respond to DDAVP by a therapeutic trial, use virally inactivated factor VIII/VWF concentrate as indicated for replacement therapy

VWD type 1 or 2 with factor VIII level of 20–50 units/dL:

- Monitor clinically, and at the time of delivery/labor administer desmopressin acetate in patients who have been previously shown to respond to desmopressin acetate or virally inactivated factor VIII/VWF concentrates to elevate the factor VIII levels >50 units/dL

VWD Type 3

- Replacement with factor VIII/VWF concentrates is necessary during and after parturition with monitoring of factor VIII and/or VWF activity
- No therapeutic role for desmopressin acetate exists in patients with type 3 VWD
- Two to four doses of factor VIII/VWF concentrate per day (40–60 units/kg VWF:RCoF) may be needed to prevent postpartum bleeding (the risk for bleeding may be higher if the dosage is lower or the duration of treatment is shorter; patients must be monitored clinically and may require additional replacement at less frequent doses for up to 3–7 days in unusual cases)

Kouides PA. Best Pract Res Clin Haematol 2001;14:381–399
Kouides PA. Haemophilia 1998;4:665–676
Lak M et al. Br J Haematol 2000;111:1236–1239
Mannucci PM. Blood 2001;97:1915–1919
Rick ME et al. Blood 1987;68:786–789

Acquired Von Willebrand Disease

General:

1. Acquired VWD is associated with a number of disease states including lymphoproliferative diseases, autoimmune diseases, malignancies, hypothyroidism, mitral valve prolapse, aortic stenosis, uremia, and drugs
2. When possible, successful treatment of the underlying disease associated with acquired VWD usually leads to resolution of the bleeding diathesis

Therapy:

For life-threatening bleeding:

- **VWF concentrates** should be used initially to attempt to reach therapeutic levels of VWF quickly. If not contraindicated, desmopressin acetate may also be administered. Although specific recommendations are not published, it is reasonable to administer factor VIII/VWF concentrate at a dose of 50–70 units/kg (VWF activity) and follow the response both clinically and with factor VIII and VWF activity levels at 1–2 hours, 4–6 hours, and 8–12 hours to assess response

For patients with bleeding that is not life-threatening:

- **Desmopressin acetate:** A trial of **desmopressin acetate** is recommended in all patients with acquired VWD
- Measure VWF and factor VIII coagulant activity at baseline, and monitor levels at intervals over the 4–6 hours after desmopressin acetate administration to evaluate the response

For patients with bleeding that is not life-threatening, but who do not have any benefit from desmopressin acetate:

- Administer either virally inactivated factor VIII/VWF concentrates or IVIG. The choice between factor VIII/VWF concentrates and IVIG should be based on the underlying cause of the acquired VWD . Patients with demonstrable antibodies to VWF are more likely to respond to IVIG than whose without antibody. (Response to IVIG may not be observed until 2–3 days after dose is administered)
    - **Virally inactivated factor VIII/VWF concentrate:** 50–60 units/kg, and monitor factor VIII coagulant activity and VWF factor levels at baseline and at intervals over the next 12 hours to assess half-life of the infused factor

    Note: Patients with demonstrable circulating antibodies (6–15% of cases) may require larger doses of factor VIII/VWF concentrate (50–100 units/kg)

    - **IVIG:** Administer 1 g/kg per day for 2 days. IVIG may have a longer duration of action than desmopressin acetate or factor VIII/VWF concentrates. Monitor factor VIII and VWF activity before and at intervals for 7–15 days after infusion for IVIG (may be effective in lymphoproliferative disorders, IgG monoclonal gammopathies)

Additional treatment options used in small number of patients with acquired VWD:

- Plasmapheresis or extracorporeal immunoadsorption for life-threatening bleeding unresponsive to other measures
- Corticosteroids, such as prednisone, beginning at 1 mg/kg and tapering over several weeks
- Other immunosuppressive agents, such as cytoxan or rituximab

Federici A. Expert Opin Investig Drugs 2000;9:347–354
Veyradier A et al. Thromb Haemost 2000;84:175–182

Alloantibodies to von Willebrand Factor

General:

1. 10–15 % of patients with type 3 VWD develop anti-VWF alloantibodies after transfusion of VIII/VWF concentrates. In some patients, factor VIII/VWF concentrates may not be effective and may cause serious or fatal anaphylaxis
2. Patients with type 3 VWD are generally not screened for alloantibodies unless there is suspicion of an antibody from a lack of response to replacement therapy, or if another family member with VWD develops an antibody

Therapy: There is limited experience in the treatment of patients with alloantibodies to VWF Treatment options include:
Recombinant activated factor VII: 90 mcg/kg intravenously every 2 hours for 2–3 doses. Assess response clinically
Recombinant factor VIII: As a continuous infusion to maintain factor VIII levels at approximately 0.5 units/dL; this may require large doses (5000–8000 units/hour in an adult). Monitor with factor VIII levels

Mannucci PM. Blood 2001;97:1915–1919
Mannucci PM. NEJM 2004;351:683–694

Treatment for Dental Procedures

General:
Prophylactic treatment depends on the type of the dental procedure to be performed

Therapy:
Routine examinations and cleaning: These can generally be performed without raising the factor VIII/VWF level. If the patient has a history of excessive bleeding with dental prophylaxis or has nonserious procedure-related bleeding, desmopressin acetate may be given prior to the procedure and/or epsilon-aminocaproic acid (Amicar®) may be administered usually for 1–3 days.

Special circumstances in which factor concentrate and/or antifibrinolytic therapy should be given before and possibly after the dental appointment:

- Deep cleaning. For patients who have heavy plaque and/or calculus accumulation in which bleeding is likely to be induced with scaling
- Block local anesthesia or mandibular block. Dependent on the severity of the patient's VWD
- Dental extractions. Before the extraction, virally inactivated factor VIII/VWF concentrate is administered to raise the level to ~50 units/mL for uncomplicated extractions or to 50–100 IU/mL for difficult or multiple extractions. Epsilon-aminocaproic acid (Amicar®) is started 4–8 hours before surgery and continued at 2–3 g 4 times daily for 5–7 days after dental work is completed. Usually, further administration of virally inactivated factor VIII/VWF concentrate is not required

57. Hemophilia

Steven J. Jubelirer, MD

Hemophilia A

Hemophilia A is a congenital X-linked recessive bleeding disorder characterized by deficient factor VIII or defective coagulant factor VIII activity (factor VIII level = factor VIII coagulant activity)

Incidence: 1 in 10,000 males
Classification: Mild hemophilia (factor VIII coagulant activity ≥5–50%)
Moderate hemophilia (factor VIII coagulant activity 2–4%)
Severe hemophilia (factor VIII coagulant activity ≤1%)

Saenko EL et al. Br J Haematol 2002;119:323–331
White GC et al. Thromb Haemost 2001;85:560

Work-Up

1. *Elevated aPPT*: Patients with hemophilia A have isolated prolongation of the activated partial thromboplastin time (aPTT), which is corrected by the addition of an equal volume of normal plasma. If the aPTT remains prolonged after the addition of an equal volume of normal plasma, consider the presence of inhibitor to factor VIII
2. A specific assay for factor VIII coagulant activity is required for definitive diagnosis

Mannucci PM, Tuddenham EG. NEJM 2001;344:1773–1779 [Erratum published in NEJM 2001;345:384]

Differential Diagnosis of Isolated Prolongation of aPTT

1. Heparin use
2. Factor VIII deficiency or inhibitor to factor VIII
3. von Willebrand disease (especially the type II N VWD)
4. Factor IX deficiency or inhibitor to factor IX
5. Factor XI deficiency or inhibitor to factor XI
6. Factor XII deficiency or inhibitor to factor XII
7. Contact factor deficiency or inhibitor
8. Lupus anticoagulant

Treatment Options

1. Factor VIII replacement
2. Desmopressin acetate
3. Antifibrinolytic therapy
4. Topical agents
5. Platelet concentrates
6. Coagulation factor VIIa (recombinant)
7. Anti-inhibitory Coagulant Complex (AICC)

REGIMEN FOR FACTOR VIII REPLACEMENT

HUMATE P®, ALPHANATE®, MONOCLATE P®, HEMOFIL® M, RECOMBINATE®, KOGENATE® FS, rAHF-PFM ADVATE®, REFACTO®

National Hemophilia Foundation, MASAC (Medical and Scientific Advisory Council) recommendation concerning the treatment of hemophilia and other bleeding disorders. 2003; No. 141
Cohen AJ, Kessler CM. In: Kitchens CS, Alving BM, Kessler CM, eds. Consultative Hemostasis and Thrombosis. Philadelphia: WB Saunders, 2002:43
Kasper CK. Haemophilia 2000;6(suppl 1):13–27
Kasper CK. Hemophilia of Georgia, USA.
Haemophilia 2000;6(suppl 1):84–93
Srivastava A. Br J Haematol 2004;127:12–25

Indications

To prevent bleeding and limit existing hemorrhage in patients with hemophilia A or factor VIII deficiency

Efficacy

Eighty-five percent of bleeding episodes are treated successfully with 1–2 infusions (rated excellent or good hemostasis)

Toxicity

1. *Infection—HIV and hepatitis C with chronic liver disease:* Seen in most patients who received old factor VIII and IX concentrates before 1985
2. *Development of an inhibitor:* 25–30%
3. *Redness at injection site:* <1%
4. *Dizziness:* <1%
5. *Hypersensitivity reaction (hives, urticaria, wheezing, chest tightness, and arthralgia):* Rare
6. *Hypotension*: Rare

Notes

1. Current practice regarding factor replacement therapy is not evidence-based. Factors contributing to this are (a) small numbers of patients seen in individual centers, (b) few multicenter studies, (c) variability in products used for treatment in terms of recovery patterns and postinfusion assays, and (d) imprecision of instruments used to measure outcome, particularly with regard to clinical and radiologic joint scores
2. Previously untreated and minimally treated patients should receive recombinant products. No recombinant product has been shown to be superior in efficacy, risk of infection, or risk of inhibitor development
3. Potential advantage of second-generation recombinant products is higher specific activity, and final formulation is stable without added serum albumin, further reducing the potential risk of human infectious agents
4. With third-generation recombinant products, animal components have been removed from the culture media. ReFacto® and rAHF-PFM ADVATE® are manufactured and formulated without human or animal protein
5. If recombinant factor VIII is not available, a plasma-derived concentrate can be used
6. Sometimes administered by continuous infusion. The national for adjusted continuous infusion is that a steady state by avoiding the peaks and troughs in clotting factor levels seen with bolus injection regimens may reduce the amount of concentrate used and be more convenient. However dosing guidelines for continuous infusion of factor VIII are not currently established and no products are currently licensed for this route of administration

Factor VIII Products

	Intermediate Purity (Humate P®, Alphanate®)	High Purity (Monoclonal-Derived) (MONOCLATE P®, HEMOFIL® M)	Recombinant Factor VIII
Viral transmission	Yes; hepatitis C in 1980s	No	No
von Willebrand factor present	Yes	No	No
Potential benefits	von Willebrand factor is present and may be used to overwhelm inhibitors	Can be used in patients already infected with HIV	Unlimited supply. Some products are human/bovine free

Recombinant Factor VIII Products

	First Generation	Second Generation Formulated in Sucrose	Third Generation B-Domain Deleted
Examples	RECOMBINATE® (Baxter Healthcare)	Kogenate® FS (Bayer)	ReFacto® (Wyeth Pharmaceutials) rAHF-PFM ADVATE® (Baxter)
Human albumin	Present	Absent	Absent
Bovine serum albumin	Yes, in culture medium	Yes, in culture medium	No
Incidence of inhibitor	Same	Same	Probably same
Assay modification	Not required	Not required	Previously required, but now packaged with more mg/unit

Administration Guidelines

Loading dose	Administer over a period of 5 minutes (maximum infusion rate 10 mL/min)
Maintenance doses	Administer over a period of 5 minutes (maximum infusion rate 10 mL/min)
Reconstitution	Reconstitute factor VIII preparations according to manufacturer's instructions

Calculating the Amount of Factor VIII Required

Initial dose

100% Plasma Factor VIII = 1 unit Factor VIII/mL Plasma

Method 1: 0.5 unit factor VIII/kg → increases factor VIII levels 1%
Amount of factor VIII required = wt (kg) × desired level (%) × 0.5
Example: Weight = 70 kg. Amount of factor VIII desired = 0.5 units/mL (50% plasma factor VIII)
70 × 50 × 0.5 = 1750 units*

Method 2: Plasma volume = 40 mL/kg
Amount of factor VIII required = 40 mL/kg × wt (kg) × desired units/mL plasma
Example: Weight = 70 kg. Amount of factor VIII desired = 0.5 units/mL (50% plasma factor VIII)
40 × 70 × 0.5 = 1400 units*

*Results would be similar if for Method 2 assume plasma volume of 50 mL/kg rather than 40 mL/kg

Maintenance dose
One-half the loading dose every 12 hours
[Biologic half-life of factor VIII is ≈12 hours. Thus, at 12 hours the plasma factor VIII level will decrease to one-half the initial level; infusion of one-half the initial dose restores the plasma factor VIII to the initial level]

Treatment of Specific Types of Bleeding Episodes

Type of Hemorrhage	Dose	% Desired Level	Dose (units/kg)[a]	Comments
Superficial laceration	None	None	None	Local pressure + apply adhesive skin closure products
Deep laceration	Single dose	50	25	Sutures after factor is given
Joint	Single dose	40	20	Second infusion (10 units/kg) may be required in 12 hours if pain and/or swelling persist *Adjunctive care:* Ice, rest, and elevation Mobilize joint when pain subsides
Muscle (not iliopsoas)	Single dose	40	20	
Iliopsas muscle	Initial bolus	80–100	40–50	Limit activity until pain resolves
	Maintenance	30–60	15–30	Every 12 hours for ≥3 days until pain or disability is resolved
CNS head	Initial bolus	80–100	40–50	Consult Neurology/Neurosurgery
	Maintenance	50	25	For ≥10–14 days if still bleeding
Throat/neck	Initial bolus	80–100	40–50	
	Maintenance	50	25	Every 12 hours for ≥7–10 days if still bleeding
Gastrointestinal	Initial bolus	80–100	40–50	Treat origin of GI bleed as indicated
	Maintenance	50	25	Every 12 hours for ≥5–7 days if still bleeding
Renal	Single dose	50	25	Avoid aminocaproic acid[b]. Order bed rest, IV hydration
Ophthalmic	Single dose	80–100	40–50	Obtain Ophthalmology consult

[a]Dose calculation based on Method 1 above

[b]Aminocaproic acid should not be used to treat hematuria because blood loss from the upper urinary tract can provoke painful clot retention and even renal failure associated with bilateral ureteral obstruction

Adapted, with permission, from Protocols for the treatment of hemophilia and von Willebrand disease. Hemophilia of Georgia USA. Hemophilia 2000:6(suppl 1):84–93.

REGIMEN

DDAVP (DESMOPRESSIN ACETATE)
(1-DEAMINO-8-D-ARGININE VASOPRESSIN)
STIMATE® (INTRANASAL PREPARATION)

Dunn AL et al. Hemophilia 2000;6:11–14
Lethagen S. Semin Thromb Hemost 2003;29:101–106

Intravenous administration
Test dose:
1. Measure factor VIII levels before the infusion
2. **Desmopressin acetate** 0.3 mcg/kg (not to exceed 20 mcg) intravenously in 50 mL 0.9% NaCl injection (0.9% NS) over 15–20 minutes
3. Measure factor VIII levels 1–2 and 4 hours after the infusion. Expect a 2- to 5-fold increase in factor VIII levels, persisting for 6–12 hours

Therapeutic dose:
Desmopressin acetate 0.3 mcg/kg (not to exceed 20 mcg) intravenously in 50 mL 0.9% NS over 30 minutes. Infusion may be repeated every 12–24 hours for 2–4 doses
Note: Tachyphylaxis with serious hyponatremia can occur with repeated doses. If possible, limit use to one dose daily to avoid tachyphylaxis. If administering more than four doses monitor daily serum sodium levels and measure VWF levels

Intranasal administration
Test dose:
Because of marked variability in response to desmopressin acetate nasal spray, all patients should be tested before therapeutic use
1. Measure factor VIII levels before administration
2. *Patient weight <50 kg:* **Desmopressin acetate** 1 spray (150 mcg) intranasally in 1 nostril
   Patient weight ≥50 kg: **Desmopressin acetate** 2 sprays (300 mcg) intranasally; 1 spray in each nostril
3. Measure factor VIII levels 2 and 4 hours after administration. Expect a 2- to 5-fold increase in factor VIII levels, persisting for 6–12 hours

Therapeutic dose:
Patient weight <50 kg: **Desmopressin acetate** 1 spray (150 mcg) intranasally in one nostril
Patient weight ≥50 kg: **Desmopressin acetate** 2 sprays (300 mcg) intranasally; 1 spray in each nostril
Administer **desmopressin acetate nasal spray** before the procedure, and repeat every 12–24 hours for 2–4 doses
Note: Tachyphylaxis with serious hyponatremia can occur with repeated doses. If possible, limit use to 1 dose daily to avoid tachyphylaxis

Subcutaneous administration*
Test dose:
1. Measure factor VIII levels before the infusion
2. **Desmopressin acetate** 0.2–0.3 mcg/kg (not to exceed 20 mcg) subcutaneously
3. Measure factor VIII levels 1 hour and 4 hours after administration. Expect a 2- to 5-fold increase in factor VIII levels, persisting for 6–12 hours

Therapeutic dose:
Desmopressin acetate 0.2–0.3 mcg/kg (not to exceed 20 mcg) subcutaneously
Note: Tachyphylaxis with serious hyponatremia can occur with repeated doses. If possible, limit use to 1 dose daily to avoid tachyphylaxis. If administering more than four doses monitor daily serum sodium levels and measure VWF levels

*Used infrequently

Indications

1. Synthetic analogue of vasopressin that indirectly releases factor VIII/VWF from endothelial cell storage sites
2. Desmopressin acetate is useful in patients with mild hemophilia,who have been shown through pretesting to be responsive to its infusion

Efficacy

On the basis of three small studies, a rise in factor VIII coagulant activity to more than 3 times baseline and normal hemostasis is seen in 80% of patients

de la Fuente B et al. Ann Intern Med 1985;103:6–14
Saulnier J et al. Oral Surg Oral Med Oral Pathol 1994;77:6–12
Warrier AL, Lusher JM. J Pediatr 1983;102:228–233

Toxicity

Usually well tolerated, desmopressin acetate has the advantage of posing no risk of transmitting blood-borne viruses
1. *Vasodilatation with associated flushing:* Occasional
2. *Headache:* Usually transient and probably dose-related, and may resolve with dose reduction
3. *Tingling:* Occasional
4. *Hypotension:* Uncommon and usually mild
5. *Hypertension*: Uncommon and usually mild
6. *Tachycardia*: Uncommon
7. *Volume overload:* Uncommon
8. *Hyponatremia:* Due to ADH

Note: Tachyphylaxis with serious hyponatremia can occur with repeated doses if desmopressin acetate is administered over a prolonged period:
1. Limit doses to once daily
2. Restrict water intake
3. Monitor daily serum sodium levels

Notes

1. A trial of desmopressin acetate at the time of diagnosis assesses the individual's response pattern
2. Once the test dose is known to be successful, desmopressin acetate can be used without further therapeutic trials
3. Adults should be advised to limit fluid intake to 1 liter in the 24 hours after desmopressin acetate

REGIMEN FOR ANTIFIBRINOLYTIC THERAPY

ANTIFIBRINOLYTIC AGENT
(EPSILON-AMINOCAPROIC ACID, EACA)
AMICAR®

Manucci PM. NEJM 1998;339:245–253
Manucci PM. Blood 2001;97:1915–1919
Amicar® product label, October 2001

Epsilon aminocaproic acid 50 mg/kg orally* every 6 hours for 7–10 days (maximum dose: 24 g per 24 hours) after dental surgery or extraction

*A liquid preparation is available and a mouthwash can be prepared

Aminocaproic acid is available in the United States as tablets containing 500 mg or 1000 mg aminocaproic acid, as a syrup and solution for oral use containing 250 mg aminocaproic acid/mL, and as an injectable product containing 250 mg aminocaproic acid/mL

Indications

1. As an antifibrinolytic agent that is often used along with factor VIII products for invasive dental work or for the treatment of mouth bleeds
2. Not recommended for treatment of most internal hemorrhages

Efficacy

In small case studies in which aminocaproic acid is given after factor VIII replacement in patients undergoing dental extractions, hemostasis was excellent in 90% of cases and good in 10%. In the studies in which aminocaproic acid is given alone in patients undergoing dental extractions, only 8% required subsequent factor replacement

Cooksey MW et al. Br Med J 1966;2:1633–1634
Djulbegovic B et al. Am J Hematol 1996;51:168–170
Reid WO et al. Am J Med Sci 1964;248:184–188
Stajcic Z. Int J Oral Surg 1985;14:339–345

Toxicity

1. Nausea: Common
2. Vomiting: Common
3. Abdominal pain: Occasional
4. Diarrhea: Occasional
5. Thrombotic complications: Rare
6. Dry ejaculation has been reported in hemophilia patients who received the drug after undergoing dental surgical procedures. This symptom resolved in all patients within 24–48 hours after completion of therapy

Notes

1. Aminocaproic acid should not be administered to a patient with evidence of an active intravascular clotting process or hematuria of upper urinary tract origin or when taken at the same time as factor IX complex concentrates or anti-inhibitor coagulant concentrates
2. Contraindicated in patients with bleeding from the upper urinary tract because dots that do not lyse may cause ureteral obstruction
3. Use intermittently since long-term use may lead to thrombosis
4. The agent's safety and effectiveness in pediatric patients have not been established

REGIMEN

TOPICAL AGENTS; PLATELET CONCENTRATES

Clinical Practice Guidelines. Hemophilia and von Willebrand's Disease: Management (edition 2, update 2 [1999-07-07])

Topical thrombin and fibrin sealants are useful for the control of localized accessible bleeding from lacerated tissues or after dental extractions **Bovine thrombin powder** reconstituted to a concentration of 100 units/mL using 0.9% NaCl injection (0.9% NS) or sterile water can be applied directly or on a gelatin sponge, especially after oral surgery. Side effects are rare and include allergic or anaphylactic reactions

Platelet concentrates are not used in hemophilia except in the rare patient with a high titer inhibitor who is bleeding and does not respond to factor concentrates, rituximab, desmopressin acetate, or other interventions

Special Therapeutic Approaches
[Any approved factor VIII product concentrate can be used]

DENTAL PROCEDURE

Considerations before dental procedure:

1. Routine examinations and cleaning generally can be performed without raising the factor VIII level
2. Adequate coverage (ie, factor VIII concentrate and/or antifibrinolytic therapy) should be given before and possibly after the dental appointment in patients who need the following:
   - Deep cleaning or scaling because of heavy plaque and/or calculus accumulation in which bleeding would be induced
   - Block local anesthesia or mandibular block
   - Dental extractions, especially multiple or other surgical procedures

Suggested therapy:

1. Multiple dental extractions or other surgery:
   - *Loading dose:* Calculate the units of **factor VIII** needed to raise the level to ≈50% in plasma. Factor VIII preparations should be reconstituted according to the manufacturer's instructions. The loading dose should be dissolved in sterile water or according to the manufacturer's instructions and administered over a period of ≤5 minutes (maximum infusion rate 10 mL/min) 1 hour before dental extraction or other surgery
   - *Maintenance dose:* Further administration of **factor VIII** is usually not required, but can be repeated every 12 hours if bleeding recurs. Factor VIII preparations should be dissolved in sterile water or according to the manufacturer's instructions and administered over a period of ≤5 minutes (maximum infusion rate 10 mL/min)
2. When surgery is performed, in addition to factor VIII:
   - *Initial dose:* Aminocaproic acid 3000 mg orally 4–6 hours after the dental procedure
   - *Maintenance dose:* Aminocaproic acid 50 mg/kg every 6 hours or 4 times per day for 7 days after dental work is completed

For additional information and indications, refer to Notes in Hemophilia A: Factor VIII Replacement

Brewer AK et al. Haemophilia 2003;9:673–677
Kasper CK. Hemophilia of Georgia, USA. Haemophilia 2000;6(suppl 1):84–93
Stajcic Z. Int J Oral Surg 1985; 14:339–345

ELECTIVE SURGERY

Considerations before surgery:

1. *Preadmission studies:* CBC, inhibitor screen
2. At least 1 week before procedure, notify the Blood Bank of approximate amount of factor VIII required
3. Notify special Hematology Department that frequent assays will be required during the week of surgery

Suggested therapy:

1. *Factor VIII bolus administration protocol:*
   - *Loading dose (approximately 2 hours before surgery):* Calculate the units of **factor VIII** needed to raise the level to ≈80–100% in plasma, dissolve in sterile water or according to the manufacturer's instructions, and administer over a period of ≤5 minutes (maximum infusion rate 10 mL/min)
   - *Maintenance dose:* Begin with approximately one-half the loading dose of **factor VIII**. Dissolve in sterile water or according to the manufacturer's instructions and administer over ≤5 minutes (maximum infusion rate 10 mL/min) every 12 hours. Adjust dose according to measured factor VIII levels to maintain factor VIII levels above 50% for the next 10–14 days or until general healing is complete. Factor VIII levels should be checked daily. Since the half-life of factor VIII is 8–12 hours, assays should be performed near the end of the 12-hour period
2. *Factor VIII continuous infusion administration protocol:*

   Rationale for adjusted continuous infusion is that a steady state, by avoiding the peaks and troughs in clotting factor levels seen with bolus injection regimens, may reduce the amount of concentrate used and be more convenient. However, dosing guidelines for continuous infusion of factor VIII are not currently established, and no products are currently licensed for this route of administration. Suggested protocol:
   - *Loading dose (approximately 2 hours before surgery):* **Factor VIII** 40–50 units/kg dissolved in sterile water or according to the manufacturer's instructions and administered intravenously per push

- *Maintenance dose (begin continuous infusion immediately after the loading dose):*
  - –**Factor VIII** 4 units/kg per hour intravenously as a continuous infusion. Dissolve factor VIII in 0.9% NaCl injection (0.9% NS). Mix an amount of factor VIII sufficient for infusion over 8 hours. Use a syringe pump with a microbore tubing
  - –One hour after the continuous infusion is started, obtain a factor VIII assay
  - –Ensure that the factor VIII level is ≥70% before sending to surgery
  - –Monitor with daily factor VIII assays
  - –Maintain factor VIII level >70% for the first 48 hours after surgery
  - –48 hours after surgery, decrease infusion to maintain a factor VIII level of 50–60%
  - –On postoperative day 5, discontinue the continuous infusion. The factor VIII level should be between 40% and 60% when infusion is discontinued
  - –When infusion is discontinued, begin intravenous bolus administration every 12 hours over a period of ≤5 minutes (maximum infusion rate: 10 mL/min) to keep levels between 40% and 60%. Continue for ≥5–7 days, depending on surgery (example: hip replacement in which physical therapy required)

Hay CR et al. Blood Coagul Fibrinolysis 1996;7(suppl 1):S15–19
Kasper CK et al. Hemophilia of Georgia, USA. Haemophilia 2000;6(suppl 1):84–93
Schulman S et al. Haemophilia 1999;5:96–100

MINOR INVASIVE PROCEDURE

Moderate or severe hemophilia A
Considerations before procedure:
Factor VIII concentrate should be infused to achieve a factor VIII level ≥50% before invasive diagnostic procedures such as lumbar puncture, arterial blood gas determinations, bronchoscopy with bushings or biopsy, colonoscopy with biopsy, upper gastrointestinal endoscopy, or cardiac catheterization
Suggested therapy:
Loading and maintenance doses: Calculate the units of **factor VIII** needed to raise the level to a value ≥50% in plasma, dissolve in sterile water or according to the manufacturer's instructions, and administer over ≤5 minutes (maximum infusion rate, 10 mL/min). The dose may be repeated 12 hours later if bleeding ensues

Mild hemophilia A
Considerations before procedure:
Desmopressin acetate can be given 60 minutes before the procedure to those who have been shown through pretesting to be responsive to its infusion
Suggested therapy:
Loading and maintenance doses: **Desmopressin acetate** 0.3 mcg/kg (not to exceed 20 mcg) intravenously in 50 mL 0.9% NS over 30 minutes. Infusion may be repeated every 12–24 hours for 2–4 doses

Kasper CK et al. Hemophilia of Georgia, USA. Haemophilia 2000;6(suppl 1):84–93
Manno CS, Larson P. Transfusion therapy for coagulation factor deficiencies. In: Hoffman R, Benz EJ Jr, Astil SJ et al, eds. Hematology: Basic Principles and Practice, 4th ed. Philadelphia: Elsevier Churchill Livingstone; 2005:2469–2480

MANAGEMENT OF A PATIENT WITH A FACTOR VIII INHIBITOR

1. Five to 10% of all patients with hemophilia A and 25–30% with severe hemophilia A have been reported to develop factor VIII inhibitor
2. Factor VIII inhibitors are IgG antibodies, predominantly of the IgG_4 subclass, which interfere with the interaction of factor VIII with its cofactors and activators. These inhibitors react slowly, and inactivation of factor VIII requires incubation with the inhibitor for 1–2 hours at 37°C. The laboratory diagnosis of a factor VIII inhibitor requires that an appropriate dilution of the patient's plasma, when mixed with normal plasma, neutralize only factor VIII and no other factor that influences the aPTT (eg, factors IX, X, XI, XII, prekallikrein)
3. Patients with hemophilia A at the highest risk for development of an inhibitor are those who have:
   - Severe hemophilia A and have received the greatest number of factor VIII concentrates
   - A noninversion gene rearrangement, especially those with large or multiple deletions
   - Positive family history for an inhibitor
   - African-American heritage
4. Some studies have suggested a higher incidence of an inhibitor with the use of recombinant products. However, the role of product type in the occurrence of an inhibitor is unresolved
5. *Assay for factor VIII inhibitors at regular intervals:* Every 3–6 months in children and annually in adults
6. Screening for an inhibitor should be done before any surgical intervention
7. Inhibitors may be:
   a. Low-response inhibitor:
      - Exposure to factor VIII produces little or no increase in inhibitor titer *or*
      - The presenting titer is ≤5 Bethesda units (BU)

b. High-response inhibitor:
- Exposure to factor VIII is followed by a rapid increase in inhibitor titer (anamnestic response) *or*
- The presenting titer is >5 BU

8. Treatment of acute bleeding in a patient with a factor VIII inhibitor depends on:
   a. Whether the patient has a high-response or a low-response inhibitor
   b. The current inhibitor titer
   c. The severity of the hemorrhagic episode
9. Both recombinant and plasma-derived factor VIII products can be used in treatment

Lloyd JM et al Haemophilia 2003;9:464–520
Schaner I et al Haemophilia 1999;1:71–76

I. Bleeding in a patient with a low-response inhibitor

Suggested therapy: [Attaining a therapeutic plasma level ≥50% is recommended]

- *Loading dose*:

  Factor VIII 100 units/kg; dissolve in sterile water or according to the manufacturer's instructions and administer intravenously over ≤5 minutes (maximum infusion rate, 10 mL/min)
- *Maintenance dose:*

  Bolus administration: **Factor VIII** 50–100 units/kg; dissolve in sterile water or according to the manufacturer's instructions, and administer intravenously over ≤5 minutes (maximum infusion rate: 10 mL/min) every 8–12 hours for 5 days

  or

  Continuous infusion administration: **Factor VIII** 10 units/kg/hour intravenously in 0.9% NaCl injection (0.9% NS) as a continuous infusion for 5 days (see continuous infusion protocol under Elective Surgery section above)

  Note: The factor VIII dose should be high enough to saturate the inhibitor and increase the plasma factor VIII activity to hemostatic levels. With an inhibitor expressed in BU, the dose needed to saturate the inhibitor may be calculated according to the following formula:

$$\text{Units factor VIII} = \frac{2 \times \text{Body weight (kg)} \times [80 \times (100 - \text{hematocrit})]}{100 \times \text{Inhibitor titer (BU)}}$$

In addition to the factor VIII bolus or infusion regimens for the management of a low-response inhibitor, aminocaproic acid 50 mg/kg per dose can be administered orally every 6 hours for 3–10 days for patients with oral mucosal or dental bleeding

II. Bleeding in a patient with a high-response inhibitor

Suggested therapy:

1. *Factor VIIa bolus dose protocol*

- *Bolus dose*[a]*:* **Coagulation factor VIIa (recombinant)** (NovoSeven®; Novo Nordisk Pharmaceuticals, Inc.) 90 mcg/kg dissolve according to the manufacturer's instructions and administer intravenously as a slow bolus injection over 2–5 minutes
- *Additional bolus doses*[b]*:* **Coagulation factor VIIa (recombinant)** (NovoSeven®) 90 mcg/kg; dissolve according to the manufacturer's instructions, and administer intravenously as a slow bolus injection over 2–5 minutes every 2–3 hours for at least 3–4 doses or longer if continued bleeding

[a]Although evidence is accumulating that higher bolus doses of recombinant factor VIIa (>200 mcg/kg) may be more efficacious for the treatment of acute bleeding, further studies are needed to test this in a prospective manner and to clarify the frequency of thrombotic events (Abshire T, Kenet G. J Thromb Haemost 2004;2:899–909)

[b]Most patients who reported adverse experiences (ie, allergic reactions or thrombotic events) received more than 12 doses

or

2. *Factor VIIa bolus dose followed by continuous infusion protocol*

- *Bolus dose*:*

  Coagulation factor VIIa (recombinant) (NovoSeven®) 90–150 mcg/kg; dissolve according to the manufacturer's instructions, and administer intravenously as a slow-bolus injection >2–5 minutes
- *Continuous infusion*:*

  Coagulation factor VIIa (recombinant) (NovoSeven®); dissolve according to the manufacturer's instructions and administer intravenously as a continuous infusion of 20–50 mcg/kg per hour

*In studies evaluating a bolus dose followed by a continuous infusion administration, targeting factor VII levels to 30–40 units/mL in the immediate postoperative period is likely to provide a margin of safety sufficient to prevent bleeding. No thrombotic events were noted in those studies

Ludlam CA et al. Br J Haematol 2003;120:808–813
Santagostino E et al. Thromb Haemost 2001;86:954–958

or

3. *Anti-inhibitor coagulant complex (AICC):*
   - **Anti-inhibitor coagulant complex (AICC)** [(FEIBA® VH [Baxter Healthcare Corporation)] 50–100 units/kg; dissolve according to the manufacturer's instructions, and administer intravenously every 12 hours for 3–4 doses, as needed or longer if there is continued bleeding. AICC should be infused slowly, at a rate of approximately 2–3 mL/minute

   Note: If headache, flushing, changes in pulse rate, or changes in blood pressure appear to be infusion-related, the rate should be decreased. In such instances, it is advisable to initially stop the infusion until the symptoms disappear, then to resume at a slower rate

III. Immune tolerance induction after acute bleeding has been controlled in a patient with a factor VIII inhibitor

Although many regimens of immune tolerance induction have been described, no single protocol has been adopted as a standard for management of patients with factor VIII inhibitors. Regimens vary with respect to inclusion criteria, schedule of factor VIII administration, specific products used, and duration of treatment.

Examples of immune tolerance induction regimens include:

1. **Factor VIII** 50 units/kg; dissolve in sterile water or according to the manufacturer's instructions, and administer intravenously over ≤5 minutes (maximum infusion rate, 10 mL/min) daily until inhibitor resolves
2. **Factor VIII** 100–200 units/kg; dissolve in sterile water or according to the manufacturer's instructions and administer intravenously over ≤ 5 minutes (maximum infusion rate, 10 mL/min) daily until inhibitor level is <1 BU or the inhibitor resolves
3. **Factor VIII** 50 units/kg kg; dissolve in sterile water or according to the manufacturer's instructions, and administer intravenously over ≤5 minutes (maximum infusion rate, 10 mL/min) daily for 3–4 weeks. Then **factor VIII** 25 units/kg; dissolve in sterile water or according to the manufacturer's instructions, and administer intravenously over ≤5 minutes (maximum infusion rate, 10 mL/min) daily until inhibitor level is undetectable using Bethesda assay

Note: Because immune tolerance induction success is better with low-titer inhibitors, occasionally plasmapheresis plus immunoadsorption (if available) is used to acutely decrease a high-titer inhibitor to a low-titer inhibitor. This improves the success of clotting factors to reverse and facilitate initiation of immune tolerance induction

4. There have been anecdotal reports using **rituximab** to reduce the inhibitor titer and increase the factor VIII level. The **rituximab** dosage used has been 375 mg/m^2 over 3–4 hours weekly for 4 weeks

Success of immune tolerance induction is defined as:

1. Disappearance of the inhibitor (ie, undetectable using the Bethesda assay)
2. Normal factor VIII kinetics after administration, with factor VIII levels >66% of normal and half-life >6 hours [kinetic study should be carried out after a treatment free washout period ≥3 days]

If the criteria for success are met:

1. Treatment can be terminated by tapering the factor VIII dose by 10–50% every month
2. Subsequent treatment, if there is no inhibitor, can either be prophylaxis (ie, 20–40 units/kg 3 times weekly) or on-demand treatment

Note: Whenever possible, hemophilia patients with inhibitors should be enrolled in prospective, randomized, well-designed national or international studies

Ananyeua NM et al. Blood Coagul Fibrinolysis 2004;15:109–124
Dimichele D et al. Haemophilia 2004;10(suppl 4):140–145
Mariani G et al. Sem Thromb Hemost 2003;29:69–76
Rodriguez-Merchan EC, Rocino A. Haemophilia 2004;10(suppl 2:22–29
Rubinger M et al. Haemophilia 2000;6(suppl 1):52–59

IV. Surgery in a patient with a high-response inhibitor

Examples of surgical procedures:

1. *Minor procedures:* Arthrocentesis, endoscopy/colonoscopy, dental extractions
2. *Intermediate procedures*: Arthroscopy, removal of osteophytes or small cysts
3. *Major procedures*: Bone fixation for fractures, hip/knee replacement, arthrodeses (joint fusions), open synovectomy, pseudotumor removal, hardware removal (plates, intramedullary nails), neurosurgery (craniotomy), general surgery (eg, appendectomy, colectomy, gastrectomy)

Anti-inhibitory Coagulant Complex (AICC) [FEIBA® VH]

	Preoperative	Days 1–5	Days 6–14
Minor procedure	50–75 units/kg	50–75 units/kg every 12–24 hours for 1–2 doses	—
Intermediate procedure or major procedure	75–100 units/kg	75–100 units/kg every 8–12 hours	75–100 units/kg every 12 hours

Coagulation Factor VIIa (Recombinant) (Novo Seven®)

	Preoperative	Days 1–5	Days 6–14
Minor procedure	90–120 mcg/kg	90–120 mcg/kg every 2 hours up to 4 doses	—
Intermediate procedure or major procedure	120 mcg/kg Pediatric dose: 150 mcg/kg	90–120 mcg/kg *Day 1*: Every 2 hours *Day 2*: Every 3 hours *Days 3–5:* Every 4 hours	90–120 mcg/kg every 6 hours
Continuous infusion	15–50 mcg/kg per hour	15–50 mcg/kg per hour	15–50 mcg/kg per hour

Adapted, with permission, from Rodriguez-Merchan EC et al. Guidelines for management: *Haemophilia* 2004;10(suppl 2):50–52

OTHER MANAGEMENT ISSUES

1. **Immunizations:** Hepatitis A and hepatitis B vaccine series should be given to all newly diagnosed patients and to those indicating no exposure to either hepatitis A or hepatitis B. Family members involved in factor replacement therapy who test negative should also receive the series. Vaccines can be given subcutaneously in the thigh or deltoid area. Antibody to hepatitis B virus should be determined following the full immunization schedule

   Makris M et al. Haemophilia 2003;9:541–546

2. **Hepatitis C and HIV testing:** Hemophilia patients should be screened for hepatitis C and should undergo HIV testing
3. **Allergic reaction to factor VIII replacement products:** To avoid the possibility of reaction, use the filters included in factor packages. Antihistamines may be used to prevent or reduce symptoms: **Diphenhydramine** 25–50 mg intravenously or orally 15–20 minutes before the administration of factor VIII

   Note: Sometimes, changing factor brand may reduce symptoms

4. **Carrier detection and prenatal diagnosis**
   - Women who are carriers usually have factor VIII levels that are 50% of those of normal women, but occasionally they have levels <30% lower and may have excessive bleeding with trauma or surgery
   - A normal level of factor VIII activity does not exclude the carrier state
   - Carrier testing is unnecessary if the individual is an obligate carrier
   - A prenatal DNA-based diagnosis is possible by performing a chorionic villous biopsy at 9–11 weeks or an amniocentesis at 12–15 weeks' gestation and extracting the DNA from fetal cells

Cohen AJ, Kessler CM. Hemophilia A and B. In: Kitchens CS, Alving BM, Kessler, CM, eds. Consultative Hemostasis and Thrombosis. Philadelphia: WB Saunders, 2002
Goodeve AC. Haemophilia 1998;4:358–364

Hemophilia B

Hemophilia B is a congenital, X-linked, recessive bleeding disorder characterized by deficient factor IX or defective coagulant factor IX activity (factor IX level = factor IX coagulant activity)

Incidence: Estimated 1 of 25,000–30,000 male births

Classification: Mild hemophilia (factor IX coagulant activity ≥5–50%)
Moderate hemophilia (factor IX coagulant activity 2–4%)
Severe hemophilia (factor IX coagulant activity ≤1%)

Bolton-Maggs PHB, Pasi KJ. Lancet 2003;36:1801–1809
White GC II et al. Thromb Haemost 2001;85:560

Work-Up

1. *Elevated aPTT.* This is corrected by the addition of an equal volume of normal plasma. If the aPTT remains prolonged after the addition of an equal volume of normal plasma, then consider the presence of inhibitor to factor IX
2. Prothrombin time is usually normal but may be prolonged in some patients if ox-brain thromboplastin is used
3. A specific assay of factor IX levels is necessary for diagnosis

White GC II et al. Thromb Haemost 2001;85:560

Differential Diagnosis of Isolated Prolongation of aPTT

1. Heparin use
2. Factor VIII deficiency or inhibitor to factor VIII
3. vonWillebrand disease (especially the type II N VWD)
4. Factor IX deficiency or inhibitor to factor IX
5. Factor XI deficiency or inhibitor to factor XI
6. Factor XII deficiency or inhibitor to factor XII
7. Contact factor deficiency or inhibitor
8. Lupus anticoagulant

Treatment Options

1. Factor IX concentrates
2. Coagulation factor VIIa (recombinant): Factor IX inhibitors

REGIMEN FOR FACTOR IX REPLACEMENT

LOW-PURITY PLASMA-DERIVED HUMAN ANTIHEMOPHILIC FACTOR IX COMPLEX CONCENTRATES (FEIBA® VH, BEBULIN® VH, PROFILNINE® SD, AND PROPLEX® T)

Very-High-Purity Plasma-derived Human Coagulation Factor IX (ALPHANINE® SD or MONONINE®) Recombinant Ultrapure Coagulation Factor IX (BeneFix®)

National Hemophilia Foundation, MASAC (Medical and Scientific Advisory Council) recommendations concerning the treatment of hemophilia and other bleeding disorders. 2003; No. 141
Cohen AJ, Kessler CM. In: Kitchens CS, Alving BM, Kessler CM, eds. Consultative Hemostasis and Thrombosis. Philadelphia: WB Saunders 2002:43
Kasper CK. Haemophilia 2000;6(suppl 1):13–27
Kasper CK. Hemophilia of Georgia, USA. Haemophilia 2000;6(suppl 1):84–93
Srivastava A. Br J Haematol. 2004; 127:12–25

Factor IX Products*

Product Class	Examples	Advantage	Disadvantage
Low-purity antihemophilic factor IX complex concentrate	FEIBA® (Baxter Healthcare Corp) PROPLEX® T (Baxter)	Only advantage is for use in the treatment of patients with an inhibitor	Less pure, higher viral risk, prothrombotic
Monoclonal product very-high-purity plasma-derived human coagulation factor IX	MONONINE® (Aventis Behring L.L.C.) ALPHANINE® SD (Grifols Biologicals, Inc)	High purity	Not recombinant derived
Recombinant factor IX	BeneFix® (Baxter)	Recombinant, effective	Only recombinant product available; high cost per unit

*All currently available factor IX concentrates are treated to inactivate viruses

Administration Guidelines

Loading dose	Administer over a period of ≤5 minutes
Maintenance doses	Administer over a period of ≤5 minutes
Reconstitution	Reconstitute factor IX preparations according to the manufacturer's instructions

Indications

For control and prevention of bleeding episodes in patients with hemophilia B (congenital factor IX deficiency), including control and prevention of bleeding in surgical settings

Efficacy

More than 90% of success in controlling bleeding on an on-demand basis or for prevention of bleeding, including soft tissue or muscle bleed and hemarthroses

Toxicity

1. Phlebitis/cellulitis at IV site
2. Alteration of taste
3. Inhibitor formation (3–5% of patients)
4. *Hypersensitivity reactions (rare):* Urticaria, dyspnea, wheezing, hypotension, tachycardia, anaphylaxis
5. Thrombosis (rare)
6. Nausea (rare)
7. Nephrotic syndrome if used for immune tolerance

Notes

1. Previously untreated and minimally treated patients should receive the recombinant product (BeneFix®). If the recombinant product is not available, then a very-high-purity plasma-derived product can be used
2. Factor IX concentrates can also be given by continuous infusion in a similar manner as that described for factor VIII for those undergoing major surgery

Calculating the Amount of Factor IX Required

Initial dose

100% Plasma Factor IX = 1 Unit Factor IX/mL Plasma

Method 1: Use for plasma-derived factor IX concentrates
1 unit factor IX/kg → increases factor IX levels 1%
Amount of factor IX required = Wt (kg) × desired level (%)
Example: Weight = 70 kg. Amount of factor IX desired = 0.5 units/mL (50% plasma factor IX)
70 × 50 = 3500 units

Method 2: Use for Ultrapure Recombinate Factor IX (BeneFix®)
Amount of factor IX required = Wt (kg) × desired level (%) × (1.2)[a]
Example: Weight = 70 kg. Amount of factor IX desired = 0.5 units/mL (50% plasma factor IX)
70 × 50 × 1.2 = 4200 units

[a]The difference in volume of distribution between the recombinant and plasma-derived products is primarily caused by a difference in charge conferred by decreased or absent phosphorylation and sulfation at two sites

Maintenance dose
One-half the loading dose every 18–24 hours
[Biologic half-life of factor IX is ≈18–24 hours. Thus, at 18–24 hours the plasma factor IX level will decrease to one-half the initial level; infusion of one-half the initial dose restores the plasma factor IX to the initial level]

Treatment of Specific Types of Bleeding Episodes

Type of Hemorrhage	Dose	% Desired Level	Dose (units/kg)	Comments
Superficial laceration	None	None	None	Local pressure + apply adhesive skin closure products
Deep laceration	Single dose	40	40	Sutures after factor given
Joint	Single dose	40	40	A second infusion (10 units/kg) may be required in 24 hours if persistent pain and/or swelling persist *Adjunctive care:* ice, rest, and elevation Mobilize joint when pain subsides
Muscle (not iliopsoas)	Single dose	40	40	
Iliopsoas muscle	Initial bolus	60–80	60–80	Limit activity until pain resolves
	Maintenance	30–60	30–60	Every 18–24 hours for ≥3 days until pain or disability is resolved
CNS/head	Initial bolus	60–80	60–80	Consult Neurology/Neurosurgery
	Maintenance	30	30	For ≥10–14 days if still bleeding
Throat/neck	Initial bolus	60–80	60–80	
	Maintenance	30	30	Every 18–24 hours for ≥7–10 days if still bleeding
Gastrointestinal	Initial bolus	60–80	60–80	Treat origin of GI bleed as indicated
	Maintenance	30	30	Every 18–24 hours for ≥5–7 days if bleeding continues
Renal	Single dose	40	40	Order bed rest, IV hydration
Ophthalmic	Single dose	60–80	60–80	Obtain Ophthalmology consult
Surgery (major)	Initial bolus	60–80	60–80	
	Maintenance	30	30	Every 18–24 hours for 10–14 days depending on the type of surgery

Adapted, with permission, from Protocols for the treatment of hemophilia and von Willebrand disease. Hemophilia of Georgia USA. Hemophilia 2000;6(suppl 1):84–93.

INHIBITORS IN HEMOPHILIA B

1. The incidence of factor IX inhibitors in hemophilia B is much lower than that found with severe hemophilia A. The estimated incidence is 3–5% of patients with severe hemophilia B
2. Factor IX inhibitors are IgG antibodies, predominantly of the IgG_4 subclass (κ light chain) that interfere with the interaction of factor IX with its cofactors and activators. Most of these inhibitors can be detected when the aPTT on a mixture of normal and patient's plasma is prolonged. In contrast to the inhibitors in hemophilia A, patient's inhibitor antibodies against factor IX are not time-dependent nor temperature-dependent; thus, it is not necessary to incubate the mixture for 2 hours at 37°C. Inhibitors to factor IX can be quantified by modifying the Bethesda method for detecting factor VIII inhibitors
3. As in hemophilia A, inhibitors primarily form in patients with gene deletions, major rearrangements, or nonsense mutations and in those who have little or no endogenous factor IX. The lower incidence of inhibitors in hemophilia B may be related to a lower incidence of patients with such severe gene defects
4. In patients with active bleeding, antihemophilic factor IX complex concentrates products (eg, FEIBA® VH, PROPLEX® T) can be given, although these can lead to continued stimulation of antibody production. Thus, recombinant coagulation factor VIIa (NovoSeven®) is the treatment of choice, particularly in those with a history of anaphylaxis to infusion therapy. [See Management of a Patient with a Factor VIII Inhibitor: Bleeding in a patient with a high-response inhibitor in the Hemophilia A section]
5. Immune tolerance induction (ITI), similar to that described above for patients with factor VIII deficiency, can be attempted. However, this approach has been less successful than in patients with factor VIII inhibitors (70%)
6. ITI therapy may be associated with the development of nephrotic syndrome with chronic factor IX administration

Note: Whenever possible, patients with factor IX inhibitors should be enrolled in prospective, randomized well-designed, national or international studies

Djulbegovic B et al. Am J Hematol 1996;51:168–170
Kasper CK. Hemophilia of Georgia USA. Haemophilia 2000;6(suppl 1):84–93
Roth DA et al. Recombinant Factor IX Study Group. Blood 2001;98:3600–3006

58. The Hypercoagulable State

Jeffrey I. Zwicker, MD, and Kenneth A. Bauer, MD

Risk Factors for Venous Thromboembolism (VTE)

Acquired* Risk Factors	Inherited Risk Factors	Mixed Risk Factors
1. Malignancy-associated 2. Antiphospholipid antibody syndrome 3. Pregnancy-associated 4. Estrogen therapy 5. Immobilization 6. Trauma 7. Nephrotic syndrome 8. Heparin-induced thrombocytopenia 9. Myeloproliferative disorders 10. Paroxysmal nocturnal hemoglobinuria 11. Prolonged air travel 12. Major surgery	1. Antithrombin deficiency 2. Protein C deficiency 3. Protein S deficiency 4. Factor V Leiden mutation 5. Prothrombin G20210A mutation 6. Dysfibrinogenemia (rare)	1. Hyperhomocysteinemia 2. Elevated factor VIII 3. Activated protein C resistance in absence of factor V Leiden 4. Elevated factor IX 5. Elevated factor XI 6. Elevated TAFI (thrombin-activatable fibrinolysis inhibitor) 7. Low free TFPI (tissue factor pathway inhibitor) 8. Low plasma fibrinolytic activity

*Some acquired risk factors may be transient

Evaluation of a Patient After a VTE

Routine Evaluation

1. History and examination to identify acquired risk factors (see above). This should include obstetric history in women because recurrent second or third-trimester fetal loss may suggest antiphospholipid antibody syndrome or hereditary thrombophilia
2. Detailed family history with inquiry regarding female family members who have taken oral contraceptives or suffered any venous thrombotic events during pregnancy
3. CBC and peripheral smear to evaluate for underlying disease (eg, myeloproliferative disorder such as essential thrombocythemia or polycythemia vera, microangiopathic hemolysis)
4. Other laboratory tests as indicated including evaluation for heparin-induced thrombocytopenia
5. Extensive screening for malignancy not recommended. Perform age-appropriate screening as indicated. Lower threshold to search for malignancy based on symptoms or signs especially in older patients with a smoking history
6. Thrombophilia screen as outlined below for idiopathic deep vein thrombosis

Laboratory Evaluation for Idiopathic VTE

Classify patient in strongly thrombophilic or weakly thrombophilic category based on the following **risk factors:**

1. Deep vein thrombosis before age 50
2. Recurrent venous thrombosis
3. Family history of VTE (in first-degree relatives)

Laboratory Testing Based on Risk Group

Strongly Thrombophilic (≥1 of the above risk factors)	Weakly Thrombophilic
1. Anticardiolipin antibodies 2. Lupus anticoagulant 3. Homocysteine 4. Factor V Leiden 5. Prothrombin G20210A mutation 6. Protein C deficiency 7. Protein S deficiency 8. Antithrombin deficiency	1. Anticardiolipin antibodies 2. Lupus anticoagulant 3. Homocysteine 4. Factor V Leiden 5. Prothrombin G20210A mutation

Laboratory Evaluation for Recurrent Arterial Thrombosis

1. Only the presence of a lupus anticoagulant/elevated cardiolipin antibody levels and hyperhomocysteinemia are risk factors for *arterial thrombosis;* the hereditary thrombophilias are not risk factors
2. Consider other disease states, including paroxysmal nocturnal hemoglobinuria, heparin-induced thrombocytopenia, occult malignancy, myeloproliferative disorders, and cocaine abuse

Acquired Risk Factors

1. Malignancy-Associated Thrombosis

General:

1. Accounts for approximately 20% of all cases of VTE
2. In some prospective studies the incidence of malignancy in the first year after diagnosis of an idiopathic VTE is >7%. However, trials have not demonstrated improved patient outcomes and cost-effectiveness of extensive screening beyond age-appropriate or symptom-directed cancer screening

Pathogenesis:

1. Etiology not clearly established
2. May be related to tissue factor elaborated by tumor cells

Management of thrombosis:

1. *Acute thrombosis:* **Heparin or low molecular weight heparin (LMWH)**
2. *Long-term therapy:* Patients with cancer have a higher risk of recurrence than individuals who suffer an unprovoked VTE in the absence of cancer. Anticoagulate a minimum of 6 months and as long as the malignancy is active. Chronic anticoagulation can be considered with **low molecular weight heparin (LMWH)** owing to high recurrence rate and potential for increased bleeding complications with anticoagulation with warfarin. In a randomized trial comparing LMWH (dalteparin) with warfarin, recurrence at 6 months was 17% in warfarin treated patients compared with 8% in the dalteparin group ($P = .0017$), although there was no significant difference in major bleeding rates

Lee AYY et al. NEJM 2003;349:146–153
Prandoni P et al. NEJM 1992;327:1128–1133

2. Antiphospholipid Antibody Syndrome

General:

1. A clinical diagnosis characterized by a thrombotic event (venous or arterial thrombosis or recurrent fetal loss) in association with a persistent lupus anticoagulant (LA) in specialized coagulation assays and/or persistently elevated titers of cardiolipin antibodies (IgG and IgM)
2. LAs are rarely associated with bleeding, but confer an increased risk for recurrent thrombosis
3. Clinical manifestations include thrombocytopenia, recurrent fetal loss, and arterial or venous thrombosis

Pathogenesis:

1. LAs result from antibodies that bind to phospholipids and plasma proteins (β_2-glycoprotein I, prothrombin) in vitro and prolong clotting times (critically dependent on the amount of phospholipid in assay)
2. LAs are often associated with:
   a. Systemic lupus erythematosus
   b. Drugs (usually not prothrombotic)
   c. Cancer
   d. Idiopathic
   e. Infections (often transient)

Management of thrombosis:

1. *Acute thrombosis:* **Unfractionated heparin or low molecular weight heparin (LMWH)**
2. *Long-term therapy:* **Warfarin** administered orally. Retrospective studies suggested that patients with antiphospholipid antibody syndrome required a target INR >3 to obtain adequate antithrombotic protection. However, subsequent prospective studies showed that an INR = 2–3 is adequate in patients with venous thrombosis

Crowther MA et al. NEJM 2003;349:1133–1138
Finazzi G et al. J Thromb Haemost 2005;3:848–853

3. Pregnancy-Associated Thrombosis

General:

1. Thrombosis is leading cause of maternal mortality in developed countries
2. The risk of thrombosis increases 5–6 times during pregnancy and the increased risk persists up to 8 weeks postpartum
3. Most (80%) of DVTs are located in the left leg due to iliac vein compression by the right iliac artery

Management (antepartum):

Warfarin is absolutely contraindicated between the 6th and 12th weeks of pregnancy when risk of warfarin embryopathy is greatest

1. *Acute thrombosis:* **Unfractionated heparin or low molecular weight heparin (LMWH)**
   - LMWH preferred for long-term anticoagulation over unfractionated heparin because of increased bioavailability and a lower incidence of osteoporosis and heparin-induced thrombocytopenia
   - When therapeutic doses are used, monitor anti-Xa levels monthly to adjust for pregnancy-associated weight changes
2. *Prophylaxis:* See **Anticoagulant prophylaxis during pregnancy** below

Management (peripartum):

Prepartum:

- Discontinue LMWH at least 24 hours before delivery to minimize bleeding risks associated with epidural anesthesia and delivery
- The decision to bridge with unfractionated heparin should be based on perceived risk of thrombosis during the time off anticoagulation
- Unfractionated heparin should be administered *if:*
  –The time interval from the episode of thrombosis has been <1 month
  –Additional prothrombotic risk factors exist or the patient is otherwise perceived as having a high risk of thrombosis
- Discontinue unfractionated heparin 4–6 hours before delivery (usually at the start of labor) to allow for normalization of aPTT

Management (postpartum):

1. Barring any bleeding complications, therapeutic anticoagulation can usually be resumed 12–18 hours after a vaginal delivery and 24 hours after cesarean section delivery

Restarting Anticoagulation Postpartum

	Vaginal Delivery	Cesarean Delivery
Prophylactic dosing	6 hours	12 hours
Therapeutic dosing	12 hours	24 hours

2. **Warfarin or LMWH,** depending on patient preference
   - Anticoagulation is recommended for at least 6 weeks postpartum (minimum 3–6 months in total after diagnosis of VTE)

Anticoagulant prophylaxis during pregnancy:

1. In women with a history of thrombosis associated with a transient risk factor, anticoagulant prophylaxis is generally not required antepartum due to low rate of recurrent thrombosis. However, short-term anticoagulation for 6–8 weeks postpartum should be considered
2. In women with history of thrombosis and a hereditary thrombophilic disorder (see below), the risk of recurrence without anticoagulation appears to be higher and anticoagulation antepartum is justified. However, the intensity of anticoagulation—therapeutic versus prophylactic—has not been established and should be based on perceived risk of thrombosis. During the postpartum period, therapeutic anticoagulation should be administered for 6–8 weeks
3. The management of asymptomatic carriers of hereditary thrombophilias is controversial. Considering that the estimated risk of thrombosis in women with the prothrombin G20210A mutation or factor V Leiden mutation is only 0.2–0.5% during pregnancy, prophylactic anticoagulation antepartum is generally not recommended. During the postpartum period, therapeutic anticoagulation can be administered for 6–8 weeks
4. In recurrent adverse pregnancy outcomes, some evidence suggests that hereditary thrombophilia, is a risk factor for recurrent fetal loss and that prophylactic LMWH may result in improved pregnancy outcomes. Additional studies are required

Brill-Edwards P et al. NEJM 2000;343:1439–1344
Dudding TE, Attia J. Thromb Haemost 2004;91:700–711
Gerhardt A et al. NEJM 2000;342:374–380
Gris J-C et al. Blood 2004;103:3695–3699

Inherited Risk Factors

Prevalence of Defects in Patients with Idiopathic VTE

Hereditary Thrombophilia	General Population	Outpatients with DVT	Relative Risk of Thrombosis (CI)	
Antithrombin Type I Type II	 1 in 2000 1 in 600	1.1%	5.0	(0.7–34)
Protein C deficiency	0.2–0.5%	4%	3.8	(1.3–10)
Protein S deficiency	Unknown	1–7%	2.4	(0.8–7.9)
Factor V Leiden	5–6%	21%	6.6	(3.6–12.0)
Prothrombin G20210A	2%	6%	2.8	(1.4–5.6)
Hyperhomocysteinemia (≥95th percentile)	5%	10%	2.5	(1.8–3.5)
Elevated factor XI (≥90th percentile)	10%	19%	2.2	(1.5–3.2)
Elevated factor VIII (≥90th percentile)	10%	25%	4.8	(2.3–10)

Adapted from Bauer KA, Zwicker JI. Natural anticoagulants and the prethrombotic state. In: Handin RI, Lux SE, Stossel TP, eds. Blood: Principles and Practice of Hematology, 2nd ed. Philadelphia: Lippincott Williams & Wilkins, 2003:1307

1. Antithrombin Deficiency

General:
Synthesized in liver and neutralizes thrombin, factors IXa, Xa, XIa, XIIa
Diagnostic assays:
Antithrombin–heparin cofactor assay to measure factor Xa inhibition (preferred); antithrombin antigen
Types of deficiency states:
1. Quantitative deficiency
2. Functional deficiency—reactive center or heparin-binding site defect

Acquired antithrombin deficiency:
1. DIC
2. Sepsis
3. Liver disease
4. Nephrotic syndrome
5. Occasionally acute thrombosis
6. Heparin therapy

Management:
1. *Acute thrombosis:* **Heparin, LMWH, rarely antithrombin concentrate with either heparin or LMWH**
   - **Heparin or LMWH.** Higher doses may be required to achieve a therapeutic aPTT. Most individuals can be successfully treated with heparin or LMWH without the addition of antithrombin concentrate
   - **Antithrombin (human) concentrate** can be used to normalize antithrombin levels in chronically anticoagulated patients in special situations that present an unacceptably high risk of bleeding with concomitant anticoagulant use, such as neurosurgery, trauma, and obstetric intervention
   - **Antithrombin (human) concentrate with either heparin or low molecular weight heparin (LMWH),** in cases of extensive or life-threatening thrombosis
2. *Asymptomatic carriers:* Anticoagulation is not routinely recommended except in high-risk situations such as surgery and possibly pregnancy. Based on familial penetrance of VTE, long-term prophylactic anticoagulation can be considered

2. Protein C Deficiency

General:
Protein C: A vitamin K-dependent protein synthesized in the liver that exerts anticoagulant activity after activation by thrombin
Diagnostic assays:
1. Protac® (Technoclone GmbH; Vienna, Austria) direct activation of protein C anticoagulant assay
2. Protac® amidolytic assay to measure active site activity
3. Protein C antigen

Types of deficiency states:
1. Quantitative deficiency
2. Functional deficiency—based on abnormal amidolytic or anticoagulant activity

Acquired protein C deficiency:
1. Warfarin
2. Liver disease
3. DIC
4. Sepsis
5. Occasionally acute thrombosis

Management:
1. *Acute thrombosis:* **Heparin, LMWH, or warfarin**

   Warfarin can be used but precaution is necessary with the initiation of warfarin due to rare occurrence of warfarin-induced skin necrosis. Keep patient fully anticoagulated with heparin when starting warfarin. The initial dose should be fairly low (2 mg for 3 days) with 2- to 3-mg increments until a therapeutic INR is achieved
2. *Asymptomatic carriers:* anticoagulation not routinely recommended except in high risk situations such as surgery

Griffin et al. J Clin Invest 1981;68:1370–1373

3. Protein S Deficiency

General:
Protein S: A vitamin K-dependent protein that enhances the anticoagulant effect of activated protein C

Diagnostic assays:
1. APC anticoagulant assay
2. Total and free protein S antigen quantification

Types of deficiency states:

	Total Protein S	Free Protein S	Protein S Activity
I	↓	↓	↓
II	↔	←	↓
III	↔	↓	↓

Acquired protein S deficiency:
1. Warfarin
2. Pregnancy (>1st trimester)
3. Oral contraception, DIC
4. Acute thrombosis
5. Liver disease
6. Inflammatory disorders

Management:
Standard therapy with **heparin and warfarin**

Comp PC, Esmon CT. NEJM 1984;311:1525–1528
Schwarz HP et al. Blood 1984;64:1297–1300

4. Factor V Leiden

General:
Arginine-506 to glutamine substitution renders factor Va relatively resistant to activated protein C

Diagnostic assays:
1. Genotyping or
2. Activated protein C (APC) resistance assay with confirmation by genotyping

Acquired factor V Leiden mutations:
None

Management:
1. *Acute thrombosis:* Standard therapy with **heparin and warfarin**
2. *Asymptomatic carriers:*
   - 5% of white population are carriers of the mutation, but it is not found among native Asian and African populations
   - Chronic anticoagulation without thrombosis is not recommended
   - Prophylactic measures should be considered during high-risk situations such as major surgery or trauma
   - Oral contraceptives containing estrogen are not recommended due to a 30-fold increased risk of thrombosis in asymptomatic carriers
   - Large-scale population screening for factor V Leiden is not cost-effective (approximately 8000 women would need to be screened to prevent a single DVT)

Bertina RM et al. Nature 1994;369:64–67
Dahlback B et al. Proc Natl Acad Sci USA 1993;90:1004–1008

5. Prothrombin G20210A Mutation

General:
Mutation at position 20210 in the 3′-untranslated region of prothrombin leads to increased efficiency of prothrombin biosynthesis without affecting the rate of transcription
Diagnostic assay:
Genotyping
Acquired prothrombin G20210A mutations:
None
Management:
1. *Acute thrombosis:* Standard therapy with **heparin and warfarin**
2. *Asymptomatic carriers:*
   - About 2% of the white population are carriers of the mutation but it is not found among native Asian and African populations
   - Chronic anticoagulation for asymptomatic carriers not recommended (see Factor V Leiden above)

Poort SR et al. Blood 1996;88:3698–3703

Mixed Risk Factors

1. Hyperhomocysteinemia

General:
Sulfur-containing amino acid involved in formation of other amino acids. Elevated levels can be due to a variety of factors, including hereditary (homozygosity for MTHFR C677T or cystathionine β-synthase 844ins68 mutations) and acquired conditions
Diagnostic assay:
1. Fasting homocysteine levels
2. Although MTHFR C677T or cystathionine β-synthase 844ins68 mutations are associated with higher homocysteine levels, testing for these mutations is not recommended

Acquired deficiencies:
1. Folate deficiency
2. Vitamin B_{12} deficiency
3. B_6 deficiency
4. Medications (eg, methotrexate, trimethoprim, cholestyramine, carbamazepine)
5. Alcohol
6. Liver failure
7. Renal failure

Management issues:
1. *Acute thrombosis*: Standard therapy with **heparin and warfarin**
2. *Asymptomatic carriers:* Lower homocysteine levels. Vitamin supplementation with low doses of folate (or replacement of B_{12} or B_6 vitamins if deficient) can substantially lower homocysteine; however, it is unclear whether lowering homocysteine translates into lower thrombosis rates

den Heijer M et al. Thromb Haemost 1998;80:874–877

Treatment of Thrombotic Events

The Seventh ACCP Conference on Antithrombotic and Thrombolytic Therapy. Buller HR et al. Chest 2004;126(3):401S–428S

Acute Treatment of Acute Thrombosis

1. Initial management not generally affected by the presence of hereditary risk factors
2. Unfractionated or low molecular weight heparin for at least 5 days
3. Unfractionated heparin should be administered in adequate dosage because failure to reach a therapeutic level of anticoagulation within the first 24 hours increases the risk for recurrence
4. Weight-based dosing for unfractionated heparin with an intravenously administered loading dose, followed by a continuous intravenous infusion
5. Warfarin can be started on day 1 with target INR = 2.0–3.0. Standard starting dose is 5–10 mg daily

Long-Term Therapy following an Acute Thrombosis: Balancing Risk of Recurrence Against Risk of Prolonged Anticoagulation

Risk of recurrence

1. Following an idiopathic event after discontinuing 3–12 months of anticoagulation: ~5–15% in the first year (25% at 5 years; 30% at 8 years)
2. After a provoked event such as surgery, pregnancy, or oral contraception, the rate of recurrence is lower (Christiansen SC et al. JAMA 2005;293:2352–2361; Baglin et al. Lancet 2003;262:523–266)
3. Generally considered higher in the following situations: (fold increased risk of recurrence in parentheses)
   - Malignancy (~3 ×)
   - Antiphospholipid antibody syndrome (~2 ×)
   - Compound heterozygosity for factor V Leiden and prothrombin G20210A mutations (~2.5 ×)
   - Homozygosity for factor V Leiden or prothrombin G20210A mutations (~2 ×)
   - Selected kindreds with strong clinical penetrance for antithrombin, protein C, or protein S deficiency
   - The presence of two or more prothrombotic risk factors (eg, factor V Leiden and protein C deficiency)

(Prandoni P et al. Blood 2002;100:3484–3488; and The Procare Group. Blood Coagul Fibrinolysis 2000;11:511–518)

4. Not increased in heterozygosity for factor V Leiden or prothrombin G20210A mutation alone

De Stefano V et al. NEJM 1999;341:801–806
Heit JA et al. Arch Intern Med 2000;160:761–768
Prandoni P et al. Ann Intern Med 1996;125:1–7

Bleeding risk with prolonged oral anticoagulation

1. Rate of major bleed is ~2% per year with a 0.4% per year fatality rate
2. The risk of bleeding is greater in patients with a history of GI bleeding, renal or liver failure, diabetes, or uncontrolled hypertension, or in those with advanced age (>75 years)

Beyth RJ et al. Am J Med 1998;105:91–99
Fitzmaurice DA et al. Br Med J 2002;325:828–831
Palareti G et al. Lancet 1996;348:423–428

Long-Term Therapy: Indications and Guidelines

Indications	Duration/Intensity of Therapy
Provoked first event with reversible or time-limited risk factor (eg, pregnancy, surgery)	3–6 months. Target INR = 2.0–3.0
Idiopathic (unprovoked) VTE, first event	6 months. Target INR = 2.0–3.0 After 6 months, consider indefinite anticoagulation
• Recurrent idiopathic VTE • High recurrence rate situations (eg, combined hereditary defects) • After a life-threatening pulmonary embolism • Thrombosis at unusual sites (eg, cerebral, mesenteric, or hepatic vein thrombosis) • Active malignancy	Indefinite anticoagulation Target INR = 2.0–3.0 (see below) Consider low molecular weight heparin (Malignancy-associated)

The Seventh ACCP Conference on Antithrombotic and Thrombolytic Therapy. Buller HR et al. Chest 2004;126(3):401S–428S; and Lee AYY et al. NEJM 2003;349:146–153

Notes: Duration and intensity of long-term therapy
Recent randomized trials evaluating strategies to prevent recurrent events after an initial idiopathic VTE have demonstrated:
- Efficacy of longer-duration therapy
- Lower intensity better than placebo but inferior to higher target INR anticoagulation after therapeutic anticoagulation for 3–6 months

	PREVENT Trial		ELATE Trial	
	Placebo	INR 1.5–2.0	INR 1.5–1.9	INR 2.0–3.0
Recurrence	7.2%	2.6%	1.9%	0.7%
Major bleed	0.4%	0.9%	1.1%	0.9%

Kearon C et al. NEJM 1999;340:901–907
Ridker P et al. NEJM 2003;348:1425–1434

Therapeutic Options For Venous Thromboembolic Events (VTE)

REGIMEN

UNFRACTIONATED HEPARIN SODIUM

Hirsh J et al. Circulation 2001;103:2994–3018

Intravenous (unfractionated) heparin sodium
Loading dose:
Heparin sodium 80 units/kg by intravenous push, *followed by:*
Maintenance dose:
Heparin sodium, begin with 18 units/kg per hour by continuous intravenous infusion diluted in a convenient volume of 0.9% NaCl injection (0.9% NS) or 5% dextrose injection (D5W)

Weight-Based Normogram for Intravenous Heparin Administration

aPPT	Bolus	Maintenance Dosing*
<1.2 × control	40 units/kg	Decrease infusion by 4 units/kg/hour
1.2–1.5 × control	20 units/kg	Decrease infusion by 2 units/kg/hour
1.5–2.3 × control	No bolus	No change in maintenance dose
2.3—3 × control	No change	Increase infusion rate by 2 units/kg/hour
>3 × control	Hold infusion for 1 hour	Increase infusion rate by 4 units/kg/hour

*Begin with 18 units/kg per hour by continuous intravenous infusion

Check aPTT every 6 hours until therapeutic range (1.5–2.5 × aPTT control) is sustained. When therapeutic range is achieved, check aPTT for 2 consecutive measurements six hours apart; then check aPPT every 24 hours

Note: Prepare heparin infusions in a standardized concentration that facilitates converting administration rates of "units/hour" to volume/time (mL/h)"; for example, heparin sodium 25,000 units in 250 mL 0.9% NS produces a concentration of 100 units/mL

Note: Intravenous (unfractionated) heparin sodium should not be used with patients who have baseline abnormal aPTT

Monitoring Therapy

Check aPTT 6 hours after starting continuous intravenous infusion and after each change in rate of administration. Maintain aPTT 1.5–2.5 × the upper limit of normal

Treatment Modifications

Adverse Event	Dose Modification
Heparin-induced thrombocytopenia (see Chapter 59)	Discontinue all heparin (including flushes). If not otherwise contraindicated, initiate therapy with direct thrombin inhibitor even with no heparin-induced thrombocytopenia
Life-threatening bleeding	Discontinue heparin

Adverse Effects

1. HIT: 1–3% of patients receiving unfractionated heparin for >1 week. (See Chapter 59)
2. Non–immune-mediated, heparin-associated thrombocytopenia (HAT): 1–30%
    - Results from temporary platelet aggregation, margination, and peripheral sequestration
    - Decreased platelet count usually mild and transient
    - Onset typically 2–4 days after start of heparin
    - Thrombocytopenia resolves despite continuing heparin administration
3. Osteopenia/osteoporosis
4. Hypoaldosteronism/hyperkalemia: 7–8% of patients
5. Increased serum free T_4 and T_3 with normal TSH
6. Increased hepatic AST and ALT
7. Increased serum triglycerides
8. Hypersensitivity reactions (rarely), including vasospasm, cutaneous effects around the injection site, conjunctivitis
9. Fever

REGIMEN: LOW MOLECULAR WEIGHT HEPARINS (LMWHs)

ENOXAPARIN SODIUM, TINZAPARIN SODIUM

Caution:

- Doses for LMWHs or unfractionated heparin cannot be used interchangeably
- Do not use any LMWH in a patient with heparin-induced thrombocytopenia

Enoxaparin sodium 1 mg/kg twice daily or 1.5 mg/kg once daily subcutaneously *only*

Tinzaparin sodium 175 anti-Xa units/kg once daily subcutaneously *only*

Toxicity

1. Increased risk of bleeding in patients who use drugs that may affect hemostasis and in those with comorbid pathologies that predispose to hemorrhage
2. Thrombocytopenia*

Incidence of HIT is less than with unfractionated heparin

Platelet Count	Incidence	LMWH Implicated
50,000–100,000/mm^3	1.3%	Enoxaparin
	1%	Tinzaparin
<50,000/mm^3	0.1%	Enoxaparin
	0.13%	Tinzaparin

*Discontinue LMWH if a platelet count decreases to <100,000/mm^3

3. Pain at injection sites/injection site hematoma
4. Reversible increase in AST, ALT + alkaline phosphatase, LDH, and CK
5. Decreases in bone mineral density and osteoporosis (but less frequent than with unfractionated heparin)
6. Other toxicities:

Enoxaparin

- Hyperkalemia
- Delayed hypersensitivity reactions
- Cutaneous necrosis and fat necrosis
- Thrombocytosis, rarely

Tinzaparin

- Increased serum free T_4 and T_3 with normal TSH
- Angioedema and allergic purpura
- Cutaneous necrosis and rashes
- Priapism, rarely

Treatment Modifications

There is cumulative anti-factor Xa activity of LMWH in patients with renal impairment, which can increase the bleeding complications of therapy. In patients with severe renal failure, anticoagulation with unfractionated heparin is recommended. If LMWH is selected, close monitoring of anti-Xa activity is recommended

Renal Impairment	
Enoxaparin Creatinine clearance <30 mL/min	Administer 1 mg/kg once daily subcutaneously
Tinzaparin Creatinine clearance (Clcr) <30 mL/min	No specific recommendation to alter tinzaparin dose or schedule

Monitoring Therapy

In most patients, no monitoring is necessary. In some circumstances such as pregnancy, renal dysfunction, obesity, and long-term therapy, a dose adjustment may be necessary. For twice-daily administration, target therapeutic range is between 0.6 and 1.0 units/mL 3–4 hours after subcutaneous dose, but for once-daily dose the target range is less well established (usually between 1.0 and 2.0 units/mL)

Notes

Advantages of LMWHs over unfractionated heparin:

1. Increased bioavailability
2. Lower incidence of osteoporosis
3. Lower incidence of heparin-induced thrombocytopenia

REGIMEN

WARFARIN SODIUM

Warfarin sodium orally once daily continually to maintain an INR of 2–3

Initiate therapy with an oral dose of 5–10 mg/day in the evening and increase dose in increments of 1–2 mg/day guided by laboratory values

Warfarin is available in the United States in many generic formulations for oral administration, including immediate-release tablets containing 1, 2, 2.5, 3, 4, 5, 7.5, and 10 mg warfarin sodium/tablet

Monitoring Therapy

Monitor INR initially 2 times per week. When stabilized, gradually reduce frequency to once per week

Adverse Effects

1. Hemorrhage: Patients with a variant polymorphism for the cytochrome P450 CYP2C9 enzyme may have an increased risk of an exaggerated response to warfarin and hemorrhage
2. Warfarin embryopathy or fetal warfarin syndrome with congenital abnormalities after exposure in utero. *Warfarin is absolutely contraindicated between the 6th and 12th weeks of pregnancy*
3. Abdominal pain, cramping, flatulence, bloating, nausea, vomiting, diarrhea
4. Increased LFTs, cholestatic liver injury, jaundice
5. Nephritis with acute renal failure
6. Urolithiasis (calcium oxalate)
7. Increased liver enzymes, hepatitis, and a syndrome that mimics viral hepatitis
8. Skin necrosis (risk factors include protein C and heparin-induced thrombocytopenia; case reports of protein S deficiency and factor V Leiden)
9. Rash, dermatitis, bullous eruptions, urticaria, pruritus, and purpuric skin eruption
10. Alopecia
11. Osteoporosis

Notes

Numerous drug and food interactions can occur with oral administration of warfarin

Drug interactions:
- Antibiotics (eg, erythromycin, metronidazole, rifampin, fluconazole)
- Antiepileptics (carbamazepine, barbiturates)
- Lipid-lowering agents (eg, clofibrate, cholestyramine, lovastatin)

Food interactions:
- Many vegetables contain high levels of vitamin K, but patients do not need to specifically avoid such foods
- Patients should be instructed to keep diet fairly uniform and adjust the warfarin dose according to INR
- Alcohol in small quantities is usually tolerated without affecting prothrombin time

Recommendations for Managing Elevated INRs or Bleeding in Patients Receiving Vitamin K Antagonists*

Condition	Description
INR above therapeutic range, but <5.0; no significant bleeding	Lower dose or omit dose, monitor more frequently, and resume at lower dose when INR is therapeutic; if only minimally above therapeutic range, no dose reduction may be required
INR ≥5.0, but <9.0; no significant bleeding	Omit next 1 or 2 doses, monitor more frequently, and resume at lower dose when INR is in therapeutic range. Alternatively, omit dose and give vitamin K[1] (≤5 mg orally), particularly if at increased risk of bleeding. If more rapid reversal is required because the patient needs urgent surgery, vitamin K[1] (2–4 mg orally) can be given with the expectation that a reduction of the INR will occur in 24 hours. If the INR is still high, additional vitamin K[1] (1–2 mg orally) can be given
INR ≥9.0; no significant bleeding	Hold warfarin therapy and give higher dose of vitamin K[1] (5–10 mg orally) with the expectation that the INR will be reduced substantially in 24–48 hours. Monitor more frequently and use additional vitamin K[1] if necessary. Resume therapy at lower dose when INR is therapeutic
Serious bleeding at any elevation of INR	Hold warfarin therapy and give vitamin K[1] (10 mg by slow IV infusion), supplemented with fresh plasma or prothrombin complex concentrate, depending on the urgency of the situation; recombinant factor VIIa may be considered as alternative to prothrombin complex concentrate. Vitamin K[1] can be repeated every 12 hours
Life-threatening bleeding	Hold warfarin therapy and give prothrombin complex concentrate supplemented with vitamin K[1] (10 mg by slow IV infusion). Recombinant factor VIIa may be considered as alternative to prothrombin complex concentrate; repeat if necessary, depending on INR

*If continuing warfarin therapy is indicated after high doses of vitamin K[1], then heparin or LMWH can be given until the effects of vitamin K[1] have been reversed and the patient becomes responsive to warfarin therapy. Note that INR values >4.5 are less reliable than values within or near the therapeutic range. Thus, these guidelines represent an approximate guide for high INRs

Chest 2004;126:204S–233S

Reproduced, with permission, from Ansell J, et al: The Pharmacology and management of the vitamin K antagonists. *Chest* 126:204s, 2004.

REGIMEN

ANTITHROMBIN III (HUMAN) (THROMBATE III)

Antithrombin III (units required[a]) intravenously over 10–20 minutes, followed by:
Antithrombin III (60% of initial dose) every 24 hours as needed (typically 2–8 days)

1. Dose should be individually determined to increase plasma antithrombin III concentration (desired [AT-III]plasma) to within a range of normal from the pre-therapy level (baseline [AT-III]plasma). Dosage may be calculated from the following formula:

$$^{a}\text{ Units required (IU)} = \frac{(\text{Desired [AT-III]}_{\text{plasma}} - \text{baseline [AT-III]}_{\text{plasma}}) \times \text{wt (kg)}}{1.4}$$

*Expressed as % normal [AT-III]plasma based on functional AT-III assay. The formula is based on an expected incremental in vivo recovery greater than baseline [AT-III]plasma of 1.4% per IU/kg administered

2. Elimination half-life is approximately 48 hours

Treatment Modifications

Infusion-related reactions	Decrease the rate of administration, or interrupt administration until symptoms abate; then resume administration at a slower rate

Adverse Effects

Infusion-related events:
1. Dizziness/light-headedness
2. Chest tightness or pain
3. Nausea
4. Dysgeusia
5. Chills
6. Cramps
7. Shortness of breath
8. Urticaria
9. Fever

Monitoring Therapy

1. Monitor peak antithrombin levels 20 minutes after infusion and trough levels just prior to next dose and adjust to keep levels above 80% of normal
2. Also recommended to check antithrombin levels 12 hours after the initial infusion
3. Simultaneous heparin administration can affect half-life and more frequent monitoring may be necessary

59. Heparin-Induced Thrombocytopenia (HIT) and HIT with Thromboembolic Syndrome (HITTS)

McDonald K. Horne III, MD

Heparin-induced thrombocytopenia (HIT) is a distinct clinicopathologic syndrome caused by platelet-activating antibodies that recognize complexes of platelet factor 4 plus heparin. HIT is associated with both arterial and venous thrombosis and, if left untreated, is associated with 20–30% mortality. HIT with thromboembolic complications is HITTS

Epidemiology

Prevalence: 0–5% of patients treated with heparin

- Surgical patients (prophylactic doses) >medical patients (therapeutic doses) >obstetrical patients
- Unfractionated bovine heparin >porcine heparin >low molecular weight heparin (LMWH) (<1%)

Mortality rate:

Isolated HIT: ~5% due to subsequent thrombosis

HITTS: ~15% due to thrombosis (higher in postoperative patients)

Male:female ratio: 1:3

Nand S et al. Am J Hematol 1997;56:12–16
Wallis DE et al. Am J Med 1999;106:629–635
Warkentin TE et al. Am J Med 1996;101:502–507
Warkentin TE. Br J Haematol 2003;121:535–555

Work-Up

The diagnosis of HIT is based on both clinical and serologic findings and thus should be considered a clinicopathologic syndrome

A. Platelet count

1. A platelet count decrease of ≥50% and/or a thrombotic event occurring between days 4 and 14 after initiation of heparin (or LMWH), even if the patient is no longer receiving heparin therapy, warrants excluding a diagnosis of HIT
2. For postoperative cardiac surgery patients, a diagnosis of HIT should be excluded if the platelet count decreases ≥50% from the highest postoperative value between postoperative days 4 and 14 (day 0 = day of cardiac surgery) and/or a thrombotic event occurs
3. No single definition of thrombocytopenia in HIT is appropriate in all clinical situations

B. Timing

1. *Typical HIT:* Thrombocytopenia occurs 5–10 days after initial exposure to heparin
2. *Rapid-onset HIT:* Platelet count falls unexpectedly within 24 hours after exposure to heparin. Affected patients have had prior heparin exposure, usually in the preceding 3 months
3. *Delayed HIT:* Thrombocytopenia and associated thrombosis occur within 3 weeks after stopping heparin

C. Clinical evaluation for thrombosis

For patients who are strongly suspected of having HIT or who have confirmed HIT, routine ultrasonography of the lower-limb veins for investigation of DVT is recommended (with or without clinical evidence of lower-limb DVT)

Adapted from seventh AACP Conference on Antithrombotic and Thrombolytic Therapy. Heparin-Induced Thrombocytopenia: Recognition, Treatment and Prevention
Warkentin TE, Greinacher A. Chest 2004; 126:311S–337S

D. Laboratory assays assessing the presence of HIT antibodies

Confirmatory laboratory assays (depending on availability)

Diagnostic Assay	% Sensitivity	% Specificity: Early Platelet Decrease (Within First 4 Days of Heparin)	% Specificity: Late Platelet Decrease (on ≥Day 5)
Platelet SRA	90–98	>95	80–97
HIPA	90–98	>95	80–97
Heparin/PF4 EIA	>90	>95	50–93
Sensitive platelet aggregation + heparin/PF4 EIA	100	>95	80–97

SRA, serotonin release assay; HIPA, heparin-induced platelet aggregation; Ag, antigen

Reproduced, with permission, from Warkentin TE, Greinacher A. Heparin-induced thrombocytopenia: Recognition, treatment, and prevention.

E. Exclusion of other causes of thrombocytopenia

Gruel Y et al. Br J Haematol 2003;121:786–792
Pouplard C et al. Am J Clin Pathol 1999;111:700–706
Rice L et al. Ann Intern Med 2002;136:210–215
Tardy B et al. Thromb Haemost 1999;82:1199–1200
Warkentin TE, Greinacher A. Chest 2004;126:311S–337S
Warkentin TE et al. Am J Med 1996;101:502–507
Warkentin TE et al. N Engl J Med 2001;344:1286–1292

Treatment Notes

1. Fifty percent of patients who develop HIT develop thrombosis (HITTS) within 30 days unless treated appropriately with nonheparin anticoagulants
2. Clinical presentation of HIT and other sequelae of HIT:
   - Deep vein thrombosis (50%)
   - Pulmonary embolism (25%)
   - Skin lesions at injection site (10–20%)
   - Acute limb ischemia (5–10%)
   - Decompensated disseminated intravascular coagulation (DIC) (5–10%)
   - Acute thrombotic stroke or MI (3–5%)
   - Acute systemic reactions after intravenous heparin bolus (~ 25% of at-risk patients)
   - Adrenal hemorrhagic infarction (rare)
   - Cerebral dural sinus thrombosis (rare)
3. Erythematous or necrotizing skin lesions at heparin or LMWH injection sites should be considered a marker for HIT. These lesions have an onset of ≥5 days after start of therapy, or earlier if HIT antibodies are present from prior heparin exposure. Seventy-five percent of these patients do not develop thrombocytopenia but may have evidence of HIT antibodies
4. An appropriate alternative anticoagulant to heparin or LMWH should not be delayed for results of HIT antibody testing in patients strongly suspected of having HIT
5. Any dose of heparin can produce HIT, even the heparin on coated intravascular devices
6. The thrombocytopenia of HIT is usually mild to moderate (eg, >50,000/mm^3)
7. Despite thrombocytopenia, bleeding is rarely a problem. Prophylactic platelet transfusions should be avoided in acute HIT/HITTS
8. LMWH is less likely than unfractionated heparin to cause HIT, but LMWH must not be substituted for unfractionated heparin in a patient who already has HIT
9. Routine HIT antibody testing in patients receiving heparin in the absence of thrombocytopenia, thrombosis, heparin-induced skin lesions, or other sequelae of HIT is *not recommended*

Alving BM. Blood 2003;101:31–37
Wallis DE et al. Am J Med 1999;106:629–635
Warkentin TE. Br J Haematol 2003;121:535–555
Warkentin TE. Thromb Haemost 1998;82:439–447
Warkentin TE, Greinacher A. In: Heparin Induced Thrombocytopenia, 3rd ed. New York: Marcel Dekker, 2004:600–601
Warkentin TE et al. Ann Intern Med 1997;127:804–812

Platelet Count Monitoring for HIT

Patient Category	Recommendation
Patients starting unfractionated heparin or LMWH and who have received unfractionated heparin within the past 100 days; those in whom recent exposure is uncertain	Obtain baseline platelet count; then repeat platelet count within 24 hours of starting unfractionated heparin or LMWH
Acute systemic reactions after intravenous unfractionated heparin: patients who experience cardiorespiratory, neurologic, or other usual symptoms and signs within 30 minutes after an intravenous unfractionated heparin bolus	Perform an immediate platelet count measurement and compare this value with recent prior platelet counts
Patients receiving therapeutic-dose unfractionated heparin	At least every-other-day platelet count monitoring until day 14 or until unfractionated heparin is stopped, whichever occurs first
Postoperative antithrombotic prophylaxsis with unfractionated heparin (HIT risk >1%)	At least, every-other-day platelet count monitoring between postoperative days 4 and 14 or until unfractionated heparin is stopped, whichever comes first
Platelet count monitoring in patients whom HIT is infrequent (0.1–1%): Medical/obstetrical patients who are receiving prophylactic-dose unfractionated heparin, postoperative patients receiving prophylactic-dose LMWH, postoperative patients receiving intravascular catheter unfractionated heparin flushes, or medical obstetric patients receiving LMWH after first receiving unfractionated heparin	Platelet count monitoring every 2 or 3 days from day 4 to day 14 (or until heparin is stopped, whichever occurs first), when practical
Platelet count monitoring when HIT is rare (<0.1%): Medical/ obstetric patients who are receiving only LMWH, or medical patients who are receiving only intravascular catheter unfractionated heparin flushes	Do not use routine platelet count monitoring

Adapted from the Seventh ACCP Conference on Thrombosis and Thrombolytic Therapy chest, 2004

Differential Diagnosis of Isolated, Acquired Thrombocytopenia

1. Pseudothrombocytopenia (ex vivo clumping)
2. Decreased production of platelets
   - Acute alcoholism, thiazide diuretics, diethylstilbestrol, cocaine, HIV
3. Increased destruction or clearance of platelets
   - Sepsis, acute viral infection
   - Drugs (abciximab, acetaminophen, amiodarone, amphotericin B, cimetidine, danazol, diclofenac, digoxin, heparin, quinidine, quinine, rifampin, sulfasalazine, trimethoprim-sulfamethoxazole, vancomycin, many others)
   - DIC, idiopathic thrombocytopenic purpura (ITP), HIV infection, cardiopulmonary bypass, antiphospholipid syndrome
4. Splenic sequestration
5. Pregnancy associated

George JN et al. Ann Intern Med 1998;129:886–890

Treatment Options for HIT/HITTS (Non-Heparin Anticoagulants)

Treatment should not be delayed pending laboratory confirmation in a patient strongly suspected of having HIT. This recommendation is supported by the reported observations from a meta-analysis of the HAT-1 and HAT-2 trials that showed a 6.1%/day incidence of thrombotic events after stopping heparin and after laboratory confirmation of HIT, but before institution of alternative anticoagulation with lepirudin (a mean treatment delay of 1.7 days)

Parenteral therapy

1. Argatroban
2. Lepirudin (a recombinant hirudin)
3. Bivalirudin (a recombinant hirudin analog): Only limited, off-label use in HIT/HITTS has been reported
4. Danaparoid (not available in the United States)

Oral therapy

Warfarin

- Delay the initiation of warfarin therapy until the platelet count has substantially recovered on alternative anticoagulation (ie, to at least 100,000/mm^3, and preferably 150,000/mm^3)
- Begin at a modest maintenance dose (maximum 5 mg/day warfarin; 6 mg/day phenprocoumon) and only during alternative parenteral anticoagulation (above) with a minimum 5-day overlap
- During co-therapy with warfarin, the alternative anticoagulant should not be discontinued until the platelet count has reached a stable plateau and the INR has been within the target prophylactic range for at least 2 consecutive days (see specific recommendations for Conversion to Warfarin with nonheparin anticoagulants for HIT)
- Venous limb gangrene has been reported with warfarin therapy in patients with HITTS, particularly with a rapid rise in the INR >3 because of persisting thrombin generation and depletion of protein C levels
- In circumstances where HIT is recognized when warfarin has already been started, oral or intravenous vitamin K (5–10 mg) is recommended to try to avert warfarin-induced microvascular necrosis or progression and to avoid aPTT prolongation due to warfarin that might lead to underdosing of alternatively therapy

Duration of treatment

- In acute HIT without thrombosis, anticoagulation should be continued until the platelet count becomes stable at its pretreatment baseline or achieves a stable plateau on alternative anticoagulation (ie, danaparoid or a direct thrombin inhibitor). Published expert opinion advises that acute HIT, by itself, is not an indication for longer-term anticoagulation (ie, 3–6 months)
- In acute HIT with thrombosis, longer-term anticoagulation (eg, 3–6 months) is often required with oral anticoagulants of the coumarin class after co-therapy with alternative anticoagulation (see above, Oral therapy: Warfarin)

Alving BM. Blood 2003;101:31–37
Greinacher A et al. Blood 2000;96: 846–851
Greinacher A, Warkentin TE. In: Heparin-Induced Thrombocytopenia, 3rd ed. New York: Marcel Dekker, 2004
Warkentin TE. Thromb Res 2003;110:73–82
Warkentin TE, Greincacher A. Chest 2004;126:311S–337S

REGIMEN

ARGATROBAN

Alving B. Blood 2003;101:33–37
Lewis BE et al. Arch Intern Med 2003;163:1849–1856
Lewis BE et al. Circulation 2001;103:1838–1843
Murray P et al. J Thromb Haemost 2003;1:1911
Verme-Gibboney CN, Hursting MJ. Ann Pharmacother 2003;37:970–975
Warkentin T. Thromb Res 2003;110:73–82
ARGATROBAN Injection prescribing information. Glaxo Smith Kline. April 2002

Mechanism of action: Direct thrombin inhibitor that reversibly binds to the thrombin active site
Half-life: 40–50 minutes
Metabolism: Hepatic clearance; no significant renal clearance

Before initiating therapy: Discontinue heparin (if ongoing administration) and allow the patient's aPTT to return to baseline

HIT or HITTS (normal liver function):
Loading dose: None
Maintenance dose: **Argatroban** 2 mcg/kg/min intravenously. Dilute **argatroban** in 0.9% NaCl injection (0.9% NS), 5% dextrose injection (D5W), or lactated Ringer's injection (LRI) to produce a concentration of 1 mg/mL (eg, 250 mg in 250 mL diluent). Two hours after starting the argatroban infusion, obtain an aPTT level and adjust the infusion rate in increments of ± 0.5 mcg/kg/min (or less in patients with hepatic impairment) to achieve a steady-state aPTT value 1.5 to 3.0 times the baseline value. Do not exceed an aPTT of 100 seconds, or an argatroban dose of 10 mcg/kg/min

HIT or HITTS (hepatic impairment)*:
Loading dose: None
Maintenance dose: **Argatroban** 0.5 mcg/kg/min intravenously. Dilute **argatroban** in 0.9% NS, D5W, or LRI to produce a concentration of 1 mg/mL

*Extent of hepatic impairment not clarified. Argatroban should be used reluctantly and cautiously whenever there is any evidence of hepatic impairment

Antidote: None. However, the drug generally disappears from the circulation within 2–4 hours. In the setting of liver disease, drug clearance time is prolonged. If such a patient were bleeding, it would be reasonable to attempt to lower the level of argatroban by plasmapheresis

Conversion to Warfarin

Note: Delay the initiation of warfarin therapy until the platelet count has substantially recovered (100–150,000/mm³)

1. Initiate warfarin at a modest daily dose (≤5 mg/day) while argatroban is continued
2. When the INR is >4 in patients taking warfarin plus >2 mcg/kg/min argatroban, the argatroban should be reduced to 2 mcg/kg/min for 4–6 hours and then the INR remeasured. If the INR has fallen below 4, the argatroban should be resumed at the higher dose. Otherwise, the sequence below should be undertaken
3. If the INR is >4 on co-therapy with warfarin and average-dose (≤2 mcg/kg/min) argatroban, discontinue argatroban and repeat the INR after 4–6 hours *if:*
   a. The repeat INR is above the prophylactic range (2–3), warfarin therapy alone is continued at a lower dose
   b. The repeat INR is below the prophylactic INR range, ≤2 mcg/kg/min argatroban is restarted, and the process repeated daily until the target INR is achieved and sustained
   c. The repeat INR is within the prophylactic range, argatroban is restarted, and the same routine is repeated the next day. If on the next day the INR on warfarin alone is again in the prophylactic range (ie, for the second day), argatroban is permanently discontinued

Efficacy

	HIT	HITTS
Thrombocytopenia	Usually resolves in 1 week	
New thrombosis	6–8%	15–20%
Thrombosis mortality	1–2%	

Toxicity

	HIT	HITTS
Major bleeding	3–5%	6–11%
% Non hemorrhagic toxicity*		
Hypotension	7.2 (2.6)	
Fever	6.9 (2.1)	
Diarrhea	6.2 (1.6)	
Nausea	4.8 (0.5)	
Vomiting	4.2 (0)	

*Percentages in HIT/HITTS patients. Numbers in parentheses are percentages in historical controls

Monitoring Therapy

Steady-state levels typically attained within 1 to 3 hours. Two hours after starting infusion, adjust dose (±0.5 mcg/kg/min or less in the setting of hepatic impairment) to give an aPTT 1.5–3-times the patient's baseline aPTT

REGIMEN

LEPIRUDIN (Hirudin, Recombinant)

Greinacher A et al. Blood 2000;96:846–851
Greincaher A et al. Circulation 1999;99:73–80
Greinacher A et al. Circulation 1999;100:587–593
Greinacher A. In: Heparin-Induced Thrombocytopenia, 3rd ed. New York: Marcel Dekker, 2004:397–436
Lubenow N et al. Blood 2004;104:3072–77
Willey ML et al. Pharmacotherapy 2002;22:492–499
REFLUDAN® [lepirudin (rDNA) for injection] prescribing information. Berlex Laboratories, Inc, October 2002

Mechanism of action: Direct thrombin inhibitor; a recombinant hirudin analogue
Half life: 0.8–1.7 hours (mean ≈80 minutes)
Metabolism: Predominantly renal clearance

Before initiating therapy: Discontinue heparin (if ongoing administration) and allow the patient's aPTT ratio (patient aPTT/median of normal aPTT range) to decline to <2.5

HIT/HITTS with normal renal function (labeled indication):
Loading dose: **Lepirudin** 0.4 mg/kg intravenously per push over 15–20 seconds
Maintenance dose: **Lepirudin** 0.15 mg/kg per hour (up to body weight of 110 kg or a maximum dose of 16.5 mg/kg per hour) intravenously in 0.9% NaCl injection (0.9% NS) or 5% dextrose injection (D5W) diluted to a concentration of 5 mg/mL. Check aPTT ratio 4 hours after starting the infusion or changing the rate and adjust rate of administration 20 to 50% to maintain a target aPTT ratio of 1.5–2.0 (HIT) or 1.5–2.5 (HITTS)

HIT or HITTS with impaired renal function (creatinine clearance ≤60 mL/min):
Loading dose: **Lepirudin** 0.2 mg/kg intravenously per push over 15–20 seconds
Maintenance dose: Administer intravenously in 0.9% NS or D5W at a final concentration of 5 mg/mL

Creatinine Clearance	Lepirudin Dose
45–60 mL/min	0.075 mg/kg per hour
30–44 mL/min	0.045 mg/kg per hour
15–29 mL/min	0.0225 mg/kg per hour
<15 mL/min	Avoid or stop infusion

Check aPTT ratio 4 hours after starting the infusion or changing the rate and adjust rate of administration 20 to 50% to maintain a target aPTT ratio of 1.5–2.0 (HIT) or 1.5–2.5 (HITTS)

Antidote: None. However, the drug clears within 2–3 hours after stopping an infusion. For patients with renal insufficiency **lepirudin** can be removed by high-flux hemodialysis with polysulfone membranes, hemofiltration or plasmapheresis

Toxicity

	HIT	HITTS
Major bleeding	6–14%	5–20%

Of the 60,000 patients treated with lepirudin, 9 patients had severe anaphylaxis in close temporal association with drug administration; all occurring within minutes of IV bolus (4 fatal outcomes)
Risk of anaphylaxis: First exposure 0.015% (5/32,500); re-exposure 0.16% (4/2500) assuming a 7.5% re-exposure occurrence
Anti-lepirudin IgG antibodies: 44% of patients with 5 or more days of therapy as early as day 4; peaked at days 8–9

Monitoring Therapy

Check aPTT ratio 4 hours after starting the lepirudin infusion and 4 hours after the rate of infusion has been changed

Target aPTT Ratio	
HIT	1.5–2.0
HITTS	1.5–2.5

Dose Adjustments	
aPTT ratio >2.5	Stop infusion for 2 hours; restart at 50% of previous dose
aPTT ratio <1.5	Increase infusion rate in 20% increments; re-measure aPTT ratio 4 hours after dosage change

Note: ~40% develop anti-lepirudin IgG antibodies after ≥5 days and require dose adjustment—usually a reduction

Conversion to Warfarin

Note: Delay the initiation of warfarin therapy until the platelet count has substantially recovered (100–150,000/mm³)

1. Initiate warfarin at a modest daily dosage (≤5 mg/day) while lepirudin is continued maintaining an aPTT ratio of 1.5–2.0
2. Once INR is in the target range (2–3) on 2 consecutive days on the combined anticoagulants, discontinue lepirudin and repeat INR ~4 hours later to confirm that it is still within the target range. If the INR falls below the target range, resume lepirudin (maintaining an aPTT ratio of 1.5–2.0) for another 24 hours and repeat the process

Efficacy

	HIT	HITTS
Thrombocytopenia	Usually resolves in 1 week	
New thromboses	2–3%	5–10%

Notes

Lepirudin is also used without the bolus dose (off-label)
HIT without thrombosis with normal renal function (off-label):
Loading dose: None
Maintenance dose: **Lepirudin** 0.1 mg/kg per hour intravenously, diluted in 0.9% NaCl injection (0.9% NS) or 5% dextrose injection (D5W) to a concentration of 5 mg/mL

REGIMEN

BIVALIRUDIN

Bartholomew JR. In: Heparin-Induced Thrombocytopenia, 3rd ed. New York: Marcel Dekker, 2004:475–507
Berilgen JE et al. Blood 2003;102:1969 [Abstract]
Francis JF et al. Blood 2003;102:571 [Abstract]
Koster A et al. Anesth Analg 2003;96:1316–1319
Reed MD et al. Pharmacotherapy 2002;22:105S–111S
Robson R et al. Clin Pharmacol Ther 2002;71:433–439
Robson R. J Invasive Cardiol 2000;12(suppl F): 33F–36F
The Medicines Company. Angiomax (bivalirudin) package insert. Cambridge, MA, 2001

Mechanism of action: Direct thrombin inhibitor; a recombinant hirudin analog
Half-life: 25–36 minutes
Metabolism: 80% proteolytic cleavage by plasma proteases; 20% renal mechanisms

Before initiating therapy: Discontinue heparin (if ongoing administration) and allow the patient's aPTT ratio (patient aPTT/median of normal aPTT range) to decline to <2.5

Dose for HIT or HITTS: (OFF-LABEL EXPERIENCE)
Loading dose: None
Maintenance dose: Bivalirudin 0.15–0.20 mg/kg per hour as a continuous intravenous infusion using a solution containing 250 mg bivalirudin in 500 mL 0.9% NaCl injection (0.9% NaCl) or 5% dextrose injection (D5W). Titrate to maintain therapeutic aPTT (1.5–2.5 × aPTT baseline); adjust in increments of 0.05 mg/kg per hour

HIT or HITTS with impaired renal function*:
Normal (≥90 mL/min): No dose reduction
Mild renal impairment (60–89 mL/min): No dose reduction
Moderate renal impairment (30–59 mL/min): 20% dose reduction
Severe renal impairment (10–29 mL/min): 60% dose reduction
*Bivalirudin dosing adjustment recommendations based on GFR for percutaneous coronary interventions

Antidote: None. Large amounts of bivalirudin can be removed by hemofiltration (65,000 Da large-pore hemofilter) or plasmapheresis

Toxicity

Bleeding is the major adverse effect of bivalirudin and occurs more frequently in patients with renal impairment
Allergic reactions: 1 in 3639 patients (0.03%) reported in clinical trials from 1993 to 1995

Monitoring Therapy

Adjust to maintain therapeutic aPTT (1.5–2.5 × baseline). Repeat aPTT at 6-hour intervals until therapeutic aPTT is reached; then daily

Conversion to Warfarin

Note: Delay the initiation of warfarin therapy until the platelet count has substantially recovered (100–150,00/mm^3)

Experience converting patients from bivalirudin to warfarin is very limited. Recommended schema:

1. Initiate warfarin at a modest daily dose (≤5 mg/day) while bivalirudin is continued, maintaining an aPTT ratio of 1.5–2.0
2. When INR is in the target range (2–3) on 2 consecutive days on the combined anticoagulants, discontinue bivalirudin and repeat INR ~ 4 hours later to confirm that it is still within the target range. If the INR falls below the target range, resume bivalirudin (maintaining an aPTT ratio of 1.5–2.0) for another 24 hours, and repeat the process

Efficacy

Although evidence suggests that the efficacy of bivalirudin in treating HIT and HITTS is comparable to that of argatroban and lepirudin, the experience with this drug is limited

Notes

1. Drugs incompatible with bivalirudin: Alteplase, amiodarone hydrochloride, amphotericin B, chlorpromazine hydrochloride, diazepam, prochlorperazine, reteplase, streptokinase, vancomycin hydrochloride
2. Bivalirudin (label indication) is used as an anticoagulant in patients with unstable angina undergoing percutaneous transluminal coronary angioplasty. In patients with renal impairment, dose reduction is recommended

REGIMEN

DANAPAROID SODIUM
(Danaparoid Sodium is not Available in the United States)

BH, Magnani HN. In: Heparin-Induced Thrombocytopenia, 3rd ed. New York: Marcel Dekker, 2004, 371–396
Chong BH, Magnani HN. Haemost 1992;22:85–91
Chong BH et al. Blood 1989;73:1592–1596
DeValk HW et al. Ann Intern Med 1995;123:1–9
Farner B et al. Thromb Haemost 2001;85:950–957
Greinacher A et al. Thromb Haemost 1992;67:545–549
Kikta MJ et al. Surg 1993;114:705–710
Magnani HN. Thromb Haemost 1993;70:554–561
Magnani HN. Platelets 1997;8:74–81

Mechanism of action: Factor Xa inhibitor; weak inhibitor of factor IIa
Anti-Xa terminal half-life: ≃25 hours
Metabolism: Predominantly renal clearance

Before initiating therapy: Discontinue heparin (if ongoing administration) and allow the patient's aPTT ratio (patient aPTT/median of normal aPTT range) to decline to <2.5

HIT and HITTS with normal renal function
Subcutaneous regimen
Loading dose: None
Maintenance dose: ≥60 kg: **Danaparoid sodium** 2250 units (3 vials) subcutaneously every 12 hours; <60 kg: **Danaparoid sodium** 1500 units (2 vials) subcutaneously every 12 hours
IV regimen
Loading dose: According to weight as follows:

<60 kg:	**Danaparoid sodium** 1500 units
60–75 kg:	**Danaparoid sodium** 2250 units
75–90 kg:	**Danaparoid sodium** 3000 units
>90 kg:	**Danaparoid sodium** 3750 units

Maintenance dose: **Danaparoid sodium** by continuous infusion. Dilute in 0.9% NaCL injection (0.9% NS) and administer as follows:
400 units/hour for 4 hours
300 units/hour for 4 hours, *then*
150–200 units/hour for ≥5 days

HIT or HITTS with impaired renal function:
In selected patients, such as those with evidence of renal dysfunction, the administration rate should be titrated to achieve a plasma anti-Xa level of 0.5–0.8 units/mL (see Therapy Monitoring)

Venous thromboembolism prophylaxsis (prior HIT): **Danaparoid sodium** 750 units subcutaneously every 8 or 12 hours

Antidote: None

Conversion to Warfarin

Note: Delay the initiation of warfarin therapy until the platelet count has substantially recovered (100–150,000/mm^3)

1. Initiate warfarin at a modest daily dosage (≤5mg/day) while danaparoid is continued maintaining and aPTT ratio of 1.5–2.0
2. Overlap both anticoagulants at least 5 days, ensuring that the INR is in the target range (2–3) for at least 2 days on the combined anticoagulants before discontinuing danaparoid therapy. Discontinue danaparoid and repeat INR ~4 hours later to confirm that it is still within the target range. If the INR falls below the target range, resume danaparoid (maintaining an aPTT ratio of 1.5–2.0) for another 24 hours and repeat the process

Efficacy

Overall success rate ~90%, as defined by normalization of platelet count and no additional thrombotic events

Toxicity

Cross-reactivity with serum heparin-associated antiplatelet antibodies	0–20%
Bleeding	Rare with HIT/HITTS
Skin hypersensitivity reaction	Rare

Monitoring Therapy

Monitoring is not required in most situations. However, anti-Xa levels should be monitored in patients with:
1. Low or high body weights
2. *Any* renal impairment
3. Life- or limb-threatening thrombosis
4. Unexpected bleeding
5. A critical illness or marked instability

In these patients, obtain anti-Xa levels at approximately 6 hours after a change in the subcutaneous or intravenous dose until a plasma anti-Xa level of 0.5–0.8 units/mL is achieved; then daily

Special Therapeutic Approaches

HIT in dialysis patients

Heparin must not be added to any flushing solution, and no heparin-coated devices should be used in this population. LMWH is also to be avoided. Argatroban is theoretically an ideal agent for this patient population because of its predominant hepatic elimination with no initial dose adjustments required based on renal dysfunction alone. However, regimens using lepirudin and danaparoid have also been published

HIT in cardiac or vascular surgery

1. For *patients with previous HIT* undergoing cardiac or vascular surgery and *who are HIT antibody–negative*, unfractionated heparin over a nonheparin anticoagulant is recommended. If indicated, pre- and postoperative anticoagulation should be administered with a nonheparin anticoagulant
2. For *patients with acute HIT* who require cardiac surgery, one of the following alternative anticoagulant approaches has been recommended (in descending order of preference; Seventh ACCP Conference on Antithrombotic and Thrombolytic Therapy, Chest, 2004):
   a. Delay surgery until HIT antibodies are negative
   b. Bivalirudin for intraoperative anticoagulation during cardiopulmonary bypass (if ecarin clotting time [ECT] available) or during off-pump cardiac surgery
   c. Lepirudin for intraoperative anticoagulation (if ECT available and normal renal function)
   d. Unfractionated heparin plus the antiplatelet agent epoprostenol (if ECT monitoring is not available or renal insufficiency precludes lepirudin use)
   e. Danaparoid for intraoperative anticoagulation (if anti–factor Xa levels are available)
3. For *patients that are HIT antibody–positive and with platelet count recovery*, delay surgery (if possible) until HIT antibody is negative then use heparin as outlined for HIT negative patients in 1 above. Alternatively, a non-heparin anticoagulant is suggested as outlined for acute HIT patients, in 2 above

HIT in patients undergoing percutaneous coronary intervention (PCI)

Bivalirudin is approved for patients with or at high risk of HIT/HITTS undergoing PCI. Bivalirudin is intended for use with aspirin in three clinical trials, subjective assessment of a satisfactory outcome was achieved in 95% of 91 patients undergoing a first PCI and in all 21 patients undergoing a repeat PCI. Secondary success, defined as absence of death, emergent bypass or Q-wave MI was achieved in 98% of initial PCI group and 100% of patients undergoing a repeat PCI. (See Dangas & Nikolsky for references and commentary)

HIT in cancer patients

Managing HIT in cancer patients can be especially complex because cancer patients are more likely to have thrombocytopenia or liver or renal dysfunction or vitamin K deficiency, all of which must be considered in selecting the anticoagulant and the dose to use as a substitute for heparin.

HIT and pregnancy

Data are limited data that describe HIT during pregnancy. Danaparoid has been used in 31 pregnant women with HIT using dosing schedules similar to those in nonpregnant women. In 19 pregnancies, no significant problems were encountered, and in 12, new thromboses occurred among whom 3 were successfully treated with increasing danaparoid doses. Danaparoid does not cross the placenta based on cord blood assessment. Fondaparinux does not cross the placenta, whereas hirudin can in low doses. If available, danaparoid (and possibly fondaparinux) is preferred for parenteral administration in pregnant patients with HIT or a history of HIT

Chong BH, Magnani HN. In: Heparin-Induced Thrombocytopenia, 3rd ed. New York: Marcel Dekker, 2004:371–396
Dangas G and Nikolsky E. J Invasive Cordiol 2003; 15:622–623
Fischer K-G. In: Heparin-Induced Thrombocytopenia, 2nd ed. New York: Marcel Dekker, 2001:409–427
Fischer K-G. In: Heparin-Induced Thrombocytopenia, 3rd ed. New York: Marcel Dekker, 2004:509–530
Greinacher A, Warkentin TE. In: Heparin-Induced Thrombocytopenia, 3rd ed. New York: Marcel Dekker, 2004:335–370
Langrange F et al. Thromb Haemost 2002;87:831–835
Lewis BE et al. Catheter Cardiovasc Interv 2002;57:177–184
O'Shea SI et al. Semin Dialysis 2003;16:61–67
Warkentin TE. NEJM 2001;344:1286–1292
Warkentin TE, Greinacher A. Ann Thorac Surg 2003;76:638–648
Warkentin TE, Greinacher A. Chest 2004;126:311S–337S

60. Autoimmune Hemolytic Anemia

James N. Frame, MD, FACP

Autoimmune hemolytic anemia (AIHA) is an acquired immunologic disease in which a patient's red blood cells are selectively destroyed or hemolyzed by autoantibodies (auto-Ab) produced by the patient's own immune system

Mack P, Freedman J. Transfus Med Rev 2000;14:223–233

Etiology

	% of Cases		
1. Idiopathic	58		
2. Secondary	42		
Neoplasia		18	
Carcinomas			25
CLL			22
NHL			18
MDS			9
Hodgkin disease			5
Drug-induced		8	
Other immune based/or miscellaneous		7	
Infection		5	
Unspecified			38
Mycoplasma pneumoniae			33
Viral/unspecified pneumonia			17
Mononucleosis			7
Collagen vascular diseases		4	
Rheumatoid arthritis			61
Systemic lupus erythematosus			37

Gehrs BC, Friedberg RC. Am J Hematol 2002;69:258–271
Pirofsky B. Semin Hematol 1976;13:251–265
Sokol RJ et al. J Clin Pathol 1992;45:1047–1052

Epidemiology

- Idiopathic AIHA is more common in women than in men (2:1) with a peak incidence in the fourth and fifth decades of life. Idiopathic AIHA is not associated with any demonstrable underlying disease
- Secondary causes have been reported in 20–80% of case series

	United Kingdom*		United States
	Incidence/Year	% of Cases	% of Cases
Overall	1/25,600	—	
Warm antibody AIHA	1/40,800	63	48–78
Cold antibody AIHA	1/87,500	29	16–32
Paroxysmal cold hemoglobinuria (PCH)	1/2,470,000	1	7–8
Mixed-type AIHA	1/370,000	7	3

*Data from a 10-year study (1982–1991) of 1834 patients evaluated for suspected AIHA or for RBC interference in blood grouping or typing from a 4.7 million population base at the Regional Blood Transfusion Center, Sheffield, UK (Sokol RJ et al. J Clin Pathol 1992;45:1047–1052)

Classification

Warm antibody AIHA

1. Idiopathic
2. Secondary type:
   a. Lymphoproliferative disorders (eg, CLL and the lymphomas)
   b. Autoimmune disorders (eg, SLE, rheumatoid arthritis, ulcerative colitis, Sjögren's syndrome)
   c. Infections
   d. Tumors (Kaposi's sarcoma, various carcinomas, teratoma, ovarian dermoid cyst), thymoma
   e. Immunodeficiency disorders (eg, AIDS, dys-/hypogammaglobulinemia)
   f. Post-transplantation

Cold antibody AIHA

1. Idiopathic
2. Secondary type (cold agglutinin syndrome):
   a. Infection (eg, *M. pneumoniae*, mononucleosis, cytometgalovirus, varicella zoster virus, HIV)
   b. Lymphoproliferative disorders (CLL, the lymphomas including Waldenström's macroglobulinemia)
   c. Tumors (squamous cell carcinoma of the lung, metastatic adenocarcinomas of the lung and adrenal gland; mixed parotid tumor)
3. Paroxysmal cold hemoglobinuria:
   a. Idiopathic
   b. Secondary: Late-onset or congenital syphilis, measles, mumps, Epstein-Barr virus, cytomegalovirus, varicella zoster virus, adenovirus, influenza A, and *M. pneumoniae, Haemophilus influenzae* infections

Mixed-type AIHA

1. Idiopathic
2. Secondary type: Autoimmune disorders (eg, systemic lupus erythematosus, lymphoproliferative disorders)

Drug-induced IHA (DIIHA)

1. Drug absorption or hapten-type (penicillin)
2. Neoantigen type (immune complex type), such as quinine, quinidine, hydralazine, cephalosporins, sulfonamides, rifampin, and isoniazid
3. Drug absorption on to RBCs, such as anti-D immune globulin sometimes used in treatment of idiopathic thrombocytopenic purpura (Gaines AR. Blood 2000;95:2523–2539)
4. True autoantibodies such as methyldopa, L-dopa, procainamide, ibuprofen, diclofenac, interferon alfa, and mefenamic acid

Notes: From 1978 to 2003 (Blood 2003; 102:2059a), most DIIHA cases were caused by cephalosporins (74%), of which cefotetan (63%) and ceftriaxone (9%) were most commonly implicated. DIIHA case reports relevant to hematology/oncology include:

a. Interferon alfa (Andriani A et al. Haematologica 1996;81:258–260)
b. Cladribine (2-chlorodeoxyadenosine) (Tetreault SA, Saven A. Leuk Lymphoma 2000;37:125–130; and Fleischman RA, Croy D. Am J Hematol 1995;48:293)
c. Fludarabine (Myint H et al. Br J Haematol 1995;91:341–344)
d. Immune globulin intravenous (human) (Okubo S et al. Transfusion 1990;30:4368)
e. Levofloxacin, with a summary of other fluoroquinolones (Oh YR et al. Ann Pharmacother 2003;37:1010–1013)
f. Pentostatin (Byrd JC et al. Ann Oncol 1995;6:300–301)
g. Ribavirin (Massoud OI et al. J Clin Gastroenterol 2003;36:367–368)
h. Rituximab (Jourdan E et al. Leuk Lymphoma 2003;44:889–909; reported to be the first case)

Serologic Findings: Autoimmune Hemolytic Anemia

Variable	Warm Antibody	Cold Antibody	PCH	Mixed
DAT (Direct antiglobulin test)	>95% DAT (+): Polyclonal IgG; more reactive at 37°C IgG only: 20–66% IgG + C3: 24–63% C3: 7–14% 2–4% DAT (−)	All DAT (+): C3 more reactive at 0–4°C IgM auto-Ab: Dissociates after C3 binding IgG or IgA auto-Ab: Rare cases	All DAT (+): C3 (IgG-positive if done at lower temperatures) Usually biphasic IgG auto-Ab that binds RBCs efficiently at 0–4°C, fixes C1 and leads to hemolysis nearer to normal body temperatures	DAT (+): "Mixed" with warm Ab AIHA *and* a cold-Ab or agglutinin Warm hemolysin: IgG, C3, and occasionally IgM or IgA
RBC eluate	**Mostly IgG_1**	**Nonreactive**	**Nonreactive**	**Variable**
Antigen targets	Rh (*e, E, C*) Band 4.1 Band 3 Glycophorin A	*Ii* (90% against *I*) *Pr, Gd, Sa Lud, Fl, Vo, M, N, D, P*	*P* antigen	*I* or *i* have been observed or no specificity
Comments	(+) DAT without AIHA reported in normal blood donors: 1:13,000 to 1:14,000	Pathogenic cold Ab AIHA: High auto-Ab titer, high thermal amplitude	Donath-Landsteiner test is used to evaluate for the biphasic hemolysin	Clinically significant cold Abs: high titer at 0-4°C (>1:1000), with thermal amplitude >30°C

Serologic Findings: Drug-Induced Immune Hemolytic Anemia[a]

Variable	Autoantibody	Drug Absorption	Neoantigen Formation
DAT	(+) for polyspecific sera/IgG C3 usually (−)	(+) for polyspecific sera/IgG; C3 usually (−)	(+) for polyspecific sera/IgG; C3 usually (−)
Serum Ab testing[b]	(±) for routine (±) for soluble drug (±) for drug-treated RBCs	(−) for routine (−) for soluble drug (+) for drug-treated RBCs	(−) for routine testing (+) for soluble drug (+) for drug-treated RBCs
RBC eluate Ab testing[b]	(+) for routine (+) for soluble drug (+) for drug-treated RBCs	(−) for routine (−) for soluble drug (+) for drug-treated RBCs	(−) for routine (−) for soluble drug (−) for drug-treated RBCs
Examples	α-Methyldopa, L-dopa, procainamide, ibuprofen, diclonfenac, interferon-α, mefenamic acid	Penicillin	Quinine, quinidine, hydralazine, isoniazid, cepahalosporins, sulfonamides, rifampin

[a]Serologically indistinguishable from warm-Ab AIHA. A presumptive diagnosis is made if there is clinical improvement after drug withdrawal

[b]Tests are as follows: Routine = indirect antiglobulin test (or indirect Coombs'); soluble drug = soluble drug added to serum Ab screening with RBCs for testing; drug-treated RBCs = RBCs treated with drug before adding to serum Ab screening system for testing

Ab, antibody; AIHA, autoimmune hemolytic anemia; DAT, direct antiglobulin test; PCH, paroxysmal cold hemoglobinuria

Buetens OW. Curr Opin Hematol 2003;10:429–433
Engelfriet CP et al. Sem Hematol 1992;29:3–12
Gehrs BC et al. Am J Hematol 2002;69:258–271
Janvier D et al. Transfusion 2002;42:1547–1552
Petz LD, Garraty G. Classification and characteristics of autoimmune hemolytic anemias. In: Petz LD, Garraty G, eds. Immune Hemolytic Anemias, 2nd ed. New York: Churchill Livingstone, 2004:61–131

Work-Up

1. Peripheral blood smear review
2. CBC with differential
3. Reticulocyte count (usually elevated unless underlying bone marrow suppression or failure is present or in earliest phase of acute hemolysis)
4. LDH
5. Total/indirect bilirubin
6. Direct/indirect antiglobulin tests (DAT, IAT); thermal amplitude of antibody
7. RBC eluate (to assess for the presence of auto- and alloantibodies)
8. Haptoglobin
9. Urine hemoglobin
10. Plasma hemoglobin
11. Ancillary testing as appropriate to the clinical setting:
    a. Bone marrow aspiration and biopsy (suggested when an underlying lymphoproliferative, plasma cell dyscrasia, or other bone marrow infiltrative disorder is suspected or when the presence of associated cytopenias requires diagnostic clarification)
    b. Renal/hepatic profile
    c. Total protein
    d. Serum/urine protein electrophoresis and immunofixation, if an underlying monoclonal gammopathy is suspected
    e. HIV testing in patients with risk factors
    f. Testing for autoimmune diseases
    g. Hemoglobin electrophoresis
    h. Pregnancy testing
    i. Assessment for underlying infection
    j. Radiographic studies
    k. Evaluation for underlying malignancy

Gehrs BC, Friedberg RC. Am J Hematol 2002;69:258–271

Treatment Overview

The level of clinical evidence supporting the management of AIHA is derived from case reports, case series, and/or expert opinion. Randomized, controlled trials of cytotoxic or immunosuppressive agents in AIHA have not been performed

Idiopathic and Secondary Warm Antibody AIHA

1. First line
    a. Single-agent glucocorticoid therapy
    b. Disease-specific treatments for secondary* etiologies ± glucocorticoids
2. Second line
    a. Splenectomy in surgical candidates who fail to benefit from glucocorticoid therapy
3. Third line:
    a. Immunosuppressive agents (cyclophosphamide and azathioprine)
    b. Danazol
    c. Cyclosporine
    d. Rituximab
    e. High-dose cyclophosphamide
    f. Immune globulin intravenous (human)
    g. Plasmapheresis
    h. Splenic irradiation (reported in CLL)
4. Mycophenolate mofetil

*In patients with secondary warm antibody AIHA due to underlying lymphoproliferative disorders or a solid tumor, therapy of the primary disorder may lead to AIHA remission

Cold Antibody AIHA [Cold-Agglutinin Syndrome (CAS)]

Idiopathic (primary) CAS

1. First line:
   a. Avoidance of cold; wearing warm clothing
2. Second line or later: Approaches that have produced responses in small groups of patients with CAS:
   a. Glucocorticoids (generally less effective than in warm Ab AIHA)
   b. Cytotoxic drugs (eg, chlorambucil)
   c. Plasma exchange
   d. Splenectomy in IgM (not IgG) CAS
   e. Rituximab
   f. High-dose cyclophosphamide
   g. Plasmapheresis

Secondary CAS

1. First line:
   a. Treat the underlying cause
   b. Provide supportive care (spontaneous remissions of secondary AIHA have been observed in patients with infectious mononucleosis and *M. pneumoniae* infections)
   c. Keep patient warm if the cold reactive antibodies demonstrate a high thermal amplitude
2. Second line or later:
   a. Glucocorticoids
   b. Rituximab
   c. Plasmapheresis

Paroxysmal Cold Hemoglobinuria (PCH)

1. First line
   a. Symptomatic therapy; avoidance of cold; wearing warm clothing
   b. Plasmapheresis if PCH is life-threatening
   c. Treatment of syphilis if present

Mixed-Type Antibody AIHA

1. First line
   a. Single-agent glucocorticoid therapy
   b. Disease-specific treatments for secondary etiologies ± glucocorticoids
2. Second line
   a. Splenectomy in surgical candidates who fail to benefit from glucocorticoid therapy
   b. High-dose cyclophosphamide
   c. Rituximab

Drug-Induced AIHA

1. First line:
   a. Discontinuation of the suspected or causative agent is indicated
   b. Supportive care
2. Second line:
   a. Glucocorticoids if hemolysis is severe

Notes: Transfusion of RBCs in patients with symptomatic life-threatening AIHA is potentially indicated at any point along the disease or treatment continuum. The early collaboration of the treating physician with their blood bank or transfusion service is indicated

REGIMEN

PREDNISONE

American College of Rheumatology Ad Hoc Committee on Glucocorticoid-Induced Osteoporosis. Arthritis Rheum 2001;44:1496–1503
Gehrs BC, Friedberg RC. Am J Hematol 2002;69:258–71
Lacy CF et al. In: LEXI-COMP'S drug information handbook, 11th ed. 2003
Murphy A et al. Sem Hematol 1976;13:323–334
Petz LD. Curr Opin Hematol 2001;8:411–416
Schwartz RS et al. Autoimmune hemolytic anemias. In: Hoffman R et al, eds. Hematology: Basic Principles and Practice, 3rd ed. Philadelphia: Churchill Livingstone, 2000:60
Petz LD, Garraty G, eds. Management of autoimmune hemolytic anemias. In: Petz LD, Garratty G, eds. Immune Hemolytic Anemias, 2nd ed. New York: Churchill Livingstone, 2004:8
Petz LD, Garraty G. Blood Transfusions in autoimmune hemolytic anemia. In: Petz LD, Garratty G, eds. Immune Hemolytic Anemias, 2nd ed. New York: Churchill Livingstone, 2004:375–400
Rosse WF. Autoimmune hemolytic anemia. In: Handin RI, Lux SE, Stossel TP, eds. Blood: Principles and Practice in Hematology. Philadelphia: Lippincott Williams & Wilkins, 2005:1859–1885

Prednisone 1–1.5 mg/kg (~40–60 mg) per day (single dose) or 0.5–0.75 mg/kg (~20–30 mg) twice per day (divided dosing) orally for a minimum of 3–4 weeks before assessing efficacy

Supportive care:
Add a **proton pump inhibitor** during prednisone therapy
Calcium and vitamin D supplementation in patients receiving long-term, low- to medium-dose glucocorticoid therapy and who have normal levels of gonadal hormones (Am Coll Rheum 2001).
Folic acid 1 mg/day orally to prevent depletion of folate stores and megaloblastic anemia resulting from chronic hemolysis
Also see Chapter 44 on bisphosphonates

Titration of prednisone in responding patients:

1. Once Hgb is ≥10 g/dL, taper prednisone by 10–15 mg/week to a dose of 20–30 mg/day. This can usually be accomplished in 4–6 weeks
2. If Hgb persists ≥10 g/dL, follow with a gradual reduction in 5-mg decrements to a dose of 10 mg/day over a period of 3 months
3. If Hgb persists ≥10 g/dL, withdraw all therapy over another 3-month period

or

1. Once Hgb is ≥10 g/dL, taper prednisone at first fairly rapidly by 20 mg/day (0.3 mg/kg/day) each week to a dose of 20 mg/day. This can usually be accomplished in 2–3 weeks. This dose is then maintained for approximately 1 month to see whether remission continues
2. If Hgb persists ≥10 g/dL, switch to an alternate day regimen over 2 months. In the first month, reduce the dose to 20 mg/day, alternating with 10 mg/day. In the second month, reduce the dose to 20 mg/every other day
3. If Hgb persists ≥10 g/dL, reduce the dose to 10 mg/every other day over the next month
4. If Hgb persists ≥10 g/dL, reduce the dose to 5 mg/ every other day over the next month
5. If Hgb persists ≥10 g/dL, withdraw all therapy over another few months

Murphy A et al. Sem Hematol 1976;13:323–334
Rosse WF. Autoimmune hemolytic anemia. In: Handin RI, Lux SE, Stossel TP, eds. Blood: Principles and Practice in Hematology. Philadelphia: Lippincott Williams & Wilkins, 2005:1859–1885

Notes:

- If the DAT is (+), a dose of 10 mg/every other day is maintained so long as remission remains
- If at any point during dose reduction exacerbation of hemolysis occurs, increase the dose to the previous level and maintain that level. If the dose exceeds 20 mg (0.3 mg/kg)/every other day, consider other therapies

Prednisone is marketed in the United States in numerous generic formulations for oral administration, including prompt-release tablets containing 1, 2.5, 5, 10, 20, and 50 mg, and in solutions and syrups

Emetogenic potential: Nonemetogenic to low

Patient Population

Initial therapy in:

- Patients with warm-antibody AIHA with clinically important signs and symptoms of anemia if there are no contraindications for its use
- Patients with mixed AIHA

Second-line therapy in others

Treatment Modifications

Note: Administer prednisone 0.6 mg/kg per day to patients >70 years or to immobilized or osteoporotic patients in the setting of active infection or other mitigating conditions

Efficacy

Response within 1 week	Most patients
Hemolysis improved within 1–3 weeks	70–80%
Lasting remissions	20–30%
Unacceptable prednisone dose/no response	10–20%
Need low-dose prednisone maintenance	50%
Response rates in idiopathic types	82%
Response rates in secondary forms	60%

Murphy A et al. Sem Hematol 1976;13:323–334

Toxicity

>10%: Insomnia, nervousness, increased appetite, indigestion
1–10%: Dizziness or lightheadedness, headache, hirsutism, hypopigmentation, glucose intolerance, diabetes mellitus, hyperglycemia, arthralgia, cataracts, glaucoma, epistaxis, diaphoresis
<1%*: Cushing's syndrome, edema, fractures, hallucinations, hypertension, muscle wasting, osteoporosis, pancreatitis, pituitary-adrenal axis suppression, seizures

*Limited to important or life-threatening

Notes

Consider splenectomy, or if the patient is not a candidate for splenectomy, other immunosuppressive therapy if:

1. Response is not achieved after 3 weeks of prednisone treatment
2. Contraindications to prednisone therapy exist
3. Patient experiences intolerable side effects
4. Prednisone doses of ≥15 mg/day are required to maintain Hgb ≥ 10 g/dL

REGIMEN

SPLENECTOMY

Akpek G et al. Am J Hematol 1999;61:98–102
Bowdler AJ. Semin Hematol 1976;13:335–348
Coon WW. Arch Surg 1985;120:625–628
Katkhouda N et al. Ann Surg 1998;228:568–578
Petz LD, Garratty G. Management of autoimmune hemolytic anemias. In: Petz LD, Garratty G, eds. Immune Hemolytic Anemias, 2nd ed. New York: Churchill Livingstone, 2004:401–458
Schwartz RS et al. Autoimmune hemolytic anemia. In: Hoffman R et al eds. Hematology Basic Principles and Practice, 3rd ed. Philadelphia: Churchill Livingstone, 2000:611–629

Open or laparoscopy splenectomy depending on the surgeon's experience or patient requirements

Before splenectomy, administer:
1. Pneumococcal vaccine
2. *Haemophilus influenzae* type b vaccine
3. Meningococcal vaccine

Supportive care:
Folic acid 1 mg/day orally to prevent depletion of folate stores and megaloblastic anemia resulting from chronic hemolysis

Efficacy

N = 9 Case Series; 308 AIHA Patients	
All patients	57.5% remission

Bowdler AJ. Semin Hematol 1976;13:335–348

N = 2 Case Series; 80 Patients	
Idiopathic AIHA (n = 55)	52.7% remission
Secondary AIHA (n = 25)	32% remission

Bowdler AJ. Semin Hematol 1976;13:335–348

N = 52	
Steroid terminated with a stable Hct ≥30%	64% (mean follow-up, 33 months).
Hct ≥30% on ≤15 mg/day of prednisone or equivalent	21% (mean follow-up, 73 months)

Coon WW. Arch Surg 1985;120:625–628

	Idiopathic (N = 11[a])	Secondary (N = 16[b])
Normal Hgb ≥6 months; no additional therapy (CR)	82%	19%
≥50% increase in Hgb; ± other therapy (PR)	18%	37%

[a]Median follow-up 18 months
[b]Median follow-up 11 months
Akpek G et al. Am J Hem 99;61:98–102

Patient Population

Recommended as second-line therapy in surgical candidates with AIHA who:

1. Do not benefit adequately from glucocorticoid therapy
2. Benefit initially from glucocorticoid therapy but suffer a relapse on taper
3. Require unacceptably high maintenance glucocorticoid doses (eg, >10–20 mg/day of prednisone) or have intractable side effects to glucocorticoid therapy

Note: Although considered ineffective in cold agglutinin syndrome (CAS) a few case reports of atypical CAS with hemolysins reactive at 37°C and responsive to splenectomy have been reported (Petz LD, Garratty G, 2004)

Toxicity

1. Overwhelming post-splenectomy infection (OPSI):
   - *Incidence*: More common in children <15 years (0.13–8.1%), adults (0.28–1.9%) but may occur at any age
   - *Risk factors*: Young age, history of hematologic disorders
   - *Timing*: Most infections occur within 2 years after splenectomy; 42% reported within 5 years
   - *Mortality*: 50–70% in older studies with >50% of deaths within the first 48 hours after hospitalization
2. Thrombocytosis
3. Deep venous thrombosis (reported increased in myeloproliferative disorders post-splenectomy)
4. Pseudohyperkalemia

Notes

1. Annual influenza vaccination is also recommended in asplenic patients
2. Patient education should include instruction as to early signs of potential overwhelming splenectomy infection and emphasis to seek early medical attention when present
3. For guidance on the prevention and treatment of overwhelming splenectomy infection and the use of vaccines in persons with altered immunocompetence, see Br Med J 1996;312:430–434; MMWR 1993;42:1–18

REGIMEN

RITUXIMAB

Berentsen S et al. Blood 2004;103:2925–2928
Frame JN et al. Blood 2004;104:3721a
Kunkel L et al. Semin Oncol 2000;27(6 suppl 12):53–61
Petz LD, Garratty G. Blood transfusions in autoimmune hemolytic anemia. In: Petz LD, Garratty G, eds. Immune Hemolytic Anemias, 2nd ed. New York: Churchill Livingstone, 2004:375–400
Wood AM. Am J Health Syst Pharm 2001;58:215–229

Premedication for rituximab:
Acetaminophen 650–1000 mg orally, +
Diphenhydramine 25–50 mg orally or intravenously 30–60 minutes before starting rituximab

Rituximab 375 mg/m^2 intravenously in 0.9% NaCl injection (0.9% NS) or 5% dextrose injection (D5W), diluted to a concentration of 1–4 mg/mL, weekly for 4 consecutive weeks (total dosage/cycle = 1500 mg/m^2)

Notes on rituximab administration:

- Infuse initially at 50 mg/hour. If hypersensitivity or infusion reactions do not occur during the first 30 minutes, increase the rate by 50 mg/hour every 30 minutes as tolerated to a maximum rate of 400 mg/hour. Subsequently, if previous administration was well tolerated, start at 100 mg/hour and increase by 100 mg/hour every 30 minutes as tolerated to a maximum rate of 400 mg/hour
- Interrupt rituximab administration for fever, chills, edema, congestion of the head and neck mucosa, hypotension, and other serious adverse events. Resume rituximab administration at a 50% reduction in rate after adverse events abate. Treat with diphenhydramine plus acetaminophen with bronchodilators and intravenous saline as indicated

Supportive care:
Folic acid 1 mg/day orally to prevent depletion of folate stores and megaloblastic anemia resulting from chronic hemolysis

Efficacy (N = 76) [Rituximab ± Other Therapy]

AIHA Type	No. of Patients	% CR[a]	% PR
Warm Ab	35 (7/28)	29 (3/7)	43 (1/14)
Cold Ab	40 (8/32)	28 (7/4)	43 (1/16)
Mixed Ab	1 (1/0)	50 (1/0)	0
Total	76 (16/60)	29 (11/11)	42 (2/30)
Mean Hgb increase	3.8 g/dL	5.6 g/dL	4 g/dL
Rituximab monotherapy		21.7	47.8
Rituximab + other therapies[b]		40	33.3
Mean time to response		22 days (5–120 days)	
Median response duration		10.5 months (1.5–42)	

[a]Numbers in parentheses refer to those with idiopathic/secondary or disease-associated AIHA
[b]IVIG, chemotherapy, or glucocorticoid

Patient Population

Off-label in the following adults with AIHA:

1. Patients with idiopathic or secondary AIHA with warm, cold, or mixed warm/cold hemolysins
2. Patients with persistent disease after immunosuppressive therapies

Rituximab alone (52%) or in combination (48%) with glucocorticoids, single or multi-agent chemotherapy (lymphoproliferative disorders; LPD), or IVIG

Treatment Modifications

Rituximab Infusion-Related Toxicities

Onset of infusion-related events (fevers, chills, rigors, edema, congestion of the head and neck mucosa, hypotension):

1. Interrupt rituximab infusion
2. For fever, chills: Give additional dose of acetaminophen 650 mg orally and diphenhydramine 25–50 mg by intravenous push
3. For rigors: Give meperidine 12.5–25 mg by intravenous push ± promethazine 12.5–25 mg by intravenous infusion in at least 10 mL 0.9% NS or D5W over 5–15 minutes. If after 15–20 minutes the response to a single dose is considered inadequate, the dose may be repeated
4. After symptoms resolve, resume rituximab infusion at 50 mg/hour and increase by 50 mg/hour every 30 minutes as tolerated up to a maximum rate of 200 mg/hour

Dyspnea or wheezing, without allergic findings (urticaria, or tongue or laryngeal edema):

1. Interrupt rituximab infusion immediately
2. Give hydrocortisone 100 mg by intravenous push (or glucocorticoid equivalent)
3. Give a histamine H_2 antagonist (ranitidine 150 mg, cimetidine 300 mg, or famotidine 20 mg) by intravenous push
4. After symptoms resolve resume rituximab infusion at 25 mg/hour with dose monitoring. Do not increase rate

Note: Medications for the treatment of hypersensitivity reactions should be available for immediate use in the event of a reaction during administration (eg, intravenous fluids, epinephrine, antihistamines, glucocorticoids, and O_2)

Toxicity (N = 92)

	% of Patients
Infusion related[a]	7.6
Headache	2.2
Pruritus	2.2
G4 WBC	2.2
Rash	1.1
Hypotension	1.1
Myalgia	1.1
Death[b]	1.1

[a]Fever, chills, rigors, nausea, vomiting, pruritus, dizziness, dyspnea, bronchospasm, sensation of tongue or throat swelling, rhinitis, flushing, hypotension, and pain at disease sites
[b]From fungal infection 3 months after rituximab

Serious infusion reactions resulting in death	0.04–0.05%
Severe mucocutaneous reactions	0.02%

Monitoring Therapy

1. *CBC with differential:* Weekly and more frequently in patients who develop cytopenias
2. Monitor renal function tests, serum calcium, phosphorus, uric acid and fluid balance and institute supportive care as indicated

REGIMEN

HIGH-DOSE CYCLOPHOSPHAMIDE

Brodsky RA et al. Ann Intern Med 2001;135:477–483
Moyo VM et al. Blood 2002;100:704–706

High-dose cyclophosphamide 50 mg/kg (ideal body weight) per day intravenously in 100–1000 mL 0.9% NaCl injection (0.9% NS) or 5% dextrose injection (D5W) over 60 minutes for 4 consecutive days on days 1–4 (total dosage = 200 mg/kg ideal body weight)
Mesna 10 mg/kg per dose intravenously, diluted to 1–20 mg mesna/mL over 15 minutes at 30 minutes before starting cyclophosphamide and 3, 6, and 8 hours after cyclophosphamide for 4 doses/day on 4 consecutive days, days 1–4 (total dosage = 160 mg/kg)
Filgrastim 5 mcg/kg per day subcutaneously, starting on day 10 (6 days after completing cyclophosphamide) and continuing beyond the ANC nadir until ANC recovers to ≥1000/mm^3

Supportive care:
Folic acid 1 mg/day orally to prevent depletion of folate stores and megaloblastic anemia resulting from chronic hemolysis

Emetogenic potential: Very high (Emetogenicity score = 5). Potential for delayed symptoms. See Chapter 39 for antiemetic regimens

Efficacy (N = 9)

Complete response (CR)[a]	67%[c]
Partial response[b]	33%
15-Month Follow-up	
Continued response	100%
Maintained without steroids	77%

[a]Normal untransfused Hgb for age/sex while taking ≤10 mg/d of prednisone with the resolution of hemolysis
[b]Hgb of ≥10 g/dL and transfusion independence
[c]Two CR patients became DAT-negative

Toxicity (N = 9)

Nausea and vomiting	Common
Transient alopecia	Common
Neutropenic fever	Common
Renal and LFT abnormalities	Infrequent
Hemorrhagic cystitis	Infrequent
SIADH	Infrequent

Parameter	Median
ANC ≥500/mm^3	16 days
Platelet transfusion independence	15 days
RBC transfusion independence	19 days
Hospital stay	21 days

Treatment Modifications

No dose modification
Treatment criteria:
1. Age ≤70 years
2. Ejection fraction >40%
3. Serum creatinine <2.5 mg/dL (220 μmol/L)
4. FVC/FEV/CO diffusion capacity at least 50% of predicted

Patient Population Studied

High-dose cyclophosphamide with mesna and filgrastim support has been reported in a limited number of patients with severe refractory AIHA, with a need for transfusions and steroids >10 mg/day despite 2 therapies for idiopathic AIHA and at least 1 for secondary AIHA. Clinical features of the enrolled patients included:

- Severe refractory AIHA (6 idiopathic; 3 secondary), warm Ab AIHA (n = 7), CAD (n = 1), mixed AIHA (n = 1)
- Median pretreatment Hgb: 6.7 g/dL (range 5–10 g/dL)
- Median number of prior regimens = 3

Notes

1. Benefits of therapy versus risks should be assessed
2. Use high-dose cyclophosphamide only by clinicians and medical centers with active experience in the use of "transplant doses" of cyclophosphamide and with the availability of appropriate ancillary clinical support and personnel

REGIMEN

RED BLOOD CELL TRANSFUSION

Branch DR, Petz LD. [editorial] Transfusion 1999;39:6–10
Buetens OW, Ness PM. Curr Opin Hematol 2003;10:429–433
Petz LD: Blood transfusion in acquired hemolytic anemia. In: Petz LD, Swisher SN, Kleinman S, Spence RK, Strauss RG (eds.) Clinical practice of transfusion medicine, 3rd ed. New York: Churchill Livingstone, 1996; 469–99
Petz LD. Hematology 2002 (Am Soc of Hematol Educational Program Book) 449–454
Petz LD. [editorial] Transfusion 2003;43:1503–1507
Petz LD, Garratty G. Blood transfusions in autoimmune hemolytic anemia. In: Petz LD, Garratty G, eds. Immune Hemolytic Anemias, 2nd ed. New York: Churchill Livingstone, 2004:375–400
Rosenfield RE, Jagathambal. Semin Hematol 1976;13:311–121

Volume and rate considerations:
Volume: The optimal volume of RBCs to be infused depends on the clinical setting. In general, the aim is to supply just enough RBCs to treat or prevent hypoxemia while avoiding overtransfusion
Rate: Administer RBCs slowly with a total volume not to exceed 1 mL/kg per hour

Monitoring considerations:
Hgb/Hct: In the setting of acute, life-threatening AIHA, the Hgb/Hct should be monitored at 2-hour intervals—at least every 12–24 hours in individuals less acutely ill
Volume status: During and after transfusion, assessments should be performed for the presence of congestive heart failure or volume overload. Particular caution is advised regarding the development of fluid overload in the elderly or those with reduced cardiac reserve. Diuretic therapy should be used as clinically indicated

Other consideration:
Cold agglutinin syndrome: The patient should be dressed warmly and should be in a warm environment

Blood Product Selection

Note: Hemoglobin-based oxygen carriers (RBC substitutes) have not received FDA approval for any indication

Warm Ab AIHA:

1. Most severe hemolytic transfusion reactions are due to anti-A or anti-B antibodies. Although a broadly reactive auto-Ab will make all units incompatible, with standard blood banking techniques the ABO type can usually be identified and permit identical or compatible ABO type blood for transfusion
2. The blood bank should assess for alloantibodies (allo-Ab) that may be present owing to prior transfusion in the past 3 months or pregnancy that may be masked by the presence of the auto-Ab. Allo-Ab have been reported to be present in 12–40% of patients with warm Ab AIHA. Allo-Ab have been reported in 209/647 (32%) sera of patients with AIHA. Failure to identify the presence of allo-Ab may lead to worsening of the hemolysis and falsely increase the perceived severity of AIHA after transfusion. The more common alloAb target antigens may include: *C, E, c, e, K*, Fy^a, Fy^b, Jk^a, Jk^b, *S* and *s*

Cold agglutinin syndrome:

1. Compatibility testing should be done at 37°C. If testing cannot be performed strictly at this temperature, then it is recommended that 1 or 2 auto-adsorptions be performed. Although high-titer cold agglutinins are not completely removed with this maneuver, reactions that occur at 37°C are likely to be eliminated
2. The specificity of cold agglutinins is often anti-*I*. Providing *I* antigen-negative blood may not be practical owing to its rarity and may not be beneficial
3. There is controversy among experts as to the worth of blood warming in this setting. In patients with severe CAS or PCH, blood warming has been advocated. When an in-line blood warmer is used, the temperature should be carefully regulated at body temperature to avoid RBC injury, which can result in lethal in vivo hemolysis. Guidelines for the use of blood-warming devices have been published by the American Association of Blood Banks (AuBuchon, JP. Guidelines for the use of blood warming devices. Bethesda: American Association of Blood Banks, 2001)

Paroxysmal Cold Hemoglobinuria
The use of *p* or p^k RBCs (lacking the *P* antigen) is not practical because of its rarity and availability only from rare donor files. In this setting, transfusion of common *P* types should be provided

Patient Population

Recommended in patients who are acutely ill with signs and symptoms compatible with acute hemolysis or in patients with progressive anemia in whom severe levels of hemolysis (eg, Hgb <5–6 g/dL) may probably be reached

General guidelines based on Hgb values and the probability of significant physiologic impairment

Note: The decision to transfuse should ultimately be guided by clinical assessments performed in the individual patient

Hgb	Probability*	Recommendation
≥10 g/dL	Low	Avoid transfusion
8–10 g/dL	Low	Avoid transfusion *or* Transfuse if improved after a transfusion trial
6–8 g/dL	Moderate	Transfuse if necessary or try to avoid transfusion
≤6 g/dL	High	Frequently require transfusion
Stable	Low	Avoid transfusion

*Probability of significant physiologic impairment

Petz LD: Blood transfusion in acquired hemolytic anemia. In: Petz LD, Swisher SN, Kleinman S, Spence RK, Strauss RG, eds. Clinical Practice of Transfusion Medicine, 3rd ed. New York: Churchill Livingstone, 1996:469–499

Efficacy

Not available. Goal of therapy was to stabilize red cell mass and reverse symptoms of acute anemia

Toxicity

Potential complications in patients with AIHA may include:

1. Volume overload and congestive heart failure with attempts to raise the hematocrit too quickly
2. Acute hemolytic transfusion reactions
3. Alloimmunization
4. Post-transfusion hemoglobinemia or hemoglobinuria, particularly with large volumes of RBCs with ongoing auto-Ab production
5. Diffuse intravascular coagulation
6. Thromboembolism
7. Death

Notes

Initial communication between the clinician and the blood bank:
At the first indication that RBC transfusion may be required, the clinician should contact the blood bank or transfusion service. This communication should include:

1. An indication of the urgency for transfusion
2. An inquiry into the compatibility testing procedures used by the blood bank to assess the safety of the selected RBCs for transfusion, and
3. Clinical information that may help in assessing the risk of alloimmunization (eg, history of pregnancy, prior blood transfusion particularly in the past 3 months)

What the clinician should expect from the blood bank—transfusion Service:

1. Notification of the diagnosis of AIHA made during compatibility testing for a requested transfusion
2. Information about the compatibility test procedures performed
3. RBCs selected for transfusion after excluding the presence of alloantibodies (eg, by adsorption techniques or by extended phenotype)
4. Assurances that the transfused cells are unlikely to cause an acute hemolytic transfusion reaction even though the RBCs cannot be expected to survive normally because of the autoantibody

REGIMEN

PLASMAPHERESIS

VA et al. J Clin Apher 1994;9:120–12
von Baeyer H. Ther Apher Dial 2003;7:127–140

Protocol for plasmapheresis alone:
Plasma exchange (PEX) and **albumin human** (HA) for IgM (IgA) Ab–mediated hemolysis and for IgG 1, 2, 4–mediated hemolysis
Daily PEX/HA at 1–1.5 × the plasma volume until the hemolysis is controlled and transfusions are no longer required

Patient Population

Therapeutic plasmapheresis in AIHA has been advocated under 2 conditions:

1. As an emergency bridging measure to eliminate auto-Ab until immunosuppressive therapy becomes effective
2. As therapy after failure of immunosuppressive therapy and splenectomy to treat relapsing hemolysis

von Baeyer H. Ther Apher Dial 2003;7:127–140

Efficacy (N = 20; 15 Cases Reports or Series of AIHA)

	% Responding
All patients (n = 20)	65
Warm-Ab (n = 10)	50
Cold-Ab (n = 6)	67
Evans syndrome (n = 4)	100
AIHA after BMT (n = 4)	25

Toxicity

Potential side effects to plasmapheresis include:

1. Complications associated with central venous catheter
2. Type I allergic hypersensitivity reactions

Notes

The American Association of Blood Banks and the American Society of Apheresis have assigned a Category III indication to plasmapheresis for AIHA, citing "insufficient data to determine the effectiveness of apheresis in which the results of clinical trials may be conflicting, or in some circumstances where efficacy has been based on uncontrolled anecdotal reports."

Smith JW et al. Transfusion 2003;43:820–822

REGIMEN FOR REFRACTORY WARM ANTIBODY AUTOIMMUNE HEMOLYTIC ANEMIA

IMMUNOSUPPRESSIVE THERAPY: AZATHIOPRINE, CYCLOPHOSPHAMIDE

American College of Rheumatology Ad Hoc Committee on Glucocorticoid-Induced Osteoporosis. Arthritis Rheum 2001;44:1496–1503
Corley CC Jr et al. Am J Med 1996;41:404–412
Cheema AR, Hersh EM. Cancer 1971;28:851–855
Habibi B et al. Am J Med 1974;56:61–9
Hitzig WH, Massimo L. Blood 1966;28:840–850
Murphy et al. Semin Hematol 1976 13:323–334
Petz LD. Curr Opin Hematol 2001;8:411–416
Petz LD, Garratty G, Management of autoimmune hemolytic anemias. In: Petz LD, Garratty G, eds. Immune Hemolytic Anemias, 2nd ed. New York: Churchill Livingstone, 2004:401–458
Rosse W et al. Challenges in managing autoimmune diseases In: Hematology 1997: Education Program, American Society of Hematology; p. 92-4 Published by American Society of Hematology
Worrledge S: Immune hemolytic anemias. In: Hardesty RM, Weatherall DJ, eds: Blood and Its Disorders. Oxford: Blackwell Scientific, 1982:479–513

Azathioprine 2 mg/kg per day orally (total dosage/week = 14 mg/kg), *or*
Azathioprine 75–200 mg/day orally (total dose/week = 525–1400 mg) *or*

Azathioprine 80 mg/m^2 per day orally (total dosage/week = 560 mg/m^2), *plus*
Prednisone 60 mg per day orally (total dose/week = 420 mg), *or*

Cyclophosphamide 60 mg/m^2 per day orally (total dosage/week = 420 mg/m^2), *plus:*
Prednisone 60 mg per day orally (total dose/week = 420 mg)

Guidelines for tapering azathioprine after 6 months of therapy:
60 mg/m^2 per day for 4 weeks; 35 mg/m^2 per day for 4 weeks; 15 mg/m^2 per day for 4 weeks; 25 mg every other day for 4 weeks; 25 mg twice weekly; discontinue

Guidelines for tapering prednisone:
30 mg/day for 1 week; 20 mg/day for 1 week; 15 mg/day for 4 weeks; 10 mg/day for 4 weeks; 5 mg/day for 4 weeks; 5 mg every other day for 4 weeks; discontinue

Guidelines for tapering cyclophosphamide after 6 months of therapy:
45 mg/m^2 per day for 4 weeks; 30 mg/m^2 per day for 4 weeks; 15 mg/m^2 per day for 4 weeks; 25 mg/m^2 every other day for 4 weeks; 25 mg/m^2 twice weekly; discontinue

Supportive care:
Add a **proton pump inhibitor** during prednisone therapy
Calcium and vitamin D supplementation in patients receiving long-term low- to medium-dose glucocorticoid therapy and who have normal levels of gonadal hormones (American College of Rheumatology Ad Hoc Committee on Glucocorticoid-Induced Osteoporosis. Arthritis Rheum 2001;44:1496–1503).
Folic acid 1 mg/day orally to prevent depletion of folate stores and megaloblastic anemia resulting from chronic hemolysis
Also see Chapter 44 on bisphosphonates

Azathioprine is marketed in the United States as tablets for oral administration containing 25, 50, 75, and 100 mg
Cyclophosphamide is marketed generically in the United States as tablets for oral administration containing either 25 mg or 50 mg anhydrous cyclophosphamide

Emetogenic potential:
Azathioprine: Low (Emetogenicity score = 2)
Cyclophosphamide: Low (Emetogenicity score = 2). See Chapter 39 for antiemetic regimens

Treatment Modifications

Adjust azathioprine and cyclophosphamide therapy to maintain a "slight degree of marrow suppression" manifested as mild thrombocytopenia or leukopenia. Although a slight degree of marrow suppression was not further defined in the studies, consider using NCI CTC grade 1 toxicity as a reasonable benchmark:
WBC: 3000/mm^3 to lower limits of normal
ANC: ≥1500/mm^3 to <2000/mm^3
Platelets: ≥75,000/mm^3 to lower limits of normal
Hemoglobin: 10 g/dL to lower limit of normal

Adverse Event	Dose Modification
If WBC <3000/mm^3 or ANC <1500/mm^3 or platelets <75,000/mm^3	Hold therapy for a minimum of 1 week. Restart only when WBC >3000/mm^3 and ANC >1500/mm^3 and platelets: >75,000/mm^3; then start with a dosage reduction for azathioprine of 0.5 mg/kg/day or 25–50 mg/day, and for cyclophosphamide of 15 mg/m^2

Patient Population

Consider immunosuppressive therapy in patients with warm Ab AIHA who:

1. Do not benefit from glucocorticoids
2. Require unacceptable maintenance doses of glucocorticoids
3. Are poor surgical candidates for splenectomy
4. Experience a relapse after splenectomy

Efficacy

Percent responding	40–60
Percent requiring low dose glucocorticoids in addition to azathioprine or cyclophosphamide	≤50

Toxicity	Monitoring Therapy	Notes
Potential side effects include: 1. Myelosuppression 2. Anemia 3. Thrombocytopenia 4. Infection 5. Renal and hepatic function abnormalities 6. Nausea and vomiting 7. Alopecia 8. Sterility 9. Secondary malignancies 10. Hemorrhagic cystitis (cyclophosphamide) 11. Syndrome of inappropriate antidiuretic hormone (cyclophosphamide)	*CBC with differential:* Weekly during the first month, weekly for a month after any dose increase; otherwise every 2 weeks until counts stabilize, then monthly	1. The rapid withdrawal of immunosuppressive agents may lead to a rebound phenomenon of hyperimmune responsiveness 2. If glucocorticoids have produced an incomplete remission before the initiation of immunosuppressive therapy, they should be continued until signs of clinical improvement

REGIMEN FOR REFRACTORY WARM ANTIBODY AUTOIMMUNE HEMOLYTIC ANEMIA

DANAZOL

Ahn YS et al. Ann Intern Med 1985;102:298–301
Pignon J-M et al. Br J Haematol 1993;83:343-5
DANAZOL® CAPSULES product label, revised February 1999, Barr Laboratories, Inc, Pomona, NY

Danazol 200 mg orally 3–4 times/day (total dose/week = 4200–5600 mg)

Notes:

- Danazol is usually added initially to any previous medication (eg, prednisone) or initiated with prednisone 1 mg/kg per day
- If a hematologic remission (HR) is attained, glucocorticoids are tapered to a minimal requirement or discontinued. If a HR is maintained for >1 month without prednisone, danazol is gradually tapered to 200–400 mg/day, and this dose is continued indefinitely as long as there is no clinically important toxicity and Hgb remains >10 g/dL

Supportive care:

Add a **proton pump inhibitor** during prednisone therapy
Calcium and vitamin D supplementation in patients receiving long-term low- to medium-dose glucocorticoid therapy and who have normal levels of gonadal hormones (American College of Rheumatology Ad Hoc Committee on Glucocorticoid-Induced Osteoporosis. Arthritis Rheum 2001;44:1496-503).
Folic acid 1 mg/day orally to prevent depletion of folate stores and megaloblastic anemia resulting from chronic hemolysis
Also see Chapter 44 on bisphosphonates

Contraindications: Undiagnosed abnormal genital bleeding, pregnancy, breast feeding, porphyria, "markedly impaired" hepatic, renal, or cardiac function

Danazol is available in the United States generically in solid formulations for oral administration that contain 50 mg, 100 mg, and 200 mg

Emetogenic potential: Nonemetogenic (Emetogenicity score = 1). See Chapter 39 for antiemetic regimens
Note: Emetic symptoms may occur in association with benign intracranial hypertension–a rare adverse event associated with danazol use

Treatment Modifications

Adverse Event	Dose Modification
≥ G2 NCI CTC LFTs	Hold danazol until LFTs ≤ G1

Patient Population

Patients with idiopathic or secondary warm antibody AIHA:

1. Refractory disease despite prior therapy with glucocorticoids, splenectomy, and immunosuppressive therapy
2. Less frequently as initial therapy with prednisone

Toxicity

Potential side effects include:

1. Virilization with facial hair growth, hair loss, and menstrual irregularities
2. Nervousness
3. Cushingoid features with glucose intolerance in patients with diabetes mellitus
4. Muscle cramps and myalgia
5. Elevations of LFTs
6. Fluid retention
7. Thromboembolism
8. Allergic skin reactions
9. Pseudotumor cerebri (benign intracranial hypertension)

Monitoring Therapy

1. Monitoring of LFTs at baseline and at least monthly or earlier as clinically indicated
2. Assessment for virilization because some signs may not be reversible

Efficacy

Up-Front Therapy with Prednisone (N = 10)	
Hgb to ≥12.5 g/dL*	80%
Complete prednisone taper	75%
Low dose every other day prednisone	25%
Mean response duration	18+ mos (14+ - 37+ mos)
Previously treated with prednisone, splenectomy and immunosuppressive therapy (N = 7)	
Excellent response	43% (14–23+ months)
Partial response	14% (77+ months)
Treatment failure	43% (7–18 months)

*With prednisone decreased to ≤5 mg/day or discontinued
Ahn YS et al. Ann Intern Med 1985;102:298–301

Idiopathic (N = 7) or Secondary Nonmalignant (N = 5) Warm Ab AIHA	
Hct increased to ≥40%	50%
Hct increased to ≥30% but less than 40%	25%
Hct increased by 6% above baseline value with 50% reduction in steroids	25%
Time to response (weeks)	1–3
Remission sustained with steroids + danazol	58%
Remission sustained with danazol alone	42%
Malignant Warm Ab AIHA (N = 3)	
Sustained remission	33%

Note: Nine of 15 patients without prior splenectomy achieved lasting remissions with addition of danazol, suggesting a splenectomy-sparing effect

REGIMEN FOR REFRACTORY WARM ANTIBODY AUTOIMMUNE HEMOLYTIC ANEMIA

CYCLOSPORINE

Emilia G et al. Br J Haematol 1996;93:341–344
Hershko C et al. Br J Haematol 1990;76:436–437
AHFS Drug Information 2004:3625–3639

Starting dosage:
Cyclosporine 2–3 mg/kg per dose orally twice daily for 6 days (total dosage/day = 4–6 mg/kg)
Maintenance dosage:
Cyclosporine 1.5 mg/kg per dose adjusted to maintain a serum cyclosporine concentration between 200 and 400 ng/mL

Alternate Schedule

Starting dosage:
Cyclosporine 1.25 mg/kg/dose orally twice daily (total dosage per week = 17.5 mg/kg)
Maintenance dosage:
If no response, increase **cyclosporine** by 0.25 mg/kg/dose (0.5 mg/kg/d) increments every 2 weeks to a maximum of 2 mg/kg/dose (4 mg/kg/day; maximum total dosage per wk = 28 mg/kg)

Note: Dosages vary with indication, and AIHA is not an approved indication. Dosage/schedules for autoimmune diseases often fall within a broad range of 0.5–4 mg/kg per dose orally every 12 hours. Generally, treatment is initiated at a low dosage and is titrated as soon as possible to the least dose that achieves a desired therapeutic effect. After that effect or a maximal response is achieved, an attempt should be made to taper the dose with the goal of discontinuing therapy

Supportive care:
Folic acid 1 mg/day orally to prevent depletion of folate stores and megaloblastic anemia resulting from chronic hemolysis

Cyclosporine is available in the United States in two encapsulated and solution formulations for oral administration: Cyclosporine (Sandimmune®; Novartis) and Cyclosporine Modified. The modified and unmodified products are distinguished by marked differences in oral bioavailability and cannot be used interchangeably without carefully monitoring cyclosporine blood concentrations and dose adjustments based on individual response. Both formulations are marketed in two strengths: 25 mg and 100 mg cyclosporine. Cyclosporine and Cyclosporine [Modified] also are available in solution formulations for oral administration.
Cyclosporine: Sandimmune® 25-mg and 100-mg capsules contain cyclosporine (Novartis Pharmaceuticals Corporation, East Hanover, NJ); Sandimmune® Oral Solution contains cyclosporine 100 mg/mL (Novartis Pharmaceuticals Corporation)
Cyclosporine [modified]: NEORAL® 25-mg and 100-mg capsules contain cyclosporine [modified] (Novartis Pharmaceuticals Corporation); NEORAL® Oral Solution contains cyclosporine [modified] 100 mg/mL (Novartis Pharmaceuticals Corporation); GENGRAF® 25-mg and 100-mg capsules contain cyclosporine [modified] (Abbott Laboratories, North Chicago, IL); GENGRAF® Oral Solution contains cyclosporine [modified] (Abbott Laboratories)

Emetogenic potential: Nonemetogenic (Emetogenicity score = 1). See Chapter 39 for antiemetic regimens

Treatment Modifications

Adverse Event	Dose Modification
First episode of serum creatinine >125% of baseline, confirmed within 2 weeks, or first episode of serum creatinine >150%	Reduce cyclosporine dosage by 25–50% for 6–10 days. If serum creatinine returns to baseline, resume original cyclosporine dosage. If serum creatinine does not return to normal, reduce cyclosporine dosage an additional 25%
Second episode of serum creatinine >125% of baseline	Reduce cyclosporine dosage by 25–50%; do not attempt to reinstitute original dosage
Third episode of serum creatinine >125% of baseline	Discontinue cyclosporine
Increase in LFTs by 25–50% above baseline	Reduce cyclosporine dosage by 25–50% for 6–10 days. If LFTs return to baseline, resume original cyclosporine dosage. If LFTs do not return to normal, reduce cyclosporine dosage an additional 25%
Second episode of LFTs 25–50% above baseline	Reduce cyclosporine dosage by 25–50%; do not attempt to re-institute original dosage
Hypertension develops in a patient with no history of hypertension	Reduce cyclosporine dosage by 25–50% for 6–10 days. If blood pressure returns to baseline with or without treatment, resume original cyclosporine dosage. Consider calcium channel blockers or β-blockers as first-line therapy
Recurrent hypertension despite multiple cyclosporine dose reductions or when adequate adjustment of antihypertensive therapy not possible	Discontinue cyclosporine

Patient Population Studied

Cyclosporine has been administered in limited numbers of patients with refractory AIHA alone or in the setting of Evans syndrome

Toxicity

	Frequency
Mild–moderate hypertension	Common
Nephrotoxicity	Common/reversible
Hepatotoxicity	Common/reversible
Cyclosporine sensitivity	Infrequent
Cremophor® EL sensitivity	Infrequent
Anaphylaxis	Infrequent (~1:1000)
Hypomagnesemia	Infrequent
Tremor	Infrequent
Hirsutism	Infrequent
Gum hypertrophy	Infrequent
Secondary malignancies	Infrequent
Hyperkalemia ± hyperchloremic metabolic acidosis	Infrequent
Thrombocytopenia and microangiopathic hemolytic anemia	Infrequent

Cyclosporine is contraindicated if the patient has a hypersensitivity to cyclosporine and/or Cremophor® EL

Efficacy (N = 5)

Coombs' (+) AIHA (3 patients)	3 Complete response
ITP + AIHA (1 patient)	1 Complete response
Evans syndrome (1 patient)	1 Partial response

Responses were dependent on continuation of cyclosporine. Two deaths (stroke and lung cancer); median follow-up of 31 months (13-62)

Coombs' (+) AIHA + CLL (2 pts)	↑ gb/↓ steroids
Coombs' (−) AIHA + CLL (1)	↑ Hgb/↓ steroids

Emilia G et al. Br J Haematol 1996;93:341–344

Monitoring Therapy

1. *Baseline:* Serum creatinine (on 2 occasions), BUN, CBC with differential, magnesium, potassium, uric acid, and lipoproteins

Note: Measurement of lipoproteins are recommended because levels may increase modestly during therapy

2. *First 3 months:* Serum creatinine, BUN and other baseline lab parameters plus blood pressure every 2 weeks; thereafter, stable patients monitored monthly

Note: Measure serum creatinine with initiation of new NSAID therapy or if a concomitantly used NSAID is increased in dose

3. *Cyclosporine levels:* Weekly for 2–3 months and then once per month

The type of cyclosporine assay used to monitor blood levels is important. Recommended trough levels for the cyclosporine parent compound depend on the type of assay used (high-performance liquid chromatography versus radioimmunoassay versus fluorescence polarization immunoassay) and vary by whole blood versus serum/plasma. Levels are based on cyclosporine monitoring in the transplant setting

Note: Monitor drug-drug interactions that may alter renal function and either increase or decrease cyclosporine concentrations

Treatment Modifications

(continued)

Tremor, headache, confusion, paresthesias, lethargy, or weakness	Reduce cyclosporine dosage by 25–50% for 6–10 days. If symptoms resolve, resume cyclosporine at the original dosage or a dosage 25% less than that in use when symptoms first appeared. If symptoms persist, reduce dosage an additional 25%

Notes

1. Every 10 months, discontinue cyclosporine for 2 weeks to evaluate for persistence of response
2. Cyclosporine levels correlating with AIHA response have not been systematically reported

REGIMEN FOR REFRACTORY WARM ANTIBODY AUTOIMMUNE HEMOLYTIC ANEMIA

IMMUNE GLOBULIN INTRAVENOUS (HUMAN) (IVIG)

Centers for Disease Control and Prevention (CDC). MMWR Morb Mortal Wkly Rep 1999;48:518–521
Epstein et al. September 29, 1999. Rockville, MD: Center for Biologics Evaluation and Research, Food and Drug Administration
Flores G et al. Am J Hematol 1993;44:237–242
Go RS, Call TG. Mayo Clin Proc 2000;75:83–85
Ratko TA et al. JAMA 1995;273:1865–1870

Hydration before immune globulin intravenous (human) (IVIG):
Ensure that patients are not dehydrated before administration. Dehydration is a risk factor for renal failure. Patients who are well hydrated do not need additional hydration

Note: Patients at an increased risk for developing ARF include those with any degree of preexisting renal dysfunction, diabetes, volume depletion, sepsis, paraproteinemia, age >65 years, and those receiving concomitant nephrotoxic drugs. The risk for renal impairment and thrombotic events associated with IVIG also correlate with administration rate and product osmolality. The best recommendation is to not exceed the administration recommendations published in the product labeling

Immune globulin intravenous (human):
0.4–0.5 g/kg per day intravenously (consult product labeling for appropriate administration rates) daily for 2–5 days

Note: For sucrose-containing products, *do not exceed* a maximum infusion rate of 3 mg sucrose/kg (patient's body weight) per minute

Supportive care:
Folic acid 1 mg/day orally to prevent depletion of folate stores and megaloblastic anemia resulting from chronic hemolysis

Patient Population

A University Hospital Consortium Expert panel on IVIG and AIHA found that:

1. IVIG *may have a role* in patients with warm-type AIHA that does not respond to glucocorticoids
2. Evidence does not exist for the routine use of IVIG in AIHA

Ratko TA et al. JAMA 1995;273:1865–1870

Efficacy (Reports and 3 case series, N = 62)

Response to therapy	54.5%
Hgb increased >2 g/dL	40%
Hgb increased >2 g/dL + peak Hgb ≥10 g/dL	14.5%
Days to achieve a response	10
Weeks Hgb elevated in responders	≥3

Monitoring Therapy

1. *Before IVIG:* BUN and serum creatinine
2. *Daily during IVIG administration:* BUN, serum creatinine, weight, and urine output monitoring

Treatment Modifications

Adverse Event or Condition	Dose Modification
Preexisting renal insufficiency	Decrease the rate of administration of the immune globulin. If permitted, dilute IVIG to decrease its osmolality. Ensure adequate hydration.
Diabetes mellitus	
Age >65 years	
Paraproteinemia	
Concomitant use of nephrotoxic drugs	
Sepsis	
Deteriorating renal function	Discontinue IVIG

Toxicity

Side effects occurring in 1–10% of patients
1. Infusion reactions[a]
2. Back or chest pain or tightness
3. Malaise and myalgia
4. Nausea and vomiting
5. Headache
6. Fever and chills
7. Renal damage[b]

Side effects occurring in <1% of patients
1. Thrombosis (myocardial infarct, stroke, spinal cord ischemia)
2. Aseptic meningitis syndrome with doses ≥2 g/kg
3. Alloimmune hemolysis

[a]Fall in blood pressure and anaphylaxis even in patients without a history of sensitivity to immunoglobulins
Note: Contraindications include a history of allergic response to thimerosal, systemic allergic response to gammaglobulin or patients with anti-IgA Ab or isolated IgA deficiency
[b]Increased serum creatinine, oliguria, or renal failure; 90% with sucrose-containing IVIG; 61% with renal predisposing factors; 100% onset in 7 days; 40% required dialysis; 10-day mean recovery time; 15% died despite therapy

REGIMEN FOR REFRACTORY WARM ANTIBODY AUTOIMMUNE HEMOLYTIC ANEMIA

MYCOPHENOLATE MOFETIL (MMF)

Howard J et al. Br J Haematol 2002;117:712–715
Zimmer-Molsberger B et al. Lancet 1997;350:1003–1004

Starting dose:
Mycophenolate mofetil 1000 mg/day orally as a single dose or 500 mg twice daily

or

Mycophenolate mofetil 1000 mg/day intravenously diluted with 5% dextrose injection (D5W) to a concentration of 6 mg/mL over at least 2 hours daily (total dose/week = 7000 mg)

Maintenance dose after 2 weeks:
Mycophenolate mofetil 1000 mg/dose orally twice daily

or

Mycophenolate mofetil 1000 mg/dose intravenously diluted with D5W to a concentration of 6 mg/mL over at least 2 hours twice daily (total dose/week = 14,000 mg)

Supportive care:
Folic acid 1 mg/day orally to prevent depletion of folate stores and megaloblastic anemia resulting from chronic hemolysis

Mycophenolate mofetil is marketed in the United States as CellCept® in the following formulations: oral capsules 250 mg, oral tablets 500 mg, oral suspension 200 mg/mL, and mycophenolate mofetil hydrochloride for parenteral injection 500 mg

Emetogenic potential: Nonemetogenic to low (Emetogenicity score ≤2). See Chapter 39 for antiemetic regimens

Patient Population Studied

MMF has been administered off-label in limited numbers of patients with AIHA treated with prior immunosuppressive regimens including glucocorticoids ± splenectomy. Concomitant medications have included prednisolone, cyclosporine, and IVIG

Efficacy

All four patients with AIHA showed a complete or good partial response to treatment with MMF

Monitoring Therapy

CBC with differential: Weekly during the first month, twice monthly during the second and third months, then monthly. Thereafter, CBC with differential monthly for the first year

Treatment Modifications

Adverse Event or Condition	Dose Modification
ANC <1300/mm³	Temporarily discontinue mycophenolate mofetil, or reduce dose and monitor as appropriate

Toxicity[a]

	%[b]
Diarrhea	30–36
Constipation	18–41
Leukopenia (dose-related)	~10
Nausea	20–55
Vomiting	12
Hypertension	28–78
Sepsis	2–5
GI bleeding	1.7–5.4
Severe neutropenia	2–3.6
Lymphoma and other malignancies	0.4–1
Weakness	20
Headache	5–20
Insomnia	10–50
Renal tubular necrosis	5–10

[a]Risk of acquiring opportunistic infections (bacterial, fungal, viral) increased by treatment with mycophenolate mofetil

[b]Patients who received mycophenolate mofetil 2000 mg/day or 3000 mg/day

Notes

Recommended for clinicians experienced in renal, hepatic, or cardiac transplantation and immunosuppressive therapy

REGIMEN FOR CYTOTOXIC THERAPY

CHLORAMBUCIL

Hippe E et al. Blood 1970;35:68–72
Petz LD, Garratty G: Blood transfusion in autoimmune hemolytic anemias. In: Petz LD, Garratty G, eds. Immune Hemolytic Anemias, 2nd ed. New York: Churchill Livingstone, 2004:375–400
Leukeran® (chlorambucil) Tablets, product label, November 2004. GlaxoSmithKline, Research Triangle Park, NC

Idiopathic Cold Agglutinin Syndrome

Chlorambucil 2–4 mg/day orally as a staring dose (total dose/week = 14–28 mg)

Notes:

- Increase dosage in 2-mg increments every 2 months until a favorable response or dose-limiting toxicity occurs
- With achievement of a favorable response, additional options include intermittent treatment as required or maintenance therapy
- Although doses as high as 8–20 mg/day may be reached, with continued therapy these may have to be reduced to as low as 2 mg/day

Supportive care:

Folic acid 1 mg/day orally to prevent depletion of folate stores and megaloblastic anemia resulting from chronic hemolysis

Chlorambucil is formulated in the United States for oral administration as tablets containing 2 mg

Emetogenic potential: Nonemetogenic at low doses, but emetogenicity correlates directly with dose. See Chapter 39 for antiemetic regimens

Treatment Modifications

Adjust chlorambucil therapy to maintain "slight degree of marrow suppression" manifested as mild thrombocytopenia or leukopenia. Although a "slight degree of marrow suppression" was not further defined in these studies, consider using NCI CTC grade 1 toxicity as a reasonable benchmark:
WBC: 3000/mm^3 to lower limits of normal
ANC: ≥1500/mm^3 to <2000/mm^3
Platelets: ≥75,000/mm^3 to lower limits of normal
Hemoglobin: 10 g/dL to lower limit of normal

Adverse Event	Dose Modification
If WBC <3000/mm^3 or ANC <1500/mm^3 or platelets <75,000/mm^3	Hold therapy for a minimum of 1 week. Restart only when WBC >3000/mm^3 and ANC >1500/mm^3 and platelets >75,000/^{3}; then starting with a dosage reduction of 25%

Patient Population Studied

Patients with idiopathic cold agglutinin syndrome producing symptomatic anemia, Raynaud's phenomenon, or cold intolerance (off-label use)

Efficacy (N = 15)

Improvement with therapy: 67% (10/15), including one patient who had improvements in acrocyanosis, thermal amplitude and cold agglutinin titer despite a falling Hgb on therapy (Petz LD, Garratty G)

Case series of 4 patients with idiopathic cold agglutinin syndrome (Hippe E et al):

Thermal amplitude:	Decreased a mean of 3.8°C
Hgb values:	Increased from 10.5 to 12.4 g/dL
IgM mean values:	Decreased from 8.8 to 2.2 g/dL
Raynaud's phenomenon:	Resolved in all patients

Toxicity

Potential side effects include:

1. Leukopenia
2. Thrombocytopenia
3. Infection
4. Oral ulcers
5. Hypersensitivity and fever
6. Hepatotoxicity
7. Infertility
8. Seizures
9. Gastrointestinal toxicity
10. Interstitial pneumonitis
11. Secondary malignancy
12. Fetal harm (contraception recommended)

Monitoring Therapy

CBC with differential: Twice per week during the first 3–6 weeks of therapy or after a dose adjustment, then weekly until counts stabilize, and then every 2 weeks

Notes

Intermittent use of chlorambucil has been reported to be beneficial in limited numbers of patients with seasonal precipitation of symptomatic idiopathic CAS where the occupational environment required cold weather exposure

61. Sickle Cell Disease: Acute Complications

James N. Frame, MD, Steven J. Jubelirer, MD, and Griffin P. Rodgers, MD

Epidemiology

Definition

Sickle cell disease (SCD) usually refers to the homozygous state of Hb SS or sickle cell anemia (SCA), but may include doubly heterozygous states in which the presence of intracellular Hb S polymerization leads to chronic hemolytic anemia, vaso-occlusive crises of varying severity and frequency with cumulative organ damage, and systemic manifestations that include impairment in growth, development, and susceptibility to infection

Incidence	
SCA	Millions worldwide
SCA	~1 in 500 African-American births (~72,000) in the United States
	1 in 1000 to 1400 Hispanic babies each year
Sickle cell trait	1 in 12 African Americans (~2 million people) in the United States
Mortality*	
US median life expectancy for Hb SS males	42 years
US median life expectancy for Hb SS females	48 years

*Mortality reductions have been attributed to several factors: development of sickle cell treatment programs, increased clinical research in SCD, and establishment of newborn screening programs combined with penicillin prophylaxis

Platt OS et al. NEJM 1994;330:1639–1644
Sickle Cell Research for Treatment and Cure. NIH Publication No. 02-5214 (2002):1–16
www.nlm.nih.gov/medlineplus.sicklecellanemia.html (Dept. of Energy, Human Genome Project)

Pathology: Major Sickle Hemoglobinopathies

	% of Patients[a]	MCV (fL)	Hb (g/dL)	% Hb A/A_2	% Hb F	% Hb S
SCD-SS	65	80–100	6–10	0/2–3	2–15	>85
SCD-SC	25	75–90	10–12	0/0	1–7	50%[b]
SCD-Sβ^+-thalassemia	8	65–75	8–12	5-30/3–6	2–10	70–90
SCD-Sβ-thalassemia	2	65–85	6–10	0/4–6	2–15	>85
SCD-S$\delta\beta$-thalassemia	<1	60–80	10–12	0/N-low[c]	10–15	>80
S-HPFH[e] pancellular	<1	80–90	12–13[d]	0/1–3	20–30	>70

[a]Approximate percentage of US patients determined by neonatal screening
[b]50% Hb C
[c]Hb A_2 normal to low
[d]Hct 38–40%
[e]HPFH, hereditary persistence of fetal hemoglobin

The Management of Sickle Cell Disease. NIH Publication No. 02-2117 (revised 2002, 4th ed) 7–14
Adams III JG. Clinical laboratory diagnosis. In: Embury SH et al. eds. Sickle Cell Disease: Basic Principles and Clinical Practice. New York: Raven Press,1994:457–468
Glader BE. Anemia. In: Embury SH et al, eds. Sickle Cell Disease: Basic Principles and Clinical Practice. New York: Raven Press, 1994:545–554
Kinney TR et al. Br J Haematol 1978;38:15–22
Murray N et al. Br J Haematol 1988;69:89–92
Sickle cell disease: clinical and epidemiologic aspects. In: Bunn HF, Forget BG, eds. Hemoglobin: Molecular, Genetic and Clinical Aspects. Philadelphia: WB Sanders, 1986:502–564

Acute Pain Syndrome

Ballas SK. Semin Hematol 2001;38:307–314
Ballas SK et al. Guidelines for Standard Care of Acute Painful Episodes in Patients with Sickle Cell Disease 2000, Pennsylvania Dept. of Health
Castro O et al. Blood 1994;84:643–649
Rees DC et al. Br J Haematol 2003;120:744–752
The Management of Sickle Cell Disease. NIH Publication No. 02-2117 (revised 2002, 4th ed) 59–74

Epidemiology

1. In SCD, pain is the most common complaint and reason for patients to consult doctors and to be admitted to the hospital
2. Among patients with SCD in the United States, an acute pain episode accounts for ~90% of visits to the ER and 70% of all hospitalizations
3. Mean rate per year of acute pain episodes:
   Hb SS (0.8)
   Hb Sβ-thalassemia (1.0)
   Hb SC (0.4)
4. The rate of painful crises increases over the first three decades of life and then declines owing to the earlier mortality of adults with higher rates of pain

Clinical Features

1. Most common type of pain
2. Unpredictably abrupt in onset
3. Sometimes migratory
4. Varies in intensity from a mild ache to a severe and debilitating pain
5. Acute pain may occur with chronic pain, and frequent episodes of acute pain can resemble chronic pain
6. In adults, about one-third of episodes are associated with a preceding or concurrent infection
7. Factors that potentate Hb S polymerization may precipitate an acute painful episode. These factors include acidosis, hypoxia, and dehydration

Treatment

Pay close attention to oxygenation, hydration and acid-base balance

Initial management in the ER, the day treatment center, or as a direct admission to the hospital:

1. **Assess** the patient for cause of **pain and complications.** Rapid pain assessment with simple self-reported pain scale
2. **Hydration** with 5% dextrose injection (D5W) or 5% dextrose injection with 0.225% NaCl (D5W/$\frac{1}{4}$ NS) at a rate not to exceed 1.5 × maintenance (volume to include any drug infusions)
3. **Institute opioids or other analgesic therapy**
   Adults >50 kg not on chronic opioid therapy:
   - **Morphine sulfate** 5–10 mg per slow intravenous push or subcutaneously every 2–4 hours, *or*
   - **Hydromorphone** 1.5 mg per slow intravenous push or subcutaneously every 3–4 hours

   Adults <50 kg not on chronic opioid therapy:
   - **Morphine sulfate** 0.1–0.15 mg/kg per slow intravenous push or subcutaneously every 2–4 hours, *or*
   - **Hydromorphone** 0.015–0.020 mg/kg per slow intravenous push or subcutaneously every 3–4 hours

   Adults currently on chronic opioid therapy:
   - Consult old records, patient, and family to identify what medications/doses have been effective
4. **Assess** degree of **pain relief** every 15–30 minutes. Add **combination therapy** as indicated
   - Anti-inflammatory medications, such as:

     Ketorolac (multiple-dose treatment)
     <65 years: **Ketorolac** 30 mg intravenously over at least 15 seconds or slowly and deeply intramuscularly every 6 hours (maximum daily parenteral dose = 120 mg)
     ≥65 years, <50 kg, or renally impaired (*see manufacturer's warnings): **Ketorolac** 15 mg intravenously over at least 15 seconds or slowly and deeply intramuscularly every 6 hours (maximum daily parenteral dose = 60 mg)

     Ketorolac (transition from IV/IM to oral)
     <65 years: **Ketorolac** 10-mg tablets, 2 tablets (20 mg) orally as a first dose followed by one 10-mg tablet every 4–6 hours (maximum dose not to exceed 40 mg/24 hours)
     ≥65 years, <50 kg, or renally impaired (*see manufacturer's warnings): **Ketorolac** 10-mg tablets, 1 tablet as first oral dose followed by 1 tablet every 4–6 hours (maximum dose not to exceed 40 mg/24 hours)

     Note: In adults, the maximum combined duration of ketorolac use (parenteral and oral) is limited to 5 days. The use of an H_2-blocker has been recommended to reduce GI side effects. (Also, see Perlin E et al. Am J Hematol 1994;46:43–47)

*Toradol® IV/IM/ORAL (ketorolac tromethamine injection/tablets). Product information. Roche Pharmaceuticals (revised Sept. 2002)

Subacute management:

1. *Moderate pain relief, acceptable toxicities:* Begin opioid analgesics on an around-the-clock (ATC) schedule
2. *Moderate pain relief, toxicities not acceptable:* Add **combination therapy** to include anti-inflammatory medications, such as **ibuprofen** 400–600 mg orally, every 6 hours (consider adding an H_2-blocker to reduce risk of GI side effects)
3. *Moderate pain relief not achieved:* Continue to adjust therapy by increasing the dose until pain is relieved. Increase dose in increments of 25–50% of the opioid analgesic loading dose

Disposition:

1. Discharge:
   - If ATC dosing and treatment are effective without complications, treat at home with oral medication to maintain adequate pain and arrange follow-up with clinician managing SCD
2. Admit:
   - If ATC dosing and treatment are not effective or with complications
   - If ATC dosing and treatment cannot be maintained at home on oral medications
   - If patient is not on ATC dosing and treatment is not effective

Supportive care:

Laxatives to avoid or treat constipation

(Rees DC et al. Br J Haematol 2003;120:744–752):
Lactulose 10 mL orally twice daily
Senna 2–4 tablets orally each day
Docusate 100 mg orally twice daily

Notes

1. **Hydration.** There is theoretical and empiric evidence that rehydration with a hypotonic solution [5% dextrose injection (D5W) or 5% dextrose injection with 0.225% NaCl (D5W/$\frac{1}{4}$NS)], unless clinically contraindicated (eg, in brain injury or severe hyponatremia), is preferable. Such therapy has been shown to swell red cells, reduce the MCHC, and thereby reduce the rate and extent of intracellular Hb S polymer formation (see: A study of induced hyponatremia in the prevention and treatment of sickle-cell crisis. NEJM 1980;303: 1138–1143)
2. **Published opioid analgesic tables vary in suggested doses that are equianalgesic to morphine.** Clinical response is the criterion that must be applied for each patient; titration to clinical response is necessary. Because there is not complete cross-tolerance among these drugs, it is usually necessary to use a lower equianalgesic dose when changing drugs and to re-titrate to response
3. **Hypovolemia should be corrected before administering ketorolac, and NSAIDS should be used with caution** in patients with congestive heart failure, dehydration, hypovolemia, and any other conditions that may compromise renal blood flow and increase the risk of developing renal toxicity. Ketorolac should be used with caution in patients with impaired hepatic function or a history of liver disease
4. **Ketorolac is contraindicated in patients with:** (1) active peptic ulcer disease (PUD), (2) recent GI bleeding or perforation, (3) a history of PUD or GI bleeding, (4) advanced renal impairment or risk for renal failure due to volume depletion, (5) previously demonstrated hypersensitivity to ketorolac, other NSAIDs, or aspirin, or patients currently receiving aspirin or NSAIDs, (6) suspected or confirmed cerebrovascular bleeding, hemorrhagic diathesis, or incomplete hemostasis. Ketorolac should not be used in nursing mothers

Acute Chest Syndrome

Ballas SK. Semin Hematol 2001;38:307–314
Bellet PS et al. NEJM 1995;333:699–703
Charache A et al. NEJM 1995;332:1317–1322
Emre U et al. J Pediatr 1993;123:272–275
Short-acting inhaled β-adrenergic agonist therapy. In: Koda-Kimble MA et al, eds. Applied Therapeutics: The Clinical Use of Drugs, 8th ed. Philadelphia: Lippincott Williams & Wilkins, 2005:23–27
The Management of Sickle Cell Disease. NIH Publication No. 02-2117 (revised 2002, 4th ed) 103–106
Vichinsky EP et al. NEJM 2000;342:1855–1865

Definition

Multicenter Acute Chest Syndrome Study (MACSS) definition: A pulmonary infiltrate consistent with consolidation, *plus at least one of the following*:

- Chest pain
- Fever >38.5°C
- Tachypnea
- Wheezing
- Cough

Associated conditions:

- Pulmonary infarction (30%)
- Pulmonary fat embolization (16%)
- Infection (33%), including chlamydia (13%), mycoplasma (12%), viruses (12%), and bacterial isolates (8%), which include *Staphylococcus aureus, Streptococcus pneumoniae, Haemophilus influenzae, Escherichia Coli and Legionella*

Vichinsky EP et al. NEJM 2000;342:1855–1865

Epidemiology

1. Acute chest syndrome is the second most common cause of hospitalization in SCD and the most common complication of surgery and anesthesia
2. **Incidence (per 100 patient-years):**
   Hb SS overall (12.8)
   Hb SS ages 2–4 years (25.3)
   Hb SS adults (8.8)
   Hb Sβ-thalassemia (9.4)
   Hb SC (5.2)
   Hb Sβ$^+$-thalassemia (3.9)
3. **In-hospital mortality:**
   9% for adults
   <2% for children

Treatment

Carefully monitor oxygenation, hydration, and acid-base balance. Obtain daily weight, input/output, CBC, and appropriate serum chemistry panels. Measure baseline and pre-/post-transfusion Hb S concentration. Follow chest x-rays until stabilization is documented

1. **Oxygen** by nasal cannula at a rate of 2 L/minute or higher if needed to maintain a PaO_2 of 70–80 mm Hg
2. **Hydration** with 5% dextrose injection (D5W) or 5% dextrose injection with 0.225% NaCl (D5W/$\frac{1}{4}$ NS) at a rate not to exceed 1.5 × maintenance (volume to include any drug infusions)
3. **Bronchodilator therapy** for patients with reactive airway disease (eg, adults with asthma):
   - **Albuterol** nebulizer solution (5 mg/mL) 2.5–5 mg by nebulizer every 20 minutes for up to 3 doses, followed by 2.5 –10 mg every 1 to 4 hours as needed **or**
   - **Albuterol metered-dose inhaler** (90 mcg/puff) 4–8 puffs every 20 minutes up to 4 hours, followed by 4–8 puffs every 1–4 hours as needed
4. **Institute opioids or other analgesic therapy** to prevent hypoventilation (see previous section on Acute Pain Syndrome)
5. **Incentive spirometry** protocol to prevent hypoventilation in patients able to perform it
6. **Transfuse packed RBCs** to achieve a Hb S concentration of <30–40% or to a stable Hb of 8–9 g/dL (See later section on Red Blood Cell Transfusion)
   Indications:
   - Poor respiratory function
   - PaO_2 <70 mm Hg on room air
   - A decline in PaO_2 of >10% from baseline in a patient with chronic hypoxia

   Note: Exchange transfusion should be undertaken in patients with a high baseline Hb and in whom transfusion of RBCs is recommended (eg, goal to reduce the Hct to <30%), signs of increasing infiltrate on chest x-ray, if the PaO_2 cannot be maintained above 70 Torr or if the patient is experiencing dyspnea or tachypnea (also see later section on Red Blood Cell Transfusion)
7. Antibiotics should be given to febrile or severely ill patients:
   A **third-generation cephalosporin:**
   Ceftriaxone 1000–2000 mg intravenously in 50 mL D5W over 30 minutes every 24 hours, *and*
   A **broad-spectrum macrolide or fluoroquinolone antibiotic:**
   Azithromycin 500 mg intravenously in 250 mL D5W over 60 minutes every 24 hours, *or*
   Ciprofloxacin 400 mg intravenously in 200 mL D5W over 60 minutes every 12 hours

Notes

1. Assess baseline oxygenation and continue to monitor ABGs as needed. The A-a gradient appears to be the best predictor of clinical severity
2. Limit hydration; avoid fluid overload
3. Incentive spirometry is encouraged because it reduces the risk of acute chest syndrome by 88% in patients hospitalized with thoracic bone ischemia/infarction.
4. The goal of transfusion therapy is to prevent progression of acute chest syndrome to acute respiratory failure. Transfusions may not be required if the decline in A-a gradient is due to chest wall splinting that corrects with adequate analgesic therapy and incentive spirometry
5. Infection is a contributing factor as cause of death in 56% of acute chest syndrome patients. Organisms include *S. pneumoniae, Escherichia. coli, H. influenzae, Legionella, S. aureus,* cytomegalovirus, and chlamydia as well as atypical microorganisms (eg, *C. pneumoniae, Mycoplasma. pneumoniae*)
6. In acute chest syndrome patients, it is often difficult to exclude a bacterial superinfection from a lung infarct

Acute Cholecystitis

Gallbladder (cholecystitis). In: Gilbert DN, Mollering RC, Sand MA. The Sanford Guide to Antimicrobial Therapy 2005, 35th ed. Hyde Park, VT: Antimicrobial Therapy, Inc, 2005:10
Nzeh DA et al. Pediatr Radiol 1989;19:290–292
The Management of Sickle Cell Disease. NIH Publication No. 02-2117 (revised 2002, 4th ed) 111–117
Walker TM et al. J Pediatr 2000;135:80–85

Epidemiology

1. *Cholelithiasis* occurs as early as 2–4 years of age; incidence progressively increases with age. ~30% of 18-year-old patients have *cholelithiasis*
2. The natural history of asymptomatic *cholelithiasis* is unknown; however, up to 30% of patients may develop symptoms or complications within 3 years. The prevalence of *cholelithiasis* appears to be lower in patients co-inheriting α- or β-thalassemia
3. Acute attacks of *cholecystitis* are difficult to differentiate from hepatic crisis
4. Patients with sickle cell trait have no increased risk of developing pigment stones

Treatment

Treatment for acute cholecystitis is similar to that of the general population

1. **Hydration (as clinically indicated)** with 5% dextrose injection (D5W) or 5% dextrose injection with 0.225% NaCl (D5W/$\frac{1}{4}$ NS) at a rate not to exceed 1.5 × maintenance (volume to include any drug infusions)
2. **Institute opioids or other analgesic therapy** as appropriate based on clinical symptoms with superimposed vaso-occlusive crises (see previous section on Acute Pain Syndrome)
3. **Antimicrobial therapy** to include:

   Piperacillin 3000 mg + **tazobactam** 375 mg intravenously in 100 mL D5W or 0.9% NaCl injection (0.9% NS) over 30 minutes every 6 hours, *or*
   Imepenem/cilastin 500 mg intravenously in 100 mL D5W or 0.9% NS over 30 minutes every 6 hours (if life-threatening)
4. **Elective cholecystectomy** is recommended several weeks after an acute episode subsides, given the greater operative risks during an episode of acute cholecystitis in SCD

   Note: Although cholecystectomy in asymptomatic patients is controversial, an aggressive surgical approach has the benefit of reducing the risk of complications arising from cholecystitis and eliminating the gallbladder as a confounding diagnosis in right upper quadrant pain. Laparoscopic cholecystectomy on an elective basis in a well-prepared patient has been reported to be the standard surgical approach to symptomatic patients

Acute Hepatic Sequestration (Right Upper Quadrant Syndrome)

Diggs LW. Am J Clin Pathol 1965;44:1–4 (AHS)
Rosse WF et al. New views of sickle cell disease: pathophysiology and treatment. In: Hematology 2000, American Society of Hematology Education Program Book:2–17
The Management of Sickle Cell Disease. NIH Publication No. 02-2117 (revised 2002, 4th ed) 111-6

Epidemiology

1. A rarely recognized complication of vaso-occlusive crisis in SCD
2. Prevalence in SCD is not well described
3. About 10% of Hb SS patients develop a transient and lesser-form of intrahepatic cholestasis that is usually self-limited

Clinical Features

- Right upper quadrant (RUQ) pain simulating acute cholecystitis
- Fever
- Jaundice
- Elevations in hepatic transaminases
- Marked elevations in serum bilirubin/alkaline phosphatase
- Progressive hepatomegaly

Note: The rapid decrease in transaminases differentiates hepatic crisis from the slower decline characteristic of acute viral hepatitis

Treatment

Carefully monitor oxygenation, hydration, and acid-base balance. Obtain daily weight, input/output, CBC, and appropriate serum chemistry panels. Measure baseline and pre-/post-transfusion Hb S concentration

1. **Hydration** with 5% dextrose injection (D5W) or 5% dextrose injection with 0.225% NaCl (D5W/$\frac{1}{4}$ NS) at a rate not to exceed 1.5 × maintenance (volume to include any drug infusions)

   Note: In the event of hypervolemia, diuretic therapy may be required
2. **Oxygen** by nasal cannula at a rate of 2 L/minute or higher if needed to maintain a PaO_2 of 70–80 mm Hg
3. **Institute opioids or other analgesic therapy** based on clinical symptoms (see previous section on Acute Pain Syndrome)
4. **Transfuse** packed RBCs to maintain Hb close to baseline and Hb S <30%

   Note: Exchange transfusion is the preferred method of transfusion, although simple transfusion may be considered. Fatal hyperviscosity syndrome may result from simple transfusion while an episode of hepatic sequestration resolves. A rapid increase in the serum Hb from sequestered RBCs accounts for this clinical finding. Patients should be carefully monitored in the recovery phase of acute hepatic sequestration for an acutely rising Hb, which could place the patient at risk for hyperviscosity. If suspected, promptly institute exchange transfusion with a goal of reducing the Hct to <30% (also see section on Acute Splenic Sequestration: Hyperviscosity)

Differential Diagnosis

Differential diagnosis of RUQ syndrome in a patient with SCD who presents with RUQ pain and abnormal LFTs includes:

- Acute cholecystitis
- Acute viral hepatitis
- Biloma
- Focal nodular hyperplasia in children
- Fungal ball
- Hepatic artery stenosis
- Hepatic infarct/abscess
- Hepatic vein thrombosis
- Mesenteric/colonic ischemia
- Pancreatitis
- Periappendiceal abscess
- Pericolonic abscess
- Pulmonary infarct/abscess
- Renal vein thrombosis

Acute Splenic Sequestration

Glader B. Anemia. In: Embury SH et al, eds. Sickle Cell Disease: Basic Principles and Clinical Practice. New York: Raven Press, 1996:548–549
Rosse WF et al. New views of sickle cell disease: pathophysiology and treatment. In: Hematology 2000, American Society of Hematology Education Program Book:2–17
Solanki DL et al. Am J Med 1986;80:985–990
The Management of Sickle Cell Disease. NIH Publication No. 02-2117 (revised 2002, 4th ed) 119–122

Epidemiology

1. Most cases occur in children <2 years of age with Hb SS. Almost all cases occur by age 6 years
2. Attacks may be associated with or preceded by bacterial or viral infections
3. Acute chest syndrome has been reported to complicate acute splenic syndrome in 20% of cases
4. Acute splenic sequestration occurs less frequently in Hb SC and Hb Sβ^+-thalassemia disease, but may occur beyond childhood because of persistent splenomegaly
5. Although rarely seen in adults, it may occur with persistent splenic function in patients with concurrent α-thalassemia
6. A mortality rate of 12% has been reported with first attacks in SCD-SS (Hb SS)
7. Recurrent episodes may occur in 50% with a mortality rate of 20%

Clinical Features

- Acutely enlarging spleen
- Decrease in steady state Hb concentration by at least 2 g/dL and evidence of increased erythropoiesis (eg, marked elevations in the reticulocyte count or nucleated RBCs)
- In more severe episodes, hypovolemic shock may complicate precipitous drops in Hb with marked splenic enlargement

Treatment

Acute management:
Carefully monitor oxygenation, hydration, and acid-base balance. Obtain daily weight, input/output, CBC, and appropriate serum chemistry panels. Measure baseline and pre-/post-transfusion Hb S concentration

Immediate treatment:

1. **Oxygen** by nasal cannula at a rate of 2 L/minute or higher if needed to maintain a PaO_2 of 70–80 mm Hg
2. **Hydration** with 5% dextrose injection (D5W) or 5% dextrose injection with 0.225% NaCl (D5W/$\frac{1}{4}$ NS) at a rate not to exceed 1.5 × maintenance (volume to include any drug infusions)
3. **Transfuse packed RBCs** by simple transfusion to maintain the patient's baseline Hb level

   Note: After transfusion therapy and correction of hypovolemia, remobilization of sequestered RBCs may result in a Hb increase greater than that predicted on the basis of the volume of administered RBCs. Because this can lead to hypervolemia, careful monitoring is indicated and use of diuretic therapy may be required. If hyperviscosity is contributing an important role in the pathogenesis of an acute complication of SCD, exchange transfusion using a mechanical device directed at reducing the hyperviscosity should be performed. The goal of this therapy would be to reduce the Hct to <30%

Chronic management:
After the acute episode of splenic sequestration, subsequent management is influenced by the high recurrence rate of this syndrome

1. Chronic transfusions are recommended in children <2 years of age after a severe episode to keep Hb S levels <30% until splenectomy can be considered after 2 years of age
2. Splenectomy is recommended in patients who experience a life-threatening episode of acute splenic sequestration shortly after being placed on a chronic transfusion program. A splenectomy can also be considered in patients with chronic hypersplenism

Acute Pain Syndrome: Priapism

Mantadakis E et al. Blood 2000;95:78–82
Rackoff WR et al. J Pediatr 1992;120:882–885
The Management of Sickle Cell Disease. NIH Publication No. 02-2117 (revised 2002, 4th ed) 129–132
Winter CC. J Urol 1978;119:227–228

Epidemiology

Definition: Sustained, painful, and unwanted erection resulting from vaso-occlusive obstruction of penile venous drainage. Priapism has been classified as:

Prolonged (>3 hours)
Stuttering (>few minutes, <3 hours)

1. Mean age of onset: 12 years
2. By age 20 years, 89% of males will have experienced one or more episodes
3. Precipitating factors include:
   - Trauma
   - Infection
   - Drug use (eg, ethanol, cocaine, sildenafil, testosterone)
   - Prolonged sexual activity
   - Full bladder with infrequent urination
4. Complications include fibrosis of the penis and impotence

Treatment

Outpatient management:

1. Encourage oral fluid intake
2. Administer oral analgesics
3. Attempt to urinate as soon as priapism develops and encourage frequent urination

Note: Instituting medication and conservative therapy within 4–6 hours of the onset of symptoms can usually lead to detumescence

Inpatient management:
Carefully monitor oxygenation, hydration, and acid-base balance. Obtain daily weight, input/output, CBC, appropriate serum chemistry panels, and baseline coagulation profile. Measure baseline and pre-/post-transfusion Hb S concentration

1. **Hydration** with 5% dextrose injection (D5W) or 5% dextrose injection with 0.225% NaCl (D5W/$\frac{1}{4}$ NS) at a rate not to exceed 1.5 × maintenance (volume to include any drug infusions)
2. **Oxygen** by nasal cannula at a rate of 2 L/minute or higher if needed to maintain a PaO_2 of 70–80 mmHg
3. **Institute opioids or other analgesic therapy** as appropriate (see previous section on Acute Pain Syndrome)
4. **A urologist can perform penile aspiration** if more conservative measures fail to achieve detumescence within 1 hour. Use a **23-gauge needle** to aspirate blood from the corpus cavernosum followed by **irrigation with a 1:1,000,000 solution of epinephrine in 0.9% NS**

   Note: This is performed within 4–6 hours of onset and under conscious sedation and local analgesia. Successful in 15 young males on 37 of 39 occasions (Mantadakis E et al. Blood 2000;95:78–82)
5. **Transfusion of packed RBCs** is considered if penile aspiration with irrigation fails to achieve detumescence. Administer packed RBCs to reduce Hb S to <30%

   Note: It is unclear whether simple transfusion is equivalent to exchange transfusion

Management of recurrent priapism:

1. Chronic simple transfusion programs have been used to maintain the Hb S at <30%

   Note: Limit this approach to 6–12 months with frequent assessments
2. Penile shunting (Winter procedure) creates a shunt between the glans penis and the distal corpora with a Tru-Cut biopsy needle. This permits penile blood to drain from the distended corpora cavernosa into the uninvolved corpus spongiosa
3. Complications of priapism and its treatment:
   - Bleeding from the holes placed in the penis as part of the penile aspiration or shunting procedures
   - Infection, skin necrosis, damage or strictures of the urethra, fistulas, and impotence

Transient Red Cell Aplasia (TRCA)

Anand A et al. NEJM 1987;316:183–186
Bell LM. NEJM 1989;321:485–491
Kurtzman G. NEJM 1989;321:519–523
Ohene-Frempong K, Steinberg MH. Clinical aspects of sickle cell anemia in adults and children. In: Steinberg MH, eds. Disorders of Hemoglobin. Cambridge, UK: Cambridge University Press, 2001:611–670
Serjeant GR et al. Lancet 1993;341:1237–1240
The Management of Sickle Cell Disease. NIH Publication No. 02-2117 (revised 2002, 4th ed) 81–82
Young NS et al. NEJM 2004;350:586–597

Epidemiology

In regions not endemic for malaria, 70–100% of episodes of TRCA are due to human parvovirus B19

Clinical Features

Characterized by a temporary suppression of erythropoiesis. Presenting manifestations may include:

- Preceding febrile illness
- Headache
- Fatigue
- Dyspnea
- More severe anemia than usual
- Reticulocytopenia* (eg, <1%)

*Reticulocytopenia begins 5 days after viral exposure and continues for 7–10 days. Hb nadir may reach values of 3–4 g/dL. Recovery is often associated with a massive increase in circulating nucleated RBCs (eg, >100 nRBC/100 WBC)

Treatment

Transfuse packed RBCs to maintain Hb close to baseline if ≥25% decrease in Hb from baseline with declining or absent reticulocyte levels and symptomatic anemia
Note: Transfuse small volumes cautiously to avoid hypervolemia and complications arising from an abrupt increase in serum viscosity

1. Although TRCA is usually self-limited with resolution over a period of 2–3 weeks, transfusion support may be required to maintain the RBC mass and blood volume during this time period (see section on Red Blood Cell Transfusion)
2. If patients show evidence of RBC production, as determined by reticulocyte count, transfusion support may not be required
3. During the earliest phases of acute illness, obtain anti-B19 parvovirus IgM and IgG levels. If initial titers are negative, repeat in 1 week to assess for recent infection manifested by a rise in IgM levels
4. If there is failure to spontaneously resolve the B19 infection, discontinuing immunosuppressive therapy (if applicable) or instituting antiretroviral therapy in patients with HIV infection (if applicable) may terminate the underlying B19 viremia
5. In patients with persistent chronic B19 viremia and anemia requiring ongoing transfusion support, intravenous immunoglobulin containing viral neutralizing antibody may lead to a prompt decline in serum viral B19 viral DNA and accompanying reticulocytosis and increased Hb production

   Immune globulin intravenous (human) 400 mg/kg per day intravenously daily for 5 consecutive days on days 1–5 (total dosage/5-day course = 2000 mg/kg)
   Note: Occasional responses to a single 400-mg/kg dose have been reported

Notes

1. Siblings and close contacts with SCD should be monitored for the development of aplastic crises
2. Complications reported to arise from TRCA in small series or single centers include bone marrow necrosis with pancytopenia, stroke, acute chest syndrome, splenic or hepatic sequestration, and glomerulonephritis
3. Most adults have acquired immunity to B19 parvovirus; however, susceptible individuals exposed to patients with active B19 parvovirus infection are at risk for contracting erythema infectiosum. Isolation precautions for pregnant staff are necessary

Stroke and CNS Disease

Albers GW et al. Chest 2004;126:483S–512S (7th ACCP Conference on Antithrombotic and Thrombolytic Therapy)
Broderick JP et al. Stroke 1999;30:905–915
Ohene-Frempong K et al. Blood 1998;91:288–294
Malinow MR et al. Circulation 1999;99:178–182
Mayberg MR et al. Stroke 1999;25:231–232
The Management of Sickle Cell Disease. NIH Publication No. 02-2117 (revised 2002, 4th ed) 83–94

Epidemiology

1. Cerebrovascular accidents (CVAs) are a leading cause of death in children and adults
2. Age-adjusted prevalence of CVAs:
   Hb SS (4.01%)
   Hb Sβ-thalassemia (2.43%)
   Hb $S\beta^+$-thalassemia (1.29%)
   Hb SC (0.84%)
3. Among Hb SS patients, first CVAs were:
   Infarctive (53.9%)
   Hemorrhagic (34.2%)
   Transient ischemic attack (TIA) (10.5%)
   Both infarctive and hemorrhagic (1.3%)
4. In all SCD patients, CVAs recur in 16% of survivors of first-time CVAs
5. Overall, the mortality rate for hemorrhagic CVA was 24–26% for Hb SS patients

Acute Complications

- CVAs
- TIAs
- Subarachnoid hemorrhage
- Intraparenchymal hemorrhage
- Intraventricular hemorrhage

Treatment

Compared with children, there is little information on the treatment and prevention of stroke in adults with SCD. Treatment and prevention recommendations for adults with SCD are therefore based primarily on current recommendations in adults without SCD. It is recommended that physicians with experience and skill in stroke management and interpretation of CT scans supervise treatment

General guidelines:

1. **Oxygen** by nasal cannula at a rate of 2 L/minute or higher if needed to maintain a PaO_2 of 70–80 mm Hg
2. **Assess** the patient for cause of **pain and complications.** Conduct a rapid pain assessment with a simple self-reported pain scale. **Institute opioids or other analgesic therapy as appropriate** (see Acute Pain Syndrome)
3. **Hydration (if required based on clinical evaluation)** with 5% dextrose injection (D5W) or 5% dextrose injection with 0.225% NaCl (D5W/$\frac{1}{4}$ NS) at a rate not to exceed 1.5 × maintenance (volume to include any drug infusions)

TIAS and CVAs:

Specifics on inclusion/exclusion criteria for- and dosing of t-PA, antiplatelet therapy, and anticoagulation are expertly presented in this guideline: The Seventh ACCP Conference on Antithrombotic and Thrombolytic Therapy: Evidenced-Based Guidelines (September 2004), section on Antithrombotic and Thrombolytic Therapy for Ischemic Stroke

Subarachnoid hemorrhage

Transfuse packed RBCs to reduce Hb S to <30%

Note: The effect of RBC transfusion on altering the course or outcome of subarachnoid hemorrhage is unknown

Notes

Without controlled trials in adults with SCD documenting the worth of transcranial Doppler and periodic transfusions in reducing the risk of brain infarction, prevention should be based on standard recommendations applicable to adults without SCD

The following URL from the NIH guidelines provides a considered approach: (http://www.scinfo.org/nihnewchap13.htm). See section on stroke and brain disease in adults

Chronic Pain Syndrome: Osteomyelitis and Septic Arthritis

Almedia A et al. Br J Haematol 2005;129:482–490
Glader B. Anemia. In Embury SH et al, eds. Sickle Cell Disease: Basic Principles and Clinical Practice. New York: Raven Press, 1996:548–549
Keeley K et al. J Pediatr 1982;101:170–175
Rao S et al. J Pediatr 1985;107:685–688
Solanki DL et al. Am J Med 1986;80:985–990
Sickle Cell Disease: Clinical and epidemiologic aspects. In: Bunn HF, Forget BG, eds. Hemoglobin: Molecular, Genetic and Clinical Aspects. Philadelphia: WB Saunders, 1986:502–564
The Management of Sickle Cell Disease. NIH Publication No. 02-2117 (revised 2002, 4th ed) 133–137

Epidemiology

1. **United States and most regions:**
   Salmonella species are the most common causative organisms of osteomyelitis in Hb SS patients (~60% or higher)
   Staphylococcus aureus is the second most common cause followed by gram-negative enteric bacilli
2. **Other regions:**
   Gram-negative organisms such as *Klebsiella* species may predominate

Treatment

1. **Assess** the patient for cause of **pain and complications.** Rapid pain assessment with simple self-reported pain scale
2. **Hydration** (as appropriate to the patient's clinical evaluation) with 5% dextrose injection (D5W) or 0.9% NaCl injection (0.9% NS) at a rate not to exceed 1.5 × maintenance (volume to include any drug infusions)
3. **Institute narcotics or other analgesic therapy** as appropriate (see previous section on Acute Pain Syndrome)
4. **Institute appropriate antibiotics**

   Adults with osteomyelitis:
   Empiric parenteral antibiotics that cover *Salmonella* species, *S. aureus,* and other gram-negative organisms until culture results are available, such as:
   Vancomycin 1000 mg intravenously in 250 mL of D5W or 0.9% NS over 1 hour every 12 hours *with*
   Ciprofloxacin 400 mg intravenously in 200 mL D5W over 1 hour every 12 hours, *or*
   Ceftriaxone 1000–2000 mg (<65 years: 2000 mg; ≥65 years: 1000 mg) intravenously in 50 mL D5W over 30 minutes every 24 hours
   Note: Definitive treatment is chosen according to sensitivity and continued for up to 6 weeks, depending on the nature and extent of the infection

   Adults with septic arthritis:
   Empiric parenteral antibiotics that cover *Salmonella* species, *S. aureus,* and other Gram-negative organisms until culture results are available (see previous section on empirical parenteral antimicrobial coverage of osteomyelitis)
   Note: Consider surgically draining the joint with the evacuation of exudates and breaking up joint loculations to reduce the risk of persistent infection and articular cartilage destruction

Notes

1. Osteomyelitis in SCD must be differentiated from acute bone infarction. Plain radiography and radionuclide bone imaging are of little or no use in differential diagnosis. However, radionuclide marrow imaging may be useful in depicting diminished uptake in infarction and normal uptake in infection
2. Despite progress made with various imaging techniques, a definitive diagnosis of osteomyelitis in SCD depends more on clinical assessment and positive blood or bone cultures obtained by aspiration or biopsy

Systemic Fat Embolization

Castro O. Hematol Oncol Clin North Am 1996;10:1289–1303
Milner PR et al. Blood 1982;60:1411–1419
The Management of Sickle Cell Disease. NIH Publication No. 02-2117 (revised 2002, 4th ed) 107
Vichinsky EP et al. NEJM 2000;342:1855–1865

Epidemiology

1. A well-documented complication in the setting of acute chest syndrome
2. Responsible for symptoms in 8.8% of patients with acute chest syndrome
3. Systemic fat embolization can occur concurrently with an infectious agent
4. Risk factors:
   - Hb SC
   - Pregnancy
   - Prior corticosteroid treatment

Treatment

A high index of suspicion is required. All acute chest syndrome patients are considered to be at risk for systemic fat embolization. Treatment should not await proof of diagnosis

1. **Oxygen** by nasal cannula at a rate of 2 L/minute or higher if needed to maintain a PaO_2 of 70–80 mm Hg. If necessary, initiate critical care supportive measures to manage respiratory insufficiency
2. **Assess** the patient for cause of **pain and complications**. Conduct a rapid pain assessment with a simple self-reported pain scale. **Institute opioids** or other analgesic therapy based on the individual patient's clinical evaluation (see previous section on Acute Pain Syndrome)
3. **Hydration** with 5% dextrose injection (D5W) or 5% dextrose injection with 0.225% NaCl (D5W/$\frac{1}{4}$ NS) at a rate not to exceed 1.5 × maintenance (volume to include any drug infusions)
4. **Transfuse packed RBCs** to reduce Hb S to <30%

   Note: Case reports suggest that exchange transfusion may prevent some deterioration (see previous sections on Acute Chest Syndrome and Red Blood Cell Transfusion)

Notes

1. Characterized by embolization of necrotic marrow and fat in the setting of massive bone marrow infarction. Respiratory insufficiency and multiorgan failure from systemic emboli may occur with clinical signs dependent on the organ(s) involved and degree of involvement
2. Clinical symptoms may include severe bone pain, fever, hypoxia, azotemia, liver damage, altered mental status or coma, progressive anemia, thrombocytopenia, and disseminated intravascular coagulation
3. Findings that prove systemic fat embolization: Fat droplets within retinal vessels or in biopsies of petechiae
4. Indirect evidence of systemic fat embolization: Positive fat stains in bronchial macrophages, lung microvesicle cells, or venous blood buffy coat
5. In the setting of acute chest syndrome, patients with systemic fat embolization have a lower oxygen saturation at presentation, are more likely to have upper lobe infiltrates during hospitalization, and have a higher incidence of vaso-occlusive events compared with patients with pulmonary infarction or infection
6. Systemic fat embolization may precipitate or coexist with acute chest syndrome (see treatment section for Acute Chest Syndrome)

Vichinsky EP et al. NEJM 2000;342:1855–1865

Acute Multiorgan Failure Syndrome

Bakanay SM et al. Blood 2005;105:545–547
Hassell KL et al. Am J Med 1994;96:155–162
Rosse WF et al. New views of sickle cell disease: pathophysiology and treatment. In: Hematology 2000, American Society of Hematology Education Program Book:2–17
The Management of Sickle Cell Disease. NIH Publication No. 02-2117 (revised 2002, 4th ed) 125

Epidemiology

1. This syndrome is most commonly reported in Hb Sβ-thalassemia but may occur in patients with classic Hb SS disease with a high hematocrit
2. Second only to acute chest syndrome as the cause of sickle cell–related mortality

Clinical Findings

Definition: Acute multiorgan syndrome is the sudden onset of severe dysfunction of 2 or more major organ systems during an acute painful vaso-occlusive episode. This syndrome may occur without an apparent predisposing event other than syncope

Initial presentation
- Fever
- Nonfocal encephalopathy
- Evidence of rhabdomyolysis
- Rapid decrease in Hb and platelet count

Organ-specific manifestations
- *Renal*: Hematuria or acute renal failure
- *Liver:* Acute hepatic necrosis or hepatic sequestration syndrome
- *Bone marrow*: Generalized necrosis with fat emboli
- *Pancreas:* Pancreatitis

Note: For associated acute chest syndrome, see previous section on Acute Chest Syndrome

Treatment

Carefully monitor oxygenation, hydration, and acid-base balance. Obtain daily weight, input/output, CBC, and appropriate serum chemistry panels. Measure baseline and pre-/post-transfusion Hb S concentration. Follow chest x-rays until stabilization is documented

1. **Oxygen** by nasal cannula at a rate of 2 L/minute or higher if needed to maintain a PaO_2 of 70–80 mm Hg. Mechanical ventilation as appropriate to the patient's clinical condition
2. **Hydration** with 5% dextrose injection (D5W) or 5% dextrose injection with 0.225% NaCl (D5W/$\frac{1}{4}$ NS) at a rate not to exceed 1.5 × maintenance (volume to include any drug infusions) with careful assessment of hydration status and fluid requirements in the setting of concomitant acute renal failure
3. **Assess** the patient for cause of **pain and complications.** Rapid pain assessment with simple self-reported pain scale, if possible, based on the underlying mental status. **Institute opioids or other analgesic therapy as appropriate** (see previous section on Acute Pain Syndrome)
4. **Perform aggressive transfusion** to reduce Hb S to <30%:

   Simple transfusion (packed RBCs) if Hb <7 g/dL and there is no evidence of hyperviscosity, *or*
   Exchange transfusion using a mechanical device, if Hb >7 g/dL or hyperviscosity is playing a role in the pathogenesis of the acute complication of SCD
   Note: Prompt initiation of transfusion therapy or exchange transfusion has the potential of reversing this syndrome
5. **Critical care** support is directed at the affected underlying organ system(s)
6. If narcosis is suspected:

   Try **naloxone** 0.4 mg in 10 mL 0.9% NaCl injection (0.9% NS), and administer 0.5 mL (0.02 mg) intravenously per push every 2 minutes, *or*
   Naloxone 0.4–2 mg per dose intravenously, subcutaneously, or intramuscularly; this may be repeated every 2–3 minutes as needed to a maximum of 10 mg
7. Empiric antibiotics, pending culture results. Antibiotics should be given to febrile or severely ill patients:

   A **third-generation cephalosporin:**
   Cefriaxone 1000–2000 mg intravenously in 50 mL D5W over 30 minutes every 24 hours, *and*
   A broad-spectrum macrolide or **fluoroquinolone antibiotic:**
   Azithromycin 500 mg intravenously in 250 mL D5W over 60 minutes every 24 hours, *or*
   Ciprofloxacin 400 mg intravenously in 200 mL D5W over 60 minutes every 12 hours

Notes

1. The pathophysiology of acute multiorgan failure syndrome has been described as arising from diffuse, small-vessel occlusion, resulting in tissue ischemia and organ dysfunction
2. There are no reported prospective trials in the management of multiorgan failure syndrome complicating SCD. Treatment approaches are based on clinical observations and expert opinion
3. Refer to the NIH suggested guidelines (http://www.scinfo.org/multiorgan.htm)

REGIMEN

HYDROXYUREA

Charache S et al. NEJM 1995;332:1317–1322
Rodgers GP et al. NEJM 1990;322:1037–1045
Steinberg MH. Hematology 2000, American Society of Hematology Education Program Book:9–13
Steinberg MH et al. JAMA 2003;289:1645–1651
The Management of Sickle Cell Disease. NIH Publication No. 02-2117 (revised 2002, 4th ed) 161–164

Initial dosing:
Hydroxyurea 10–15 mg/kg per day (based on actual or ideal body weight; whichever is less) orally in a single daily dose for 6–8 weeks

Initial dose adjustment based on renal function

CrCl ≥60 mL/min[a]	No dose adjustment
CrCl <60 mL/min[a]	50% reduction
End-stage renal disease[b]	50% reduction

[a]CrCl: Creatinine clearance
[b]Treatment should be given following hemodialysis

Maintenance therapy:

1. Adjust hydroxyurea dosage in increments of 2.5–5 mg/kg per day per guidelines in Treatment Modifications. If no major toxicity is observed, escalate hydroxyurea dosage by 5 mg/kg per day every 12 weeks until a maximum tolerated dose (the highest dose that does not produce toxic blood counts over a 24-week period) or 35 mg/kg per day is reached.

   Note: In the MSH trial, 33% and 51% received maximal doses of hydroxyurea (35 mg/kg per day) at 6 and 21 months, respectively
2. A trial period of 6–12 months without transfusion support is adequate, provided the patient does not suffer an intercurrent illness that suppresses erythropoiesis
3. Because hydroxyurea is a teratogen and its effects in pregnancy are unknown, contraception should be practiced by both women and men. Patients should be instructed to notify their physician if they plan to or become pregnant so that treatment can be discontinued

Hydroxyurea is marketed in the United States as capsules for oral administration containing hydroxyurea 200 mg, 300 mg, and 400 mg (Droxia®), and as capsules for oral administration containing hydroxyurea 500 mg (Hydrea®)
DROXIA® (hydroxyurea capsules) Package Insert. Bristol-Myers-Squibb Co, Princeton, NJ. June 2003
HYDREA® (hydroxyurea capsules) Package Insert. Bristol-Myers-Squibb Co, Princeton, NJ. June 2003

Note: Droxia® has a labeled indication for use in SCA to reduce the recurrent moderate-to-severe painful crises and blood transfusions in adults. Hydrea® *does not* carry SCA as a labeled indication

Emetogenic Potential: Non-emetogenic (Emetogenicity score = 1). See Chapter 39 for antiemetic regimens

Treatment Modifications

Adverse Event	Dose Modification
ANC ≥2500/mm³, platelet count ≥95,000/mm³, Hb >5.3 g/dL, and reticulocytes ≥95,000/mm³ if the Hb is <9 g/dL	Escalate dosage by 5 mg/kg/day every 12 weeks until a maximum tolerated dose (the highest dose that does not produce toxic blood counts over a 24-week period) or 35 mg/kg/day is reached
ANC 2000–2500/mm³ or platelet count 80,000–95,000/mm³ or reticulocytes 80,000–95,000/mm³ if the Hb is <9 g/dL	Continue with same hydroxyurea dosage
ANC <2000/mm³ or platelet count <80,000/mm³ or reticulocytes <80,000/mm³ if the Hb is <9 g/dL	Stop hydroxyurea until ANC >2000/mm³ and platelet count >80,000/mm³ and reticulocytes >80,000/mm³ if the Hb is <9 g/dL; then restart hydroxyurea at a dosage 2.5 mg/kg/day lower*
Hematologic toxicity twice on one dosage	Do not administer or exceed this dosage again
Abnormal LFTs	There are no data that specifically guide dosage adjustment. Monitor hematologic parameters closely and adjust according to hematologic guidelines

*Subsequent doses may be titrated up or down every 12 weeks in 2.5 mg/kg per day increments, until the patient is at a stable dose for 24 weeks that does not result in toxicity

Patient Population Studied

A landmark prospective, double-blind, placebo-controlled dose-escalation trial evaluating the effect of hydroxyurea on the frequency of painful vaso-occlusive crises in adults with SCD and ≥3 painful crises per year. This trial confirmed earlier studies and established hydroxyurea as the first clinically acceptable drug to prevent painful crises in adults with SCA. Enrolled were 148 males and 151 females; 75% of patients took 80% of their capsules

Charache S et al. NEJM 1995; 332:1317–1322
Rodgers GP et al. NEJM 1990; 322:1037–1045

Efficacy

- Median rates of vaso-occlusive crises were reduced by 44% with hydroxyurea
- There were no differences between the 2 arms in the rates of death, stroke, or hepatic sequestration

Event	HU (n = 152)	Placebo (n = 147)	*P* value
Median time in months to first crisis[a]	3	1.5	.01
Median time in months to second crisis[a]	8.8	4.6	<.001
Requirement for transfusion[b]	48	73	.001
Units of blood transfused	336	586	.004
Acute chest syndrome[b]	25	51	.001
Median number of acute pain crisis/year	2.5	4.5	<.001
Discontinued treatment[b]	14	6	

[a]Definition of painful crisis = visit to a medical facility that lasted >4 hours for sickling-related pain that was treated with a parenterally or orally administered opioid

[b]In number of patients

Charache S et al. NEJM 1995; 332:1317–1322

Toxicity

1. Almost all patients had treatment temporarily stopped owing to myelosuppression with counts usually recovering within 2 weeks
2. Leukemia has been reported in 3 patients with SCD treated with hydroxyurea; 2 reported after 6 years and 8 years of treatment

Charache S et al. NEJM 1995;332:1317–1322
Steinberg MH et al. JAMA 2003;289:1645–1651

Monitoring Therapy

Treatment end points include:

- Less pain
- Improved well-being
- Increase in Hb F to 15–20%
- Increased Hb level if severely anemic
- Acceptable myelotoxicity

Laboratory monitoring

1. *Baseline:* CBC with differential, RBC indices, % Hb F, serum creatinine, BUN, LFTs, renal panel, and pregnancy test in females
2. *After initiation:*
   - Every 2 weeks: CBC with differential
   - Every 2–4 weeks: Serum creatinine, BUN, LFTs, and renal panel
   - Every 6–8 weeks: % Hb F
3. *After a stable and nontoxic dose is reached:* Every 4–8 weeks obtain a CBC with differential as long as ANC $\geq$2000/mm^3 and platelets/reticulocytes $\geq$80,000/mm^3

Notes

1. *Mechanism of action*: Hydroxyurea is a ribonucleotide reductase inhibitor that blocks ribonucleoside conversion to deoxyribonucleotides and interferes with DNA synthesis. It induces Hb F expression by a mechanism of erythroid regeneration that induces F-cell production. In adults, F cells are rare erythrocytes that contain small amounts of Hb F. Enhanced concentrations of Hb F in F cells can inhibit Hb S polymerization and RBC sickling and improve the course of SCD
2. *Hydroxyurea has been recommended in the following settings* (Management of SCD, NIH Publication No. 02-2117, 2002):
   - Adults, adolescents, or children with SCD after consultation with parents and physician
   - Hb Sβ thalassemia and frequent pain episodes
   - History of acute chest syndrome, other severe vaso-occlusive events, or severe symptomatic anemia
3. *Duration of therapy*: A long-term observational follow-up study of mortality in patients with SCD in the original MSH trial (Multi-center Study of Hydroxyurea) was conducted from 1996 to 2001. Of the original 299 patients, 233 (77.9%) were enrolled in the MSH Patients' Follow-up: 52% and 16% received hydroxyurea for ≥1 year and <1 year, respectively. When analyzed according to original assignment (treatment versus placebo) and regardless of a patient's treatment choice in the post-randomization phase, the mortality rates were similar (23.7% versus 26.5%). Twenty-five percent of patients (n = 75) died during the original trial or during follow-up. Of these, 28% died from pulmonary disease and 12% during SCD crisis

   Cumulative mortality in the MSH trial analyzed according to clinical events and laboratory measurements at the conclusion of randomized treatment showed the following:

Clinical Variable at Conclusion of MSH Trial	Cumulative Mortality (%) at 9 Years	*P* value[a]
Hb F[b]: <0.5 g/dL versus >0.5 g/dL	28 versus 15	.03
Acute chest syndrome: presence versus absence	32 versus 18	.02
Acute chest syndrome: ≥3 versus <3 episodes/year	27 versus 17	.06
Reticulocytes: <250,000/mm^3 versus >250,000/mm^3	37 versus 18	.001

[a]*P* values are reported as indicators of association, not tests of a priori hypotheses
[b]Hb F expressed as absolute levels (g/dL) = Hb F (%) × Hb concentration (g/dL)

Recommendations:

- Continue treatment indefinitely in patients who benefit from therapy and have no toxicity
- If Hb F (or MCV) does not increase, consider poor compliance or biological inability to respond. A trial period of 6–12 months without transfusion support is adequate, provided that the patient does not suffer an intercurrent illness that suppresses erythropoiesis

Steinberg MH et al. JAMA 2003; 289:1645–1651

REGIMEN

RED BLOOD CELL TRANSFUSION

Hemolytic Transfusion Reactions. In: Petz L, Garratty G, eds. Immune Hemolytic Anemias, 2nd ed. Philadelphia: Churchill Livingstone, 2004
Ohene-Frempong K. Semin Hematol 2001;38:5–13
The Management of Sickle Cell Disease. NIH Publication No. 02-2117 (revised 2002, 4th ed) 153–160
Vichinsky EP et al. NEJM 1995;333:206–213

Most appropriate RBC product

1. Phenotypically matched, sickle-negative, leuko-depleted packed RBCs
2. Administer washed RBCs if a patient had an allergic reaction to prior transfusions
3. Irradiation of RBCs is recommended in patients who are likely candidates for BMT

Methods of transfusion

1. Simple transfusion
   - Acute transfusion
     Note: Volume overload can occur when a large volume of blood is transfused too quickly. The administration of intravenous diuretics, slowing the rate of transfusion or partial removal of red cell supernatant fluid can help to prevent this complication
   - Chronic transfusion: Simple transfusion every 2–4 weeks to maintain a Hb A level at 60–70%. The pretransfusion Hct should be between 25% and 30% and post-transfusion Hct ≤36% to prevent hyperviscosity
2. Partial exchange transfusion: The final Hb should not exceed 10–12 g/dL
3. RBC apheresis

Review transfusion goals before starting

1. Assess for appropriate indication
2. Set goals for final post-transfusion hematocrit or Hb and % Hb S (avoid Hct >36%)
   - Major surgery: Hb 10 g/dL, Hb S ~60% or less
   - Sudden severe illness: maintain Hb S <30%

Toxicity

1. *Alloimmunization.* The highest incidence is reported to be associated with SCD and autoimmune hemolytic anemia. In a summary of 12 reports of 2818 transfused SCD patients, alloimmunization occurred in 8–35% (mean and median 25%)
   - Sickle cell hemolytic transfusion reaction: Manifestations of an acute or delayed hemolytic transfusion reaction where serologic studies may not provide an explanation for the hemolytic transfusion reaction
   - Development of symptoms suggestive of a sickle cell pain crisis that develop or are intensified by the hemolytic reaction
   - Development of a more severe anemia after transfusion than was previously present, with exacerbation of subsequent transfusions
   - Difficulty in finding compatible RBC units due to alloantibodies ± autoantibodies
2. *Delayed hemolytic transfusion reaction*: Four series in SCD reported an incidence of 4–22%; an incidence 10 times higher than that for randomly transfused patients. This reaction occurs 5–20 days after transfusion. Results from RBC antibodies are not present at the time of compatibility testing
3. Transfusion iron overload
4. Transmission of B19 parvovirus occurs in 1:40,000 RBC units (see Chapter 45, Transfusion Therapy)
5. Precipitation of pain episodes, strokes, acute pulmonary insufficiency
7. Hyperviscosity
8. Volume overload in which a large volume of blood is transfused too quickly

Patient Population

Indications

1. Acute pain episodes complicated by sufficient physiologic derangement to result in heart failure, dyspnea, hypotension, or marked fatigue
2. Acute chest syndrome, systemic fat embolization, and stroke
3. Acute splenic sequestration
4. Multiorgan failure syndrome
5. Transient red blood cell aplasia or "aplastic crisis"
6. Severe anemia in patients with serious and potentially life-threatening infection
7. Hyperhemolysis in which a Hb level after transfusion is lower than that before transfusion; generally proposed to result from an increased rate of destruction of a patient's own RBCs. This may occur:
   - As a component of delayed hemolytic transfusion reactions or occasionally from an underlying glucose-6-phosphate dehydrogenase deficiency
   - As a consequence of occult splenic sequestration or aplastic crises detected during a period of resolving reticulocytosis

   (Petz LD et al. Transfusion 1997;37:382–392)
8. Before major surgery
9. Considered for pregnant patients with complications such as preeclampsia, severe anemia, increasing frequency of pain episodes and women with previous pregnancy losses or who have multiple gestations

Controversial indications

1. Priapism
2. Leg ulcers
3. Preparation for infusion of hypertonic contrast media (gadolinium and nonionic contrast media lower the risk of RBC sickling)
4. Management of silent cerebral infarct and/or neurocognitive damage

Inappropriate indications and contraindications

1. Chronic steady-state anemia
2. Uncomplicated acute pain episodes
3. Uncomplicated infection
4. Minor surgery that does not require prolonged anesthesia (eg, myringotomy)
5. Aseptic necrosis of the shoulder or hip (except when surgery is required)
6. Uncomplicated pregnancies

Notes

In a randomly-assigned cohort of 551 patients with SCD undergoing 604 operations, a conservative transfusion regimen (designed to increase preoperative Hb to 10 g/dL, regardless of Hb S) was found to be as effective as an aggressive transfusion regimen (designed to maintain a preoperative Hb at 10 g/dL; Hb S ≤30%) in preventing serious complications (35% versus 31%) and the development of acute chest syndrome (each regimen 10%), but was associated with half as many transfusion-associated complications

Vichinsky EP et al. NEJM 1995;333:206–213

62. Aplastic Anemia

Michael M. Boyiadzis, MD, MHSc, Neal S. Young, MD

Aplastic anemia (AA) is a distinct entity characterized by peripheral blood cytopenias and bone marrow hypocellularity. Aplastic anemia can be acquired or congenital. **Acquired aplastic anemia** is distinguished from iatrogenic marrow aplasia, which is the common occurrence of marrow hypocellularity after intensive cytotoxic chemotherapy for cancer

Epidemiology

Incidence: 2 per 1 million of population per year (Europe)
Male/female ratio: 1:1

Kaufman DW et al: The Drug Etiology of Agranulocytosis and Aplastic Anemia. New York: Oxford University Press, 1991:159–169

Pathology

Severe aplastic anemia

- Bone marrow cellularity <25% of normal or 25–50% of normal with <30% residual hematopoietic cells
- Two out of three criteria:
  (1) neutrophils $<500/mm^3$;
  (2) platelets $<20,000/mm^3$;
  (3) reticulocytes <1%

Very severe aplastic anemia

- Bone marrow cellularity <25% of normal or 25–50% of normal with <30% residual hematopoietic cells
- Neutrophil count $<200/mm^3$ and platelets $<20,000/mm^3$; or reticulocytes <1%

Moderate (nonsevere) aplastic anemia

- Conditions that do not fulfill the above criteria

Historically, patients with severe aplastic anemia had a poor prognosis. In the early 1970s, 80–90% of patients died of complications of pancytopenia within 12–18 months. However, with the introduction of bone marrow transplantation and later the use of antithymocyte globulin (ATG), the 5-year survival is 75%

Bacigalupo A et al. Br J Haematol 1988;70:177–182
Bacigalupo A et al. Semin Hematol 2000;37:69–80
Camitta BM et al. Blood 1976;48:63–70
Rosenfeld S et al. JAMA 2003;289:1130–1135

Etiology and Classification

I. **Acquired aplastic anemia**
  A. Idiopathic causes (two-thirds of all cases)
  B. Secondary causes
    1. Drugs
      a. Cytotoxic chemotherapeutic agents
        (1) Alkylating agents (busulfan cyclophosphamide, melphalan)
        (2) Antimitotics (vincristine, vinblastine)
        (3) Antimetabolites (antifolate compounds, nucleotide analogues)
      b. Idiosyncratic:
        (1) Chloramphenicol
        (2) Antiprotozoal agents (quinacrine, chloroquine)
        (3) Nonsteroidal anti-inflammatory drugs: ibuprofen, indomethacin, sulindac, diclofenac, naproxen, phenylbutazone
        (4) Anticonvulsants: hydantoins, carbamazepine, phenacemide, ethosuximide
        (5) Gold and arsenic
        (6) Sulfonamides
        (7) Antithyroid drugs (methimazole, methylthiouracil, propylthiouracil)
        (8) Oral hypoglycemic agents (tolbutamide, carbutamide, chlorpropamide)
        (9) Penicillamine
        (10) Mesalazine
    2. Chemicals: benzene, insecticides
    3. Radiation
    4. Viral infections
      a. Parvovirus (rare, usually cause transient aplastic crisis, pure red cell aplasia)
      b. Hepatitis virus (non-A, non-B, non-C hepatitis)
      c. Epstein-Barr virus
      d. Human immunodeficiency virus
    5. Immune disorders
      a. Eosinophilic fasciitis
      b. Systemic lupus erythematosus
      c. Graft-versus-host disease, transfusion associated
      d. Hypoimmunoglobulinemia
      e. Thymoma and thymic carcinoma
    6. Paroxysmal nocturnal hemoglobinuria
    7. Pregnancy

II. **Inherited aplastic anemia**
  A. Fanconi's anemia
  B. Dyskeratosis congenita
  C. Shwachman-Diamond syndrome
  D. Amegakaryocytic thrombocytopenia

Young NS. In: Young NS, ed. Bone Marrow Failure Syndromes. Philadelphia: WB Saunders, 2000:1–46

Differential Diagnosis of Pancytopenia

Pancytopenia with hypocellular bone marrow
1. Acquired aplastic anemia
2. Inherited aplastic anemia
3. Myelodysplasia syndromes (rare)
4. Aleukemic leukemia (rare)
5. Lymphomas of bone marrow (rare)

Pancytopenia with cellular bone marrow

Primary bone marrow diseases:
1. Myelodysplasia syndromes
2. Paroxysmal nocturnal hemoglobinuria
3. Myelofibrosis
4. Hairy cell leukemia
5. Myelophthisis
6. Bone marrow lymphoma

Secondary to systemic diseases:
1. Systemic lupus erythematosus
2. Sjögren's syndrome
3. Hypersplenism
4. Vitamin B_{12} deficiency, folate deficiency
5. Alcoholism
6. Brucellosis
7. Ehrlichiosis
8. Sarcoidosis
9. Tuberculosis and atypical mycobacteria

Hypocellular bone marrow with or without cytopenia
1. Q fever
2. Legionnaires' disease
3. Toxoplasmosis
4. Mycobacteria
5. Tuberculosis
6. Anorexia nervosa, starvation
7. Hypothyroidism

Work-Up

(It is important to exclude other disorders that may present with pancytopenia and a hypoplastic bone marrow)

CBC with differential	• All cell lineages may not be affected; bicytopenias or monocytopenias may occur • Decreased reticulocyte count • Red blood cells usually are normocytic, but occasionally erythrocyte macrocytosis may be present • In the peripheral blood smear the remaining elements, while reduced, are morphologically normal
Bone marrow biopsy and aspiration	• The degree of bone marrow hypocellularity may not correlate with the peripheral blood count • Marrow morphology is usually normal or may have erythroid megaloblastoid changes • The marrow space is composed of fat cells and marrow stroma • Malignant infiltrates or fibrosis are absent
Cytogenetic analysis of marrow cells	• Usually normal in AA in contrast to MDS • However, presence of cytogenetic clones does not exclude AA • Most common associated cytogenetics abnormalities with AA are monosomy 7 and trisomy 8
Flow cytometry	• To investigate for paroxysmal nocturnal hemoglobinuria; expression of the glycosylphosphatidylinositol-anchored proteins CD55 and CD59
HLA typing	• For patients <55 years old and their siblings • Consider HLA typing for older patients with good performance status
Serology	• Hepatitis profile if liver function abnormalities and human immunodeficiency virus if clinically indicated

Treatment Options

First line of therapy	Immunosuppression with antithymocyte globulin (ATG) + cyclosporine *or* Allogeneic hematopoietic stem cell transplantation
Second line of therapy	Supportive care, androgens, enrollment into clinical trials

Notes:
- Allogeneic hematopoietic stem cell transplantation should be consider as first line of therapy for younger patients who have HLA-matched sibling donors. All other patients should receive ATG with cyclosporine
- If a patient does not respond to ATG + cyclosporine, options include: a second cycle of ATG + cyclosporine, androgen therapy or enrollment in a clinical trial

Young NS. In: Young NS, ed. Bone Marrow Failure Syndromes. Philadelphia: WB Saunders, 2000:1–46

REGIMEN

ANTITHYMOCYTE GLOBULIN (ATG) [LYMPHOCYTE IMMUNE GLOBULIN] + CYCLOSPORINE

Rosenfeld S et al. JAMA 2003;289:1130–1135
Rosenfeld S et al. Blood 1995;85:3058–3065

Premedication:
Acetaminophen 650 mg orally 60 minutes before each ATG treatment *and*
Diphenhydramine 25–50 mg orally 60 minutes before each ATG treatment

Antithymocyte globulin* [equine] 40 mg/kg through a high-flow (central) vein, vascular shunt, or arteriovenous fistula in a volume of 0.9% NaCl injection, (0.9% NS), 5% dextrose injection (D5W), 0.225% NaCl injection (.225% NS), or 5% dextrose and 0.45% NaCl injection (D5W/.45% NS) sufficient to produce a solution with ATG concentration ≤4 mg/mL over at least 4 hours on days 1–4 (total dosage/course = 160 mg/kg)

Notes:
1. The initial infusion rate should be 10% of the total volume/hour. For example, for a total volume of 500 mL, start at 50 mL/hour for the first 30 minutes. If there are no signs of an adverse reaction, the infusion rate can be increased to complete the infusion within 4 hours
2. Always administer ATG through an in-line filter with pore size 0.2–1 μm
3. *Atgam® (ATG [equine]) product labeling recommends skin testing before administration

Methylprednisolone 1 mg/kg per day orally or intravenously for 10 consecutive days; taper the dose to discontinue by day 14

Cyclosporine (initially) 6 mg/kg per dose for adults; 7.5 mg/kg per dose for children, administer orally twice daily, continually for 6 months, commencing on day 1

Note: Cyclosporine doses should be adjusted to maintain a serum level of 200–400 ng/mL, while monitoring for any renal and hepatic toxicity

Emetogenic potential: Nonemetogenic (Emetogenicity score = 1). See Chapter 39 for antiemetic regimens

Cyclosporine is available in the United States in two encapsulated formulations for oral administration: cyclosporine (Sandimmune®; Novartis) and Cyclosporine Modified
The products are distinguished by marked differences in oral bioavailability and cannot be used interchangeably without carefully monitoring cyclosporine blood concentrations and dose adjustments based on individual response. Both formulations are marketed in two strengths, containing 25 mg or 100 mg cyclosporine. Cyclosporine and Cyclosporine Modified also are available in solution formulations for oral administration

Cyclosporine: Sandimmune® 25-mg and 100-mg capsules contain Cyclosporine (Novartis Pharmaceuticals Corporation, East Hanover, NJ), Sandimmune® Oral Solution contains Cyclosporine 100 mg/mL (Novartis Pharmaceuticals Corporation)
Cyclosporine Modified: NEORAL® 25-mg and 100-mg capsules contain Cyclosporine [Modified]
(Novartis Pharmaceuticals Corporation); NEORAL® Oral Solution contains Cyclosporine, [Modified] 100 mg/mL
(Novartis Pharmaceuticals Corporation); GENGRAF® 25-mg and 100-mg capsules contain Cyclosporine [Modified]
(Abbott Laboratories, North Chicago, IL); GENGRAF® Oral Solution contains Cyclosporine [Modified] (Abbott Laboratories)

Methylprednisolone is available generically in solid formulations for oral administration, including products containing 2, 4, 8, 16, 24, and 32 mg methylprednisolone

Patient Population Studied

A study of 122 patients with severe aplastic anemia (31 patients ≤18 years, 91 patients >18 years). Patients were not excluded if they had received prior ATG or cyclosporine

Efficacy (N = 122)

Hematologic Response[a]	
At 3 months	60%
At 6 months	61%
At 1 year	58%
Relapse[b]	
Cumulative 5-year relapse among responders	35%
Survival	
Overall survival at 7 years	55%
5-year survival in patients with response at 3 months	86%
5-year survival in patients without response at 3 months	40%

Disease Evolution

- 13 patients evolved to a new hematologic disease, mainly associated with monosomy 7 (AML and MDS)
- PNH developed in 7 patients within 6 months after diagnosis

[a] *Response:* Defined as no longer meeting blood cell count criteria for severe AA in the absence of recent blood transfusions and filgrastim administration
[b] *Relapse:* Not defined by blood cell counts but by any reinstitution of immunosuppressive therapy

Toxicity

1. Severity and frequency of toxicities (rigors, fevers, oxygen desaturation, hypotension, nausea, vomiting, anaphylaxis) are greatest during the first day of infusion and diminish with each subsequent day. Toxicities generally subside after treatment is complete
2. Adverse effects generally can be managed while continuing the ATG infusion (see table below, Infusional Toxicities of ATG)
3. Most patients receiving ATG develop fever. Most fevers are not infectious in origin
4. Serum sickness consisting of fever, rash, and arthralgia develops in most patients between 7 and 14 days after ATG start of treatment

Monitoring Therapy

1. *During ATG infusion:* CBC with differential, LFTs, electrolytes, mineral panel, and serum creatinine
2. *After ATG therapy:* CBC monitoring is dependent on blood counts. If they are stable, CBC with differential can be as infrequent as once every 2–3 weeks. Patients requiring platelets may need more frequent CBCs, but not more than twice weekly and usually only once weekly
3. *Six months after the start of therapy:* Bone marrow biopsy and aspiration. If patients are stable based on blood counts, bone marrow biopsy may not need to be repeated
4. *Laboratory monitoring while on cyclosporine:* Cyclosporine levels: When initiating cyclosporine treatment and after any dose adjustments monitor cyclosporine trough concentrations (sampled at the end of a dosing interval) every 4–7 days until stable concentrations are achieved. For patients on a stable cyclosporine regimen, monitor trough levels every 2 weeks. More frequent cyclosporine monitoring is recommended whenever dosage adjustments are made or the serum creatinine increases

   Serum creatinine: Should be monitored every 2 weeks for the first 6 weeks and, if stable, monthly thereafter

Notes

1. Avoid other nephrotoxic drugs concurrent with cyclosporine treatment
2. Avoid medications that alter cyclosporine metabolism by cytochrome P450 CYP3A subfamily enzymes
3. Patients should receive monthly prophylaxis against *Pneumocystis carini* with aerosolized pentamidine during cyclosporine treatment
4. Granulocyte-colony-stimulating factors should be administered as clinically indicated, usually for evidence of infection, such as fever or localized inflammation in the setting of severe inflammation
5. **Guidelines for administering ATG**

   Allergy skin testing before ATG administration:

   - Advise patients to avoid using H_1-receptor antagonists for 72 hours before skin testing
   - ATG [equine] is freshly diluted (1:1000) with 0.9% NaCl injection (0.9% NS), to a concentration of 5 mcg/0.1 mL and administered intradermally
   - Administer 0.1 mL 0.9% NS intradermally in a contralateral extremity as a control
   - Observe every 15–20 minutes over the first hour after intradermal injection
   - A local reaction ≥10 mm with a wheal, erythema, or both, ± pseudopod formation and itching or a marked local swelling is considered a positive test. For a positive test, consider desensitization before therapy
   - If ATG is administered after a locally positive skin test, administration should only be attempted in a setting where intensive life support facilities are immediately available and with the attendance of a physician familiar with the treatment of potentially life-threatening allergic reactions
   - Systemic reactions such as generalized rash, tachycardia, dyspnea, hypotension, or anaphylaxis preclude ATG administration

   Monitoring during ATG administration:

   - Patients should remain under continual surveillance
   - Assess peripheral vascular access sites for thrombophlebitis every 8 hours
   - Monitor vital signs and assess for adverse reactions (flushing, hives, itching, SOB, difficulty breathing, chest tightness) before starting administration

     During initial dose: Continually during the first 15 minutes, then every 30 minutes × 2, then at least every hour until administration is completed

     During subsequent doses: 30 minutes after initiating infusion

Infusional Toxicities of ATG

Adverse Events	Interventions
Rigors	Antihistamines (eg, diphenhydramine 25–50 mg intravenously or orally every 6 hours as needed) Meperidine 12.5–50 mg intravenously every 3–4 hours as needed
Nausea, vomiting	Antiemetic rescue. Give antiemetic primary prophylaxis during subsequent ATG treatments
Anaphylaxis[a]	Immediately *stop* administration; administer steroids; assist respiration; and provide other resuscitative measures. *Do not* resume treatment
Thrombocytopenia, anemia	Blood product transfusions as needed[b]
Fever and neutropenia[c]	Broad-spectrum antibiotics empirically, if ANC <500/mm^3; may give acetaminophen 650 mg orally every 4 hours
Hypotension	Fluid resuscitation
Refractory hypotension	May indicate anaphylaxis. Stop ATG infusion and stabilize blood pressure. Intensive Care Unit support
Oxygen desaturation	Oxygen therapy
Refractory desaturation	Discontinue ATG. Intensive Care Unit support
Respiratory distress	Discontinue ATG. If distress persists, administer an antihistamine, epinephrine, corticosteroids
Rash, pruritus, urticaria	Administer antihistamines and/or topical steroids for prophylaxis and treatment
Serum sickness-like symptoms[d]	Administer prophylactic glucocorticoids
Hepatotoxicity[e]	Monitor LFTs

[a]Anaphylaxis (<3% of patients) more frequently occurs within the first hour after starting ATG infusion. After the first hour, adverse effects occur as a result of a delayed immune response and generally can be managed while continuing ATG infusion

[b]Concomitant administration of blood products should be avoided with ATG infusions to avoid confusing transfusion reactions with reactions to ATG

[c]Most patients who receive ATG develop fever as a result of the drug. Most fevers are not infectious in origin

[d]Type II hypersensitivity reactions/serum sickness consisting of fever, rash, and arthralgia develops in approximately 85% of patients between 7 and 14 days after ATG treatment has begun. These symptoms can be managed with corticosteroids

[e]An isolated increase in serum alanine transaminase frequently has no clinical significance. Generally, liver function abnormalities are transient and return to normal within 1 month

Bevans MF, Shalabi RA. Clin J Oncol Nurs 2004;8:377–382

REGIMEN

ANDROGENS

Bacigalupo A et al. Br J Haematol 1993;83:145–151
Besa EC. Semin Hematol 1994;31:134–145
Heimpel H. Acta Haematol 2000;103:11–15
Najean Y. Am J Med 1981 71:543–551

Oxymethalone 0.25–4 mg/kg per day orally, continually
Nandrolone phenpropionate 1 mg/kg intramuscularly every 2 weeks
Nandrolone decanoate 1.5–2 mg/kg per dose by deep intramuscular injection weekly
Danazol 600–800 mg per day orally, continually

Oxymethalone is a schedule III controlled substance that is marketed in the United States as tablets for oral administration containing 50 mg oxymethalone (ANADROL®-50; Unimed Pharmaceuticals, Inc, Marietta, GA). ANADROL®-50 (oxymethalone) 50-mg Tablets product label, September 2004. Unimed Pharmaceuticals, Inc, Marietta, GA
Nandrolone decanoate injection (in oil) is a schedule III controlled substance that is marketed in the United States in two concentrations: 100 mg/mL and 200 mg/mL. Both products are formulated in oil and are for *administration only by deep intramuscular injection.* Nandrolone Decanoate Injection product label, Watson Pharmaceuticals, Corona, CA
Danazol is available generically in the United States in solid formulations for oral administration that contain 50, 100, and 200 mg danazol. Danocrine® (danazol) product label, February 2003. Sanofi-Synthelabo Inc, New York, NY

Emetogenic potential: Nonemetogenic (Emetogenicity score = 1). See Chapter 39 for antiemetic regimens

Toxicity

Common toxicities: Acne, seborrhea, edema, emotional lability, nervousness, flushing, sweating, hair loss, hirsutism, menstrual disturbances, vaginal dryness and irritation, voice change, weight gain, changes in libido
Serious side effects: Cholestatic jaundice, peliosis (hemorrhagic liver cysts), hepatic tumors. Peliosis hepatis and hepatic adenomas may be silent until complicated by acute, potentially life-threatening intra-abdominal hemorrhage. Hepatotoxicity occurs less frequently with parenteral preparations

Oxymethalone: Decreased serum HDL ± increased LDL. Cholestatic hepatitis and jaundice ± pruritus at low doses may be associated with acute hepatic enlargement and right upper quadrant pain. Continued therapy has been associated with hepatic coma and death

Danazol: Thromboembolism, thrombotic and thrombophlebitic events, including sagittal sinus thrombosis and life-threatening or fatal strokes; benign intracranial hypertension (pseudotumor cerebri)

Monitoring Therapy

1. *Twice weekly to every 2–3 weeks:* CBC monitoring is dependent on blood counts. If they are stable, a CBC with differential can be obtained as infrequently as once every 2–3 weeks. Patients requiring platelet counts may need more frequent CBCs, but not more than twice weekly and usually only once weekly
2. *Monthly:* LFTs
3. *Periodic:* Serum HDL and LDL (anabolic steroids have been reported to lower the level of high-density lipoproteins and raise the level of low-density lipoproteins. These changes usually revert to normal on discontinuation of treatment)
   Serum iron and iron binding capacity (Because iron deficiency anemia has been observed in some patients treated with steroids. If iron deficiency is detected, it should be appropriately treated with supplementary iron)
4. *Every 6 months:* X-ray examinations of bone in prepubertal patients to determine the rate of bone maturation and drug effects on the epiphyseal centers

Patient Population Studied

Patients with aplastic anemia who are not candidates for HSCT or who did not respond to immunosuppressive therapy

Efficacy

Response rate at 6 months	35–60%
5-year survival rate	25–50%

Notes

1. A trial of 3–6 months is recommended to evaluate a patient's response to androgens
2. Patients may respond to different androgen preparations. An alternative product may be used if the initially chosen androgen was not effective or no longer produces a therapeutic benefit
3. Hypoglycemic drug regimens may need to be adjusted in diabetic patients who receive anabolic steroids
4. Anabolic steroids may suppress clotting factors II, V, VII, and X and increase prothrombin times
5. Danazol may produce symptoms of benign intracranial hypertension (papilledema, headache, nausea, vomiting, and visual disturbances). Advise patients who exhibit these symptoms to immediately discontinue danazol, and refer them to a neurologist for further diagnosis and care
6. Contraindications to the use of androgens include undiagnosed abnormal genital bleeding, impaired hepatic function, impaired renal function, impaired cardiac function, pregnancy, porphyria, breast cancer in women with hypecalcemia, prostate cancer

REGIMEN

ALLOGENEIC HEMATOPOIETIC STEM CELL TRANSPLANATATION

1. Allogeneic hematopoietic stem cell transplantation from a histocompatible-matched donor can be curative and should be recommended for young patients who have HLA-matched sibling donors
2. The outcome of allogeneic stem cell transplantation for patients with severe aplastic anemia has improved considerably over the last two decades, mostly because of the reduction of early mortality
3. Survival data after HLA-matched allogeneic stem cell transplantation ranges from 66% to 80%
4. Survival is age-dependent; 75% for patients younger than 20 years, 68% for patients 20–40 years, and 35% for patients older than 40 years in an analysis of 1699 patients in the International Bone Marrow Registry between 1991 and 1997, largely because the incidence of GVHD increases with age
5. Only 20–30% of patients in North America and Europe with severe aplastic anemia have an HLA genotypically identical sibling. Patients who receive a transplant from donors other than an identical sibling have a poor prognosis with at best a 50% survival rate of 5 years. The principal reasons for this poor outcome are graft rejection and GVHD

Bacigalupo A et al. Acta Haematol 2000;103:19–25
Horowitz MM. Semin Hematol 2000;37:30–42
Young NS. Ann Intern Med 2002;136:534–546

Supportive Care in AA

Transfusion recommendations

RBC transfusions

1. Transfuse patients with symptomatic anemia to keep Hgb >7 g/dL (>9 g/dL in patients with cardiopulmonary compromise)
2. Consider iron chelation in patients with:
   a. A transfusion burden >20 to 50 units of packed RBCs
   b. Ferritin levels consistently >2500 ng/mL
   c. A reasonable expectation of survival
3. Leukocyte depletion minimizes allosensitization. To avoid alloimmunization family donors should not be used
4. If a patient is a potential HSCT candidate, irradiation of blood products is also indicated (The risk of rejection is 5% in patients who did not receive transfusions before allogeneic transplantation and increases to 15% for 1–40 units and >25% for >40 units.)
5. Do not withhold RBC transfusions from patients who are not candidates for stem cell transplantation

Platelet transfusions

1. Prophylactic platelet transfusions are controversial. Adjust to the individual patient; a goal of maintaining platelet counts $>10{,}000/mm^3$ is reasonable
2. Platelet collection by cytopheresis and leukocyte reduction by UV light or filtration and single-donor rather than pooled platelets reduce alloimmunization

Growth factors

Growth factors are used empirically for infections that do not respond to parenteral antibiotics and antifungal agents. Neutrophil response is usually transient, which necessitates continuous administration of hematopoietic growth factors

Heimpel H. Acta Haematol 2000;103:11–15
Young NS. JAMA 1999;282:271–278 [published erratum appears in JAMA 2000;283:57]
Young NS. In: Young NS, ed. Bone Marrow Failure Syndromes. Philadelphia: WB Saunders, 2000:1–46

63. Thrombotic Thrombocytopenic Purpura/Hemolytic Uremic Syndrome (TTP/HUS)

Kiarash Kojouri, MD, MPH, and James N. George, MD

Thrombotic thrombocytopenic purpura (TTP) is defined clinically by the abnormalities caused by systemic thrombotic microangiopathy: thrombocytopenia and microangiopathic hemolytic anemia. Additional clinical features may include neurologic abnormalities, renal failure, and gastrointestinal symptoms

Hemolytic-uremic syndrome (HUS) is another clinical presentation of thrombotic microangiopathy. Like TTP, HUS is manifested by thrombocytopenia and microangiopathic hemolytic anemia with the additional abnormality of renal failure.

Although it is commonly stated that HUS is manifested primarily by renal failure whereas TTP is manifested primarily by neurologic abnormalities, these two syndromes cannot be distinguished clinically because many patients have both renal failure and severe neurologic abnormalities, or neither. Often these conditions are referred to by the comprehensive term, TTP-HUS

Amorosi EL, Ultmann JE. Medicine 1966;45:139–159
George JN. Blood 2000;96:1223–1229

Epidemiology

Incidence:

Inherited: Very rare; described in isolated case reports

Acquired: Estimated 3.7 cases/10^6 population per year, based on an analysis of death certificate data and is therefore uncertain, because TTP has no specific defining clinical features.

Male/female ratio: 1:2

Age: Rare in children; occurs in the complete age range of adults

Mortality rate: Untreated, TTP is fatal in 90% of patients. With effective treatment, mortality is approximately 15%

Amorosi EL, Ultmann JE. Medicine 1966;45:139–159
Torok TJ et al. Am J Hematol 1995;50:84–90
Vesely SK et al. Blood 2003;102:60–68

Classification

Congenital:

Patients with congenital TTP, presumably caused by inherited abnormalities of the *ADAMTS13* gene, may present in early childhood or as adults or may remain asymptomatic

Acquired:

1. *Idiopathic:* Most patients with TTP present without an associated condition or apparent cause
2. *Allogeneic hematopoietic stem cell transplantation:* Although there are reports describing TTP as a specific complication of allogeneic hematopoietic stem cell transplantation, this may not exist as a specific entity. In most patients diagnosed with TTP after allogeneic hematopoietic stem cell transplantation, the clinical features suggesting thrombotic microangiopathy are caused by systemic infection (eg, *Aspergillus* infection, cytomegalovirus), regimen-related toxicity, or acute graft-versus-host disease
3. *Pregnancy/postpartum:* Pregnancy is a risk factor for developing TTP, particularly in patients with congenital TTP. Congenital and acquired TTP typically occur near term or postpartum. Other pregnancy-related complications, such as severe preeclampsia and the HELLP (**h**emolysis, **e**levated **l**iver function tests, and **l**ow **p**latelets) syndrome, may have clinical features identical with those of TTP
4. *Drug-associated, immune-mediated:* Hypersensitivity reactions to drugs can cause the complete syndrome of TTP. Most frequent is quinine hypersensitivity; also reported are ticlopidine, clopidogrel
5. *Drug-associated dose-dependent toxicity:* The clinical and pathologic features of TTP can be caused by dose-dependent toxicity of chemotherapeutic agents, most commonly mitomycin, and by immunosuppressive agents, most commonly cyclosporine
6. *Shiga toxin:* Enterohemorrhagic infections producing Shiga toxin, characteristically *Escherichia coli* 0157:H7, can cause all clinical features of TTP. Shiga toxin causes the characteristic HUS of young children, and may also cause TTP in adults, with or without renal abnormalities
7. *Association with established autoimmune disorders:* In some instances, the clinical syndrome of TTP occurs in a patient with an established diagnosis of an autoimmune disorder, such as systemic lupus erythematosus or the antiphospholipid antibody syndrome. Whether TTP is merely an additional manifestation of the established autoimmune disorder or whether TTP should be considered as a distinct entity is never clinically clear
8. *High-titer inhibitor of ADAMTS13:* Consistent with an autoimmune etiology

George JN et al. Semin Hematol 2004;41:60–67
George JN et al. Transfusion 2004 ;44:294–304
Kojouri K et al. Ann Intern Med 2001;135:1047–1951
Vesely SK et al. Blood 2003;102:60–68

Pathology

The clinical syndrome of TTP is caused by disseminated platelet thrombi obstructing arterioles and small vessels. The characteristic histologic pattern is described as thrombotic microangiopathy. TTP, like other thrombotic and vascular disorders, is the result of multiple causes and risk factors:

1. ADAMTS13 deficiency. Best-described etiology is a congenital or acquired deficiency of the plasma von Willebrand factor–cleaving protease, ADAMTS13. Severe deficiency of ADAMTS13 results in an accumulation of unusually large von Willebrand factor multimers that can cause platelet agglutination in regions of high-shear stress, resulting in platelet–von Willebrand factor thrombi
2. Shiga toxin damage of endothelial cells
3. Drug-dependent antibodies directed against platelets, granulocytes, and endothelial cells
4. Dose-dependent drug toxicity
5. Additional risk factors include factor V Leiden, female gender, African-American race, and obesity

Moake JL. NEJM 2002;347:589–600
Raife TJ et al. Blood 2002;99:437–442
Vesely SK et al. Blood 2003;102:60–68

Differential Diagnosis

The diagnosis of TTP is based on the observation of thrombocytopenia and microangiopathic hemolytic anemia without another clinically apparent cause. In rare instances, even these two cardinal features may not be present, as for example, patients with previously diagnosed episodes of TTP who subsequently have acute neurologic symptoms without thrombocytopenia or anemia and are documented to have severe ADAMTS13 deficiency. **Classically, TTP was diagnosed by the pentad of clinical features: thrombocytopenia, microangiopathic hemolytic anemia, neurologic abnormalities, renal insufficiency, and fever. However, in the current era, urgency of diagnosis is required to initiate effective treatment. Therefore, only thrombocytopenia and microangiopathic hemolytic anemia without another clinically apparent cause are sufficient to establish the diagnosis.** The differential diagnosis includes all conditions associated with the clinical features of TTP

1. **Systemic infections**
   - Systemic fungal infections. Aspergillosis and other angioinvasive fungi can cause all clinical features of thrombotic microangiopathy
   - Viral infections. Disseminated CMV infection can cause all clinical features of thrombotic microangiopathy. HIV infection can also mimic TTP, typically related to additional opportunistic infections
   - Rickettsial infections. For example, Rocky mountain spotted fever
   - Bacterial sepsis, especially bacterial meningitis
2. **Systemic malignancy**
   Disseminated micrometastatic malignancies may mimic all clinical features of TTP without evidence by imaging studies. Although disseminated intravascular coagulation can occur in patients with disseminated malignancy, systemic small vessel metastases causing obstruction and thrombosis can occur without evidence of DIC. A syndrome mimicking TTP may occur with breast cancer, pancreatic cancer, gastric cancer, and non–small cell lung cancer
3. **Complications of pregnancy**
   Severe preeclampsia and the HELLP syndrome may mimic all clinical features of TTP
4. **Malignant hypertension**
   Severe hypertension may cause all clinical features of TTP including thrombocytopenia, severe microangiopathic hemolysis, renal failure, and acute central nervous system abnormalities
5. **Autoimmune disorders**
   Patients with acute systemic symptoms related to systemic lupus erythematosus, antiphospholipid antibody syndrome, acute systemic sclerosis, polyarteritis nodosa, and other autoimmune disorders can have all clinical features of TTP

Downes KA et al. J Clin Apheresis 2004;19:86–90
George JN et al. Seminars Hematol 2004;41:60–67
McMinn JR et al. J Clin Apheresis 2001;16:202–209

Work-Up

1. *CBC:* Thrombocytopenia and anemia should be present; the white blood cell count is typically normal
2. *Peripheral blood smear* should demonstrate polychromasia consistent with a high reticulocyte count and fragmented red blood cells
3. *Serum chemistry profile:* Most remarkable should be the increased LDH level, a manifestation of severe systemic tissue ischemia as well as hemolysis. An elevated indirect bilirubin level indicates hemolysis. Elevated creatinine is commonly present
4. *Urinalysis:* Proteinuria and microscopic hematuria are nearly always present
5. *Imaging studies:* X-rays and scans are typically normal. Pulmonary manifestations are uncommon. Even in the presence of severe central nervous system abnormalities, the head CT scan is typically normal because abnormalities are caused by diffuse small vessel disease
6. *Microbiology:* Cultures and serologic tests for infectious causes should be negative in patients with TTP, although these studies are an essential part of the evaluation to exclude infections as an alternative etiology for the presenting signs and symptoms. Patients presenting with bloody diarrhea need a stool culture on special media to detect *E. coli* 0157:H7
7. *Plasma sample for assay of ADAMTS13 activity and ADAMTS13 inhibitor activity:*
   - These measurements remain research investigations. Results do not currently affect management decisions.
   - Normal values for ADAMTS13 activity do not exclude the diagnosis of TTP and do not suggest that plasma exchange treatment is not indicated.
   - A severe deficiency of ADAMTS13 activity may be specific for TTP, but may also occur in asymptomatic individuals. Therefore, demonstration of absent ADAMTS13 activity does not exclude the possibility of systemic infections or other causes of the signs and symptoms suggesting TTP.
   - The demonstration of severely decreased ADAMTS13 activity in association with a high-titer inhibitor is consistent with an autoimmune etiology and may predict a prolonged and severe course of illness.
   - ADAMTS13 circulates for several days in the plasma; therefore, levels can be falsely elevated due to previous transfusions; patients with TTP are commonly transfused with red cells and platelets upon initial emergency room evaluation, and therefore plasma samples for ADAMTS13 activity are frequently inaccurate

Furlan M, Lammle B. Best Prac Res Clin Haematol 2001;14:437–454
George JN. Blood 2000;96:1223–1229
Zheng XL et al. Blood 2004;103: 4043–4049

Treatment Options

Congenital TTP

Plasma infusion

Congenital TTP due to abnormality of the *ADAMTS13* gene is caused by a deficiency of ADAMTS13 activity. These rare patients can be treated simply with plasma infusion to restore ADAMTS13 activity. Once the diagnosis of congenital TTP is established, regular infusions of 10 mL/kg of fresh frozen plasma given at intervals of approximately 2–3 weeks are appropriate lifetime prophylactic treatment. Whole fresh frozen plasma and cryoprecipitate-poor plasma are equivalent

Acquired TTP

Plasma exchange treatment

Plasma exchange treatment is the key element for management of TTP. It is the one treatment with documented effectiveness by a randomized controlled clinical trial that compared plasma exchange with plasma infusion. Plasma exchange is urgently indicated in all patients with a clinical diagnosis of TTP. Although there are no data that clearly support the efficacy of glucocorticoids, they are commonly given in addition to plasma exchange since acquired TTP is commonly thought to have an autoimmune etiology. Many other immunosuppressive agents have been used in the treatment of TTP, such as cyclophosphamide and vincristine. These are used in patients with disease refractory to plasma exchange and glucocorticoids. Recently, rituximab has been frequently used to induce durable remissions in patients with severe and prolonged courses involving multiple exacerbations and relapses

Transfusion therapy

Most patients with TTP require red cell transfusions during their acute illness. Several well-publicized anecdotes of individual patients have suggested that platelet transfusions may be harmful in patients with TTP. The rationale for this suggestion is strong because the pathogenesis of TTP involves platelet thrombi. However, many patients with TTP have received platelet transfusions appropriately given for overt bleeding or for invasive procedures without complications. Aspirin may be used in patients with TIA or stroke symptoms, as in patients without TTP, in a dose of 81–325 mg/day. It is prudent to avoid aspirin in patients with platelet counts less than 20,000/μL

Barbot J et al. Br J Haematol 2001;113:649–651
George JN. Blood 2000;96:1223–1229
Zheng X et al. Ann Intern Med 2003;138:105–108

REGIMEN

PLASMA EXCHANGE (WHOLE FRESH FROZEN PLASMA OR CRYOPRECIPITATE-POOR PLASMA)

Rock G et al. NEJM 1991;325:393–397

Before therapy:
Insert a double-lumen dialysis catheter. Placed in internal jugular, subclavian, or femoral vein. Percutaneously at bedside when an elective procedure is not feasible, or when time and conditions allow, tunneled in the subclavian or internal jugular vein with sterile operating room conditions

Plasma exchange:
Use **whole fresh frozen plasma or cryoprecipitate-poor plasma** to exchange one plasma volume per treatment each day. Continue daily exchanges until the platelet count reaches the normal range, indicating a hematologic response. Then discontinue exchanges either abruptly or gradually, depending on the patient's condition

Patients whose illness is responding slowly or who develop acute neurologic complications while on daily plasma exchange:
Use **whole fresh frozen plasma or cryoprecipitate-poor plasma** to exchange 1.5 plasma volumes per treatment each day or one plasma volume twice daily

Indications

Plasma exchange is urgently indicated in all patients with a clinical diagnosis of TTP

Efficacy

1. Effectiveness documented in a randomized controlled clinical trial that compared plasma exchange with plasma infusion
2. Although some advocate cryoprecipitate-poor plasma because it is depleted of von Willebrand factor, one small, randomized clinical trial found equivalent clinical outcomes with whole fresh frozen plasma and cryoprecipitate-poor plasma
3. Although the postulated mechanism for effectiveness of plasma exchange is removal of antibodies to ADAMTS13 by apheresis and replacement of ADAMTS13 by plasma infusion, plasma exchange probably has additional mechanisms for its effectiveness. Patients have been reported to achieve complete and durable remissions with plasma exchange treatment in spite of persistent severe ADAMTS13 deficiency and persistent inhibitor activity

Toxicity

Insertion and maintenance of central venous catheters are associated with significant morbidity

McMinn JR et al. Transfusion 2003;43:415–416
Rizvi MA et al. Transfusion 2000;40:896–901

Notes

Exacerbations of continuing disease requiring resumption of daily plasma exchange are common

REGIMEN

GLUCOCORTICOIDS

Bell WR et al. NEJM 1991;325:398–403

Initial therapy:
Methylprednisolone 125 mg per dose twice daily intravenously per push or as an infusion in 10–50 mL 0.9% NaCl injection (0.9% NS) or 5% dextrose injection (D5W) over 5–15 minutes

When a clinical response begins as evidenced by a sustained rise in the platelet count:
Prednisone 0.5–2 mg/kg per day orally until the platelet count reaches the normal or near-normal range, indicating a hematologic response; then taper the dose gradually over 10 days to 2 weeks

Prednisone is marketed in the United States in numerous formulations for oral administration, eg, 1-mg, 2.5-mg, 5-mg, 10-mg, 20-mg, and 50-mg tablets, and in solutions and syrups for oral administration

Indications

As an adjunct to plasma exchange in the initial therapy of *acquired* TTP

Efficacy

Although no data clearly support the efficacy of glucocorticoids, they are commonly given in addition to plasma exchange because acquired TTP is commonly thought to have an autoimmune etiology

Toxicity*

Weight gain, facial swelling, hypertension, hyperglycemia, osteoporosis, cataracts, and mood and behavioral abnormalities

*Incidence and severity depend on the dose administered and the cumulative duration of administration

Notes

Glucocorticoids are important adjunctive therapy for patients with ADAMTS13 deficiency caused by autoantibody inhibitors

REGIMEN

OTHER IMMUNOSUPPRESSIVE AGENTS: CYCLOPHOSPHAMIDE AND VINCRISTINE

Zheng XL et al. Blood 2004;103:4043–4049

Cyclophosphamide 1–2 mg/kg per day to maximum dose of 150 mg/day orally, *in the morning*, until platelet count reaches normal or near-normal range. Ensure that patients consume plenty of liquids (64–80 ounces [1900–2400 mL] of nonalcoholic fluid) during the day to prevent hemorrhagic cystitis

Cyclophosphamide is generically marketed in the United States as tablets for oral administration containing either 25 mg or 50 mg

Emetogenic potential: Low. See Chapter 39 for antiemetic regimens

or

Vincristine 1–2 mg by intravenous push over 1–3 minutes once per week until platelet count reaches normal or near-normal range (total dose/week = 1–2 mg)

Emetogenic potential: Low. See Chapter 39 for antiemetic regimens

Indications

Adjunct to plasma exchange when disease does not respond to glucocorticoids or at a subsequent relapse

Efficacy

Although no data clearly support the efficacy of cyclophosphamide and vincristine, they are commonly given to patients whose disease does not improve with glucocorticoids in addition to plasma exchange, since acquired TTP is commonly thought to have an autoimmune etiology

Toxicity

Cyclophosphamide*

1. Dose-related marrow suppression
2. Teratogenicity
3. Infertility
4. Alopecia
5. Hemorrhagic cystitis in 10% of patients
6. A risk for development of AML

*Serial blood counts should be monitored: Weekly CBC initially, then CBC every other week

Vincristine

1. Inflammation/thrombophlebitis at infusion site
2. Dose-related peripheral neuropathy
3. Constipation

Notes

Immunosuppressive agents may be effective to suppress autoantibodies to ADAMTS13

REGIMEN

RITUXIMAB

Zheng XL et al. Blood 2004;103:4043–4049

Premedication: Primary prophylaxis with:
Acetaminophen 650–1000 mg *and*
Diphenhydramine 50–100 mg orally 30 minutes to 1 hour before rituximab administration to mitigate infusion reactions
Rituximab 375 mg/m^2 intravenously in 0.9% NaCl injection (0.9% NS) or 5% dextrose injection (D5W) diluted to a concentration within the range of 1–4 mg/mL, once weekly for 4 weeks (total dosage/4-week course = 1500 mg/m^2)
Infusion rate:

- Initially at 50 mg/hour. If hypersensitivity or infusion reactions do not occur during the first 30 minutes, increase the rate by 50 mg/hour every 30 minutes to a maximum of 400 mg/hour
- Subsequently, if previous administration was well tolerated, start at 100 mg/hour and increase by 100 mg/hour every 30 minutes to a maximum of 400 mg/hour

Emetogenic potential: Low (Emetogenic score = 2). See Chapter 39 for antiemetic regimens

Toxicity

Common Side Effects (Generally limited to time of infusion and may be of greatest severity during initial administration)
1. Fever
2. Chills
3. Rigors
4. Nausea
5. Vomiting
6. Diarrhea
7. Headache
8. Asthenia
9. Hypotension
10. Cardiac arrhythmias

Black Box Warnings (For severe infusion reactions)
1. Hypotension
2. Angioedema
3. Bronchospasm

Hematologic Toxicities
1. Lymphopenia > neutropenia
2. Thrombocytopenia
3. Anemia

Rare, Fatal Mucocutaneous Reactions
1. Stevens-Johnson syndrome
2. Vesiculobullous dermatitis
3. Lichenoid dermatitis
4. Toxic epidermal necrolysis

Indications

Adjunct to plasma exchange when disease does not respond to glucocorticoids or at a subsequent relapse

Efficacy

In patients with high-titer inhibitors to ADAMTS13, rituximab has induced long-term remissions

Notes

1. Chimeric murine/human monoclonal antibody directed against CD20, a surface antigen on B lymphocytes
2. Management of rituximab infusion related toxicities:

Rituximab Infusion-Related Toxicities

Onset of infusion-related events (fevers, chills, rigors, edema, congestion of the head and neck mucosa, hypotension):

1. Interrupt rituximab infusion
2. For fever, chills: Give additional dose of acetaminophen 650 mg orally and diphenhydramine 25–50 mg by intravenous push
3. For rigors: Give meperidine 12.5–25 mg by intravenous push ± promethazine 12.5–25 mg by intravenous infusion in at least 10 mL 0.9% NS or D5W over 5–15 minutes. If after 15–20 minutes the response to a single dose is considered inadequate, the dose may be repeated
4. After symptoms resolve, resume rituximab infusion at 50 mg/hour and increase by 50 mg/hour every 30 minutes as tolerated up to a maximum rate of 200 mg/hour

Dyspnea or wheezing, without allergic findings (urticaria, or tongue or laryngeal edema):

1. Interrupt rituximab infusion immediately
2. Give hydrocortisone 100 mg by intravenous push (or glucocorticoid equivalent)
3. Give a histamine H_2 antagonist (ranitidine 150 mg, cimetidine 300 mg, or famotidine 20 mg) by intravenous push
4. After symptoms resolve resume rituximab infusion at 25 mg/hour with dose monitoring. Do not increase rate

Note: Medications for the treatment of hypersensitivity reactions should be available for immediate use in the event of a reaction during administration (eg, intravenous fluids, epinephrine, antihistamines, glucocorticoids, and O_2)

REGIMEN

SPLENECTOMY

Kremer-Hovinga TK et al. Haematologica 2004;89:320–324

Before splenectomy:

1. To enhance operative hemostasis, platelet transfusion can be considered if the platelet count is <20,000/mm^3
2. At least 2 weeks before surgery immunize with:
   - **Polyvalent pneumococcal vaccine**
   - ***Haemophilus influenzae*** **b (Hib) vaccine**
   - **Quadrivalent meningococcal polysaccharide vaccine**
3. Preoperative platelet transfusions are inappropriate if platelet count is >100,000/mm^3 Splenectomy can be performed by **open laparotomy** or **laparoscopy**, depending on surgeon's experience

Prognosis After Recovery

1. **Risk for relapse:**

   Recurrent episodes of TTP occur almost exclusively in patients with severe ADAMTS13 deficiency without acute renal failure. In patients with severe ADAMTS13 deficiency, the rate of relapse may approach 50% within 5 years. Most relapses occur within the first year after recovery. Most patients have only one relapse. The occurrence of repeated relapses is uncommon
2. **Chronic renal failure:**

   Patients who have acute renal failure as part of their initial acute episode commonly develop persistent renal failure. Even patients who initially recover may develop renal insufficiency and hypertension years later
3. **Cognitive deficits:**

   Although no published data have documented long-term cognitive deficits, patients who appear to completely recover from an acute episode of TTP commonly describe symptoms
4. **Risk of future pregnancies:**

   Because pregnancy appears to be a risk factor for the development of TTP, the safety of future pregnancies is a common issue. However, with the exception of a rare female with congenital TTP, recurrence during subsequent pregnancy is uncommon. Women who have congenital TTP inevitably appear to have exacerbations of their recurrent episodes during pregnancy and require more frequent plasma infusion prophylaxis

Howard MA et al. J Clin Apheresis 2003;18:16–20
Vesely SK et al. Blood 2003;102:60–68
Vesely SK et al. Transfusion 2004;44:1149–1158

Indications

Recurrent episodes of TTP in a patient whose disease has failed to respond to immunosuppressive treatment, including rituximab

Efficacy

Efficacy is documented only in case reports. However, the decreasing frequency of relapses over time may confound the interpretation of efficacy

Toxicity

Laparoscopic splenectomy has less operative mortality and morbidity, as well as more rapid postoperative recovery

Notes

The mechanism for the effect of splenectomy is unknown, but may be related to removal of a major site of autoantibody production

64. Idiopathic Thrombocytopenic Purpura

Kiarash Kojouri, MD, MPH, and James N. George, MD

Idiopathic thrombocytopenic purpura (ITP) is defined as isolated thrombocytopenia with no other clinically apparent associated conditions or causes of thrombocytopenia caused by accelerated destruction of platelets by antiplatelet autoantibodies

British Committee for Standards in Haematology, General Haematology Task Force. Br J Haematol 2003;120:574–596
George JN et al. Blood 1996;88:3–40

Epidemiology

Incidence: 1.6–3.2/10^5 per year, based on platelet count <50,000/mm^3. Incidence increases among the elderly, reaching 4.6/10^5 per year in persons >60 years old

Median age: 56 years

Female/male ratio: 1.2–1.7/1; however, in the elderly, males and females are equally affected

Mortality rate: The 10-year relative risk of mortality compared with the general population is 1.5 (95% CI: 1.1–2.2) for patients with diagnosis of ITP and 4.2 (95% CI: 1.7–10.0) for the subgroup with persistent thrombocytopenia despite treatment 2 years after diagnosis. Most deaths are due to unrelated causes or complications of treatment, rather than to hemorrhage

Frederiksen H et al. Blood 1999;94:909–913
Neylon AJ et al. Br J Haematol 2003;122:966–974
Portielje JEA. Blood 2001;97:2549–2554

Classification

Childhood ITP: Usually an acute, self-limited disorder that characteristically resolves within 6 months with supportive care only. Males and females are equally affected, with a peak age at diagnosis of 2–4 years

Adult ITP: Usually a chronic disorder, with insidious onset of symptoms that rarely resolves spontaneously

Differential Diagnosis

1. Pseudothrombocytopenia (platelet clumping in the presence of EDTA by naturally occurring autoantibodies to normally concealed epitopes on GP IIb/IIIa)
2. Drug-induced thrombocytopenia
3. Secondary autoimmune thrombocytopenia (CLL, SLE, antiphospholipid antibody syndrome)
4. Infectious disorders (HIV, HCV, EBV)
5. Bone marrow failure (myelodysplasia)
6. Congenital/hereditary nonimmune thrombocytopenia
7. Occult liver disease
8. Incidental thrombocytopenia of pregnancy

British Committee for Standards in Haematology, General Haematology Task Force. Br J Haematol 2003;120:574–596
George JN et al. Blood 1996;88:3–40
George JN et al. Ann Intern Med 1998;129:886–890

Work-Up

Objectives are to assess type, severity, and duration of bleeding and to exclude other causes

1. *CBC:* Pseudothrombocytopenia from EDTA-dependent platelet agglutination occurs in ~0.1% of adults
2. *Peripheral blood smear:* Findings consistent with the diagnosis of ITP include thrombocytopenia with normal-sized or slightly larger than normal platelets, and normal red and white blood cell morphology
3. *Bone marrow examination:* The American Society of Hematology guidelines recommend bone marrow examination as appropriate to establish diagnosis in patients over age 60 because of the higher incidence of myelodysplasia in older persons, in those with atypical features in peripheral blood smear, and in patients considering splenectomy. This view has been supported in two recent case series
4. *HIV serology:* Patients with HIV risk factors should be screened for HIV infection
5. *Autoimmune profile:* If suggested by history and physical findings (ANA, antiphospholipid antibodies)

If history, physical examination, and examination of peripheral blood smear are consistent with diagnosis of ITP and no atypical features are present, no further tests are necessary for diagnosis

British Committee for Standards in Haematology, General Haematology Task Force. Br J Haematol 2003;120:574–596
George JN et al. Blood 1996;88:3–40
Mak YK et al. Clin Lab Haematol 2000;22:355–358
Westerman DA et al. Med J Australia 1999;170:216–217

Treatment Overview

1. The goal of treatment is to achieve a *safe platelet count* while minimizing the side effects of therapy. Achievement of a *normal platelet count* is not a goal of treatment
2. Observation is recommended for patients with platelet counts ≥30,000/mm^3 unless they are undergoing a procedure likely to induce blood loss, such as surgery or dental extraction or delivery
3. Glucocorticoids are considered the initial line of therapy in a patient with a platelet count <30,000/mm^3 or a platelet count of 30,000–50,000/mm^3 in the presence of clinically important bleeding.
4. Splenectomy is recommended for patients with persistent thrombocytopenia despite steroids or for those who require steroids (>5 mg prednisone per day) for prolonged periods (>6 weeks) to maintain safe levels of platelet count (≥30,000/mm^3), but it is considered inappropriate as initial therapy or if the platelet count is >30,000/mm^3.
5. Patients with persistent thrombocytopenia despite prior therapy with glucocorticoids and a prior splenectomy can be treated with a variety of agents. Most of these second-line therapies can variably induce complete remission and partial remission in 20–70% of patients after glucocorticoids and splenectomy have failed. However, most of these remissions are not durable. In some cases, responses occur slowly over few months and treatment needs to be continued for several months before being considered a failure

Emergency Treatment

Hospitalization is required for severe, life-threatening bleeding, regardless of the platelet count. Emergency treatment in addition to general supportive care measures includes:

1. Platelet transfusions
2. High-dose parenteral glucocorticoids, such as **methylprednisolone** 1000 mg intravenously in 50–1000 mL of 0.9% NaCl injection (0.9% NS) or 5% dextrose injection (D5W) over at least 30 minutes daily for 3 consecutive days
3. **Immunoglobulin, intravenous (IVIG)** 1000–2000 mg/kg given intravenously as a single dose (1000 mg/kg) or in divided doses (1000 mg/kg per day for 2 days or 400 mg/kg per day for 5 days) (total dosage per 1- to 5-day course = 1000–2000 mg/kg)

These modalities are given either alone or in combination

British Committee for Standards in Haematology, General Haematology Task Force. Br J Haematol 2003;120:574–596
George JN et al. Blood 1996;88:3–40

REGIMEN

OBSERVATION

British Committee for Standards in Haematology, General Haematology Task Force. Br J Haematol 2003;120:574–96
Cortelazzo S et al. Blood 1991;77:31–33
George JN et al. Blood 1996;88:3–40
Provan D et al. Br J Haematol (2002) 118:933–944

Indications

Patients with platelet counts $>30{,}000/mm^3$ unless they are undergoing a procedure likely to induce blood loss, such as surgery or dental extraction or delivery

Notes

Patients with lower platelet counts ($<30{,}000/mm^3$) may also be managed with observation alone if they have no or minimal bleeding symptoms

Toxicity

None

Efficacy

In a consecutive series of 117 patients, no major hemorrhages occurred among 49 patients with platelet counts $>30{,}000/mm^3$ who did not receive treatment and were followed up for a median of 30 months

REGIMEN

GLUCOCORTICOIDS

Ben-Yehuda D et al. Acta Haematol 1994;91:1–6
British Committee for Standards in Haematology, General Haematology Task Force. Br J Haematol 2003;120:574–596
Cheng Y et al. NEJM 2003;349:831–836
George JN et al. Blood 1996;88:3–40
Pizzuto J et al. Blood 1984;64:1179–1183
Provan D et al. Br J Haematol 2002[118:933–944]
Stasi R et al. Am J Med 1995;98:436–442

Prednisone 1 mg/kg per day (0.5–2 mg/kg per day) orally for not more than 4–6 weeks (usually 2–4 weeks), after which it should be tapered slowly to the lowest effective dose or discontinued if there is no improvement in platelet count. The lowest effective dose can be continued for 4–6 weeks before further attempts are made to slowly taper and discontinue steroids. Splenectomy should be considered if steroids are required for prolonged periods to maintain safe levels of platelet count

Prednisone is marketed in the United States in numerous formulations for oral administration, such as 1-, 2.5-, 5-, 10-, 20-, and 50-mg tablets, and in solutions and syrups for oral administration

or

Dexamethasone 40 mg per day orally for 4 consecutive days as a single dose

Dexamethasone is marketed in the United States in numerous formulations for oral administration, such as 0.25-, 0.5-, 0.75-, 1-, 2-, 4-, and 6-mg tablets, and in elixirs (which contain alcohol) and solutions for oral administration

In patients with severe, life-threatening bleeding, such as intracranial hemorrhage:
Methylprednisolone 1000 mg/day intravenously in 100–250 mL 0.9% NaCl injection (0.9% NS) or 5% dextrose injection (D5W) over at least 30 minutes daily for 3 days

Toxicity

Weight gain, facial swelling, hypertension, hyperglycemia, osteoporosis, cataracts, and mood and behavioral abnormalities

Note: Incidence and severity depend on dose administered and duration of glucocorticoud administration

Efficacy

Prednisone:

1. Two randomized studies found equal efficacy between lower vs. higher doses of glucocorticoids (Prednisone: 0.5 versus 1.5 mg/kg/day and 0.25 versus 1 mg/kg/day)
2. In one large study, the incidence of prolonged complete remission was the same for patients treated 4–6 weeks compared with those treated for >3 months
3. About two-thirds to three-fourths of patients initially respond, but long-term remission without maintenance treatment occur only in 10–30% following cessation of therapy

Dexamethasone:
In a consecutive cohort of 125 newly diagnosed adult ITP patients, 85% of patients had an initial response; half of those had a sustained platelet count of >50,000/mm^3 and required no further treatment during 2–5 years of follow-up

Methylprednisolone:
High-dose parenteral glucocorticoids are reserved for severe, life-threatening bleeding, such as intracranial hemorrhage (see Emergency Treatment)

Indications

Glucocorticoids are considered the initial line of therapy in a patient with:
1. Platelet count <30,000/mm^3
2. Platelet count 30,000–50,000/mm^3 in the presence of clinically important bleeding

Notes

Glucocorticoids are the least toxic and least expensive initial treatment. A short course of dexamethasone may be less toxic and more effective than prolonged prednisone treatment

REGIMEN

SPLENECTOMY

British Committee for Standards in Haematology, General Haematology Task Force. Br J Haematol 2003;120:574–596
George JN et al. Blood 1996;88:3–40
Kojouri K et al. Blood 2004;104 (in press)
Pizzuto J et al. Blood 1984;64:1179–1183

Before splenectomy:
To enhance operative hemostasis if the platelet count is ≤20,000/mm³, preoperative **intravenous immunoglobulin, (IVIG)** 1000–2000 mg/kg given as a single intravenous dose (1000 mg/kg) or in divided doses (1000 mg/kg per day for 2 days or 400 mg/kg per day for 5 days; total dosage/1- to 5-day course = 1000–2000 mg/kg)

or

Prednisone 1 mg/kg/day orally as a single dose for 5–7 days if the platelet count is <20,000/mm³.

or

Dexamethasone 40 mg/day orally as a single dose for 4 days if the platelet count is <20,000/mm³

At least 2 weeks before surgery immunize with:
- **Polyvalent pneumococcal vaccine**
- ***Haemophilus influenzae*** b (Hib), *and*
- **Quadrivalent meningococcal polysaccharide vaccine**

Note: Preoperative platelet transfusions are inappropriate if platelet count is >100,000/mm³
Splenectomy can be performed by **open laparotomy** or **laparoscopy**, depending on surgeon's experience

Indications

Recommended in patients with:
1. Platelet counts <10,000/mm³, 6 weeks after initiation of medical therapy
2. Platelet counts <30,000/mm³, 3 months after initiation of medical therapy

Considered inappropriate:
1. As initial therapy
2. If the platelet count is >30,000/mm³

Efficacy

66%	Long-term normalization of platelet count without maintenance medical therapy (complete remission)
10–15%	Safe platelet count level with or without further medical therapy (partial remission)

Toxicity

Laparoscopic splenectomy has lower operative mortality and morbidity rates, as well as more rapid postoperative recovery.

Notes

1. Splenectomy is the most effective treatment for achieving long-term complete remissions in adults with ITP
2. Consider in patients whose disease:
   - Does not respond to glucocorticoids
   - Recurs after an initial response
   - Requires continued steroid treatment to maintain safe platelet counts

REGIMEN

ACCESSORY SPLENECTOMY

British Committee for Standards in Haematology, General Haematology Task Force. Br J Haematol 2003;120:574–596
Vesely SK et al. Ann Intern Med 2004;140:112–120

Before accessory splenectomy:
To enhance operative hemostasis if the platelet count is ≤20,000/mm³, preoperative **intravenous immunoglobulin (IVIG)** 1000–2000 mg/kg given as a single dose (1000 mg/kg) or in divided doses (1000 mg/kg per day for 2 days or 400 mg/kg per day for 5 days) intravenously (total dosage/1- to 5-day course = 1000–2000 mg/kg)

or

Prednisone 1 mg/kg/day orally as a single dose for 5-7 days if the platelet count is <20,000/mm³

or

Dexamethasone 40 mg/day orally as a single dose for 4 days if the platelet count is <20,000/mm³

Note: Preoperative platelet transfusions are inappropriate if the platelet count is >100,000/mm³

Indications

Many hematologists feel that accessory splenectomy is never indicated. However, in patients who fail to respond to splenectomy, or suffer relapse after an initial response, imaging studies to detect an accessory spleen have been suggested by some clinicians

Efficacy

Some case reports have described success with accessory splenectomy. However, these reports are difficult to evaluate, and the experience of many hematologists is that accessory splenectomy is not effective

Toxicity

Laparoscopy may not be appropriate to identify and remove small accessory spleens

Notes

Accessory spleens are present and removed in 15% of ITP patients undergoing splenectomy

REGIMEN

INTRAVENOUS IMMUNOGLOBULIN (IVIG) (POOLED NORMAL HUMAN IMMUNOGLOBULIN)

British Committee for Standards in Haematology, General Haematology Task Force. Br J Haematol 2003;120:574–596
George JN et al. Blood 1996;88:3–40
Godeau B et al. Blood 1993;82:1415–1421
Provan D et al. Br J Haematol 2002;118:933–944

IVIG 400 mg/kg per day by intravenous infusion for 5 consecutive days (total dosage/course = 2000 mg/kg)

or

IVIG 1000 mg/kg per day by intravenous infusion for 2 consecutive days (total dosage/course = 2000 mg/kg)

or

IVIG 1000 mg/kg by intravenous infusion as a single dose (total dosage/course = 1000 mg/kg)

Note: Refer to individual IVIG product labeling for information about product preparation (reconstitution and dilution when appropriate), initial administration rates and rate escalation, and advice about in-line filtration during administration

Toxicity

Side effects are common, occurring in 15–75% of patients and may be severe. Hepatitis C infection has not been reported with viral-inactivated products

Common	Rare
1. Headache	1. Aseptic meningitis
2. Backache	2. Alloimmune hemolysis
3. Nausea and vomiting	3. Acute renal failure
4. Fever and chills	4. Pulmonary insufficiency
	5. Thrombosis

Efficacy

1. Seventy-five percent of patients respond to IVIG by increasing their platelet count
2. About 50% achieve normal platelet counts
3. In almost all patients, the platelet count returns to pretreatment levels in 3–4 weeks
4. Five-day, 2-day and single-dose regimens are equally efficacious

Indications

1. As a temporary measure to increase platelet count
2. In a patient with a platelet count <50,000/mm³ in the presence of severe, life-threatening bleeding
3. In a patient with a platelet count <30,000/mm³ before splenectomy (or another major operation) to achieve hemostasis during surgery

Treatment Modifications

Adverse Event or Condition	Dose Modification
Preexisting renal insufficiency	Decrease the rate of administration of the immune globulin. If permitted, dilute IVIG to decrease its osmolality. Ensure adequate hydration.
Diabetes mellitus	
Age >65 years	
Concomitant use of nephrotoxic drugs	
Sepsis	
Deteriorating renal function	Discontinue IVIG

Monitoring Therapy

1. *Before IVIG:* BUN and serum creatinine
2. *Daily during IVIG administration:* BUN, serum creatinine, weight, and urine output monitoring

Notes

The mechanism of action of IVIG remains largely unknown but is reported to involve Fc receptor blockade on macrophages, the presence of anti-idiotype antibodies in IVIG that block autoantibody binding to circulating platelets, and immune suppression

REGIMEN

RHO(D) IMMUNGLOBULIN IV (HUMAN) [RHO(D) IVIG]

British Committee for Standards in Haematology, General Haematology Task Force. Br J Haematol 2003;120:574–596
Gaines AR. Blood 2000;95:2523–2529
George JN et al. Am J Hematol 2003;74:161–119
Scaradavou A et al. Blood 1997;89:2689–2700

Rho(D) IVIG 50–75 mcg/kg *only* by the intravenous route over 3–5 minutes after reconstitution in diluent containing 0.8% NaCl plus 10 mmol/L sodium phosphate

Dosing Guidelines

Pretreatment Hemoglobin	Rho(D) IVIG Dosage
<10.0 g/dL	50 mcg/kg
≥10.0 g/dL	75 mcg/kg

Reconstitution Guidelines

1 microgram (mcg) = 5 International Units (units)

Vial Contents	Diluent	Final Concentration
120 mcg	2.5 mL	48 mcg/mL
300 mcg	2.5 mL	120 mcg/mL
1000 mcg	8.5 mL	117.6 mcg/mL

Indications

Rho(D) IVIG is used to transiently elevate the platelet count in Rho(D)-positive patients who have a spleen

Efficacy

In a single-institution experience with Rho(D) IVIG, 70% of adult ITP patients had an increased platelet count of $\geq$20,000/mm^3 within 2 days. In 50% of those patients, the response lasted 3 weeks or more

Toxicity

1. The only clinically important adverse effect is alloimmune hemolysis. All Rho(D)-positive patients develop a positive direct antiglobulin test result after treatment, accompanied by a transient (1–2 weeks) decrease in hemoglobin concentration of about 0.5–2 g/dL
2. Severe intravascular hemolysis with acute renal failure has been reported as an adverse effect of Rho(D) IVIG

Notes

The mechanism of action is destruction of Rho(D)-positive red blood cells, which are preferentially removed by the spleen and thus sparing autoantibody-coated platelets through Fc receptor blockade

REGIMEN FOR REFRACTORY ITP

AZATHIOPRINE, CYCLOPHOSPHAMIDE

British Committee for Standards in Haematology, General Haematology Task Force. Br J Haematol 2003;120:574–596
George JN et al. Blood 1996;88:3–40
George JN et al. Semin Hematol 2000;37:290–298
McMillan R. Ann Intern Med 1997;126:307–314
Quiquandon I et al. Br J Haematol 1990;74:223–228
Vesely SK et al. Ann Intern Med 2004;140:112–120

Azathioprine 1–2 mg/kg per day orally to a maximum of 150 mg/day, given continuously if a response occurs

Azathioprine is generically marketed in the United States as tablets for oral administration containing 25, 50, 75, or 100 mg

Emetogenic potential: Low. See Chapter 39 for antiemetic regimens

or

Cyclophosphamide 1–2 mg/kg per day to a maximum of 150 mg/day given continuously if a response occurs, orally *in the morning.* Ensure that patients consume plenty of liquids (64–80 ounces [1900–2400 mL] of nonalcoholic fluid) during the day to prevent hemorrhagic cystitis

Cyclophosphamide is generically marketed in the United States as tablets for oral administration containing either 25 mg or 50 mg

Emetogenic potential: Low. See Chapter 39 for antiemetic regimens

Toxicity*

Azathioprine: Generally well tolerated
Potential side effects:
Reversible leukopenia
Small, but possibly significant risk of developing a malignancy
Teratogenicity

Cyclophosphamide
Potential side effects:
Dose-related marrow suppression
Teratogenicity
Infertility
Alopecia
Hemorrhagic cystitis in 10% of patients
A risk for development of AML

*Serial blood counts should be monitored during therapy with these agents: Weekly CBC initially, then CBC every other week

Indications

Persistent thrombocytopenia despite prior therapy with glucocorticoids and a prior splenectomy

Efficacy

1. Can induce complete remission in 15–20% and partial remission in another 30–50% of patients after glucocorticoids and splenectomy have failed
2. Responses occur slowly over a few months. Treatment should continue up to 4 months before being considered a failure

Monitoring Therapy

CBC with differential: Weekly during the first month, weekly for a month after any dose increase; otherwise every 2 weeks until counts stabilize, then monthly

Notes

1. Adjust dose to induce mild neutropenia

   Note: Although dose that induces mild neutropenia have not been further defined in most studies, consider using NCI CTC grade 1 toxicity as a reasonable benchmark:

   WBC: 3000/mm^3 to lower limits of normal
   ANC: ≥1500/mm^3 to <2000/mm^3
2. Reduce dose when platelet count response occurs, while maintaining a safe platelet count

REGIMEN FOR REFRACTORY ITP

CYCLOSPORINE

British Committee for Standards in Haematology, General Haematology Task Force. Br J Haematol 2003;120:574–596
McMillan R. Ann Intern Med 1997;126:307–314
Vesely SK et al. Ann Intern Med 2004;140:112–120

Cyclosporine 1.25–2.5 mg/kg per dose orally every 12 hours (total dosage/day = 2.5–5 mg/kg) given continuously if a response occurs

Cyclosporine is available in the United States in two encapsulated and solution formulations for oral administration: Cyclosporine (Sandimmune®; Novartis) and Cyclosporine Modified. The modified and unmodified products are distinguished by marked differences in oral bioavailability and cannot be used interchangeably without carefully monitoring cyclosporine blood concentrations and dose adjustments based on individual response. Both formulations are marketed in two strengths: 25 mg and 100 mg cyclosporine. Cyclosporine and Cyclosporine [Modified] also are available in solution formulations for oral administration.
Cyclosporine: Sandimmune® 25-mg and 100-mg capsules contain cyclosporine (Novartis Pharmaceuticals Corporation, East Hanover, NJ); Sandimmune® Oral Solution contains cyclosporine 100 mg/mL (Novartis Pharmaceuticals Corporation)
Cyclosporine [modified]: NEORAL® 25-mg and 100-mg capsules contain cyclosporine [modified] (Novartis Pharmaceuticals Corporation); NEORAL® Oral Solution contains cyclosporine [modified] 100 mg/mL (Novartis Pharmaceuticals Corporation); GENGRAF® 25-mg and 100-mg capsules contain cyclosporine [modified] (Abbott Laboratories, North Chicago, IL); GENGRAF® Oral Solution contains cyclosporine [modified] (Abbott Laboratories)

Emetogenic potential: Low. See Chapter 39 for antiemetic regimens
Cyclosporine can be given in combination with:
Prednisone 0.5–2 mg/kg per day orally for not more than 4–6 weeks (usually 2–4 weeks) followed by slow taper and continuation of lowest effective dose for up to 4–6 weeks. Discontinue prednisone if there is no improvement in platelet count
Prednisone is marketed in the United States in numerous formulations for oral administration, such as tablets containing 1, 2.5, 5, 10, 20, and 50 mg, and as solutions and syrup for oral administration

Toxicity

Common	Frequent/Serious
1. Headache	1. Nephrotoxicity
2. Hirsutism	2. Hepatotoxicity
3. Nausea	3. Hypertension
4. Vomiting	
5. Diarrhea	
6. Tremor	
7. Fatigue	
8. Paresthesias	

Measure serum creatinine[a], LFTs[b], and cyclosporine levels[c] periodically, and adjust dose as needed in increments or decrements of 0.5–0.75 mg/kg per day

[a]*Serum creatinine:* Every week, then every other week
[b]Every week, then every other week
[c]For patients without hepatic impairment on an "every-12-hour" administration regimen, obtain sample just before the fifth or seventh dose after starting treatment or altering dose. A general range of 100–200 ng/mL (HPLC) can be used as the reference. Blood level monitoring is not a substitute for renal and liver function test monitoring

Indications

Patients with persistent thrombocytopenia despite prior therapy with glucocorticoids and a prior splenectomy

Efficacy

Cyclosporine has been reported to induce rates of remissions comparable to those induced with azathioprine and cyclophosphamide, with complete remission in 15–20% and partial remission in another 30–50% of patients
Responses occur slowly over a few months. Treatment should continue up to 4 months before being considered a failure

Monitoring Therapy

1. *Baseline:* Serum creatinine (on 2 occasions), BUN, CBC with differential, magnesium, potassium, uric acid, and lipoproteins

Note: Measurement of lipoproteins are recommended because levels may increase modestly during therapy

2. *First 3 months:* Serum creatinine, BUN and other baseline lab parameters plus blood pressure every 2 weeks, thereafter, stable patients monitored monthly

Note: Measure serum creatinine with initiation of new NSAID therapy or if a concomitantly used NSAID is increased in dose

3. *Cyclosporine levels:* Weekly for 2–3 months and then once per month

The type of cyclosporine assay used to monitor blood levels is important. Recommended trough levels for the cyclosporine parent compound depend on the type of assay used (high-performance liquid chromatography versus radioimmunoassay versus fluorescence polarization immunoassay) and vary by whole blood versus serum/plasma. Levels are based on cyclosporine monitoring in the transplant setting

Note: Monitor drug-drug interactions that may alter renal function and either increase or decrease cyclosporine concentrations

Notes

Because of serious side effects, cyclosporine should be used cautiously

REGIMEN FOR REFRACTORY ITP

MYCOPHENOLATE MOFETIL

Hou M et al. Eur J Haematol 2003;70:353–357

Mycophenolate mofetil 750–1000 mg orally twice daily for a minimum of 12 weeks (total dose/day: 1500–2000 mg)

Mycophenolate mofetil is marketed in the Untied States for oral administration in several formulations, including: capsules containing 250 mg, tablets containing 500 mg, an extended-release tablet formulation containing 180 mg or 360 mg, and a powder for reconstitution as a suspension

Emetogenic potential: Low. See Chapter 39 for antiemetic regimens

Toxicity

1. Constipation
2. Diarrhea
3. Nausea
4. Vomiting
5. Headache
6. Hypertension
7. Peripheral edema
8. Myelosuppression
9. Weakness
10. Insomnia

Efficacy

Therapy for a minimum of 12 weeks in a series of 21 ITP patients produced an overall response rate of 62% (13/21), including 24% (5/21) complete responses. Responses occurred after 4–10 weeks (median 8 weeks) of therapy. However, only 14% (3/21) maintained response after discontinuation of treatment

Indications

Patients with persistent thrombocytopenia despite prior therapy with glucocorticoids and a prior splenectomy

Monitoring Therapy

CBC with differential: Weekly during the first month, twice monthly during the second and third months, then monthly. Thereafter, CBC with differential monthly for the first year

Notes

1. Monitor CBC weekly, then every other week
2. If no response occurs, discontinue after 12 weeks; if a response occurs, continue further until peak platelet count, and then taper slowly and discontinue

REGIMEN FOR REFRACTORY ITP

VINCA ALKALOIDS

British Committee for Standards in Haematology, General Haematology Task Force. Br J Haematol 2003;120:574–596
George JN et al. Semin Hematol 2000;37:290–298
George JN et al. Blood 1996;88: 3–40
McMillan R. Ann Intern Med 1997;126:307–314
Vesely SK et al. Ann Intern Med 2004;140:112–120

Vincristine 1–2 mg by intravenous push over 1–3 minutes once per week for 4–6 weeks (total dosage/week: 1–2 mg)

Emetogenic potential: Low. See Chapter 39 for antiemetic regimens

or

Vinblastine 5–10 mg by intravenous push over 1–3 minutes once per week for 4–6 weeks (total dosage/week: 5–10 mg)

Emetogenic potential: Low. See Chapter 39 for antiemetic regimens

Toxicity

Vincristine and Vinblastine
Tissue ulceration and necrosis after soft tissue extravasation
Cumulative dose-related peripheral neuropathies (vincristine >> vinblastine) *Early:* ↓ DTRs and sensory neuropathies *Late:* Motor and autonomic neuropathies (occur after sensory neuropathies, but onset is variable)
Constipation → paralytic ileus (vincristine > vinblastine)
Syndrome of inappropriate antidiuretic hormone (SIADH)
Muscle weakness, myalgias (vincristine >> vinblastine)
Leukopenia >> thrombocytopenia (vincristine << vinblastine)
Alopecia

Indications

Patients with persistent thrombocytopenia despite prior therapy with glucocorticoids and a prior splenectomy

Efficacy

1. Either vincristine or vinblastine can achieve a transient increase in platelet count, usually lasting 1–3 weeks in about 50% of patients with persistent thrombocytopenia after splenectomy
2. Sustained responses are observed in <10% of patients
3. Results are comparable with both drugs and methods of administration

Monitoring Therapy

1. PE with attention to neurosensory exam
2. CBC with differential before every dose of vinblastine

Notes

Vincristine should be discontinued after 4–6 weeks or after dose-related peripheral neuropathy occurs—whichever is earlier

REGIMEN FOR REFRACTORY ITP

DANAZOL

British Committee for Standards in Haematology, General Haematology Task Force. Br J Haematol 2003;120:574–596
George et al. Semin Hematol 2000;37:290–298
George et al. Blood 1996;88: 3–40
McMillan R. Ann Intern Med 1997;126:307–314
Vesely SK et al. Ann Intern Med 2004;140:112–120

Danazol 200 mg orally 2–4 times per day continuously
Danazol is generically marketed in the United States as capsules for oral administration containing 50 mg, 100 mg, and 200 mg

Emetogenic potential: Low. See Chapter 39 for antiemetic regimens

Toxicity

1. Weight gain
2. Headaches
3. Amenorrhea
4. Breast tenderness
5. Rash
6. Liver function abnormalities*
7. Drug-induced thrombocytopenia

*Liver function tests should be checked monthly

Efficacy

1. Danazol, a weak androgen, can raise the platelet count >50,000/mm^3 in 60% of patients while they are receiving the medication
2. Treat for at least 4 months, because responses are often slow

Indications

1. As a glucocorticoid-sparing agent in patients who benefit from glucocorticoids and receive longer-term treatment
2. May be contraindicated in patients with preexisting liver disease. Use with caution

Monitoring Therapy

1. Monitoring of LFTs at baseline and at least monthly or earlier as clinically indicated
2. Assessment for virilization because some signs may not be reversible

Notes

Danazol must be discontinued if liver function abnormalities develop. Using NCI CTC criteria, consider holding danazol if LFTs ≥ G2. Resume only when LFTs ≤ G1.

REGIMEN FOR REFRACTORY ITP

HIGH-DOSE DEXAMETHASONE

Andersen et al. NEJM 1994;330:1560–1564
British Committee for Standards in Haematology, General Haematology Task Force. Br J Haematol 2003;120:574–596
Vesely SK et al. Ann Intern Med 2004;140:112–120

Dexamethasone 40 mg orally on days 1–4 every 4 weeks for 6 cycles (total dosage/cycle = 160 mg/kg)
Dexamethasone is marketed in the United States in numerous formulations for oral administration, such as in 0.25, 0.5, 0.75, 1, 2, 4, and 6 mg tablets and in elixirs (which contain alcohol) and as solutions for oral administration

Toxicity

Weight gain, facial swelling, hypertension, hyperglycemia, osteoporosis, cataracts, and mood and behavioral abnormalities

Efficacy

1. The regimen increased platelet counts >100,000/mm^3 in all 10 patients who were refractory to prior interventions, including 6 who had undergone a splenectomy. Responses were sustained ≥6 months after therapy was discontinued
2. However, all other case series have been unable to duplicate these results and have reported serious adverse events with the regimen
3. A systematic review found the regimen induced complete remissions in only 10% of patients after failure of glucocorticoids and splenectomy

Indications

Patients with persistent thrombocytopenia despite prior glucocorticoid therapy and prior splenectomy

Notes

Complete responses have been reported in only one article

REGIMEN FOR REFRACTORY ITP

RITUXIMAB

British Committee for Standards in Haematology, General Haematology Task Force. Br J Haematol 2003;120:574–596
Stasi R et al. Blood 2001;98:952–957
Vesely SK et al. Ann Intern Med 2004;140:112–20

Premedication: Primary prophylaxis with: **Acetaminophen** 650–1000 mg *and* **Diphenhydramine** 50–100 mg orally 30 minutes to 1 hour before rituximab administration to mitigate infusion reactions

Rituximab 375 mg/m² intravenously in 0.9% NaCl injection (0.9% NS) or 5% dextrose injection (D5W), diluted to a concentration within the range of 1–4 mg/mL once weekly for 4 weeks (total dosage/4-week course = 1500 mg/m²)
Infusion rate:
- Initially at 50 mg/hour. If hypersensitivity or infusion reactions do not occur during the first 30 minutes, increase the rate by 50 mg/hour every 30 minutes to a maximum of 400 mg/hour
- Subsequently, if previous administration was well tolerated, start at 100 mg/hour, and increase by 100 mg/hour every 30 minutes to a maximum of 400 mg/hour

Indications

Patients with persistent thrombocytopenia despite prior therapy with glucocorticoids and a prior splenectomy

Efficacy

1. In a 25-patient series, rituximab induced 5 complete, 5 partial, and 3 minor responses, for an overall response rate of 52%. In 7 patients, responses were sustained for >6 months. Only 8 patients previously had splenectomy
2. A recent systematic review of chronic refractory ITP, reported complete remissions in 24% (10/41) of patients treated with rituximab

Toxicity

Common Side Effects

(Generally limited to time of infusion and may be of greatest severity during initial administration)

Fever	Diarrhea
Chills	Headache
Rigors	Asthenia
Nausea	Hypotension
Vomiting	Cardiac arrhythmias

Black Box Warnings

(Severe infusion reactions)

Hypotension	Bronchospasm
Angioedema	

Hematologic Toxicities

Lymphopenia >> neutropenia
Thrombocytopenia Anemia

Rare, Fatal Mucocutaneous Reactions

Stevens-Johnson syndrome
Vesiculobullous dermatitis
Lichenoid dermatitis
Toxic epidermal necrolysis

Monitoring Therapy

1. *CBC with differential:* Weekly and more frequently in patients who develop cytopenias
2. Monitor renal function tests, serum calcium, phosphorus, uric acid and fluid balance and institute supportive care as indicated

Notes

1. Chimeric murine/human monoclonal antibody directed against CD20, a surface antigen on B-lymphocytes
2. Management of rituximab infusion related toxicities:

Rituximab Infusion-Related Toxicities

Onset of infusion-related events (fevers, chills, rigors, edema, congestion of the head and neck mucosa, hypotension):

1. Interrupt rituximab infusion
2. For fever, chills: Give additional dose of acetaminophen 650 mg orally and diphenhydramine 25–50 mg by intravenous push
3. For rigors: Give meperidine 12.5–25 mg by intravenous push ± promethazine 12.5–25 mg by intravenous infusion in at least 10 mL 0.9% NS or D5W over 5–15 minutes. If after 15–20 minutes the response to a single dose is considered inadequate, the dose may be repeated
4. After symptoms resolve, resume rituximab infusion at 50 mg/hour and increase by 50 mg/hour every 30 minutes as tolerated up to a maximum rate of 200 mg/hour

Dyspnea or wheezing, without allergic findings (urticaria, or tongue or laryngeal edema):

1. Interrupt rituximab infusion immediately
2. Give hydrocortisone 100 mg by intravenous push (or glucocorticoid equivalent)
3. Give a histamine H_2 antagonist (ranitidine 150 mg, cimetidine 300 mg, or famotidine 20 mg) by intravenous push
4. After symptoms resolve resume rituximab infusion at 25 mg/hour with dose monitoring. Do not increase rate

Note: Medications for the treatment of hypersensitivity reactions should be available for immediate use in the event of a reaction during administration (eg, intravenous fluids, epinephrine, antihistamines, glucocorticoids, and O_2)

REGIMEN FOR REFRACTORY ITP

INTERFERON ALFA-2B

British Committee for Standards in Haematology, General Haematology Task Force. Br J Haematol 2003;120:574–596
Dubbeld J et al. Eur J Haematol 1994;52:233–235
George JN et al. Blood 1996;88:3–40
Vesely SK et al. Ann Intern Med 2004;140:112–120

Premedication: None. Symptomatic treatment and secondary prophylaxis only
Interferon alfa-2b 3 million units/dose subcutaneously 3 times each week for 4 weeks (total dose/week = 9 million units)

Emetogenic potential: Low (Emetogenicity score = 2). See Chapter 39 for antiemetic regimens

Toxicity

Acute*

1. Fever and flulike symptoms (headache, chills, rigors, myalgias, malaise, fatigue)
2. Blood pressure changes

*May be lessened by acetaminophen and graduated dose escalation

Chronic*

1. Fatigue
2. Anorexia/weight loss
3. Depression

*May be related to weekly cumulative doses and persist for as long as therapy is continued

Sporadic

1. Nausea
2. Diarrhea
3. Emesis
4. Abdominal pain
5. Peripheral and central neurologic and neuropsychiatric effects
6. Granulocytopenia and thrombocytopenia (mild to moderate)
7. Exacerbation of preexisting autoimmune disorders or de novo induction of autoimmunity
8. Binding and neutralizing antibodies
9. Clinically significant cardiovascular adverse effects (infrequent)
10. Increased LFTs
11. Alopecia

Indications

Patients with persistent thrombocytopenia despite prior therapy with glucocorticoids and a prior splenectomy

Efficacy

1. The largest case series reported 2 complete remissions and 8 partial remissions in 21 patients, with severe thrombocytopenia after glucocorticoids and splenectomy. Both patients with complete responses subsequently relapsed
2. In a systematic review of chronic refractory ITP, complete remissions were reported in only 8% (3/40) of patients treated with interferon alfa-2b

Notes

1. Its mechanism of action is unknown, but may be due to modulation of effector B lymphocytes involved in the autoimmune process
2. The British Society of Haematology guidelines recommends against its use in managing ITP

65. Polycythemia Vera

Celia L. Grosskreutz, MD, and Steven Fruchtman, MD

Polycythemia vera (PV) is a typically clonal disorder involving a multipotent hematopoietic progenitor cell in which there is accumulation of phenotypically normal red cells, granulocytes, and platelets, and no recognizable physiologic stimulus

Epidemiology

Incidence: 2 per 100,000 people per year

Mean age: 60 years (range 20–85 years)

Survival: Symptomatic patients without treatment: ~6–18 months
Symptomatic patients with appropriate therapy: >10 years

Causes of death: Thrombosis (29%)
Hematologic malignancies (23%)
Nonhematologic malignancies (16%)
Hemorrhage (7%)
Myelofibrosis with myeloid metaplasia (3%)

Ania BJ et al. Am J Hematol 1994;47:89–93
Berk PD et al. In: Wasserman LR, Berlin NI, eds. Polycythemia Vera and the Myeloproliferative Disorders. Philadelphia: WB Saunders, 1995:166
Berlin NI. Semin Hematol 1975;12:339–351

Proposed Modified Diagnostic Criteria

A1	Red cell mass >25% above mean normal predicted value, or packed cell volume ≥0.60 in males or ≥0.56 in females
A2	Absence of cause of secondary erythrocytosis
A3	Palpable splenomegaly
A4	Marker of clonality, ie, acquired abnormal marrow karyotype
B1	Thrombocytosis (platelet count >400,000/mm^3)
B2	Neutrophil leukocytosis (neutrophil count >10,000/mm^3; >12,500/mm^3 in smokers)
B3	Splenomegaly demonstrated on isotope or ultrasound scan
B4	Characteristic BFU-E growth or reduced serum erythropoietin

PV = A1 + A2 + (A3 or A4) or
PV= A1 + A2 + two of B

Pearson TC. Baillieres Clin Haematol 1998;11:695–720

Work-Up

Exclude secondary erythrocytosis caused by physiologically appropriate or inappropriate erythropoietin (EPO)

CBC	• Elevated hematocrit and RBC mass (almost all patients) • Platelet count >400,000/mm^3 (60%) • WBC >12,000/mm^3 (40%)
Serum EPO level	• Low or normal EPO production (secondary to negative feedback) *vs.* Secondary erythrocytosis: Elevated EPO levels
Red cell mass	• Raised red cell mass (>25% above mean normal predicted value) *or* Raised packed cell volume ≥0.60 in males or ≥0.56 in females
BM aspirate and biopsy	• Bone marrow cellularity increased in 90% • Iron stores absent in 95% • Cytogenetics

Other Causes of Secondary Erythrocytosis

Congenital

1. Mutant high oxygen affinity hemoglobin
2. Congenital low 2,3-diphosphoglycerate
3. Autonomous high erythropoietin production
4. Truncation of the erythropoietin receptor

Acquired

1. Arterial hypoxemia (high altitude, cyanotic congenital heart disease, chronic lung disease)
2. Other causes of impaired tissue oxygen delivery (smoking)
3. Renal lesions (tumors, cysts, diffuse parenchymal disease, hydronephrosis, renal artery stenosis, transplantation)
4. Endocrine lesions (adrenal tumors)
5. Miscellaneous tumors (cerebellar hemangioblastoma, uterine fibroids, bronchial carcinoma)
6. Drugs (androgens)
7. Hepatic lesions (hepatoma, cirrhosis, hepatitis)

Berlin NI. Semin Hematol 1975;12:339–351

Treatment Options

Phlebotomy	• Reduces thrombotic events by reducing the RBC mass
Cytoreduction	• Cytoreductive drugs to control the number of circulating blood elements • Indicated when phlebotomies are problematic, in patients with a history of thrombosis, in patients with symptomatic or progressive splenomegaly and in elderly patients who are more prone to thrombotic disease
Allogeneic stem cell transplantation	• Only potentially curative therapy • Consider only in: (1) Patients who develop high-risk postpolycythemic myeloid metaplasia with myelofibrosis, *or* (2) Patients whose disease transforms to acute leukemia
Antithrombotic therapy	• Major thrombotic events can happen in 15% of patients and include: (1) Cerebrovascular accidents (2) Superficial thrombophlebitis (3) Pulmonary emboli (4) Mesenteric thrombosis (5) Myocardial infarction (6) Deep venous thrombosis (7) Budd-Chiari syndrome

Berk PD et al. In: Wasserman LR, Berlin NI, eds. Polycythemia Vera and the Myeloproliferative Disorders. Philadelphia: WB Saunders, 1995:166

Note: Manage reversible Thrombotic risk factors aggressively (eg, smoking, hypertension, hypercholesterolemia and obesity) Campbell DJ and Green AR, Hematology 2005; American Society of Hematology Education Book: 201–208

REGIMEN

PHLEBOTOMY

Streiff MB et al. Blood 2002;99:1144–1149

Phlebotomy

Indications

- Prevents thrombosis by reducing the RBC mass. Indicated for all patients to normalize hematocrit
- Treatment of choice for patients <50 years and all women of childbearing years

Goal

- Achieve and maintain a hematocrit of 40–45 (Hct <45% in men and <42% in women)

Therapy

Initial:

- Most patients: 250–500 mL every other day to achieve a hematocrit of 40–45%
- *Elderly and those with hemodynamic compromise:* 250–300 mL twice weekly

Maintenance:

- CBC every 4–8 weeks: Phlebotomy if hematocrit >45% in men; >42% in women

Limitations

- Phlebotomy unable to control leukocytosis, hyperuricemia, hypermetabolism, pruritus, and complications of splenomegaly seen in PV patients
- Patients treated with phlebotomy alone have a higher incidence of serious thrombotic complications during the first 3 years of therapy compared with patients treated with myelosuppression. This is especially true in the elderly (>60 years old)
- Elderly should be treated with cytoreduction in addition to phlebotomy

REGIMEN FOR CYTOREDUCTIVE THERAPY

HYDROXYUREA

Fruchtman SM et al. Semin Hematol 1997;34:17–23 [Editorial. Haematologica 1999;84:673–674

Nonemergent presentation:
Initial and maintenance dose: **Hydroxyurea** 15 mg/kg orally every day after meals as single dose or divided into 2 doses

Emergency situations: Decreased cerebral perfusion in setting of an elevated hematocrit or marked thrombocytosis:
Phlebotomy: Daily to a hematocrit of 45% in men and 42% in women
Initial (loading) dose: **Hydroxyurea** 30 mg/kg orally every day after meals as single dose or divided into 2 doses for 7 days, *followed by:*
Maintenance dose: **Hydroxyurea** 15 mg/kg orally every day after meals, as single dose or divided into 2 doses with close monitoring of CBC

Chronic therapy:
Optimal dose: Determined **empirically**, with frequent monitoring of CBC (eg, once weekly when adjusting dose*). Increase total daily dosage by 25–50%, and assess effect after 7 days before further escalation. Hydroxyurea 500–1000 mg/day is sufficient for most patients; however, the total daily dose is extremely variable

*When the peripheral blood count is maintained within acceptable range on stable dose of hydroxyurea, lengthen interval to 2 weeks and then to 4 weeks

Therapeutic goal (very high doses carry risk of prolonged aplasia):

1. Control the hematocrit without causing leukopenia (<3500/mm^3) or thrombocytopenia (<100,000/mm^3). This may require significantly higher or lower doses than the initial dose
2. For patients requiring frequent phlebotomies or those with platelet counts >600,000/mm^3, increase hydroxyurea dosage by 5 mg/kg per day at monthly intervals, with frequent monitoring until control is achieved
3. Supplemental phlebotomy is preferable to increased myelosuppression to control the hematocrit

Hydroxyurea is marketed in the United States as capsules for oral administration containing hydroxyurea 200 mg, 300 mg, and 400 mg, Droxia™ (hydroxyurea capsules); and as capsules for oral administration containing hydroxyurea 500 mg, Hydrea® (hydroxyurea capsules)

Emetogenic potential: Nonemetogenic (Emetogenicity score = 1). See Chapter 39 for antiemetic regimens

Toxicity

Hematologic side effects

1. Neutropenia is common; thrombocytopenia is rare
2. Cytopenias are usually rapidly reversible (within 3–4 days)
3. High doses and/or failure to stop treatment despite cytopenia may result in prolonged aplasia

Relatively common nonhematologic side effects

1. Gastrointestinal symptoms (stomatitis, anorexia, mild nausea/vomiting, diarrhea)
2. Acute skin reactions (rash, lower extremity ulcerations, dermatomyositis-like changes, erythema, nail discoloration)

Rare, nonhematologic side effects

1. Chronic skin reactions (hyperpigmentation, atrophy of skin and nails, skin cancer, alopecia)
2. Headache, drowsiness, convulsions
3. Fever, chills, asthenia
4. Renal and hepatic impairment

The leukemogenic risk of hydroxyurea is controversial. The sequence of administration of drugs is important in this regard. Hydroxyurea after ^{32}P or alkylating agents has a high risk of leukemogenic potential. A patient who is started on hydroxyurea and needs further treatment should receive either anagrelide HCl or interferon alfa

Treatment Modifications

Hematologic Toxicity	
WBC <3500/mm^3 or platelets <100,000/mm^3	Hold hydroxyurea until WBC >3500/mm^3 and platelets >100,000/mm^3, then restart hydroxyurea at 50% of prior dose
Nonhematologic Toxicity	
G1	No dose modifications
G2/3	Hold hydroxyurea until toxicity ≤G1; restart at prior dose
Recurrent G2/3	Hold hydroxyurea until toxicity ≤G1; restart at 75% of prior dose
G4	Hold hydroxyurea until toxicity ≤G1; restart at 50% of prior dose
Recurrent G4	Discontinue hydroxyurea.

Patient Population Studied

Patients with Philadelphia-positive and Philadelphia-negative myeloproliferative disorders have been studied

Efficacy

Eighty percent of patients will achieve control of blood counts with hydroxyurea and phlebotomy. The other 20% of patients will have refractory disease, will not tolerate therapy, or will develop a leukopenia, preventing further dose escalation

Monitoring Therapy

Frequent monitoring is necessary to prevent excessive marrow suppression

1. *During period of initial dose adjustment:* Weekly CBC
2. *When the peripheral blood count is maintained within an acceptable range on a stable dose of hydroxyurea:* Lengthen the evaluation interval for a CBC to 2 weeks, then to 4 weeks

REGIMEN FOR CYTOREDUCTIVE THERAPY

INTERFERON ALFA 2B

Silver RT. Semin Hematol 1997;34:40–50

Primary antipyretic prophylaxis:
Acetaminophen 650–1000 mg orally 1 hour before interferon administration, then every 4 hours for a total of 3 doses, *or*
Ibuprofen 400–600 mg orally 1 hour before interferon administration, then every 4 hours for a total of 3 doses
Secondary antiemetic prophylaxis:
If needed, use as primary prophylaxis with subsequent doses
Note: Have patients take interferon at bedtime, so that they sleep through the period of most severe symptoms

Initial dose: **Interferon alfa** 3 million units per dose subcutaneously 3 days/week [MWF] (total dose/week = 9 million units)

Maintenance dose: Increase **interferon alfa** in increments of 1 million units per dose to a dosage of 5 million units 3 days per week. Dose adjustments should be performed no more frequently than once every 8 weeks
Interferon alfa 5 million units per dose subcutaneously 3 days/week [MWF] (total dose/week = 15 million units *or*
Interferon alfa 3 million units per dose subcutaneously 5 days/week [MTWTF] (total dose/week = 15 million units)

Emetogenic potential: Low (Emetogenicity score = 2). See Chapter 39 for antiemetic regimens

Patient Population Studied

Multiple single-investigator reports of over 100 patients

Efficacy

Full benefit of therapy with interferon alfa 2b usually requires 6 months to 1 year
Control of erythrocytosis is achieved in approximately 76% of patients receiving subcutaneous interferon alfa in doses ranging from 4.5 to 27 million units per week. Similar degree of benefit has been seen regarding reduction in spleen size and relief from pruritus

Monitoring Therapy

1. *Every 3 to 4 weeks:* CBC with differential, LFTs, and serum glucose
2. *During therapy:* Ophthalmologic examination in patients with changes in visual acuity or visual fields
3. *If clinically indicated during treatment:* Chest x-ray (interferon alfa has been associated with pulmonary infiltrates)

Notes

1. Although most pregnant women do not have an indication for cytoreduction and CBC may normalize during pregnancy, interferon alfa doesn't cross the placenta and may be used in pregnancy if cytoreduction is indicated
2. Interferon alfa can aid in the treatment of pruritus

Berlin N, Berlin NI. Hematol Oncol Clin North Am 2003;17:1191–1210

Treatment Modifications

Adverse Event	Dose Modification
ANC $<750/mm^3$; platelets $<50,000/mm^3$	Discontinue interferon alfa until CBC normalizes; then reduce dose by 50%
LFTs >5 × upper limits of normal	Discontinue interferon alfa; resume treatment at 50% of original dose after LFTs normalize
Life-threatening or persistent, severe toxic reactions	Discontinue therapy
WHO G ≥3 toxicity	Stop treatment. Resume when toxicity G ≤1 at original dose
Recurrent WHO G ≥3 toxicity	Stop treatment. Resume when toxicity G ≤1 with interferon-alfa dose decreased by 50%

Toxicity

Acute Symptoms During Induction Therapy	% Occurence
Nonhematologic	
Flu like symptoms*	92%
Fever*	88%
Joint pain*	47%
Depression	28%
LFT abnormalities	5%
Hematologic	
Leukopenia	20%
Thrombocytopenia	27%
Symptoms Following Long-Term Administration	
Mild weight loss	Reversible after discontinuing therapy
Alopecia	Reversible after discontinuing therapy
Thyroiditis and hypothyroidism	Autoimmune disorders
Hemolytic anemia	Autoimmune disorders

*Can be controlled with acetaminophen. Up to 35% of patients discontinue therapy because of side effects such as fever, malaise, nausea, and vomiting

REGIMEN FOR CYTOREDUCTIVE THERAPY

ANAGRELIDE HCl

Fruchtman SM et al. Annual Meeting of the American Society of Hematology, Philadelphia, 2002; [Abstract #256]
Storen EC, Tefferi A. Blood 2001;97:863–866
Fruchtman SM et al. Leuk Res 2005; 29:481–491

Note: Anagrelide specifically targets megakaryocytes and is used to treat Thrombocytopenia

Initial dose: **Anagrelide HCl** 0.5 mg orally 2 (preferable) or 4 times daily

Maintenance dose: **Anagrelide HCl** 0.5–1 mg/dose orally, 2–4 doses/day to provide a total daily dose of 2–2.5 mg/day (doses need not be equal). To attain maintenance dose, increase dose at weekly intervals. Increment in dose should not exceed 0.5 mg per day

Optimal dose: Determined **empirically**, with frequent monitoring of platelet count (eg, 5–7 days when adjusting dose). Increase total daily dose by 0.5 mg if after 5–7 days platelet count does not begin to drop. Typically steady state doses are 2.2–2.5 mg daily. *Total anagrelide doses should not exceed 10 mg/day or 2.5 mg/dose*

Anagrelide HCl is available in the United States in capsules for oral administration containing 0.5 mg or 1 mg anagrelide. Product labeling, Argrylin® (anagrelide hydrochloride) Capsules; Shire Pharmaceutical Corp, Wayne, PA

Emetogenic potential: Low (Emetogenicity score = 2). See Chapter 39 for antiemetic regimens

Patient Population Studied

Over 2000 patients with both Philadelphia-positive and Philadelphia-negative myeloproliferative diseases have been studied

Efficacy

Over 75% of patients will achieve good platelet control. The remaining 25% will be either intolerant or have disease that is refractory to anagrelide

Toxicity

Hematologic	
↓ Hematocrit	36%
↓ WBC	—
Leukemogenic	(2.6%)[a]

Nonhematologic		
Palpitations[b]	26%	Administer carefully to elderly; avoid in patients with cardiac disease
Fluid retention[b]	20%	
Dizziness	15%	Usually within 2 weeks of start of therapy; often diminishes in severity or resolves in 2 weeks with continued therapy
Headaches	43%	
Diarrhea[c]	25%	
Nausea	17%	
Abdominal pain	16%	

[a]All patients who developed acute leukemia were previously exposed to other cytoreductive agents. No patients who transformed were exposed only to anagrelide

[b]Related to drug's vasodilatory and inotropic properties. Minimize by starting with a low dose (0.5 mg twice daily), gradually increasing dose until control of the platelet count is achieved

[c]Occurs in patients with lactose intolerance due to its packaging with lactose

Treatment Modifications

Hematologic Toxicity	
Platelet count <100,000/mm^3	Hold anagrelide until platelet count >100,000/mm^3; restart at 50% of prior dose

Nonhematologic Toxicity (>initial 2 weeks)	
G1	No dose modifications
G2/3	Hold anagrelide until toxicity ≤G1; restart at prior dose
Recurrent G2/3	Hold anagrelide until toxicity ≤G1; restart at 75% of prior dose
G4	Hold anagrelide until toxicity ≤G1; restart at 50% of prior dose
Recurrent G4	Discontinue anagrelide

Monitoring Therapy

Frequent monitoring is necessary to prevent excessive marrow suppression

1. *During period of initial dose adjustment:* Platelet count every 5–7 days
2. *When the peripheral blood count is maintained within acceptable range on stable dose of anagrelide:* Lengthen interval to 2 weeks, then to 4 weeks

Notes

1. Anagrelide, an oral quinazoline derivative, has a profound effect on the maturation of megakaryocytes, resulting in a reduction of platelet production. Also reported to cause a minimal decrease in hematocrit
2. Anagrelide HCl currently is not advised for use during pregnancy
3. Because anagrelide specifically targets the megakaryocytes, the increase in red cell mass seen in PV must be managed independently with phlebotomy
4. Symptoms improved with reduction in platelet count to 450,000–550,000/mm^3
5. A platelet count ≤ 450,000/mm^3 may *lead to* greater protection from thrombosis than reduction to a level ≤ 600,000/mm^3. Because no randomized trials support this, if a platelet count ≤ 450,000 mm^3 is not achievable owing to poor compliance or toxicity, continuing therapy and accepting a platelet count in the 600,000/mm^3 range are acceptable

REGIMEN

ALLOGENEIC STEM CELL TRANSPLANTATION

Deeg HJ, Appelbaum FR. Stem cell transplantation for myelofibrosis. NEJM 2001;344:775–776
Rondelli D et al. ASH Meeting 2003[Abstract # 695]

With standard fully ablative preparative regimens, a proportion of patients may be cured, but the peritransplantation mortality, especially in patients >45 years is high. Most patients are not candidates for this procedure, and the risks are greater than the risks from their underlying disease. However, some high-risk patients with myelofibrosis, or post-PV myelofibrosis, have, based on anemia, cytogenetics, or the level of the WBC, such a poor prognosis that an allogeneic transplant is a consideration if a match is available. Recently, outcomes have been improved using reduced-intensity regimens, but further studies must be performed

REGIMEN

ANTITHROMBOTIC THERAPY

Landolfi R et al. NEJM 2004;350:114–124

Patients with a history of thrombosis or cardiovascular disease:

1. **Low dose aspirin** 80–100 mg orally once daily, continuously. The results of the ECLAP study (European Collaboration Low Dose Aspirin in PV) *suggest* that unless a contraindication to ASA exists, patients with PV should be treated with low-dose ASA to prevent thrombotic complications. In addition, aspirin is effective for the treatment of erythromelalgia and other microvascular, neurologic, and ocular disturbances

   Note: The ECLAP study enrolled 518 patients with polycythemia vera with no clear indication for aspirin treatment and no contraindication to such treatment in a double-blind, placebo-controlled trial to assess the efficacy and safety of prophylaxis with low–dose aspirin (100 mg daily). Cytoreductive therapies (aspirin group vs. placebo group) included phlebotomy (69.2% vs. 74.3%), any cytoreductive drug (58.9% vs. 54.7%) and hydroxyurea (46.2% vs. 42.3%). Compared with placebo (n = 265 pts.) at a mean follow-up of 3 years, treatment with aspirin (n = 253 pts.):

- Reduced the risk of the combined end point of nonfatal myocardial infarction (MI), nonfatal stroke, or death from cardiovascular causes (relative risk, RR; 0.41; p = 0.09)
- Reduced the risk of the combined end point of nonfatal MI, pulmonary embolism, major venous thrombosis, or death from cardiovascular causes (RR, 0.40; p = 0.03)
- Reduced the risk of a thrombobotic event (RR, 0.42; p = 0.42) by intention-to-treat principle
- Did not significantly reduce overall mortality and cardiovascular mortality (RR, 1.62)

Safety. In the aspirin group versus the placebo group, there were non-significant increases in the risk of any bleeding episode (9.1% vs. 5.3%), a major bleeding episode (1.2% vs. 0.8%) and a minor bleeding episode (7.9% vs. 4.5%). At the completion of the study, 30.6% of the placebo group and 24.5% of the aspirin group had stopped taking the study drug. Discontinuation of therapy due to side-effects was reported in 6.4% of the placebo group and 6.4% of the aspirin group. The most frequent side effects leading to therapy discontinuation in the placebo group vs. aspirin group were gastrointestinal intolerance (4.5% vs. 2.8%) and bleeding (1.5% vs. 4.4%)

Landolfi R, et al. N Engl J Med 2004;350:114–124

2. Cytoreduction

Patients with PV who continue to have thrombotic or vascular symptoms, despite aspirin and good control of the hematocrit and platelet count with phlebotomy and myelosuppression:

1. **Clopidogrel** 75 mg orally once daily, continuously, *or*
2. **Ticlopidine** 250 mg orally twice daily, continuously

Note: These agents have not been studied in PV in a controlled fashion, but have been used by clinicians in these circumstances

Clopidogrel (Plavix® is marketed in the United States as capsules for oral administration containing 75 mg
Ticlopidine (Ticlid®) is marketed in the United States as capsules for oral administration containing 250 mg

66. Essential Thrombocythemia

Celia L. Grosskreutz, MD, and Steven Fruchtman, MD

Essential thrombocythemia (ET) is a chronic myeloproliferative disorder characterized by a sustained proliferation of megakaryocytes, which leads to increased numbers of circulating platelets. It is typically a clonal disorder originating at the level of the pluripotential hematopoietic stem cell

Epidemiology

Incidence: 2.38/100,000 per year
Average age at diagnosis: 50–60 years
Male/female ratio: 1:2

Survival: 10-year survival—64–80%
Principal cause of death: Thrombotic complications.
Leukemic transformation ranges from 3% to 10%, depending on treatment received

Mesa RA et al. Am J Hematol 1999;61:10–15

Work-Up

CBC	• Platelet count: 450,000–1,000,000/mm^3 • Hemoglobin normal (normal red cell mass) • Normal WBC • Absent *BCR/ABL* rearrangement
Peripheral smear	• Megathrombocytes
Bleeding time	• Prolonged in 10–20% of patients
Bone marrow aspirate and biopsy[a]	• Marrow may be normal • Increased marrow cellularity (90%) • Enlarged megakaryocytes with multilobulated nuclei clustering in small groups along sinuses is the hallmark of ET
Platelet aggregation[b]	• Frequently abnormal with impaired aggregation in response to epinephrine, ADP, and collagen, but not to arachidonic acid and ristocetin
von Willebrand factor[b]	• Laboratory features of acquired von Willebrand syndrome simulating type II von Willebrand factor deficiency (seen with marked increase in platelet numbers)

[a]Bone marrow study is necessary at initial evaluation. The following should be performed:
1. Histologic evaluation of the megakaryocyte lineage
2. Cytogenetics studies to rule out myelodysplastic syndrome and CML
3. Reticulin stains to rule out myelofibrosis
4. Iron stains

[b]Laboratory features of acquired von Willebrand syndrome (simulating type II von Willebrand factor deficiency) may be associated with a platelet count >1,000,000/mm^3. An enhanced thrombotic risk in ET patients has been associated with a reduction in the concentration of protein S, antithrombin III, protein C, and resistance to activated protein C resulting from an associated genetic defect in Factor V Leiden. Platelet aggregation studies and a screen for von Willebrand syndrome are recommended only in patients with a bleeding tendency

Finazzi G et al. Leuk Lymphoma 1996;22(suppl 1):71–78
Georgii A et al. Leuk Lymphoma 1996;22(suppl 1):15–29
Ruggeri M et al. Am J Hematol 2002;71:1–6

Criteria for Diagnosis of ET

1. Platelet count >600,000/mm^3 on two different occasions, separated by a 1-month interval
2. Hemoglobin normal or normal red cell mass (males <36 mL/kg; females <32 mL/kg)
3. Stainable iron in marrow, normal peripheral blood iron studies, or failure of iron trial (<1 g/dL rise in hemoglobin after 1 month of iron therapy) if appropriate to perform
4. Collagen fibrosis of marrow:
   a. Absent *or*
   b. <1/3 biopsy area without both splenomegaly and leukoerythroblastic reaction (typically seen in myelofibrosis)
5. Absence of the Philadelphia chromosome and/or the fusion *bcr/abl* gene by PCR
6. Absence of clonal cytogenetic abnormalities associated with myelodysplastic disorders
7. Absence of identifiable cause of reactive thrombocytosis

Murphy S et al. Semin Hematol 1997;34:29–39

Other Causes of Thrombocytosis

1. Iron deficiency anemia
2. Hyposplenism
3. Postsplenectomy*
4. Malignancy
5. Collagen vascular disease
6. Inflammatory bowel disease
7. Infection
8. Hemolysis
9. Rebound (cessation of ethanol intake, correction of vitamin B_{12} or folate deficiency)
10. Hemorrhage
11. Polycythemia vera
12. Idiopathic myelofibrosis
13. Essential thrombocytosis
14. Chronic myeloid leukemia
15. Idiopathic sideroblastic anemia
16. Myelodysplasia (5q− syndrome)
17. Postsurgery

*If platelet-count >2 million/mm³, cause is most likely a myeloproliferative disorder

Treatment Notes

1. The optimal therapy for patients with ET remains uncertain
2. Treatment of choice is based on patient age, ease of administration, comorbidities, and drug-related toxicity
3. Lacking a well-tolerated agent that is safe for long-term use, "no therapy" is acceptable if patient is asymptomatic and <60 years of age, although many clinicians use **low-dose aspirin (81–100 mg)** for patients in this category
4. A **cytoreductive agent** is indicated in high-risk patients to avoid the **high risk** of thrombosis and/or hemorrhage:

Cytoreductive agents
1. Hydroxyurea
2. Anagrelide
3. Interferon alfa
4. Busulfan

High-risk patients
1. ≥60 years of age
2. Prior thrombotic episode, including erythromelalgia, transient ischemic attacks, an large vessel thrombosis
3. Platelet count ≥1.5 million/mm³
4. Acquired von Willebrand syndrome

Recommended Treatment

	<60 Years and Asymptomatic	<60 Years and Symptomatic	≥60 Years
First choice	No therapy	Anagrelide	Hydroxyurea[a]
Second choice	Aspirin	Hydroxyurea	Anagrelide
Third choice	—	Interferon alfa	Interferon alfa
Fourth choice	—	Busulfan[b]	Busulfan[§]

1. Doses of each agent required for disease control depend on the target platelet level. A strict control to a platelet count ≤450,000/mm³ may lead to greater protection from thrombosis than reduction to a level ≤600,000/mm³. Although no randomized trials support this approach, it is easier to achieve this objective with anagrelide or interferon alfa than with agents from previous eras because of the avoidance of neutropenia
2. In younger patients, if a platelet count ≤450,000/mm³ is not achievable owing to poor compliance or toxicity, continuing therapy and accepting a platelet count in the 600,000/mm³ range are acceptable. **Low-dose aspirin (81 mg/day)** is also recommended in patients who suffer from thrombotic episodes, especially episodes involving the microcirculation or large vessels
3. **Low-dose aspirin (81 mg/day)** can also be considered in patients who cannot achieve better platelet control with cytoreductive therapy. Contraindications for aspirin, such as bleeding and peptic ulcer disease, should be considered before initiating aspirin. Concern regarding combination with anagrelide needs further studies, but this regimen should not be considered standard of care

[a]Patients who initially receive hydroxyurea and who no longer respond to this agent or suffer toxicity and require another agent *should not* receive long-term ^{32}P or melphalan therapy. This sequence of administration is associated with an extremely high risk of leukemic transformation. Patients who have had a trial of hydroxyurea and require further treatment should receive either anagrelide or interferon alfa

[b]Busulfan therapy is reserved for patients older than 60 years of age and those refractory or intolerant to other treatment approaches. Busulfan can precipitously lower platelet numbers, and patients treated with busulfan must be monitored closely. Rarely an elderly patient who cannot tolerate oral agents or does not have reliable access to laboratory monitoring may benefit from ^{32}P, which can be administered on a yearly basis by an expert

Finazzi G, Barbui T. Pathol Biol (Paris) 2001;49:167–169
Finazzi G et al. Br J Haematol 2000;110:577–583
Finazzi G et al. [Letter] Blood 2003;101:3749. [Comment on: Blood 2001;97:863–866]
Hanft VN et al. Blood 2000;95:3589–3593
van Genderen PJ et al. Br J Haematol 1997;97:179–184

REGIMEN FOR CYTOREDUCTIVE THERAPY

HYDROXYUREA

Cortelazzo S et al. NEJM 1995;332:1132–1136

Initial dose: **Hydroxyurea** 15 mg/kg per day orally after meals *or*

Hydroxyurea 7.5 mg/kg twice daily orally after meals

Optimal dose: Determined **empirically**, with frequent monitoring of CBC (eg, once per week when adjusting dose*). Increase total daily dose by 25–50%, and assess effect after 7 days before further escalation. Hydroxyurea 500–1000 mg/day is sufficient for most patients; however the total daily dose is extremely variable.

Therapeutic goal: Achieve a target platelet count <600,000/mm^3 (greater protection from thrombosis if platelet count <450,000/mm^3), with care to avoid the development of significant leukopenia

*When peripheral blood count is maintained within acceptable range on stable dose of hydroxyurea, lengthen monitoring interval to 2 and then to 4 weeks

Hydroxyurea is marketed in the United States as capsules for oral administration containing hydroxyurea 200, 300, and 400 mg Droxia™ (hydroxyurea capsules); and as capsules for oral administration containing hydroxyurea 500 mg, Hydrea® (hydroxyurea capsules)

Emetogenic potential: Nonemetogenic (Emetogenicity score = 1). See Chapter 39 for antiemetic regimens

Patient Population Studied

A study of 56 patients with essential thrombocythemia with median platelet count of 788,000/mm^3

Efficacy

Patients treated with hydroxyurea had lower incidence of thrombotic events compared with patients who received placebo. Hydroxyurea is not universally successful in controlling thrombocytosis. Resistance to hydroxyurea has been reported in 11–17% of cases

Toxicity

Hematologic

1. Neutropenia is common; thrombocytopenia is rare
2. Cytopenias are usually rapidly reversible within 3–4 days
3. High doses and/or failure to interrupt treatment despite cytopenia may result in prolonged aplasia

Relatively common nonhematologic

1. Gastrointestinal symptoms (stomatitis, anorexia, mild nausea/vomiting, diarrhea)
2. Acute skin reactions (rash, lower extremity ulcerations, dermatomyositis-like changes, erythema, nail ridging or discoloration)

Rare, nonhematologic

1. Chronic skin reactions (hyperpigmentation, atrophy of skin and nails, skin cancer, alopecia)
2. Headache, drowsiness, convulsions
3. Fever, chills, asthenia
4. Renal and hepatic impairment

The leukemogenic risk of hydroxyurea is controversial. The sequence of administration of drugs is important in this regard. Hydroxyurea followed by ^{32}P or alkylating agents has a high risk of leukemogenesis. A patient who is started on hydroxyurea and needs further treatment should next receive either anagrelide or interferon alfa

Treatment Modifications

Hematologic	
WBC < 3500/mm^3 or platelets <100,000/mm^3	Hold hydroxyurea until WBC >3500/mm^3 and platelets >100,000/mm^3, then restart hydroxyurea at 50% of prior dose
Nonhematologic	
G1	No dose modifications
G2/3	Hold hydroxyurea until toxicity ≤G1; restart at prior dose
Recurrent G2/3	Hold hydroxyurea until toxicity ≤G1; restart at 75% of prior dose
G4	Hold hydroxyurea until toxicity ≤G1; restart at 50% of prior dose
Recurrent G4	Discontinue hydroxyurea

Monitoring Therapy

Frequent monitoring is necessary to prevent excessive marrow suppression

1. *During period of initial dose adjustment:* Weekly CBC
2. *When the peripheral blood count is maintained within an acceptable range on a stable dose of hydroxyurea:* Lengthen the evaluation interval for a CBC to 2 weeks, then to 4 weeks

REGIMEN FOR CYTOREDUCTIVE THERAPY

ANAGRELIDE HCl

Anagrelide Study Group. Am J Med 1992;92:69–76
Storen EC, Tefferi A. Blood 2001;97:863–866
Tomer A. Blood 2002;99:1602–1609

Initial dose:
Anagrelide HCl 0.5 mg orally two times daily

Usual maintenance dose: **Anagrelide HCl** 0.5–1 mg/dose orally 2–4 doses per day to provide a total daily dose of 2–2.5 mg per day (doses need not be equal)

Optimal dose: Determined **empirically**, with frequent monitoring of platelet count (eg, 5–7 days when adjusting dose). Increase total daily dose by 0.5 mg if after 5–7 days platelet count does not begin to drop. Typically steady state doses are 2.2–2.5 mg daily. *Total anagrelide doses should not exceed 10 mg/day or 2.5 mg/dose*

Therapeutic goal: Achieve a target platelet count of <450,000–600,000/mm^3

Anagrelide HCl is available in the United States in capsules for oral administration containing 0.5 mg or 1 mg anagrelide. Product labeling, Argrylin® (anagrelide hydrochloride) Capsules; Shire Pharmaceutical Corp., Wayne, PA

Emetogenic potential: Low (Emetogenicity score = 2). See Chapter 39 for antiemetic regimens

Treatment Modifications

Hematologic Toxicity	
Platelet count <100,000/mm^3	Hold anagrelide until platelet count >100,000/mm^3; restart at 50% of prior dose
Nonhematologic Toxicity >Initial 2 Weeks	
G1	No dose modifications
G2/3	Hold anagrelide until toxicity ≤G1; restart at prior dose
Recurrent G2/3	Hold anagrelide until toxicity ≤G1; restart at 75% of prior dose
G4	Hold anagrelide until toxicity ≤G1; restart at 50% of prior dose
Recurrent G4	Discontinue anagrelide

Patient Population Studied

The Anagrelide Study Group included 335 patients with essential thrombocythemia

Anagrelide Study Group. Am J Med 1992;92:69–76

Efficacy

In a major study of 577 patients, among 335 patients with ET anagrelide HCl in low doses was effective in lowering the platelet count in 94% of patients. Most important, it was effective despite disease resistance to previous therapy. Anagrelide HCl was effective in lowering the platelet counts in 93% of patients treated previously with myelosuppressive agents alone (N = 169); and in 92% of patients treated with myelosuppressive agents plus interferon (N = 13). The time to a 50% reduction in platelet numbers was 11 days. The mean dose over time was 2.3–2.5 mg/day (median 2.0 mg/day). The median treatment duration was >31.4 months. Over 5 years, 16% of patients discontinued treatment because of side effects. An objective response was defined as a reduction of the platelet count from pre-treatment levels by 50% or to below 600,000/mm^3 (for those with baseline counts <1,200,000/mm^3) for at least 4 weeks.

Anagrelide Study Group. Am J Med 1992;92:69–76

Toxicity[a]

	%	Comment
Hematologic		
↓Hematocrit	36	—
↓WBC	—	—
Leukemogenic	(2.6)[b]	—
Nonhematologic		
Palpitations[c]	26	Administer carefully to elderly; avoid in patients with cardiac disease
Fluid retention[c]	20	
Dizziness	15	
Headaches	43	Usually within 2 weeks of start of therapy; often diminishes in severity or resolves in 2 weeks with continued therapy
Diarrhea[d]	25	
Nausea	17	
Abdominal pain	16	

[a]Not to be used during pregnancy
[b]All patients who developed acute leukemia were previously exposed to other cytoreductive agents. No patients transformed who were exposed only to anagrelide
[c]Related to drug's vasodilatory and inotropic properties. Minimize by starting with a low dose (0.5 mg twice daily) and gradually increasing dose until control of the platelet count is achieved
[d]Occurs in patients with lactose intolerance due to its packaging with lactose

Monitoring Therapy

Frequent monitoring is necessary to prevent excessive marrow suppression

1. *During period of initial dose adjustment:* Platelet count every 5–7 days
2. *When the peripheral blood count is maintained within acceptable range on stable dose of anagrelide:* Lengthen interval to 2 weeks, then to 4 weeks

Notes

1. Anagrelide, an oral quinazoline derivative, has a profound effect on the maturation of megakaryocytes, resulting in a reduction of platelet production
2. Anagrelide HCl is currently not advised for use during pregnancy
3. A platelet count ≤450,000/mm^3 may lead to greater protection from thrombosis than reduction to a level ≤600,000/mm^3. However because no randomized trials support this, if a platelet count ≤450,000/mm^3 is not achievable owing to poor compliance or toxicity, continuing therapy and accepting a platelet count in the 600,000/mm^3 range are acceptable

REGIMEN FOR CYTOREDUCTIVE THERAPY

INTERFERON ALFA 2B

Elliott MA, Tefferi A. Semin Thromb Hemost 1997;23:463–472
Sacchi S. Leuk Lymphoma 1995;19:13–20
Sacchi S et al. Ann Hematol 1991;63:206–209

Primary antipyretic prophylaxis:
Acetaminophen 650–1000 mg orally 1 hour before interferon administration, then every 4 hours for a total of 3 doses *or*
Ibuprofen 400–600 mg orally 1 hour before interferon administration, then every 4 hours for a total of 3 doses
Secondary antiemetic prophylaxis:
If needed, use as primary prophylaxis with subsequent doses
Note: Have patients take interferon at bedtime, so that they sleep through period of most severe symptoms

Initial dose: **Interferon alfa** 3 million units per dose subcutaneously 3–5 days/week [MTWTF] (total dose/week = 15 million units)* *or*
Interferon alfa 3 million units per dose subcutaneously 3 days/week [MWF] (total dose/week = 9 million units)

Maintenance dose: Usually 3 million units 3 times per week for most patients, but some require only 3 million units once per week (total dose/week = 3 to 9 million units)

Emetogenic potential: Low (Emetogenicity score) = 2). See Chapter 39 for antiemetic regimens

Patient Population Studied

Patients with essential thrombocythemia

Efficacy (N = 212)

In a total of 212 patients treated in 11 different clinical trials, a response rate of approximately 90% has been reported. At 3 million units per dose administered subcutaneously 5 days per week, the median time to complete response is 3 months

Sacchi S et al. Leuk Lymphoma 1995;19:13–20

Toxicity (N = Variable)

Acute Symptoms During Induction Therapy	
Fever	Frequently controlled with acetaminophen
Bone and muscle pain	
Fatigue	
Lethargy	
Depression	
Symptoms Following Long-term Administration	
Mild weight loss	Reversible after discontinuing therapy
Alopecia	
Thyroiditis and hypothyroidism	Autoimmune disorders
Hemolytic anemia	

Treatment Modifications

Adverse Event	Dose Modification
ANC <750/mm^3; platelets <50,000/mm^3	Discontinue interferon alfa until CBC normalizes then reduce dose of interferon alfa by 50%
ANC <500/mm^3; platelets <25,000/mm^3	Discontinue interferon alfa
LFTs ≥3–5 × upper limits of normal	Discontinue interferon alfa; resume treatment at 50% of original dose after LFTs normalize

Monitoring Therapy

1. *Every 3 to 4 weeks:* CBC with differential, LFTs, and serum glucose
2. *During therapy:* Ophthalmologic examination in patients with changes in visual acuity or visual fields
3. *If clinically indicated during treatment:* Chest x-ray (interferon alfa has been associated with pulmonary infiltrates and pneumonia)

REGIMEN FOR CYTOREDUCTIVE THERAPY

BUSULFAN

Van de Pette E et al. Br J Haematol 1986;62:229–237

Busulfan 4 mg orally, daily, until platelet count drops below 400,000/mm^3, *followed by*
Busulfan 4 mg orally, daily, for 2 weeks when the platelet count rises above 400,000/mm^3 (total dosage/2-week cycle: 56 mg)

Busulfan is manufactured in the United States in tablets for oral administration containing busulfan 2 mg. Myleran® (busulfan) Tablets product label, GlaxoSmithKline, Research Triangle Park, NC

Emetogenic potential: Nonemetogenic if <4 mg/day (Emetogenicity score = 1). Moderately high if ≥4 mg/day (Emetogenicity score = 4). See Chapter 39 for antiemetic regimens

Patient Population Studied

A study of 37 patients with essential thrombocythemia

Efficacy (N = 37)

Given on the mentioned doses, busulfan is a tolerable and effective regimen. These conclusions were based on a lengthy examination of the course of 37 patients. Among 24 patients followed for at least 4 years, a "controlled phase" with a platelet count of <400,000/mm^3 for a period of at least one year, was achieved in 76%. The "controlled phase" was achieved either without maintenance therapy or with only one two week course of busulfan. The median dose of busulfan required to achieve control was 589 mg with a median "controlled phase" duration of 164 weeks.

Toxicity (N = 37)

	%/Comment
Myelosuppression, all cell lines are equally affected*	Platelets can drop precipitously*
G1/2 nausea	>80%
G1/2 vomiting	>80%
G1/2 diarrhea	>80%
Skin hyperpigmentation	5–10%
Insomnia	Rare
Anxiety	Rare
Dizziness	Rare
Depression	Rare
Elevated LFTs	Rare
Pulmonary symptoms, cough, dyspnea and fever	Seen with long-term use in <5% of patients
Increased risk of secondary malignancy, especially AML	Seen with long-term use in <5% of patients

*Failure to stop busulfan treatment may result in bone marrow failure with severe, prolonged pancytopenia. Pancytopenia is potentially reversible, but recovery may take from 1 month to 2 years

Treatment Modifications

Adverse Event	Dose Modification
WBC* <4000/mm^3, but >3500/mm^3	Reduce busulfan dose by 50%
WBC* <3500/mm^3	Discontinue busulfan
LFTs 2–3 × upper normal limits	Reduce busulfan dose by 50%
LFTs >3 × upper normal limits	Hold busulfan until LFTs have returned to baseline values

*Regarding WBC, the product labeling for Myleran® states: "WBC counts typically decrease in response to busulfan, but its onset may be delayed by 10 days to 2 weeks after starting treatment. After decreasing WBC counts become apparent, the decline tends to continue exponentially if the busulfan dose and schedule is maintained. Decisions to change busulfan doses must be based on absolute hematological values *and* the rate at which the values are changing in response to treatment. Plotting a weekly WBC on semi-logarithmic graph paper (WBC counts on the log axis; time on the linear axis) may aid in planning when to discontinue therapy"

Monitoring Therapy

1. *Weekly:* CBC with differential and platelet count; LFTs during period of busulfan therapy

   Note: Because sudden, unexpected marrow suppression may occur, frequent CBC monitoring is mandatory
2. *Chest x-ray as indicated:* For insidious onset of cough, dyspnea, and low-grade fever after months to years of therapy, consider busulfan-related lung toxicity in differential diagnosis

Notes

Busulfan therapy is reserved for patients older than 60 years of age and for those refractory or intolerant to other approaches

Special Therapeutic Approaches

Surgery

1. Surgery can increase the risk of thrombosis. Under elective circumstances, the platelet count should be lowered to approach the normal range of ≤450,000/mm^3. There are no trials to compare the optimal cytoreductive agent in this setting, and either **anagrelide HCl** or **hydroxyurea** can be used. Therapy can be discontinued when a patient is ambulatory and the thrombotic risk is minimized
2. Patients who require emergency surgery must proceed to receive the surgical care they require despite elevated platelet numbers

Elliott MA et al. Curr Hematol Rep 2004;3(5):344–351

Pregnant Patients with ET

1. **Low-dose aspirin (81 mg/day)** therapy is the first treatment option and should be started during the first trimester. Some low-risk patients can be followed up with no therapeutic intervention. Aspirin should be discontinued 1 week before delivery to avoid bleeding complications during delivery or during the postpartum period. Cesarean section delivery is not routinely required for these patients
2. If a patient develops symptoms as a result of thrombosis within the vasculature, platelet reduction therapy is necessary and **interferon alfa** therapy is the treatment of choice. Since interferon alfa does not cross the placenta, it likely will not be teratogenic
3. **Hydroxyurea, anagrelide HCl, and busulfan** have been successfully used to treat myeloproliferative disorders during pregnancy, but they are probably teratogenic if used during the first trimester. If such agents are mandatory, they should be instituted after the first trimester, but ideally should be avoided. Patients already on these agents before pregnancy should have them stopped, and they should be managed with either **interferon alfa** or aspirin, depending on the clinical situation

Griesshammer M et al. Leuk Lymphoma 1996;22(suppl 1):57–63
Wright CA, Tefferi A. Eur J Haematol 2001;66:152–159

Patients with a Serious Acute Hemorrhagic Event

1. The site of bleeding should be determined immediately and antiplatelet aggregating agents stopped. Although the platelet count may be high, these platelets should be considered to be qualitatively abnormal, leading to defective hemostasis
2. The patient may be suffering from acquired von Willebrand syndrome. In these patients, desmopressin acetate (DDAVP) or factor VIII concentrates containing von Willebrand factor can be used immediately as chemotherapy is being administered
3. If acquired von Willebrand syndrome is not present, the transfusion of normal platelets is suggested. In patients with persistent hemorrhage, immediate reduction of the platelet count can be achieved by platelet pheresis
4. Alternately, **hydroxyurea 2000–4000 mg/day for 3–5 days should be administered immediately, then reduced to 1000 mg/day.** Any patient receiving hydroxyurea should be monitored for granulocytopenia and/or thrombocytopenia. Reduction of platelet counts is usually observed within 3–5 days after starting hydroxyurea treatment

Michiels JJ et al. Leuk Lymphoma 1996;22(suppl 1):47–56

Patients with Acute Arterial Thrombosis

1. These patients require immediate institution of platelet anti-aggregating agents. **Aspirin 81–100 mg/day** is suggested. Patients with erythromelalgia or transient ischemic attacks will have a rapid cessation of symptoms after the use of low-dose aspirin
2. In a patient with a life-threatening arterial thrombosis, the platelet count should be lowered with either a combination of **apheresis and hydroxyurea** or with **hydroxyurea alone**, depending on the severity of the event. Clinical judgment must be used. Surgical intervention may also be required, and, depending on the site, thrombolytic therapy can be used
3. If the arterial thrombosis involves the microcirculation and is not life-threatening (transient ischemic attacks or erythromelalgia), immediate **low-dose aspirin therapy (81 mg/day)** is indicated and platelet reduction therapy **(hydroxyurea, anagrelide HCl, or interferon alfa)** can be initiated using standard doses and schedules

van Genderen PJ et al. Br J Haematol 1997;97:179–184

Settings in Which to Consider Platelet Pheresis

Patients with life-threatening thrombotic complications or hemorrhage can be considered for emergency platelet reduction with **platelet pheresis.** When platelet pheresis is used, it should always be used in combination with a cytoreductive agent to suppress further platelet production. Frequency and volumes of platelet pheresis are decided after discussion with consultant. Consider platelet pheresis in:

1. Acute stroke
2. Myocardial infarction
3. Infarction of an organ other than the heart
4. Budd-Chiari syndrome

ET with von Willebrand Syndrome

Platelets have receptors for von Willebrand multimers. Thus, in the presence of markedly elevated platelet numbers, these multimers can be absorbed by platelets and an acquired deficiency created. This von Willebrand deficiency can contribute to a bleeding diathesis. Some clinicians believe acquired von Willebrand syndrome is an indication for platelet reduction therapy.

67. Myelodysplastic Syndromes

Michael M. Boyiadzis, MD, MHSc, and Neal S. Young, MD

Myelodysplastic syndromes (MDS) are clonal disorders characterized initially by ineffective hematopoiesis and subsequently by the development of acute leukemias. Peripheral blood cytopenias in combination with a hypercellular bone marrow exhibiting dysplastic changes are the hallmark of MDS

Epidemiology

Incidence: Increases with age	
Mean age:	68 years
Overall:	4.1 per 100,000
Ages 50–59:	5.3 per 100,000
Ages 60–69:	15 per 100,000
Ages 70–79:	49 per 100,000
Ages >80:	89 per 100,000
Male/female ratio:	1:1

Survival

Overall median survival	2 years
Median Survival Based on the International Prognostic Scoring System (IPSS)	
Low risk	5.7 years
Intermediate-1 risk	3.5 years
Intermediate-2 risk	1.2 years
High risk	0.4 years

Dunbar CE, Saunthararajah Y. In: Young NS, ed. Bone Marrow Failure Syndromes. Philadelphia: WB Saunders, 2000:69–98
Greenberg P et al. Blood 1997;89:2079–2088

Who Classification of Myelodysplastic Syndromes

Category	Peripheral Blood	Bone Marrow
RA	Anemia No or rare blasts —	Erythroid dysplasia only Blasts <5% Ringed sideroblasts <15%
RARS	Anemia No blasts	Erythroid dysplasia only Blasts <5% Ringed sideroblasts ≥15%
RCMD	Cytopenias (bi- or pancytopenia) No or rare blasts Monocytes <1000/mm³ — No Auer rods	Dysplasia ≥10% of cells in two or more myeloid cell lines Blasts <5% — Ring sideroblasts <15% No Auer rods
RCMD-RS	Cytopenias (bi- or pancytopenia) No or rare blasts Monocytes <1000 mm³ — No Auer rods	Dysplasia ≥10% of cells in two or more myeloid cell lines Blasts <5% — Ring sideroblasts ≥15% No Auer rods
RAEB-I	Cytopenias Blasts <5% Monocytes <1000 mm³ No Auer rods	Unilineage or multilineage dysplasia Blasts 5–9% — No Auer rods
RAEB-II	Cytopenias Blasts 5–19% Monocytes <1000/mm³ Auer rods±	Unilineage or multilineage dysplasia Blasts 10–19% — Auer rods±
MDS-U	Cytopenias No or rare blasts No Auer rods	Unilineage dysplasia in granulocyte or megakaryocytes Blasts <5% No Auer rods
MDS, isolated del (5q)	Blasts <5% Platelets: normal or increased Anemia	Isolated del (5q), blasts <5% Megakaryocytes: normal or increased —

RA, refractory anemia; RAEB, RA with excess blasts; RARS, RA with ringed sideroblasts; RCMD, refractory cytopenia with multilineage dysplasia; RCMD-RS, RCMD with ringed sideroblasts; MDS-U, Myelodysplastic syndrome, unclassified

Germing U et al. Leuk Res 2000;24:983–992
Harris NL et al. Histopathology 2000;36:69–86
Harris NL et al. JCO 1999;17:3835–3849
Vardiman JW et al. Blood 2002;100:2292–2302

Work-Up

1. CBC with differential	Leukocytes:	ANC <2500/mm^3: 50% of patients at presentation ANC <1500/mm^3: 20–35% of patients at presentation ↑ WBC: Rare (except patients with chronic myelomonocytic leukemia)
	Erythrocytes:	Hgb <10 g/dL: 80% Anemia as an isolated cytopenia: 30–35%
	Platelets:	Thrombocytopenia: 25–50% of patients at presentation
2. Peripheral blood smear	Peripheral blood smear abnormalities are a hallmark of MDS: 1. Hypogranulated neutrophils with abnormal nuclei 2. Giant platelets 3. Polychromasia 4. Macrocytosis and anisopoikilocytosis 5. Reticulocytosis (rare)	
3. Bone marrow biopsy and aspiration with iron stains	• Marrow cellularity is usually normal or increased • No single characteristic feature of marrow morphology distinguishes MDS • Dysplastic features seen in MDS marrow: 1. Megaloblastoid changes 2. Ringed sideroblasts 3. Micromegakaryocytes 4. Abnormal megakaryocyte nuclei 5. Increased myeloblasts 6. Hypogranular promyelocytes 7. Increased monoblasts	
4. Cytogenetic analysis of bone marrow cells	• Clonal cytogenetic abnormalities: 30–79% of patients at presentation 1. Deletions are more common than translocations 2. Most common chromosomal aberrations in MDS patients:	

Numericals	(%)	Translocations	(%)	Deletions	(%)
+8	19	inv 3	7	del(5q)	27
−7	15	t(1;7)	2	del(11q)	7
+21	7	t(1;3)	1	del(12q)	5
−5	7	t(3;3)	1	del(20q)	5
		t(6;9)	<1	del(7q)	4
		t(5;12)	<1	del(13q)	2

−, loss of chromosome; +, additional chromosome; inv, inversion; t, translocation; del, deletion

5. HLA typing	• For patients <60 years and their siblings • Consider HLA typing for older patients with good performance status
6. Serology	HIV testing if clinically indicated
7. Chemistry	RBC folate, serum B_{12}, serum iron/TIBC/ferritin, serum erythropoietin level (before RBC transfusion)

Dunbar CE, Saunthararajah Y. In: Young NS, ed. Bone Marrow Failure Syndromes. Philadelphia: WB Saunders, 2000:69–98
Hofmann W-K et al. Hematol J 2004;5:1–8

International Prognostic Scoring System (IPSS)

	Score Value				
Prognostic Variable	**0**	**0.5**	**1**	**1.5**	**2**
BM blasts (%)	<5	5–10	—	11–20	21–30
Karyotype[a]	Good	Intermediate	Poor	—	—
Cytopenias[b]	0–1 lineage	2 or 3 lineages	—	—	—

[a]Good = normal, −Y, del(5q), del(20q)
Poor = complex (≥3 abnormalities) or chromosome 7 abnormalities
Intermediate = all other abnormalities
[b]Cytopenias defined as: hemoglobin level <10 g/dL; ANC <1800/mm^3; Platelet count <100,000/mm^3

IPSS Risk Group	Total Score	No. of Years for 25% of Patients to Evolve to AML
Low	0	9.4
Intermediate-1	0.5–1	3.3
Intermediate-2	1.5–2	1.1
High	≥2.5	0.2

Greenberg P et al. Blood 1997;89:2079–2088 [Erratum in Blood 1998;91:1100]

Differential Diagnosis of Hypoproductive Cytopenias

Hematologic Conditions

1. Congenital
   - Hereditary sideroblastic anemia
   - Congenital dyserythropoietic anemia
   - Fanconi's anemia
   - Diamond-Blackfan syndrome
   - Shwachman syndrome
   - Kostmann's syndrome
2. Nutritional
   - Vitamin B_{12} deficiency
   - Folate deficiency
   - Iron deficiency
3. Aplastic anemia
4. Paroxysmal nocturnal hemoglobinuria
5. Systemic mastocytosis
6. Hairy cell leukemia
7. Large granular lymphocyte disease
8. Myeloproliferative syndromes
   - Idiopathic myelofibrosis
   - Polycythemia vera
   - Chronic myelogenous leukemia
   - Essential thrombocytosis

Nonhematologic Conditions

1. Toxins
   - Alcohol
   - Post-chemotherapy or radiation
   - Medications
2. Chronic diseases
   - Renal failure
   - Collagen-vascular diseases
   - Chronic infections
3. Viral infections
   - Parvovirus B19
   - Cytomegalovirus
   - Human immunodeficiency virus
4. Malignancy
   - Marrow infiltration
   - Paraneoplastic syndrome

International Working Group Treatment Response Criteria for MDS

Complete remission (CR)	• <5% myeloblasts with normal maturation of all cell lines • No evidence of dysplasia • Hemoglobin >11 g/dL (untransfused, patient not on cytokine support) • Neutrophils ≥1500/mm^3 (patient not on cytokine support) • Platelets ≥100,000/mm^3 (patient not on cytokine support)
Partial remission (PR)	Same as CR except blast decreased by 50% or more over pretreatment
Stable disease	Failure to achieve at least PR, but without evidence of progression for at least 2 months

Hematologic Improvement

Erythroid response

Major	Pretreatment hemoglobin <11g/dL	>2 g/dL increase in hemoglobin
	RBC transfusion-dependent patients	Transfusion independence
Minor	Pretreatment hemoglobin <11g/dL	1–2 g/dL increase in hemoglobin
	RBC transfusion-dependent patients	50% decrease in transfusion requirement

Platelet response

Major	Pretreatment platelet count <100,000/mm^3	Absolute increase of ≥30,000/mm^3 in platelet count
	Platelet transfusion-dependent patients	Stabilization of platelet counts and transfusion independence
Minor	Pretreatment platelet count <100,000/mm^3	≥50% increase in platelet count with a net increase of 10,000/mm^3–30,000/mm^3

Neutrophil response

Major	Pretreatment ANC <1500/mm^3	≥100% increase in ANC, or an absolute increase of >500/mm^3 whichever is greater
Minor	Pretreatment ANC <1500/mm^3	≥100% increase in ANC, but absolute increase <500/ mm^3

Cytogenetic response

Major	No detectable cytogenetic abnormality, if preexisting abnormality was present
Minor	50% or more reduction in abnormal metaphases

Cheson BD et al. Blood 2000;96:3671–3674

Treatment Options

1. *Supportive care:* Transfusions and cytokine support (See Supportive Care section)
2. *Low-intensity therapy:* Agents in this group should be used preferably in the context of a clinical trial because little is known about their efficacy, optimal doses, toxicity, and the appropriate selection of patients. Azacitidine and decitabine have has been approved by the FDA for treatment of MDS, and lenalidomide for patients with MDS associated with a deletion 5q cytogenetic abnormality. Other agents that have shown some efficacy include antithymocyte globulin (ATG), thalidomide, amifostine, cyclosporine, vitamin D analogues, farnesyltransferase inhibitors, arsenic trioxide.
3. *High-intensity therapy:*
   - Hematopoietic stem cell transplantation (HSCT) *or*
   - Intensive chemotherapy

Treatment Recommendation depends on:
Patient's IPSS Risk Group, age, performance status and comorbid conditions

Therapy for Lower Risk Patients (IPSS Low/Intermediate-1)

- Supportive care and consider low intensity therapy
- Patients with del(5q) abnormality should receive lenalidomide

Therapy for Higher Risk Patients (IPSS Intermediate-2/High)

- HSCT or intensive chemotherapy
- If patient is not candidate for high intensity therapy consider supportive care and low intensive therapy

Supportive Care

Transfusion recommendations

RBC transfusions:

1. Transfuse patients with symptomatic anemia on a regular schedule that allows normal activity
2. Consider iron chelation in patients with:
   a. A transfusion burden >20 to 30 units of packed RBCs
   b. Ferritin levels consistently >2500 ng/mL
   c. Sideroblastic anemia, because they hyperabsorb iron and present with iron overload even before RBC transfusions
   d. Chelation therapy is not indicated in patients with a very poor prognosis who are unlikely to die of iron overload
3. Leukocyte depletion minimizes allosensitization
4. If a patient is a potential HSCT candidate, irradiation of blood products is also indicated

Platelet transfusions:

1. Most patients with MDS do not require platelet transfusion despite severe thrombocytopenia
2. Platelet dysfunction may predispose to bleeding even at platelet counts >20,000/mm^3. In such patients, prophylactic or therapeutic transfusions may be appropriate, regardless of platelet count
3. Consider aminocaproic acid or other antifibrinolytic agents for bleeding refractory to platelet transfusion or profound thrombocytopenia
4. Leukocyte depletion minimizes allosensitization

Cytokine support recommendations

1. Epoetin is not recommended if the endogenous serum erythropoietin levels >500 units/L, because of low erythroid response
2. Iron repletion must be verified before initiating epoetin therapy
3. Erythroid response of epoetin (150–300 units/kg per day subcutaneously) generally occurs within 6–8 weeks after starting treatment
4. If a patient is started at a low dose of epoetin and/or no response occurs within the first 6–8 weeks, the epoetin dose should be increased and the patient reassessed after an additional 6- to 8-week period
5. If response occurs, then either maintain the epoetin dose or reduce the number of weekly epoetin treatments stepwise from daily to 5 days → 4 days → 3 days per week at 4-week intervals to the lowest dose that maintains an acceptable response
6. If no response occurs with epoetin alone, consider adding filgrastim
7. Filgrastim and epoetin synergistically increase the erythroid response rate to 34–38%
8. Low filgrastim dosages (0.3–3 mcg/kg per day subcutaneously) are generally needed for the synergistic erythropoietic effect. Filgrastim doses should be escalated weekly to normalize the neutrophil count in initially neutropenic patients; or double the neutrophil count in patients who are initially normal
9. If a response to combined therapy occurs, then consider reducing filgrastim to 3 ×/week and epoetin from daily to 5 days → 4 days → 3 days per week at 4-week intervals to the lowest dose that maintains an acceptable response
10. If no response occurs within 6–8 weeks, then combined treatment should be discontinued
11. Patients with RARS have a lower response to epoetin. Consider combination therapy with epoetin and filgrastim from the outset
12. Filgrastim should be consider for neutropenic MDS patients with recurrent or resistant infections

Bowen D et al. Br J Haematol 2003;120:187–200
Dunbar CE, Saunthararajah Y. In: Young NS, ed. Bone Marrow Failure Syndromes. Philadelphia: WB Saunders, 2000:69–98
Hellström-Lindberg E et al. Br J Haematol 2003;120:1037–1046
Hellström-Lindberg E et al. Br J Haematol 1995;89:67–71

REGIMEN FOR LOW-INTENSITY THERAPY

AZACITIDINE

Silverman LR et al. JCO 2002;20:2429–2440
Vidaza ® (Azacitidine) product labeling

Recommended starting dose:
Azacitidine 75 mg/m^2 per day* subcutaneously for 7 days on days 1–7 every 4 weeks (total dosage/cycle = 525 mg/m^2)

*The dose may be increased to 100 mg/m^2 per day for 7 days if no beneficial effect is seen after two treatment cycles and if no toxicities occurred other than nausea and vomiting

Emetogenic potential: Nonemetogenic (Emetogenicity score = 1). See Chapter 39 for antiemetic regimens

Indications

1. Refractory anemia
2. Refractory anemia with ringed sideroblasts (if accompanied by neutropenia, thrombocytopenia, or transfusions requirement)
3. Refractory anemia with excess blasts
4. Refractory anemia with excess blasts in transformation
5. Chronic myelomonocytic leukemia

Efficacy (Randomized, N = 191)

	Supportive Care (n = 92)	Azacitidine 75 mg/m^2/day (n = 99)
Overall response	5%	60%
Complete response	—	7%
Partial response	—	16%
Improved	5%	37%
Median time to leukemia or death	13 months	21 months
AML transformation as first event	38%	15%

Monitoring Therapy

1. *Every week for 4 months then every 2 weeks:* CBC with differential
2. *Before beginning each treatment cycle:* LFTs, serum creatinine, and electrolytes
3. *At 2 and 4 months:* Bone marrow aspiration and biopsy to evaluate response

Treatment Modification

Adjustments Based on Hematology Values

For patients with pretreatment WBC ≥3000/mm^3, ANC ≥1500/mm^3, and platelets ≥75,000/mm^3, adjust azacitidine dosage based on nadir counts

Nadir Count ANC (/mm^3)	Nadir Count Platelets (/mm^3)	% Dosage in Next Cycle
<500	<25,000	50
500–1500	25,000–50,000	67
>1500	>50,000	100

For patients with pretreatment WBC <3000/mm^3, ANC <1500/mm^3, and platelets <75,000/mm^3, adjust azacitidine dosage based on nadir counts and bone marrow biopsy cellularity at the time of the nadir*

% Decrease in WBC or Platelet Nadir from Baseline	BM Biopsy % Cellularity at Nadir	% Dosage in Next Cycle
50–75	30–60	100
50–75	15–30	50
50–75	<15	33
>75	30–60	75
>75	15–30	50
>75	<15	33

If a nadir as defined above occurs, next cycle should be given 28 days after the start of preceding course, provided both WBC and platelet counts are >25% above the nadir and rising.
If by day 28 counts are not yet >25% above nadir, reassess every 7 days. If a 25% increase is not seen by day 42, then patient should be treated with 50% of scheduled dose

Note: If there is a clear improvement in differentiation at time of the next cycle, then continue current treatment dose. Improvement is defined as a greater percentage of mature granulocytes and ANC than were present before a treatment cycle commenced

Adjustment Based on Renal Function and Serum Electrolytes

Adverse Event	Modification
Unexplained reductions in serum bicarbonate to <20 mEq/L	Reduce dosage in next cycle by 50%
Unexplained elevations of BUN or serum creatinine	Delay next cycle until values normalize or return to baseline; then resume with dosage decreased by 50%

Toxicity (N = 99)

Hematologic

	% G3/4
Leukopenia	43
Granulocytopenia	58
Thrombocytopenia	52

Common Nonhematologic

Nausea, vomiting, diarrhea, fatigue, pyrexia, irritation at the site of injection, and constipation

Notes

1. It is recommended that patients be treated for a minimum of 4 cycles. However, complete or partial response may require more than 4 treatment cycles
2. Treatment may be continued as long as a patient continues to benefit

REGIMEN FOR LOW-INTENSITY THERAPY

ANTITHYMOCYTE GLOBULIN (ATG) [LYMPHOCYTE IMMUNOGLOBULIN]

Molldrem JJ et al. Ann Intern Med 2002;137:156–163
Molldrem JJ et al. Br J Haematol 1997;99:699–705
Atgam® (antithymocyte globulin [equine]) product labeling

Premedication:
Acetaminophen 650 mg orally 60 minutes before each ATG treatment *and*
Diphenhydramine 25–50 mg, orally 60 minutes before each ATG treatment
Prednisone 1 mg/kg per day orally (minimum dose: 40 mg on days 1–10) for 10 consecutive days on days 1–10, and then taper the dose to discontinue prednisone by day 17

Antithymocyte globulin [equine]* 40 mg/kg through a high-flow (central) vein, vascular shunt, or arteriovenous fistula in a volume of 0.9% NaCl injection (0.9% NS), 5% dextrose injection (D5W), 0.225% NaCl injection (0.225% NS), or 5% dextrose and 0.45% NaCl injection (D5W/.45% NS) sufficient to produce a solution with ATG concentration ≤4 mg/mL over at least 4 hours on days 1–4 (total dosage/course = 160 mg/kg)

Notes:
1. The initial infusion rate should be 10% of the total volume/hour. For example, for a total volume of 500 mL, start at 50 mL/hour for the first 30 minutes. If there are no signs of an adverse reaction, the infusion rate can be increased to complete the infusion within 4 hours
2. Always administer ATG through an in-line filter with pore size 0.2–1 micrometer
3. *Atgam® (antithymocyte globulin, [equine]) product labeling recommends skin testing before ATG administration

Emetogenic potential: Nonemetogenic (Emetogenicity score = 1). See Chapter 39 for antiemetic regimens

Patient Population Studied

A single-treatment, prospective study of 61 patients with MDS

Efficacy (N = 61)

Transfusion (Tx) Independence (N = 61)	
Tx independent in ≤8 months	34% (21)
Median time to Tx independence	10 weeks
Median duration of Tx independence	36 months[a]

Platelet Response (Sustained without Transfusion) (Initial Platelets ≤20,000/mm^3) (n = 21)	
Platelets[b] 25,000–217,000/mm^3	76%

Neutrophil Responses (Initial ANC ≤500/mm^3) (n = 11)	
Sustained ANC >1000/mm^3	55%

[a]In 17/21(81%) responders
[b]16/21 including 12 responders and 4 nonresponders

Toxicity (N = 61)

1. Severity and frequency of toxicities are greatest during the first day of infusion and diminish with each subsequent day. Toxicities generally subside after completing treatment
2. Adverse effects usually can be managed while continuing the ATG infusion (see table below, Infusional Toxicities of ATG)
3. All patients developed some degree of serum sickness (consisting of fever, rash, and arthralgia) between 7 and 14 days after treatment
4. Two patients had a 5-fold elevation of alanine aminotransferase and aspartate aminotransferase, and 1 patient had cardiovascular instability
5. No other immediate or delayed toxicity resulted from ATG treatment

Monitoring Therapy

1. *During ATG infusion:* CBC with differential, LFTs, and electrolytes
2. *After ATG therapy:* CBC monitoring is dependent on blood counts. If they are stable, CBC with differential can be as infrequent as once every 2–3 weeks. Patients requiring platelets may need more frequent CBCs, but not more than twice weekly and usually only once weekly
3. *Six months after the start of therapy:* Bone marrow biopsy and aspiration. If patients are stable according to blood counts, bone marrow biopsy may not need to be repeated

Notes

ATG has been shown most efficacious in MDS patients with HLA-DR 15 histocompatability type Saunthararajah et al. Blood 2002;100:1570–1574

Guidelines for administering ATG

Allergy skin testing before ATG administration:
- Advise patients to avoid using H_1-receptor antagonists for 72 hours before skin testing
- Antithymocyte globulin [equine] is freshly diluted (1:1000) with 0.9% NaCl injection (0.9% NS) to a concentration of 5 mcg/0.1 mL and administered intradermally
- Administer 0.1 mL 0.9% NS intradermally in a contralateral extremity as a control
- Observe every 15–20 minutes over the first hour after intradermal injection
- A local reaction ≥10 mm with a wheal, erythema, or both ± pseudopod formation and itching or a marked local swelling is considered a positive test result. For a positive test result, consider desensitization before therapy
- If antithymocyte globulin is administered after a locally positive skin test, administration should be attempted only in a setting where intensive life support facilities are immediately available and with the attendance of a physician familiar with the treatment of potentially life-threatening allergic reactions
- Systemic reactions eg, generalized rash, tachycardia, dyspnea, hypotension, or anaphylaxis preclude antithymocyte globulin administration

Monitoring during ATG administration
- Patients should remain under continual surveillance
- Assess peripheral vascular access sites for thrombophlebitis every 8 hours
- Monitor vital signs and assess for adverse reactions (flushing, hives, itching, SOB, difficulty breathing, chest tightness) before starting administration, then:

  During initial dose: Continually during the first 15 minutes, then every 30 minutes × 2, then at least every hour until administration is completed
  During subsequent doses: 30 minutes after initiating infusion

Infusional Toxicities of ATG

Adverse Events	Interventions
Rigors	Antihistamines (eg, diphenhydramine 25–50 mg intravenously or orally every 6 hours as needed) Meperidine 12.5–50 mg intravenously every 3–4 hours as needed
Nausea, vomiting	Antiemetic rescue. Give antiemetic primary prophylaxis during subsequent ATG treatments
Anaphylaxis[a]	Immediately *stop* administration; administer steroids; assist respiration; and provide other resuscitative measures. *Do not* resume treatment
Thrombocytopenia, anemia	Blood product transfusions as needed[b]
Fever and neutropenia[c]	Broad-spectrum antibiotics empirically, if ANC <500/mm^3. May give acetaminophen 650 mg orally every 4 hours
Hypotension	Fluid resuscitation
Refractory hypotension	May indicate anaphylaxis. Stop ATG infusion and stabilize blood pressure. Intensive Care Unit support
Oxygen desaturation	Oxygen therapy
Refractory desaturation	Discontinue ATG. Intensive Care Unit support
Respiratory distress	Discontinue ATG. If distress persists, administer an antihistamine, epinephrine, corticosteroids
Rash, pruritus, urticaria	Administer antihistamines and/or topical steroids for prophylaxis and treatment
Serum sickness–like symptoms[d]	Administer prophylactic glucocorticoids
Hepatotoxicity |[e]	Monitor LFTs

[a]Anaphylaxis (<3% of patients) more frequently occurs within the first hour after starting ATG infusion. After the first hour, adverse effects occur as a result of a delayed immune response and generally can be managed while continuing the ATG infusion

[b]Concomitant administration of blood products should be avoided with ATG infusions to avoid confusing transfusion reactions with reactions to ATG

[c]Most patients who receive ATG develop fever as a result of the drug. Most fevers are not infectious in origin

[d]Type II hypersensitivity reactions/serum sickness consisting of fever, rash, and arthralgia develop in approximately 85% of patients between 7 and 14 days after treatment. These symptoms can be managed with corticosteroids

[e]An isolated increase in serum alanine transaminase frequently has no clinical significance. Generally, liver function abnormalities are transient and return to normal within 1 month

Bevans MF, Shalabi RA. Clin J Oncol Nurs 2004;8:377–382

REGIMEN FOR LOW INTENSITY THERAPY

LENALIDOMIDE

List AF, et al. Proc Am Soc Clin Oncol 2005;23:2S
REVLIMID® product label, December 27, 2005

REGIMEN

Note: Lenalidomide is indicated for the treatment of patients with transfusion-dependent anemia due to Low- or Intermediate-1-risk myelodysplastic syndromes associated with a deletion 5q cytogenetic abnormality with or without additional cytogenetic abnormalities
Lenalidomide 10 mg/day, administer orally, continually (total dose/week = 70 mg)
In the USA, lenalidomide is available as prompt-relase capsules for oral administration containing either 5 mg or 10 mg. REVLIMID® product label, December 27, 2005. Celgene Corporation, Summit, NJ Information about REVLIMID® and the RevAssist℠ program can be obtained by calling the Celgene Customer Care Center toll-free at 1-888-423-5436

Emetogenic Potential = Non-emetogenic (Emetogenicity score = 1). See Chapter 39 for antiemetic regimens

Patient Population Studied

148 patients (median age, 71 years) with del 5q31 low- or intermediate-1-risk MDS who had RBC transfusion-dependent anemia (≥ 2 Units of RBCs within 8 weeks prior to study treatment), absolute neutrophil counts (ANC) ≥500 cells/mm^3, and platelet counts ≥50,000/mm^3

Efficacy

- Transfusion independence (≥56 days RBC transfusion-free and ≥1 g/dL Hgb increase): 64% of transfusion dependent patients
- Median Hgb increase 3.9 g/dL
- Cytogenetic responses (≥50% decrease in abnormal cells in metaphase): 76% of transfusion independent patients with 55% cytogenetic complete responses
- Pathologic CR: 29% of evaluable pts

Toxicity

	% All grades	%G3/4
Neutropenia	59	53
Thrombocytopenia	62	50
Diarrhea	49	–
Pruritus	42	–
Pneumonia	N/A	8
Rash	36	7
Anemia	N/A	6
Leukopenia	N/A	6
Fatigue	31	5
Dyspnea	N/A	5
Back pain	N/A	5
Febrile neutropenia	N/A	4

Monitoring Therapy

1. *Weekly for the first 8 weeks of treatment and monthly thereafter to monitor for cytopenias:* CBC with differential
2. *Every two weeks for the first 8 weeks and then monthly:* BUN and creatinine

Treatment Modifications

If thrombocytopenia develops within 4 weeks after starting 10 mg daily and if baseline platelet count was ≥100,000/mm³	
Platelets <50,000/mm³	Interrupt therapy
Platelets ≥50,000/mm³	Resume lenalidomide at 5 mg daily
If thrombocytopenia develops within 4 weeks after starting 10 mg daily and if baseline platelet count was ≤100,000/mm³	
Decrease to 50% of the baseline value	Interrupt therapy
If baseline platelet count was ≥60,000/mm³ and returns to ≥50,000/mm³	Resume lenalidomide at 5 mg daily
If baseline platelet count was ≤60,000/mm³ and returns to ≥30,000/mm³	Resume lenalidomide at 5 mg daily
If thrombocytopenia develops more than 4 weeks after starting 10 mg daily	
<30,000/mm³ or <50,000/mm³ and requiring platelet transfusions	Interrupt therapy
Return to ≥30,000/mm³ (without hemostatic failure)	Resume lenalidomide at 5 mg daily
If thrombocytopenia develops during treatment at 5 mg daily	
<30,000/mm³ or <50,000/mm³ and requiring platelet transfusions	Interrupt therapy
Return to >30,000/mm³ (without hemostatic failure)	Resume lenalidomide at 5 mg every-other-day
If neutropenia develops within 4 weeks after starting 10 mg daily and if baseline ANC ≥1000/mm³	
ANC decrease to <750/mm³	Interrupt therapy
ANC recovers to ≥1000/mm³	Resume lenalidomide at 5 mg daily
If neutropenia develops within 4 weeks after starting 10 mg daily and if baseline ANC <1000/mm³	
ANC decrease to <500/mm³	Interrupt therapy
ANC recovers to ≥500/mm³	Resume lenalidomide at 5 mg daily
If neutropenia develops within 4 weeks after starting 10 mg daily	
<500/mm³ for ≥7 days, or <500/mm³ associated with fever ≥38.5°C (≥101.3°F)	Interrupt therapy
Return to ≥500/mm³	Resume lenalidomide at 5 mg daily
Patients who experience neutropenia at 5 mg daily should have their dose adjusted as follows:	
<500/mm³ for ≥7 days, or <500/mm³ associated with fever ≥38.5°C	Interrupt therapy
ANC recovers to ≥500/mm³	Resume lenalidomide at 5 mg every-other-day

*The dose of lenalidomide was reduced or interrupted at least once due to an adverse event in 118 (79.7%) of 148 patients; the median time to the first dose reduction or interruption was 21 days (mean, 35.1 days; range, 2 – 253 days)

Notes

1. Lenalidomide is an analogue of thalidomide. Thalidomide is a known human teratogen that causes severe life-threatening human birth defects. If lenalidomide is taken during pregnancy, it may cause birth defects or death to an unborn baby. Females should be advised to avoid pregnancy while taking lenalidomide. Because of this potential toxicity and to avoid fetal exposure, lenalidomide is available only under a special restricted distribution program named RevAssist℠. Under the RevAssist℠ program, only prescribers and pharmacies registered with the program are able to prescribe and dispense the product, respectively. In addition, lenalidomide must only be dispensed to patients who are registered and meet all the conditions of the RevAssist℠ program
2. Before prescribing lenalidomide, females of childbearing potential should have 2 negative pregnancy tests (sensitivity of at least 50 mIU/mL). The first test should be performed within 10–14 days, and the second test within 24 hours prior to prescribing lenalidomide
3. Because it is not known whether lenalidomide is present in the semen of patients receiving the drug, males receiving lenalidomide must always use a latex condom during any sexual contact with females of childbearing potential even if they have undergone a successful vasectomy.
4. It is not known whether prophylactic anticoagulation or antiplatelet therapy used in conjunction with lenalidomide may lessen the potential for venous thromboembolic events. A decision to use antithrombotic prophylaxis should be done carefully after an assessment of an individual patient's underlying risk factors.

REGIMEN

DECITABINE

Kantarjian H, et al. Cancer 2006; 106:1794–80

Dacogen™ (decitabine) for Injection product label, May 2006. MGI Pharma, Inc., Bloomington, MN

Note: Decitabine is indicated for treatment of patients with MDS including previously treated and untreated, *de novo* and secondary MDS of all FAB subtypes or IPSS groups

Decitabine 15 mg/m^2 per dose, administer intravenously diluted in sufficient 0.9% Sodium Chloride Injection (0.9%NS), 5% Dextrose Injection (D5W), or Lactated Ringer's Injection to produce a concentration of 0.1−1.0 mg/mL, over 3 hours, every 8 hours for 3 consecutive days, every 6 weeks (total dosage/cycle = 135 mg/m^2)

Emetogenic Potential: Low (Emetogenicity score = 2). See Chapter 39 for antiemetic regimens

Patient population studied

A total of 180 patients with MDS were randomized to receive either decitabine (n = 89) or best supportive care (n = 81)

Efficacy

	Decitabine (n = 89) %	Supportive care (n = 81) %
Complete response (CR)	9	0
Partial response (PR)	8	0
Overall response (CR + PR)	17	0
Major hematologic improvement	13	6
Minor hematologic improvement	0	1
Response by IPSS risk subgroup		
Intermediate-1	14	0
Intermediate-2	18	0
High risk	17	0
Response according to cytogenetics		
5q abnormality	13	0
5q not present	16	0
7q abnormality	21	0
7q not present	14	0
Response according to MDS therapy		
Yes	15	0
No	17	0
Response according to MDS status		
de novo	17	0
Secondary	17	0

Treatment modifications

Adverse Effects	Treatment Modification
If the duration of hematological recovery (ANC ≥1000/mm^3 and platelets ≥50,000/mm^3) after a previous decitabine cycle is >6 weeks, but <8 weeks	Delay decitabine for up to 2 weeks, then resume at 11 mg/m^2 per dose, every 8 h for 3 days*
If the duration of hematological recovery (ANC ≥1000/mm^3 and platelets ≥50,000/mm^3) after a previous decitabine cycle is >8 weeks, but <10 weeks	Assess for disease progression. If assessment is negative, delay decitabine for up to 2 weeks, then resume at 11 mg/m^2 per dose, every 8 h for 3 days*
Serum creatinine ≥2 mg/dL (≥177 µmol/L)	Delay decitabine until toxicity is resolved
ALT (SGPT) or bilirubin ≥2 times ULN	
Active or uncontrolled infection	

*Maintain or increase decitabine dosage during subsequent cycles as clinically indicated

Toxicity*

	Decitabine (n = 83)		Supportive care (n = 81)	
	% G3	% G4	% G3	% G4
Neutropenia	10	77	25	25
Thrombocytopenia	22	63	27	16
Anemia	11	1	14	1
Febrile neutropenia	17	6	4	0
Leukopenia	8	14	5	2
Pyrexia	5	1	0	1
Hyperbilirubinemia	5	1	0	0
Pneumonia	13	2	7	2
Nausea	1	0	4	0
Constipation	2	0	1	0
Diarrhea	0	0	1	1
Abdominal pain	2	0	4	0
Oral mucosal petechiae	2	0	1	0

*NCI Common Toxicity Criteria, version 2.0

Monitoring Therapy

1. *At least before each cycle and as needed to monitor response and toxicity:* CBC with differential
2. *Prior to initiation of each treatment cycle:* LFTs and serum creatinine

Notes

Decitabine is indicated for treatment of patients with MDS including previously treated and untreated, *de novo* and secondary MDS of all FAB subtypes or IPSS groups

REGIMEN FOR HIGH-INTENSITY THERAPY

HEMATOPOIETIC STEM CELL TRANSPLANTATION (HSCT)

Benesch M, Deeg HJ. Mayo Clin Proc 2003;78:981–990
Deeg HJ, Appelbaum FR. Curr Opin Oncol 2000;12:116–120
Estey EH et al. Blood 2001;98:3575–3583
Oosterveld M, de Witte T. Blood Rev 2000;14:182–189

Efficacy

Allogeneic HSCT is the only potentially curative option for patients with MDS. However, most patients are not candidates because of advanced age and/or coexisting health problems

Results of Hematopoietic Stem Cell Transplantation (HSCT): % Blasts in Marrow

Patient Group	HSCT Donor	Survival/Remission	Probability of Relapse
Less advanced MDS (<5% blast in the marrow)	HLA identical related and HLA identical unrelated	3-year survival 65–75%	<5%
Advanced MDS (≥5% blasts in the marrow)	HLA identical related	>3-year remission 35–45%	10–35%
Advanced MDS (≥5% blasts in the marrow)	HLA identical unrelated	>3-year remission 25–30%	10–35%

International Prognostic Scoring System (IPSS) Risk Groups

Patient Group	Survival/Remission
Low and intermediate-1 risk	5-year DFS 60%
Intermediate-2 risk	5-year DFS 36%
High risk	5-year DFS 28%

DFS, disease-free survival